OUTPATIENT PSYCHIATRY
Diagnosis and Treatment
Treatment
Second Edition

OUTPATIENT PSYCHIATRY
Diagnosis and Treatment

Second Edition

Aaron Lazare, M.D., *Editor*

Professor and Chairman
Department of Psychiatry
University of Massachusetts Medical Center
Worcester, Massachusetts

Consultant in Psychiatry
Massachusetts General Hospital
Boston, Massachusetts

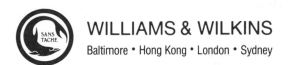

WILLIAMS & WILKINS
Baltimore • Hong Kong • London • Sydney

Editor: Michael Fisher
Associate Editor: Carol Eckhart
Copy Editor: Debbie Klenotic
Design: Saturn Graphics
Illustration Planning: Lorraine Wrzosek
Production: Charles E. Zeller
Cover Design: Dan Pfisterer
Cover Illustration: John Meyers

Accurate indications, adverse reactions, and dosage schedules for drugs are provided in this book, but it is possible that they may change. The reader is urged to review the package information data of the manufacturers of the medications mentioned.

Printed in the United States of America

First Edition 1979

Library of Congress Cataloging in Publication Data

Outpatient psychiatry.

　　Includes bibliographies and index.
　　1. Psychiatry.　2. Psychotherapy.　I. Lazare, Aaron,
1936–　　.　[DNLM: 1. Mental Disorders—diagnosis.
2.　Mental Disorders—therapy. WM 100 094]
RC480.087　　1988　　　　616.89　　　　88-146
ISBN 0-683-04851-1

　　　　　　　　　　　　　　　　　　　87　88　89　90　91
　　　　　　　　　　　1　2　3　4　5　6　7　8　9　10

Dedicated to the Memory of my Mother and Father

Anne Storfer Lazare

and

H. Benjamin Lazare

Foreword to the First Edition

Of the making of medical textbooks, there is no end; most are pedestrian, rehashing what has been said before and forcing the variability and richness of clinical experience into abstract categories which bear only a tenuous relationship to the problems patients present. Hence springs the intellectual excitement of one's encounter with the book Aaron Lazare has edited.

Here, for the first time, is a scholarly book about outpatient psychiatry, one which corresponds to the actuality of medical practice, which is enhanced by research data, and which draws on the relevant literature in a way that illuminates rather than confounds understanding. Although this book can be of value to all mental health professionals, it has particular relevance to the education of a psychiatrist, whether he or she be in training or in practice.

A psychiatrist should be, above all, a physician, in the fullest meaning of that term. In a trivial sense, that statement reduces to the occupational requirement of psychiatric practice: a medical degree, residency training, state licensure and Board certification. However, it is not the formal but the connotative meaning which is emphasized here, namely, the medical imperatives of the physician's role: *always* to care for the patient, *insofar as possible* to mitigate distress and to restore function, and *sometimes* to cure. Nowhere in this role defini-

tion is there mention of theory or method. These matter, but they matter only insofar as they are in the service of the primary functions of care, relief, and cure.

As I see it, this belief inspirits this excellent book, unique in its focus on patient needs and how they can be met. The reader is assisted in assimilating a variety of ways of conceptualizing patient problems and in mastering a broad array of techniques for minimizing those problems. The authors mine the crude ore of a vast and contradictory psychiatric and behavioral science literature in order to extract those ideas and those methods which may be of help for particular patients in particular kinds of distress.

In choosing to emphasize the psychiatrist as a "physician," I deliberately put forward an idealized version of the medical calling; I stress what the physician should be and should do, even though I recognize that not all attain that goal. In so doing, I recognize that I invite criticism at a time when the "medical model" of psychiatric disorder is under sharp attack. Much of the criticism stems from a deliberately narrowed conception of the medical model. More accurately put, the critics mistake the current "biomedical" model of disease for a more broadly conceived understanding of the physician's role in health and illness. Curiously enough, those who contend that psychiatric disorders are primarily sociogenic and therefore ill-suited to medical management do so by assigning other medical disorders rather cavalierly to biological causes alone.

No illness problems are simply matters of disordered biology; relatively few are without biological concomitants. The very concern for psychosocial matters that should inform the physician who cares for schizophrenic patients is no less fundamental to the one who cares for diabetics. Though we know less of the pathophysiology of schizophrenia than we do of diabetes, knowledge of pathophysiology, though essential, provides only a partial and limited guide for the care of the patient. The diabetic, no less than the schizophrenic, has thoughts and feelings about his illness, is subject to functional limitation because of its characteristics, and is responsive to familial and social pressures. The mere prescription of diet, exercise, and medication provides no assurance of improved outcome unless the prescription makes sense to the patient as the logical consequence of his understanding of the nature of the illness, unless its aims are viewed as being in accord with the patient's own goals, and unless its impact on daily activities is compatible with the patient's life-style. Furthermore, the course of diabetes, like that of all illnesses, can be exacerbated by social stress and mitigated by social support. Thus, the role of the internist is in principle no different from that of the psychiatrist in the need to be alert to psychosocial factors and to be sophisticated in the use of community resources to moderate their influence. Neither the internist nor the psychiatrist need be the sole agent for assisting the patient in carrying out the therapeutic program; indeed, social workers, psychologists, counselors, and others may be far more skilled in particular aspects of management, but the physician must have a comprehensive view of the necessary ingredients of total care in order to prescribe an appropriate regimen.

Thus, although the focus throughout this book is on the patient and on patient problems, terms which place the issues within the framework of medical care, its orientation is quite the opposite of medical imperialism. No biological flag is staked out on foreign territory. Quite the opposite. Because patient problems are identified as the resultant of psychological and social, as well as biological, determinants, the turf reserved for biomedicine in the strict sense is sharply reduced.

The conceptual scheme Professor Lazare has employed in organizing this book will serve to make its readers aware that the meaning of the clinical encounter is understandable only in a framework that includes the perspective of the patient as well as that of the physician. In recent years, the patient perspective has been slighted in relation to physician preoccupation with the biological mechanisms of disease. To ascribe this narrow medical focus to the perversity or insensitivity of doctors is to mistake consequence for cause. It is best understood as an undesirable side effect of the technological revolution that has, in other ways, been of significant benefit to health care. Because biomedical technology has contributed to therapeutic power, it has come to dominate professional ideology. It would be absurd to abandon the gains it has brought with it. The challenge is to add an understanding of the patient's illness to an understanding of the patient's disease.

Diagnostic precision can make an important difference for the patient when it leads to the identification of disorders for which powerful remedies exist. In consequence, the diagnosis of disease has pre-empted medical consciousness. When the "work-up" fails to uncover biological malfunction, the physician is ill-prepared to cope with the complaints of the patient which are no less "real" for being psychosocial in origin. The virtue of the conceptual framework Aaron Lazare has embodied in this book is that it opens new avenues to the understanding and management of the complaints that bring the patient to the doctor: personal distress and an inability to fulfill expected social roles. The negotiated (customer) approach is not presented in opposition to standard and still essential steps in medical diagnosis, but as an enlargement of them. It adds to the clinician's effectiveness by increasing his or her sensitivity to illness as the personal experience which motivates the search for help.

Contemporary psychiatry, like the rest of medicine, has shared in biomedical progress. A generation ago, psychiatric diagnosis had little other value for the clinician and for the patient than in formulating prognosis. We now possess moderately effective remedies which are relatively disorder-specific. Distinguishing one disorder from another has important implications for prescribing appropriate treatment. Thus, a significant part of this textbook is devoted to the strategies for making diagnostic distinctions and for the use of available therapeutic regimens. Speculations about cause and underlying pathophysiology are not ignored, but they are always balanced by keeping clinical actualities and the pragmatics of care in the forefront.

In stressing the originality of the concepts that underlie the organization of this book, I do not wish to suggest that the framework is in any way complete or that later editions (of which I anticipate many) will not require continuous revision. Psychiatry still lacks a comprehensive theory of behavior that permits adequate translation from one level of behavioral organization to another. When, and if, that will be achieved remains uncertain. For the present, the best we can do is to hold simultaneously in mind a set of hypotheses, in part complementary and in part contradictory, in order to identify the points of maximum leverage to promote better function for a particular patient.

I consider myself privileged in having been invited to prepare a foreword to a book that will become a landmark in psychiatry. It is a tribute both to high intelligence and to hard work. It provides a firm foundation for the approach to the care of ambulatory psychiatric patients. It is without peer.

Leon Eisenberg, M.D.
Presley Professor of Social Medicine
and Professor of Psychiatry
Harvard Medical School
Boston, Massachusetts

Preface to
the Second Edition

My interest in editing this textbook of general outpatient psychiatry emerged from my responsibilities as clinician, teacher, and administrator in a variety of ambulatory settings. These included the walk-in and other outpatient psychiatric clinics at the Massachusetts General Hospital and the public-sector psychiatry ambulatory clinics at the University of Massachusetts Medical Center. In all of these settings there was a general sense of confusion, frustration, and exhaustion on the part of clinicians, trainees, teachers, and administrators. There was considerable disappointment that work and learning were not as intellectually gratifying and emotionally satisfying as had been expected.

This unhappiness and dissatisfaction on the part of outpatient professionals can be understood in large part as a result of the radical changes that have occurred in outpatient practice during the past three decades.

First, during this time the varieties of effective treatments, both biologic and psychosocial, have increased dramatically. This has led to ideologic and empirical debates over what is the best treatment for a given patient. The development of DSM-III and DSM-III-R have further fueled the controversy as to whether and under what circumstances the patient should be understood as a person suffering from a DSM-III-R diagnostic category, or whether and under what circumstances formal DSM-III-R diagnostic categories should be abandoned in favor of perceiving the person as a unique individual.

Second, the types of clinical settings have expanded to include walk-in/emergency clinics, community mental health centers, student counseling services, health maintenance organizations, and subspecialty clinics. Many of these new settings are tied to a financing of care which includes more state and federal funding as well as increased support from private insurers. As a result of these new clinical settings and broader financing, together with legislative and policy changes that have brought about deinstitutionalization, the patients who seek ambulatory care have increased dramatically both in number and in heterogeneity. They now include people from all social classes whose suffering covers the range of psychosocial problems of everyday life to acute and chronic severe mental disorders. This range includes those referred to as the "worried well" to those referred to as the "deinstitutionalized state hospital patient." Thus we see many patients with complex psychosocial problems and functional disabilities that do not easily lend themselves to official diagnostic categories or psychodynamic formulations. As a result, outpatient professionals are often unprepared by their training for the day-to-day tasks that they face.

Finally, this heterogeneous population of patients is now being served by an ever increasing number and diversity of mental health care professionals. The diversity of training is a source of ongoing conflicts over (*a*) the importance of a medical/biologic approach; (*b*) the importance of other possibly competing approaches such as the psychodynamic and behavioral; (*c*) the nature of the professional relationship between patient and clinician (and even whether the patient should now be called "client"); (*d*) and the nature and leadership of the treatment team, including the delegation of clinical responsibilities.

The above problems of ambulatory practice are addressed in this book by means of seven integrating themes.

1. A patient should be understood simultaneously from biologic, psychodynamic, sociocultural, and behavioral perspectives. This approach recognizes that no one of these four perspectives alone is adequate to understand most patients (Chapters 2–6).
2. Although none of these four perspectives should be ignored, the clinician must be ever vigilant to the importance of the biologic/medical approach because of the high incidence of medical illness in psychiatric patients and the significance of biologic treatments for many patients (Chapters 3, 15, 17–30).
3. The clinician must be cognizant of both the power and the limitations of diagnostic systems in understanding heterogeneous outpatient populations. In practice this can be accomplished by approaching each patient both as a member of a diagnostic category and as a unique individual (Chapter 8).
4. In order to apply our knowledge of the four conceptual paradigms and the categorical/individualistic perspective described above, a hypothesis-testing approach should be applied to the clinical interview. More specifically, it is proposed that the clinician consider, for each patient, a closed system of clinical hypotheses (partial formulations) based on biomedical, psychodynamic, sociocultural, and behavioral paradigms. This approach helps the clinician become more comprehensive while offering for trainees and teachers the method and language of hypothesis testing to facilitate discussions of diagnostic and treatment skills (Chapter 7).
5. In order to systematically consider the various clinical hypotheses, the clinician must be an acute observer both of the patient and of him- or herself. This requires a careful description of important clinical observations that are important and the various means of collecting clinical data (Chapters 12–16).
6. In contemporary ambulatory settings, neither traditional authoritarian clinician/patient relationships nor egalitarian relationships, commonly associated with a kind of pseudointimacy, can be generally effective. This book proposes a negotiated relationship which assumes that differences in perspective (conflict) between patient and clinician are inherent in most clinical encounters. An essential task of the clinician is to determine these conflicts and to resolve them, whenever possible, by clinical negotiations (Chapters 9 and 10).
7. The concepts described above can be applied to each clinical syndrome and patient population by analyzing the three major functions of the clinical interview: determining the nature of the problem, developing and sustaining a therapeutic relationship, and educating and recommending treatment plans to the patient. The multidimensional approach, methods of hypothesis testing, assessment techniques, and negotiation techniques constitute many of the clinical skills necessary to accomplish these three functions for each interview (Chapters 11, 31, 33, 34, 36–41).

The rationale for this second edition of *Outpatient Psychiatry* is the significant conceptual and empirical advances in the field since the first edition was published in 1979. In addition, public-sector psychiatry has assumed greater importance in American psychiatry during the past decade. The 2nd edition consists of 50 chapters. It builds on the theoretical foundation of the 1st edition, has 13 chapters which are entirely new, and has 37 chapters which are significantly revised from the 1st edition. New conceptual chapters are the reformulation of "The Biologic Approach," "Dilemmas in Psychiatric Diagnosis: A Perspective From the History of Medicine," and "Three Functions of the Clinical Interview." New chapters for data assessment are "The Use of the Laboratory in Outpatient Psychiatry" and "Psychology Testing for Mental Disorders." The new chapter for the section on the organic/medical differential diagnosis of psychiatric presentations is a review of "Medical Disorders in Psychiatric Populations." The new syndromal chapter is "Anorexia Nervosa and Bulimia Nervosa." The new chapters in public-sector psychiatry are "The Mentally Retarded/Mentally Ill,"

"The Chronic Mentally Ill," "Psychosocial Rehabilitation," and "Legal Issues in Outpatient Psychiatry." Finally, there are new treatment chapters entitled "The Psychology of Psychopharmacology" and "The Individual Psychotherapies: Efficacy, Syndrome-Based Treatments, and the Therapeutic Alliance." Because of space limitations, there is no discussion of children and adolescents, and certain topics uncommon in ambulatory practice are omitted. There is no definitive chapter on psychopharmacology because comprehensive coverage of this topic would require a book in itself. Psychopharmacologic treatment is included in the chapters on the biologic approach and in the syndromal chapters.

It is hoped that this book will be useful for psychiatrists, residents in psychiatry, nonpsychiatric physicians, psychologists, psychiatric social workers, and psychiatric nurses, as well as medically and nonmedically-oriented family practitioners.

Acknowledgments

I would like to express my appreciation to Paul Barreira, M.D., Mai-Lan Rogoff, M.D., and William Vogel, Ph.D., for their suggestions in the planning of this book and the preparation of many of the chapters; to Tom Manning, M.A., for the added administrative responsibilities he assumed in the Department of Psychiatry while I worked on the manuscript; to Denise George for her tireless secretarial and administrative assistance, both for the book and for the Department of Psychiatry; to my wife Louise Lazare for her creativity, support, and encouragement; and to my children Jacqueline, Samuel, Sarah, Thomas, Hien, Robert, David, and Naomi for their tolerance and support.

I would also like to thank mentors and teachers who were responsible for the development of my career: Beatrice Harelick, who first awakened my interest in ideas and writing; Ralph H. Turner, Ph.D., J. Milton Yinger, Ph.D., George Simpson, Ph.D., and Luke Steiner, Ph.D., who introduced me to the fields of psychology, sociology, anthropology, and chemistry; John L. Caughey, M.D., Benjamin Spock, M.D., Leston Havens, M.D., Ives Hendrick, M.D., and Eric R. Kandel, M.D., for their dedication to teaching during my medical school years; Elvin Semrad, M.D., who taught me the empathic approach to patients; Gerald L. Klerman, M.D., who introduced me to and encouraged my scholarly activities in psychiatry; John Stoeckle, M.D., who nurtured my interest in the clinical interview and clinician/patient relationships with medical patients; Sherman Eisenthal, Ph.D., a mentor and collaborator on research issues in clinician/patient relations: Tom Scheff, Ph.D., who has been a continuing source of intellectual stimulation; and especially Leon Eisenberg, M.D., who has nurtured my career at every turn for the past 20 years.

Contributors

STEVEN A. ADELMAN, M.D. Assistant Professor of Psychiatry and Director of Ambulatory Psychiatry Service, University of Massachusetts Medical Center, Worcester, Massachusetts

ANNE ALONSO, Ph.D. Staff Psychologist, Department of Psychiatry, Massachusetts General Hospital, Boston; Assistant Professor of Psychiatry, Harvard Medical School, Boston, Massachusetts

PAUL S. APPELBAUM, M.D. A. F. Zeleznik Professor of Psychiatry and Director of Law and Psychiatry, University of Massachusetts Medical Center, Worcester, Massachusetts

PAUL J. BARREIRA, M.D. Assistant Professor of Psychiatry and Director of Psychiatry Residency Training Program, University of Massachusetts Medical Center, Worcester, Massachusetts; Director of Clinical and Professional Services, Worcester State Hospital, Worcester

DAVID M. BEAR, M.D. Associate Professor of Psychiatry and Neurology, Director of Division of Neuropsychiatry, Department of Psychiatry, Vanderbilt University School of Medicine; Director of Psychiatry, Vanderbilt University Hospital, Nashville, Tennessee

SHELDON BENJAMIN, M.D. Associate Professor of Psychiatry and Neurology, University of Massachusetts Medical Center, Worcester, Massachusetts; Director of Neuropsychiatry, Westboro State Hospital, Westboro, Massachusetts

ALINE L. BISGAIER, B.A. Research Coordinator, Eating Disorders Unit, Massachusetts General Hospital, Boston

BRUCE BONGAR, Ph.D. Assistant Professor, Department of Psychology, College of the Holy Cross, Worcester, Massachusetts; Adjunct Assistant Professor of Psychiatry, University of Massachusetts Medical Center, Worcester

ANTHONY J. BOUCKOMS, M.D. Associate Professor of Psychiatry, Harvard Medical School

ANDREW W. BROTMAN, M.D. Assistant Professor of Psychiatry at Harvard Medical School; Chief, Freedom Trail Clinic, Massachusetts General Hospital, Boston

DENNIS S. CHARNEY, M.D. Adjunct Director, Clinical Neuroscience Research Unit, Connecticut Mental Health Center; Chief of Psychiatry, West Haven VA Medical Center, Yale University School of Medicine

ARNOLD COHEN, Ph.D.   Coordinator of Group Development, Boston Institute of Psychotherapies, Inc., Boston

GEORGE L. DION, Sc.D.   Assistant Professor of Psychiatry, University of Massachusetts Medical Center; Director of Psychiatric Rehabilitation, Worcester State Hospital, Worcester, Massachusetts

JOHN P. DOCHERTY, M.D.   Medical Director, Nashua Brookside Hospital, Nashua, New Hampshire

SHERMAN EISENTHAL, Ph.D.   Associate Professor of Psychology, Department of Psychiatry, Massachusetts General Hospital, Harvard Medical School, Boston

MILTON K. ERMAN, M.D.   Director of the Sleep Disorders Center, Scripps Clinic and Research Foundation, Lajolla, California; Clinical Associate Professor of Psychiatry, University of California at San Diego, Lajolla

WILLIAM E. FALK, M.D.   Staff Psychiatrist, Clinical Psychopharmacology, Wang Ambulatory Care Center, Massachusetts General Hospital, Boston

ARLENE FRANK, Ph.D.   Instructor in Psychology, Department of Psychiatry, Harvard Medical School, Boston; Director of Research, Nashua Brookside Hospital, Nashua, New Hampshire

JEFFREY L. GELLER, M.D., M.P.H.   Associate Professor of Psychiatry and Director of Public Sector Psychiatry, University of Massachusetts Medical Center, Worcester, Massachusetts

DAVID GITLIN, M.D.   Resident in Psychiatry, University of Massachusetts Medical Center, Worcester, Massachusetts

SHIRLEY M. GLYNN, Ph.D.   Staff Research Associate, Department of Psychiatry, University of California at Los Angeles

WAYNE K. GOODMAN, M.D.   Assistant Professor of Psychiatry, Chief, Obsessive–Compulsive Disorder Clinic, Connecticut Mental Health Center, New Haven, Connecticut

THOMAS G. GUTHEIL, M.D.   Associate Professor of Psychiatry, Harvard Medical School; President Program in Psychiatry and the Law, Massachusetts Mental Health Center, Boston

DAVID B. HERZOG, M.D.   Associate Professor of Psychiatry, Harvard Medical School; Chief, Eating Disorders Unit, Massachusetts General Hospital, Boston

STEVEN K. HOGE, M.D.   Assistant Professor of Psychiatry, Director of Forensic Consultation Service, University of Massachusetts Medical Center, Worcester, Massachusetts

MERLE INGRAHAM, M.D.   Assistant Professor of Psychiatry, University of Massachusetts Medical Center, Worcester, Massachusetts

MARTIN B. KELLER, M.D.   Associate Professor of Psychiatry, Harvard Medical School; Director of Outpatient Research Department of Psychiatry, Massachusetts General Hospital, Boston

HERBERT D. KLEBER, M.D.   Professor of Psychiatry, Substance Abuse Treatment Unit, Yale University School of Medicine, New Haven, Connecticut

THOMAS R. KOSTEN, M.D.   Assistant Professor of Psychiatry, Substance Abuse Treatment Unit, Yale University School of Medicine, New Haven, Connecticut

JOHN H. KRYSTAL, M.D.   Assistant Professor of Psychiatry and Associate Inpatient Unit Chief, Clinical Neuroscience Research Unit, Yale University; Director, Traumatic Stress Disorders Program, West Haven VA Medical Center, Yale University School of Medicine

AARON LAZARE, M.D.   Professor and Chairman, Department of Psychiatry, University of Massachusetts Medical Center, Worcester, Massachusetts

TED LAWLOR, M.D.   Assistant Professor of Psychiatry, University of Massachusetts Medical Center, Worcester, Massachusetts, Clinical Director of Admission Unit, Worcester State Hospital

ROBERT PAUL LIBERMAN, M.D.   Professor of Psychiatry, UCLA School of Medicine, Chief of Rehabilitation, Brentwood Veterans Administration Medical Center, Los Angeles, California

THEO C. MANSCHRECK, M.D.   Associate Professor of Psychiatry, Massachusetts General Hospital and Harvard Medical School; Clinical Director, Harbor Area, Erich Lindemann Mental Health Center, Boston

ANN OHM MASSION, M.D.   Assistant Professor of Psychiatry, University of Massachusetts Medical Center, Worcester, Massachusetts

GARY S. MOAK, M.D.   Assistant Professor of Psychiatry, University of Massachusetts Medical Center, Worcester, Massachusetts; Director of Psychogeriatric Unit, Worcester State Hospital

KIM T. MUESER, Ph.D.   Assistant Professor of Psychiatry, Medical College of Pennsylvania at Eastern Pennsylvania Psychiatric Institute, Philadelphia, Pennsylvania

GENE R. MOSS, M.D.   President of Behavioral Medicine Associates, Inc., Beverly Hills, California; Director of Psychiatry, Somerset Medical Center, Somerville, New Jersey

LINDA GAY PETERSON, M.D.   Associate Professor of Psychiatry and Family and Community Medicine, Director of Consultation/Liaison Service, University of Massachusetts Medical Center, Worcester, Massachusetts

MAI-LAN ROGOFF, M.D.   Associate Professor of Psychiatry, Director of Student Counseling Service, Associate Director of Residency Training, University of Massachusetts Medical Center, Worcester, Massachusetts

J. SCOTT RUTAN, Ph.D.   Director, Center for Group Therapy, Massachusetts General Hospital, Boston

WILLIAM VOGEL, Ph.D.   Associate Professor of Psychiatry, Director of Family and Couples Therapy, University of Massachusetts Medical Center, Worcester, Massachusetts

ROGER D. WEISS, M.D.   Director, Alcohol and Drug Abuse Treatment Center, McLean Hospital, Belmont, Massachusetts, Associate Professor of Psychiatry, Harvard Medical School

SCOTT W. WOODS, M.D.   Assistant Professor of Psychiatry, Chief, Anxiety Disorders Clinic, Connecticut Mental Health Center, New Haven, Connecticut

LINDA ZAMVIL, M.D.   Resident in Child Psychiatry, Massachusetts General Hospital, Boston; Clinical Fellow in Psychiatry, Harvard Medical School

Contents

Section II. Data for Assessment

Section III. Differential Diagnosis of Psychiatric Presentations With Known Organic Causes

Section IV. Selected Problems in Outpatient Practice

Section V. Aspects of Treatment in Outpatient Practice

Section I
Conceptual Approaches for Clinical Practice

1

Current Issues in Outpatient Psychiatry

Aaron Lazare, M.D.

This chapter attempts to describe the extensive changes that have occurred in ambulatory psychiatric practice during the past three decades. These changes are organized into five related and overlapping categories: (*a*) available treatments, (*b*) clinical settings, (*c*) patients, (*d*) care providers, and (*e*) financing. I then analyze the impact of these changes on diagnosis, clinician–patient relationships, and treatment.

RECENT DEVELOPMENTS IN OUTPATIENT PSYCHIATRY

Available Treatments

The range of available treatments for use in ambulatory settings has increased dramatically. Of great importance has been the development of modern psychopharmacologic agents. The use of neuroleptics and mood-altering drugs for the seriously mentally ill has reduced the time of stay of hundreds of thousands of patients on inpatient units or made hospitalization unnecessary. These medications, also effective in mild to moderate conditions, such as some of the depressive and anxiety disorders, have resulted in positive clinical outcomes in outpatient settings where earlier treatments had little effect.

In addition to biologic treatments, a wide range of psychosocial treatments have assumed an important role in the outpatient care of virtually all of the so-called functional psychiatric disorders. These include short-term, intermediate, and long-term behavioral, cognitive, and psychodynamic treatments for individuals, couples, families, and groups. Finally, refinements in psychiatric diagnosis have led to the prescription of specific treatments for particular disorders, including the combination of psychologic and biologic treatments.

Clinical Settings

Just two to three decades ago, ambulatory care was provided predominantly in the private offices of psychiatrists and psychologists and in clinics subsidized by teaching hospitals, state departments of mental health, the Veterans Administration, and various charitable and nonprofit organizations. A significant number of patients are now seen in community mental health centers, health maintenance organizations, student counseling services, group practices, and single private practices of various mental health professionals where patients may be seen by appointment or on a walk-in basis. A recent trend, particularly in teaching hospitals, has been to organize clinics on the basis of diagnostic categories, such as eating disorders, mood disorders, and anxiety disorders. Alternatively, clinics have been organized around treatment modalities such as psychopharmacology, behavioral treatments, and psychodynamic psychotherapy. Large numbers of patients with primary psychiatric problems are seen in the offices of internists and family practice physicians. In all of the settings described above, patients may be seen from once a month (or even less frequently) for psychologic support or medication evaluation to 4 or 5 days a week for psychoanalysis. The greater diversity of clinical settings and the increased amount of service they provide are undoubtedly a result of the effectiveness of new treatments, deinstitutionalization, innovations in the delivery of mental health services (community mental health centers and health maintenance organizations), and new mechanisms for financing mental health care.

Patients

Closely related to the availability of new treatments and the increased number and diversity of outpatient facilities are the number and type of outpatients. During the past 30 years, there has been a dramatic increase in the number of ambulatory psychiatric visits as well as a marked increase in the ratio of outpatient episodes to inpatient episodes. Between 1955 and 1977, the number of outpatient episodes in the United States increased from 391,000 to 4,830,000, a 12-fold increase. This excludes care provided by private practice mental health professionals (1, 2). In addition, the patient population has become more diverse, representing people from all social classes who suffer from acute and chronic severe mental illness as well as less disabling mental distress. The increase in the ambulatory patient population is a direct result of new treatment modalities, deinstitutionalization, increased insurance coverage, and diminished stigmatization of those seeking mental health services.

Care Providers

In response to the increased number of people seeking ambulatory psychiatric treatment, there has been an increase in the number and variety of mental health practitioners who serve them. In addition to psychiatrists and doctoral-level clinical psychologists, there are now large numbers of master's-level psychologists, psychiatric social workers, master's-level psychiatric nurses, family and marital therapists, alcohol counselors, clergy, and other mental health professionals. Nonpsychiatric physicians working in medical settings see more patients with psychiatric disorders than do psychiatrists. The mental health practitioners described above vary considerably in the type and duration of their training and consequently in the quality and methods of their clinical practice.

Financing

The wide range of fiscal mechanisms that finance ambulatory mental health influences where and by whom the patient will be seen and the duration of treatment. The decision, for instance, to use a health maintenance organization, a Veterans Administration clinic, a community mental health center, or a private therapist is often determined by the nature of insurance or financial coverage. During recent years, insurers and prepaid health providers have been exerting increasing control over the utilization of ambulatory care. They determine what conditions may be covered, the duration of treatment, and the requirements for documentation.

Implications

There is much that is positive about the current state of outpatient psychiatry. Greater numbers of patients from all social strata, with psychiatric disorders ranging from the serious to minor problems in living, are receiving mental health care. This has diminished the numbers of patients in psychiatric hospitals and reduced mental suffering overall. In addition, there is growing evidence that ambulatory mental health care contributes to cost offsets for medical care. As a result of (or at least concomitant with) these developments, the stigma formerly associated with seeking and receiving mental health care has been diminished. Much of our population now shares a cultural attitude that legitimizes, supports, and encourages treatment for serious mental illness as well as for self-actualization and the common distresses of living: marital crisis, sexual dysfunction, stress, and self-defeating and maladaptive behaviors. Yet, this proliferation and organization of ambulatory services raises serious clinical questions that may be usefully organized around three central issues: diagnosis, clinician–patient relationships, and treatment.

These issues are less problematic in inpatient settings where there is greater control and predictability over the kinds of patients who are admitted, the fiscal arrangements, the physical plant, the usual treatments, and the mix and qualifications of the professional staff. Any deficiencies or major deviations from standard practice are continuously reviewed by hospital committees and accrediting agencies responsible for maintaining standards.

CLINICAL PROBLEMS IN OUTPATIENT PSYCHIATRY

Diagnosis

Outpatient clinicians vary markedly in the importance they place on the diagnostic process. Some regard accurate diagnosis as the cornerstone of treatment, whereas others regard it as a useless exercise only necessary because of the requirement for reimbursement. In inpatient settings, in contrast, patients are screened prior to admission for more clear-cut syndromes and dysfunctional behaviors, and treatment plans are commonly based on established diagnoses. In addition, inpatient settings afford the opportunity to establish more valid and reliable diagnoses. There is generally more time to observe

the patient, more opportunity to gather biographical data from families, more opportunity for corroborative input from other clinicians, and greater access to medical assessment including laboratory data.

The most serious diagnostic problem in outpatient settings, I believe, is the detection of medical disease that coexists with or is in itself a cause of psychiatric symptoms. Nineteen studies of medical disease in psychiatric populations reveal that from 7 to 46% of psychiatric patients have medical diseases that are directly related to psychiatric symptoms, such as anxiety, depression, and mania. (See Chapter 17 for a discussion of the problem of medical disease in psychiatric populations.) Many mental health professionals, in my opinion, are inadequately trained to recognize these organic conditions. The limited amount of time available for assessment in some clinical settings further complicates this problem. In addition, routine medical referral to "rule out medical disorder" often results in an inadequate medical evaluation.

A second important diagnostic problem in outpatient settings is the adequate assessment of *Diagnostic and Statistical Manual of Mental Disorders* (*Third Edition-Revised*) (DSM-III-R) Axis I disorders, as well as disorders early in their clinical development that do not yet meet the diagnostic criteria. For example, it is common in outpatient settings for anxiety disorders, mood disorders, and substance abuse disorders to be overlooked, particularly in their early stages before the symptom picture is typical or complete, especially by clinicians who are either inadequately trained and/or who regard categorical diagnoses as irrelevant.

A third diagnostic problem in ambulatory practice is the difficulty in describing, assessing, and conceptualizing the problems of stress and maladaptive behaviors and personality patterns. Many of these problems do not fit into DSM-III-R diagnostic categories, and when they do, the diagnoses (particularly the personality disorders) are of limited clinical value. Psychologically oriented clinicians of varying disciplines and theoretical orientations are apt to formulate these problems in ways that defy classification and confuse other clinicians. Psychodynamic and behavioral therapists, for example, rely on complex individualistic formulations or assessments rather than categorical diagnoses.

Clinician–Patient Relations

In the past, there were two primary types of relationships between mental health professionals and psychiatric patients. The first has been referred to as the "diagnostic" or "medical" model. With this approach clinicians are seen to have superior knowledge, which they use to establish diagnoses and recommend treatment. The patient's role is to cooperate with the diagnostic process and follow the treatment recommendations. In the second approach, the clinician assesses the prospective patient's suitability for psychodynamic psychotherapy and then enters into a particular type of therapeutic relationship in which the therapist assumes a more passive and less direct role than in the medical model. In both, the clinician has considerably more power than the patient. Although both continue to have their value, I believe that a more encompassing model of the clinician–patient relationship is now required. This need is a consequence of (a) the altered power relationships between clinician and patient resulting from the current methods of financing of mental health care and (b) the broad range of treatment modalities and combinations that may be useful in any given case. As a result, patients need to assume active roles in the diagnostic process and treatment planning and need to work cooperatively with the clinician toward developing a negotiated consensus (3). Such a relationship is particularly important in outpatient settings where, in contrast to inpatient settings, the illness is less severe and treatment is voluntary.

Of great concern in the clinician –patient relationship is the style of practice of pro-

fessionals from widely varied training backgrounds, which sometimes permits any kind of relationship that feels "right" to the clinician. Such relationships vary along the dimensions of degree of physical and social intimacy that are regarded as permissible with patients. Inappropriate and unprofessional intimacy, in the opinion of the most highly respected clinicians, may result in irreparable damage to both the patient and the profession.

A final problem in clinician–patient relationships in outpatient settings is the triangular relationship involving the patient, his or her nonmedical therapist, and the psychiatrist/psychopharmacologist. Problems inevitably arise as to who is in charge and how each clinician is to assess the clinical data without full knowledge of the impact the other clinician is having.

Treatment, Patient Education, and Communication of Information

There are several aspects of outpatient treatment that are distinctive to the setting. First, there are a wide range of treatments and combination of treatments from which to choose. These choices are often made according to the preference and expertise of the practitioner rather than on the evidence of efficacy of treatment and as a result of a negotiated exchange. Clinical options are further subject to financial and organizational constraints. Membership in a health maintenance organization or coverage by particular insurance plans, for instance, may significantly limit treatment options. Second, treatment and patient management often center around entry and discharge from the hospital. Finally, an important aspect of treatment and management is the communication of information to and education of the patient. This is an area of growing interest and importance in ambulatory medicine. I believe that this function of clinical care is equally important in ambulatory psychiatry where patient compliance and self-help are highly important.

SUMMARY

During the past three decades, there have been significant changes in outpatient practice as evidenced by a wide variety of available treatments, a diversity of clinical settings, a heterogeneity of patients and care providers, and new mechanisms for finanancing mental health care. While these changes have improved the care of the mentally ill in ambulatory settings, they have also led to serious problems over the importance of diagnosis, the nature of clinician–patient relations, and the nature of patient education and treatment. This book attempts to address these three issues.

References

1. National Institute of Mental Health: *Mental Health, United States, 1985.* Taube CA, Barrett SA (eds). DHHS Pub. No. (ADM) 85-1378. Washington, D.C., Government Printing Office, 1985.
2. American Psychiatric Association: *Economic Fact Book for Psychiatry.* Washington, DC, American Psychiatric Press, 1983.
3. Levinson DJ, Merrifield J, Berg K: Becoming a patient. *Arch Gen Psychiatry* 17:385-406, 1967.

2

A Multidimensional Approach to Psychopathology[a]

Aaron Lazare, M.D.

Many clinicians find it difficult to understand how their colleagues, teachers, and students, select relevant clinical data, formulate a case, and develop a treatment plan. In the patient who is psychiatrically ill or in psychologic distress, is it the cluster of symptoms, the unconscious conflict, the abnormal family interaction, or the behavioral reinforcer that holds the key to case formulation and decision making? How is it that one clinician will emphasize electroconvulsant therapy or tricyclic antidepressants, another individual psychodynamic psychotherapy, a third family therapy, and a fourth behavior modification for similar patients? Why is it apparently easier to formulate and implement a treatment plan for a patient suffering from a medical illness such as congestive heart failure?

One major reason for the difficulty in understanding clinical thinking is that in the clinical formulation several different conceptual approaches are implicitly used, but are rarely identified as such. The four most common are the biologic, the psy-

chodynamic, the sociocultural, and the behavioral. The kind of history obtained, the meaning assigned to certain historical facts, and the treatment modalities most often chosen depend on which approach or combination of approaches the clinician employs. These points are illustrated by four case histories of the same middle-aged depressed patient. For heuristic reasons, each history is presented in terms of one of the four conceptual approaches to the exclusion of the other three.

FOUR CASE HISTORIES

Biologic Approach

Mrs. J., a 53-year-old widow, gave a history of depressive syndrome. During the past few months she had lost 9.1 kg in weight, had early morning awakening, and had a diurnal variation in mood manifested by feeling better as the day went on. She described herself as feeling hopeless, helpless, and worthless. There was some retardation of speech. She felt life was not worth living although she denied suicidal intent. There was no evidence of delusions or paranoid ideation. There was no prior history of manic or hypomanic symptoms, although 23

[a] Adapted with permission from Lazare A: Hidden conceptual models in clinical psychiatry. *N Engl J Med* 288:345–351, 1973. Copyright 1973, *New England Journal of Medicine*.

years previously a similar episode of depression had remitted spontaneously. The patient has a sister who was hospitalized for a depressive illness that responded positively to electroconvulsive treatments. A recent physical examination and routine laboratory tests including those for thyroid function were normal. Both the dexamethasone suppression test (DST) and the thyrotropin-releasing hormone (TRH) test were positive for depression.

Psychodynamic Approach

Mrs. J., a 53-year-old widow, presented with a history of depression since the death of her husband a few months ago. Although the marriage seemed happy at times, there were many stormy periods in their relationship. There had been no visible signs of grief since his death. Following the funeral, she became depressed and lost interest in her surroundings. For no apparent reason she blamed herself for traits that characterized her husband more than herself. She had had a similar reaction to the death of her mother 23 years previously, at which time she and her mother had been living together. From the family history, it could be inferred that their relationship was characterized by hostile dependency. Six months after her mother's death, the patient had married. She seemed intelligent and motivated for treatment and said she had considered psychotherapy in the past to gain a better understanding of herself.

Sociocultural Approach

Mrs. J., a 53-year-old widow, presented with depression which began with the death of her husband a few months ago. He had been the major figure in her life, and his loss left her feeling lonely and isolated. After his death, she moved to a small apartment, which was some distance from her old neighborhood. Although she was satisfied with her new quarters, she experienced the community as unfriendly. Furthermore, she did not have access to public transportation, which would have enabled her to visit her old friends, children, and grandchildren. Since her husband's death, old strains between the patient and her children had been aggravated.

Behavioral Approach

Mrs. J., a 53-year-old widow, gave a history of depressive behaviors of anorexia and insomnia, and reported feelings of hopelessness, helplessness, and worthlessness. These symptoms had begun shortly after the death of her husband. Throughout the marriage, he had been a continuous source of reinforcement to the patient. This quality of the husband's interaction with his wife had been evident since the beginning of the marriage, at a time when the patient was still depressed following her mother's death. The family stated that the husband had always ignored the patient's demands and pleas of helplessness while responding actively to the more positive aspects of her personality. After his death, she began to complain to her children about her loss of appetite and her sense of helplessness. She verbalized to them negative conceptions about her own self-worth. They responded to these complaints with frequent visits and telephone calls, which only seemed to worsen the depressive behaviors.

These four histories could each have been elicited from the same patient by four different clinicians, each employing a different conceptual approach to understand the case. It can be seen from the case material above how the clinician, by using one approach to the exclusion of the other, unnecessarily limits the data base and the treatment options. This problem is particularly serious in ambulatory practice because of the great diversity of clinical problems and heterogeneity of clinicians. Both these factors lend themselves to the use of and need for multiple perspectives.

This chapter first describes the four most frequently employed conceptual approaches for the understanding and treatment of psychiatric disorders and psychologic distress by reference to the histories cited above. It then shows how in everyday practice, the decision to use one or a combination of approaches is implicitly determined by the interplay of clinician, patient, and clinical situation. Finally, the integration of these conceptual approaches into a multidimensional, pluralistic framework for clinical practice is discussed.

FOUR MAJOR APPROACHES

The Biologic Approach

The biologic approach views psychiatric disorders as diseases like any others. Even in the absence of known etiology, it is assumed that a relatively uniform syndrome with a predictable natural history identifies the disease. For each disease, it is believed that there eventually will be found a specific cause (or causes) related to the functional anatomy of the brain (1). The clinician using the biologic approach is concerned with etiology, pathogenesis, signs and symptoms, differential diagnosis, treatment, and prognosis. Genetic causation is pursued. Blood testing for trait and state markers, when available, is performed. Every effort is made to rule out known organic causes for the syndrome. Treatment is primarily of a biologic nature when there is one available—either medications or electroconvulsive treatment. The clinician relates to the patient as any other physician would to his or her medical patient—with respectful support but with appropriate distance to preserve objectivity.

Although the biologic approach can be traced to Hippocrates, the modern period in psychiatry begins with Kraepelin's attempts to classify psychiatric disorders by identifying the natural history of symptom clusters. Antidepressant and antipsychotic medications were introduced in the late 1950s, and major strides in the understanding of the biology of mental illness were initiated in the 1960s. (Although the discovery of syndromes and the pursuit of their biologic causes have been an important part of the biologic approach in medicine and psychiatry, in Chapter 8 I show that syndromal phenomena can have psychologic antecedent explanatory models and that biologic explanatory models are relevant to nonsyndromal phenomena. In other words, a syndromal approach and the biologic model should not be considered to be synonymous.)

Consider the case history according to the biologic approach. The clinician observes a group of symptoms consistent with the syndrome of major depression. The current syndrome, the earlier episode of depression, the family history, the positive DST and TRH tests, and the normal medical findings make the diagnosis of major depression most probable. The patient's relation with her family, her ambivalence toward her dead husband, and her motivation to understand her illness are interesting but not central to the recognition and treatment of the disorder. Antidepressant medications or electroconvulsive therapy are the treatment of choice. The patient will be told that she is suffering from depression, a psychiatric illness that is common in her age group. With proper treatment the disorder will probably be time limited and have a favorable prognosis.

The Psychodynamic Approach

According to the psychodynamic approach, the developmental impasse, the early deprivation, the distortions in early relations, and intrapsychic conflict lead to the adult neuroses and vulnerabilities to certain stress. As a result of these psychologic determinants, we see patients who distort reality, who are prone to depression, who avoid heterosexuality, or who fear success. Psychotropic drugs may be given, the social setting may be changed, and behaviors may be extinguished. The abnormality remains, however, because the personality structure is abnormal.

Therapy consists of resolving conflict and strengthening the ego by various psychologic techniques. In the process, the patient is given the opportunity to experience appropriate feelings and to bear intolerable feelings. The psychologic meanings of thoughts, feelings, and behaviors are clarified and put into adult perspective. It is the strength of the therapeutic alliance between therapist and patient that will enable the patient to remember what he or she has not wanted to remember and to abandon familiar but pathologic ways of coping. The transference neurosis—the patient's recreation of pathologic relations to the therapist—will give him or her the opportunity to resolve conflicts and discover new ways of relating.

The psychodynamic approach has exerted considerable influence not only on American psychiatry but also on everyday thinking. Its derivative, psychodynamic psychotherapy, has become a commonly accepted treatment, particularly for the neuroses and personality disorders. Advocates of the psychodynamic approach have been able to translate the clinical insights derived from classical psychoanalysis, ego psychology, object relations theory, and self psychology into concepts that large numbers of clinicians can use in the understanding of many psychiatric patients.

Returning to the case history: The clinician first takes note of the problems in the marital relation. Special attention is paid to the absence of grief, which suggests the presence of psychic conflict and is related to her ambivalent feelings toward her husband. The history of marital conflict is predictive of pathologic grief (2). A similar reaction after her mother's death suggests the possibility of a psychologic connection between feelings toward her husband and mother. This is supported by the history that she married only 6 months after the death of her mother. The patient's criticism of herself in terms that she had used to criticize her husband suggests Freud's concept of introjection of the lost object (3) or Horowitz's activation of latent negative self-images (4). Since the primary modality of treatment is psychotherapy, it is a favorable sign that she is motivated to gain a better understanding of herself.

The Sociocultural Approach

The sociocultural approach to psychiatric illness focuses on the way in which the individual functions in his or her social system. Symptoms are traced not to conflicts within the mind and not to manifestations of psychiatric disease, but to the "relationship of the individual to his manner of functioning in social situations, i.e., in the type and quality of his 'connectedness' to the groups which make up his life space" (5). Symptoms may therefore be regarded as a sign that the social support system is inadequate. Accordingly, when a socially disruptive event occurs, such as a son's leaving home, a wife's death, a geographic displacement by urban renewal, a war, or an economic depression, the resultant symptoms may be seen as stemming from the social disorder (6).

Treatment consists of reorganizing the patient's relation to the social system or reorganizing the social system. If others do not seem to care, how can she get them to care? If the patient's behavior is irrational, how can she learn to stop acting irrationally, or how can her family better tolerate the behavior? If the therapist wants to restructure the nuclear social system, he or she may see the patient with her family or with significant relationships. If the therapist wants to affect the broader social system, he or she may attempt to influence major social issues such as housing or education.

The sociocultural approach, like the biologic and psychodynamic, was reawakened in the 1950s. Since that time the psychiatric ward has been viewed as a social system (7, 8), the relation between social class and mental illness has been established (9), and federal legislation to provide psychiatric care for catchment areas in the community has been enacted (10). During these years, various treatment modalities have succeeded as treatment for mentally ill patients, with minimal separation from their social milieu.

The clinician using the sociocultural approach observes that the patient's social matrix has been altered in two ways. First, she has permanently lost the one person from whom she received the most support. Second, by moving, she has placed herself in a situation where she has lost access to her remaining social support system. In individual or group therapy, one could temporarily provide a substitute or transitional social system. Simultaneously, the therapist might attempt to reestablish a social network in which the patient could be comfortable after discharge. To this end, the therapist might encourage Mrs. J. to move to a home where she could have better access to family and old friends, work with the family to repair any estrangement, or suggest a return to work. Continued individual or group therapy might help the patient acquire social skills that she might never have developed in the marital situation.

The Behavioral Approach

According to the behavioral approach, both neurosis and psychosis are examples of abnormal behaviors that have been learned as a result of aversive events and are maintained either because they lead to positive effects or because they avoid deleterious ones. The overt symptoms are the ones that require treatment, since they themselves are the problem and are not secondary manifestations of disease or unconscious conflict. The typical therapeutic course includes (a) determining the behaviors to be modified, (b) establishing the conditions under which the behaviors occur, (c) determining the factors responsible for the persistence of the behaviors, (d) selecting a set of treatment conditions, and (e) arranging a schedule of retraining. The conditions that precede the behaviors may be modified by such techniques as desensitization, reciprocal inhibition, conditioned avoidance, and cognitive restructuring. The conditions that result from the behaviors may be modified by positive reinforcement, negative reinforcement, aversive conditioning, and extinction.

The behavioral approach, resting on theoretical foundations from the early 20th century, began its period of rapid growth in the late 1950s. Its derivative, behavior therapy, has enjoyed considerable interest in the clinical field during the relatively brief period of its existence. Behavior therapists are hopeful of offering several advantages to other forms of treatment, including shorter duration of treatment and applicability to a broader range of patients.

Regarding the case of Mrs. J., the behavioral clinician first identifies the pathologic behaviors of anorexia and insomnia and the feelings of helplessness. He or she then determines the empirical relation between the depressive behaviors and the antecedent and consequent environmental events that precipitate and maintain the depression. The death of the husband, when one considers the history of the marriage, is interpreted as a sudden withholding of positive reinforcement of adaptive behaviors. The attention received from family members reinforces the depressive behaviors.

Treatment consists of reinforcing adaptive behaviors incompatible with depression, extinguishing depressive behaviors, or correcting cognitive distortions. The clinician may accomplish these therapeutic goals by teaching the family to respond positively to the adaptive behavior instead of the depressive behavior, by purposefully encouraging the patient to express feelings incompatible with depression, or by cognitive restructuring.

CHOICE OF CONCEPTUAL APPROACH

The clinician implicitly uses one or a combination of conceptual approaches in evaluating and treating the patient by the process referred to as clinical judgment. This may be based on empirical data ("That is what research shows"), on ideologic grounds ("That is what I believe"), or on practical grounds ("This is the only available treatment; let's make the best of it"). In this section some of the variables that determine the choice of conceptual model in clinical practice are described.

Ideology of the Therapist and Other Cognitive Factors

Studies of the attitudes of psychiatrists toward the understanding of mental illness have concluded that several ideologies exist (I have been unable to find similar studies for other mental health professionals). Ideology here refers to a coherent system of ideas subscribed to by a subgroup of the profession as a whole. Armor and Klerman point out that ideologic factions are most likely to occur when the codified knowledge base is markedly incomplete and ambiguous about the means to be used to attain a professional goal (11). This has been the position of psychiatry for many decades. Fortunately, this has been much less true for the past decade.

Studies of psychiatric ideologies describe three basic orientations: biologic (objective, descriptive, medical, somatotherapeutic, and directive–organic), psychodynamic (psychotherapeutic and analytic–psychologic), and social (sociotherapeutic) (11–15). These studies do not explore the behavioral orientation, which, in contrast to the other three, has received its greatest impetus from psychologists. Of the ideologies described above, it must be remembered that only a small number of clinicians can be rigidly classified into a single ideology. More commonly, the clinician is committed in various degrees to more than one ideology.

Yager has reviewed some of the cognitive factors that may be involved in the choice of theoretical orientation, the perception of data, and the diagnosis selected (16). These include the views of the senior, prestigious members of the treatment team (17); the order in which the information is presented (18); the clinician's age (19); the personality of the clinician, with its influence on the "style" in reaching a diagnosis (20) and the manner in which data are distorted (21); and, finally, attitudinal variables such as, in Strupp's words, "tolerance, humaneness, and permissiveness, or, in contrast, disciplinarian, moralistic, and harsh qualities" (22).

Diagnosis and the Effectiveness of Somatic Treatment

Other things being equal, particular psychiatric syndromes are apt to be viewed more by one model than by another. Schizophrenia and bipolar disorder are apt to be conceptualized primarily as biologic illness. This is supported by the mounting evidence of genetic transmission of the schizophrenias and some of the mood disorders and by the clear-cut efficacy of phenothiazines and butyrophenones for the treatment of the acute symptoms of schizo-

phrenia, of lithium and carbamazine for the treatment of bipolar disorder, and of the tricyclics, monoamine oxidase inhibitors, and electroconvulsive therapy for the treatment of many depressions. In current practice, psychosocial treatments are combined with the biologic approaches described above for the best results. The zeal for psychotherapy as the only intervention for these syndromes, particularly mania and the schizophrenias, has radically diminished over the past decades.

The personality disorders are more apt to be treated by psychodynamic and behavioral approaches, although some clinicians maintain a biologic model. For these disorders, syndromes are less clearly distinguishable, there is minimal evidence of genetic transmission, and medication has less specific effects. Furthermore, the efficacy of the psychotherapies in these disorders is gaining support from clinical research (23, 24).

Social Class and Other Attributes of the Patient

A number of studies have demonstrated the importance of the patient's social class in the application of psychotherapy (25–27). Patients of the middle and upper social classes are more apt to be accepted for, and to continue in, psychotherapy. Patients of the lower and lower-middle classes, in contrast, have a poorer chance of being accepted for therapy and drop out of treatment at higher rates (28). Other patient characteristics that determine the use of psychotherapy include responsibility, verbal intelligence, psychologic-mindedness, the capacity for forming a close personal relation, young adult age, history of effective adaptation before the current difficulty, likeability, and attractiveness (29). In addition, patients treated by psychotherapy are apt to continue in treatment when their expectations are congruent with those of the therapist (30).

Such a patient population, presenting as they often do as relatively healthy people who want help in achieving personal fulfillment (greater psychologic strength, more satisfactory relationships, comfort with their sexual identity, etc.), may be rejected by those who adhere to the biologic approach as "not mentally ill."

Although psychotherapeutically oriented clinicians may attempt to explain and understand most or all of the pathologic and normal behavior by psychodynamic theory, they may be reluctant to take patients into treatment if they want medication or advice, if they have had previous psychiatric hospitalization, if they are vulnerable to psychosis, if they are psychotic or older, or if they present a multitude of somatic complaints (29). A welcome countertrend to this position is the increasing interest of psychodynamic clinicians, particularly those of the object relations school, in treating more seriously ill patients.

Available Services

The available treatment resources are an important determinant of the choice of conceptual model. Psychotherapy clinics, especially when not overcrowded, attempt to apply the psychodynamic approach to the understanding of patients. Walk-in and emergency clinics of general hospitals and community mental health centers, in responding to large numbers of patients in crisis, approach the patient from sociocultural and biologic perspectives that usually require less time from the professional but are effective for many clinical conditions. Specialty clinics that deal with problems such as stress, eating disorders, and marital conflict commonly apply a single orientation to all patients according to the ideology of its leadership.

AN INTEGRATION FOR CLINICAL PRACTICE

It is unfortunate that the conceptual approaches have remained so separate from each other. To the degree that this occurs, communication between professionals is impaired, progress requiring a broad focus is slowed, and treatment options are limited. Nevertheless, there have been promising and exciting attempts to provide an integration for these and other apparently disparate approaches.

Vertical Integration

Vertical reasoning in science refers to thinking about the objects and processes under study in descending or ascending order according to the size and complexity of the units. A vertical hierarchy, for instance, may range from culture to family to person to nervous system to organ to tissue to cells to molecules to atoms (31).

The most common and successful process of integration of the various phenomena in the vertical hierarchy for the physical and biological sciences is *reductionism*. This refers to the process by which (and the belief that) various phenomena are explained by mechanisms at a lower level in the scientific hierarchy. In other words, social phenomena are to be explained by or reduced to the specific terms and laws of psychology, while psychologic phenomenon are to be explained by or reduced to the specific terms and laws of the nervous system—its biology, chemistry, and physics (32, 33). Reiser (34) has recently reviewed the pioneering neurobiologic work of Kandel (35) and Goldman and Rakic (36), who offer reductionist explanations for certain aspects of learning and psychoanalytic theory.

The problem with the reductionist integration in clinical psychiatry and medicine is that many of the phenomena under investigation require simultaneous explanations from various hierarchical levels for adequate understanding. Furthermore, optimal explanation and clinical intervention may require the use of higher rather than lower levels in the vertical hierarchy. For example, a child's maladaptive behavior may be best explained and treated by an understanding of family psychopathology rather than individual psychology or biology.

Many psychiatrists, psychologists, and internists oppose the philosophic premise of reductionism. While admitting that many behavioral phenomena will eventually be reduced to meaningful subunits, they argue that there are other important phenomena that are not reducible. The philosophic basis of this reasoning can be understood through the notion of *emergence*, which refers to the appearance of new properties of the phenomena in question as one moves up the vertical hierarchy toward larger and more complex units (31–33). For example, once the atoms of hydrogen and oxygen combine to form the molecule of water, new properties emerge such as viscosity, density, and transparency which cannot be described and explained by the language and explanatory models of atomic physics. From a different perspective, reducing a Cezanne painting to a molecular examination of the paint pigments does not provide a more profound or basic analysis of the work as art. In clinical psychiatry, understanding how people function in groups requires explanatory models of group interaction that individual psychology or biologic psychiatry cannot provide. Although there undoubtedly is a biology of the experience of shame, its clinical understanding requires a psychologic and social understanding of a shame-inducing event, a personal vulnerability to shame based on past experience, and a social context for the shame experience (37). In individual psychology, concepts such as self, meaning, purpose, and hope have emergent qualities which require psychologic language and explanation. On the basis of the above analysis, it seems inappropriate to refer to the more biologic sciences as *basic* in contrast to the behavioral sciences (38). The biologic sciences are more reductionistic in the sense of attempting to explain phenomena on the basis of smaller units, but not more basic in the sense of being necessarily more profound, more scientific, more fundamental, or more useful.

Spiegel's transactional approach (39) and Engel's biopsychosocial approach (40, 41), based on von Bertalanffy's general systems theory (42), are attempts to integrate phenomena of the behavioral sciences from several vertical levels of knowledge. The systems integration studies the various levels of integration, their interrelations, and the relationship of each level to the whole. It admits to the occurrence of emergence (33). Such integrations attempt to avoid two major pitfalls of the behavioral sciences: brainlessness (a psychology devoid of neuroscience) and mindlessness (a neuroscience devoid of personal and social meaning (33, 43).

Horizontal Integration

Within a given level in the hierarchy, particularly at the psychologic level, there are several competing explanatory models, such as the psychodynamic, the behavioral, and the existential. Each model may further contain several alternative approaches. For example, the psychodynamic model includes ego psychologic, object relational, and self psychologic approaches. Walsh and Peterson have described two types of horizontal integration for the above models (44). They refer to the first as single school expansionism in which adherents of one school attempt to expand their concepts to include those of other schools while remaining faithful to their basic theoretical premises. The incorporation by ego psychologists of environmental and social dimensions into the psychodynamic approach (45, 46) and the incorporation by some behaviorists of intrapersonal, cognitive phenomena into the behavioral approach (47, 48) are examples of this form of integration. The second form of integration, referred to as *cross-school integration*, attempts to combine "the strengths of different schools into a new, superior hybrid" (44). The works of Marmor and Woods (49) and Wachtel (50), for example, propose to integrate psychoanalysis and behaviorism.

A Multidimensional Approach

Although the vertical and horizontal integrations described above represent significant theoretical contributions, they are difficult to translate into clinical practice. Neither systems theory nor behavioral/psychodynamic hybrids provide guidelines that help a clinician decide for a given clinical situation (*a*) at what level(s) of the vertical hierarchy and with what model in a given horizontal level to begin, (*b*) what approaches should be combined, and (*c*) when to switch. Given these clinical problems, the most effective clinical integration of various conceptual points of view or paradigms at both horizontal and vertical levels can be best accomplished, in my view, by an approach referred to as multidimensional, perspectival, pluralistic, or eclectic. This is consistent with my understanding of the positions of McHugh and Slavney (51), Eisenberg (43), Yager (16), Abrams (52), Simon (53), Strauss (54), and Walsh and Peterson (44). In a multidimensional approach, the clinician attempts to understand the problems of each patient through each of several frames of reference. Yager refers to this process as the "eclectic mental operation," the application of different perspectives to the specific situation, "as if they were a series of different colored lenses and filters flashing one after another" (16) before the clinician's eyes. Following the optical metaphor, only one perspective can be put into clear focus at a given moment in time. The others blur in the periphery. de Bono talks about "approaching the available information from several points of entry and repatterning the information in an attempt to see alternative possibilities" (55). Finally, McHugh and Slavney describe the material of psychiatric practice "as a fabric of distinct themes: a warp of constructs— tied together by a woof of explanatory methods" (51). The study and practice of psychiatry, they conclude, is the study of separate and interlocking constructs and explanatory methods.

In sum, the clinician needs to view human beings simultaneously and separately through alternative horizontal and vertical frames of reference. (The four models presented in this chapter are both vertical and horizontal. That is, the behavioral and psychodynamic approaches are horizontal to each other, while the social, psychodynamic, and biologic are on a vertical hierarchy.) The use of each approach and combinations of approaches should be considered according to empirical evidence for efficacy, the patient's requests and expectations, and the feasibility of providing the treatment. Each clinical situation requires a fresh problem-solving approach. This and much more is what is referred to as clinical judgment.

References

1. Slater F, Roth M: *Clinical Psychiatry*, ed 3. Baltimore, Williams & Wilkins, 1969.
2. Parkes CM, Weiss RS: *Recovery from Bereavement*. New York, Basic Books, 1983.
3. Freud S: Mourning and melancholia. In *Collected Papers*, vol 4 (1917). New York, Basic Books, 1959, pp. 152–170.
4. Horowitz M, Wilner N, Marmar C, et al: Pathological grief and the activation of latent self-images. *Am J Psychiatry* 137:1157–1162, 1980.
5. Thomas CS, Bergen BJ: Social psychiatric view of psychological misfunction and role of psychiatry in social change. *Arch Gen Psychiatry* 12:539–544, 1965.
6. Weiss RJ, Bergen BJ: Social supports and the reduction of psychiatric disability. *Psychiatry* 31:107–115, 1968.
7. Caudill WA: *The Psychiatric Hospital as a Small Society*. Cambridge, MA, Harvard University Press, 1958.
8. Stanton AH, Schwartz MS: *The Mental Hospital: A Study of Institutional Participation in Psychiatric Illness and Treatment*. New York, Basic Books, 1954.
9. Hollingshead AB, Redlich FC: *Social Class and Mental Illness: A Community Study*. New York, John Wiley & Sons, 1958.
10. Weston WD: Development of community psychiatry concepts. In Freedman AM, Kaplan HI, Sadock BJ (eds): *Comprehensive Textbook of Psychiatry*. Baltimore, Williams & Wilkins, 1975, pp 2310–2323.
11. Armor DJ, Klerman GL: Psychiatric treatment orientations and professional ideology. *J Health Soc Behav* 9:243–255, 1968.
12. Sharaf MR, Levinson DJ: Patterns of ideology and role definition among psychiatric residents. In Greenblatt M, Levinson DJ, Williams RH (eds): *The Patient and the Mental Hospital*. Chicago, Free Press of Glencoe Illinois, 1957, pp 263–285.
13. Gilbert DC, Levinson DJ: Ideology, personality, and institutional policy in the mental hospital. *J Abnorm Soc Psychol* 53:263–271, 1956.
14. MacIver J, Redlich FC: Patterns of psychiatric practice. *Am J Psychiatry* 115:692–697, 1959.
15. Ehrlich D, Sabshin M: A study of sociotherapeutically oriented psychiatrists. *Am J Orthopsychiatry* 34:469–480, 1964.
16. Yager J: Psychiatric eclecticism: a cognitive view. *Am J Psychiatry* 134:736–741, 1977.
17. Lehmann HE, Banta DM: Rating the rater. *Arch Gen Psychiatry* 13:67–75, 1965.

18. Gauron EF, Dickinson JK: The influence of seeing the patient first on diagnostic decision making in psychiatry. *Am J Psychiatry* 126:199–205, 1969.
19. Katz MM, Cole JO, Lowery HA: Studies of the diagnostic process: the influence of symptom perception, past experience, and ethnic background on diagnostic decisions. *Am J Psychiatry* 125:937–947, 1969.
20. Guaron EF, Dickinson JK: Diagnostic decision making in psychiatry. II. Diagnostic styles. *Arch Gen Psychiatry* 14:233–237, 1966.
21. Raines GN, Rohrer JH: The operational matrix of psychiatric practice. I. Consistency and variability in interview impressions of different psychiatrists. *Am J Psychiatry* 111:721–733, 1955.
22. Strupp HH: *Psychotherapists in Action.* New York, Grune & Stratton, 1960.
23. Luborsky L, Singer B, Luborsky L: Comparative studies of psychotherapies. *Arch Gen Psychiatry* 32:995–1008, 1975.
24. Smith ML, Glass GV: Meta-analysis of psychotherapy outcome studies. *Am Psychologist* 32:752–760, 1977.
25. Lief HI, Lief, VF, Warren CO, et al: Low dropout rate in a psychiatric clinic: special reference to psychotherapy and social class. *Arch Gen Psychiatry* 5:200–211, 1961.
26. Schaffer L, Myers JK: Psychotherapy and social stratification: an empirical study of practice in a psychiatric outpatient clinic. *Psychiatry* 17:83–93, 1954.
27. Myers JK, Schaffer L: Social stratification and psychiatric practice: a study of an out-patient clinic. *Am Sociol Rev* 19:307–310, 1954.
28. Overall B, Aronson H: Expectations of psychotherapy in patients of lower socioeconomic class. *Am J Orthospsychiatry* 33:421–430, 1963.
29. Levinson DJ, Merrifield J, Berg K: Becoming a patient. *Arch Gen Psychiatry* 17:385–406, 1967.
30. Heine RW, Trosman H: Initial expectations of the doctor–patient interaction as a factor in continuance in psychotherapy. *Psychiatry* 23:275–278, 1960.
31. Blois MS: Medicine and the nature of vertical reasoning *N Engl J Med* 318:847–851, 1988.
32. Hempel CG: *The Philosophy of Natural Science.* Englewood Cliffs, NJ, Prentice-Hall, 1966.
33. Bunge M, Ardila R: *Philosophy of Psychology.* New York, Springer-Verlag, 1987.
34. Reiser MF: *Mind, Brain, and Body: Toward a Convergence of Psychoanalysis and Neurobiology.* New York, Basic Books, 1984.
35. Kandel ER: Psychotherapy and the single synapse: the impact of psychiatric thought on neurobiologic research. *N Engl J Med* 301:1028–37, 1979.
36. Goldman PS, Rakic PT: Impact of the outside world upon the developing primate brain. *Bulletin of the Menninger Clinic* 43:20–28, 1979.
37. Lazare A: Shame and humiliation in the medical encounter. *Arch Intern Med* 147:1653–1658, 1987.
38. Engel GL: Enduring attributes of medicine relevant for the education of the physician. *Ann Intern Med* 78:587–593, 1973.
39. Spiegel J: *Transactions: The Interplay Between Individual, Family and Society.* New York, Science House, 1971.
40. Engel GL: The need for a new medical model: a challenge for biomedicine. *Science* 196:129–130, 1977.
41. Engel GL: The clinical application of the biopsychosocial model. *Am J Psychiatry* 137:535–544, 1980.
42. von Bertalanffy L: *General Systems Theory.* New York, Braziller, 1968.
43. Eisenberg L: Mindlessness and brainlessness in psychiatry. *Br J Psychiatry* 148:497–508, 1986.
44. Walsh BW, Peterson LE: Philosophical foundations of psychological theories: the issue of synthesis. *Psychotherapy* 22:145–153, 1985.
45. Mahler MS: *The Psychological Birth of the Human Infant.* Chicago, University of Chicago Press, 1978.
46. Blanck G, Blanck R: *Ego Psychology II.* New York, Columbia University Press, 1979.
47. Meichenbaum D: *Cognitive Behavior Modification.* New York, Plenum, 1978.
48. Mahoney MJ: *Cognition and Behavior Modification.* Cambridge, MA, Ballenger, 1974.
49. Marmor J, Woods SM: *The Interface Between the Psychodynamic and Behavioral Therapies.* New York, Plenum Press, 1980.
50. Wachtel PL: *Psychoanalysis and Behavior Therapy.* New York, Basic Books, 1977.
51. McHugh PR, Slavney PR: *The Perspectives of Psychiatry.* Baltimore, MD, John Hopkins University Press, 1986.
52. Abrams GM: The new eclecticism. *Arch Gen Psychiatry* 20:514–523, 1976.
53. Simon RH: On eclecticism. *Am J Psychiatry* 131:135–139, 1974.
54. Strauss JS: A comprehensive approach to psychiatric diagnosis. *Am J Psychiatry* 132:1193–1197, 1975.
55. de Bono E: *The Mechanism of Mind.* New York, Simon & Schuster, 1969.

3

The Biologic Approach

Mai-Lan Rogoff, M.D.
Aaron Lazare, M.D.

This chapter presents an overview of five aspects of biologic psychiatry for the practicing clinician. We refer to them collectively as the biologic approach. They include (a) the relationship of medical disease to psychiatric symptoms, (b) psychologic and social influences on biologic processes and disease, (c) biologic treatments for psychiatric disorders, (d) the syndromal approach, and (e) presumed biologic mechanisms in the etiology and pathogenesis of psychiatric disorders. Each of these aspects of the biologic approach has its own history, research base, and clinical application. This diversity may explain, in part, the differences in focus, emphasis, and expertise among clinicians who espouse the biologic approach. We conclude this chapter by attempting to provide a synthesis of these five dimensions of the biologic approach through their application to clinical practice and training.

THE RELATIONSHIP OF MEDICAL DISEASE TO PSYCHIATRIC SYMPTOMS

The types of relationships between medical disease and psychiatric symptoms and disorders can be classified in the following manner: (a) There are psychiatric symptoms and medical disorders which share a common symptomatology, resulting in medical conditions mimicking psychiatric conditions or psychiatric conditions mimicking medical conditions. Examples of the first situation are symptoms of anxiety caused by hyperthyroidism or manic behavior caused by steroids. Examples of the second situation are symptoms of medical disorders which are manifestations of conversion symptoms or somatization disorder. (b) Medical disease may exacerbate or precipitate psychiatric disorders in vulnerable individuals. Depression secondary to medical disorders and conversion symptoms secondary to neurologic disease are examples. (c) Psychiatric conditions may have a causal relationship to medical disorders. Examples include the increased cardiovascular vulnerability, particularly in men, following bereavement and the obvious medical complications of anorexia nervosa and substance abuse. (d) Medical disease and psychiatric symptoms or disorders may coexist independently in the same patient with no etiologic or pathogenic link. An example is a patient who has schizophrenia and a myocardial infarction. Interactions between the two conditions still exist in that the patient's thought disorder will influence how he or she interprets and responds to the pain of coronary insufficiency (1).

17

Of the four kinds of medical/psychiatric relationships described above, the one that is of greatest interest to the biologic psychiatrist and behavioral neurologist is the relationship of psychiatric symptoms to known medical conditions. The literature on this subject can be organized in three categories: the incidence of medical disease in various types of psychiatric practice, the incidence of misdiagnosed conversion symptoms which ultimately are determined to be caused by or associated with known medical disease, and the psychiatric manifestations of specific medical disorders or the differential diagnosis of psychiatric symptoms.

Incidence of Psychiatric Disease in Psychiatric Populations

We have found 19 studies of the incidence of medical disease in psychiatric populations. (These are reviewed in Chapter 17.) Five were conducted in the 1960s, seven in the 1970s, and five in the 1980s. Only two were conducted prior to 1960. The settings include eight inpatient units, six outpatient units, one brief-stay observation unit, one day hospital, one emergency clinic, one community support program, and one outpatient rehabilitation program. On psychiatric inpatient services, 34% to 84% of patients were noted to have physical diseases. In these studies, the range of patients with physical disease previously undiagnosed ranged from 10% to 80%. The range of patients whose physical disease caused or contributed to the psychiatric presentation ranged from 12% to 46%. On the outpatient services, 26% to 51% of patients were noted to have physical disease, with 13% to 35% previously undiagnosed. The range of outpatients whose physical disease caused or contributed to the psychiatric presentation ranged from "a few" to 36%.

Conversion Symptoms and Known Medical Disease

Two aspects of the relation between organic illness and conversion symptoms are of vital importance in clinical diagnosis. The first is the high incidence of concomitant medical disease in patients with conversion symptoms. The second is the substantial percentage of patients whose initial diagnosis of conversion symptoms is changed to medical disease (2).

The frequent association of conversion symptoms with organic disease has been noted for more than 100 years. Specific lesions and diseases mentioned by Merskey include frontal lobe lesions, epilepsy, multiple sclerosis, head injury, encephalitis, and Klinefelter's syndrome (3). Whitlock, in a study of hysteria-diagnosed patients in psychiatric inpatient units in Australia and England found that 63.5% of patients had coexisting or antecedent organic brain disorders, compared with only 5.5% in a control group. This association suggests that in the evaluation of patients presenting with conversion symptoms, even with psychologic validating criteria, the possibility of a concomitant organic illness must not be overlooked (4).

There are six noteworthy studies of the incidence of misdiagnosed conversion symptoms based on follow-up studies of up to 20 years (5–10). From these studies it can be concluded that of all hospitalized patients who receive a diagnosis of conversion reaction, 13% to 30% will subsequently be found to have organic illness which accounts for the presumed functional etiology. These studies offer some evidence that spontaneous improvement, improvement following amytal, or conversion patterns on the Minnesota Multiphasic Personality Inventory do not necessarily confirm the diagnosis of conversion rather than organic disease. There are two limitations of these studies. First, they were performed before certain diagnostic procedures such as computerized tomographic scanning became available. Second, they are based primarily on inpatient populations. It is highly unlikely that such high percentages of outpatient conversion symptoms will ultimately be diagnosed as organic in origin.

Psychiatric Manifestations of Specific Medical Disorders and the Differential Diagnosis of Psychiatric Symptoms

Perhaps the first book on the psychiatric aspects of neurologic disease was *Psychiatric Aspects of Neurologic Disease*, edited by Benson and Blumer (11). The first edition appeared in 1975 and the second volume in 1982 (12). The next major book on the psychologic manifestations of medical disorders was *Organic Psychiatry*, written by Lishman in 1978 (13). This 999-page compendium containing more than 2000 references is now in its second edition (1986) (14). This book was followed by five more brief clinically oriented works: Hall's *Psychiatric Presentations of Medical Illness* in 1980 (15), Jefferson and Marshall's *Neuropsychiatric Features of Medical Disorders* in 1981 (16), Cummings's *Clinical Neuropsychiatry* in 1985 (17), Extein and Gold's *Medical Mimics of Psychiatric Disorders* in 1986 (18), and Soreff and McNeil's *Handbook of Psychiatric Differential Diagnosis* in 1987 (19). In 1979, the first edition of *Outpatient Psychiatry* devoted more than 100 pages in 14 chapters on the differential diagnosis of psychiatric symptoms with known medical conditions (20). The present edition continues this practice. All of the above books have reviewed, organized, and integrated the research literature, predominantly from the 1960s and 1970s, for clinical practice for the 1980s. It is of historical interest that the late Norman Geschwind wrote the forward to the Benson and Blumer book, that Benson was Geschwind's first behavioral neurology fellow, and that Benson was mentor to Cummings.

A Historical Perspective

There are several possible reasons for the appearance of these articles and books in the last three decades: First, the rapid expansion of outpatient psychiatric services during these decades brought new patient populations to psychiatric attention, many of whom had medical disorders which were causative of or coexisted with psychiatric conditions. The limited amount of time available for assessment in these clinical settings made careful but rapid medical diagnosis essential. Second, biologic psychiatry was at that time in its ascendency. This was a result of the impressive gains in biologic treatments for psychiatric disorders, studies of the biology of mental illness, and new diagnostic tests for medical and neurologic disorders. Third, of added significance was the rapid increase in nonmedical mental health clinicians (psychologists, social workers, and mental health workers) trained in the psychosocial treatments. This influenced many psychiatrists to reaffirm their medical identity as diagnosticians of medical and psychiatric conditions.

PSYCHOLOGIC AND SOCIAL INFLUENCES ON BIOLOGIC PROCESSES AND DISEASE

The study of the psychologic influence of conflict or stress on human biology has taken two distinct directions over the past 40 years. The first may be referred to as the specificity hypothesis and the second as the nonspecific stress hypothesis.

Specificity Theory

Specificity theory, which flourished in the 1950s (21–23), developed out of a psychoanalytic tradition and initially emphasized a limited number of "psychosomatic" diseases. These included asthma, hypertension, peptic ulcer, rheumatoid arthritis, thyrotoxicosis, ulcerative colitis, migraine, and eczema. Theories linking psyche and soma in these disorders suggested that specific unconscious emotional conflicts led to disorders related to that conflict. For example, conflicts over dependence/independence were felt to be associated with intestinal disorders, expression/suppression of rage or anxiety with cardiovascular problems or vascular headaches, and panic at feared object loss with asthma, hyperthyroidism, and rheumatoid arthritis.

Critiques of specificity theory have focused on (a) the underlying assumptions of specificity theory (psychoanalytic principles and consideration of illnesses with varying etiologies as if they had a uniform pathophysiology), (b) methodology (use of inference, retrospective studies, lack of adequate controls), (c) failure to appreciate the difference between correlation and causation, (d) the failure of controlled studies to validate the theory, and (e) the existence of animal models for most of these illnesses despite the fact that animals are unlikely to possess the symbolic thought necessary for the production of complex psychoanalytic mechanisms.

These arguments do not suggest that emotional state is unrelated to illness, merely that biology and psychology are related in more complex ways than originally envisioned. Actually, Franz Alexander, whose name is most linked with specificity theory, felt that specific psychologic conflicts are not sufficient to account for disease and suggested that an organ vulnerability is also necessary. Weiner, in his extensive summary of research in the psychosomatic illnesses (24), concluded that if there is any role for specific conflicts in illness production, it can only be in the presence of organ vulnerability.

Nonspecific Stress Hypothesis

Work with life events scales such as that by Holmes and Rahe (25) has shown that life crises often precede the onset of physical illness. The same stressor has different effects on different people, however, because of the different meanings of stressors to individuals. Stress is thus conceived of as transactional rather than unidirectional, not the result of specific psychologic conflicts, but rather resulting from an imbalance between the demands of a situation and the individual's ability to respond. Selye's General Adaptation Syndrome (GAS) (26) and Cannon's fight-or-flight theories (27) proposed that continued activation of compensatory mechanisms by chronic emotional stress is harmful to the body.

The cardiovascular system has been extensively studied in this context, mainly through research in hypertension, myocardial infarction, and cardiac arrhythmias. Cardiac arrhythmias, for example, may be provoked by psychologic stress in the laboratory in vulnerable subjects (28, 29). A more controversial question has been whether a specific personality style, such as the "Type A personality," might lead to increased risk of physical illness. The Type A behavior pattern has been defined as "a characteristic action–emotion complex which is exhibited by those individuals who are engaged in a chronic struggle to obtain an unlimited number of poorly defined things from their environment in the shortest period of time and, if necessary, against the opposing efforts of other things or persons in this same environment" (30). While some support for the concept of Type A behavior as a risk factor in coronary artery disease has been developed (31), several subsequent studies have failed to bear out this hypothesis (32–34). Ruberman found that neither Type A personality nor depression were important variables in sudden death after myocardial infarction unless they were also associated with a poor social network (35). Current interest in this issue focuses on attempts to define aspects of the Type A personality (such as hostility) which might be correlated with increased risk.

Similar difficulties have been encountered in looking for a personality style associated with cancer. The hypothesis has been that individuals who repress and deny emotional stress and have slow recovery from depression after loss are more vulnerable to cancer. Inconsistencies in studies looking at spontaneous remission or 5-year survival rates versus personality style have prevented a definitive at-risk personality from being defined.

One concept present in both specificity and nonspecific stress hypotheses of the "psychosomatic" illnesses is the importance of the maintenance of bonds between people. Writers in specificity theory tended to conceptualize only the exaggeration of these bonds as "dependence" or "self-objects required to prevent fragmentation." Alexander referred to patients with psychosomatic disorders as having a "regressive need to be loved and helped" (21). Support for a more general role of human attachments in decreasing vulnerability to illness has been provided by research into the effects of bereavement.

Real or imagined rupture of human relationships has been shown in many studies to lead to increased illness and mortality (36, 37). This has been true of the classic "psychosomatic" illnesses, as well as of cancer, diabetes mellitus, cardiac arrhythmias, congestive heart failure, and adverse outcome of surgical operations (24). Social bonds are also important in social animals other than man. Separating young monkeys from their mothers produces marked psychologic and physical effects. The adverse effect of isolation is not limited to higher primates; isolation rearing is also used as a standard stressor in rat studies. In humans, on the other hand, social and community ties have been associated with lower mortality in bereavement (38, 39), decreased complications after childbirth (40), decreased risk of death in cardiac illness (35), reduced joint swelling in arthritis (41), and with reduction in need for steroids in asthma (42). High social support or even the mere presence of a confidant also reduces clinical depression (43).

Proposed Physiologic Mechanisms

The mechanisms which translate emotional experience into physiologic change and disease are still being developed, as are the mechanisms which translate physiologic input back into emotional experience. Stress may exert both direct and indirect biologic effects. An example of an indirect biologic effect of stress might be changed behavior such as increased alcohol drinking or cigarette smoking, in turn contributing to disease. Studies of the direct effects of stress are generally divided into those which examine ways in which

early exposure to stress may induce chronic vulnerabilities to subsequent stressors, and studies which look at the immediate effects of stress.

Immediate Effects of Stress

Much of the work on the biologic effects of stress has been done on the immediate effects of stress or bereavement. Stress causes a broad range of physiologic changes, including changes in hormone levels, 24-hour rhythms, elevated levels of 17-OH corticosteroids, epinephrine, and norepinephrine. Acute changes in sympathetic tone may be responsible for a variety of effects, such as increased heart rate, body temperature changes, and cardiac arrhythmias; increased sleep latency and sleep disruption have also been described, in nonhuman primates as well as in humans (44, 45). Graboys has suggested that sudden changes in sympathetic adrenergic tone may change levels of catecholamines and other neurotransmitters leading to acute alteration of cellular automaticity and excitability (46). Increased sympathetic activity may raise blood fatty acid levels and lead to atherosclerosis (47), or acute increases in blood pressure may lead to increased production of connective tissue in arterial walls for support, leading to hypertension (48).

Neuroendocrine changes following stress have been well described. Acute stress provokes the release of catabolic hormones adrenocorticotropic hormone, growth hormone, and thyroid stimulating hormone. These hormones promote increases in blood sugar and free fatty acids. There is a reciprocal inhibition of anabolic hormones (sex hormones, insulin) which may rebound during the recovery phase from acute stress. Plasma cortisol increases acutely, not always in correlation with the degree of behavioral disturbance shown by the subject, and remains elevated for a period of time after the cessation of the trauma in both animal and human studies (49, 50).

As stress becomes more intense and then chronic, the shifts in hormone and catecholamine production which occur are more complex. Rises in urine 17-OH corticosteroids, epinephrine, and norepinephrine are followed by different rates of fall after the cessation of acute stress: thyroid level rises followed by a slow fall, insulin decreases during stress followed by a rise, sex hormones fall and remain low next day, and urine volume decreases (51, 52). The fall in norepinephrine and epinephrine levels with chronic stress may be a result of synthesis falling behind utilization, while corticosterone is increased as the activity of the hypothalamic–pituitary–adrenal axis increases. Under continuous stress, neurochemical adaptation occurs and many of these changes are no longer seen. The limbic–midbrain circuit probably functions as the intermediary between the hypothalamus/pituitary, the autonomic nervous system, and the cerebral association cortex. A central endorphin system has also been suggested. Endorphins are concentrated in sites known to be involved in mood and hormone regulation (limbic system, pituitary, and brainstem).

The large number of studies which show increased rates of morbidity and mortality after bereavement have led to the suspicion that immune functioning also may be compromised after acute stress. High doses of exogenous steroids are known to have an immunosuppressive effect (via both cellular and humoral response); thyroid, sex hormones, growth hormone, and insulin are all necessary for the development of the immune response and are all affected by stress. Studies have described both decreases and exaggeration of immune functioning following stress. These changes have been found in both humoral and cellular immune systems (53, 54). In addition, decreases in the concentration of adenosine cyclic monophosphate (cAMP) or increases in the relative concentration of cyclic guanosine monophosphate (cGMP) over cAMP could have an effect on allergic disease by facilitating the release of histamine from mast cells. It is also interesting to note that immune system dysfunction has been implicated in most of the original "psychosomatic" illnesses.

Thus there are multiple physiologic changes which accompany acute and chronic stress and which seem to vary by intensity and duration of the stressor but not by specificity of the conflict. The specificity may lie not in the psychologic conflict but in a vulnerable organ system which reacts physiologically to nonspecific physical and emotional stressors in a more intense and sustained fashion, resulting in disease.

Delayed Effects of Early Life Stress

In this more speculative area of research into the effects of stress, various mechanisms have been proposed. Increased subsequent vulnerability to illness following early life stress may be induced through biologic or psychologic factors or, most likely, through some combination of the two. Genetic or induced changes in physiology, for example, may interact with the environment to alter personality development. An infant with a tendency to increased gastric secretion might feel constantly hungry and inconsolable regardless of mothering, leaving him vulnerable to oral dependency needs and peptic ulcer (55). Early experiences have also been shown to change subsequent behavior and physiologic response in animals (56). The effect of early life stress may depend on the timing and type of stressor as well as of the subsequent challenge. For example, various social stresses increased susceptibility to a virus to which a mouse strain was normally resistant but made no difference in susceptibility to a virus to which the mice were normally susceptible (57). Handling and shock stress may increase or decrease susceptibility to injected Walker Sarcoma virus, depending on the type of stress and its timing (58).

Loss of social supports has been shown to produce biologic effects in both humans and animals. Reaction to separation in animals depends on species characteristics, on the characteristics of their natural social groups, and on strong individual variation in the response to separation (59, 60). This individual variation raises the interesting question of which innate or learned factors may enable coping in the animal or human. Harlow's monkeys separated from their mothers showed temperamental differences; monkeys which adjusted to the parting generally showed less fear and anxiety when confronted with other novel situations; these differences were apparent as early as the first month of life and held true until 4 years and even adulthood (61). It is unclear whether the monkey's lower physiologic arousal in the face of stress was a cause or a result of their enhanced coping. High-reactivity monkeys also had high-reactivity relatives and the first-borns of high-reactivity mothers were often abused or neglected. The appearance of differences in response to stress so early in life has led to speculation about the effect of prenatal stress on subsequent adaptation; however, this work has remained highly conjectural.

Other biologic mechanisms may operate to facilitate the development of illness through earlier experiences. Early life experiences could condition physical responses which would then predispose to certain illnesses. For example, increased crying in infancy might lead to subsequent hypertension through mechanisms of conditioning (62). Early life experiences might also cause structural alterations, as has been shown to occur for the visual system (63, 64), or may alter hormonal or enzymatic functioning. Environmental changes have been shown to change postsynaptic membrane response or to increase synaptic connections (65). Early handling of mice changes their glucocorticoid receptor status and affects the development of cognitive deficits in mouse senescence (66). Adult rats stressed as infants have a more marked adrenocortical response to cold or shock than unhandled litter mates (67, 68) and are more vulnerable to adjuvant-induced arthritis (69). Early experience with social isolation or crowding changes the subsequent hormonal and neurotransmitter response as well as degree of blood pressure rise to restraint stress in mice (70–74). These effects of early adverse experiences in animals may be evident only under later stress and provide a biologic insight into the clinical observation that human individuals who function adequately under normal circumstances may still be unusually vulnerable to stress.

Another way in which early life stress may predispose to illness is by altering subsequent immune functioning. Genetics, experience, and stress interact in the formation of amyloid deposits, which are chains of immunoglobulins. Classical conditioning of the immune response has been demonstrated, using saccharin paired with cyclophosphamide (which depresses immune response). A subsequent challenge with a previously sensitized allergen and saccharin led to partial reduction of the immune response even in the absence of cyclophosphamide (75). There is also some evidence of neurohumoral connection between the brain and immune system, suggesting the possibility of reciprocal influence: alpha- and beta-adrenergic, cholinergic, and other neurotransmitter receptors are present on lymphocytes, and damage to the anterior hypothalamus has an ameliorating effect on experimentally induced anaphylaxis in animals (76).

Early life experience thus may increase vulnerability to subsequent illness. It is likely that early experience interacts with maturational processes of the brain to produce different effects at different ages, or effects which may not become manifest until a later maturational age. These changes in brain structure or function may alter the way in which subsequent experiences are perceived or integrated. Illness results from an imbalance in dynamic regulatory mechanisms and also has multiple rather than unitary causation on both psychodynamic and physiologic bases.

BIOLOGIC TREATMENTS FOR PSYCHIATRIC DISORDERS[a]

The modern era of biologic treatments in psychiatry began during the 10-year period from 1949 to 1959, during which time the modern antipsychotic, antidepressant, and antianxiety agents were discovered and established as effective. The specific drugs introduced during this period in-

---

[a] This section is based on three sources (77–79).

clude lithium, reserpine, chlorpromazine (Thorazine), the tricyclic antidepressants, the monoamine oxidase inhibitors (MAOIs), chlordiazepoxide (Librium), and meprobamate. Prior to this time, biologic treatments for the mentally ill included the barbiturates, amphetamines, narcotics, anticholinergic drugs such as scoploamine, various shock treatments (with insulin, convulsive drugs, and electricity), and neurosurgical techniques.

Electroconvulsive Therapy

Electroconvulsive therapy (ECT) is the only biologic treatment in common use in clinical psychiatry that was developed in the first half of the century. Its development was based on the erroneous belief that schizophrenia and epilepsy were incompatible. On the basis of this belief, causing convulsions in schizophrenic patients was hypothesized to be curative. In 1934, Meduna, a Hungarian psychiatrist, induced seizures using camphor which was eventually replaced by its synthetic derivative Metrazol. Cerletti and Bini in 1938 reported successful results using electrical seizures, which had many advantages over its chemical predecessors.

Electroconvulsive therapy has its greatest effectiveness in the treatment of major depression, especially with melancholic and psychotic features. It is also effective in the treatment of acute mania and some schizophrenic disorders. It is usually used in drug-resistant cases or when the risk of drugs is too great. As of 1976, 90,000 courses of ECT were administered in the United States.

The therapeutic effect of ECT is likely to be related to electrical, neurochemical, and neuroendocrinologic changes that also occur with antidepressant medications.

Psychosurgery

Psychosurgery was initiated in 1936 by Moniz, a Portuguese psychiatrist. Up to the 1950s the frontal lobes were the only sites of surgery. Since that time, surgery has been limited to the limbic system. The treatment is presumed to be effective for long-standing severe depression that does not respond to any other treatments, for severe obsessive–compulsive conditions, and for incapacitating anxiety and phobic conditions. Because of the absence of comprehensive, scientific data as to efficacy, psychosurgery is not currently regarded as an established and accepted therapy.

Antipsychotic Medications

The first antipsychotic phenothiazine, chlorpromazine (Thorazine), was used in 1951 as a preanesthetic sedative by a French surgeon who noticed that it produced behavioral effects of indifference to surroundings in the context of retention of consciousness. By 1952 and 1953 Delay and Deniker (80) reported the effectiveness of this agent in psychiatric patients. Since that time more than 20 phenothiazines have been used clinically. Alteration of the tricyclic core of the molecules led to a second group of antipsychotic agents called the thioxanthenes which include chlorprothixene (Taractan) and thiothixene (Navane). In 1959 the butyrophenones were developed during a search for derivatives of meperidine as a better analgesic agent. Haloperidol (Haldol) is the only butyrophenone in regular clinical use in the United States as an antipsychotic agent. Finally, there are a miscellaneous group of antipsychotic agents which include molindone, loxapine, and sulpiride.

Most of the above drugs are remarkably similar in their overall effects and efficacy. They are useful for a variety of psychiatric conditions including schizophrenia, mania, psychotic depression, senile psychoses, the agitation of organic dementia, acute brain syndromes, and reactions to hallucinogens. These drugs are most effective for acute cases with anxiety and agitation. The major differences among the antipsychotic medications are in their side effects. Drug selection is commonly made on this basis.

Antipsychotic agents are generally considered to be dopamine antagonists whose action is the blocking of postsynaptic dopamine receptors. Antiserotonin or antiadrenoceptor actions may also contribute to their therapeutic effects.

The use of antipsychotic agents has had a revolutionary impact on clinical practice. Because of these medications, psychotic patients are more apt to be managed on open wards, in general hospitals, at home, and in outpatient settings, as opposed to overcrowded inpatient facilities. The problems that remain are the side effects of the medications and the lack of efficacy for chronic psychosis or "negative" symptoms. There is still no cure for schizophrenia.

Antimanic Agents

In 1949 Cade (81) reported the dramatic response of manic patients to lithium salts. Following convincing studies in England and on the continent, lithium was finally accepted into American psychiatric practice in 1970. Its primary clinical use is for the treatment of acute mania and the prevention of mania and depression in bipolar illness. Less common uses of lithium include major depression, cyclothymic personality disorder, and cluster headache. Its profound clinical value has had an important effect on psychiatric nosology, particularly in the United States. Whereas before the use of lithium, there was a tendency to diagnose most functional psychosis as schizophrenia, now the tendency is for American psychiatrists to follow the European tradition of diagnosing psychotic states with predominant mood disturbances as manic–depressive disorders. Problems in the use of lithium include side effects, delay of therapeutic action, and nonresponsiveness to treatment. Although the mechanism of action of lithium in affective disorders is ill defined, research has focused on its effects on neurotransmitters and cell membranes.

Alternatives to lithium for bipolar disorders include certain anticonvulsant drugs such as carbamazepine (Tegretol), valproate (Depakene), and clonazepam (Klonopin). Both lithium and the group of anticonvulsants have also been used in other psychiatric conditions. One such current use is in the managment of agitation and aggression in patients with organic brain dysfunction.

Antidepressant Agents

In the early 1950s iproniazid, a structural analogue of nicotinic acid developed for the treatment of tuberculosis, was found to have mood-elevating and behaviorally activating properties. It was also found to be a potent inhibitor of monoamine oxidase, an amine-catabolizing enzyme. The current MAOIs in use in the United States are phenelzine (Nardil), tranylcypromine (Parnate), and isocarboxazid (Marplan). A third group of antidepressants are the sympathomimetic stimulants, which include dextroamphetamine and methylpenidate. Finally, a fourth heterogeneous group of antidepressant drugs—the so-called second-generation antidepressants—include amoxapine, maprotiline, and trazodone.

Tricyclic antidepressants have documented usefulness for the treatment of major depression, secondary depression, panic disorder, bulimia, and chronic pain. If the tricyclic fails, it is common to administer one of the MAOIs, usually phenelzine. The stimulants may be used for reactive depressions in medical/surgical patients and for attention deficit disorder. Problems in the use of antidepressants include delay of therapeutic onset, side effects, and the failure of these medicines to work on certain groups of affective disorders.

The tricyclic antidepressants act by blocking neuronal uptake of the neurotransmitter amines into nerve terminals; the MAOIs act by preventing the enzymatic inactivation of monoamine neurotransmitters.

Antianxiety Agents

Most modern antianxiety or sedative–hypnotic agents, introduced during the 1960s, are members of the benzodiazepine class of agents. Chlordiazepoxide (Librium) was the first. Subsequent preparations include diazepam (Valium), oxazepam (Serax), alprazolam (Xanax), lorazepam (Ativan), and temazepam (Restoril). During the first half of this century, prior to the introduction of the benzodiazepines, the main antianxiety agents were the bromides, paraldehyde, chloral hydrate, the barbiturates, and meprobamate (Miltown, Equinal). The benzodiazepines became the preferred antianxiety agents because they were safer than their predecessors with regard to withdrawal as well as addictive and depressant (central and respiratory) qualities. In contrast to the antipsychotic agents, the benzodiazepines do not affect the extrapyramidal system and do not cause tardive dyskinesias. Other drugs used in anxiety include the beta-blocking agents such as propranolol, nadolol and atenolol, and buspirone, a recently available nonbenzodiazepine anxiolytic agent. Advantages of these agents include lack of apparent addictive potential, decreased sedation, and decreased effects on cognition and memory. Disadvantages include the cardiac and bronchoconstrictor effects of the beta-blockers as well as questions about the range of efficacy of both beta-blockers and buspirone.

The benzodiazepines are most useful in the short-term treatment of transient forms of anxiety and tension, as preoperative sedatives, as hypnotics, and for alcohol detoxification. They may also be helpful in severe anxiety disorders, for temporarily sedating acutely agitated psychotic and manic patients, and as an adjunct to antidepressants in treating the anxiety of depressions. Some benzodiazepines have mood elevating effects but there are no antipsychotic effects. All the benzodiazepines have similar anxiolytic, sedative–hypnotic, and anticonvulsive effects. Pharmacokinetic differences determine their clinical use. The limitations of the benzodiazepines are the development of tolerance to antianxiety and sedative effects and the risk of psychiatric habituation and physical dependence. In addition, the range of conditions that they treat is limited. It is believed that the benzodiazepines and barbiturates exert their therapeutic action through the modification of the function of gamma-aminobutyric acid (GABA), an inhibitory neurotransmitter in the central nervous system.

THE SYNDROMAL APPROACH

The psychopharmacologic revolution gave rise to a renewed interest in the care-

ful description of clinical symptoms and syndromes and in the distinction between diagnostic catgories. The reasons for this renewed interest are easy to understand. The dramatic response of symptoms of acute schizophrenia to the phenothiazines and of the affective disorders to the tricyclics and MAOIs supported Kraepelin's initial classification and confirmed the importance of distinguishing the various psychiatric syndromes. It further suggested that biologic causation may be of central importance in explaining the mechanisms of these disorders. It was anticipated at that time that future research would determine symptom profiles and homogeneous syndromes responsive to particular drugs or classes of drugs.

The history of this movement has been well described by Klerman, who has aptly named it the "neo-Kraepelinian revival" (82). The early contributors to this approach in the United States came from the Department of Psychiatry in Washington University in St. Louis and include Eli Robbins, Samuel Guze, George Winokur, Paula Clayton, and Robert Woodruff. One of their early contributions was the definition, clarification, and partial validation of the psychiatric disorder referred to initially as hysteria, later as Briquet's syndrome, and now as somatization disorder. The textbook *Psychiatric Diagnosis*, written by Woodruff, Goodwin, and Guze in 1974 (83) and now in its 3rd edition, has had a significant influence on psychiatric training and practice in this country. British support for objective descriptive psychiatry can be traced to the early 1950s in the influential textbook authored by Mayer-Gross, Slater, and Roth (84).

Guze and Helzer (85) apply this neo-Kraepelinian postition to what they refer to as the "medical model" in psychiatry:

The medical model implies that psychiatric disorders are best approached in the same way that physicians approach all illnesses. Diagnosis and differential diagnosis are the indispensable first steps . . . which is the physician's attempts to categorize and classify the disorders of patients into relatively discrete groups.

One of the major tasks for contemporary psychiatry, according to Guze and Helzer, is the diagnostic validation of psychiatric disorders. For most conditions, validity is still incomplete and must rest on clinical data such as clinical course, response to treatment, and patterns of the disorder in families. As new knowledge becomes available about etiology and pathogenesis and their biologic mechanisms, continued reclassification will occur.

Beginning in the 1960s, there was a convergence of the neo-Kraepelinian interest in the precise description of discrete diseases or syndromes with the methods and skills of psychometricians and biostatisticians. This collaboration resulted in the Research Diagnostic Criteria (RDC) and Schedule for Affective Disorders and Schizophrenia (SADS), research tools for the diagnosis of psychopathology. Both these instruments were precursors to the *Diagnostic and Statistical Manual of Mental Disorders (Third Edition)* (86).

This categorical/medical approach has challenged the psychodynamic approach which had gained ascendency in the United States during the 1940s and 1950s. According to the psychodynamic approach, psychopathology is best described and explained in psychologic terms by etiologic mechanisms and processes common to all conditions. Detailed phenomenologic descriptions and sharp differences between patients are minimized. The diagnosis in the psychodynamic approach, in contrast, is a complex formulation unique to each individual.

The neo-Kraepelinian revival has made many positive contributions to clinical practice. Most important, the syndromal or disease paradigm of Sydenham and Kraepelin has been rigorously applied to diagnosis and taxonomy in psychiatric practice. As a result, clinicians are more precise in observing and describing what they see and are more effective in making syndromal diagnoses. Researchers now have reliable instruments to record psychopathology as they attempt to improve the reliability and validity of their categories. Drug research has been facilitated and

the quest for biologic markers for particular syndromes has been enhanced.

There is a conceptual problem in equating the search for discrete syndromes with a biologic etiology. The presence of a clearcut syndrome can not logically be assumed to be associated with primary biologic causation. The bereavement response, for instance, is a syndromal response to a psychosocial stressor. Furthermore, the centrality of biologic etiology and pathogenesis are not necessarily associated with syndromal responses. Some neuroendocrine approaches to psychopathology bear this out. In sum, whether pathology is best described in syndromal, dimension, or individualistic modes is not necessarily related to whether the primary explanatory model is biologic or psychologic. (See Chapter 8 for discussions of the dialectic between syndromal and individualistic approaches to psychopathology and for the relationship of the biologic approach to categorical thinking.)

PRESUMED BIOLOGIC MECHANISMS IN THE ETIOLOGY AND PATHOGENESIS OF DISORDERS

Information from psychopharmacologic advances and the renewed interest in the syndromal approach have fueled a search for biologic mechanisms of mental disorder which dates back at least to Freud, whose neurologic background influenced his research into the "structures" of the mind. Kraepelin, the father of the syndromal approach, gathered a number of distinguished neuroscientists at the Psychiatric Clinic of Munich University, including Alzheimer, Brodmann, and Nissl, to search for the biologic basis of psychiatric disorders. Nineteenth-century descriptions of changes in long-term motivation and impulse control following damage to the orbital frontal cortex (87) and Broca's original description of the limbic system (88), were also harbingers of a rapid increase of information about biologic mechanisms in the 20th century. Despite the important contributions of these men, the "information explosion" regarding biologic mechanisms in psychiatry has only come about within the past 30 years. Several major events have facilitated this development; most significantly, these are (a) the development of psychopharmacologic treatments, which gave rise to research about their actions, and (b) the availability of brain imaging techniques which permit in vivo examination not only of static anatomy but also of metabolic events. Areas which have been investigated in the interest of clarifying underlying biologic mechanisms of mood and behavior include genetics, structural/neuropsychiatric disorders, neurotransmitters, and hormones. Current research into neural networks and artifical intelligence, while running far behind the brain's capabilities, may one day help model ways in which processes become disordered and guide the search for analogous biologic mechanisms.

Genetics

Children of psychiatrically disturbed parents are at a higher risk for the development of psychopathology. Almost three times as many children attending a child psychiatry department had a parent with a history of psychiatric disorder as a matched group of pediatric and dental patients (89). An increased incidence of a variety of psychiatric disorders in the children of depressed or schizophrenic mothers has been described, including conduct disorders, difficulties with relationships, lack of attachments, hostility, impulse control problems, and attentional disorders (90–93).

While it is clear that having a psychiatrically ill parent places an individual at higher risk, the relative contribution of genetics and environment to the production of illness is less clear. Various strategies for examination of the genetic contribution have been utilized (94, 95). In the classic literature, epidemiologic trials have predominated. Adoption studies include examination of incidence of the disorder among adoptive versus biologic parents of

psychotic probands, cross-fostering studies, and studies of the prognosis of adopted-away infants of psychotic mothers versus those who remained in their biologic families. Studies of twins include examination of incidence of the disorder among monozygotes versus dizygotes, identical twins reared apart, and family incidence. The existence of a genetic contribution to the development of schizophrenia, affective disorders (particularly bipolar illness), and alcoholism has been fairly well established. The majority of cases continue to arise de novo, however, suggesting that the genetic contribution is only one factor in vulnerability.

Current genetic investigations have broadened into (a) the epidemiologic examination of a variety of disorders, most notably major personality disorders (antisocial, borderline), alcoholism, eating disorders, and anxiety disorders; (b) investigation of differences in response to pharmacologic agents which may be genetically based; (c) mathematical and computer models for polygenic inheritance and incomplete penetrance, and (d) the methods of molecular genetics, such as use of restriction fragment length polymorphisms and linkage studies. Examples of new research directions made possible by advances in molecular genetics include the recent discovery of a genetic marker for manic–depressive illness and the suggestion that autosomal maternal and paternal genes may contribute differentially to phenotypic expression (96, 97).

While the vulnerability to some psychiatric disorders may be genetically transmitted, its expression appears to be mediated by the effects of environment. Major psychiatric disorders can and do present in patients with no known family history. Nevertheless, the existence of a genetic vulnerability strongly suggests a biologic substrate at least to some psychiatric disorders.

Structural

Considerable information regarding the neurology of emotional processing, based on studies in both animals and man, has accumulated over the past two decades. Particular neural structures such as the hypothalamus, amygdaloid complex, and prefrontal cortex have been implicated in specific aspects of emotional and behavioral control. Classical observations include the phenomenon of sham rage produced by stimulation of the posterior lateral hypothalamus (98), and taming, change in sexual behavior, and loss of social affiliation following bilateral anterior temporal lobectomy (99). Seminal theoretical concepts, such as Geschwind's theory of sensory–limbic disconnection (100) have advanced the understanding of these and other observations. It appears that characteristic organic behavioral disorders may result from localized structural, chemical, or electrophysiological abnormalities of the central nervous system (CNS). Interest has increased in phenomena of cerebral lateralization, such as the apparent localization of the right hemisphere for comprehension of emotional gesturing, speech inflection, and comprehension of facial affects (101). Possible disorders of brain development during embryogenesis and early extrauterine life in relationship to later appearing disorders, such as schizophrenia, are also being investigated. Specific organic syndromes such as the localized degeneration of the caudate nucleus in Huntington's disease illustrate important structure–function relations relevant to the neurology of emotion; such illnesses may serve as models for understanding currently obscure psychiatric disorders.

The neocortex receives and processes information from lower centers such as the cranial nerves and spinal nerves and from higher centers such as internal productions of the neocortex itself. There are extensive interconnections between the limbic system and the neocortex, particularly frontal and temporal lobes. The hypothalamus is the central passageway for many limbic system circuits and is the major link in the passageway between the limbic system and midbrain. Nuclei in the hypothalamus also contain peptide-producing neurons which affect the release of hormones from the pituitary gland and may also have a direct effect on CNS receptors. Limbic structures have connections to beta-endorphin and encephalin-producing neurons which are thought to have effects on mood. The limbic system, composed of multineural interconnected circuits, thus participates in the modulation of behavioral expression by linking the sensory and integrative functions of the neocortex with the automatic brain functions of the brainstem and pituitary.

The line between neuroanatomy and neurophysiology is rapidly blurring as immunocytochemical techniques facilitate the study of the tracts in which various neurotransmitters lie. These functional circuits do not always correlate with classical structural circuits. Rapid developments in imaging techniques such as magnetic resonance imaging (MRI) and CT have improved studies of structural alterations in psychiatric disorders. Techniques such as positron emission tomography (PET), single photon emission computed tomography (SPECT) and regional blood flow studies have also permitted the study of functional rather than purely structural changes. Less invasive studies, such as brain electrical activity mapping (BEAM), may in the future offer similar insights into the functional organization of the brain.

Neurotransmitters

Neurotransmitters allow communication between nerve cells by permitting the electrical signal to pass between cells. Many biologic theories of the etiology of mental illness focus on the alteration and modification of these signaling compounds. More than 40 neurotransmitters and neuropeptides have been identified in the mammalian central nervous system. These neurotransmitters are released in response to the depolarization of one cell, bind to specific receptors on another cell, and are removed from the synaptic cleft by metabolism or reuptake. These three processes—presynaptic transmitter synthesis and release, postsynaptic receptor mechanisms, and metabolism or reuptake of neurotransmitter in the cellular cleft—have been the focus of inquiry into disturbance in neurotransmitter function. Interest in neurotransmitter receptors has burgeoned as the availability of radioactively labeled high-affinity ligands has enabled the study of receptor location and pathways. Binding studies are supplemented by more traditional pharmacologic studies in order to establish that the receptor under investigation is the active receptor. Neurotransmitters may function as depolarizers of the next cell or may have a modulating effect. This appears to be particularly true of the peptide neurotransmitters.

The synthesis of a neurotransmitter may be altered by (a) changing the amount of necessary enzyme synthesized, (b) changing the rate of enzyme activity by removing some inhibiting factor, or (c) altering enzyme activity by metabolic alteration of the enzyme such as changing its affinity for cofactors and inhibitors. Receptors may be affected by a change in their absolute number or by changes in their ability to bind to a ligand, for example because they have previously bound to another molecule. Receptors are said to be "up-regulated" when their functional effect is to be more active and "down-regulated" when their sensitivity is reduced.

Norepinephrine and Serotonin

Clinical interest in monoamines began in the 1950s, with the observation that drugs such as reserpine, MAOIs, and heterocyclic antidepressants, which affect monoamine systems, can affect mood. Serotonin, which was initially investigated as a possible agent in psychosis because of similarities in its structural and binding affinity to hallucinogenic compounds, is currently being examined for its possible role in affective illness, aggression and violent suicide, autism, and illnesses affected by circadian rhythms such as sleep and seasonal affective illness. Both serotonin and norepinephrine appear to be involved in affective disorders, though their relative contribution to depression in general or to any specific patient's depression in particular has remained unclear. In addition, the

originally proposed mechanism of action of the heterocyclic antidepressants (reuptake inhibition) does not adequately explain their actions. Some of the newer antidepressants (mianserin and trazodone) also seem to exert their effect through mechanisms other than reuptake blockade or change in metabolism, intensifying the search for other biologic models of depression.

A major focus of current interest is in the monoamine receptor. Down-regulation of the beta-adrenergic receptor has been investigated in all known treatments for depression, including ECT. While norepinephrine is generally thought of as an excitatory neurotransmitter, at least in some instances it may function to inhibit firing by a slow hyperpolarizing response, resulting in increased membrane resistance. This inhibitory effect appears to be mediated by beta-adrenergic receptors. Tricyclics are also known to down-regulate the presynaptic alpha-2 receptor, thus removing an inhibitory influence on norepinephrine production. Pathologic decreased activity of the alpha-2 inhibitory receptor in the locus ceruleus is thought to be responsible for increased norepinephrine activity in panic attacks (102). This may explain the effect of clonidine, an alpha-2 agonist, in relieving panic attacks induced by lactate. The partial release of the inhibitory effects of alpha-2 and beta-receptors may be one mechanism of action of heterocyclic antidepressants. Down-regulation of the serotonin receptor has also been proposed as a mechanism of action of some antidepressants. This presupposes that in depression, a decrease in serotonin production has been followed by pathologic up-regulation and supersensitivity of the serotonin receptor. Unquestionably, simple theories of etiology of affective illness involving too little or too much of a particular neurotransmitter require reexamination.

Dopamine

Suggestions that variations in dopamine level or metabolism might be involved in psychosis began in the 1950s with investigations of the amphetamine psychosis as a model for schizophrenia, after earlier transmethylation models had failed to provide an adequate simulation of psychosis. All of the major antipsychotics interact with dopamine as blockers or antagonists, further contributing to the proposed role of this system in the etiology of psychoses. Cells using dopamine as a transmitter are not as widely distributed in the central nervous system as norepinephrine and serotonin-containing cells and run mainly in three projections: nigrostriatal, mesolimbic/mesocortical, and tuberohypophyseal. The mesolimbic/mesocortical system, which connects the ventral tegmentum to the limbic system and cortex, is probably involved in psychosis, and there has been a search for a "magic bullet" neuroleptic which would have specific effects on this tract.

As with affective illness, research has shifted from interest in absolute levels of dopamine to work on its receptors. This work has identified two dopamine receptors, D1 and D2. Clinical neuroleptic potency is highly correlated with butyrophenone binding to D2 receptors, and some studies have shown increased D2 receptors in the basal ganglia and limbic regions of patients with schizophrenia (103). Milligram potency is not, however, a measure of effectiveness of treatment, and the possibility that increased D2 receptors are an effect of treatment for schizophrenia rather than a causal factor has not been eliminated. Evidence for the involvement of dopamine in psychosis has remained pharmacologic rather than direct.

Amino Acid Neurotransmitters

The most well known of the amino acid neurotransmitters is GABA, which, along with glycine and taurine, is an inhibitory neurotransmitter. A very widely distributed neurotransmitter, GABA is found in highest concentration in the basal ganglia and in lowest concentration in the cerebellar cortex. Benzodiazepines increase the affinity of the GABA receptor for GABA and, together with the benzodiazepine receptor and chloride ion chan-

nels, act to decrease the activity of an anxiety-producing system which may not be mediated by norepinephrine (104). Further work in clarifying the systems which mediate anxiety is being carried out.

Cholinergic Mechanisms

Although acetylcholine was the first neurotransmitter described and identified, psychiatric interest in this neurotransmitter is relatively recent. Cholinergic neurons have a very widespread distribution in the brain, both in long tracts and as intermediary neurons. The areas of cholinergic nuclei currently under investigation are located in the base of the forebrain, in and around the nucleus basalis of Meynert, because of their apparent role in Alzheimer's disease. A role for cholinergic mechanisms in affective disorder has also been proposed (105).

Neuropeptides

Neuropeptides are one of the most actively studied families of neurotransmitters because of current interest in the possible role of endorphins in relief of pain, stress, dysphoria, and syndromes from premenstrual tension to runner's "high." There are many peptides which have been shown to function as neurotransmitters; more than 30 have been identified in mammalian neurons. They are generally thought to function in a modulatory role over longer distances and with a longer time course than classical neurotransmitters.

Hormones

Hormones act to influence mood and behavior both through endocrine activity and by acting as short neurotransmitters in the CNS. There are several ways in which hormones may affect behavior (106):

1. By altering the general energy state of the individual;
2. By altering the state of some effector organ (for example, making muscle contraction weaker or stronger);
3. By changing the state of a sensory-receptor area, such as smell; and

4. By changing the state of the CNS, for example, by retarding or facilitating growth of dendrites, interacting with neurotransmitters, or directly altering CNS function.

The hypothalamic–pituitary–adrenal axis has been one of the most extensively studied hormonal systems and appears to be involved in stress response and in affective disorders. Since hormonal systems involve self-regulatory feedback loops, adrenal hormones also affect the functioning of the pituitary, which in turn influences hypothalamic release. Other endocrine systems have also been examined for their ability to affect psychiatric symptoms. The effect of disturbances of thyroid and parathyroid function on mood is well known. Hyperprolactinemia is associated with sexual dysfunction and depression in males (107). Current interest in premenstrual syndrome and in aggression has produced renewed interest in the effects of sex hormones on behavior, without conclusive results. The relationship of progesterone levels and beta-endorphins to premenstrual syndrome is currently under investigation. Investigations of the correlation between testosterone level and aggression have been inconclusive.

APPLICATION TO CLINICAL PRACTICE

In applying the biologic approach to clinical practice, we follow the multidimensional, pluralistic position described in Chapter 2. To review briefly, although all behaviors and emotions are reflections of biologic mechanisms, many clinical phenomena are best explained and influenced by psychologic and social explanatory models. Each patient, therefore, needs to be understood simultaneously from biologic as well as from other approaches in the vertical hierarchy such as the psychologic and sociocultural. There are not as yet a general set of rules that determine for a given patient which of the conceptual models should be applied and when in the course of treatment to switch.

Clinical Hypotheses

We believe the biologic approach reviewed in this chapter can be applied to the care of a particular patient by considering the following five clinical hypothesis. (a) Can, and to what degree, the patient's problem be understood as a syndromal diagnosis as described in Axes I and II in the *Diagnostic and Statistical Manual of Mental Disorders* (*Third Edition-Revised*). These diagnoses are important because the literature relating to etiology, epidemiology, course, prognosis, and treatment is diagnosis based. The clinician should be aware, however, that validity and reliability varies from diagnosis to diagnosis; that certain kinds of psychologic distress do not readily lend themselves to the categorical approach; and that the information the diagnosis contributes about a given patient is quite variable. (b) The patient's psychiatric presentation may be caused by one or more known organic/medical diseases. (c) The patient may be suffering from a concomitant physical condition. (d) The patient may be suffering from a stress-induced biologic condition. (e) The patient's condition may be known to be treatable, in part, by biologic treatments. Whether or not the clinician elects to use such a treatment depends on the efficacy of the treatment, the risks of treatment, and the efficacy and safety of alternative treatments.

Biologic Approaches and the Clinical Interview

Testing the above hypotheses requires an approach in which the clinician actively questions the patient about the presence or absence of various symptoms, observes carefully for physical signs, and considers the possible diagnostic value of a physical examination and laboratory data. This differs from the behavioral approach in which the questioning concerns a different content and from the psychodynamic approach in which much of the critical data emerges from the collection of a different quality of historical data, an observation of the spontaneous flow and content of the patient's activity, and the subjective impact of the patient on the clinician.

The nature of the relationship between clinician and patient and patients' attitude toward their disorder may be influenced by the choice of conceptual approach. With the biologic approach, patients may attempt to define the problem as a disease which entitles them to the sick role, a problem which is thrust upon them rather than one for which they are responsible, and a problem for which the cure will be offered from external sources. They are apt to perceive the clinician as someone in authority who makes the diagnosis and prescribes treatment. In an extreme example, the patient (using a biologic model) tells us he has a depression caused by some metabolic abnormality. The same patient (using a psychodynamic model) tells us he feels depressed because he is having trouble coping with a loss. In actual practice, both psychiatric and medical patients with known biologic disturbances are taking on more responsibility for the management of their disorders.

In the caricature of the biologic interview, the clinician limits his or her activities to an interrogation of the patient over the symptoms and associated syndromal history in order to establish the syndromal and/or medical diagnosis. The clinician is in authority and the patient passively responds. This caricature differs markedly from the approach of psychiatrists who have expertise in the biologic approach. Such clinicians determine what is wrong with the patient by simultaneously considering biologic with other social and psychologic approaches. In addition they carry out two more functions of the interview: (*a*) developing and maintaining a therapeutic relationship with the patient and (*b*) educating and communicating information to the patient. These suggestions for the integration of biologic approaches into an effective interview apply equally to the surgical, neurological, and medical interview. The most highly regarded clinicians in these fields interview comprehensively and do not limit themselves to the exploration of the biologic hypotheses.

Given the most effective attempts at integration of the biologic with other approaches as described above, there may be irreconcilable differences. For example, in the psychotherapy of a neurotic condition, the patient develops some of the symptoms of major depression. Is this to be understood as a predictable regression from the stressful issues of psychotherapy or the first sign that the patient is suffering from a biologic syndrome, a major affective disorder? The clinician must make a choice which, in turn, will influence the nature of the therapeutic relationship, the patients' image of him- or herself and the nature of the intervention.

CONCLUSIONS

On the basis of the evidence presented in this chapter and elsewhere in this book, knowledge of biologic mechanisms in medical and psychiatric disorders is essential for responsible clinical practice. This includes knowledge of the relationship between medical disease and psychiatric symptoms and disorders, the effect of stress on biologic processes, the response of psychiatric symptoms and syndromes to biologic treatments, the importance of clinical description and the identification of discrete syndromes, and the biology of psychiatric disorders. Clinicians' failure to understand these biologic mechanisms can lead to serious misdiagnoses and missed opportunities to relieve distress and even save life.

The application of the biologic approach is an essential but not a comprehensive part of clinical psychiatry. Limiting psychiatric procedures to symptom and syndromal diagnoses and their biologic treatments is ineffective clinical practice. Such a practice will fail in developing and maintaining a therapeutic relationship and in addressing many of the patient's psychologic problems. The integration of knowledge from the biologic, psychologic, and social approaches to psychopathology and its application to practice may be the greatest challenge facing the clinician.

(The biologic approach is introduced in Chapter 2, "A Multidimensional Approach to Psychopathology." It is further discussed in Chapter 7, "Clinical Hypothesis Testing"; Chapter 8, "Psychiatric Diagnosis"; Chapter 15, "The Use of the Laboratory in Outpatient Psychiatry"; and Chapters 17 through 30, "Differential Diagnosis of Psychiatric Presentations with Known Medical Causes." In addition, the chapters on the various syndromes discuss the presumed biologic theories and treatments.)

Acknowledgments. The authors wish to thank Dr. David Bear for his suggestions in the preparation of this chapter.

References

1. Pincus HA, Rubinow DR: Research at the interface of psychiatry and medicine. In Pincus HA, Pardes H (eds): *The Integration of Neuroscience and Psychiatry.* Washington, DC, American Psychiatric Press, 1985, pp 77–94.
2. Lazare A: Conversion symptoms. In Sederer LI (ed): *Inpatient Psychiatry: Diagnosis and Treatment.* Baltimore, Williams & Wilkins, 1983, pp 157–167.
3. Merskey H: *The Analysis of Hysteria.* London, Bailliere, Tindall, 1979.
4. Whitlock FA: The aetiology of hysteria. *Acta Psychiatr Scand* 43:144–162, 1967.
5. Ziegler GK, Paul N: On the natural hysteria in women: follow-up study of twenty years after hospitalization. *Dis Nerv Syst* 15:301–306, 1954.
6. Gatfield PD, Guze SB: Prognosis and differential diagnosis of conversion reactions: a follow-up study. *Dis Nerv Syst* 23:623–631, 1962.
7. Slater ETO, Glithero E: A follow-up of patients diagnosed as suffering from "hysteria." *J Psychosom Res* 9:9–13, 1965.
8. Raskin M, Talbott JA, Meyerson AT: Diagnosed conversion reactions: predictive value of psychiatric criteria. *JAMA* 197:530–534, 1966.
9. Stefansson JG, Messina JA, Meyerowitz S: Hysterical neurosis, conversion type: clinical and epidemiological considerations. *Acta Psychiatr Scand* 53:119–138, 1976.
10. Watson CG, Buranen C: The frequency and identification of false positive conversion reactions. *J Nerv Ment Dis* 167:243–247, 1979.
11. Benson DF, Blumer D (eds): *Psychiatric Aspects of Neurologic Disease.* New York, Grune and Stratton, 1975, pp 219–265.
12. Benson DF, Blumer D (eds): *Psychiatric Aspects of Neurologic Disease,* vol 4. New York, Grune and Stratton, 1982.
13. Lishman WA: *Organic Psychiatry: The Psychological Consequences of Cerebral Disorder.* London, Blackwell Scientific Publications, 1978.
14. Lishman WA: *Organic Psychiatry: The Psychological Consequences of Cerebral Disorder,* ed 2. London, Blackwell Scientific Publications, 1986.
15. Hall RCW: *Psychiatric Presentations of Medical Illness: Somatopsychic Disorders.* New York, SP Medical & Scientific Books, 1980.
16. Jefferson JW, Marshall JR: *Neuropsychiatric Features of Medical Disorders.* New York, Plenum Medical Book Company, 1981.
17. Cummings JL: *Clinical Neuropsychiatry.* New York, Grune and Stratton, 1985.
18. Extein I, Gold MS (eds): *Medical Mimics of Psychiatric Disorders.* Washington, DC, American Psychiatric Press, 1986.
19. Soreff SM, McNeil GN: *Handbook of Psychiatric Differential Diagnosis.* Littleton, MA, PSG Publishing Company, 1987.
20. Lazare A (ed): *Outpatient Psychiatry: Diagnosis and Treatment.* Baltimore, Williams & Wilkins, 1979.
21. Alexander F: *Psychosomatic Medicine: Its Principles and Applications.* New York, W.W. Norton, 1950.
22. Deutsch F (ed): *The Psychosomatic Concept in Psychoanalysis.* New York, International Universities Press, 1953.
23. Dunbar F: *Emotions and Bodily Changes,* ed 4. New York, Columbia University Press, 1954.
24. Weiner H: *Psychobiology and Human Disease.* New York, Elsevier, 1977.
25. Holmes TH, Rahe RH: The social readjustment rating scale. *J Psychosom Res* 2:213–218, 1967.
26. Selye H: *The Stress of Life.* New York, McGraw Hill, 1956.
27. Cannon WB: *The Wisdom of the Body.* New York, Newton, 1939.
28. Lown B, DeSilva RA, Lenson R: Roles of psychologic stress and autonomic nervous system changes in provocation of ventricular premature complexes. *Am J Cardiol* 41:979–985, 1978.
29. Lown B, DeSilva RA, Reich P, et al: Psychophysiologic factors in sudden cardiac death. *Am J Psychiatry* 137:1325–1335, 1980.
30. Friedman M: *Pathogenesis of Coronary Artery Disease.* New York, McGraw-Hill, 1969.
31. Jenkins CD: Recent evidence supporting psychologic and social risk factors for coronary disease. *N Engl J Med* 294:1033–1038, 1976.
32. Case RB, Heller SS, Case NB, et al: Type A behavior and survival after acute myocardial infarction. *N Engl J Med* 312:737–741, 1985.
33. Shekelle R et al: Multiple risk factor intervention trials group. Cited in Ruberman W, Weinblatt E, Goldberg JD, et al: Psychosocial influences on mortality after myocardial infarction. *N Engl J Med* 311:552–559, 1984.
34. Marmot MG: Socio-economic and cultural factors in ischaemic heart disease. *Adv Cardiol* 29:68–76, 1982.
35. Ruberman W, Weinblatt E, Goldberg JD, et al: Psychosocial influences on mortality after myocardial infarction. *N Engl J Med* 311:552–559, 1984.

36. Young M, Benjamin B, Wallis C: The mortality of widowers. *Lancet* 2:454–456, 1963.
37. Adamson JD, Schmale AH Jr: Object loss, giving up, and the onset of psychiatric disease. *Psychosm Med* 27:557–576, 1965.
38. Berkman LF, Syme L: Social networks, host resistance, and mortality: a nine-year follow-up study of Alameda County residents. *Am J Epidemiol* 109:186–204, 1979.
39. Blazer DG: Social support and mortality in an elderly community population. *Am J Epidemiol* 115:684–94, 1982.
40. Nuckolls KB, Cassel J, Kaplan BH: Psychosocial assets, life crisis, and the prognosis of pregnancy. *Am J Epidemiol* 95:431–441, 1972.
41. Cobb S: Social support as a moderator of life stress. *Psychosom Med* 38:300–314, 1976.
42. De Araujo G, Dudley DL, Van Arsdel PP Jr: Psychosocial assets and severity of chronic asthma. *J Allergy Clin Immunol* 50:257–263, 1972.
43. Brown GW, Andrews B, Harris T, Adler Z, et al: Social support, self-esteem and depression. *Psychol Med* 16:813–831, 1986.
44. Reite M, Short R, Kaufman IC, et al: Heart rate and body temperature in separated monkey infants. *Biol Psychiatry* 13:91–105, 1978.
45. Reite M, Stynes AJ, Vaughn L, et al: Sleep in infant monkeys: normal values and behavioral correlates. *Physiol Behav* 16:245–251, 1976.
46. Graboys T: Stress and the aching heart (editorial). *N Engl J Med* 311:594–595, 1984.
47. Carruthers ME: Aggression and atheroma. *Lancet* 2:1170–1171, 1969.
48. Wolinsky H: Effects of estrogen and progestogen treatment on the response of the aorta of male rats to hypertension. Morphological and chemical studies. *Circ Res* 30:341–349, 1972.
49. Levine S, Coe CL, Smotherman WP: Prolonged cortisol elevation in the infant squirrel monkey after reunion with mother. *Physiol Behav* 20:7–10, 1978.
50. Gunnar MR, Fisch RO, Korsvik S, et al: The effects of circumcision on serum cortisol and behavior. *Psychoneuroendocrinology* 6:269–275, 1981.
51. Mason JW, Kenion CC, Collins DR: Urinary testosterone response to 72-hour avoidance in the monkey. *J Psychosom Med* 30:721–732, 1968.
52. Breese GP, Smith RD, Mueller RA, et al: Induction of adrenal catecholamine synthesizing enzymes following mother–infant separation. *Nature: New Biology* 246:95–96, 1973.
53. Stein M, Schiavi RC, Camerino M: Influence of brain and behavior on the immune system. *Science* 191:435–440, 1976.
54. Stein M, Schleifer SJ, Keller SE: *Immune disorders.* In HI Kaplan, BJ Sadock (eds): *Comprehensive Textbook of Psychiatry,* ed 4. Baltimore, Williams & Wilkins, 1985, pp 1206–1211.
55. Mirsky IA: Physiologic, psychologic, and social determinants in etiology of duodenal ulcer. *Am J Digest Dis* 3:285–314, 1958.
56. Turkkan JS, Brady JV, Harris AH: Animal studies of stressful interactions: behavioral–physiological overview. In L Goldberg, S Breznitz (eds): *Handbook of Stress.* New York, Macmillan, 1982, pp 153–182.
57. Friedman SB, Ader R, Glasgow LA: Effects of psychological stress in adult mice inoculated with Coxsackie B viruses. *Psychosom Med* 27:361–368, 1965.
58. Ader R, Friedman SB: Differential early experiences and susceptibility to transplanted tumor in rat. *J Comp Physiol Psychol* 59:361–364, 1965.
59. Kaufman IC, Rosenblum LA: The reaction to separation in infant monkeys: anaclitic depression and conservation–withdrawal. *Psychosom Med* 29:648–675, 1967.
60. Hinde RA, Spencer-Booth Y: Individual differences in the responses of rhesus monkeys to separation from their mothers. *J Child Psychol Psychiatry* 11:159–176, 1970.
61. Mineka S, Suomi SJ: Social separation in monkeys. *Psychol Bull* 85:1376–1400, 1978.
62. Reiser MF: Theoretical considerations of the role of psychological factors in pathogenesis and etiology of essential hypertension. *Biol Psychiatry* 144:117–124, 1970.
63. Hubel DH, Weisel TN: Receptive fields, binocular interaction and functional architecture in the cat's visual cortex. *J Physiol* 160:106–154, 1962.
64. Hubel DH, Weisel TN: Binocular interaction in striate cortex of kittens reared with artificial squint. *J Neurophysiol* 28:1041–1059, 1965.
65. Kandel ER, Schwartz JH: Molecular biology of learning: modulation of transmitter release. *Science* 218:433–443, 1982.
66. Meaney MJ, Aitken DH, VanBerkel C, et al: Effect of neonatal handling on age-related impairments associated with the hippocampus. *Science* 239:766–768, 1988.
67. Levine S, Alpert M, Lewis GW: Differential maturation of an adrenal response to cold stress in rats manipulated in infancy. *J Comp Physiol Psychol* 51:774–777, 1958.
68. Levine S, Lewis GW: Critical period for effects of infantile experience on maturation of stress response. *Science* 129:42–43, 1959.
69. Amkraut AA, Solomon GF, Kramer HC: Stress, early life experience and ajuvant induced arthritis in the rat. *Psychosom Med* 33:203–214, 1971.
70. Welch AS, Welch BL: Effect of stress and p-chlorophenylalanine upon brain serotonin, 5-hydroxyindoleacetic acid and catecholamines in grouped and isolated mice. *Biochem Pharmacol* 17:699–708, 1968.
71. Welch AS, Welch BL: Differential activation by restraint stress of a mechanism to conserve brain catecholamines and serotonin in mice differing in excitability. *Nature* 218:575–577, 1968.
72. Henry JP, Meehan JP, Stephens PM: The use of psychosocial stimuli to induce prolonged systolic hypertension in mice. *Psysom Med* 29:408–432, 1967.
73. Henry JP, Stephens PM, Axelrod J, et al: Effect of psychosocial stimulation on the enzymes involved in the biosynthesis and metabolism of no-

radrenaline and adrenaline. *Psychosom Med* 33:227–237, 1971.

74. Axelrod J, Mueller RA, Henry JP, et al: Changes in enzymes involved in the biosynthesis and metabolism of noradrenaline and adrenaline after psychosocial stimulation. *Nature* 225:1059–1060, 1970.

75. Ader R, Cohen N: Behaviorally conditioned immunosuppression. *Psychosom Med* 37:333–340, 1975.

76. Schiavi RC: Effect of hypothalmic lesions on histamine toxicity in the guinea pig. *Am J Physiol* 211:1269–1273, 1966.

77. Baldessarini RJ, Cole JO: Chemotherapy. In Nicoli AM (ed): *The New Harvard Guide to Psychiatry*. Baltimore, Williams & Wilkins, 1988, pp 481–533.

78. Davis JM: Organic therapies. In Kaplan HI, Sadok BJ (eds): *Comprehensive Textbook of Psychiatry*, ed 4. Baltimore, Williams & Wilkins, 1985, pp 1481–1513.

79. David JM: Antidepressant drugs: In Kaplan HI, Sadok BJ (eds): *Comprehensive Textbook of Psychiatry*, ed 4. Baltimore, Williams & Wilkins, 1985, pp 1513–1537.

80. Delay J, Deniker P, Harl J: Utilization therapeutique psychiatrique d'une phenothiazine d'action centrale elective (4560 RP). *Ann Med Psychol* 110:112–117. 1952.

81. Cade JFJ: Lithium salts in the treatment of psychotic excitement. *Med J Aust* 2:349–352, 1949.

82. Klerman G: The neo-Kraepelinian revival in American psychiatry: its history, promise and prospect. Presented at scientific symposium honoring Dr. Eli Robins by the Department of Psychiatry, Washington University School of Medicine, St. Louis, MO, 1977.

83. Woodruff RA Jr, Goodwin DW, Guze SB: *Psychiatric Diagnosis*. New York, Oxford University Press, 1974.

84. Mayer-Gross W, Slater E, Roth M: *Clinical Psychiatry*. London, Bailliere, Tindall and Cassele, 1954.

85. Guze SB, Helzer JE: The medical model and psychiatric disorders. In Michels R, Cavenar JO Jr, Brodie HKH, et al (eds): *Psychiatry*. Philadelphia, J.B. Lippincott, 1986, vol 1, chap 51, pp 1–8.

86. Klerman GL: Historical background. In Michels R, Cavenar JO Jr, Brodie HKH, et al (eds): *Psychiatry*. Philadelphia, J.B. Lippincott, 1986, vol 1, chap 52, pp 1–23.

87. Harlow JM: Recovery from the passage of an iron bar through the head. *Mass Med Soc* 2:329–346, 1868.

88. Broca P: Anatomic Comparee Circonvolutions Cerebrales. Le Grand Lobe Limbique et la Scissure Limbique. *Revue Anthropologie* (Ser. 2) 1384–1349, 1898.

89. Rutter M: Children of sick parents: an environmental and psychiatric study (Maudsley Monograph No. 16). London, Oxford University Press, 1966.

90. El-Guebaly N, Offord DR, Sullivan KT, et al: Psychosocial adjustments of the offspring of psychiatric inpatients: The effect of alcoholic, depressive, and schizophrenic parentage. *Canadian Psychiatric Assoc J* 23:281–289, 1978.

91. Grunebaum H, Cohler BJ, Kauffman C, et al: Children of depressed and schizophrenic mothers. *Child Psychiatry Human Dev* 8:219–228, 1978.

92. Reider RO: The offspring of schizophrenic parents: a review. *J Nerv Ment Dis* 157:179–190, 1973.

93. Schulsinger H: A ten year followup of children of schizophrenic mothers: clinical assessment. *Acta Psychiatr Scand* 53:371–386, 1976.

94. Gershon ES, Mathysse S, Breakefield XO, et al (eds): *Research Strategies for Psychobiology and Psychiatry*. Pacific Grove, CA, Boxwood Press, 1981.

95. Gottesman II, Shields J: *Schizophrenia: The Epigenetic Puzzle*. Cambridge, England, Cambridge University Press, 1982.

96. Egeland JA, Gerhard DS, Pauls DL, et al: Bipolar affective disorders linked to DNA markers on chromosome 11. *Nature* 325:783–787, 1987.

97. Marx JL: A parent's sex may affect gene expression. *Science* 239:352–353, 1988.

98. Bard P: A diencephalic mechanism for the expression of rage with special reference to the sympathetic nervous system. *Am J Physiol* 84:490–515, 1928.

99. Kluver H, Bucy PC: Preliminary analysis of functions of the temporal lobes in monkeys. *Arch Neurol Psychiatry* 42:979–1000, 1939.

100. Geschwind N: Disconnection syndromes in animals and man. *Brain* 88:237–294, 1965.

101. Kupfermann I: Hemispheric asymmetries and the cortical localization of higher cognitive and affective functions. In Kandel ER, Schwartz JH (eds): *Principles of Neural Science*, ed 2. New York, Elsevier, 1985, pp 673–687.

102. Redmond DE Jr, Huang YH: Current concepts. II. New evidence for a locus coeruleus-norepinephrine connection with anxiety. *Life Sci* 25:2149–2162, 1979.

103. Seeman P, Ulpian C, Bergeron C, et al: Bimodal distribution of dopamine receptor densities in brains of schizophrenics. *Science* 225:728–731, 1984.

104. Insel TR, Ninan PT, Aloi J, et al: A benzodiazepine receptor-mediated model of anxiety. Studies in nonhuman primates and clinical implications. *Arch Gen Psychiatry* 41:741–750, 1984.

105. Janowsky D, El-Yousef K, Davis M, et al: A cholinergic–adrenergic hypothesis of mania and depression. *Lancet* 2:632–635, 1972.

106. Leshner AI: *An Introduction to Behavioral Endocrinology*. New York, Oxford University Press, 1978.

107. De la Fuente R, Rosenbaum A: Prolactin in psychiatry. *Am J Psychiatry* 138:1154–1160, 1981.

4

The Psychodynamic Approach

Anne Alonso, Ph.D.

The psychodynamic approach is a comprehensive theory of personality that describes both normal and abnormal development. The term *psychodynamic* includes Freud's (1) original theory of psychoanalysis as well as the main branches of psychologic thought that evolved from and expanded his classical theory. Psychodynamic therapy is the application of these theories for the treatment of certain kinds of psychologic suffering. While the psychodynamic theories are a valid way of thinking of all human behavior, the derivative treatments are applicable to specific situations that shall be discussed later in this chapter.

The basic assumptions of the psychodynamic approach have been so interwoven into Western society that it is difficult to remember that they have been in existence for less than a century. There is now common acceptance of psychodynamic concepts such as the importance of the unconscious process, the meanings of dreams, the awareness of intrapsychic conflict, and the importance of early childhood development. Literature, art, journalism, and common jargon are imbued with aspects of psychodynamic theory.

There have been numerous elaborations of Freud's theories since the turn of the 20th century. Four of the major schools are discussed in this chapter: Freud's classical drive theory, Anna Freud's ego psychology (2), Melanie Klein's object relations theory (3), and the self psychology of Heinz Kohut (4) (see Table 4.1). The neoanalysts such as Sullivan (5), Adler (6), and Horney (7) made major contributions as well; although they are mostly omitted from this chapter for the sake of brevity, their work has had a profound impact on psychodynamic thought and practice.

The aim of this chapter is to examine the basic assumptions of psychodynamic thought, describe the various theories that are subsumed under the psychodynamic approach, and explore the treatment implications and methods that emerge logically from the above.

BASIC ASSUMPTIONS OF THE PSYCHODYNAMIC APPROACH

Five fundamental ideas form the basis for all the branches of psychodynamic thought:

1. Psychologic determinism;
2. The existence of unconscious processes;
3. The dynamic, goal-directed quality of human motivation;
4. Epigenetic development;
5. Functions of the mind at work at a given point in time.

37

Table 4.1 Comparison of Psychodynamic Theories

Theory	Primary Theorists	Structure of Mind	Energic Source	Development	Pathology	Curative Process	Role of Therapist
Structural (classical)	S. Freud, H. Deutsch, S. Ferenczi, O. Fenichel, M. Gill, C. Brenner	Id, Ego, Superego	Libido/aggression (dual instincts)	Oral, anal, phallic, and oedipal stages	Unresolved sexual conflict	Interpretation of unconscious transference leads to resolution of conflict	Interpretation of transference
Ego psychology	A. Freud, H. Hartmann, E. Kris, R. Loewenstein, G. Blanck & R. Blanck, E. Erickson	Id/ego/superego; mechanism of ego defense	Libido/aggression id/ego conflict	Primitive to sophisticated ego defenses	Irreconcilable tension between id demands and environmental pressures	Restore conscious aims by providing defenses that neutralize primary process materials; leads to higher degree of conflict-free ego functioning	Analysis of defenses and affirmation of executive ego functions
Object relations	M. Klein, W. Fairbairn, D. Winnicott, H. Guntrip, M. Mahler, A. Modell, E. Jacobson, J. Greenberg, S. Mitchell	Modified id/ego/superego	Klein–death instinct; after Klein leads to attachment drive for object relatedness	Schizoid, paranoid, depressive positions	Disruption in capacity for object relation and formation of true self	Analysis of therapeutic relationship; containment leads to structure	Interpretation of false self formation; containment of longings for the object
Self psychology	H. Kohut, A. Ornstein, P. Ornstein, J. Teicholz	Id/ego/superego replaced by cohesive self	Idealized self/object	Object relation and narcissistic lines run parallel; fragmented to cohesive self	Fragmentation; disintegration of self	Restoration of self via transmuting internalizations in relationship with empathic mirroring object	Functions as self/object; empathic mirroring
Neoanalytic	A. Adler, H. Sullivan, K. Horney, O. Rank, T. Reik, E. Fromm, F. Fromm-Reichman, C. Thompson	Ego	Ego and environment (culture)	Multivaried social accommodation of "true" authentic self	Culture impinging on blank slate	Real relationship with therapist leads to recovery of overly accommodated self; this leads to autonomy	Interpersonal clarification and support for internal perspective on external reality

Psychologic Determinism

Psychologic determinism is the assumption that every manifestation of the human mind is lawfully connected with every other manifestation of that mind, that there is a rational explanation of human behavior, that all human behavior makes sense. Even that which appears accidental, irrational, or self-defeating follows the rule of psychologic determinism. This notion helps to explain the meanings of apparently maladaptive behaviors, symptoms, bizarre dreams, irrational thoughts, and conflicting motives.

The concept of determinism in psychoanalysis is to be distinguished from the philosophic debate between determinism and free will. It assumes that the content of the mind determines all mindful activity and can be explained ultimately by knowing that person better. It is further assumed that much of what is contained in the mind has been stored, rearranged, disguised, and fashioned into a tolerable story of the individual's life.

Psychologic concepts are rarely absolute and concrete. If we say that nothing is accidental, we do not mean to say that a truck careening out of control because of a slick highway is not accidental. Rather, we mean that it is imperative even in this case to examine all the possible meanings, including the possibility that the driver was asleep, or drunk or suicidal, as well as acknowledging that, indeed, the road was slick, and the disaster could not have been prevented. Too narrow and mechanistic a stance moves us away from common sense. But to move too quickly into commonsense explanations may prematurely truncate the psychodynamic inquiry.

The Existence of Unconscious Processes

In order to explain the logic underlying the apparent illogic in human thought and behavior, Freud introduced the concept of unconscious process. For efficient mental functioning, the mind selects those thoughts and feelings that will serve the present needs of the person and deletes from present awareness those thoughts and feelings that threaten to disequilibrate and interfere with the goals of the moment. The *unconscious* is the term used to describe a process of storing out of awareness all the data that are not relevant or tolerable; it is not a place or an anatomic structure of the mind.

Access to the unconscious process of the mind is found through the process of free association, dream analysis, exploration of fantasies, slips of the tongue, and other mental "accidents" that point the way to hidden logic and allow the person to "know again" what was too difficult to remember. The present can now be perceived on its own terms and not simply as a symbolic reminder of all prior related experience. If one had difficult and abandoning parents, that person's view of men and women in the present is apt to be colored by expectations set by the repressed memories of the past. If these memories are brought out of repression the person may be freed from the burden of having current perceptions corrupted by the template of the past. Not all women have to be experienced as a condensation of all infantile maternal memories—not every good-bye is a paternal abandonment. The energy that was previously expended to keep something repressed is now available to use for the person's conscious goals.

The concept of unconscious process assumes that nothing is forgotten. All the experiences of an individual from birth until death are indelibly fixed in memory. Although some small portion of early experience and feelings are available to conscious recall, the greater portion is stored away unconsciously, either for economic or for psychologic reasons. At any given moment in time, the total awareness of current facts and feelings would overwhelm the attention and concentration of an individual. For example, it is unlikely that one would remember the lyrics of a pop tune from many years past, but should that tune reappear in a current film, the words might spontaneously reemerge, although the viewer had not thought of them in years.

The economical storage of facts in this example is less an avoidance of difficult memories than it is a housekeeping function of keeping "clutter" out of the way until the material is needed again. The facts and feelings here are presumably not emotion laden and are easily retrievable when the occasion dictates.

Other memories, especially emotionally laden ones, are stored away in order to preserve the person's emotional equilibrium. This method of avoiding anxiety is called *repression*, and it occurs at a point in time when the person feels emotionally threatened. This may happen for developmental reasons, at times when the infant is not mature or resilient enough to manage the distress, or when the adult is overwhelmed by a current agony that feels too huge to bear. For example, should we find that the forgotten song mentioned above is one that was heard just prior to the departure of a loved one who was going off to perish in the war, then the "forgetting" takes on a quite different cast. Now the listener might be awash in tears upon being forced to hear the words again. This unconscious forgetting makes a certain kind of psychologic sense: The person avoids mourning in order to avoid facing the permanency of the loss of the loved one.

Another major characteristic of the unconscious is that it is timeless. In the course of any single journey through life, poignant memories of conflicted yearnings and unresolved losses are frozen in time and repressed. Like Sleeping Beauty, they maintain their pristine freshness, to be awakened in full passion at the moment of a present and compelling stimulus. This uncovering of lost memories lends continuity to a life. Without it, life can feel like a series of meaningless and disjointed incidents that are random and chaotic.

At the moment of reawakening, an incident from decades past may elicit the fullness of affect that was experienced originally. For example, one might still blush at the memory of a terrible faux pas committed during one's awkward adolescence, even so simple a one as plunging one's fork into a piece of meat only to have it land in one's lap at a formal dinner party. But if in addition one's childhood was riddled with humiliating criticism from an overly harsh family, the incident may distill an accumulation of shame and generate rage, bitterness, and a retaliatory wish in the present. Similarly, a memory of a hard-won but delicious victory over adversity may fill one with the same glow of pride and self-esteem at a moment of victory in the present. Thus both humiliation and pride are cumulative over time and define a person's self-esteem in a profound way that far transcends any given incident in present life.

Dynamic Motivation

Psychodynamic theory rests on the assumption that the mind is propelled by the drives. If one ascribes to the Freudian concepts, libido and aggression are the dual drives or instincts that propel a person toward pleasurable discharge, by finding a person who serves as a target for the drives. If, on the other hand, one is an object relationist, the developmental thrust is powered by an innate instinct for attachment to an important other. In any case, psychodynamic theory assumes that the mind is inevitably goal directed, seeking pleasure and attachment and avoiding pain according to instinctual drives.

Epigenetic Development

All psychodynamic approaches postulate developmental lines that define a sequential path from infancy to maturity. An epigenetic model is one in which past experience accumulates like a series of building blocks that then support and influence the next layer of growth. Major emphasis is placed on early years. The child's primary motivational forces are seen as undergoing major transformation as a result of the maturational processes.

In this sense, it can be said that the past is a prologue. The earliest infantile experiences are the foundations of all later experiences. Theorists such as Anna Freud (2), Margaret Mahler (8), and Erik Erikson (9) have proposed the concept of lines of development, elaborating a series of sequential milestones that build upon one another from infancy to maturity. In the course of any human life, there will be interferences in development that will compromise the individual's growth. Sometimes these are understood as fixations that are specific to certain stresses that occurred at a point in the child's life in such a way as to mute further development of that particular skill or aptitude; other interferences are thought of as deficits and are more commonly postulated in people who have not ever had the chance to develop certain capacities, because of the absence of an enabling maturational environment.

A critically important correlate of the epigenetic model of development is that growth can be resumed if the missing building blocks can be recalled and/or developed anew. If the repressed can be reawakened, then we are left with an ultimately optimistic view of human possibilities. If the conscious, goal-directed ego of the individual is compromised by the unknown turbulence in the unconscious, it follows that making the unconscious conscious can liberate the mind. If, on the other hand, development failed to occur at an earlier age, it is possible to set in place new "structures" to compensate for the deficit in earlier maturation. The dual goals of freeing the person from repression and establishing new compensatory psychologic functions are the primary functions of psychodynamic treatment; together, they provide the person with broader opportunities for autonomy and fulfillment.

Functions of the Mind at Work

All psychodynamic approaches assume that there are distinct functions of the mind that may be in conflict. They are managed by an internal structure that theorists have postulated to explain the process of how the mind works in the here and now. By structure, we mean stable and predictable mental states—clusters of thinking that are permanent or change very slowly, and that organize and manage conflicting ideas and competing impulses. Structures are a way

of explaining simultaneous and opposing thoughts and impulses in an individual. In psychodynamic theory, structures of the mind are heuristically divided into id, ego, superego, and, later, the self. Classically, the id is seen as the repository of primitive instinct, in search of gratification. The superego is the internalization of the civilizing strictures as imposed by the parents as representatives of the external world, and the ego mediates between the demands of the id and the superego, via a set of defenses that allow compromise solutions of the intrinsic conflicts. More recently, self psychologists conceptualize the self as a structure of the mind, although this remains a very controversial matter in the field.

COMPARISONS AND CONTRASTS IN THEORIES

The differences among the theorists grew and were elaborated in response to Freud's orthodox theory; however, they are still firmly rooted in Freudian thought.

The history of psychoanalysis has been marked by innovation and controversy. Freud began the tradition of innovation by his own constant revision of his theories throughout his career. Although Freud was receptive to ideas advanced by his associates, he was also adamant about preserving the conceptual pillars upon which his psychoanalytic theory rested. When his followers' innovations went too far afield, Freud initially attempted to help them see the error of their ways, then eventually considered them outside the fold and cut them off from the psychoanalytic movement.

Much of the early controversy centered around the dual instinct theory and the role of the drives. Freud's emphasis on the primacy of drives became the point of departure for many of those who followed him more or less loyally, despite his resolute distancing from the "heretics" in the psychoanalytic movement. Although most remained loyal to his structural concepts, they tended to part with him over his mechanistic/biologic energic focus and moved instead toward the importance of the child's need to attach and relate to important people as the main force motivating development. Even among those remaining within the ranks of loyal followers, frequent and passionate controversy has accompanied and fueled divergent strains of thought, all of which can nonetheless be subsumed under the heading of psychodynamic theories.

Such a controversy occurred in the British Psychoanalytic Society in the 1920s in a disagreement between Melanie Klein and Anna Freud. Over the next two decades, this disagreement developed into a major ideologic schism. Klein and her followers went on to form the object relations school, while those loyal to Anna Freud evolved the theory of ego psychology. Still later, Kohut posited a psychology of the self, which combined some of the tenets of drive theory and also borrowed from object relations theory. He went on to develop a mixed-model theory for understanding the development of the self from the earliest narcissistic phase to later more mature states of being.

As a group, these analysts trace the evolution of psychodynamic thought from

1. Sigmund Freud's dual instinct theory, which posits the drives as primary while the people in the infant's world serve as the initially impersonal target of the drives, to
2. Anna Freud's ego psychology, which emphasizes adaptation and accommodation between the inner and outer world, as perceived through the defensive operations and the functioning of the ego, to
3. Melanie Klein's object relations theory, which places the infant's needs for attachment to the mother as primary, to
4. Heinz Kohut's self psychology, which is primarily interested in the development of an integrated self via the infant's access to a mirroring and holding environment, and finally to
5. the neoanalysts, who deemphasize the role of the instincts and stress the impact of external environment on the in-

trapsychic maturation of the individual. Alfred Adler, Karen Horney, and Harry Stack Sullivan are some of the many representatives of this largely varied group.

All these theories maintain a commitment to the basic psychodynamic assumptions delineated earlier and thus are properly subsumed under the psychodynamic approach. Consistent with its theoretical beliefs, each has a model of the mind that emphasizes some aspects of general psychodynamic theory and deemphasizes others. In particular, they all maintain some of Freud's constructs, while debating the existence or importance of others. At times the differences in theory emerged in response to patient populations that were not adequately explained by orthodox thinking. One example is found in the work of Klein and others who studied children; later still, some of the neoanalyst writers attempted to explain female development in ways that felt truer to the realities of their patients. In the following section, the major schools are briefly reviewed to illustrate first the Freudian model and then the divergences and similarities of the more modern proponents of psychodynamic thought.

Freud's Classical Dual Instinct Theory

In the last year of his life, Freud (1) wrote,

The concept of the unconscious has long been knocking at the gates of psychology and asking to be let in. Philosophy and literature have often toyed with it, but science could find no use for it. Psycho-analysis has seized upon the concept, has taken it seriously and has given it a fresh content.

Freud proceeded from an assertion of the importance of unconscious process to posit the unconscious contents, namely the dual instincts of libido and aggression. He further postulated that the language of the unconscious is basically dreamlike, fantastic, and disconnected; the interpretation of dreams and fantasies is the path to this infantile mode of instinctual existence. He wrote early and fundamentally about the interpretation of dreams as a way to make contact with what he called the *primary process*, by which he meant the irrational, noncivilized, and atavistic impulses that are common to primitive beings, in order to understand the person at a more rational level of secondary process. *Secondary process*, then, refers to the conscious and deliberate part of the individual's life and behaviors that conforms to the mores of the world around him or her.

The pleasure principle and the emphasis on infantile sexuality distinguish Freud's work from his followers in some fundamental ways. He maintained that the psyche seeks to avoid stimulation that can cause pain; instead, it seeks gratification of hungers that he referred to as sexual hungers. The damming up of these hungers produced pain. He expanded the notion of sexuality beyond genital gratification to encompass all bodily pleasure. He located sexual pleasure in specific body zones and described the infant's development as proceeding from oral to anal to phallic and genital levels. He reiterated often that his constructs were metaphors, not to be taken literally and concretely.

Over time, Freud changed his mind about how the instincts were to be contained and how they interacted within the person. Initially he proposed a hydraulic or topographic theory: The instincts moved along toward gratification like water along a pipe. At each point of trauma in the child's life, the pipe was constricted, thereby narrowing the child's options for continued development. Later he superimposed a structural theory upon the earlier topographic theory; he called these structures the *id*, *ego*, and *superego*. The id contained all the sexual energy in primitive form: The dual instincts of libido and aggression were located in the id and propelled the person through life. The superego developed as an accommodation to the civilizing influences of the parents and the culture. The ego, through a hierarchical set of defenses, mod-

ulated the expression of the drives by generating a set of defenses for sublimating the primitive instincts into modulated and creative activity. But the ego is always only partially successful at this compromise. For example, we might say that Lady Macbeth had successfully sublimated her phallic drives by marrying a powerful man and vicariously gratifying her needs through his ambition. But when she urges him to kill the King only to find that her husband now repudiates her, sublimation fails, and we find her compulsively washing off her bloody shame; she loses her capacity to symbolize her dirty wishes and instead tries to literally cleanse herself in her madness. The instinctual press may be too intense because of earlier trauma, genetic endowment, or present stress coming from within or without the individual; the conflict remains in part irreconcilable and generates anxiety.

Freud identified two kinds of anxiety: primary anxiety and signal anxiety. *Primary anxiety* results from the frustration of the child's libidinal drive toward gratification, i.e., the wish to seek pleasure and avoid pain. For example, the hungry child will begin to experience anxiety and displeasure if the mother is absent and will seek to suckle to experience bodily relief from hunger and enjoy the mother as a gratifying source of pleasure. *Signal anxiety* is a learned response that points to the near emergence of a painful conflict and at the same time distracts and defends the person from that conflict. Signal anxiety emerges from the child's relationships with important others in the course of development. The child has now moved from purely solitary preoccupation with the self to the wish and capacity to relate to important others and to anticipate their response, either positive or negative. The source and focus of anxiety then change as well, from those of physical unpleasure to those of loving and hating, being ashamed and guilty, or being excited and intimately engaged with the family and with the world at large. For example, the child learning bowel and bladder control will seek the admiration of his or her parents around toilet training and may experience signal anxiety as he or she feels the need to eliminate without the assurance that he or she can control his functions in order to comply with their wishes. The child anticipates their displeasure and feels anxious. This anxiety in turn motivates the child to control his or her bodily functions and avoid shame and censure.

Those wishes and drives that are not managed by the ego in present reality will be suppressed and ultimately repressed so that the individual can continue to function and grow. They are essentially unreconciled areas of conflict and may simply remain repressed for life. They form the compromise solutions by which we manage despite an imperfect world. However, if these are too many, or too early in life, they accumulate to the extent of interfering with the person's capacity to manage an adult life. These form the basis for neurosis. *Neurosis* is defined as a set of compromise formations that permitted survival at one point in life but later may emerge as anachronistic interferences with the more current needs of the ego and its aims. For example, the child anxious to comply with toilet training as described above may have experienced too little support or too harsh and unattainable a set of demands. His or her conflicts around the anal level of development may remain largely unresolved and may appear now in the form of an obsessional neurosis. This same child may grow into an adult banker who is unable to manage tally sheets in a calm and timely way; always anxious about losing control, he or she may have to compulsively repeat the count long after everyone else in the office has left for home. This person's workaholic symptoms would plague his or her present functioning, interfering with the capacity for pleasure or competence.

Ego Psychology

The notable theorists in the area of ego psychology—Anna Freud (2); Hartmann, Kris, and Loewenstein (10); and Blanck and Blanck (11)—are often difficult to distinguish from the more classical Freudians.

In fact, the theories of all of these individuals lie on a continuum with Freudian theory. But the ego psychologists remain closer to the id–ego model, with less attention to the importance of the superego, while insisting that the inner life is known by the workings of the ego, which are observable via its functions. It is the incompatibility of the demands of the id with the demands of the environment that necessitates the formation of ego defenses. For example, the banker in the example above may use intellectual defenses that will lead to computerizing his or her work in order to accommodate to the needs of the environment. In ego psychology, the ego is defined as having both a conscious and an unconscious aspect and to have at its disposal repression as well as nine other defenses: regression, reaction formation, undoing, introjection, identification, projection, tuning against the self, reversal, and sublimation. But any list of defenses is incomplete; some of the more commonly added ones are intellectualization and rationalization, and there are many others as well.

All the defenses are in the service of allowing the person to function and adapt. According to Hartmann (12), "Adaptation is primarily a reciprocal relationship between the human organism and its environment." He coined the term "average expectable environment" for the typical situation and defined the process of changing one's self as "autoplastic" activity. In contrast, changing the environment is "alloplastic" activity.

The duality in ego psychology is at two levels: The individual is seen as both biologically and psychologically driven and motivated, and in addition, the person and the environment act reciprocally to change one another. The reality principle (ego activity) replaces the pleasure principle (drive expression of classical theory) through a process of environmentally mediated learning. The child becomes aware of probable changes in the environment in interaction with the mother. Furthermore, the child learns that to behave in a certain way causes her to react in a certain way.

The child develops capacities for establishing objective criteria and using them in thought and action. The sum of these capacities is designated as ego function. This step becomes possible when the child is able to substitute future gratification for immediate gratification. Hartmann et al. state "Experience with those whom the child loves is no longer exclusively in terms of indulgence or deprivation. The child's attachment to them can outlast deprivation and they gain characteristics of their own that the child tries to understand" (10). In other words, the child can see both good and bad and can tolerate present frustrations for the long-term gain of identification with the parents.

Object Relations Theory

All psychodynamic theorists adhere to the importance of the internal representation of the earlier people in the child's life, but few have so clearly elaborated the internal fantasy of infants as did Melanie Klein and her followers. Her developmental schema is consistent with the primacy she gives to "object relationships," by which she means the partially incorporated parental images that reside in the individual in split-off and incomplete memories. The remembered mother of the adult often bears little resemblance to the white-haired elderly lady of the present. Instead, she lives in caricature and undigested fantasy that bears some truth and some distortion in the mind of the adult. We react to people as adults on the basis of these internal and partially fantastic emotional memories from childhood.

It is important from the onset to define object relations theory as that theory which stresses the importance of internal and partial representations of the important people in the child's early environment. This is to be distinguished from real relationships in the person's present life. More recent theorists dispute this view and extend the meaning of object relations theory. Greenberg and Mitchell (13) describe object relations as encompassing both the internal object representations as well as the important external relationships of the individual.

With the exception of the earliest writings of Melanie Klein, object relations theory repudiates the concept of libido and aggression as primary instinctual forces. Instead it stresses as primary the drive toward attachment to another person. Aggression is secondary and is understood as a result of a perceived threat to attachment. Winnicott (14) most dramatically states this position when he writes, "there is no such thing as a baby" (15). By this he means that the baby exists only in relationship with the mother and knows itself only as it is known and responded to by the mother.

Klein's developmental theory is consistent with her belief in the richness of the child's fantasy life. The infant here moves from the "schizoid," to the "paranoid," to the "depressive" position. In the earliest schizoid position, the child lives in a fantasy of omnipotent fusion with the mother. As it develops and is forced to confront the reality that the mother can move away, that fantasy bursts and a primitive defense known as splitting occurs. This is a mental phenomenon in which the child copes with opposing realities by seeing only one at a time, and denying the other. Klein refers to this as good-breast/bad-breast oscillations, in which the mother is magnificent one moment and monstrous the next. The child is endowed with a rich fantasy life from birth on and uses these fantasies as defenses against overwhelming anxiety. The primary defense here is defined as *projective identification,* a term much in use currently to describe a clinical phenomenon that arises in the treatment of certain disturbed patients. Eventually, these oscillations in the child become less violent, given an adequate maturational environment, and the child begins to contain the ambivalent feelings more consciously. This stage is the depressive position, and it contains the melancholy acceptance of compromise and a capacity to grieve the loss of the idealistic and unrealizable grandiosity of the earlier stages. The mother evolves from perfect/horrid to "good enough," as does the child's view of the self as well. From a lack of differentiation, the child incorporates parts of the important people and makes them a part of his or her inner life.

Self Psychology

Self psychologists, led by Heinz Kohut, position the self as the fundamental and supraordinate structure in mental functioning. To be sure, earlier psychodynamic theorists had written of the self, notably Freud and Hartmann, but it was left to Kohut to define the formation of a stable self as a line of narcissistic development separate from the structural line of id, ego, and superego development. For instance, Teicholz (16) says that by the phrase "narcissistic development" Kohut meant the development of a stable, coherent, accurately perceived, and esteemed sense of self as a center of experience and a center of initiative, with attainable ideals that serve to guide, enhance, and inspire the person toward ever higher levels of development throughout the life cycle (17). At the core of Kohut's theory is the experience of the relation between the self and the empathic self-object. *Self-objects* is the term for the child's partially fused view of the self and others. It is a word coined by Kohut to describe the child's internal perception of those people in his or her environment who serve functions that will later be performed by the individual's own psychic structure. For example, the parental applause for the baby's first step will be replaced by the child's own pride in finding that he or she can run very fast. The child that is to survive psychologically is born into an empathic–responsive human milieu consisting of people who are in tune with his or her psychologic needs and wishes. When this happens, the child experiences a merger with the omnipotent self-object; to the extent that the latter is calm, the child's anxieties, needs, and rage are calmed, and he or she experiences the rudiments of a stable self. As life proceeds, and the people must necessarily disappoint the desires of the infant, this moment of "optimal frustration"—also known as empathic failure—leads to the formation of structure or stable psychologic function within the child to cope with the disappointment. To the extent that the failure is kept at the capacity of the child to manage it, this is a healthy push toward maturation; if the empathic failure occurs too early or too violently, then the stability of the self is compromised, and the child is threatened with anxiety that is disintegrative and overwhelming. It can lead to a diminished capacity to function in the world and a subsequent loss of self-esteem.

Kohut subdivided disorders of the self into primary and secondary disturbances, primary ones being the result of the child's never having experienced a calm and mirroring environment, and secondary disturbances being the acute or chronic reactions of a consolidated, firmly established self to the vicissitudes of life. Kohut insisted that any understanding of fluctuations of self-esteem and of normal feelings of joy or rage is oversimplified or irrelevant if the psychology of the self is not considered. In contrast to Freud's emphasis on infantile sexuality and the place of the drives, Kohut stesses the importance of the mirroring and empathic environment from which the infant internalizes a stable sense of self.

In sum, a narcissistic disorder results from early empathic failure on the part of the primary objects. This produces a lack of cohesion in the child's sense of self. Rage, autoerotic preoccupations, splits, projections, and delusional restitutive attempts are the sequelae of the above. To treat these interferences one must resolve the early deficits in development that interfere with the adult's capacity to deal with the frustrations that are part and parcel of every-day life.

The Neoanalysts

As a group, the neoanalysts maintain some vital connections with the traditional analysts but depart from them in some important respects. Major emphasis is placed on the importance of the environment on the internal development of the individual. The environment is defined as the family and later the culture at large. The neoanalysts focus on interpersonal communications (5), on the importance of inferiority versus superiority (6), and on the emphasis given to the birth trauma as the beginning of a dialectic between union and separation (18). Karen Horney (7) was a member of Freud's inner circle but parted with him on the primacy of the oedipal complex. Her publication on female sexuality presaged the writings of the more modern feminist analysts, such as Jean Baker-Miller (19) and Janine Chasseguet-Smirgel (20).

THE CLINICAL PROCESS

Earlier in this chapter the psychodynamic approach was defined and the main branches of current psychodynamic theory briefly reviewed. Now let us consider the application of the psychodynamic process to the treatment of patients with psychological distress.

Who Should Be Treated by a Psychodynamic Approach?

Psychodynamic theory offers a rich opportunity for understanding all human motives and behaviors; however, the application of this or any theory should be considered as part of the overall treatment planning for the best care of a particular patient. Many clinical approaches are useful for the treatment of psychologic distress. Still, some conditions lend themselves better to resolution by the psychodynamic method, either primarily or in conjunction with other models of treatment. Since psychodynamic psychotherapy has as its goal the uncovering of early repressed conflict and the resolution of characterologic pathology, it is especially applicable with those patients whose goals are congruent with these aims or whose problems will be more seriously intractable without this kind of exploration.

Three categories of patients are the primary candidates for treatment by the psychodynamic method: (a) patients seeking insight and needing to resolve conflicts they are aware of but are unable to solve by more conscious logical means; (b) patients suffering from major pathologies that may be treated by biologic therapies, but who nonetheless are left with difficult personality problems that have developed and existed concurrently; and (c) clinicians who intend to practice in this model and therefore will need to have as full an awareness of their own inner conflicts and the effectiveness of the method as possible if they are to legitimize, experientially, what they are learning didactically.

Originally, these treatments had been recommended primarily for relatively healthy patients. In the past 25 years or so, largely because of the community mental health legislation, a much larger population of patients, some very disabled, have found access to the dynamic treatments. Very disturbed patients have been a source of stimulation to the development of object relations theory, self psychology, and even ego psychology. Now, many psychodynamic clinicians treat the very disturbed patients, including the narcissistic and borderline patients, and are finding increasing validation for the effectiveness of the theory with these newer patient populations.

Diagnosis and Formulation

Let us examine the case of a star athlete who stumbles and breaks his leg just at the beginning of his last season in college. He has become depressed after his fall and has found himself anxiously distracted, unable to concentrate on his school work. He has quarreled with his girlfriend and is considering dropping out of school. His coach persuades him to seek psychotherapy, and he presents himself for evaluation. How should the potential patient be greeted, evaluated, and diagnosed? How should the clinician decide about the appropriateness of the psychodynamic method for him should it appear that treatment is in order? If treatment does begin, what are the parameters that will support the model? What are the expectable factors that will emerge in the course of treatment?

How will the methods differ in each theoretical approach? How will the clinician and the patient know when to terminate treatment and assess its relative success or lack thereof?

It will not suffice to refer only to categorical nosology for the dynamic method. Given the developmental and epigenetic underpinnings of the theory, a descriptive symptom approach will leave the clinician with few roadmaps for the resolution of infantile conflict in the adult. To be sure, it is necessary to take into account all the axes developed for the *Diagnostic and Statistical Manual of Mental Disorders* (*Third Edition-Revised*) (DSM-III-R), such as levels of stressors, character traits, etc. but the psychodynamic clinician will need to examine the genesis of the symptoms and behaviors given the presumption that they are expressions of intrapsychic conflict and infantile defensive operations.

A host of general philosophic and attitudinal values define the psychodynamic method and influence the stance of the psychodynamic clinician. This philosophy informs the theory of technique and cuts across the range of theoretical branches and forms of psychodynamic treatment, such as psychoanalysis, individual psychotherapy, group psychotherapy, couple therapy, etc. Together they constitute a culture that is designed to provide the patient with a climate that is optimal for the resolution of neurotic conflicts as defined earlier in this chapter. For the purposes of this discussion, the terms *analysis, analytic therapy,* and *psychodynamic therapy* are used interchangeably. They apply to the general approach and not to the more specific treatment context.

From the point of view of the psychodynamic clinician, nonrational intuition and rational theorizing are equally important in the work with the patient. He or she must be able to think intuitively *in* the hour and to think formally and theoretically *about* the hour. Theoretical abstractions are connected with observations of the patient. No simple, unidimensional view of the patient is complete in itself. Past, present, and transference must all receive the free-floating attention that is central to the analytic function. As Fenichel (21) pointed out decades ago, it is the content of analysis that is irrational, not its method.

In beginning to arrive at a formal diagnosis, it is important to remember that people come to treatment and present us with their solutions, not their problems. By this it is meant that their problems are the underlying and unconscious conflicts that are causing them to feel or act in a way that makes them unhappy. The neurotic solutions that they have devised to cope with life have now failed them, and it is precisely these failed solutions that constitute the "chief complaint" of the patient who first enters treatment. For instance, the patient who says she is very lonely may mean that she feels terrible living alone after the loss of her husband, or that she is a solitary person living in the midst of a devoted family and circle of friends. Each complaint has very different psychodynamic implications. The psychodynamic investigation of the chief complaint sets the stage for the entire treatment. Consistent with a philosophy of epigenesis, the diagnostician begins with an assessment of the here-and-now dilemma, moves to an investigation of the antecedents of the dilemma in the recent and remote past, and finally derives a psychodynamic formulation that explains the here and now in terms of the there and then. "After placing the presenting problem in the context of the patient's life and identifying non-dynamic determinants of the psychopathology, the formulation explains the development of central conflicts and their repetitive effect on the patient's behavior. It concludes by describing how these conflicts will be manifested in treatment" (22).

To return to our injured athlete, the analyst will begin by studying the content as well as the process by which the patient expresses his chief complaint. Is he fearful, dejected, despairing, relieved? Does he approach the doctor diffidently, arrogantly, or suspiciously? Does he expect to be helped? The focus here is on what he is saying, but no less on how he is saying it.

From the beginning encounter, the capacity of the patient to trust the doctor, to question beneath the surface, to tolerate the anxiety generated by the more neutral and abstinent stance of the clinician, will help diagnose the severity of present and past trauma in the patient's life. Let us suppose that our athlete is severely depressed, is losing sleep, and is contemplating a bleak and downward-spiraling life. As he speaks further, his despair is generated in part by the fact that he really meant to prove his father wrong when the father felt the boy would never amount to much of anything if he "wasted time" playing instead of studying. In addition, it turns out that the father retired early from the military and has failed at several business ventures since leaving the army. Now the diagnosis begins to take more ominous aspects, with strong hints that the boy's victories were to be won "over the father's dead body." If we learn later that the boy was quite accident prone in childhood, and that his mother and he spent many a precious hour with her reading to him when he stayed home with an injury, we infer again that the present symptom has strong ties to a regressive situation in the past. The injury then might be seen as an unconscious attempt to regain both parents' approval—by staying home with mother (girlfriend) and living up to father's legacy. When the girlfriend failed to cooperate with his unconscious effort to recreate his early family situation, the compromise failed and he became depressed.

But it is not enough to diagnose pathology and formulate present and prior dynamic explanations. Equally important is an understanding of the patient's defenses—his way of coping with the disappointments that occur in any life. We note of our athlete that he can study, he can succeed at athletics, he can form intimate if conflicted relationships. When pressed, he can rationalize and at times projects onto the others in the team some of the causes of his failure. The diagnosis and formulation then emerge around the patient's strengths and weaknesses, both internal and external resources, and on his capacity to engage the clinician in a manner that is reciprocally inviting.

From dual instinct theory, we might see our athlete as demonstrating castration anxiety related to the too easy victory over his father and his too intimate relationship with his mother (libido and aggression). As he is about to complete his education and begin an adult and sexually committed life, he symbolically hurts himself in a guilty preempting of the fantasied paternal revenge. Libido and aggression are fused around this conflict, and his sublimations fail.

From an object-relational point of view, he might be perceived as arrested at a stage of competing dyads (sex, or study, or athletics) in an unblended way (paranoid position). His attachments to the external world are reflections of his internal objects, which in turn exert competing pulls that are difficult for him to reconcile. The loss of the girlfriend activates his internal dread of the loss of the parental objects and results in the attenuation of his capacity to love, to play, and to work, all at the same time, and in some harmony. He regresses to a schizoid set of fantasies and contemplates withdrawing from the world.

From an ego psychology perspective, we might look at his defenses as having failed because of the press of the unresolved id conflicts. He is no longer able to cope with the world in a way that can compromise the demands of the id with the goals of the ego, and he is left to regress to more primitive levels of defense, such as projection and isolation.

Self psychology would argue that our athlete has met with a serious challenge to his narcissistic grandiosity, related to the injury and the loss of the girlfriend. He loses the mirroring relationships that sustained him—the applauding bleachers and the loving girlfriend which have been his organizing self/objects, and experiences a disintegration of the self that leaves him withdrawn and empty. The ensuing self-denigration fuels his fantasy of dropping out of the world.

These brief and oversimplified comparisons of theoretical formulations are hardly meant to be comprehensive or deep; they are offered merely as illustrations of some of the different ways that psychodynamic theoreticians have of organizing the patient's data. A fuller diagnosis will await the data from the biologic and cultural realities of the patient, as well as the effects that the clinician has on the data being gathered. Together, all these factors are important for the accuracy and completeness of the diagnosis and formulation of the case of our athlete. Once this is accomplished, the clinician will arrive at a treatment plan to propose to and negotiate with the patient.

Some psychodynamic clinicians will interpret all of the data from one of the four perspectives described in this chapter and then plan treatment according to that perspective. Others will "mix and match" perspectives according to the available data and the clinician's skills. The dilemmas resulting from this richness of theory are similar to those described in Chapter 2 of this book in which the clinician must come to terms with biologic, sociocultural, behavioral, and psychodynamic approaches to interpreting clinical data and planning treatment.

The Psychodynamic Contract

The parameters of the working agreement are designed to facilitate the psychodynamic process. Once the diagnosis and the formulation are derived, the contract is negotiated in a way that makes explicit a base of operations for the work. Aspects such as time, fees, frequency, and the rule of free association are explained and agreed to, as well as the invitation to present dreams, fantasies, and feelings or attitudes that the patient may develop toward the clinician. This contract serves a number of functions. It protects the patient from undue humiliation that he or she may encounter in the process of learning to become a patient and offers a predictable, externally enforced environment, like a tight box in which it is safe for the patient to spill the contents of a chaotic inner life. It also serves as a baseline from which to notice and then examine those

deviations from the agreement that may arise later as resistances to the treatment.

The Analytic Stance

Some of the more scathing biases about therapists derive from a misunderstanding of the clinical stance: It is often portrayed in caricature—a silent and cold analyst dozing behind the couch while the patient blithely pours out his or her heart in naive and misguided innocence. Nothing could be further from the truth. The analytic stance demands that the clinician be extremely active, as distinct from verbal; neutral as distinct from judgmental; devotedly analytic as opposed to directive of the patient's behavior. The activity of the clinician takes place in his or her own mind. In addition to a hovering attention to the patient's manifest and latent meanings, to the mood and other nonverbal aspects of the hour, and to relating these factors to the patient's early history, the clinician constantly monitors his or her own internal states for feelings, fantasies, personal associations that will further deepen the way in which the patient and the clinician reciprocally resonate and make contact at the less conscious levels of human dialogue.

The abstinent verbal stance of the clinician is aimed at giving primacy to the patient's productions. The clinician is not so much the conductor of the orchestra but more the accompanist—encouraging, playing subtle background themes, and holding the tone when words fail and the patient's courage falters. Like Occam's razor, the parsimony of the clinician's words is the most effective and simplest way to keep out of the patient's way, and to turn up the inner volume in both parties to the interaction.

Nonjudgmental empathy is the sine qua non of the analytic attitude. The analyst's dedication to entering the patient's experience without prejudice is a goal that can only be approximated, since no one can really set aside all of the internal biases and moral judgments of his or her own life. No one is value free; indeed, to be so would require an amoral stance that would diminish the clinician's humanity. It would be strange to have no moral position on the patient's past abusive acts toward her child, or on a revelation of the patient's plan to defraud a third-party payer! What matters is that the clinician know what his or her moral position is and without applying those standards in a judgment about the patient. Instead, the goal is to promote a personal sense of values in the patient, according to his or her life situation and goals.

But the intense analytic stance is of little comfort to the patient unless the clinician can somehow establish a climate in which the patient feels warmly regarded and respected. The patient must be contained in a climate of nonpossessive caring that the clinician struggles to maintain. How to express warmth and regard for the patient without interfering with the patient's needs to be hateful and cold, or to recreate the feeling of being unloved by the doctor as by the world at large . . . this balance is the greatest challenge to the artful practice of dynamic psychotherapy.

Since analytic neutrality and perfect empathy remain an ideal, the burden is on the therapist to acknowledge and circumscribe the limitations of that empathy and to avoid the narcissistic fantasy of Godlike omnipotence. It is not the failure of empathy that damages the patient; rather, it is the inability of either party to live and deal with the doctor's limitations that threatens the alliance and the ultimate outcome of the work. Left unexamined, these ruptures erode the ultimate needs of the patient to accept the melancholy reality of an imperfect but good enough therapist and an imperfect, but good enough self.

Finally, the analytic method stands on the belief that to give voice to feelings is healing in and of itself. The ego functions by channeling the tumult of the primitive life into symbolic language that moves an individual out of isolation, and enables him or her to form bonds with another. As Shakespeare said in *Macbeth*,

> Give sorrow words;
> The grief that does not speak
> Whispers the o'erfraught heart
> And bids it break.

The Rule of Free Association

To the extent that the patient can give voice to confusion, anguish, and wrath, the feelings separate themselves from the mass of undifferentiated distress into more manageable particles of cognitively recognizable affects. Freud and others conceived of a process of free association that became a rule of the analytic treatment at that time and remains largely so to this day. The patient is encouraged to say whatever comes to mind, in as uncensored a flow of associations as possible. In effect, this shakes the patient free of the constraints of conscious logic and begins to illuminate the unconscious logic that dictates the associative stream of ideas. For example, from an observation that the person leaving the waiting room just prior to her entering the doctor's office looked pretty sick, the patient may move to talking about a lunch with her sister, and to a comment about flowers on the doctor's desk. She might then remember picking wildflowers with her father on the day that her sister was born, and of the bee sting she sustained at the same outing. Since nothing is accidental, the juxtaposition of ideas that compose the patient's free associations is a clue to the internal and unconscious logic that is occurring simultaneously with the more conscious mental activity of which the patient is aware. The more proximate sting of jealousy about the competing "sibling" in the form of the other patient would lead to the feelings of earlier jealousy toward the sister at the competition for their father's love and attention, and the concomitant wish that the sister might have become ill and died. The patient may indeed find some important insight into why she always reaches for the luncheon check, although her sister is far wealthier at this point in time.

Establishing the Alliance

The process of free association is facilitated by the presence of a trusted other. Just as a blind person might wish very dearly to walk through the forest again to smell forgotten scents and feel forgotten branches, so the patient might yearn to travel again the regions of a dimly remembered childhood. But both will find more courage for the journey if there is a trusted guide who nudges them along the overgrown path and is there to help them avoid the perils of too great a drop. To ask the patient to free associate is to ask that he or she be willing to grope in the dark of the unconscious. It is precisely the therapist's trusted presence that can make this a tolerable experiment.

The therapist must earn the patient's trust by establishing an alliance based on respect, genuine interest, empathy, and tact. The earliest alliance is forged around the therapeutic stance and the working contract. Here and later, the emphasis must remain on negotiation from mutually respectfully positions. "Somewhere between the image of psychoanalysis as suggestion and psychoanalysis as unearthing is that of analysis as negotiation. This is a picture of a mutual construction of reality by analyst and patient (which) allows for a reciprocal input of the participants and a possible change in both" (23). An attitude of negotiation permeates the entire process of treatment, from the analyst's theory to the rules of the work and the goals of the work. In this spirit of negotiation the clinician begins to gather the history—not along a mechanistically derived symptom checklist that ignores the patient's initiative, but in a more complex and gentle channeling of the material so that the clinician can make early assessments about the patient's safety and the appropriateness of the psychodynamic model to the case at hand (see Chapters 9 and 10 for a further discussion of negotiation).

At this stage patient and therapist begin to negotiate the real and the transferential relationship. Does the patient have the capacity to be psychologically minded? This is a somewhat ineffable quality that implies the capacity to look within, to be curious about latent meanings, to work in the world of symbols. Is the doctor's personality one that the patient can like and respect, or are there aspects that are expe-

rienced as intolerable and that will interfere with the patient's ability to want to expose old wounds and explore new risks? Is the therapist too young, too old, too culturally divergent, too cold, too inexperienced? Although they are rarely voiced, these aspects of the real relationship lend cement to the contractual agreements and pave the way for the transferential relationship that will follow.

Transference and Countertransference

It is axiomatic in psychodynamic work that as soon as the rational alliance is formed, the patient begins to feel and behave in irrational ways.

Transference has evolved in its definition from the earliest days of Freud and Breuer (24), who describe a distortion in the connections the patient makes between present to past. More currently, transference is defined both as a distortion that arises in the excavation of repressed conflicts and as a defense against some painful realities. "A more accurate formulation than distortion is that the real situation is subject to interpretations other than the one the patient has reached" (25). The latter is a more interactive stance, in which the patient is invited to note what has been omitted from the present view of reality. For example, if the patient is convinced that the doctor is distracted, he or she might assume that this is because of the patient's rudeness the prior week; in this case the patient might be invited to ponder alternate explanations of present reality, such as the fact that the doctor obviously has a cold. Still, whichever definition of transference we prefer as fundamental assumptions that there are things that the patient does not see because they are too difficult to see and that it is the goal of the analyst to interpret the transference and thereby enlarge and buttress the patient's access to the inner reality of his or her mind and the outer reality of his or her world.

By definition, transference is unconscious and is a process by which the individual is reliving feelings, yearnings, and conflicts originally experienced with earlier figures and now directed toward the therapist or the clinical situation. For example, our injured athlete may stumble when leaving the doctor's office after learning that the doctor is about to take a vacation. Depending on the history, this could be interpreted as a self-directed vengeful act related to the abandonment of the disappointing "doctor/parent." Even in the first hours, the precursors of the transference may emerge, as in the earlier example of the woman noticing the flowers on the analyst's desk. Gradually, the patient begins to perceive the analyst in some distortion or to act toward the treatment in ways quite different from his or her usual mode of being in the world. For example, the conscientious banker may neglect to sign the check he mailed to the analyst; the modest clergywoman starts to wear a lot of perfume to the analytic hour. The patient may become uncharacteristically inarticulate or sarcastic. All of these peculiarities are outside the awareness of the patient and are assumed to be transference reactions.

The clinician experiences a similar resonance and amplification of his or her own unresolved conflicts in a set of responses to the patient. This process is known as the countertransference. For example, the doctor whose own childhood was spent in denying any dependency feelings may react to the extremely dependent patient with a resentful overindulgence; unconsciously, the clinician is doing for the patient what he wishes had been done for him, without having to acknowledge this infantile wish in the self. In fact, he or she may misjudge the patient's capacity to function autonomously, choosing instead to foster the illusion of being indispensable to the patient. Again, it is the unconscious aspect of these distortions that composes the countertransference, and not the whole range of reactions to the patient, most of which will, it is hoped, be in the clinician's awareness. The latter are often reactions to the patient's transference or to the objectively difficult aspects of the

work, such as sitting with the boring patient or the menacing one.

It has become commonplace to refer to all the feelings and attitudes toward the therapist as transference and to all those toward the patient as countertransference. This is inaccurate and often misleading. Many reactions of the therapist and the patient are essentially subjective responses to the personality of the other, are usually quite conscious, and form part of the real relationship, but not the transferential one.

Regression

At the core of long-term, open-ended psychoanalytic psychotherapy is the concept of regression. "What we call regression . . . refers to a very considerable retrograde process of personality functioning. There is a regression to earlier and more primitive ways of feeling, experiencing, and behaving. There is a constriction in the field of attention, a preoccupation with the self, and a simplification or reduction in the structural complexity of functioning. Primary processes emerge and secondary processes diminish in importance" (26). This regression is stimulated by the vulnerable patient's response to the dependent patient position. It is further increased by the clinician's stance, which violates "polite" social rules and frustrates the patient's more civilized expectations. The patient's anxiety is increased, and he or she reverts to earlier modes of functioning under stress. This allows the clinician to help the patient note his regressive behavior, to become curious about its effects in the present, and ultimately to seek out its origins.

Let us suppose that our athlete finds himself yearning for an intense relationship such as he once had with his mother and in which he found solace as a child. To the extent that he remains unconscious of this yearning, he cannot directly discuss or understand it; instead, he develops headaches. After biologic causes are ruled out, it becomes clear that this is a psychosomatic regression that has emerged with the increasing force of his desperate need for infantile attachment and should yield to the interpretation of the transference. As the symptoms abate, the patient has been brought face to face with the power of his primitive wishes and fears and gains greater mastery over his poorly channeled libido. It can be said that psychodynamic treatment involves a series of frequent encounters with the beast within, and a yoking of its energies in the service of ego.

The onus is on the therapist to avoid too early or too activist an intervention that would disallow the necessary regression. It is always a matter of careful clinical judgment to assess the highest tolerable levels of anxiety while still conducting an ethical and safe practice. But the psychodynamic clinician must be willing and able to tolerate the ambiguity and fears that are similar to those we ask our patients to bear, and to trust in the ultimate strength of the healing relationship and the patient's own ego.

An interesting debate is now in progress concerning the method of short-term psychodynamic therapy and the place that regression occupies in that modality. It remains an open question as to whether regression occurs in short-term work and whether regression does, indeed, occupy such a central place in the curative process.

Remembering, Repeating, and Working Through

As patients delve into the narrative of their life, they will begin to feel with the therapist many of the characteristic conflicts that they experience elsewhere in their life. This is a kind of emotional remembering of earlier conflicts. In many respects, character is tenacious and habitual. The very neat child is probably going to grow into a neat adult. The avoidant child is going to struggle hard to overcome a phobic tendency at times of conflict as an adult. So will the adult repeat emotional states in dealing with the adults in his or her life, including the therapist.

There is a tendency to try to resolve unconscious conflict by repeating the early dilemma, in the hopes that it will "work out better this time." Freud called this the *repetition compulsion.* It is a magical fantasy that is doomed to fail, but explains how an otherwise rational person can be caught time and again in a maze of repetitious self-destructive behaviors. For example, a patient may marry several times and each time find himself or herself with a spouse that closely resembles the prior ones in fundamental ways that generate the old marital problems anew. On the other hand, this repetition compulsion is also an expression of a blindly optimistic thrust toward health; the conflict seeks resolution as surely as an infant seeks the breast.

And so, the patient will tend to express repressed conflicts by repeating them in the transference neurosis that develops with the clinician. As the transference is interpreted, the patient becomes aware of the archaic danger with which he or she is trying to cope. In effect, the bogeymen of the past are exposed to the light of the adult's day; the defenses appropriate to an infant of age one or three can now be replaced by the defenses and options of an adult. The truly ominous parent of one's childhood is replaced by the "make-believe" parent in the figure of the therapist, and the patient is always aware at some level that he or she can walk away from the office should he or she choose to. It is precisely the partially make-believe quality of the transference relationship that allows for the old terrors to be brought forth repeatedly and resolved a bit more each time. Working through involves the patients' actively translating the insights derived from the analyst's interpretations into their own metaphors and in their own actions—in other words, by transforming some aspects of the new ideas into their own and discarding the rest.

With each unshackling from the encumbrances of the past patients find they have more conflict-free ego available to make informed decisions about life and to feel the full range of their affect in terms of the present rather than the past.

Resistance

The rather idyllic evolution of the treatment described above is hardly realistic, since things rarely progress so geometrically and systematically. The early conflicts were repressed specifically because they were felt to be extremely threatening, and the patient has developed a set of defenses and character patterns that have helped him or her to get through life with some modicum of success. Even the pain of the patient's life has been largely syntonic, that is, a familiar and personal devil that may be preferable to a new devil that may prove to be dystonic or outside of one's capacity to keep at bay. Binstock states, "It is obvious why the patient is not wholly allied with what is, after all, an undertaking that he face what frightens him honestly. If there is a lion in the room, it might be more comfortable to close one's eyes, but this use of denial precludes one's knowing when the lion springs. It is often more comfortable in the short run not to know, but it is safer in the long run to know" (25). However, anyone who has tried to convince himself or herself that the snake is really not slimy and is in fact warm to the touch knows how hard it is to reconcile conscious resolve with unconscious and irrational terror.

With the deepening of the transference, and the return of the repressed, the patient begins to experience some of the archaic anxiety and to resist the treatment. Appointments are forgotten or business meetings somehow occur in conflict with the therapy time. The patient's dreams are no longer remembered or reported. The patient manages to convince the spouse that the therapy is destructive to their relationship, and the distress is reported as a reason to stop treatment. Free association is blunted, long silences ensue, and the patient begins to keep secrets from the doctor. These resistances are referred to as "acting out," a somewhat pejorative term that means that the anxiety generated in the clinical situation is being discharged outside the agreements of the treatment; the cause for the anxiety is then lost to analytic investigation.

Defenses

Theoretically, anxiety is emerging because the patient's defenses are failing and earlier, more regressed ones are taking over the functions of keeping the instincts in some control. Thus, for example, the obsessive–compulsive patient who keeps every appointment in perfect order may misplace his appointment book, feel extreme anxiety at this loss, and decide instead that his wife hid it to get even. He becomes paranoid and projects his own unconscious malicious intent onto her. This projection allows him to avoid the awareness of his wish to punish the therapist for real or imagined slights during the prior hour.

Defenses are psychic ways of not knowing or not acknowledging ownership of impulses that the patient experiences as too threatening or too humiliating to bear. The incapacity may be a developmental one—a child does not yet have the ego to manage opposing and simultaneous feelings—or it may be related to superego shame and guilt, in which the gap between the patient's ego ideal and self-image is too disparate to allow for an adequate maintenance of self-esteem. Extremes of externally induced trauma such as rape or combat in war may also require the patient to develop defenses in order to survive. The analysis of resistance paves the way for an analysis of the defense and ultimately, of the instinct that underlies them both. To return to our athlete, he might find that the resistance that caused him to stumble and reinjure himself might have had as its goal his avoidance of treatment for the next few meetings. He could then avoid and deny the furious wish to injure the analyst (and his father) by injuring himself instead. Injuring himself here is perceived as the defense of displacement, in which he positions himself in lieu of his father as the target of his aggressive instinct.

This patient will cycle through his circular dilemma time and again, under the sway of the repetition compulsion and in the transference with the analyst. Each time he does so, the clinician will interpret the resistance, then the defense, and then the underlying instinct that is being played out in the transference; each time, this conflict is repeated, emotionally remembered, and worked through or partially resolved.

Termination

The patient who entered treatment as a stranger is not the patient from whom the therapist will ultimately part company. Both the patient and therapist are changed in the process of the "irrational involvement" that has formed the matrix for change. Criteria are difficult to assess. Originally, analysts insisted that orgastic potency must be established if a treatment is to be judged complete. Since then, many vague criteria such as a sense of well-being, a sense of coping better with the vicissitudes of life, and a capacity to examine one's inner life and befriend the "beast within" are all rather poetic goals. "One swallow does not make a summer. The clinical improvement of . . . patients represented by the successive abandonment of the phases of regression is like birds returning in the spring" (26). The patient has learned to love and believes the self to be lovable. He or she is active where previously passive in the face of pain, and trusts internal resources. There is no longer the feeling that the patient's ego is disintegrating under stress. Attachments are valued, and the patient's life history is now rewritten in shades of pastel, to replace the tyranny of black and white judgments from a sadistic superego. Self-image approaches ego ideal. As this happens, the patient begins to wonder why he or she is coming to the therapist when the therapist now resides within. The patient decides that the visits to the therapist are more out of affection than need, and develops dreams or fantasies of replacing him- or herself in the doctor's practice. The patient may refer a friend to the therapist or dream that the patient and the doctor are really

colleagues about to give a lecture together. The patient may wonder what all the fuss was about that brought him or her in to treatment in the first place, since that early self no longer seems to be around. Finally, the patient and therapist begin to negotiate a termination of treatment.

The deepening of the good-bye is no different from the deepening of the resolution of any other conflict, and it brings with it the inevitable cycles of regression and progress. Freud said, "after the first death, there is no other." Each current loss resonates and awakens the pain of the earliest loss of the attachment to the symbiotic mother. Each current loss is also an opportunity to recall from repression former unresolved losses and to make peace with the archaic grief from the past. "It is always a race," said Searles (27), "between the analyst and the patient as to who will cure whom first." Each time the patient works through a conflict, the clinician too is faced with a renewal of his or her own resonating conflicts and arrives at some resolution alongside the patient.

TRAINING THE PSYCHODYNAMIC CLINICIAN

Supervision is the cornerstone in the training of the psychodynamic psychotherapist. In addition to gathering data and understanding theory, the clinician has ultimately only the self to rely upon as the tool for the work. It is imperative to know the self in relation to the patient. Just as the patient needs the therapist to enable his self-exploration, so too does the student need the supervision to help think about the hour, and feel in the hour, while maintaining a grip on the boundaries between the doctor and the patient.

The unusual aspect of the supervision of the psychodynamic clinician derives from the essentially private nature of the clinical hour. While the apprentice surgeon can watch the senior surgeon perform in the surgery, or the case worker can accompany the supervisor in community organization, the apprentice psychotherapist rarely if ever watches a senior clinician work; for that matter, it is rare that the supervisor has any intimate view of the trainee at work. Fortunately, there are some breaks in this tradition with the use of live observation and video and audiotapes, but for the most part, the only way the supervisor can "know" what the student is doing and feeling with the patient is by gauging what the supervisor can know and feel with the student in the supervisory hour.

As the trainee presents notes from the clinical hour and discusses the patient, a parallel process takes place in which the trainee will tend to replicate in the process of the supervisory hour those attitudes, mood states, and styles of interaction obtained in the hour with the patient. This parallel process allows the supervisor some access, however derivative, to the inner workings of the hour. Most importantly, psychodynamic supervision makes the point that a combination of cognitive depth and emotional immersion together are conducive to growth and change. The medium is the message. It is always desirable that the clinician engage in his or her own psychotherapy to deal with the more personal intrapsychic issues, but it is left for the supervisor to help the student become sensitive to the theoretical manifestations as they are elaborated in the field of emotions that is generated by the therapeutic dyad working in the hour.

The supervisor's capacity to educate, to nurture, to tolerate ambiguity, and to challenge and contain the clinician and honor the struggle will ultimately be transformed, via the parallel process, to the work with the patient, in whose best interest they both work.

References

1. Freud S: An outline of psychoanalysis. In Strachey J (ed): *Standard Edition of the Complete Psychological Works of Sigmund Freud*. London, Hogarth Press, 1964 (originally published 1949), pp 1–87.
2. Freud A: *The Writings of Anna Freud. Volume 2. The Ego and the Mechanisms of Defense*. New York, International Universities Press, 1966.
3. Klein M: *Contributions to Psychoanalysis 1921–1945*. London, Hogarth Press, 1948.
4. Kohut H: *The Analysis of the Self*. New York, International Universities Press, 1971.
5. Sullivan HS: *Conceptions of Modern Psychiatry*. New York, W.W. Norton, 1953.
6. Adler A: Adler's individual psychology. In Wolman BB (ed): *Psychoanalytic Techniques: A Handbook for the Practicing Analyst*. New York, Basic Books, 1967, pp 14–28.
7. Horney K: *New Ways in Psychoanalysis*. New York, W.W. Norton, 1939.
8. Mahler MS: *On Human Symbiosis and the Vicissitudes of Individuation*. New York, International Universities Press, 1968.
9. Erikson E: *Childhood and Society*. New York, W.W. Norton, 1950.
10. Hartmann H, Kris E, Loewenstein RM: Comments on the formation of psychic structure. *Psychoanalytic Study of the Child* 2:11–38, 1946.
11. Blanck G, Blanck R: *Ego psychology*. New York, Columbia University Press, 1974.
12. Hartmann H: Comments on the scientific aspects of psychoanalysis. In *Essays on Ego Psychology*. New York, International Universities Press, 1964, pp 297–317.
13. Greenberg J, Mitchell S: *Object Relations in Psychoanalytic Theory*. Cambridge, Harvard University Press, 1983.
14. Winnicott DW: *Collected Papers: Through Pediatrics to Psychoanalysis*. New York, Basic Books, 1958.
15. Guntrip H: My experience of analysis with Fairbairn and Winnicott. *International Review of Psychoanalysis* 2:145–156, 1975.
16. Teicholz J: A selective review of psychoanalytic literature on theoretical conceptualizations of narcissism. *J Am Psychoanal Assoc* 26:831–862, 1978.
17. Teicholz JG: *Kohut and His Critics*. Presented at the Kohut Colloquium, Massachusetts School of Professional Psychology, Boston, 1982.
18. Rank O: *The Trauma of Birth*. New York, Harcourt Brace and Co., 1929.
19. Baker-Miller J: *Psychoanalysis and Women*. New York, Penguin Books, 1973.
20. Chasseuet-Smirgel J: *The Ego Ideal* (Barrow P, trans). London, Free Association Books, 1973.
21. Fenichel O: *The Psychoanalytic Theory of Neurosis*. New York, W.W. Norton, 1945.
22. Perry S, Cooper A, Michels R: The psychodynamic formulation: its purpose, structure, and clinical application. *Am J Psychiatry* 144:5, 1987.
23. Goldberg A: Psychoanalysis and negotiation. *Psychoanal Q* 56:109–129, 1987.
24. Breuer J, Freud S: *Studien uber Hysterie*. Leipzig, Franz Deuticke, 1895.
25. Binstock W: The mind as conflict. In Lazare A (ed): *Outpatient Psychiatry*. Baltimore, Williams & Wilkins, 1979.
26. Menninger K, Holzman P: *Theory of Psychoanalytic Technique*, ed 2. New York, Basic Books, 1973.
27. Searles H: *Collected Papers on Schizophrenia and Related Subjects*. New York, International Universities Press, 1965.

Additional Readings

Alonso A: *The Quiet Profession: Supervisors of Psychotherapy.* New York, MacMillan, 1985.

Brenner C: *The Mind in Conflict.* New York, International Universities Press, 1982.

Deutsch H: *The Psychology of Women.* New York, Grune and Stratton, 1944.

Eagle M: *Recent Developments in Psychoanalysis.* New York, McGraw Hill, 1984.

Ferenczi S: Thalassa: a theory of genitality. *Psychoanal Q* 2:361–403, 1924.

Fromm E: *The Forgotten Language.* New York, Grove Press, 1951.

Fromm-Reichmann F: *Principles of Intensive Psychotherapy.* Chicago, University of Chicago Press, 1950.

Gill M: *Analysis of Transference* (Psychological Issues, Monograph 53). New York, International Universities Press, 1982.

Goldberg A: *The Psychology of the Self: A Casebook.* New York, International Universities Press, 1978.

Modell A: Denial and the sense of separateness. *J Am Psychoanal Assoc* 9:533–547, 1961.

Ornstein P (ed): *The Search for the Self: Selected Writings of Heinz Kohut: 1950–1978.* New York, International Universities Press, 1978.

Thompson C: *Psychoanalysis: Evolution and Development.* New York, Grove Press, 1950.

5

The Behavioral Approach

Shirley M. Glynn, Ph.D.
Kim T. Mueser, Ph.D.
Robert Paul Liberman, M.D.

Behavioral psychotherapy is first and foremost an empirical approach to understanding and treating clinical problems. In the initial step of behavioral therapy, psychopathology and associated functional disabilities are specified and measured, with special attention being paid to identifying environmental determinants of behavior. Second, treatment goals are operationalized and interventions are aimed at improving the frequency, quality, or context of adaptive functioning. Goal setting in behavior therapy is multimodal; that is, therapeutic objectives are formulated in the relevant spheres of human experience—affect, instrumental skills, social relations, cognition and imagery, and psychophysiology.

In contrast to psychodynamic therapists, behavioral psychotherapists do not conceptualize patients' problems in terms of inferred mental events, unconscious conflicts, or underlying personality traits. Rather, behavioral psychotherapists view the deviance and dysphoria of patients as acquired behavioral excesses or deficits that are inappropriate to specific contexts and thus preclude optimal functioning. Each patient requires a behavioral analysis of his or her problems, tailored to his or her assets, deficits, excesses, culture, and

environmental resources. Behavioral analysis is firmly entrenched in measurement of the multimodal behaviors of clinical interest; in fact, adherence to specification of problems and goals is the characteristic that most distinguishes behavioral therapy from other psychotherapies. Behavioral analysis provides guidelines for assessing the nature, severity, and frequency of targeted problems, as well as for teasing apart the functional relationships between the patient's behavior and its environmental antecedents and consequences.

The behavioral psychotherapist and his or her patient mutually agree on ways to arrange the immediate therapeutic and natural environments to bring about favorable changes in the patient's behavior. Behavioral psychotherapists attempt to influence behavior by changing the environment, especially the interpersonal milieu of the patient. This often requires interventions carried out with the mediation of relatives, teachers, friends, and natural support groups. Thus, behavioral psychotherapy can be more aptly termed "environmental modification," with therapeutic gains occurring only as a function of changes in the interaction between the patient and a responsive environment. Since behavior and the environment influence each other reciprocally, behavioral psychotherapists encourage their patients to take an active role in modifying their environments and the contingencies of reinforcement that impinge upon them.

Behavior analysis is a critical aspect of behavioral psychotherapy. Regardless of the specific treatment interventions used, all behavioral psychotherapists are committed to determining the efficacy of their treatments as objectively as possible. By collecting and monitoring behaviorally based data, behavioral clinicians continually evaluate the utility of their interventions and are thus provided with opportunities to strengthen effective interventions and modify ineffective ones. This dynamic interplay of behavior analysis and intervention is the sine qua non of behavioral psychotherapy.

THEORETICAL PREMISES

The evolving nature of behavioral psychotherapy makes identifying its defining features a complex task. Twenty years ago, it would have been appropriate to describe behavioral psychotherapy as the systematic application of empirically derived principles of learning to the analysis and treatment of disorders and behavior. This definition has become outmoded, however, as the range of behavioral techniques, targeted behaviors, and behavioral theory has broadened. Today, clinical studies establishing the utility of a behavioral procedure are often conducted concurrently with laboratory studies testing the underlying learning-based premises for these procedures. Similarly, behavioral interventions are being used effectively with an ever-widening array of psychiatric problems, including those such as personality disorders that may have no laboratory analogue. Finally, cognitions and emotions, as well as motoric behaviors, are now considered appropriate targets for behavioral intervention.

Regardless of the specific techniques used, individuals committed to behavioral psychotherapy share the following assumptions as the foundation of their work (1):

1. Abnormal behavior that is not a result of specific brain dysfunction or biochemical disturbance is assumed to be governed by the same principles that regulate normal behavior. Even deviant behavior stemming from biologic disturbances can be affected by environmental influences.

2. Abnormal behavior is not viewed solely as a superficial "symptom" or manifestation of an underlying disease process, but also as the patient's problem in living. The target behavior is considered not a substitute for a conflict or an unconscious expression of a blocked desire, but rather a learned response that has detrimental consequences for the patient and his or her environment, regardless of how it was acquired.

3. Most abnormal behavior is assumed to be acquired and maintained through the same biopsychosocial mechanisms as normal behavior and can be treated through the application of behavioral procedures.

4. Behavioral assessment focuses on the current determinants of behavior rather than the post hoc analysis of possible historical antecedents.

5. Interventions are focused on rendering improvement in measurable, specifiable *behavior*. Interventions may be directed to alleviating subjective states of distress (e.g., anxiety, depression), but each of these internal states is considered to have observable manifestations (e.g., avoidance of places or situations, sleep difficulties) that must be specified and monitored in order to evaluate treatment effectiveness.

6. Specificity is the hallmark of behavioral assessment and treatment, and it is assumed that the person is best understood and described by what he or she does in a particular situation.

7. Treatment requires a fine-grain analysis of the problem into components or subparts and is targeted at these components specifically and systematically.

8. Treatment strategies are individually

tailored to different problems in different individuals.

9. Understanding the development of a psychologic problem is not essential for producing behavior change; conversely, success in changing a problem behavior does not imply knowledge about its etiology.
10. Since behavior change occurs in a specific social context, therapeutic interventions may result in side effects, i.e., changes in behaviors that were not the focus of treatment. These are not necessarily deleterious effects or a product of "symptom substitution." More often than not, these broader treatment effects are positive outcomes.
11. Behavioral psychotherapy involves a commitment to an applied science approach. This includes the following characteristics:
    • an explicit, testable conceptual framework;
    • treatment that is either derived from, or at least consistent with, the content and method of experimental–clinical psychology;
    • therapeutic techniques that can be described with sufficient precision to be measured objectively and replicated;
    • the experimental evaluation of treatment methods and concepts.

HISTORIC BACKGROUND OF BEHAVIORAL PSYCHOTHERAPY

Just as behavioral psychotherapists share a common set of scientific assumptions, so they share a rich historic tradition. Although reports exist in the clinical literature dating back to the 19th century and before of the application of behaviorally oriented treatments such as reinforcement, aversive conditioning, and reciprocal inhibition (2, 3), these isolated successes made a negligible contribution to the development of behavior therapy because they did not embrace any widely accepted principles of learning or behavior. As a result, the origins of behavior therapy as a cohesive set of therapeutic principles

and procedures are relatively modern, and can be traced to the first rigorous attempts to establish laws of learning by the Russian school of reflexology in the 19th and 20th centuries.

Sechenov (4) is regarded as the father of reflexology and is credited with developing the theory that behavior could be explained by simple and complex reflexes that were acquired through the repeated pairings of environmental stimuli and muscular movements. This theory served as a general guide for the research of Pavlov (5) and Bechterev (6), who provided the first strong empirical evidence in support of Sechenov's hypothesis.

Pavlov is best known for his work in establishing that glandular secretions in animals could be elicited by environmental stimuli through the learning process of classical conditioning (also known as Pavlovian or respondent conditioning). He showed that the secretion of gastric juices (unconditioned response) in dogs that occurred when presented with food (unconditioned stimulus) could be elicited by ringing a bell (conditioned stimulus) after the two stimuli had been repeatedly presented together. This principle of learning continues to be important in many modern behavioral conceptualizations of the development of anxiety disorders, in which anxiety is viewed as an unconditioned response that has become conditioned to incidental stimuli in the environment that were initially paired with internal or environmental fear-provoking stimuli.

Pavlov worked primarily with animals and for the most part did not attempt to extend his findings to human behavior. Bechterev, on the other hand, attempted to apply principles of conditioning to explain a broader range of human behavior and to propose methods for treating abnormal behavior as a function of environmental events. In this regard, Bechterev's writings were more influential than Pavlov's in establishing the behaviorism movement in the United States in the early 20th century.

Watson (7, 8) was the most forceful advocate of behaviorism, which eschewed the use of introspection and subjective data in preference for the objective study of overt behavior. Watson's contribution to behavior therapy stems from his persuasive rejection of mentalistic or cognitive processes (which could not be objectively observed) to account for human behavior, and his experimental approach of developing causal hypotheses to explain abnormal behavior. In a now famous extension of classical conditioning with a child, Little Albert, Watson showed that the pairing of a loud noise (unconditioned stimulus) with an innocuous white rat (conditioned stimulus) resulted in a fear response to the rat which subsequently generalized to other white objects. In one of the first trials of behavior therapy, Watson's student Jones (9, 10) demonstrated that fears in children could be treated (i.e., deconditioned) by exposing them to the feared stimulus while engaging in a positive behavior such as eating or having them observe another fearless child in the presence of the stimulus. These treatment techniques did not become widely adapted until Wolpe (11) developed the theory of reciprocal inhibition, which states that responses incompatible with anxiety which occur in the presence of the anxiety-evoking stimulus will decrease the bond between the stimulus and the anxiety response. This theory led directly to the development of systematic desensitization for the treatment of anxiety and the use of relaxation and pleasant imagery as tools with which to aid the deconditioning of fear to the conditioned stimuli.

The Russian school of reflexology and Watson's early brand of behaviorism addressed how existing responses could become conditioned to novel stimuli. By comparison, Thorndike (12) studied how new responses were learned that did not previously exist in the animal's repertoire. He proposed that learning takes place through trial and error and that the acquisition of behaviors is determined by the law of effect, which states that behaviors that are followed by "satisfying consequences" (positive reinforcement) are more likely to occur again, whereas behaviors followed by "annoying consequences" (negative reinforcement or punishment) are less likely to recur. Thorndike's law of effect helped to distinguish between classical conditioning and purposive, goal-directed behavior learned through operant or instrumental conditioning.

Skinner's (13, 14) work on schedules of reinforcement and discriminative learning built on Thorndike by developing an approach to assessing and altering behavior referred to as the experimental analysis of behavior. This approach, which Skinner has argued is theoretical, involves the identification of environmental antecedents and consequences to behavior that affect its frequency of occurrence. Consequent stimuli (i.e., reinforcers) that increase or decrease the rate of response can be manipulated to shape new behaviors via positive reinforcement of successive behavioral approximations, or to extinguish behaviors by removing a positive reinforcer or imposing a negative reinforcer. Unlike Thorndike, Skinner was very influential in highlighting the potential for operant conditioning to modify abnormal behavior as well as to improve the social behavior of humans in general. The principles of operant conditioning were critical to the development of a diverse range of behavioral interventions, including the token economy, self-reinforcement strategies, and selective reinforcement or extinction of childrens' problematic classroom behavior.

The clinical application of the principles of operant conditioning primarily led to methods of behavior modification through the manipulation of the consequences of behavior. Bandura (15, 16) demonstrated that learning could occur through vicarious reinforcement, without prior engagement in the behavior or the experience of direct reinforcement. Thus, an individual who observes another person engage in a behavior (i.e., model the behavior) which is subsequently positively reinforced will be more likely to engage in that behavior. This method of learning is referred to as observational or imitative learning, and is particularly useful in teaching new interpersonal skills.

Bandura's work on observational learning was preceded by and paralleled others who developed new methods for teaching interpersonal skills. Salter (17) described methods for facilitating the self-expression of mildly disturbed persons, which he believed would help them overcome problems such as depression and anxiety. Lazarus (18, 19) introduced the term *behavioral rehearsal* to describe a combination of modeling and role playing (engaging in a simulated social encounter) aimed at improving the assertive behavior of patients. The method of behavioral rehearsal coupled with verbal reinforcement from other patients and/or the therapist was originally termed *assertiveness training*, but has since been expanded to a broader range of interpersonal skills and is currently referred to a social skills training (20). This technique has been applied to remediate a range of maladaptive behaviors and to improve the functioning of persons with anxiety, depression, schizophrenia, anger control problems, and social inadequacy, as well as distressed marital and family relationships.

The growing prominence of "cognitions" in the domain of behavioral psychotherapy is highlighted in Bandura's work on observational learning. Skinner (21) originally argued that cognitions are unobservable, private events that are not subject to reliable measurement, but more recently, behavioral psychotherapists have developed innovative methods for incorporating cognitions into behavioral frameworks. For example, Bandura (22) hypothesized that all psychotherapy achieves its primary benefits by increasing patients' self-perceptions that they can perform necessary behaviors adequately to achieve desired goals. These cognitions are labeled self-efficacy; self-efficacy theory has been successfully used to explain behavioral improvements in such diverse patient groups as snake phobics (23), unassertive adolescents (24), agoraphobics (25), and cigarette smokers in cessation clinics (26). In another vein, Meichenbaum (27) emphasized the

importance of self-verbalizations on behavior and has developed a cognitive–behavioral intervention labeled "self instructional training" that involves modifying these internal verbalizations in order to help patients gain better control over impulsive behaviors.

Today, behavioral psychotherapists use eclectic combinations of respondent, operant, and cognitive–behavioral techniques to remediate behavioral excesses and deficits. Drawing on the rich tradition of vigorous empiricism and tests of real-world utility, behavioral psychotherapists have developed a wide array of effective techniques that enhance patients' adaptive functioning in an efficient manner.

ETHICAL CONSIDERATIONS

Any comprehensive presentation of behavioral psychotherapy must address the criticism that behavioral interventions are mechanistic, Machiavellian, and manipulative. While there has been an increasing acceptance of behavioral psychotherapy over the past 30 years, a contingent of clinicians and policymakers continue to hold that behavioral approaches violate humanistic and ethical principles. Generally, the ethical criticism of behavioral psychotherapy centers on the issue of behavioral control.

In contrast to psychodynamic and humanistic writers, behaviorists openly raise the issue of *control* of behavior and have attempted to identify the variables (internal and external stimuli) that systematically influence behavior. In a culture that values "freedom of choice," the concept of behavioral control seems, at first, almost repugnant. However, behavioral psychotherapists envisage behavioral control in an entirely different light. Within the behavioral model, *all* behavior (desirable and undesirable) is determined by antecedent stimuli and subsequent consequences, and thus behavioral psychotherapy simply involves acknowledging and making use of the obvious. By incorporating positive and negative consequences in behavioral treatment regimens, behaviorists are actively replicating "real world" circumstances to increase the probability that these interventions will yield desired changes that are maintained in nontreatment settings.

It is important to recognize, however, that the process of behavior therapy mandates *shared* control. Patients consult behavioral psychotherapists for relief of distress. Integral to the development of an effective behavioral treatment plan to alleviate that distress is a mutual decision by the therapist and the patient as to the specific therapeutic goal and the techniques to be used in achieving that goal. Unlike more traditional psychotherapies, behaviorists have a heterogeneous array of therapeutic procedures at their disposal, and it is incumbent upon them to present patients with a variety of potential treatment alternatives, from which the patient may help select the ones to be used.

As is true for all psychotherapeutic approaches, the quality of the patient–therapist relationship is a critical aspect of behavioral psychotherapy. Without a positive, therapeutic alliance between the clinician and patient, successful intervention becomes unlikely. Behavioral interventions may involve suggestions to generate specific activities and interaction, demonstrations by the clinician for modeling purposes, and differential feedback or reinforcement on directly observed or indirectly reported behaviors. The clinician is an effective instructor and reinforcer only to the extent that he or she is valued, respected, esteemed, and liked. The therapeutic relationship exerts a pervasive and profound influence on the process and outcome of any therapy, and behavioral psychotherapy is no exception (see Chapters 9, 10, and 45).

Behavioral psychotherapy requires obtaining informed consent from competent adult patients. Children, prisoners, and acutely psychotic and/or developmentally disabled individuals, all of whom may be unable to give informed consent, present a complex ethical dilemma for behavioral and nonbehavioral therapists. Decisions pertaining to therapeutic goals and procedures can no longer be fully shared by the

therapist and patient. Behaviorists are still committed to sharing as much decision-making power with these patients as they possibly can. Behavioral psychotherapists strive at all times to improve the quality of the patient's life. When a responsible third party advocates therapeutic goals or procedures not in the patient's best interest, the behavioral psychotherapist must follow his or her mandate to help the patient achieve the highest level of adaptive functioning using the most effective procedures possible. In cases of conflict, a special review board should be available for final decisions (28).

The ultimate treatment goal for the behavioral psychotherapist is in accordance with the highest ethical standards—to enhance the patient's control of his or her own life. As Bandura (15) well said, behavioral interventions promote individuals' control over their behavior by widening their behavioral repertoires and thus increasing their freedom of choice. Individuals enter therapy when they perceive their options are limited; that is, because of inhibitions, fears, or behavioral excesses or deficits, they are unable to achieve what they desire. Behavioral psychotherapy is educative, leading to the development of new skills and behaviors that result in higher adaptive functioning and a greater probability of achieving desired goals.

OBSTACLES AND SOLUTIONS TO DISSEMINATION AND ADOPTION OF BEHAVIORAL PSYCHOTHERAPY

As is discussed more fully in Chapter 48, behavioral interventions have been used to great advantage on a variety of psychiatric disorders, including alcoholism (29), schizophrenia (30), depression (31), obsessive–compulsive disorder (32), obesity (33), and phobias and anxiety (34). Although the efficacy of behavioral interventions has been empirically demonstrated, behavioral psychotherapy is still viewed with skepticism by many mental health professionals. A recent survey of all 152 Veterans Administration (VA) medical centers with psychology services revealed that only 20 had a "behavior modification unit/token economy" program of any kind (35). In answering questions regarding why such programs are so few, VA respondents cited staff resistance and shortage, lack of support from administrators, high cost, lack of training, and concerns about patients' rights and explanations.

These concerns are genuine. A full 30 years after the initiation of behavioral treatments for psychiatric disorders, training in behavioral psychotherapy is still the exception rather than the rule in medical, psychology, and social work graduate schools. Without adequate exposure and training, mental health professionals are understandably reluctant to provide behavioral treatment. Philosophical conflicts and concerns about additional costs accruing from behavioral intervention serve as additional impediments to its widespread implementation. However, each of these obstacles can be successfully overcome:

Lack of Knowledge and Skill. Mental health professionals tend to use the techniques acquired in their formal instruction, and most clinicians have not had training to competence in behavioral psychotherapy. Although enrollment in continuing education has become an integral part of many state's professional licensing requirements, few professionals implement the new procedures learned in this training (36, 37). Successful adoption of innovative techniques requires a provision for ongoing consultation and supervision until the new practitioner demonstrates mastery of the skill.

Confronted with an ever expanding technology, administrators and leaders in mental health movements must assume assertive stances in ensuring that their staffs are provided with the time, resources, and incentives to develop new skills. In these days of uncertain funding for mental health initiatives, upgrading skills and developing new competencies often have low priority. Nevertheless, new technologies using training videotapes, computer-assisted instruction, and on-site consulta-

tion can greatly increase the availability of learning opportunities and provide for improved patient treatment.

Concerns over Cost. Behavioral psychotherapy greatly differs from traditional psychotherapy. Behavioral sessions may be held in patients' homes, places of work, public meeting places, or settings that patients have identified as distressing (e.g., elevators, tall buildings). In vivo sessions are frequently not limited to the 50-minute hour, and behavioral psychotherapists sometimes use reinforcers (e.g., consumables, community outings) that require money. The financial requirements of these nontraditional activities often dampen initial enthusiasm over behavioral interventions.

Although behavioral interventions may require more financial support initially, when compared to traditional psychotherapy, their greater efficacy renders them more cost-effective in the long term. A large-scale study conducted by Paul and Lentz (30) illustrates this point. The authors randomly assigned 84 long-term, schizophrenic patients to state hospital units using social learning, milieu therapy, or traditional custodial care approaches. The social learning program employed a highly specific token economy with many hours of structured educational activities throughout the day. Patients were positively reinforced with praise and tokens for productive, appropriate behavior (e.g., cleaning rooms, attending classes, grooming) and were fined tokens and/or ignored for inappropriate activities (e.g., yelling, assaults). They could exchange tokens for backup reinforcers such as consumables (e.g., food, cigarettes) and privileges (e.g., access to ground). Patients were held accountable for behavior and were provided with training in social skills to equip them for community living.

The milieu program was based on a therapeutic community structure wherein all patients were members of a 9- to 10-person "living groups," which were assigned the tasks of identifying problems and promoting change among individual members. The major vehicle for promoting change was the social and group pressure exerted by living groups on its members. Just as in the social learning group, patients were scheduled to spend the majority of their time in structured life skills or academic classes. Patients in both programs were scheduled to be in formal treatment 85% of the time.

Across all measures, the social learning intervention achieved superior results to the milieu or traditional care intervention. By the end of treatment, social learning patients spent less time in the hospital, achieved greater discharge rates, were maintained longer in the community, and required less psychotropic medication than either of the two comparison groups. All differences were statistically significant. Importantly, the social learning program was clearly the most cost-effective as well when decreased need for continued hospitalization was included in cost calculations. While the social learning and therapeutic community were both slightly more expensive than custodial care on a daily basis ($10.47 versus $10.29 in 1970 dollars) the social learning program resulted in shorter hospital stays, such the average cost (in 1970 dollars) over length of stay was $11,794 for social learning patients, $15,252 for therapeutic community patients, and $17,506 for custodial care patients.

While the Paul and Lentz results demonstrate the cost-effectiveness of inpatient behavioral interventions for schizophrenia, a recent study on outpatient behavioral therapy for schizophrenics and their families (38) substantiates its economic benefits. Briefly, Falloon, Boyd, and McGill randomly assigned 36 recently discharged schizophrenic patients to receive either traditional after-care or behavioral-oriented family therapy conducted on the patients' home. Actual client contact hours were equivalent in both groups, and pharmacotherapy was provided for all patients. Psychosocial treatment was provided weekly during the first 3 months of the study, biweekly for the next 6 months, and monthly thereafter.

The behavioral family intervention was clearly the most advantageous, both clinically and economically. At 9 months, only two (11%) of the behavioral family therapy patients had been readmitted to the hospital, while nine (50%) of the traditional after-care patients had. Patients in the behavioral family therapy group demonstrated significantly less psychopathology and better social functioning than the traditional after-care patients as well.

In terms of economic costs, in-home family treatment was initially more expensive than traditional after-care. However, missed and extra appointments, as well as emergency phone calls, were disproportionately greater in the traditional after-care group; extra costs due to these ad hoc interventions matched 63% of the additional funding initially required for in-home treatment. When the additional costs of rehospitalization and community resources (e.g., law enforcement involvement) were taken into account, in-home behavioral family treatment resulted in a 19% cost savings over traditional after-care.

These findings substantiate the cost-effectiveness of many behavioral interventions. Although the initial financial outlay may be greater than for traditional care, the improved treatment results clearly support the early expenditures. Considering long-term results, behavioral interventions provide for better patient care at lower cost.

Philosophical Conflicts. The greatest barrier to the dissemination and implementation of behavioral psychotherapy is philosophical. Psychoanalysis preceded the development of behavioral psychiatry by 50 years. It is so embedded in our culture that phrases such as "unconscious" and "oedipal complex" are part of the common parlance. Psychoanalysis rests on the assumption that changing the present requires comprehending the past, while behavioral psychotherapy posits that changing the present requires modification of the present. Such a dramatic shift in conceptualization naturally results in conflict and misconception, as has most scientific development (39).

Preconceptions and misconceptions about

behavioral psychotherapy abound. Because the animal lab served as the foundation for many of the procedures later used by clinicians on humans, many naive clinicians may believe that behavior modification necessitates treating people like animals. Similarly, the scientific language developed to describe behavioral techniques precisely (e.g., "extinction," "punishment," "aversive conditioning") does not have the emotional appeal of traditional psychotherapeutic terms such as "unconditional positive regard," "insight," and "accurate empathy." Unfortunately, the negative connotations associated with the nonprofessional use of words such as "punishment" overshadow the value that the so labeled procedures have in bringing about positive behavioral change.

The clear solution to this problem involves continued education about behavioral psychotherapy to correct these misconceptions. Chapters such as this are directed to that end, as are investigations aimed at testing for untoward effects of behavioral psychotherapy that might be predicted using the psychoanalytic framework. For example, many psychoanalysts have argued that behavioral interventions will result in symptom substitution and are thus antitherapeutic. Support for this argument has been difficult to find, as most desired behavioral changes result in accompanying positive (not negative) outcomes. This can be illustrated in a study on childhood enuresis conducted by Baker (40). Baker found that a behavioral intervention (bell and pad wake-up device) was more effective than a parents' wake-up call or no treatment in curing the bed-wetting. Contrary to psychodynamic prediction, the children whose bed-wetting was eliminated showed improvements in school functioning and on projective tests. Symptom substitution did not occur.

SUMMARY

Our goal in this chapter was to describe the theoretical foundation of behavioral therapy and the ethical concerns and obstacles to its implementation. As has been outlined, behavior therapy does not stem from a unitary learning theory, but instead reflects a diverse set of conceptual and technical approaches. Behavior therapy is primarily an empirical and operational strategy for the understanding and treatment of clinical problems. With the measurement of behavior as a means for initial assessment and continuing monitoring of progress, behavior therapy has within its methods and procedures a self-correcting informational feedback loop whereby effective techniques gradually emerge by trial and error for both the individual patient and the field as a whole.

It is unlikely that any one set of general principles will very satisfactorily explain the onset, duration, and amelioration or remission of psychiatric problems. We must accept the overriding fact of individual differences and learn to tolerate the untidy likelihood that for the wide range of individuals presenting with signs and symptoms, many different biologic and environmental factors are responsible and many different biologic and environmental interventions will be necessary. Since the complexity of brain neurochemistry and neurophysiology easily matches the variability in individuals' life experiences, we may also find the search for "common biochemical pathways" for psychiatric syndromes illusory. Nevertheless, behavioral psychotherapy, in conjunction with judicious types and doses of psychotropic drugs, offers an effective framework to remediate the full spectrum of psychiatric disorders (41).

References

1. Taylor CB, Liberman RP, Agras WS, et al: Treatment evaluation and behavior therapy. In Lewis J, Usdin G, (eds): *Treatment Planning in Psychiatry.* Washington, DC, American Psychiatric Press, 1982, pp 151–224.
2. Franks CM: Introduction: behavior therapy and its Pavlovian origins—review and perspectives. In Franks CM (ed): *Behavior Therapy: Appraisal and Status.* New York, McGraw-Hill, 1969, pp 1–26.
3. Wolpe J: *The Practice of Behavior Therapy,* ed 2. New York, Pergamon, 1973.
4. Sechenov IM: *Reflexes of the Brain: An Attempt to Establish the Physiological Basis of Psychological Pro-*

cesses (Belsky S, trans). Cambridge, MIT Press, 1965.

5. Pavlov IP: *The Work of the Digestive Glands* (Thompson WH, trans). London, Charles Griffin, 1902.

6. Bechterev VM: *General Principles of Human Reflexology: an Introduction to the Objective Study of Personality* (Murphy E, Murphy W, trans). New York, International Publishers, 1932.

7. Watson JB: Psychology as the behaviorist views it. *Psychol Rev* 20:158–177, 1913.

8. Watson JB: *Behaviorism*. Chicago, University of Chicago Press, 1924.

9. Jones MC: The elimination of children's fears. *J Exp Psychol* 7:382–390, 1924.

10. Jones MC: A laboratory study of fear: the case of Peter. *Pedagogical Seminary* 31:308–315, 1924.

11. Wolpe J: *Psychotherapy by Reciprocal Inhibition*. Stanford, CA, Stanford University Press, 1958.

12. Thorndike EL: *Human Learning*. New York, Century, 1931.

13. Skinner BF: *The Behavior of Organisms*. New York, Appleton-Century-Crofts, 1938.

14. Skinner BF: *Science and Human Behavior*. New York, Free Press, 1953.

15. Bandura A: *Principles of Behavior Modification*. New York, Rinehart & Winston, 1969.

16. Bandura A, Ross D, Ross SA: Vicarious reinforcement and imitative learning. *J Abnorm Soc Psychol* 67:601–607, 1963.

17. Salter A: *Conditioned Reflex Therapy*. New York, Farrar, Straus & Giroux, 1949.

18. Lazarus AA: Behavior rehearsal vs. nondirective therapy vs. advice in effecting behavior change. *Behav Res Ther* 4:109–212, 1966.

19. Lazarus AA: New methods in psychotherapy: a case of study. *S Afr Med J* 32:664–669, 1958.

20. Hersen M, Eisler PM: Social skills training. In Craighead WE, Kazdin AE, Mahoney MJ (eds): *Behavior Modification: Principles, Issues and Applications*. Boston, Houghton-Mifflin, 1976, pp 361–375.

21. Skinner BF, Solomon HC, Lindsley OR: *Studies in Behavior Therapy* (Status Report I). Waltham, MA, Metropolitan State Hospital, 1953.

22. Bandura A: Self-efficacy: Toward a unifying theory of behavioral change. *Psychol Rev* 84:191–215, 1977.

23. Bandura A, Adams NE: Analysis of self-efficacy theory of behavioral change. *Cognitive Therapy and Ressearch* 1:287–310, 1977.

24. Pentz M, Kazdin A: Assertion modeling and stimuli effects on assertive behavior and self-efficacy and adolescents. *Behav Res Ther* 20:365–371, 1982.

25. Bandura A, Adams NE, Hardy A, et al: Tests of the generality of self-efficacy theory. *Cognitive Therapy and Research* 4:39–66, 1980.

26. Condiotte MM, Lichtenstein E: Self-efficacy and relapse in smoking cessation programs. *J Consult Clin Psychol* 49:648–658, 1981.

27. Meichenbaum D: *Cognitive–Behavior Modification*. New York, Plenum Press, 1977.

28. O'Leary KD, Wilson GT: *Behavior Therapy: Application and Outcome*, ed 2. Englewood Cliffs, NJ, Prentice-Hall, 1987.

29. Chaney E, O'Leary M, Marlatt GA: Skill training with alcoholics. *J Consult Clin Psychol* 46:1092–1104, 1978.

30. Paul GP, Lentz RJ: *Psychosocial Treatment of Chronic Mental Patients: Milieu vs. Social Learning Programs*. Cambridge, Harvard University Press, 1977.

31. Lewinsohn PM, Sullivan JM, Grosscup SJ: Behavioral therapy: clinical applications. In Rush AJ (ed): *Short-term Psychotherapies for the Depressed Patient*. New York, Guilford Press, 1982, pp 271–302.

32. Marks I, Hodgson R, Rachman S: Treatment of obsessive–compulsive neuroses by in vivo exposure. *Br J Psychiatry* 127:349–364, 1975.

33. Wadden TA, Stunkard AJ, Brownell KD, et al: Treatment of obesity by behavior therapy and very low calorie diet: a pilot investigation. *J Consult Clin Psychol* 52:692–694, 1984.

34. Barlow DH, Cohen AJ, Waddell MT, et al: Panic and generalized anxiety disorders: Nature and treatment. *Behav Ther* 15:431–499, 1984.

35. Boudewyns PA, Fry TJ, Nightingale EJ: Token economy programs in VA medical centers: Where are they now? *The Behavior Therapist* 6:126–127, 1986.

36. Kuehnel TG, Flanagan SG: Training professionals: guidelines for effective continuing education workshops. *The Behavior Therapist* 7:85–87, 1984.

37. Kuehnel T, Marholin D, Heinrich R, et al: Evaluating behavior therapists' continuing education activities: the AABT 1977 Institutes. *The Behavior Therapist* 1:5–8, 1978.

38. Falloon IRH, Boyd JL, McGill CW: *Family Care of Schizophrenia: A Problem-Solving Approach to the Treatment of Mental Illness*. New York, Guilford Press, 1984.

39. Kuhn TS: *The Structure of Scientific Revolutions*. Chicago, University of Chicago Press, 1962.

40. Baker BL: Symptom treatment and symptom substitution in enuresis. *J Abnorm Psychol* 74:42–49, 1969.

41. Liberman RP, Bedell J: Behavior therapy. In Kaplan S, Sadock B (eds): *Comprehensive Textbook of Psychiatry V*. Baltimore, Williams & Wilkens, in press.

6

The Sociocultural Approach[a]

Sherman Eisenthal, Ph.D.

Humans are social beings. Social groups, large and small, shape, direct, orient, and validate human behavior and experience. Clinicians know these facts, yet clinical theory and practice relegate this "outer" sociocultural reality to a place of secondary concern, compared to the "inner" world of psychologic defense, neuroanatomy, and biochemistry. This state of affairs is understandable for three reasons. First, clinicians are trained predominantly in the psychodynamic and biologic models (described in Chapter 2), which provide them with the language and concepts suitable for understanding the inner world of the patient, but not the outer social world. The phenomenologic self and the biologic workings of the organism are clearly in focus in these models. Second, most investigators of the social and cultural influences on mental illness and illness behaviors are not clinicians. The questions they ask, therefore, are not couched in clinical language, and their findings, though clinically relevant, seldom appear in the clinical journals. Third, there is no single, coherent sociocultural approach to diagnosis and treatment. Instead, a variety of influences and distinct models exist—from that of

Adolph Meyer on accumulated life events to Harry Stack Sullivan on interpersonal relationships to Maxwell Jones on the therapeutic community, Gerald Caplan on prevention and consultation, and Alexander Leighton on disintegrated social communities. The conceptual continuum is thus broad, ranging from interpersonal relationships at one end to community integration at the other.

Even if one turns to the field known as social psychiatry, there is diffusion of content, lack of direction, and professional rivalries (1). This framework has been claimed by different professional groups and assigned different areas of application. The term "'social psychiatry" was first used in 1917 in the writings of E. E. Southard, chief of psychiatry at the Boston Psychopathic Hospital, who regarded it as an interdisciplinary field, a subspecialty of both psychiatry and social work. During that time, social psychiatry was taught by some of the major figures in psychiatry in schools of social work—James Jackson Putnam, Adolph Meyer, E. E. Southard, and A. A. Brill. After this period of initial interest and involvement by leaders in psychiatry, development of the field among psychiatrists slackened, though sociologists continued to show an interest in it. In 1955 Thomas Rennie (2), a psychiatrist,

---

[a] The section "Symptoms as Social Communication" was coauthored by Leonard Solomon, Ph.D.

wrote the lead article in the new journal *Social Psychiatry*, in which he described the field as "the study of etiology and dynamics of persons seen in their total setting." Subsequent conflicts over the concept of social psychiatry have revolved around (*a*) whether the content should include service, training, research, or some combination of the three; and (*b*) how and whether social psychiatry should be distinguished from other fields such as community psychiatry or psychiatric sociology. Unlike psychoanalysis or behavioral theory, social psychiatry has not set for itself the task of providing a comprehensive theory of human behavior.

As a result of the absence of a coherent sociocultural approach and the inaccessibility of sociocultural data with specific clinical application, clinicians evaluate and respond to patients in ways that limit therapeutic possibilities. In certain situations, patients may be viewed from their social matrix as if they were independent of it. Social data, when collected, are used for background, out of a need to be "thorough," not to help the clinician in making more informed decisions regarding diagnosis or treatment. In other situations, the clinician makes major social decisions without fully appreciating the basis upon which the decision was made or the impact of the decision on the patient's social system. For instance, the clinician may not be aware that hospitalizing a patient may significantly change (for better or worse) the manner in which the family perceives and responds to the patient, or that hospitalization may be the only way to engage the family and thereby define the problem as a family problem. In suggesting couple therapy for certain individuals, the clinician may not appreciate that certain social goals not possible with individual therapy become available, while other goals unique to individual therapy may be lost. In providing individual psychodynamic psychotherapy, the clinician may not appreciate that he or she may be the patient's entire social support system and that the outcome of treatment depends more on the success of that social support system than on intrapsychic change.

For clinical practice in outpatient settings, the sociocultural approach will be defined in terms of how the individual functions in his or her social system. Whether or not a person defines him- or herself or is defined by others as "ill," neurotic, or a mental patient depends not so much on the person's biology, intrapsychic structure, or behavior as on social influences such as the person's status, support systems, sociocultural group, and community.

Diagnoses by self, by family, or by a professional are conferred on the individual and are not necessarily inherent in the individual's behavior. Hearing voices, for example, has very different meanings in different sociocultural contexts. Al-Issa (3) describes considerable sociocultural variation in the meaning attached to hallucinations. In Western society, where rationality and control have great significance, especially in view of their close behavioral relationship, hallucinations are feared cues to the presence of serious disorder. However, in societies with different forms of rationality and emphasis on emotional response in social situations, hallucinatory experiences are often sought after (4). Symptoms and maladaptive personality traits may be traced to the "relationship of the individual to his manner of functioning in social situations, i.e., in the type and quality of his 'connectedness' to the groups which make up his life space" (5). Symptoms themselves may be attempts to communicate indirectly to others in the social system to restore social equilibrium.

In fashioning treatment to fit the needs of the individual in his or her community, the clinician needs sociocultural data relevant to etiology, entry into the health care system, definition of the problem, orientation and motivation for treatment, treatment expectations, requests for help, maintenance of the disorder, and an individual's potential for engaging in the change process. The clinician cannot negotiate effectively without understanding both the patient's perspectives and his or her own (including assumptions, value judgments, and distortions), and these perspectives are in large part based on sociocultural factors. The sociocultural approach, therefore, can have profound effects on diagnosis and treatment.

This chapter describes selected aspects of a sociocultural approach to outpatient psychiatry. It includes an introduction to the rich and varied literature on sociocultural influences on symptoms, societal response to mental symptoms and disorder, social stress, social integration–disintegration, social isolation, family dynamics, the concept of symptoms as social communication, and patienthood. The sociocultural approach to clinical states of depression and schizophrenia is selected for more detailed discussion.

Subsequent chapters on group therapy, couple therapy, bereavement and unresolved grief, suicide, and mood disorders provide clinical applications of the sociocultural approach.

SOCIOCULTURAL DETERMINANTS OF MENTAL DISORDER

The search for social causes has been the dominant aim of most of the social research on mental disorder in the last 40 years. In the 1930s, Faris and Dunham (6) linked schizophrenia to the psychologic effects of living in the central city slums of Chicago. Social isolation, a crucial aspect of slum existence, was proposed as a condition for the development of schizophrenia in that setting. During the 1950s, two very influential projects on social causation began. Leighton and his colleagues (7) investigated the relationship between community disorganization and the development of mental disorder in a rural setting (the Stirling County Study). Somewhat later, Srole and his colleagues (8) launched a massive epidemiologic study of mental disorder in an urban setting (the Midtown Manhattan Study). In the 1960s, social stress, embodied in life change events, became a major focus of research led by Holmes and Rahe

(9) and Brown and Birley (10). In the 1970s and 1980s attention was directed to social support, coping style, vulnerability, and other resources that effect response to stress (11–14).

The work on social causation can be divided into three major areas: (*a*) social stress, (*b*) social integration–disintegration, and (*c*) family dynamics. We shall review work in these areas and pay special attention to schizophrenia and depression.

Social Stress

Hans Selye (15), a pioneer in the field of stress, defined stress as a response that sets off a biologic process—the adaptation syndrome—that is a nonspecific, bodily response to a variety of physical and psychosocial stimuli, either pleasant or unpleasant, that signals the preparation of the organism for an adaptive response of either fight or flight. Dohrenwend and Dohrenwend (16) adapted Selye's paradigm to a social–psychologic framework and defined social stressors as "objective events that disrupt or threaten to disrupt the individual's usual activities." Stressful life events thus induce a state of strain that sets into motion the individual's adaptive capacities (17). In a more subjective view, an event is qualified as stressful when the individual perceives a discrepancy between the demands placed on him or her by life events and his or her potential response to meet these demands (18, 19). The degree of stress thus depends on subjective evaluation, rather than on objective threat. Parkes (20) sees stress as losses or gains that challenge the individuals assumptions about self and world.

Descriptive Dimensions

Stressors can be described according to dimensions of time, content, intensity, and motivational base. Among the clinically salient features of the time dimension are recency, duration, predictability, clustering, and life stage. In the initial interview, clinicians generally attend to relatively recent, discrete life change events, looking for recent precipitating events separating the situational from the characterologic and biologic. The clinical inquiry is facilitated by attention to life stage—the status and resolution of predictable problems and conflicts for a given age. The content of most social stressors can be subsumed in six categories: marital and parental (both often identified as interpersonal), health, work–achievement, financial–economic, and neighborhood. The intensity dimension varies from mild to extreme. This category is susceptible to confusion by interchangeable usage of objective and subjective criteria. Crisis is a case in point, reflecting a strong subjective response to events that may not be objectively extreme, e.g., a child's leaving home. The motivational base refers to the positive or negative goals—the reward versus punishment aspect—of the change situation. Although stress is usually associated with negative or undesirable life changes, positive change nonetheless makes adaptive demands, as in the case of marriage, a promotion, or a birth.

Weiss (12) provides a clinically useful threefold schema for describing stress: crisis (sudden onset, threat, limited duration), transition (changes in personal relations that alter life assumptions), and deficit situation of enduring excessive demands. He posits a sequential order (crisis, transition, deficit) as likely if effective resolution does not occur at each stage.

Techniques of Measurement

One of the most simple and direct approaches to the description and evaluation of stress is identification of discrete life change events, either positive (such as a promotion) or negative (a demotion). This approach was the basis for measurement used by Holmes and Rahe (9) in the extensively used Social Readjustment Rating Scale (SRRS). An impetus for their research came from the work of Adolph Meyer (21) on the influence of life events. Life change events were classified according to four categories: (*a*) familial (such as death of a spouse), (*b*) personal (such as major personal injury or illness), (*c*) work (e.g., being dismissed from a job), and (*d*) financial

(major change in financial state). A number of efforts have been made to improve the SRRS. One example is the PERI Life Events Scale developed by Dohrenwend et al. (22).

A second approach focuses on role change, entailing and yielding a more process-oriented and complex level of analysis than can be obtained from examining discrete change events. Ilfeld (23) developed an instrument to measure change in five social roles: marital, parental, job, financial–economic, and neighborhood. Since roles constitute a basic unit of participation in the social structure, changes in roles (and associated status) have vast implications for subsequent social behavior.

The use of inventories such as the SRRS have potential weaknesses such as inaccurate dating of onset of distress and lack of independence of life event from psychiatric symptoms. Brown and Harris (24) prefer a semistructured interview for these reasons.

Social Stress and Mental Dysfunction

The relationship between social stress and mental dysfunction depends on properties of the stressful event and on a number of mediating variables, some internal and some external. Caplan (11) and Weiss (12) have recognized the role of social support. Lazarus and his colleagues (25, 26) have systematically investigated coping styles and stress. Zubin and Spring (17) elaborate on the role of personal vulnerability, especially in schizophrenia. Antonovsky (27) describes a number of "resistance resources" to counter the effects of stress such as flexibility, ties to others, and ties to the community. The clinical understanding of the influence of stress, therefore, requires analysis of both the stressful event and the social and person-centered mediating variables.

Social stress may induce "a bad day" or months and years of psychiatric disturbance and psychosomatic disorder. Generally, the episodes of psychiatric disturbance are transient (28–30). Enduring effects of life events account for a small percentage (8 to 10%) of the variance in psychopathology (31). However, a large percentage (20 to 40%) of those exposed to a crisis (rape, serious surgery) continue to have symptoms and never fully recover (32).

The features of life events most associated with psychopathology are undesirability, magnitude (intensity), and time clustering (31). Several investigators have proposed that threat—the undesirability of change—constitutes the core of stress (33–35). Undesirable life change events in normal persons correlated significantly with emotional disturbances such as depression, paranoid thinking, suicidal proclivity, and anxiety, but desirable life change events did not (34). Depressed patients differed significantly from controls only in the undesirable event category (35). The undesirable events included death of a family member, separation, and demotion.

Among the first dimensions of stress evaluated by clinicians is intensity. Most clinical studies use the SRRS or a similar instrument to measure the intensity of life change events. Scores are based on normative ratings by judges; death of a spouse, for example, is scored 100, being fired from work is scored 47, and a wife starting or ending work is scored 26.

Intensity of stressful life events correlated in a number of studies with the manifestation of symptoms (29, 36–40). Although intensity did not correlate with configuration of symptoms, Uhlenhuth and Paykel (40) found that it did correlate with magnitude of psychiatric disturbance. All the patients in their study, whether outpatients, inpatients, or day-care patients, exhibited higher stress scores than did nonpatients, even when demographic variables were controlled statistically. They concluded that the amount of life stress during a defined time period served to determine both the time of the onset and the magnitude of symptoms in a patient population.

Life stage is an especially useful frame of reference in evaluating stress. A common view is that the damaging effect of extreme stress is likely to be greatest during the critical developmental periods of the early years of life and adolescence. Loss of a parent at a critical early age is an instance of a trauma which Zilboorg (41) proposed as the underlying cause in many adult suicides. Maternal deprivation early in life has been cited by Bowlby (42) for its severely damaging effects on personality. There are qualifications, however, on the irreversible effects of early trauma. Bronfenbrenner (43) reports that the effects of maternal deprivation may be transitory if the child is subsequently placed in a favorable environment, and Sullivan (44) talks about "reparative effects" during the preadolescent period of ages 8 through 11, during which "chumship" can overcome previous malevolent influences.

Relationship of Stress to Depression and Schizophrenia

Stressful life events have been found to precede the onset of both depression and schizophrenia by 2 to 3 months (24). According to Paykel (45), within 6 months of experiencing a major life stress, the relative risk increases sixfold for depression and three- to fourfold for schizophrenia. Brown and Harris (24) concluded that stress plays a formative role etiologically in depression and a triggering role (exacerbating a predisposition) in schizophrenia.

The role of loss in depressive disorders is not resolved. In some studies of depressive patients, loss was particularly prominent (46–48). Brown and Harris reported that psychotic depression was associated with loss by death and neurotic depression with loss by separation. In other studies, loss was not a frequent precipitant of depressive disorders (40, 49). For example, Leff et al. (49) reported that loss ranked tenth in a list of 20 stresses of clinical depression.

In addition to cases of diagnosed depression, a number of investigators have found that stressful life events precede the onset of depressive symptoms in the general population (36, 50, 51). Ilfeld (36) investigated the effect of stressful life experiences (role changes) in the general population and found that marital changes ranked first in relationship to depressive symptoms, followed by parental, job, and financial role stresses. Least related to depressive symptoms were neighborhood stresses (e.g., safety, friendliness, type of people).

Two common examples of interpersonal stresses conducive to depressive symptoms in a normal population are physical disability and bereavement. Physical disability in the family may induce social constriction, which in turn induces depressive mood. From a behavioral point of view, depression would be related to a reduction in positive social reinforcement. Rosenbaum and Najenson (50) compared the social adjustment of wives of severely brain-injured soldiers with that of paraplegic and normal individuals. The wives of severely brain-injured soldiers experienced fewer pleasant activities (greater constriction) and more depressive mood than did the other groups. Bereavement has long been linked to depressive symptoms. Parkes (46) reports that for a period of 6 months after the death of their husband, wives under 65 years were much more likely to consult their general practitioner for psychiatric symptoms, especially depression. The decrease in consultation after 6 months is consistent with the transiency of such depressive symptomatology.

Repeated efforts have failed to demonstrate that endogenous and reactive depressions differ in exposure to a precipitating social stress (51). The precipitating stress is thus not sound as a diagnostic indicator of endogenous versus reactive depression. Paykel (53) concludes that "although most depressions bear some relationship to life events, the proportion of variance and causation which can be attributed to the life event is relatively small. The event falls on some kind of fertile soil, and a host of factors modify the reaction to it."

Social Support

It is widely observed that the effects of exposure to stress are quite variable and do not automatically result in psychiatric symptoms or disorder. Resistance resources such as social support mediate between stress and maladaptive response and partially account for this variability. Social support can be described in terms of structure and function. The structure of support—the social network, has been described in terms of size, close friends, percentage of relatives, interconnected members, frequency of contact, and living arrangement (54). The social networks of psychiatric patients have been found to differ from normals (55). Neurotic individuals have networks that are loose and sparse compared to those of normals; psychotic individuals have tight but almost exclusively kin-based networks (55). Caplan (11) and Weiss (12) described the functions of support in terms of emotional, cognitive, and material aid (also see House [13] and Heller and Swindle [56]).

There have been many studies of the buffering effects of social support on stress. Emotional support is especially helpful. For example, several investigators report that married women with children (a high-risk group for depression) are more vulnerable when they lack a supportive, intimate relationship (24). The highest incidence of depression among these women was not associated with the highest frequency of stress—it was related to emotional support. The claim that work is a stress buffer for married women with children was not supported except when emotional support was available, as Parry (57) reports. Thoits (31) cautions that social support is not necessarily beneficial; it can have undesirable effects.

Social Integration— Disintegration

In assessing the stressful effects of changes in an individual's social milieu, the unit of analysis is relatively discrete, involving life change events or role change events. The French sociologist Emile Durkheim, though not interested in mental disorder, was the first to propose in 1897 that suicide was influenced by the quality of social integration (58). The social systems dimension of social integration entails a higher and more complex level of analysis than do life change events. Four variables associated with the quality of integration of individuals in their community are reviewed in this section: (*a*) urbanization and poverty, (*b*) social isolation, (*c*) lower social class status, and (*d*) social disintegration.

Urbanization and Poverty

Faris and Dunham (6), in their pioneering epidemiologic study of first admissions of schizophrenic patients to mental hospitals, found that the incidence rate of schizophrenia was highest in urban slums; as one moved out toward the suburbs, the rate of schizophrenia decreased. The findings of Faris and Dunham have been replicated many times over (15). Explanations of this phenomenon fall into two main categories: social stress and social selection. Initially, Faris and Dunham favored a social stress explanation, the notion that central city social conditions facilitated social isolation, which furthered the development of distorted personalities. The impoverished and transient life-style conditions of central city slums associated with boarding houses and run-down neighborhoods were seen to minimize positive and enduring social contact and relationships. More recently, Dunham (59) has revised this interpretation in favor of a social selection explanation. The interpersonal factors associated with poverty fail to explain the geographic distribution of schizophrenia.

Analysis of the process of social selection has resulted in two different explanations: social drift and social residues. In the downward social drift explanation, schizophrenic individuals tend to find their way to city slums because of their inability to sustain the level of economic existence required elsewhere. The social residues explanation is based on the notion that competent individuals who grow up in the city slums tend to leave and those who remain are incompetent—the social residues (60).

The social stress explanation still have very forceful supporters. Among the foremost proponents of this interpretation are investigators associated with the Midtown Manhattan study (8), who view poverty, role disturbances, and stigmatization as causative factors in the etiology of mental disorder. However, even when the causal role of social stress in mental disorder is accepted, there is disagreement about the effect of factors such as poverty and urbanization (61). Thus Leighton and his group, in their research on Stirling County (7) and Yoruba (62), proposed that social systems factors contribute to the etiology of mental disorder but did not find that poverty or socioeconomic status per se is the significant factor.

Social Isolation

The hypothesis that social isolation is a significant antecedent of schizophrenia has been popular since the work of Faris and Dunham (6). Others have also found a significant correlation between schizophrenia and social isolation (63, 64). In a highly regarded study designed to test the causal role of social isolation, Kohn and Clausen (65) found no evidence that the individuals who developed schizophrenia had been prevented from interacting because of social factors such as the lack of playmates, parental attitudes, or residential mobility. Social isolation was not a cause, they concluded, but rather a result of the schizophrenic reaction; that is, individuals predisposed to schizophrenia tended to avoid and isolate themselves from other people. The avoidance may derive from fear of social censure and/or from the dysphoric consequences of being observably different in social and school settings—because of being socially and cognitively deficient (66).

Although social isolation may not be an antecedent condition of schizophrenia, it is nonetheless a stressful condition that has disruptive psychologic consequences and may well contribute further to the maintenance of the schizophrenic adjustment. In other conditions, such as neuroses and personality disorders, the usual forms of loneliness and social isolation have a direct and significant effect (67). The extreme form of social isolation resulting from sensory deprivation (68) indicates that most normal individuals, when prevented from having regularly patterned stimulation, will develop hallucinatory experiences and other signs of personality disorganization, such as interference with attention, concentration, and memory. The social isolation associated with "brainwashing" also provides evidence of the role of group interaction and support in psychologic function (69).

Social Class

One of the most consistent findings in epidemiologic studies of the incidence and prevalence of mental disorder, particularly schizophrenia, has been the relatively high rates in the lower classes.

In a review of community studies, the lowest social class had the highest rate of mental disorder in 28 of 33 communities (15). The most consistent relationship was for personality disorders. The pattern also held up for schizophrenia, but not for manic–depressive psychosis or neuroses. In an analysis of social class and psychiatric symptoms, Derogatis et al. (70) report consistent findings regarding this inverse relationship for two symptoms: somatization and anxiety. The inverse relationship between social class and depression appears to hold only for less severe forms of depressive disorder (52, 71). Kohn (72) concludes that "rates of mental disorder, particularly of schizophrenia, are highest at the lowest socioeconomic levels, at least in moderately large cities, and this probably is not just a matter of drift, inadequate indices, or some other artifact of the methods we use." Kessler et al. (73) report in their review that up to the 1970s, the dominant interpretation of this inverse relationship was that lower social classes had greater exposure to adversity than the middle or upper class. Now the dominant interpretation is class-linked vulnerability. One current explanation is that the least competent members of society drift down to the lower classes. Another explanation is that there is less effective socialization in coping skills in the lower classes as manifested by lower class "fatalism" and intellectual inflexibility.

Lower class persons have to adjust to stressful events without the social resources and support available to the middle-class persons. The family unit, often broken or discordant instead of being a resource, is often a stressor (74). Komarovsky (75) reports that even in intact lower class families, the marital partners offer little psychologic support to each other.

Social Disintegration

One of the major studies on the role of social disintegration in the development of mental disorder has been the study of Stirling County, Nova Scotia, led by Alexander Leighton (7). Leighton proposed that communities with widespread disintegration become sources of stress because such social conditions interfere with "essential strivings" for psychological well-being. The result is the development of psychologic, psychophysiologic, and physical dysfunction. What Leighton calls social disintegration, sociologists in the past have called social disorganization (76).

Mental disorder was associated with interference blocking the achievement of socially valued goals by legitimate means, with limitations on the giving and receiving of love, with interference with spontaneity, and with interference with the individual's sense of membership in the moral order. This latter point has been identified by other investigators as anomia (8, 77, 78). No support was found for the hypothesis that social disintegration fostered psychiatric disorder by interfering with either physical security (such as needs for food, shelter, and clothing) or the individual's orientation regarding his place in society or sense of membership in a definite human group.

The excessive social control over the expression of aggression has been linked to the development of depressive symptoms—the high rate of depression in women (79) and psychiatric patients who appear to have strongly repressed hostility (80) and among the Hutterites (81) (who strongly suppress aggression).

In addition to the excessive social control of aggression, another social condition linked to the manifestation of depression is the loss of a crucial social role, which alters one's social integration. In three psychologic theories of depression, loss takes a central position: psychoanalytic theory (loss of an ambivalently loved object), ego psychology (loss of ego ideals), and existential theory (loss of meaning). In sociologic theory the concept of loss is linked to concepts of role and self. Rose (82) proposed that the loss of salient roles leads to "a mutilated self." Positive regard for the self is regulated by the adequacy of one's role performances and experiences. For women, for example, loss of the marital and maternal roles reduces or eliminates contact with significant others, which often deflates self-esteem and may precipitate feelings of uselessness, unattractiveness, and depreciated self-value. Role loss was investigated for 533 middle-aged (ages 40 to 59) women hospitalized for the first time, who carried a diagnosis of depression (51). Three role losses were investigated: maternal role loss (at least one child not living at home), marital role loss (separation, divorce, or widowhood), and occupational role loss (becoming unemployed prior to the symptom onset). Depression was found to be associated with any role loss, and especially with maternal role loss. Housewives who were overinvolved and overprotective of their children were likely to become depressed when their children left. The symptom of depression (in women not carrying a diagnosis of depression) was associated most strongly with maternal but not other forms of role loss. Among Jewish women, as compared to Black and Anglo-Saxon women, Bart (51) found that the ethnic socialization patterns made the maternal role most salient and therefore most likely to induce depression when maternal role loss occurred.

Family Dynamics

For many theorists, the period of childhood provides the single most important set of influences in the etiology of psychopathology. This tenet is documented by a vast literature on the role of maternal deprivation (42), poor maternal care (83), foster home placement (84), and adoptive home placements (85).

Three different theoretical approaches were identified by Mischler and Waxler (86) as having considerable importance in a study of the impact of family experience in the formation of severe psychopathology, especially schizophrenia: that of the Bateson group (87) on the double-bind hypothesis, that of the Lidz group (88) on schismatic and skewed families, and that of Wynne and Singer (89) on amorphous–fragmented family systems. Each approach emphasizes a different aspect of the functioning of the family, but all three focus in important ways on communication with the family unit.

In the double-bind hypothesis, attention is directed to the communicative act and not to the content of the communications or to the nature of the social roles and interactions. Schizophrenia is seen as resulting from exposure to pathologic communication. Repeated exposure of the child to such communication, in which the child cannot ask questions about its contradictory nature and in which punishment is included, is believed to encourage the child to develop pathologic communication also. The key pathologic feature, however, may not be paradoxical communications, which are neither rare nor limited to disturbed individuals (90), but rather the quality of its repetition and the requirement of restraint on leaving the scene. The child then learns that the best choice available is to avoid making a coherent communication as a means of avoiding punishment.

Lidz and his colleagues (88) investigated marital conflict and discord. The approach, derived from psychoanalytic theory, attempts to demonstrate that children who are exposed to parents whose marital relationship is disturbed suffer psychologic dysfunction. Such parents are defective role models for the child; they disturb appropriate age- and sex-role behavior and engage the child in coalitions of one parent against the other. Two types of distorted or deviant marital relationships have been identified: skewed and schismatic. In both, a pathologic distortion in role reciprocity occurs. In the schismatic relationship, one finds continuous conflict, discord, and undercutting, in which the parents fail to present themselves as capable of sharing and problem solving. Appropriate ego development and identity formation are thereby impaired. In the skewed family arrangement, open conflict is avoided by one parent taking a passive role and the other a dominant one, the latter usually having more severe psychopathology. Female schizophrenic patients tend to come from schismatic marital pairs, whereas male schizophrenic patients tend to come from skewed marital pairs in which the mother tends to be the dominant figure.

A third model of family relationship, studied by Wynne and Singer, focuses less on the content of role relationships and more on formal qualities of the family system. Their general hypothesis is that schizophrenic behavior is a product of a characteristic family social organization. They align family transactions on a continuum from amorphous to fragmented. The amorphous pattern is one in which family discussion is characterized by a drifting quality of attention; references are vague and nonspecific and tend to produce blurred, irrelevant meanings. The fragmented pattern of interaction and communication has a primary process quality: It is poorly integrated and is distorted. Wynne and Singer stress that the entire family system, and not specific members, is the model of defective communication. Another factor in the family system is the erratic response to affectional distance, being either too close or too far. The research of this group has been identified also with the concept of "pseudomutuality," which implies that families strive assiduously to maintain harmony at any price: They erect the image of mutuality when in fact there is a disregard for the identities of individual family members.

In the past, studies of the etiologic role of family interaction in schizophrenia have yielded few consistent results. Jacob (91) found no consistent differences between schizophrenic and normal family interactions with regard to three of four variables: conflict, dominance, and affect. With regard to the fourth variable, communication, some consistent differences were found. In families with schizophrenic children, communication lacked clarity and accuracy. However, a causal relationship between family interaction and schizophrenia has not been demonstrated. Liem (92) investigated the role of intrafamilial communication in schizophrenic and normal families. The purpose was to evaluate whether parental communication caused or was a response to the distorted communication patterns of the schizophrenic child. The results did not support the etiologic contention. The communications by parents or schizophrenic children were not more disordered or more adverse in effect than those of normal parents.

In recent prospective etiologic studies (93–95), the causal effect of family experience depended on a vulnerability to schizophrenia. Family experience alone was not a sufficient cause. In the University of California at Los Angeles (UCLA) Family Project Study (93, 94), 15-year follow-up of 64 disturbed adolescents indicated that parental behavior affected outcome. The parental communication style lacked clear focus, fitting the amorphous–fragmented continuum described by Wynne et al. (89). The affective style of their verbal behavior was negative–critical and guilt inducing. The expressed emotion (EE) measure (96, 97) (critical, emotionally overinvolved) was high (93, 94).

Exposure to stress, especially from the family, has been found to affect the relapse rate of schizophrenic patients (96, 97). Expressed emotion, a complex measure of critical and hostile family behavior (indicative of chronic rather than acute stress), has been used in these studies. Outpatients were more likely to relapse if EE was high (51%) than if it was low (13%). In intervention studies, where high EE was reduced, the relapse rate dropped (98, 99).

The value and efficacy of neuroleptic treatment of schizophrenic outpatients were also found to be related to the level of EE in the family (100). Without neuroleptic treatment, patients had a high relapse rate if their family had a high level of EE or if they were exposed to other stressful life events. With neuroleptic treatment, patients had a high relapse rate only if their family was high in EE *and* they experienced recent stressful life events.

In a 20-year follow-up study in Israel, Mirsky et al. (101) reported that the impact of early socializing experience was complex and apparently inconsistent with the findings of the UCLA (93, 94) and Finnish (95) longitudinal studies. Contrary to expectation, vulnerable children raised in a Kibbutz had twice as high a rate of schizophreniform disorders as those raised in an urban family setting. Furthermore, the Kibbutz children had a much higher rate of affective disorders. Mirsky et al. attempt to resolve the inconsistency between their results and the other two longitudinal studies by concluding that although a Kibbutz reduced contact with schizophrenic parents, this community acted as a hypercritical extended family likely to be intolerant of the manifest deviance of the vulnerable children.

SOCIOCULTURAL INFLUENCES OF PATIENTHOOD

In all cultures, dysfunctional behavior initiates a pattern of social reactions. Between complaints and patienthood, there is usually an extended period of time. This time period can be divided into a series of overlapping stages or processes, starting with the initial evaluative reactions to the symptoms of self, family, friends, and others (prior to the official consultation for diagnosis of the symptom) and proceeding stepwise to recognition of dysfunction and need for help, the help-seeking process, the labeling process, the diagnostic and treatment process, and outcome.

Once the initial reactions to symptoms have occurred, the first group of stages is patient centered and includes the recognition, help-seeking, and labeling processes. These are followed by the clinician-centered processes—diagnosis, treatment, and prognosis.

Patient-Centered Processes

In this section, I shall delineate the stages of recognition, help seeking, and labeling. These stages constitute an overlapping temporal sequence. Labeling, for example, may be both a consequence of help seeking, as Phillips (102) has pointed out, and a social cue for help seeking. The material is organized from the perspective of the patient (or, more aptly, the applicant for services) and the significant others in his or her life. A detailed description of this process is provided, in the hope that the clinician will become more attuned to this clinically rich and essential source of data. When a person comes for help, it signifies that a complex social negotiation is in process over the reality of dysfunction and appropriate means of treatment. The clinician joins the negotiation process at the point of entry and needs to know the details of this process. Sometimes the process is very apparent, as when the patient is brought to the clinic by another person rather than coming alone. Even in this case, clinicians often neglect to discuss the situation with the accompanying person.

Recognition Process

The recognition of disordered behavior appears to be influenced by the interplay of a number of variables: the behavior displayed, the social identity of the individual, the roles played and the statuses occupied by the individual, the effects of role failure or dysfunction, the immediate context of the disordered behavior, the individual's community and cultural group, cultural beliefs regarding the nature and etiology of disordered behavior, and cultural beliefs and practices regarding treatment and prognosis.

First, let us focus on factors that facilitate recognition. Recognition is contingent on role failure or dysfunction, especially with regard to major social roles. For this reason recognition almost always occurs first in the family. The more important and essential an individual's role in the family, the more salient the disordered behavior (the role failure) and the more likely that action will be taken (103–105).

Role failure has different consequences according to status, relationship factors in the primary group, and social identity in the community. If the marital relationship has a long history of dissatisfaction and discontent, then the recognition process may be prolonged. Sampson et al. (106) reported that recognition of mentally disordered wives was retarded in marriages in which mutual withdrawal had occurred early. Husbands were oblivious or indifferent to the bizarre behavior and disordered thinking of their wives; failure in the nurturant role had little salience, since it had lost its significance. If, on the other hand, the marital relationship was characterized by closeness, mutual respect, and communication, recognition would be without a long delay (104). Recognition, however, does not necessarily lead to seeking professional help. It may lead to supportive reactions from family and friends that may in fact obviate the need for professional help (11, 107, 108).

If an individual's deficient role performance is linked to a physical illness or disability, then social standards are lowered and social supports provided, circumventing lowered regard from others and from self. Weiss and Bergen (108) hypothesized that the relatively infrequent psychiatric hospitalization of rheumatoid arthritis patients results from their occupying a chronic sick role that legitimizes gratification of dependency needs without loss of self-esteem.

In addition to disruption of normal role functioning, Mechanic (109) states that symptoms are recognized according to visibility to others, perceived seriousness, and social embarrassment. Social visibility seems to be an organizing principle in the recognition of mental disorder in our society. Cultural alertness to appearance is reflected in the assigning of greater seriousness to disruptive behavior than withdrawing behavior. If the residual norm (behavior so basic as to be unstated, e.g., looking at a conversational partner) that is violated is overt and thereby socially visible (being troublesome, bizarre, or destructive), then that individual is more likely to be re_ognized than if his or her behavior is less overt (as in withdrawn, quiet, deluded behavior). The work of Lemkau and Crocetti (110) on public attitudes toward mental disorder demonstrates this visibility phenomenon. In a similar study, psychiatrists were found to rate 20 case vignettes more on the basis of social visibility than on the severity of the symptomatology presented (111).

Now I shall consider factors that impede recognition. Denial is the most pervasive response to indications of disorder (112). Even when individuals have mild to serious physical disorders, they are frequently not recognized as ill, nor are they encouraged, or likely, to seek treatment for their dysfunction (113). Sociocultural variation in the denial of symptoms seems related to prevalence. Zola (114) reports that the signs of physical disorder are often ignored when they are widespread, for example, diarrhea, sweating, and coughing among Mexicans; trachoma among Greeks; lower back pain among lower class American women.

Indifference to deviance has been associated with social class. Some investigators (115) claim that the unresponsiveness of lower socioeconomic status (SES) individuals is more a matter of indifference than of tolerance: They are likely to deny symptoms of withdrawal and not consider antisocial behavior indicative of mental disorder. Their conception of mental disorder seems to be less inclusive than that of middle-class individuals. However, once a person is identified as a disordered, the consequences are more likely to be severe rejection.

The recognition process is also impeded by the fear of the social consequences of recognition—the likelihood of social rejection (101, 116). Fears of stigma and rejection (abandonment in a state hospital) contribute to the fears that disturbance may be present. The strength of these fears was demonstrated in a study of attitude change by Cumming and Cumming (117) in a small Canadian community. The investigators used an educational campaign to increase public recognition and tolerance of mental illness. The title of their book, *Closed Ranks*, depicts the consolidated community opposition and rejection of their approach. The community feared normalizing mental disorder, placing it on a continuum of possible human conditions: The implication that anyone could become "insane" was unacceptable to the community. Despite considerable media attention to mental disorder since the 1950s, gains in public recognition of mental disorder have not occurred. Crocetti et al. (118) argue that recognition has increased; Sarbin and Mancuso (119) argue that it has not. In a repeat study of the population studied by Cumming and Cumming 20 years later, D'Arcy and Brockman (120) found no evidence of public attitude change.

The public has resisted the efforts of the mental health movement to apply the medical sick role to those who are mentally disordered. Despite continuing campaigns to identify alcoholism as an illness, the reaction of the general public is still to place this disorder in an evaluative and moral framework. Blackwell (121) found that the criteria for societal agreement regarding assignment to the medical role decreased with the number of social and psychologic characteristics associated with the complaint. A number of investigators have reported that society does not treat the patienthood of those who are identified as mentally ill in a similar manner to those who are identified as physically ill. The same exemptions from social responsibility are not applied. Although the mentally ill are expected to seek professional help, they are not seen as exempt from responsibility for their condition (122).

Although the general cultural orientation to mental illness is negative and tinged with fear, there are variations in beliefs and attitudes regarding its nature that may

in turn cause variations in social response. Cohen and Struening (123) found five attitudinal factors, only two of which involved negative and fearful qualities. Cox et al. (124) reported that the public orientation to mental disorder can be sorted into three organizing beliefs: (*a*) social inadequacy, characterized by difficulties ranging from drug abuse to family discord; (*b*) personal inadequacy, characterized by such difficulties as lack of confidence; and (*c*) psychotic involvement, characterized by such behavior as excessive religiosity and bizarre sensations. It is doubtful that behavior in the first two categories is sufficiently deviant to be labeled as mental disorder, unless the individual seeks help (102).

Help Seeking

The help-seeking process can be described in terms of three components: (*a*) the nature and severity of the problem, (*b*) the society's orientation to illness and treatment, and (*c*) the nature of the treatment system.

Kadushin (125) reports on the *kind of problem*. He has found that the more specific the symptoms, the more likely they are to be recognized and acted on. The specific symptoms are somatic, sexual, marital–interpersonal, and occupational–role. In contrast, the nonspecific diffuse symptoms are cognitive (disordered thinking), cathectic (related to mood and energy), and depreciated self-regard. Even in regard to the specific symptoms, only the sexual ones were consistently recognized as being a reason for seeking professional help. A deflated sense of self-regard is not a universal cue for seeking help; it is more specifically associated with overall education and psychologic sophistication. Individuals having low self-regard were most likely to seek help if they read mental health books and belonged to the "friends and supporters of psychotherapy." The high incidence of self-reported somatic symptoms of lower SES persons in psychiatric settings, despite the actual incidence being unrelated to class, suggests that somatization is both a socially acceptable way of expressing emotional difficulties and a legitimate and concrete manifestation of dysfunction that justifies help seeking. Impulsive and antisocial behavior is more likely to provoke help-seeking action by middle-class than by lower class parents.

Although one would expect severity of symptoms to correlate with help seeking, this is not the case. The more severely disturbed individuals have been found to be less likely to recognize the need for help and to seek treatment (126). If the individuals can recognize the need, then the acuteness of the symptoms is more likely to lead to action (125). Irrespective of patient recognition of need, the severity of symptomatology does not prompt greater accessibility of outpatient treatment. Levinson et al. (127) investigated this relationship. If clinicians subscribed to the medical model, then medical decision making would be based on need, and severity then would be a major basis for psychiatric treatment dispositions. This is not the case. Clinicians tend to choose patients suitable for psychotherapy. Thus, the mild to moderately disturbed individuals were most likely to be accepted for treatment.

Help seeking has been empirically associated with certain sociocultural attributes and orientations. Females recognize, report, and seek help earlier than do men (128–130). Individuals with relatively high education, from urban or suburban settings, who are low in religious identification, except for those who are Jewish, are more likely to recognize and seek help early (125, 131). Middle- and upper-class males are more likely to react to instrumental role failure by seeking help. As stated earlier, a facilitating factor in the help-seeking process is alliance with a group of individuals who have had psychotherapy—"the friends of psychotherapy" (125). In order to maintain perspective, it is essential to realize that only one-third of individuals with symptoms seek help (132).

Help seeking is influenced by the treatment expectations and goals of the patient and significant others in his or her life. In the 1960s a series of studies were initiated on patient expectation and goals (133–135). The impetus for this research was the fact that many patients were leaving therapy prematurely. Expectations were investigated with regard to the kind of treatment (talking versus drugs) and the patient–therapist roles (active and advice giving versus nondirective and insight oriented). Lower class individuals were reported to seek help expecting the therapist to be active and directive and to provide somatic treatments. In subsequent reviews of the materials on treatment expectations, the social class differences in expectations have been found to be exaggerated and negligible (132, 136).

In addition to expectations and goals, Lazare et al. have investigated patient requests. They reported in a series of studies that a majority of patients coming to a walk-in clinic have specific ideas about how they hope the clinician will help them (137–140). The three highest ranking requests were for clarification, psychologic insight, and psychologic expertise, (141, 142). Social class differences in requests were found to be negligible (136).

Help-seeking behavior is strongly influenced by the physical and psychologic accessibility of the health delivery system and the kind of services provided. Individuals seeking help start first with their support system (family, friends, and peers); they then turn to other mental health resources, primarily the family physician and social agencies, then to their minister, priest, or rabbi, and last, to psychiatric clinics or caretakers (143). They may go no further than informal or formal self-help groups. Barriers to accessibility of mental health treatment include physical location; economic cost for care; cultural, ethnic, and racial differences between clinic staff and the clients; and administrative practices, particularly the waiting lists and complex instructions necessary to make an appointment. Psychologic, economic, and administrative barriers to the outpatient treatment of lower SES patients have been described by Hollingshead and Redlich (144) and Myers and Schaffer (145). An effort to lower these barriers has been associated with the efforts of community mental health innovations; treatment centers are located closer to the individual's home, length of stay is shortened, treatment personnel are more similar to the clients, and the community is included in the control of the operation of the clinic and hospital. Professional mental health consultation to community resources has been a promising alternative to direct treatment (146).

Labeling

In the 1960s, in addition to social causation another mode of viewing social dimensions of mental disorder was gaining momentum. This approach focuses on how the reaction of others influences the persistence of symptoms and the character of mental disorder. Following from the key assumption within this framework—that disordered behavior develops and is formed in response to social reinforcement—social stigma and "labeling" are viewed as two of the most powerful social influences for what is referred to as "career training" in mental disorder. Thus, the reaction of others to the "disordered" behavior becomes as important as the reasons that led to the disorder. Mischler and Waxler (86) refer to this approach to explaining mental disorder as a "responsive" theory rather than an "etiological" theory. Some of the leading investigators using an approach based on the importance of social responsiveness are Lemert (147), Goffman (148), Scheff (149), and Mechanic (150). Their message to clinicians was to heed the major role of reaction to psychosocial difficulties in the development and maintenance of mental dysfunction.

An observable social fact is that deviant behavior is not a sufficient reason for labeling. Most individuals who violate norms are not labeled as mentally ill or criminal (149, 151, 152). Two key aspects of societal reactions are (a) the conditions under which labeling occurs, and (b) the effect of labeling on the stabilization of mental symptoms. If others ignore or deny the norm violations associated with mental symptoms, then, Scheff (149) states, "the rule breaking will be transitory, compensated for, or channeled in socially acceptable forms." If the social reaction labels the individual as deviant, then rule breaking will persist and the individual will be launched on a career of "chronic mental illness." Lemert (147) states that if an individual is labeled as deviant during the process of socialization, that deviant role is often irreversible. Labeling theorists thus believe that social reaction has a causal and not just a confirmatory effect on mental dysfunction.

The very nature of mental illness is thus put in question. A central proposition of this approach is that mental illness does not inhere in the primary deviance, i.e., in rule-breaking behavior or symptoms. Rather, it is conferred on the individual by his social group. Labeling theorists do not address primary deviance, that is, the initial instances of rule breaking associated with mental disorder. They focus on secondary deviance or the behavior associated with playing the role, often a stereotype, of the mentally ill individual.

Not all norm violations have the same implications for labeling. Scheff distinguishes between violations of most norms and violations of residual norms. Most norm violations are explicit, easily identified, and do not carry serious social sanctions, since they are easily controlled within the social group. However, a residual norm violation (rule breaking) is "unnameable" and "unmentionable" and has more serious consequences in initiating the labeling process. Examples of residual rule breaking range from minor instances, such as not looking at your conversational partner, to major instances, such as muttering, hallucinating, and posturing. Violation of residual rules, when attributed to alcohol, drugs, stress, or physical illness, is not a sufficient condition for labeling. Scheff notes the general tendency to deny the significance of residual deviance. A number of investigators report that residual deviance may be manifested for years in a family without the person being labeled as mentally ill (104, 153, 154). Fletcher et al.

(154) report that families of psychotic individuals normalize the deviant behavior by using organic explanations ("It's nerves") or situational explanations ("It's overwork"). Families usually find the behavior of the family member not so extreme as the public stereotype and are thereby able to deny illness.

In the transition from violating residual rules to labeling, there is disagreement about the point of labeling. Frequently threatening or dangerous behavior, when added to other instances of residual rule breaking, leads to labeling. Even the case of admission to a mental hospital is not sufficient to confer the label of mental illness (155, 156).

There is disagreement regarding the conditions under which an individual may be labeled as deviant. More important, there is serious question regarding the consequences of labeling. Gove (157) reviewed the evidence for stabilization of mental symptoms through labeling and found it to be scant. He states that Scheff's evidence tends to be indirect, based on the important fact that mental disorder is often diagnosed on the basis of incomplete and questionable information. This indirect evidence, Gove asserts, does not support the proposition that carrying an inappropriately assigned label leads to the stabilization of symptoms.

Aside from the question of symptom stabilization, there is evidence that labeling has adverse effects. Doherty (158) compared the response to psychiatric hospital treatment of acceptors, rejectors, and deniers of the mental illness label. Contrary to the staff expectation that acceptors would fare the best, the rejectors did best. Though the public negative attitude toward the mentally ill has been reported to be diminishing (118), Page (159) reports that the stigma of mental illness still has effects, such as refusal to rent rooms. In sum, there is good reason to believe that social reaction to deviant behavior has powerful, though not fully understood, effects both before and after entry into the mental health system.

Clinician-Centered Processes

In this section the stages in the response process shall be examined starting with entry into the mental health system and focusing on diagnosis, treatment, and prognosis—the clinician-centered processes. A special effort is made to consider the implications of the sociocultural approach for modification and expansion of the existing approach to diagnosis, treatment, and prognosis.

Traditional Diagnosis

There are two propositions regarding traditional diagnosis: (*a*) Sociocultural variations in the form and kind of mental disorder are minor in extent and seldom disrupt or distort the diagnostic process; and (*b*) sociocultural factors can be identified that bias and distort diagnosis.

Schizophrenia is found in all cultures and societies (15). In a standard assessment of schizophrenia in nine societies, Sartorius et al. (160) report that schizophrenic patients shared similar characteristics and could be differentiated from other mental disorders. The clinical subforms of schizophrenia also occur in all societies. However, variations among cultures in the incidence of subforms have been reported. Wittkower and Dubreuil (161) report that catatonic states in chronic schizophrenia are common in India and Asia but rare in Europe and America, and they explain this finding on the basis of the acceptability of social and emotional withdrawal in the Hindu and Buddhist religions. They also infer that the diagnosis of simple schizophrenia will be rare in those communities in which standards of work and performance are low, since this diagnosis is tied often to marginal social and occupational adjustment. Deficient role performance associated with simple schizophrenia cannot be distinguished from normative behavior. Parsons (162) reported that social withdrawal does not commonly occur in schizophrenic individuals in southern Italy, because of the high cultural value accruing to gregariousness and sociability. In Japan an increase in paranoid schizophrenia has been reported since the country's defeat in World War II, with fewer delusions connected with the Emperor (163).

In contrast to schizophrenia, cultural variations are found in the genesis of depressive disorders, including manic–depressive illness. In Western society, the incidence of manic–depressive illness has been showing a steep decline (164); for example, the rate of manic–depressive illness between 1928 and 1947 declined by two-thirds in New York state, whereas the depressive disorders in general have been found to be increasing.

Cohen (165) hypothesized that "psychotic depression is generally more frequent among those persons who are more cohesively identified with their families, kin groups, communities, and other significant groupings." Further, Cohen stated, "Depression is more likely to be found predominantly (1) in societies characterized by highly traditionalized and tightly knit social groupings, (2) in the higher socioeconomic statuses of communities/societies, (3) among professional and executive groups in the society, and (4) among women—to the extent that they are found to be more closely identified with family and kin than men in the same society." Murphy et al. (166) found support for Cohen's hypothesis in a cross-cultural survey.

Cross-cultural data provide useful insight into some diagnostic issues regarding depression, especially the generality of particular symptoms. Murphy et al. (166) collected questionnaires on psychotic depressive symptoms on 98 patient samples throughout the world. Respondents were asked to report on a cluster of four core symptoms: depressive mood, diurnal mood change, insomnia with early morning awakening, and loss of interest in the external environment. Where the depressive cluster was above average in frequency, respondents also reported a more than average frequency of anorexia, weight loss, self-accusation, loss of sexual interest, and fatigue, and the patients tended to be European and middle or upper class. Where the depressive cluster was less than

average in frequency, they found self-neglect, semimutism, and religious preoccupation to be characteristic of the sample, but did not find the symptoms of anorexia, weight loss, and so on found in the above-average group. An explanation for the divergence in the incidence of the four core symptoms was related to social cohesion, not to culture, religion, social class, or residence. The prevalence of the four core symptoms is greater in cohesive communities where the individuals feel freer to express hostility (less social constraint) and thus are less frequently depressed and less self-punitive when they are depressed.

Another important and related diagnostic finding concerns the relationship of guilt to depression. Murphy et al. (166) found that guilt was greater with exposure to Christian and Judeo-Christian traditions— the more involvement in these religions, the greater self-depreciation and guilt. In Moslem samples, guilt was uncommon, as was suicide ideation. They inferred that for Moslems the bad internal objects are projected onto the external world, manifested in ideas of influence and possession. Collomb (167), in a review of the incidence of depression in Africa, asserts that depression is present, but that "the depressive frame of mind" is reflected by projection (persecution) and by somatic hypochondriacal complaints. Field (168) reports that depression was not found by some investigators because they looked in the wrong place; she found an abundance of clinically depressed individuals at religious shrines, but not in hospitals.

With regard to the second proposition, bias is found in the diagnosis of lower class patients by middle-class psychiatrists. There is greater likelihood for lower class than middle-class patients to be diagnosed psychotic and to be assigned other "tough" diagnoses (125). The diagnosis of chronic alcoholism has been found to be much more likely the primary diagnosis for lower than for middle-class problem drinkers (169). Diagnosis is biased not only by the socioeconomic status of the patient, but also by the treatment ideology of the clinic. Kadushin (125) reports in his study of five clinics in New York City that the diagnosis of schizophrenia was two and three times higher in some clinics than in others and that differences in the patient population could not account for this difference in diagnostic decisions.

Bias may be subtle, embedded in unstated ideologic and value positions. It has been observed in a series of studies, for example, that English and American psychiatrists differed in their diagnosis of depressive and schizophrenic disorders. The Americans were more ready to diagnose schizophrenia than were the English, and the English were more ready to diagnose depressive disorders than were the Americans, especially manic–depressive illness (170–173).

The diagnostic significance and evaluation of hallucinations are influenced by sociocultural conditions. Edwards (174) reported that American psychiatrists used a broader definition than did British psychiatrists, often failing to distinguish hallucinatory experiences from pseudohallucinations and hypnogogic and hypnopompic imagery. The American psychiatrists also assigned greater significance to hallucinations in diagnosing schizophrenia and were less aware of its occurrence in other psychiatric conditions. Strauss (175) found almost as many questionable and pseudohallucinations as definite ones in American hospitalized schizophrenics. Zigler and Phillips (176) report not only that hallucinations were distributed among other diagnostic groups in addition to schizophrenics, but also that the percentage of hallucinations among schizophrenics (35%) was lower than had been expected.

Social Diagnosis

Because effective intervention requires sorting out of the contribution of social processes in the formation and maintenance of current dysfunction, clinicians should examine ways of assessing the patient's social environment. A basic assumption in social diagnosis is that treatment interventions should be directed toward the sociocultural environment, whether emphasis is on the family, neighborhood, or employer. Unfortunately, current diagnostic procedures are of little help for such aims, since they ignore for the most part the role of the sociocultural environment and operate as if behavior were a function of the person alone, rather than a function of the interaction of the person with his environment.

There are four basic descriptive goals in social diagnosis. One goal is to evaluate the stressful life processes as described earlier in this chapter. In more global terms, this would involve assessing the state of community disintegration, which Leighton (7) has identified as causing mental disorder. A second goal is to identify the social contents of maladaptive behavior, whether in the family, work, neighborhood, or some other setting. Identifying the social context of drinking, for example, is of value in the treatment of alcoholism (177, 178). A third goal is to assess the understanding and explanations made by the patient and family regarding the patient's dysfunctional behavior. The social group's evaluation of dysfunctional behavior is of crucial significance in planning future interventions. Understanding the causal attributions regarding the presenting problem has become a topic of clinical and research interest in recent years (179). At the most basic level, the requests, expectations, and goals of the patient and family in treatment will depend on what they believe to be the cause of the dysfunction. Finally, assessment of the patient's social resources—the nature and accessibility of support groups—is essential in evaluating and treating dysfunction.

Treatment

Sociocultural variables have been implicated in the acceptance of patients for treatment, early termination, treatment effectiveness, and prognosis. The most widely investigated sociocultural variable in regard to treatment is social class. It has been reported that lower class individuals are less likely to be accepted for psychotherapy (144, 180), and if accepted for treatment in an outpatient setting, they are less likely to be treated by experienced therapists (181) and more likely to be treated with organic therapies (182).

Sociocultural factors significantly affect the treatment process. Baekeland and Lundwall (183) reviewed 57 studies of premature termination and found that in 35 (61%), SES was a significant predictor: Lower class individuals dropped out more frequently than did middle-class patients. Meltzoff and Kornreich (184) claim this effect is strongest in psychoanalytic clinics. Efforts to explain this result include the divergence between the patient and therapist in a number of regards, especially social class. One aspect is a discrepancy between lower and middle-class orientations to time; Hollingshead (185) reported that lower class patients were more "present" oriented than were middle-class patients and therapists. Being on time, keeping appointments, and staying for a prolonged treatment process has been claimed to be more consistent with the time orientation of the middle class than with that of the lower class. Kluckhohn (186) developed a framework for analysis of value orientations, including time. Papajohn and Spiegel (187) find a "present" over "future" orientation in a study of working-class Puerto Rican families and rural Greek and Italian families.

In addition to time, a number of investigators have noted discrepancies over role expectations. Patients of lower SES tend to expect therapy to be directive, concrete, and organic and the therapist to be active, which contrasts with the patient role norms held by the therapist (133, 135, 144, 188–190). Many of these discrepancies in role expectations that applied in the 1950s may no longer apply to the same degree in the 1970s (132). Frank et al. (136) report minimal class difference in treatment requests. Garfield (191), in an analysis of patient–therapist expectations, points out that misconceptions regarding therapy tend to apply across social classes. Most individuals, irrespective of class, want more directive treatment, more advice. They also expect treatment to be much shorter than it actually turns out to be.

Attitudes and beliefs about the efficacy of treatment (prognostic expectation) are socially conditioned and affect treatment outcome. Goldstein (135) reports that treatment benefit obtains when the patient's prognostic expectations are moderate and the therapist's expectations are high. For lower class patients this pattern does not hold—patients expect too much and the therapist too little (134, 192). Goldstein (193) suggests that such a patient–therapist discrepancy over prognosis constitutes a condition for early termination.

In evaluating factors that influence early termination and treatment effectiveness, sociocultural attributes of a therapist are more important than are those of the patient. Baekeland and Lundwall (183) report on a number of therapist variables, including ethnocentrism, which have a strong effect in producing early termination. Efforts have been made to correct for negative effects on treatment, stemming from social class differences of patient and therapist regarding roles in treatment, nature of treatment, and social attributes. One strategy has been "anticipatory socialization": to educate and prepare the patient for appropriate treatment expectations (194–196). Another strategy has been to modify the kind of treatment itself. Treatment has been made shorter, more problem centered, and more action oriented through the use of such techniques as role-playing. Behavior therapy has been identified as distinctively effective with low-income patients (197). A third strategy has been to increase the sensitivity of the residents and staff to the problems and needs of patients of lower SES. The importance of acceptance and sensitivity is demonstrated in the study by Kandel (198), in which premature termination was less likely to occur when the social class origins of both the patient and therapist were similar. With this in mind, residents have been trained to be more receptive to the social stresses in the patient's life, less rigidly adherent to a purely psychodynamic formulation, and more sensitive to the cultural orientation of the lower class patients (199, 200).

Social ideologies have also influenced

the nature of treatment. In the past century one can see how the care of patients has varied with changing ideologies. The moral therapy of the mid-19th century reflected a shift from the segregation and incarceration of the 18th century (201). In moral therapy man was seen as perfectable, and mental disorder was viewed as the result of the destructive effects of society. With the influx of immigrants to the United States in the late-19th century and a consequent rise in the numbers of people committed to mental institutions, the humanistic approach of moral therapy shifted to institutional control. Folta and Schatzman (202) hypothesized that custodial care of the past century was due to the ascendence of Social Darwinism that invited disregard for the unfit. One might speculate that this change in treatment philosophy was able to occur because it was with an "outgroup" population.

The greatest 20th century ideologic influence on psychotherapy has come from Freudian theory. Freud's emphasis was almost exclusively on the intrapsychic problem and the intrapsychic response, dissociating the reality of social problems and social injustice from treatment.

Bart (203) sees the culture-bound and quietistic nature of psychiatry in the recent past as coming from the psychotherapeutic pessimism of Freud. This is now changing and there are advocates of more activist treatment approaches (204, 205). One of the first steps toward the recognition of the role of the social environment was the work on crisis intervention. Along with Lindemann (206) and Caplan (146), Fried (207) proposed that situations of change and transition can provide the opportunity for different ways of coping that are not necessarily negative or maladaptive. These situations may provide for (*a*) a reorganization of old patterns and development of new adaptive processes, (*b*) stabilization of existing modes of adaptation alerted to meet the present circumstances, and (*c*) retrenchment, in the face of new expectations, in a retreat to past patterns. Most investigators report that the timing of treatment is crucial during crises in order to

provide support necessary to prevent or retard damaging effects and to provide treatment when the individual is more open than usual to change (208).

Weiss (12) for example, in his sequential theory of stress (crisis, transition, and deficit), claims that different kinds of support apply best in this temporal sequence: emotional support for crisis, cognitive support for transition, and material support for deficit. Jacobson (209) describes the role of timing of support in crisis situations such as serious illness, grief, and marital problems.

Group therapy and psychodrama have been the established treatment modes that incorporate social reality directly into treatment. Brief therapies represent a more recent serious effort toward the recognition of the social environment in treatment. Normand et al. (200) have developed a systematic approach to brief therapy with lower income patients. They integrate the dynamic- and situational-centered goals. Residents are trained to modify the traditional diagnostic model. They are encouraged to collect dynamic material tailored to the patient's current life situation; current symptoms have priority over past history. After making a dynamic formulation, the next step is to make a blueprint for action, incorporating the intrapsychic and situational factors into an action formulation. Goldstein (199) devised a behavioral therapy to be effective with the poor. A short-term interpersonal psychotherapy has been developed by Klerman, Weissman, and their colleagues (210, 211) for the treatment of depression that is highly sensitive to sociocultural factors. This therapy explicitly addresses current psychosocial problems as they are embedded in interpersonal relationships and the social context, the interplay of acute and chronic stressors, and the individuals social resources. They cite three broad areas of application: abnormal grief reactions, role disputes, and role transitions.

Prognosis

Comparison of two very different cultures regarding prognosis of schizophrenia reveals striking evidence of the role of crucial sociocultural factors. Waxler (212) found that the prognosis of schizophrenia was better in the peasant society of Mauritius than in the complex industrial society of Great Britain in her comparison of two longitudinal studies, one in each society. Waxler stated, "Almost all the findings support the conclusion that clinical and social outcome for treated schizophrenics is better in the peasant society of Mauritius than Great Britain." Similar findings on prognosis in schizophrenia was reported by Sartorius et al. (160) in a comparison of four undeveloped countries with five developed countries.

Waxler (212), taking a labeling theory approach, proposed that the difference in prognosis was due to differences in the cultural beliefs, family response to illness, and the impact of bureaucracy. In Mauritius, where causes of illness tend to be attributed to external factors, patients are not held responsible for their disorder, the self is not seen as being changed by the symptoms, and return to normal functioning is expected in a short time. The family, in addition, plays a greater role in negotiations over the disorder with treatment personnel in Mauritius than in Great Britain. They could challenge "poor" prognoses and have them revised. In Great Britain patients are more likely to see themselves as being changed by having symptoms and to have to negotiate with an impressive bureaucracy regarding the permanency of occupying any sick role. Waxler (212) concludes that bureaucracies have an investment in maintaining patients in the sick role and transmit messages that confirm sickness rather than recovery. This is less the case in Mauritius, where the treatment system is less organized.

In sum, patienthood is a sociocultural phenomena. Symptoms and complaints in social isolation constitute a myopic view. Diagnosis and treatment cannot be effectively conducted without full appreciation of the complex sociocultural processes that influence entry and the very process of diagnosis and treatment planning itself. The problems of noncompliance and premature termination of treatment are aversive reminders of the sociocultural reality. The clinician needs to clinically integrate both the patient's and his or her own sociocultural perspective on the problem and on appropriate treatment. We have documented how recognition and help seeking are complex social processes affecting the definition of the problem, expectations, goals, and requests in treatment. Important prognostic factors are how individuals define themselves vis-à-vis the dysfunctional behavior and how it affects their personal identity. The reaction of others influences not only the help-seeking process, but also the maintenance and change of dysfunction. Labeling one's personal identity reflects the influence of significant others, mental health professionals, their bureaucracies, and oneself. Some patients "seal over" the issue of their dysfunctional behavior (their sanity), whereas others are painfully aware and continuously evaluating and responding to cues from significant others regarding their status. Clinicians need to be aware that biasing factors extend from social class differences between clinician and patient to the ideology of the organization of which they are functionaries. Treatment decisions, such as whether to hospitalize, are often influenced by biases in organizational values that affect staffing and range of treatment. It is clinically useful to negotiate differences or conflicts over the problem, the treatment, and the relationship, recognizing that both the patient and clinician have constituencies overseeing their actions.

In the next section, the symptom is used as a starting point for understanding the embeddedness of dysfunction in the social system. The thesis is that symptoms have communicative significance for significant others.

SYMPTOMS AS SOCIAL COMMUNICATION

In the previous two sections of this chapter, symptoms and "mental illness" were discussed as responses to social stress influenced by the repertoire of behavioral possibilities provided by the sociocultural matrix, by the amount and quality of social support, and by the societal and professional response that influence help seeking, patienthood, and outcome. From the sociocultural perspective, symptoms can also be understood as transactional phenomena—nonverbal parts of a dialogue or extranormative means of communication about relationships. To understand these communications, one needs to look at the entire cast of actors and the transactional episode in which they are embedded. Unfortunately, in diagnostic treatment efforts, the communicative nature of symptomatic behavior is generally neglected and relegated to the background. In the initial encounter in mental health settings, attention is predominantly directed to psychodynamic and biologic considerations.

The communication aspects of symptoms, nonetheless, merit serious consideration by clinicians, since they carry invaluable information for treatment. To obtain this information the clinician is required to act as if he or she were a translator of a foreign language. In the analysis of dreams (which quite legitimately may be viewed as a foreign language), Freud aimed to decode significant intrapsychic conflicts of his patients by searching for wish fulfillment in the dream content and using the patient as a resource for further exploration of associated mental events. In the social analysis of symptoms, the aim is to decode the interpersonal content of the symptoms. The clinician searches for the interpersonal meanings in this mode of communication, looking to the individual for data on the individual's relationship to significant others. To gather such data the clinician should suspend, at least momentarily, the search for the biologic causes or unconscious conflicts that may underlie the symptomatic behavior and should treat the symptoms as primary data, not as derivative phenomena. The clinician should view the symptoms as a medium of communication suited to the perceived social requirements of allusion, hinting, and disguises, rather than as a direct, precise, and overt expression of feelings and thoughts about one's relationships.

Patterns of Communication with Diagnostic Groupings and Symptoms

There appears to be distinct general interpersonal messages associated with the symptoms in different clinical disorders. In this section symptomatic communications associated with hysteria, suicidal behavior, schizophrenia, and depression are described.

In the studies on hysteria by Breuer and Freud (213), Freud observed that the choice of a particular bodily complaint conveyed expressive interpersonal information. Freud's interest and attention were directed to the conversion of the energy of the intrapsychic conflict into the physical manifestation—the symptom—rather than to the social communication aspects of the symptom. His focus was on the path of blocked energy and on the repression of thoughts, feelings, and impulses, not on the communication to a significant other. For example, Freud described the case of a woman who complained of facial neuralgia and who said later, after some analytic work, that the pain was like a "slap in the face." She associated her symptom with being severely insulted by her husband: The verbal act is equal to a physical act. When she made the connection between the facial pain and the verbal "slap," Freud reports that the patient was able to give up the symptom. One can see that the symptom was a form of disguised communication between the wife and her husband. Freud focused on the internal mechanism of symptom formation and explained this behavior as a "conversion" reaction. The social significance of the symptom was recognized but relegated to a secondary position. In the concept of secondary gain, Freud identified and evaluated the status of the interpersonal communication carried by the symptom. The primary gain lay in the reduction of anxiety bound to a symptom; the secondary gain lay in the use to which the woman put the symptom. This distinction partitions the intrapsychic from interpersonal aspects and focuses treatment on intrapsychic rather than on interpersonal factors. Some clinicians believe this distinction to be excessively sharp.

One of the foremost proponents of an interpersonal analysis of symptoms is Thomas Szasz (214). In his view, hysterical conversion is the prototype of symptomatic communication. Bodily symptoms signify learned ways of coping with interpersonal relationships, ways learned and developed in response to social rules presented in the guise of biologic ones. Child-rearing practices in our society teach us the obligation to help the helpless, to care for the sick. The game plan of hysteria is to use these rules by impersonating the physically ill in order to achieve, maintain, or regain control over an interpersonal relationship. Hysteria is thus likened to game playing organized around the rules of coercion and deceit. It is a counterfeit game, since it exploits by deceit the complementary rules of helplessness and helpfulness. The communication is clearly analogical; the individual acts as if he or she is beset with a physical disorder. The generalized message is "treat me as if I am ill." Illness disguises the real message: "I am helpless and need your care." In addition to the general message "I am ill," the symptom also carries more specific information, embedded in the specific dysfunction being enacted, about the relationship which is sought after.

According to Szasz (214), the "illness" game is learned in childhood and linked to the socially appropriate conditions for exhibiting weakness and helplessness. With changes in status from infant to child, the nurturance, care, and support appropriate to the infant is gradually withdrawn. When feeling hurt, needy, or helpless, the child is more and more likely to be told "Don't be a cry baby," but the child learns an exception—the illness status. When ill, the child may legitimately seek nurturance and support. In physical illness the interpersonal stance resembles that of early childhood: helplessness, weakness, and fragility. The child not only learns the privileges associated with being ill, but also learns that the cues distinguishing physi-

cal illnesses from feelings of helplessness are vague and often private. Being ill can become playing ill. The social conditions for gaining access to nurturance and support thus appear to invite deception. The admission of weakness and helplessness outside of illness provokes humiliation and shame, except in the very young.

Illness behavior is under social regulation resulting in personal and social barriers to playing ill. When evaluated from a personal perspective, individuals learn to regard illness as a form of weakness and self-indulgence, a cue for negative self-regard. When considered from a social perspective, the individual must legitimate this status by seeing a physician and by efforts to become well (215). The individual risks being shamed if the claim is false. It is commonplace for children to be tested for the physical reality of their complaint. When the individual is feeling insecure, weak, or helpless, the social choice available thus seems to be between the shame of admitting such feeling or the deception to self and others by playing the illness game.

Symptomatic communication is a special case of indirect communication commonly found in normal social discourse. The basic features of indirect communication are social disguise and pretense. In verbal behavior it is found in hinting, allusion, and metaphor. In nonverbal behavior, it is found in "putting on a face" (216). One can see indirect communication in the rituals and rules of conduct in social games. In nonsymptomatic games the rules of disguise are understood by the role players when playing these games. Hinting and allusion thus serve a useful protective social function, permitting interaction in which the individual is less exposed to potential aversive social consequences, ranging from rebuff and rejection to unforeseen obligation and commitment. Self-protection is thus the strong and pervasive social motivation underlying indirect communication.

The referential ambiguity in indirect communication, the hinting and allusion, can be illustrated by social games such as the "dating game" in which the individual disguises his or her intentions by following social rules of pretension. Pretense in these games differs from that in the "illness" game. Unlike the impersonated sick role, both of the role players in the "dating game" understand that the game is "on." The participants can regulate the interaction by using scripts that maintain safe distances; the costs of breaking contact are minimal. Unlike these sanctioned varieties of indirect communication, hysteria is more costly than beneficial. It is self-defeating, on the one hand, since the hysteric cannot claim credit for his or her successes. On the other hand, the recipient, exploited and coerced to act in a helping way, is unlikely to continue to act helpful if the truth becomes known. Thus, the desired relationship continues at the price of maintaining the symptom. The desired progression from indirect to direct communication can occur in normal relations, but not in relationships dominated by symptomatic communication.

Even more strongly than Szasz, others such as Carson (217), Sarbin (218), and Adams (219) view traditional psychodynamic or biologic interpretation of symptoms as unfortunate and misleading, diverting attention from the fundamental consideration in "mental" symptoms, the interpersonal process. In their view, symptoms, such as hysteria, are extranormative efforts, exaggerations of normal strivings, to achieve or protect a secure relationship with significant others.

Suicidal Behavior

In most suicidal behavior the basic message is a cry for help (220). Such behavior is often seen as a coercive effort to control a significant other person, often a departing lover. Suicidal individuals express this message of desperation by their statements and acts: "If you leave, if you do not help me, I will die." The threatened rupture of a love relationship is made analogous to death by the suicidal act. Among diverse symptomatic communications, suicidal behavior represents an extreme effort to regain control over an endangered rela-

tionship. In some cases, clinicians believe that the communication is between the suicidal individual and an already lost significant other, usually a parent lost during early childhood (41). In that case, the suicidal activity signifies a communication of a desire for reunion. Others, such as Weiss (221) have discussed the suicide attempt as a communication with God (or some powerful other), as a test of God's love, a gamble with death—"If God does not care, I will die."

In both observational and experimental studies of suicidal behavior (222, 223), the targets of the suicidal communication most often ignore the communication and act as if it has not been made. In some cases the target person will try to argue the suicidal individual out of the idea and into seeking professional help. When the suicidal communication is not a threat but an attempt, the response of others is often to modify the patient's social field and to accept the interactive burden (224, 225).

Schizophrenia

In schizophrenia, where the symptoms are most often chronic, one can see a variety of social communications. The metacommunication is often to deny any relationship or influence (226). The individual communicates to others by his or her symptoms the wish to retain a mistrusting, degraded, submissive, and often self-punitive interpersonal stance vis à vis others. The intentional "craziness" in schizophrenic behavior was documented by studies conducted by Braginsky and Braginsky (227). The authors hypothesized that the communications of hospitalized chronic schizophrenic patients are under the patient's control and are used to support the goals of remaining in the hospital and retaining an open-ward status. Three groups of patients, randomly selected, were told that they were about to be interviewed, but for the following different purposes: (a) to be evaluated for discharge, (b) to be evaluated for retaining open-ward privileges, and (c) to be evaluated for their general level of functioning, implying their being evaluated for discharge. Tapes of these interviews were presented to psychiatrists unaware of the experimental conditions. The results were clear. The patients varied their symptomatic "communications" to fit their objectives of staying in the hospital and keeping their open-ward privileges. For the discharge condition, they appeared "crazy," and for the open-ward evaluation condition, they appeared intact and organized.

Some researchers have investigated whether the aim of schizophrenic symptoms is to avoid emotional warmth or self-disclosure. Shimkunas (228) found support for the avoidance of intimacy hypothesis, whereas Levy (229) found both factors applicable. He found that individuals with paranoid schizophrenia were most likely to emit bizarre symptoms when threatened by mutual intimacy.

Depression

Depressive symptoms have been associated with communications regarding self-degradation, helplessness, and hopelessness. Somewhat different views have been found regarding the message in depressions. One view is that they signify a learned negative self-appraisal, part of a negative cognitive set: "I am helpless, worthless, and hopeless" (230, 231). In this view, depressive symptoms are not instrumental responses but rather are response deficits, or learned maladaptive reactions, and the downward depressive spiral is not due to interaction and communication with others. In another view, Greenwald (232) and Hill (233) state that depressive symptoms are instrumental responses; they are interpersonal maneuvers aimed at influencing self and significant others— promotive forms of expression. The depressive symptoms proclaim, "Help me, tell me I am not as bad as I think." In this view, the presentations of worthlessness, hopelessness, and helplessness are indirect statements of need. The individual does not directly communicate his or her need or reaction to not receiving fulfillment of that need. Anger and reproach for loss or removal of love and support are indirectly communicated by the overt display

before others of suffering, helplessness, and sadness, and by insistently not asking for anything. The message is "You can see how helpless I feel; if you care you will help me, stay with me, appreciate my suffering."

A third view, also taking an interpersonal approach, is that the pattern of repetitive depressive behavior without receptivity to feedback from others conveys mistrust to the help providers, contributes to the erosion of the helping relationship, and ultimately supports the depressive individual's negative world view. This pattern of communication with caretakers thus serves to maintain and amplify the patient's depressive spiral (224). Coyne (234) sees lack of relevant social skills as contributing to maintenance of the depressive spiral.

Therapeutic Implications

In the conduct of the initial interview, certain factors should be taken into consideration in order to most effectively decipher the social communication of symptoms. At the outset one can divide the task into two parts: (a) decoding the manifest content of the message (symptom), and (b) decoding the metacommunication regarding the relationship to the receiver. For example, in the case of the hysterical paralysis cited earlier, the manifest content is the complaint of painful facial paralysis. This content is a repetitive analogical presentation of the experience of psychological attack, namely, that of being insulted. The message conveyed is more than "I am sick"; it is also "I am in pain and am hurt." At a less obvious level, the symptom represents "having been slapped" and signifies, on a metacommunication level, "I will be passive, self-effacing, and masochistic in our relationship, allowing you to attack me, but not letting you forget when you hurt me." The prime source of information on the metacommunication is the reaction of the significant other to the symptom. The focus is less on content and more on relationship. In the case mentioned the husband becomes solicitous.

In order to decipher the underlying meaning of the social communication in a symptom, it is necessary to establish temporal and contextual social facts. Important considerations are (a) the setting, (b) the social group context (family, friends, group, and so forth), (c) the specific target person or persons to whom the symptom is directed, (d) the nature of the past relationship with the target person, and (e) the reaction of the significant others to the symptom. The last point is central to understanding the social significance of the symptoms. In most circumstances the symptom cannot be understood without reference to the social group in which it is manifested.

In all social groups the individuals learn to form specific interpersonal arrangements as a means of making their social world predictable and secure. The pursuit of system stability is embodied in a number of concepts, such as norms, contracts, and games. Extreme efforts at retaining or regaining stable patterns of interpersonal relationships are identified as fraudulent contracts (217). Symptoms are such fraudulent contracts. The role of contextual factors in understanding the social communication in symptoms is presented in Jackson's (235) concept of family homeostasis, wherein symptoms, or self-defeating behaviors, play an essential part in the maintenance of stability within a disturbed family system. Rosman et al. (236) describe how an adolescent girl could defy, manipulate, and defeat her powerful parents with her anorexic symptoms. With the use of a treatment technique developed by Minuchin (237), the Family Lunch Session, the problem was translated from the psychosomatic symptom to one of interpersonal relationships. The therapy took the "symptomatic" child out of the spotlight and obliged the parents to disengage from using the symptom as a "conflict-detouring device." In her anorexic behavior, the girl acts as if she is powerless in her defiance of her parents. She does not have to say that she will disobey their unreasonable demands and thereby face their unreasonable retribution; she stops eating and becomes "ill." She gains a degree of autonomy only when the intent of her behavior is disguised and disowned. By eating together, the symptomatic communication very quickly becomes accessible to observation as an interpersonal communication. The therapist can "deoralize" the symptom, transforming it by his or her comments from an eating problem to an interpersonal one. The family that maintained homeostasis by using this symptom as a detour from significant conflicts is now obliged to face the actual issues.

In some cases, the essential social group is the dyad, such as a marital pair. Individual symptoms in a marriage are often adaptations to an intolerable dyadic situation that the partners are unable to discuss. A case example cited by Freud (238) fits this analysis very well. It also presents data for divergent interpretations. In "The Disposition to Obsessional Neurosis," Freud describes a patient who fell ill when she learned that it was impossible for her to have any children by her husband, whom she loved very much. After rejecting fantasies of being sexually seduced, which could fulfill her wish for a child, she reacted with anxiety hysteria. In Freud's own words:

She now did all she could to prevent her husband from guessing that she had fallen ill owing to the frustration of which he was the cause. But I have good reason for asserting that everyone possesses in his own unconscious an instrument with which he can interpret the utterances of the unconscious of other people. Her husband understood, without any admission or explanation on her part, what his wife's anxiety meant; he felt hurt without showing it, and in turn reacted neurotically by—for the first time—failing in sexual intercourse with her. Immediately afterwards he started on a journey. His wife believed he had become permanently impotent, and produced her first obsessional symptoms on the day before his expected return.

In this example, Freud suggested than an unconscious communication existed between the marital partners. An interpersonal analysis would not need to introduce the concept of an "unconscious instrument" to explain such symptomatic behavior. Rather, it would stress the avoidance by both partners of an intolerable situation that they could not discuss. In all likelihood the fear was that discussion would lead to irreparable damage in the relationship.

Let us consider another example of marital conflict. Haley (226) cites the example of a wife who developed obsessive hand washing that effectively contravened the dominating behavior of her rigid and authoritarian husband. Once she engaged in her obsessive hand washing, he was obliged to respond according to the rules of the sickness game. When he wanted to dominate her, this symptom could control his behavior. He could not, however, assign responsibility to her for such behavior. The metacommunication to her husband was "I am not opposed to doing what you wish, but I cannot help not complying with this wish due to my symptoms." The husband's reaction indicated that he could accept the wife's failure to submit under the conditions dictated by symptomatic communication. However, he could not accept direct, overt, and open expression of such an intention. One can see that the husband rewards indirect (symptomatic) communication and punishes direct communication. The problem is obviously not the wife's alone.

The temporal history of the symptom is essential to understanding its communication value. If the symptom is acute, we assume the purpose of the communication is to react against a recent change, to restore a previous equilibrium. One is thus led to ask what recent changes in interpersonal relationships have occurred.

In the context of chronic symptoms, however, some special additional condition must have occurred in order for the social group or the individual to press for change. Often what is new is a violent or aggressive threat to person or property in the social group (153, 239).

The acute–chronic distinction has important implications for making effective treatment plans. A paradox of chronic symptomatology that has a profound effect on treatment is that the social group usually does not want the symptoms to change. A number of clinicians have commented on this issue in the conduct of family therapy with disturbed adolescents. With improvement in the disordered behavior of the adolescent, the family often undermines this kind of change. The parents may not be able to tolerate each other without a helpless child at home. The adolescent's symptoms serve to maintain the family's disturbed equilibrium. Some clinicians such as Erickson, as noted by Haley (240), make a concerted effort when dealing with the parents of adolescents to treat the parents concurrently.

SUMMARY

I have attempted in this chapter to synthesize from psychiatry, psychology, sociology, and anthropology a sociocultural approach to understanding and dealing with the psychiatric outpatient. One major purpose is to call to the clinician's attention the "outer" social reality of the patient. Clinicians, I propose, will find their work more satisfying and effective when they integrate the sociocultural along with the psychodynamic, behavioral, and biologic data. Selection of material for this chapter was based on clinical need and relevance. Three areas were selected for review: the development of mental disorder, the process of becoming a patient, and the social communication value carried by symptoms. Chapter 7 proposes five sociocultural hypotheses for the clinical interview based on the material presented in this chapter.

References

1. Bell NW, Spiegel JP: Social psychiatry: vagaries of a term. *Arch Gen Psychiatry* 11:373–345, 1966.
2. Rennie TAC: Social psychiatry—a definition. *Int J Soc Psychiatry* 1:5–13, 1955.
3. Al-Issa I: Social and cultural aspects of hallucinations. *Psychol Bull* 84:570–587, 1977.
4. Wallace AFC: Anthropology and psychiatry. In Freedman AM, Kaplan HI, Sadock BJ (eds): *Com-*

prehensive Textbook of Psychiatry II. Baltimore, Williams & Wilkins 1975, vol 1, pp 336–373.

5. Thomas CS, Bergen BJ: Social psychiatric view of psychological misfunction and role of psychiatry in social change. *Arch Gen Psychiatry* 12:539–544, 1965.

6. Faris REL, Dunham HW: *Mental Disorders in Urban Areas: An Ecological Study of Schizophrenia and Other Psychoses.* Chicago, University of Chicago Press, 1939.

7. Leighton AH: *My Name is Legion. Volume I. The Stirling County Study of Psychiatric Disorder and Sociocultural Environment.* New York, Basic Books, 1959.

8. Srole L, Langner TS, Opler MK, et al: *Mental Health in the Metropolis: The Midtown Study.* New York, McGraw-Hill, 1962, vol 1.

9. Holmes TH, Rahe RH: The Social Readjustment Rating Scale. *J Psychosom Res* 11:213–218, 1967.

10. Brown GW, Birley JL: Crises and life changes and the onset of schizophrenia. *J Health Soc Behav* 9:203–214, 1968.

11. Caplan G: *Support Systems and Community Mental Health.* New York, Behavioral Publications, 1974.

12. Weiss RS: Transition states and other stressful situations: their nature and programs for their management. In Caplan G, Killilea M (eds): *Support Systems and Mutual Help: Multi-disciplinary Explorations.* New York, Grune and Stratton, 1976, pp 213–232.

13. House JS: *Work Stress and Social Support.* Reading MA, Addison-Wesley, 1981.

14. Thoits PA: Conceptual, methodological, and theoretical problems in studying social support as a buffer against life stress. *J Health Soc Behav* 23:145–159, 1982.

15. Selye H: *The Stress of Life.* New York, McGraw-Hill, 1956.

16. Dohrenwend BP, Dohrenwend BS: Social and cultural influences on psychopathology. *Annu Rev Psychol* 25:417–452, 1974.

17. Zubin J, Spring B: Vulnerability—a new view of schizophrenia. *J Abnorm Soc Psychol* 86:103–126, 1977.

18. Mechanic D: Invited commentary on self, social environment and stress. In Appley MH, Trumbull R (eds): *Psychological Stress.* New York, Appleton-Century-Crofts, 1967, pp 199–202.

19. French AP, Steward MS: Adaptation and affect. Towards a synthesis of Piagetian and psychoanalytic psychologies. *Perspect Biol Med* 18:464–474, 1975.

20. Parkes CM: Psycho-social transitions: a field for study. *Soc Sci Med* 5:101–115, 1971.

21. Meyer A: The life chart and the obligation of specifying positive data in psychopathological diagnosis. In Winters EE (ed): *The Collected Papers of Adolph Meyer. Volume III. Medical Teachings.* Baltimore, Johns Hopkins University Press, 1951, pp 52–56.

22. Dohrenwend BS, Krasnoff L, Askenasy AR, et al: Exemplification of a method for scaling life events: the PERI life events scale. *J Health Soc Behav* 19:205–229, 1978.

23. Ilfeld FW Jr: Characteristics of current social stressors. *Psychol Rep* 39:1231–1247, 1976.

24. Brown GW, Harris TO: *Social Origins of Depression.* New York, Free Press, 1978.

25. Lazarus RS, Launier R: Stress-related transactions between person and environment. In Pervin LA, Lewis M (eds).: *Perspectives in Interactional Psychology.* New York, Plenum Press, 1978, pp 287–327.

26. Lazarus RS, Folkman S: Stress, Appraisal and Coping. New York, Springer, 1984.

27. Antonovsky A: Breakdown: a needed fourth step in the conceptual armamentarium of modern medicine. *Soc Sci Med* 6:537–544, 1972.

28. Gunderson EKE, Rahe RH: Life Stress and Illness. Springfield, IL, Charles C. Thomas, 1974.

29. Myers JK, Lindenthal JJ, Pepper MP: Life events and psychiatric impairment. *J Nerv Ment Dis* 152:149–157, 1971.

30. Janis IL: *Air War and Emotional Stress.* New York, McGraw-Hill, 1951.

31. Thoits PA: Dimensions of life events that influence psychological distress: an evaluation and synthesis of the literature. In Kaplan HB (ed): *Psychosocial Stress: Trends in Theory and Research.* New York, Academic, 1983, pp 33–103.

32. Silver RL, Wortman CB: Coping with undesirable life events. In Garber J, Seligman MEP (eds): *Human Helplessness: Theory and Applications.* New York, Academic, 1980, pp 279–375.

33. Gersten JC, Langner TS, Eisenberg JG, et al: Child behavior and life events: undesirable change or change per se? In Dohrenwend BS, Dohrenwend BP (eds): *Stressful Life Events: Their Nature and Effects.* New York, John Wiley & Sons, 1974, pp 159 170.

34. Vinokur A, Selzer ML: Desirable versus undesirable life events: their relationship to stress and mental distress. *J Pers Soc Psychol* 32:329–337, 1975.

35. Paykel ES, Myers JK, Dienelt MN, et al: Life events and depression: a controlled study. *Arch Gen Psychiatry* 21:753–760, 1969.

36. Ilfeld FW Jr: Current social stressors and symptoms of depression. *AM J Psychiatry* 134:161–166, 1977.

37. Wyler AR, Masuda M, Holmes TH: Magnitude of life events and seriousness of illness. *Psychosom Med* 22:115–122, 1971.

38. Fontana AF, Marcus JL, Noes B, et al: Prehospitalization coping styles of the psychiatric patients: the goal directedness of life events. *J Nerv Ment Dis* 155:311–321, 1972.

39. Morrice JKW: Life crisis, social diagnosis and social therapy. *Br J Psychiatry* 125:411–413, 1974.

40. Uhlenhuth EH, Paykel ES: Symptom intensity and life events. *Arch Gen Psychiatry* 28:473–477, 1973.

41. Zilboorg G: Differential diagnostic types of suicide. *Arch Neurol Psychiatry* 35:270–291, 1936.

42. Bowlby J: *Maternal Care and Mental Health.* New York, Schocken Books, 1952.

43. Bronfenbrenner U: Early deprivation in animals and man. In Newton G (ed): *Early Experience and Behavior*. Springfield IL, Charles C. Thomas, 1968, pp 627–664.

44. Sullivan HS: Preadolescence. In Perry HS, Gawel ML (eds): *The Interpersonal Theory of Psychiatry*. New York, WW Norton, 1953, pp 245–262.

45. Paykel ES: Recent life events in the developments of the depressive disorders. In Depue RA (ed): *The Psychobiology of the Depressive Disorders: Implications of the Effects of Stress*. New York, Academic Press, 1979, vol 22, pp 245–262.

46. Parkes CM: Effects of bereavement on physical and mental health—a study of the medical records of widows. *Br Med J* 2:274–279, 1964.

47. Parkes CM: Unexpected and untimely bereavement: a statistical study of young Boston widows and widowers. In Schoenberg B, Gerber I, Wiener A, et al (eds): *Bereavement: Its Psychosocial Aspects*. New York, Columbia University Press, 1975, pp 119–138.

48. Parkes CM, Weiss RS: *Recovery from Bereavement*. New York, Basic Books, 1983.

49. Leff JJ, Roatch JF, Bunney WE Jr: Environmental factors preceding the onset of severe depression. *Psychiatry* 33:293–311, 1970.

50. Rosenbaum M, Najenson T: Changes in life patterns and symptoms of low mood as reported by wives of severely brain injured soldiers. *J Consult Clin Psychol* 44:881–888, 1976.

51. Bart PB: The sociology of depression. In Roman PM, Trice HM (eds): *Explorations in Psychiatric Sociology*. Philadelphia, F. A. Davis, 1974, pp 139–157.

52. Bebbington PE: Psychosocial etiology of schizophrenia and affective disorder. In Michels R (ed): *Psychiatry*. New York, Lippincott, 1985, pp 1–22.

53. Paykel ES: Recent life events and clinical depression. In Gunderson EKE, Rahe RH (eds): *Life Stress and Illness*. Springfield, IL, Charles C. Thomas, 1974, pp 134–163.

54. Mueller DP: Social networks: a promising direction for research on the relationship of the social environment to psychiatric disorder. *Soc Sci Med* 14A:147–51, 1980.

55. Levy RL: Social support and compliance: a selective review and critique of treatment integrity and outcome measurement. *Soc Sci Med* 17(8): 1329–1338, 1983.

56. Heller K, Swindle R: Social networks, perceived social support and coping with stress. In Felner RD, Jason LA, Moritsugu J, et al (eds): *Prevention Psychology: Theory, Research and Practice in Community Intervention*. New York, Pergamon, 1983, Farber SS (eds) pp 87–103.

57. Parry G: Paid employment, life events, social support and mental health in working-class mothers. *J Health Soc Behav* 27:193–208, 1986.

58. Durkheim E: *Suicide: A Study in Sociology* (Spaulding J, Simpson G, trans.), New York, Free Press, 1951 (first published 1897).

59. Dunham HW: Society, culture and mental disorder. *Arch Gen Psychiatry* 33:147–156, 1976.

60. Gruenberg EM: Socially shared psychopathology. In Leighton AH, Clausen JA, Wilson RN (eds): *Explorations in Social Psychiatry*. New York, Basic Books, 1957, pp 201–229.

61. Murphy JM: Social causes: the independent variables. In Kaplan BH, Wilson RN, Leighton AH (eds): *Further Explorations in Social Psychiatry*. New York, Basic Books, 1976, pp 386–506.

62. Leighton AH, Lambo TA, Hughes CC, et al *Psychiatric Disorder Among the Yoruba*. New York, Cornell University Press, 1963.

63. Jaco EG: The social isolation hypothesis and schizophrenia. *Am Sociol Rev* 19:567–577, 1954.

64. Hare EH: Mental illness and social conditions in Bristol. *J Ment Sci* 102:349–357, 1956.

65. Kohn ML, Clausen JA: Social isolation and schizophrenia. *Am Sociol Rev* 20:265–273, 1955.

66. Mirsky AF, Duncan CC: Etiology and expression of schizophrenia: neurobiological and psychosocial factors. *Annu Rev Psychol* 37:291–319, 1986.

67. Weiss RS: *Loneliness: The Experience of Emotional and Social Isolation*. Cambridge, MA, MIT Press, 1973.

68. Bexton WH, Heron W, Scott TH: Effects of decreased variation in the sensory environment. *Can J Psychol* 8:70–76, 1954.

69. Lifton RJ: "Thought reform" of Western civilians in Chinese communist prisons. *Psychiatry* 19:173–195, 1956.

70. Derogatis LR, Yevzeroff H, Wittelsberger G: Social class, psychological disorder and the nature of the psychopathologic indicator. *J Consult Clin Psychol* 43:183–191, 1975.

71. Bagley C: Occupational class and symptoms of depression. *Soc Sci Med* 7:327–339, 1973.

72. Kohn ML: Social class and schizophrenia: a critical review and reformulation. In Roman PM, Trice HM (eds): *Explorations in Psychiatric Sociology*. Philadelphia, F. A. Davis, 1974, pp 113–137.

73. Kessler RC, Price HR, Worthman CB: Social factors in psychopathology: the social support and coping process. *Annu Rev Psychol* 36:531–572, 1985.

74. Bernard J: Marital stability and patterns of status variables. *Journal of Marriage and the Family* 28:421–439, 1966.

75. Komorovsky M: *Blue-Collar Marriage*. New York, Random House, 1962.

76. Dunham HW: Theories and hypotheses in social psychiatry: an analysis of the evidence. In Zubin J, Freyham F (eds): *Social Psychiatry*. New York, Grune & Stratton, 1968.

77. Srole L: Social integration and certain corollaries: an exploratory study. *Am Sociol Rev* 21:709–716, 1959.

78. Reinhardt AM, Gary RM: Adjustment to society: interrelations among anomia, social class and psychiatric impairment. In Roman PM, Trice H (eds): *Explorations in Psychiatric Sociology*. Philadelphia, F. A. Davis, 1974, pp 185–207.

79. Silverman C: *The Epidemiology of Depression*. Baltimore, Johns Hopkins University Press, 1968.

80. Huston PE: Psychotic depressive reaction. In Freedman AM, Kaplan HI, Sadock BJ (eds): *Comprehensive Textbook of Psychiatry II*. Baltimore, Williams & Wilkins, 1975, vol 1, pp 1043–1055.

81. Eaton JW, Weil RJ: *Culture and Mental Disorders*. New York, Free Press, 1955.

82. Rose A: A socio-psychological theory of neurosis. In Rose A (ed): *Human Behavior and Social Processes*. Boston, Houghton-Mifflin, 1962, pp 537–549.

83. Yarrow LJ: Separation from Parents during Early Childhood. In Hoffman ML, Hoffman LW (eds): *Review of Child Development Research*. New York, Russell Sage Foundation, 1964, vol 1, pp 89–136.

84. Eisenberg L: The sins of the father: urban decay and social pathology. *Am J Orthopsychiatry* 32:5–17, 1962.

85. Witmer H: *Independent Adoptions*. New York, Russell Sage Foundation, 1963.

86. Mischler E, Waxler N: *Interaction in Families: An Experimental Study of Family Processes and Schizophrenia*. New York, John Wiley & Sons, 1968.

87. Bateson G, Jackson DD, Haley J et al: Toward a theory of schizophrenia. *Behav Sci* 1:251–264, 1956.

88. Lidz T, Fleck S, Cornelison AR, et al: The intrafamilial environment of the schizophrenic patient. II. Marital schism and marital skew. *Am J Psychiatry* 114:241–248, 1957.

89. Wynne LC, Singer MT: Thought disorder and family relations of schizophrenics. II. A classification of forms of thinking. *Arch Gen Psychiatry* 9:199–201, 1963.

90. Arieti S: Recent conceptions and misconceptions of schizophrenia. *Am J Psychother* 14:3–29, 1960.

91. Jacob T: Family interaction in disturbed and normal families: a methodological and substantive review. *Psychol Bull* 82:33–65, 1975.

92. Liem JH: Effects of verbal communications of parents and children: a comparison of normal and schizophrenic families. *J Consult Clin Psychol* 42:438–450, 1974.

93. Goldstein MJ: *The UCLA Family Project*. Presented at the National Institute of Mental Health High-Risk Consortium, San Francisco, 1985.

94. Doane JA, West KL, Goldstein MJ, et al: Parental communication deviance and affective style: predictors of subsequent schizophrenia-spectrum disorders in vulnerable adolescents. *Arch Gen Psychiatry* 38:679–685, 1981.

95. Tienari P, Sorri A, Lahti I, et al: *Interaction of Genetic and Psychosocial Factors in Schizophrenia: The Finnish Adoptive Family Study*. Presented at the National Institute of Mental Health High-Risk Consortium, San Francisco, 1985.

96. Brown GW, Birley JLT, Wing JK: Influences of family life on the course of schizophrenic disorders: A replication. *Br J Psychiatry* 121:241–258, 1972.

97. Vaughn CE, Leff JP: The influence of family and social factors on the course of psychiatric illness: a comparison of schizophrenic and depressed neurotic patients. *Br J Psychiatry* 129:125–137, 1976.

98. Leff JP, Kuipers L, Berkowitz R, et al: A controlled trial of social intervention in schizophrenic families. *Br J Psychiatry* 141:121–134, 1982.

99. Falloon IRH, Boyd JL, McGill CW, et al: Family management in the prevention of exacerbations of schizophrenia: a controlled study. *N Engl J Med* 306:1437–1440, 1982.

100. Leff JP, Kuipers L, Berkowitz R, et al: Life events, relatives' expressed emotion and maintenance neuroleptics in schizophrenic relapse. *Psychol Med* 13:799–806, 1983.

101. Mirsky AF, Silberman EK, Latz A et al: Adult outcomes of high-risk children: differential effects of town and kibbutz rearing. *Schizophr Bull* 11:150–154, 1985.

102. Phillips D: Rejection: a possible consequence of seeking help for mental disorders. *Am Sociol Rev* 28:963–978, 1963.

103. Hammer M: Influence of small social networks as factors in mental hospital admission. *Human Organization* 22:243–251, 1963–1964.

104. Clausen JA, Huffine CL: Sociocultural and social–psychological factors affecting social responses to mental disorder. *J Health Soc Behav* 16:405–420, 1975.

105. Dean A: The social system deviance and treatment efforts. In Kaplan BH, Wilson RN, Leighton AH (eds): *Further Explorations in Social Psychiatry*. New York, Basic Books, 1976, pp 75–93.

106. Sampson H, Messinger SL, Towne RD: Family processes and becoming a mental patient. *Am J Sociol* 67:88–96, 1962.

107. Cobb S: Social support as a moderator of life stress. *Psychosom Med* 38:300–314, 1976.

108. Weiss RJ, Bergen BJ: Social supports and the reduction of psychiatric disability. *Psychiatry* 31:107–115, 1968.

109. Mechanic D: Stress, illness, and illness behavior. *J Hum Stress* 2:2–6, 1976.

110. Lemkau PB, Crocetti GM: An urban population's opinion and knowledge about mental illness. *Am J Psychiatry* 118:692–700, 1962.

111. Manis JG, Hunt CL, Brawerm MJ, et al: Public and psychiatric conceptions of mental illness. *J Health Hum Behav* 6:48–55, 1965.

112. Wallace AFC: Anthropology and psychiatry. In Freedman AM, Kaplan HI, Sadock BJ (eds): *Comprehensive Textbook of Psychiatry II*. Baltimore, Williams & Wilkins, 1975, vol 1, pp 336–373.

113. Koos E: *The Health of Regionville*. New York, Columbia University Press, 1954.

114. Zola JK: Culture and symptoms: an analysis of patients presenting complaints. *Am Sociol Rev* 31:615–630, 1966.

115. Dohrenwend BP, Chin-Shong E, Egri G, et al: Measures of psychiatric disorder in contrasting class and ethnic groups: a preliminary report of on-going research. In Hare EH, Wing JK (eds): *Psychiatric Epidemiology. An International Sympo-*

sium. New York, Oxford University Press, 1970, pp 159–202.

116. Farina A, Felner R, Boudreau L: Reactions of workers to male and female mental patient job applicants. *J Consult Clin Psychol* 51:363–372, 1973.

117. Cumming E, Cumming J: *Closed Ranks. An Experiment in Mental Health Education*. Cambridge, MA, Harvard University Press, 1957.

118. Crocetti G, Spiro H, Siassi I: *Contemporary Attitudes Towards Mental Health*. Pittsburgh, University of Pittsburgh Press, 1974.

119. Sarbin TR, Mancuso JC: Failure of a moral enterprise: attitudes of the public toward mental illness. *J Consult Clin Psychol* 35:159–173, 1970.

120. D'Arcy C, Brockman J: Changing public recognition of psychiatric symptoms? Blackfoot revisited. *J Health Soc Behav* 17:302–310, 1976.

121. Blackwell BL: Upper middle class adult expectations about the sick role for physical and psychiatric dysfunctions. *J Health Soc Behav* 8:83–95, 1967.

122. Erickson K: Patient role and social uncertainty: a dilemma of the mentally ill. *Psychiatry* 20:263–274, 1957.

123. Cohen J, Struening EL: Opinions about mental illness in the personnel of two large mental hospitals. *J Abnorm Soc Psychol* 64:349–360, 1962.

124. Cox G, Coctango PR, Coci JD: A survey instrument for the accessment of popular conceptions of mental illness. *J Consult Clin Psychol* 44:901–909, 1976.

125. Kadushin C: *Why People Go to Psychiatrists*. New York, Atherton Press, 1969.

126. Calhoun L, Dawes AS, Lewis PM: Correlates of attitudes toward help-seeking in outpatients. *J Consult Clin Psychol* 38:153, 1972.

127. Levinson DJ, Merrifield J, Berg K: Becoming a patient. *Arch Gen Psychiatry* 17:385–406, 1967.

128. Mechanic D: The concept of illness behavior. *J Chron Dis* 15:189–194, 1962.

129. Horwitz A: The pathways into psychiatric treatment: some differences between men and women. *J Health Soc Behav* 18:169–178, 1977.

130. Phillips DL, Segal B: Sexual status and psychiatric symptoms. *Am Sociol Rev* 29:679–187, 1969.

131. Gurin G, Veroff J, Feld S: *Americans View Their Mental Health*. New York, Basic Books, 1960.

132. Lorion RP: Patient and therapist variables in the treatment of low-income patients. *Psychol Bull* 81:344–354, 1974.

133. Overall B, Aronson H: Expectations of psychotherapy in patients of lower socioeconomic class. *Am J Orthopsychiatry* 33: 421–430, 1963.

134. Borghi JH: Premature termination of psychotherapy and patient–therapist expectations. *Am J Psychotherapy* 22:460–473, 1965.

135. Goldstein AP: *Therapist–Patient Expectancies in Psychotherapy*. New York, Pergamon Press, 1962.

136. Frank A, Eisenthal S, Lazare A: Are there social class differences in patients' treatment conceptions? *Arch Gen Psychiatry* 35:61–69, 1978.

137. Lazare A, Cohen F, Jacobson AM et al: The walk-in patient as a 'customer': a key dimension in evaluation and treatment. *Am J Orthopsychiatry* 42:872–883, 1972.

138. Lazare A, Eisenthal S, Wasserman L: The customer approach to patienthood: attending to patient requests in a walk-in clinic. *Arch Gen Psychiatry* 32:553–558, 1975.

139. Eisenthal S, Lazare A: Specificity of patients' requests in the initial interview. *Psychol Rep* 38:739–748, 1976.

140. Eisenthal S, Lazare A: Expression of patients' request in the initial interview. *Psychol Rep* 40:131–138, 1977.

141. Lazare A, Eisenthal S, Wasserman L, et al: Patient requests in a walk-in clinic. *Compr Psychiatry* 16:467–477, 1975.

142. Lazare A, Eisenthal S: Patient requests in a walk-in clinic. *J Nerv Ment Dis* 165:330–340, 1977.

143. Cumming E: *Systems of Social Regulation*. New York, Atherton Press, 1968.

144. Hollingshead AB, Redlich FC: *Social Class and Mental Illness: A Community Study*. New York, John Wiley & Sons, 1958.

145. Myers JK, Schaffer L: Social stratification and psychiatric practices: a study of an out-patient clinic. *Am Sociol Rev* 19:307–310, 1954.

146. Caplan G: *Principles of Preventive Psychiatry*. New York, Basic Books, 1964.

147. Lemert EM: *Social Pathology*. New York, McGraw-Hill, 1951.

148. Goffman E: *Asylums: Essays on the Social Situation of Mental Patients and Other Inmates*. Garden City, NY, Doubleday, 1961.

149. Scheff TJ: *Being Mentally Ill: A Sociological Theory*. Chicago, Aldine Publishing, 1966.

150. Mechanic D: *Medical Sociology—A Selective View*. New York, Free Press, 1968.

151. Lemert EM: *Human Deviance, Social Problems and Social Control*. Englewood Cliffs, NJ, Prentice-Hall, 1967.

152. Becker HS: *The Outsiders*. New York, Free Press, 1963.

153. Yarrow MR, Schwartz CG, Murphy HS, et al: The psychological meaning of mental illness in the family. *J Soc Issues* 11:12–24, 1955.

154. Fletcher CR, Manning PK, Reynolds LT, et al: The labeling theory and mental illness. In Roman PM, Trice HM (eds): *Explorations in Psychiatric Sociology*. Philadelphia, F. A. Davis, 1974, pp 43–62.

155. Gove WR: The labeling versus psychiatric exploration of mental illness: a debate that has become substantively irrelevant. *J Health Soc Behav* 20:301–304, 1979.

156. Weinstein RM: Labeling theory and attitudes of mental patients: a review. *J Health Med Behav* 24:70 –84, 1983.

157. Gove W: Societal reaction as an explanation of mental illness: an evaluation. *Am Sociol Rev* 35:873–884, 1970.

158. Doherty EG: Labeling effect in psychiatric hospitalization. *Arch Gen Psychiatry* 32:562–568, 1975.

159. Page S: Effects of the mental illness label in attempts to obtain accommodation. *Canadian Journal of Behavioral Science* 9:85–90, 1977.

160. Sartorius N, Jablensky A, Shapiro R: Cross cultural differences in the short-term prognosis of schizophrenic psychoses. *Schizophr Bull* 4:102–113, 178.

161. Wittkower ED, Dubreuil G: Psychocultural stress in relation to mental illness. *Soc Sci Med* 7:691–704, 1973.

162. Parsons A: Some comparative observations on ward social structure: Southern Italy, England and the United States. *Review and Newsletter: Transcultural Research in Mental Health Problems.* 10:65–67, 1961.

163. Asai T: The contents of delusions of schizophrenic patients in Japan: comparison between periods 1941–1961. *Transcultural Psychiatric Research* 1:27–28, 1964.

164. Mendels J: *Concepts of Depression.* New York, John Wiley & Sons, 1970.

165. Cohen YA: *Social Structures and Personality.* New York, Holt, Rinehart & Winston, 1961.

166. Murphy HBM, Wittkower ED, Chance NA: Crosscultural inquiry into the symptomatology of depression: a preliminary report. *Int J Psychiatry* 3:6–22, 1967.

167. Collomb H: Assistance psychiatrique en Afrique: experience Senegalaise. *Psychopathol Africaine* 1:11–84, 1965.

168. Field MJ: *Search for Security: An Ethno-Psychiatric Study of Rural Ghana.* Evanston, IL, Northwestern University Press, 1960.

169. Wolf I, Chafetz ME, Blane HT et al: Social factors in the diagnosis of alcoholism. *Q J Stud Alcohol* 26:72–79, 1965.

170. Sandifer MG, Hordern A, Timbury GC, et al: Psychiatric diagnosis: a comparative study in North Carolina, London and Glasgow. *Br J Psychiatry* 114:1–9, 1968.

171. Cooper JE, Kendell RE, Gurland BJ, et al: Cross-national study of diagnosis of the mental disorder: some results from the first comparative investigation. *Am J Psychiatry* 125:Supplement 21–29, 1969.

172. Katz MM, Cole JO, Lowery HA: Studies of the diagnostic process: the influence of symptoms perception, past experience, and ethnic background on diagnostic decisions. *Am J Psychiatry* 125:937–947, 1969.

173. Kramer M: Some problems for international research suggested by observations on differences in first admission rates to mental hospitals of England and Wales and of the United States. In *Proceedings of the Third World Congress of Psychiatry.* Toronto/Montreal, University of Toronto Press/McGill University Press, 1961, vol 3, pp 153–160.

174. Edwards G: Diagnosis of schizophrenia: an Anglo-American comparison. *Br J Psychol* 120:385–390, 1972.

175. Strauss JS: Hallucinations and delusions as points on continua function. *Arch Gen Psychiatry* 21:581–586, 1969.

176. Zigler E, Phillips L: Psychiatric diagnosis and symptomatology. *J Abnorm Soc Psychol* 63:69–75, 1961.

177. Harford TC: *Some Notes on the Development of a Contextual Drinking Model.* Presented at National Institute of Alcohol Abuse Workshop on Conceptual and Methodological Aspects of Drinking Contexts. Washington, DC, 1978.

178. Hanna EZ: *Towards a Contextual Understanding of the Development of Problem Drinking.* Presented at National Institute of Alcohol Abuse Workshop on Conceptual and Methodological Aspects of Drinking Contexts. Washington, DC, 1978.

179. Antaki C, Brewin C (eds): *Attributions and Psychological Change: Application of Attributional Theories to Clinical and Educational Practice.* London, Academic Press, 1982.

180. Rosenthal D, Frank JD: The fate of psychiatric clinic outpatients assigned to psychotherapy. *J Nerv Ment Dis* 127:330–343, 1958.

181. Schaffer L, Myers JK: Psychotherapy and social stratification. An empirical study of practice in a psychiatric outpatient clinic. *Psychiatry* 17:83–93, 1954.

182. Robinson HA, Redlich FC, Myers JK: Social structure and psychiatric treatment. *Am J Orthospsychiatry* 24:307–416, 1954.

183. Baekeland F, Lundwall L: Dropping out of treatment: a critical review. *Psychol Bull* 82:738–783, 1975.

184. Meltzoff J, Kornreich M: *Research in Psychotherapy.* Chicago/New York, Adeline Publishing Co./Atherton Press, 1970.

185. Hollingshead AB: *Elmtown's Youth.* New York, John Wiley & Sons, 1949.

186. Kluckhohn FR: Dominant and Varient Value Orientations. In Kluckhohn C, Murray HA, Schneider DM (eds): *Personality in Nature: Society and Culture.* New York, Alfred A. Knopf, 1956, pp 342–357.

187. Papajohn J, Spiegel J: *Transactions in Families.* San Francisco, Jossey-Bass, 1975.

188. Heine RW, Trossman H: Initial expectations of the doctor–patient interaction as a factor in the continuance of psychotherapy. *Psychiatry* 23:275–278, 1960.

189. Aronson H, Overall B: Treatment expectations of patients in two social classes. *Soc Work* 11:35–42, 1966.

190. Williams HV, Lipman RS, Uhlenhuth EH, et al: Some factors influencing the treatment expectations of anxious neurotic outpatients. *J Nerv Ment Dis* 145:208–220, 1967.

191. Garfield SL: Research on client variables in psychotherapy. In Bergin AE, Garfield S (eds): *Handbook of Psychotherapy and Behavior Change.* New York, John Wiley & Sons, 1971, pp 271–298.

192. Goldstein AP: *Psychotherapeutic Attraction.* New York, Pergamon Press, 1971.

193. Goldstein AP: *Structured Learning Therapy. Toward a Psychotherapy for the Poor.* New York, Academic Press, 1973.

194. Orne MI, Wender PH: Anticipatory socialization for psychotherapy: method and rationale. *Am J Psychiatry* 124:1202–1212, 1968.

195. Strupp HH, Jenkins JJ: The development of six motion pictures simulating psychotherapeutic situations. *J Nerv Ment Dis* 136:317–328, 1963.

196. Jacobs D: Preparation for treatment of the disadvantaged patient: affects on disposition and outcome. *Am J Orthopsychiatry* 42:667–674, 1972.

197. Lazarus AA: *Clinical Behavior Therapy.* New York, Brunner Mazel, 1972.

198. Kandel D: Status homophily, social context, and participation in psychotherapy. *Am J Sociol* 71:640–650, 1966.

199. Baum OE, Feltzer SB, D'zmura FL, et al: Psychotherapy, dropouts and lower socioeconomic patients. *Am J Orthopsychiatry* 36:629–635, 1966.

200. Normand WC, Fensterhelm H, Schrenzel S: A systematic approach to brief therapy for patients in a low socioeconomic community. *Community Ment Health J* 3:349–354, 1967.

201. Foucault M: *Madness and Civilization.* New York, Pantheon, 1965.

202. Folta Jr, Schatzman L: Trends in public urban psychiatry in the United States. *Social Problems* 16:60–72, 1968.

203. Bart PB: Ideologies and utopias of psychotherapy. In Roman PM, Trice HM (eds): *The Sociology of Psychotherapy.* New York, Jason Aronson, 1974, pp 9–57.

204. Duhl L: What mental health services are needed for the poor? *Psychiatr Res Rep* 21:72–78, 1967.

205. Geiger HJ: Of the poor, by the poor, or for the poor: the mental health implications of social contact of poverty programs. *Psychiatr Res Rep* 21:55–71, 1967.

206. Lindemann E: Symptomatology and management of acute grief. *Am J Psychiatry* 101:141–148, 1944.

207. Fried M: Grieving for a lost home. In Duhl LF (ed): *The Urban Condition.* New York, Basic Books, 1963, pp 151–171.

208. Kelly JG, Snowden LR, Munoz RF: Social and community interventions. *Annu Rev Psychol* 28:303–361, 1977.

209. Jacobson DE: Types and timing of social support. *J Health Soc Behav* 27:250–264, 1986.

210. Klerman GL, Weissman MM, Rounsaville BJ, et al: *Interpersonal Psychotherapy of Depression.* New York, Basic Books, 1984.

211. Weissman MM, Klerman GL, Rounsaville BJ, et al: Short-term interpersonal psychotherapy (IPT) for depression: description and efficacy. In Anchin TC, Keisler DJ (eds): *Handbook of Interpersonal Psychotherapy.* New York, Pergamon Press, 1982.

212. Waxler NE: Culture and mental illness: a social labeling perspective. *J Nerv Ment Dis* 159:379–395, 1974.

213. Breuer J, Freud S: Studies on hysteria. In Strachey J, Freud A (eds): *Standard Edition of the Complete Psychological Works of Sigmund Freud.* London, Hogarth Press, 1955, vol 2, pp 3–17.

214. Szasz TD: *The Myth of Mental Illness. Foundations of a Theory of Personal Conduct.* New York, Harper & Brothers, 1961.

215. Parsons T: Definitions of health and illness in the light of American values and social structure. In Jaco EG (ed): *Patients, Physicians, and Illness.* Glencoe, IL, Free Press, 1958, pp 165–187.

216. Goffman E: *The Presentation of Self in Everyday Life.* Garden City, NY, Doubleday, 1959.

217. Carson RC: *Interaction Concepts of Personality.* Chicago, Aldine Publishing, 1969.

218. Sarbin TR: On the futility of the proposition that some people should be labeled "mentally ill." *J Clin Consult Psychol* 31:447–453, 1967.

219. Adams HB: "Mental illness" or interpersonal behavior? *Am Psychol* 19:191–197, 1964.

220. Farberow NL, Schneidman ES: *The Cry for Help.* New York, McGraw-Hill, 1961.

221. Weiss JMA: The gamble with death in attempted suicide. *Psychiatry* 20:17–25, 1957.

222. Rudestam KE: Stockholm and Los Angeles: a cross-cultural study of the communication of suicidal intent. *J Consult Clin Psychol* 36:82–96, 1971.

223. Cowgell VG: Interpersonal effects of a suicidal communication. *J Consult Clin Psychol* 45:592–599, 1977.

224. McPartland TS, Hornstra RK: The depressive datum. *Compr Psychiatry* 5:253–261, 1964.

225. Moss L, Hamilton DM: The psychotherapy of the suicidal patient. *Am J Psychiatry* 112:814–820, 1956.

226. Haley JJ: *Strategies of Psychotherapy.* New York, Grune & Stratton, 1963.

227. Braginsky BH, Braginsky DD: Schizophrenic patients in the psychiatric interview: an experimental study of their effectiveness at manipulation. *J Consult Psychol* 31:543–547, 1967.

228. Schimkunas AM: Demand for intimate self-disclosure and pathological verbalization in schizophrenia. *J Abnorm Psychol* 80:197–205, 1972.

229. Levy SM: Schizophrenia symptomatology: reaction or strategy? A study of contextual antecedents. *J Abnorm Psychol* 85:435–445, 1976.

230. Seligman ME: *Helplessness: On Depression, Development, and Death.* San Francisco, W. H. Freeman, 1975.

231. Beck AT: *Depression: Clinical, Experimental and Theoretical Aspects.* New York, Paul B. Hoeber, 1967.

232. Greenwald H: Depression and an interpersonal maneuver. *Journal of Contemporary Psychology* 2:110–116, 1970.

233. Hill D: Depression: disease, reaction or posture. *Am J Psychiatry* 125:37–49, 1968.

234. Coyne JC: Toward an interpersonal description of depression. *Psychiatry* 39:28–40, 1976.

235. Jackson DD: The question of family homeostatis. *Psychiatr Q* (Suppl) 31:79–90, 1957.

236. Rosman BL, Minuchin S, Liebman R: Family lunch session: an introduction to family therapy in anorexia nervosa. *Am J Orthopsychiatry* 45:846–853, 1975.

237. Minuchin S: *Anorexia Nervosa: Interaction Around the Family Table.* Presented to the Institute for Juvenile Research, Chicago, IL, 1971.

238. Freud S: The Disposition to Obsessional Neuro-sis, in Strachey J, Freud A (eds): *Standard Edition of the Complete Psychological Works of Sigmund Freud.* London, Hogarth Press, 1958, vol 12, pp 1911–1913.

239. Lowenthal MF: *Lives in Distress: The Path of the Elderly to the Psychiatric Ward.* New York, Basic Books, 1964.

240. Haley J: *Uncommon Therapy—The Psychiatric Techniques of Milton H. Erickson, M.D.* New York, W. W. Norton & Co., 1973.

7

Clinical Hypothesis Testing[a]

Aaron Lazare, M.D.

This chapter attempts to integrate the previous five chapters on the multidimensional approach for application to clinical practice. Two concepts central to this clinical integration shall be presented: (a) the application of a closed system of hypotheses to formulate the patient's problem and (b) the clinical process of hypothesis testing.

THE INTERVIEW AS HYPOTHESIS TESTING

Clinicians initially learn the techniques of interviewing and assessment by collecting and recording large numbers of observations from patients whom they see over extended periods of time. The data are then organized in some fashion such as chief complaint, present illness, family history, developmental history, sexual history, occupational history, medical history, and mental status examination. Finally, the clinician sorts out symptoms, syndromes, and processes in order to establish a diagnosis, formula-

[a] Adapted with permission from Lazare A: The psychiatric examination in the walk-in clinic: hypothesis generation and hypothesis testing. *Arch Gen Psychiatry* 33:96–102, 1976. Copyright 1976, American Medical Association.

tion, or assessment in order to develop a plan for treatment.

As clinicians gain experience, they change their interview strategies from the collection and assimilation of large amounts of data to the generation and testing of various hypotheses. This enables them to make rapid decisions and provide competent care for more patients per unit of time. This skill is particularly useful in ambulatory settings such as walk-in clinics, emergency settings, health maintenance organizations, community mental health centers, and busy private practices. In these settings, clinicians must decide, within a limited amount of time, whether a patient is suicidal, in need of psychotropic agents, in need of hospitalization, can be helped in a few sessions, or has a chronic illness that will require ongoing care.

A growing number of investigators in medicine and psychiatry have demonstrated that during clinical encounters, hypothesis testing is, in fact, an essential aspect of the interview process (1–6). They have observed that the clinician generates a limited number of provisional diagnoses, formulations, or hypotheses that explain, in part, the patient's problem and then suggests a treatment plan. The clinician, by thinking in terms of hypotheses, avoids being bombarded or overloaded with large

103

amounts of unstructured data, an experience shared by all beginners. Each new piece of data can now be considered in terms of its relevance to a limited number of hypotheses under consideration, instead of being one of thousands of possible observations or facts.

T.C. Chamberlin, a geologist, eloquently described in 1890 the importance of working hypotheses in scientific thinking (7). He begins by advocating the use of the *working hypothesis* over the common tendency toward what he calls *ruling theories.* The two differ, Chamberlin maintains, in that "the working hypothesis . . . is used as a means of determining facts, and has for its chief function the suggestion of lines of inquiry; the inquiry being made, not for the sake of the hypothesis but for the sake of facts. Under the method of the ruling theory, the stimulus was directed to the finding of facts for the support of the theory"(7). Chamberlin goes on to advocate the use of multiple working hypotheses to minimize the possibility of reductionistic thinking. Here the effort of the investigator is to "bring up into view every rational explanation of new phenomena, and to develop every tenable hypothesis respecting their cause and history"(7). He goes on to argue that "adequate explanation often involves the co-ordination of several agencies, which enter into the combined result in varying proportions. . . . Such complex explanations of phenomena are specially encouraged by the method of multiple hypotheses, and constitute one of its chief merits. We are so prone to attribute a phenomenon to a single cause, that, when we find an agency present, we are liable to rest satisfied therewith, and fail to recognize that it is but one factor, and per chance a minor factor, in the accomplishment of the total result."

In psychiatric practice, clinicians bring to the interview partial formulations based on their previous experience. A formulation is defined here as a concept that organizes, explains, or makes clinical sense out of large amounts of data and influences treatment decisions. These concepts include syndromes, personality styles, social situations, and behavioral conditions. Such concepts may be apples and oranges, but they do represent clusters of information that clinicians find useful in understanding patients. In Weisman's terms, "This is the nature of communication between people—to operate on many levels at once with different words, different objects, and different meaning" (2). These concepts are partial formulations, because any one alone is insufficient to provide adequate understanding of any given patient. In the process of bringing these partial formulations to the interview for consideration, they become hypotheses to be tested.

A CLOSED SYSTEM OF CLINICAL HYPOTHESES

Two problems immediately arise in applying the clinical approach described above to the psychiatric interview. The first is that in considering a few hypotheses usually generated early in the interview, the clinician may come to premature closure, thereby ignoring more relevant hypotheses. The second is that given the rich and varied data and theoretical approaches that are available, there could be an unmanageable number of possible hypotheses or ways of organizing the data. A solution to both problems would be the development of a manageable list of hypothesized partial formulations based on current psychiatric knowledge that would organize most of the observations that might relate to decision making. The entire range of hypotheses could then be considered, at least briefly, during each interview. The composition of such a list might vary with the clinical setting and would undoubtedly change with advances in the field.

This chapter presents 20 clinical hypotheses that my colleagues and I have found useful in evaluating and treating patients in our outpatient practices. They are described under the four major headings referred to in Chapters 2 through 6: biologic syndromal, psychodynamic, sociocultural, and behavioral. The rationale for the joining of the biologic and syndromal hypotheses is described in Chapters 3 and 8. This joining does not mean that *Diagnostic and Statistical Manual of Mental Disorders (Third Edition-Revised)* (DSM-III-R) diagnoses are necessarily best explained by biologic pro cesses or that biologic phenomena necessarily produce clinical phenomena that are syndromal.

In any clinical situation, several partial formulations will usually be necessary to approach a comprehensive understanding of the patient's problem. For example, the syndromal hypothesis of conversion disorder is a partial formulation or "diagnosis" for a given patient. Add to this the sociocultural formulation of the symptom as social communication, the psychodynamic formulation of a symptom as a manifestation of unresolved grief (identification with the symptom of the deceased), and the behavioral formulation of conditions that reinforce the presenting symptom. These additional partial formulations provide the clinician with considerably more power to understand and treat the patient. According to this approach, several clinical hypotheses can be confirmed for a given patient even in the absence of a DSM-III-R diagnosis.

The clinical integrative approach described above is consistent with that described by McHugh and Slavney in *The Perspectives of Psychiatry* (8). In their words, "Each construct and explanatory method has its own set of premises, store of facts, and mode of progression. . . . But each must be woven into a comprehensive design in every clinical encounter."

CLINICAL HYPOTHESES (HYPOTHESIZED PARTIAL FORMULATIONS)

The following 20 clinical hypotheses are derived from the four conceptual approaches described in Chapters 2 through 6.

Biologic/Syndromal Hypotheses

1. *The patient's condition can be understood in part as one or more DSM-III-R Axis I disorders.* These include organic mental dis-orders, substance use disorders, sleep disorders, schizophrenia, mood disorders, anxiety disorders, somatoform disorders, dissociative disorders, and others. Many of these syndromes or disorders are discussed in Sections III and IV of this book.

2. *The patient's condition can be understood in part as a DSM-III-R Axis II disorder.* These include paranoid, schizoid, schizotypal, histrionic, narcissistic, antisocial, borderline, avoidant, dependent, obsessive–compulsive, and passive–aggressive personality disorders.

3. *The patient's psychiatric presentation may be caused in part by one or more known organic/medical diseases.* Section III of this book discusses 13 common psychiatric symptoms or behaviors that may be caused by known organic conditions. These include anxiety, depression, manic behavior, disturbances in thinking, perceptual disturbances, disturbances in higher intellectual functions, disturbed motor disturbance, pain, sexual dysfunction, disturbances of sleep and arousal, disturbances of eating and body weight, violent and aggressive behavior, and organic personality syndromes.

4. *The patient's condition and treatment may be affected, in part, by a concomitant physical condition.* Many patients with psychiatric disorders have concomitant physical conditions that may be important in optimal psychological management. These conditions are often overlooked in psychiatric patients. The physical condition is listed in Axis III of DSM-III-R.

5. *The patient's condition is known to be treatable, in part, by psychopharmacologic agents or other biologic treatments.*

Psychodynamic Hypotheses

The five psychodynamic hypotheses that follow must be viewed in the context of which of three psychodynamic models of the mind the clinician believes to be most appropriate for a particular patient: the classical/ego psychological, the object relational, or the self psychology. Chapter 4 describes and distinguishes these three psychodynamic models of the mind.

1. *The patient's problem can be understood, in part, through knowledge of the precipitating event and its psychodynamic meaning.* It is essential to learn the stress or precipitating event (when present) that precedes the onset of symptoms. Simultaneously, one attempts to understand the psychological meaning of the event. Does the event mean to the patient that he or she is now hopeless, weak, powerless, out of control, destructive, bad, a failure, unreal, unloved, alone, attacked, penetrated, damaged, overwhelmed, smothered, ridiculed, humiliated, insulted, cheated, or abandoned? Is the reaction to the precipitation event evidence of a recurrent neurotic theme? Understanding the psychological meaning of the event and sharing this understanding with the patient improves rapport between clinician and patient. In addition, the clinician may now know with considerable specificity the therapeutic work that needs to be done.

2. *The patient's problem can be understood, in part, as a result of unresolved or pathologic grief.* This hypothesis is a variation on the previous one when it is determined, for instance, that the symptoms followed a loss that the patient inadequately mourned. The grief hypothesis is worth considering for several reasons: (*a*) The symptom picture may not follow a discrete stress but may occur after an anniversary of a loss, a holiday, or a minor event symbolizing the loss; (*b*) the symptom picture of unresolved grief often presents as a discreet clinical phenomenon; (*c*) specific methods must be employed to elicit the necessary observations to confirm or refute the hypothesis; and (*d*) there is, in my opinion, a relatively high incidence of patients coming to outpatient treatment for whom unresolved grief is an important issue (see Chapter 32).

3. *The patient's problem can be understood, in part, as a crisis of adult development.* When it is difficult to understand the patient's presentation as a reaction to a discrete event, the problem may be better understood as part of a developmental crisis. Using this approach, the clinician considers the constellation of issues that patients at this age are apt to be struggling with. For instance, a 50-year-old woman may well be struggling simultaneously with menopause, children leaving home, strains in the marital relationship, and the death of a parent. With the development crisis hypothesis in mind, the clinician can elicit specific historical data that may clarify the clinical problem.

4. *The patient's problem can be understood, in part, by an assessment of his or her character or personality.* An understanding of psychodynamic aspects of character may be important in determining developmental deficits, characteristic conflicts, defensive posture, quality of object relations, and the like. Such knowledge can be useful in planning both short- and long-term interventions. This represents a different perspective on personality from the syndromal perspective (see Chapter 35).

5. *The patient's condition is known to be treatable, in part, by psychodynamic therapeutic approaches.* These treatments may be individual, family, or group, and they may be short term or long term.

Sociocultural Hypotheses

1. *The patient's problems can be understood in part by cultural factors.* It is important to consider to what degree cultural factors influence perceptions, beliefs, values, behavioral norms, and expectations that give clues as to the choice, expression, and seriousness of symptomatology. Cultural factors also influence the choice of an attitude toward treatment and even the basic communicative processes between clinician and patient.

2. *The patient's problem can be understood, in part, in terms of the nature and social impact of stressful life events.* The clinician investigates the content, intensity, amount, temporal onset, and duration of stress, noting whether the change is desirable or undesirable, whether it is predicted or unpredicted, and whether there is an entrance or exit from the social field. This analysis helps provide a cognitive map of the patient's social field, thereby helping the patient see his or her reactions as meaningful and somewhat within his or her control.

3. *The patient's problem can be understood in terms of the extent, nature, and accessibility of social support.* The clinician should review members of the patient's social support system, including friends, relatives, working relations, and religious affiliations. The assessment should include the nature of the available social support as well as recent changes in membership or access of the social support system.

4. *The patient's problem can be understood, in part, as a social communication.* The symptom or even the clinic visit can be understood as an attempt to influence or to communicate something to some person, social group, or institution. This hypothesis, like the previous one, can be determined by reviewing the persons or groups in the patient's life space. The questions to ask are, Who wants what from whom, and who is doing what to whom? Sometimes the communication can be discerned by watching the patient with a relative or friend in the waiting room or at a family conference.

5. *The patient's problem is treatable, in part, by social interventions.* These treatments may include interpersonal therapeutic approaches, a supportive therapeutic relationship, family therapy, or intervention with members of the patient's broader social network.

Behavioral Hypotheses

1. *The patient's problem can be understood in part as disordered thinking, feeling, or acting causally related to antecedent events.* The clinician, in considering this hypothesis, studies the varying situations in the patient's daily life that appear to be causally related to the occurrence of the disordered behavior from the time the symptoms first appeared until the patient presents to the clinician.

2. *The patient's problem can be understood as disordered thinking, feeling, or acting resulting from reinforcing consequences of the behavior.* The clinician determines, for this hypothesis, the events that maintain or reinforce the disordered behavior. The reinforcing events may be the changes produced in the behaviors of those with whom the patient is interacting. They may also be avoidance of anxiety or discomfort by escaping from adverse conditions.

3. *The patient's problem can be understood as disordered thinking, feeling, or acting in response to sociocultural and biologic events.* The clinician explores to what degree cultural, social, and biologic conditions determine the immediate stimulus condition activating the disordered behavior, the experiences a patient is subject to in the present, and how the individual expects to behave in a given situation in the future.

4. *The patient's problem can be understood in part as a deficit of behavior in the areas of thinking, acting, and feeling.* The clinician considers for this hypothesis that the individual never acquired the necessary repertoire for functioning effectively in his or her environment. The deficits may include areas of cognition, emotional responsiveness, and motor skills. Anxiety is conceptualized here as a secondary reaction to the lack of skills rather than a primary causative factor.

5. *The patient's condition is known to be treatable, in part, by specific behavioral techniques.* These techniques, include relaxation, systematic desensitization, flooding, and cognitive restructuring.

THE DYNAMICS OF HYPOTHESIS GENERATION AND TESTING

Hypothesis generation and testing can be thought of as a three-step mental process repeated many times throughout the interview by which the clinician (*a*) collects data (makes observations); (*b*) generates, confirms, and refutes hypotheses on the basis of data collected; and (*c*) employs clinical methods or strategies to elicit further data, which will generate new hypotheses and conform or refute old ones.

Data Collection

The observations or data that lead to hypothesis generation, confirmation, and refutation may come from the following:

1. Outside the patient (previous records, clinic face sheets, the family or school);
2. The patient's biographical reconstructions;
3. The mental status examination (behavioral observations made during the interview);
4. The physical examination and laboratory data;
5. Psychodynamic material including history, dreams, fantasies, memories, associations, recurrent themes, and transference and countertransference reactions;
6. Social interactions in waiting rooms, family conferences, homes, or neighborhoods;
7. Standardized psychologic and biologic assessments.

What there is to observe is the result of the clinician's methods, the patient's pathology, and other dimensions of the clinical situation such as the size of the room, the position of the chairs, the duration of the wait, the time of day, etc. Clinicians' abilities to perceive observations depend on what they think is important and on their ability to observe.

Hypothesis Generation and Testing

Although clinicians can briefly consider all of the hypotheses on the list, it is usually possible to explore only a few in depth. The selection of these few is best determined by several criteria.

1. One considers hypotheses that are most probable on the basis of available data. For example, fastidious dress may lead to consideration of an obsessional style; recurrent presentations on the same date may lead to consideration of unresolved grief. Visual hallucinations suggest organic psychoses.
2. One considers those hypotheses that are most serious, even though they may not be highly probable. These include mood disorders, organic mental disorders, and schizophrenic disorders.

3. One gives special consideration to those hypotheses which have a high probability of being reversed with treatment, such as mood disorders, unresolved grief, and acute brain syndromes.
4. One considers those hypotheses for which there are adequate treatment resources.
5. One considers those hypotheses that the patient believes are relevant and are consistent with his or her own theoretical orientation. Patients are often right, and if they are wrong, it will be important that they know that their concerns and perspectives have been taken seriously (see Chapter 9).
6. Which hypotheses clinicians test depends not only on the priorities listed above, but also on an awareness of the range of hypotheses to be tested and on an ability to relate specific data to the formation, refutation, and confirmation of hypotheses. For instance, clinicians must know that delusions may be part of schizophrenia, affective disorders, or organic brain disease if this symptom is to alert them to test these hypotheses.

Strategies

After clinicians generate several hypotheses on the basis of the available observations, they develop a strategy to test these hypotheses. To do this, they must know what further data are required to confirm or refute any given hypothesis. They then set out to collect this data by methods such as direct questioning, sitting in silence, encouraging free associations, speaking to the family, testing the patient's memory, paying attention to their own subjective responses, stressing the patient, using sodium amytal, evaluating the response of a trial medication or performing a behavioral assessment. Many of these methods can be traced to the four basic conceptual frameworks previously described. The effectiveness of the method will depend on choosing the proper one for the particular hypothesis, on the skill of the clinician, and on the responsiveness of the patient.

The Conduct of the Interview

In conducting the interview, the clinicians proceed in the usual manner by first asking the patient what brought him or her to treatment and then by elaborating the events, symptoms, and issues of the present illness. It is neither necessary nor desirable to systematically ask questions about each successive hypothesis. Such a procedure would reduce the interview to a disjointed interrogation. Clinicians, in gathering the relevant information, are active and directive as necessary for diagnostic completeness. At the same time, they remain as nondirective as possible to preserve the free flow of the patient's thoughts.

Many of the hypotheses can be tested without the clinician's interfering at all with the flow of the interview. For instance, one can refute with relative certainty the idea that the patient is suffering from an organic illness with disturbed sensorium when the presentation is psychologically understandable, when there is no obvious thought or affective disorder, when the patient appears in good physical health, and when there is no evidence of intellectual impairment. All of these observations can be made with little or no verbal activity on the part of the clinician. Much of the evidence about personality style is derived in a similar fashion. Even when hypotheses require direct questioning for their confirmation, the questions can often become a part of the natural flow of the interview.

I find it useful to review the complete list of hypotheses in two specific circumstances during the clinical examination. The first is when the data that become available during the first 10 to 15 minutes of the interview fail to make clinical sense or generate useful hypotheses. The review becomes a source of new ideas, new approaches, and new meanings for previously discarded observations. The second circumstance is 5 to 10 minutes prior to completion of each interview. This provides the opportunity to be certain that all of the major diagnostic and therapeutic possibilities have been considered. It is surprising how often such an approach leads to the consideration of hypotheses and the elicitation of data that significantly supplement the working case formulation. For example, during a 30-minute interview, I elicited data that led to the following partial formulation: The patient, a 38-year-old Roman Catholic female, reported mild depressive symptomatology beginning 12 months previously, at which time she had divorced her alcoholic husband. She had considerable ambivalence about the decision, was now in a situation of relative social isolation, and was feeling guilty about the possibility of renewed heterosexual contacts. These explanations for her clinical condition combining psychodynamic, sociocultural, and biologic hypotheses "felt right." Before completing the interview, I reviewed in my mind the entire list of hypotheses to ensure at least brief consideration of each. After pondering the unresolved grief hypothesis, I asked the patient whether anyone important to her had died. She immediately burst into tears as she told me of her father-in-law's death 6 months previously. Her father-in-law, she explained, was a source of constant support to her. He shopped for her, listened to her troubles, and cared for her "more than my own husband." His relationship to her never faltered, even after the divorce. There was no one to support her in her grief over this seemingly distant relationship. The patient then recalled that she had been depressed for the 6 months since her father-in-law's death, not for the 12 months since the divorce. Without reviewing the unresolved grief hypothesis, this new historical data with its added partial formulation might have been omitted.

DISCUSSION

Mental health professionals in outpatient settings have set for themselves the task of delivering care that requires rapid assessment and decision making. One step in accomplishing this goal is the reorganization of clinical knowledge acquired from long-term in-depth work with patients and clinical research and its reapplication and transmission to new clinical settings. The hypothesis generation and testing approach, together with the development of a closed system of multiple hypotheses, is offered as one way of reorganizing ideas. This approach is not intended to oversimplify the enormously complex clinical process. Rather, it attemps to analyze and make explicit what experienced clinicians already do.

In our own clinics and practices my colleagues and I have found that the language of hypothesis testing raises several important questions:

1. For a particular setting, what is the best way to organize data into hypotheses that are intellectually manageable and clinically useful?
2. What clinical observations should lead to the generation of a given hypothesis?
3. Conversely, what hypotheses should be generated by a given observation?
4. What data are necessary to confirm or refute any given hypothesis?
5. What strategies may be employed to collect data necessary for the confirmation and refutation of a given hypothesis?

These questions are seldom asked or answered in textbooks of psychiatry. Clinicians, nevertheless, deal with them im-plicitly in deciding what to look for, how to look, and when to look. Such skills and processes are the heart of clinical practice. We learn them from teachers and from clinical experience, and we pass them on by the oral tradition. I believe that it is useful to make these processes explicit so that what we now call clinical skill or intuition can more effectively be communicated by the written word. Our ability to learn from each other will then be enhanced, and what we believe to be true can become open to scientific inquiry.

References

1. Elstein AS, Schulman LS, Sprafka SA: *Medical Problem Solving: An Analysis of Clinical Reasoning.* Cambridge, MA, Harvard University Press, 1978.
2. Weisman AD: The psychodynamic formulation of conflict. *Arch Gen Psychiatry* 1:288–309, 1959.
3. Erikson EH: *Insight and Responsibility.* New York, WW Norton, 1964.
4. The Royal College of General Practitioners: *The Future General Practitioner.* Lavenham, England, Lavenham Press, 1972.
5. Like R, Reeb KG: Clinical hypothesis testing in family practice: a biopsychosocial perspective. *J Fam Pract* 19:517–523, 1984.
6. Kassirer JP: Teaching clinical medicine by iterative hypothesis testing: let's preach what we practice. *N Engl J Med* 309:921–923, 1983.
7. Chamberlin TC: The method of multiple working hypotheses. *Science* 14:754–759, 1965.
8. McHugh PR, Slavney PR: *The Perspectives of Psychiatry.* Baltimore, Johns Hopkins University Press, 1986.

8

Dilemmas in Psychiatric Diagnosis:
A Perspective from the History of Medicine

Aaron Lazare, M.D.

In ambulatory settings, patients present with a wide range of problems ranging from lack of personal fulfillment to maladaptive habits and behaviors to marital and family discord to disabling depression. Clinicians who assess and treat these patients vary considerably as to professional discipline, theoretical ideology, and amount of training. This understandably leads to difficulty in achieving consensus over how to make a diagnosis, what kinds of diagnoses one should use, and even the desirability of making diagnoses. In inpatient settings, these problems are considerably diminished: The kinds of presenting problems and diagnoses are more limited; clinicians can usually agree that one of the *Diagnostic and Statistical Manual of Mental Disorders (Third Edition-Revised)* (DSM-III-R) diagnostic categories captures the essence of the problem; and a consensus over the specific diagnosis is usually easy to achieve. (In Sederer's *Inpatient Psychiatry: Diagnosis and Treatment* (1), only eight diagnostic categories are described, presumably because the vast majority of inpatient disorders fall into one or more of these eight categories.) Yet, in outpatient settings, diagnosis is essential

for prescribing treatment, communicating information from one clinician to another, conducting research, and receiving reimbursement from insurance companies.

This chapter attempts to provide a historic and philosophic perspective to the problem of psychiatric diagnosis. It first reviews the basic concepts of disease, diagnosis, and taxonomy. It then reviews both the importance of DSM-III-R in clinical psychiatry and the source of controversy between its advocates and critics. The controversy has to do with the relative merits of categorical versus idiographic or individualistic approaches to patients. I shall attempt to show that this 3000-year-old controversy has considerable relevance for medicine as well as psychiatry. This chapter closes with some of the implications of this history review for outpatient clinicians.

DISORDER, DIAGNOSIS, AND TAXONOMY

A disorder or disease is a concept, an abstraction, not an objective entity with an independent material existence (2, 3). This concept attempts to capture or circumscribe a set of real, natural relationships in order to facilitate their explanation, prediction, and control. For example, depressed mood, insomnia, suicidal ideation, and weight loss are real phenomena that often occur together. The disorder called major depression is the abstraction that circumscribes the relationships between these behaviors so they can more effectively be understood and treated. Over the centuries diseases have changed because methods of observation have become more sophisticated (so that there has been more to observe), more treatments have become available (so diagnostic entities could be found in the phenomena that responded to treatment), and new conceptual paradigms have become available (so observed phenomena could be organized in different ways).

For symptoms, behaviors, or syndromes to qualify as diagnostic entities they must be associated with subjective distress or important functional impairment. In addition, they must be considered by society to be a disease or illness. Normal bereavement, pregnancy, and normal aging are all conditions that are the legitimate subject of scientific study, and all of them may produce psychologic and/or physical distress. None, however, are granted disease status. Historic content and social values may influence the decision as to what will be called a disease. In past centuries, for instance, masturbation was regarded as a disease (4). In 1851, it was proposed that running away of slaves was a disease, which was given the name drapetomania, a Greek derivation for mad or crazy runaway slave (5). In the 1980s there has been active debate as to whether and under what conditions homosexuality should be considered a disorder.

The word *diagnosis* comes from the Greek *dia* (two or apart) and *gignoskein* (to know or perceive). The combined meaning is to know apart, distinguish, or differentiate (3, 6). The diagnosis in medicine or psychiatry is that which distinguishes or differentiates the problems of patients.

When the diagnosis takes the form of a word or phrase that is part of an official classification, it is referred to as a formal diagnosis. When it takes the form of a more lengthy and complex statement that attempts to provide a more comprehensive picture of an individual, it is referred to as a diagnostic assessment, a diagnostic workup, or a diagnostic formulation (6).

Taxonomy refers to an organization of diagnostic categories. The most widely used taxonomy for psychiatric disorders in the United States is the DSM-III-R. The ninth edition of the *International Classification of Diseases* (ICD-9) enjoys broad usage in other parts of the world.

DSM-III and DSM-III-R

The most significant contribution to diagnosis and taxonomy in psychiatry in several decades is DSM-III and DSM-III-R. The national and international response to this manual has been very positive (7). This work, first published in 1980, was the product of 5 years of scientific input, field trials involving large numbers of clinicians, and negotiations among various groups within psychiatry and between psychiatrists and other mental health professionals. Taking an approach that is for the most part descriptive and atheoretical, its specific accomplishments include

1. Greater specificity and precision of criteria necessary for making diagnoses;
2. Critera that are derived from research;
3. Improved reliability in diagnostic practices as compared with DSM-I and DSM-II;
4. A multiaxial system that allows for greater "comprehensiveness and recording of non-diagnostic data that are valuable in understanding possible etiologic factors and in treatment planning and prognosis"(8).

Despite the broad acceptance of DSM-III and DSM-III-R, some psychiatrists, psychologists, and nonpsychiatric physicians have been critical of the choice, definition, naming, and validity of some of the categories (7, 9). As part of a healthy debate, this is all to the good. A more serious source of opposition to DSM-III comes from a large body of clinicians, the great majority of whom work in ambulatory settings, who strongly believe that the diagnostic categories have little relevance to a significant portion of patients in their practice.

In my opinion, the most substantive aspect of the controversy over DSM-III has to do with its assumption of a categorical paradigm and taxonomy. (Synonyms for *categorical* have been *medical*, *disease*, and *Kraepelinian*.)

CATEGORICAL VERSUS INDIVIDUALISTIC APPROACHES

Spitzer and Guze are among the most articulate proponents of the categorical approach, and they are central figures in the development of nosologic systems in contemporary psychiatry. Spitzer et al. (10) in their guiding principles for DSM-III state,

We regard the medical model as a working hypothesis that there are organismic dysfunctions which are relatively distinct with regard to clinical features, etiology, and course. No assumption is made regarding the primacy of biological over social or environmental etiologic factors.

Similarly, Guze (11) states,

The medical model requires no assumptions about etiology or effective treatment. It assumes only that there are different psychiatric disorders with different clinical pictures, natural histories, etiologies, and mechanisms and that different disorders will respond best to different treatments. This assumption results in efforts to divide psychiatric disorders into homogeneous groups based upon common etiology, pathogenesis, clinicial features, and response to treatment. Features that patients have in common are the major focus of concern. Diagnosis is the medical term for this kind of classification. Its essential role is implicit in the medical model. Physicians have traditionally worked to recognize and characterize different illnesses and to distinguish one from another.

The categorical paradigm described above may be contrasted to the individualistic or idiographic, which is represented in contemporary psychiatry by four major diagnostic paradigms: psychodynamic, behavioral, sociocultural, and psychometric or dimensional.

The psychodynamic paradigm understands behavior as indicative of unconscious conflicts, drive derivatives, defense mechanisms, developmental arrests, and fixations. Presumed causation is described in psychologic/developmental terms. The resultant pathologic behaviors are conceived as quantitative deviations from the normal that may be found in all individuals, not just those who become dysfunctional and/or present for treatment. Generally, a diagnostic formulation is preferable to a formal diagnosis. This provides a unique, idiographic, individualistic diagnostic assessment for each patient.

In the behavioral paradigm, diagnosis is based on the assessment of the pathologic behavior in the context of its antecedent and reinforcing events in the current environment. Unlike the medical paradigm, the behavioral lacks an organized taxonomy. The assessment for each patient is idiographic or individualistic (6, 12).

The sociocultural paradigm has received the least attention from clinical investigators. There have been, however, attempts to understand human distress from an analysis or diagnosis of the social condition—of the couple, the family, or the society (13).

The dimensional or psychometric paradigm assesses each patient according to a finite number of variables that are presumed to be important in understanding the patient's problem. Quantitative scores are obtained for each dimension and then compared to various reference groups. The Minnesota Multiphasic Personality Inventory is an example of a dimensional diagnostic instrument. The dimensional concept has also been elaborated in studies of personality by Eysenck, Cattell, and Guilford (6).

Advocates for all four approaches described above believe that the syndromal approach of DSM-III-R is too limited and ill suited to provide meaningful diagnostic assessments and taxonomies for the patients they treat and study.

Categorical–individualistic debates can become bitter. The categorical group regard their adversaries (particularly the psychodynamic group) as sloppy and imprecise in clinical observation, too speculative in their theoretical framework, prone to giving nonspecific or similar treatments to a wide variety of diagnostic categories, too interested in the "whole patient," too interested in patients with minimal pathology, and not appreciative of the importance of specific diagnosis. They are concerned that students are taught theories that are far removed from clinical observation.

The individualistic group, on the other hand, believe their adversaries are rigid and authoritarian, interested in diseases not patients, not attentive to critical individual differences, and obsessed with some ill-defined notion of being "medical." They believe the diagnostic categories of DSM-III-R are too numerous, inappropriately conceived, and poorly named, and they assert that "psychiatric classification of mental illness, bound and constricted by the medical diagnostic model, does not transpose satisfactorily to diagnoses of emotional problems"(14). They are concerned that students will use DSM-III-R as a textbook and devote their energy to an endless classification of patients' diseases rather than to studying psychologic processes.

A PERSPECTIVE FROM THE HISTORY OF MEDICINE

The intellectual roots of this debate in medicine can be traced as far back as Hippocrates. It has been chronicled by medical historians Faber (15), Cohen (16, 17), Temkin (18), and Engle (19). This is the ongoing debate over which of two concepts best explains the nature of medical disease. The first concept is referred to as individualistic, biographic, or historic since its main interest is the meticulous study of the varied manifestations of disease in individual patients. It is based on the Aristotelian interest in the world of the senses and the individual. It is also referred to as Hippocratic, after the great physician founder of the school; Coan, from the site of its temple at Cos; humoralist, after the belief that pathology resides in the humors of the body; and physiologic, after its proponents of the 19th century and the interest in function over structure. Physicians representing this approach are Hippocrates, Galen, Virchow (at least in his early years), and Wunderlich. Representative psychiatrists are Benjamin Rush, Adolph Meyer, Sigmund Freud, and Karl Menninger (see Table 8.1).

The second concept may be referred to as the categorical approach. It is based on the Platonic belief that reality resides in universal ideas rather than in individual objects of our senses. It is also referred to as Cnidian, from the site of its temple at Cnidos; solidist, after the belief that pathology resides in anatomic structures; and

Table 8.1   Names Applied to Approaches to Disease

Historical Perspective	Individualistic Approach	Categorical Approach
After the great philosophers	Aristotelian	Platonic
After the great physicians	Hippocratic	Paracelsian
From the site of the main temples	Coan	Cnidian
From the doctrines of pathology	Humoralist	Solidist
From the great 19th century debate	Physiologic	Ontologic
Representative physicians	Hippocrates	Paracelsus
	Galen	Sydenham
	Virchow	deSauvages
Representative psychiatrists	Benjamin Rush	Karl Kahlbaum
	Sigmund Freud	Emil Kraepelin
	Adolph Meyer	
	Karl Menninger	

ontologic, indicating the independent nature of disease running a predictable course and with a natural history of its own. Physicians representating this approach are Paracelsus, Sydenham, deSauvages, and Laennec. Representative psychiatrists are Kahlbaum and Kraepelin.

The Hippocratic Physicians

The views of Hippocrates (460–375 B.C.) or the Hippocratic physicians, passed on through Galen (130–200 A.D.), represented a departure from earlier notions that disease is the invasion of a demon, an external entity, or a foreign body. According to the Hippocratic view, disease resides in the very nature of man. There is one basic general disease with many forms, one common general disturbance that gives rise to various symptom pictures. Health is the condition of perfect equilibrium, and sickness is the state of disequilibrium. It is only within this context that individual diseases are identified and named. Hippocrates initiated the bedside method of clincial study and advocated the meticulous study of individuals, each of whom was to be treated differently, not subject to rigid categories (15, 19, 20).

Celsus (30 B.C.–50 A.D.), a Roman physician who lived during the reign of Tiberius Caesar, illustrated the Hippocratic approach in his discussion of the importance of ongoing care of the patient. The physician, he says, can only know what is wrong with the patient by being the patient's friend and knowing him intimately over long periods of time. He contrasts this type of care to the categorical approach, an inferior clinical method used by veterinarians, foreigners, and physicians working in large hospitals:

For in like manner those who treat cattle and horses, since it is impossible to learn from dumb animals particulars of their complaints, depend only upon common characteristics; so also do foreigners, as they are ignorant of reasoning subtleties, look rather to common characteristics of disease. Again, those who take charge of large hospitals, because they cannot pay full

attention to individuals, resort to these common characteristics. (18)

The Hippocratic approach competed successfully with the Cnidian emphasis on the exact classification of disease and categories. Cnidos, for instance, described 7 diseases of the bile and 12 of the bladder (19).

The Hippocratic view evolved during the course of many centuries into hazy, speculative, unscientific chemical theories that ignored the method of careful clinical observation as practiced by Hippocrates (15).

Sydenham and deSauvages

There was no major breakthrough in medicine until Thomas Sydenham (1624–1689) brilliantly reintroduced the categorical approach to medicine. His hope was that

all diseases be reduced to definite and certain *species*, and that, with the same care which we see exhibited by botanists in their phytologies; since it happens, at present, that many diseases, although included in the same genus, mentioned with a common nomenclature, and resembling one another in several symptoms, are, notwithstanding, different in their natures, and require a different medical treatment. (21)

To achieve his goal Sydenham returned to the Hippocratic method of studying disease by careful observation at the bedside of the sick person. He acknowledged Hippocrates' contribution by referring to him as the "Romulus of Medicine." Sydenham's admirers referred to him, in turn, as the "English Hippocrates." There was, however, a fundamental difference in the goals of these two men: Hippocrates used the clinical method to study sick people; Sydenham used it to study disease entities.

Sydenham's laboratory was the city of London. In 1665 the plague killed 100,000 of its inhabitants (15% of the population). By 1667 the plague had ceased, but 1300 died of smallpox, 2000 of cholera, and 3000 of tuberculosis, while only 1000 died of old age. He discovered in this population that certain symptoms invariably occurred with others and that together they followed a predictable natural history. With this method, he was able to provide impressive descriptions of small pox, dysentery, cholera, and the plague. He was the first to distinguish measles from scarlatina and gout from rheumatism (15).

Sydenham's hope that there would be a specific treatment for each disease was not realized in his time. There was then only quinine for malaria. The treatment of other diseases was still of a general nature: bleeding, vomiting, purging, and diaphoresis.

Sydenham's greatest accomplishment lay in his study of acute diseases that were ultimately discovered to be infectious in origin. He was close to the truth in his belief that acute diseases were caused by the invasion of a person's body by atmospheric miasmata that developed in the humours of the body. Sydenham sensed that his categorical approach could not easily be applied to chronic diseases, which he believed had their origin in "unhealthy ways of living, eating, and drinking" (21–23).

Perhaps Sydenham's receiving the degree of doctor of medicine at age 52 and his prior army career in which he achieved the rank of captain in Cromwell's cavalry while fighting against royalist forces spared him the indoctrination of medical myths and prepared him for combat against the archaic medical doctrines of his day. "Our modern Doctrine," he said, "is a contrivance of the word-catchers, the art of talking rather than the art of healing"(21).

In his continued attack on the individualistic approach, Sydenham stated,

No man can state the errors that have been occasioned by these physiological hypotheses. Writers . . . have saddled diseases with phenomena which existed in their own brains only; . . . if by chance some symptom really coincided accurately with their hypothesis, and occur in the disease whereof they describe the character, they magnify it beyond all measure and moderation; they make it all and in all; the molehill becomes a mountain; whilst if it fails to tally with the said hypothesis, they pass it over either in perfect silence or with only an inciden-

tal mention, unless, by means of some philosophical subtlety, they can enlist it in their service, or else, by fair means or foul, accommodate it in some way or other to their doctrines. (21)

Sydenham's work was continued by Francois Boissier deSauvages (1706–1762), a botanist and a physician. In his main work, published in 1763, which exerted a world-wide influence, he catalogued and grouped 2400 species of "diseases" into classes, orders and genera. These included 18 kinds of angina, 19 of asthma, 20 of pleurodynia, 20 of phthisis, 29 of vomiting, and 12 of nausea. The work of deSauvages and those who followed in his example merely catalogued and grouped symptoms. They missed the essence of Sydenham's contribution to nosology (15).

19th Century French and German Schools

Let us review one additional era, French and German medicine of the 19th century, because of the clarity with which the opposing issues are stated. French medicine, referred to as the pathologico–anatomical school, was categorical in orientation. Its great physicians were Pinel (the anatomic classification of acute inflammation), Bichat (the study of pathologic involvement of separate tissues), and Laennec (the idea of indirect ascultation resulting in the invention of the stethoscope and the discovery that all forms of tuberculosis were a unitary disease). The French, later joined by the English (Addison, Bright, Hodgkin, Parkinson, and others) described a whole series of new diseases characterized by pathognomonic symptoms and characteristic signs. The philosophic position of this school was to "set aside all incidental and individual phenomena to arrive at the typical picture of disease" (15).

The French categorical school was opposed by the German individualistic school, whose physicians were Schwann, Wunderlich, Traube, Virchow, Helmholtz, Brucke, and others. Their goal was to go beyond the description of phenomena by describing their interrelation, their genesis and development. "Pathology," according to Wunderlich, "is only the physiology of diseased man"(15). This group resisted all attempts to establish or describe definite clinical pictures or individual diseases. Wunderlich commented in an article for the *Archiv Fur Physiologische Heilkunde,*

To the most widespread and the most dangerous consequences of ontology belongs the practice of setting up species of diseases which have been grouped in classes in the same way as plants. By raising them to the dignity of species these ontological personifications received, as it were, the sanction of natural history . . . But to the ontologist the assumed disease is a dogma; the group once collected, it becomes a concept, an entity. (15)

The eminent neurologist Lasegue criticized the individualistic German physiologists in language similar to Sydenham's:

They observe little, and they observe badly. They explain much, or rather, they explain everything, and they pass quickly from hypothesis to practice. But after the most adventurous excursions they all end peacefully at the same point, the point which had already been reached, and medicine proceeds undisturbed, though with caution, on its onward march.(15)

The individualistic, physiologic physicians, according to Englehardt, were attempting to make the following three points: (*a*) The concept of disease is a general, not a specific notion; diseases were functions of the general laws of physiology rather than "functions of the more particular laws of the pathology of specific diseases." (*b*) There should be a "greater appreciation of the individuality of illnesses so that every particular disease-state could be understood in terms of its particular departures from general physiological norms." And (*c*) ontological concepts of disease must be avoided; diseases are not real things but rather the result of various physiologic forces; they are more contextual than substantial (24).

The physiologic school of the 19th century made significant contributions to medical science. They introduced graphic, microscopic, and chemical methods of investigation to medicine while providing great impetus to the developing fields of experimental physiology and pathogenic anatomy. At the same time, by failing to comprehend important nosologic accomplishments of their time, they developed a dual conception of tuberculous phenomena and refused to accept the established relationship between croup and pharyngeal diptheria. Because of the dogmatic positions of both the physiologic (individualistic) and the anatomic (categorical) schools, progress in medicine requiring the application of physiologic and categorical methods to the study of disease was delayed (15).

ONE HUNDRED YEARS OF PSYCHIATRY[a]

Kraepelin

The categorical approach of Thomas Sydenham was skillfully applied to psychiatric disorders by the German psychiatrist Emil Kraepelin (1856–1926). Like Sydenham, he traced the natural history of symptoms and syndromes to their final outcome in order to separate and identify independent clinical entities. In doing so he, like Sydenham, replaced metaphysical and symptomatic systems of nosology. Integrating his own observations with those of such predecessors as Hecker, Kahlbaum, Morel, Griesinger, and Krafft-Ebing, he produced nine editions of a premier textbook which spanned the years 1883 through 1929. Kraepelin's accomplishments mark the beginning of modern psychiatry. His nosology was the intellectual precursor of DSM-III (25).

Meyer

The person most influential in bringing Kraepelin's categorical approach into the

---

[a] This discussion of individualistic psychiatric approaches is limited to Meyer's psychobiology and the psychodynamic approach.

mainstream of American psychiatry was the great individualistic psychiatrist Adolph Meyer (1866–1950). Meyer, Swiss born and German speaking, traveled to Europe in 1896 on a 6-week leave from his responsibilities at Worcester State Hospital. He spent this time in Heidelberg as a visitor and pupil in Kraepelin's clinic, just before the publication of the important fifth edition of Kraepelin's textbook, which Meyer later referred to as "revolutionary" and "the greatest challenge that had ever come to psychiatry in the form of a text." It was in this edition that Kraepelin proclaimed the need for the nosologic principles of course, prognosis, and outcome rather than symptom description. On his return to Worcester, Meyer became the first to introduce Kraepelin's conceptions into American hospital practice, "but with reservations which mitigated the dogmatic assumption of 'one man, one disease' and the exclusive specificity of the entities, and with adequate room for . . . a dynamic genetic formulation"(26).

From the start, Meyer admired Kraeplin's courage and wisdom in replacing the metaphysic or symptomatic systems with one based on sound clinical empiricism, and he appreciated the practical value of bringing order to nosology. Having acknowledged this, he noted how the fixed nosologic system of Kraepelin "leads to such a deplorable limitation of concepts and a lack of appreciation of the facts presented by the patient." Nosology, he said, is a preference for concepts over facts to be controlled. The disease is a naively conceived enemy or intruder. Kraepelin's nosologic approach, continued Meyer, "is the bald expression of the dogma, impressive and simple, but not altogether convincing or satisfying." He "bends the facts of psychiatric observation to the concept of disease processes." In commenting on the general concept of diagnosis, Meyer states,

Can we not use general principles and valuable deductions without pulling them into the service of a vicious attitude of mind, the attitude of that medical conceit which delights in sur-

rounding the diagnosing and prescribing with a mystic halo so much adored by the patients trained to see wonders in the wise terms? Why not regard the 'diagnosis' as merely a convenient term for the actually ascertained facts which do or do not tell a clear and plain story, and, accordingly, are or are not especially gratifying data of medical insight? (27)

Meyer's own clinical perspective and contribution consisted of his meticulous biographic study of the individual. Psychologic, sociocultural, and biologic factors were all taken into account. Symptoms were understood as being interactive with the person's psychologic and biologic functioning, as being reactions to stress rather than manifestations of disease. Meyer's influence was manifested through many of his students who went on to become leaders of American and British psychiatry. Although skeptical of psychoanalysis, Meyer provided the fertile intellectual soil for the development of psychoanalysis in contemporary American psychiatry (28).

Freud and Psychoanalysis

Sigmund Freud (1856–1939), a contemporary of Kraepelin and Meyer, was the founder of the psychoanalytic movement. Freud's intellectual connection to Hippocrates was noted by O. Temkin, a medical historian, and by A. A. Brill, one of Freud's translators. Temkin points out that Freud and his followers rely on the biographic approach and the detailed case history, look for the vicissitudes of an individual's neurosis in his or her biography, and impute neuroses—more or less—to everyone (18). Brill comments that both Hippocrates and Freud proceed from the general concept to the specific, focusing on individual patients and how they deviate from the normal. "We know, indeed that the neurotic or psychotic struggle is in itself an effort at adjustment, or in the Hippocratic sense, an effort to re-establish the former equilibrium or harmony"(29). This very point became the subject of Karl Menninger's book on psychiatric nosology, appropriately entitled *The Vital Balance* (30).

The psychoanalytic notion of lines of development, initially developed by Ferenczi (31), elaborated by Anna Freud (32), and valued by most psychodynamic psychiatrists, clarifies in part why psychoanalytic theory is an individualistic approach to emotional distress. Human psychologic development is conceived of as proceeding along several continuous and coexisting developmental lines or sequences of behavior. These include libidinal development (33), ego and object relations development (10, 34), narcissistic development (35), and self development (36). Developmental arrests or distortions or suboptimal growth resulting from genetic predisposition, parental deprivations or excess, or mismatches between childhood needs and parental resources are possibilities for everyone. Personality formation and psychopathology in any individual represents the unique outcome of the interplay between the multiple early developmental vicissitudes described above, later environmental events, and biologic variables. Although diagnostic labels may be attached to nodal points on developmental continua, comprehensive individualistic formulations provide the only meaningful diagnoses.

Psychodynamic psychiatry was the school of greatest influence in the United States throughout the middle of this century until the early 1960s, when biologic, behavioral, and social psychiatry gained momentum. It is now one of several key approaches in understanding psychopathology. Its major interest has been the neuroses and personality disorders (37).

The Neo-Kraepelinians

The categorical approach to psychiatry in the United States during the late 1940s and 1950s was regarded by leaders in major academic centers as rigid, sterile, pessimistic, and undynamic. This situation changed radically in the late 1950s with the introduction of the new psychopharmacologic agents and subsequent advances in brain chemistry. The need to study the efficacy of these drugs served as an impetus for the development of rating scales, checklists and sophisticated mathematical techniques for the evaluation of patients entering research trials. These techniques were eventually applied to "problems of descriptions, reliability, and validity of categorical diagnostic categories by a group referred to as neo-Kraepelinians"(38, 39). This group emphasized the importance of defining, distinguishing, and validating specific syndromes of mental disorders. Their efforts led to the development of Research Diagnostic Criteria (RDC) for mental disorders and finally to DSM-III. The major clinical areas of interest of the categorical group have been the schizophrenias, the depressive disorders, and some of the neuroses.

The categorical approach has been furthered in recent years by reasons of a sociopolitical nature. Health insurers insist on a categorical diagnosis (25) as a condition of payment. Furthermore, with the diagnosis-related group concept, acceptable duration of treatment and payment are directly related to diagnosis. While accommodating the bureaucratic demands for diagnosis, individualistic physicians such as primary care specialists and psychodynamic psychiatrists believe that such an approach detracts from the personal care of patients.

IMPLICATIONS

Controversy as Dialectic

This review has attempted to show that the current controversy between the critics and supporters of DSM-III is embedded, in part, in the debate between individualistic and categorical approaches to disease and nosology. Each approach has achieved positions of intellectual dominance, lost it, and then regained it. This process has been more than swings of a pendulum. It is a dialectic in which two opposing forces come together, clash, then separate after significantly influencing each other: the Hippocratic physicians and Sydenham, the German physiologists and French anatomists, humoral pathology and solidist pathology, Meyer and Kraepelin, the psychodynamic school and DSM-III.

The DSM-III itself reflects the impact of individualistic approaches and attempts to avoid the mistakes of earlier categorical approaches. It disclaims the assumption "that each mental disorder is a discrete entity with sharp boundaries (discontinuities) between it and other mental disorders, as well as between it and No Mental Disorder"(40). It asserts that this is a classification of mental disorders, not individuals. And it employs a multiaxial system to capture some individualistic dimensions of patients. In contemporary psychoanalytic thinking, there are increasing attempts to reliably define and validate theoretically important personality types (41), to obtain precision in the measurement of discrete ego functions (42), and to add a psychodynamic axis to DSM-III (43).

Dialectic thinking in medicine is ubiquitous. The great historical figures presented in this chapter as examples of one approach all make use of the opposing approach. A patient who comes to his or her physician with an undiagnosed problem hopes that his or her symptoms are part of a category of diseases (benign, it is hoped) that the physician has been taught to recognize. At the same time the patient fears that his or her condition is so unique, it may defy diagnosis and require uncommon medical skills. In the words of T. S. Eliot, "all cases are unique and very similar to others"(44).

Biologic Versus Psychologic

Since modern psychopharmacology has been a major force in the development of diagnostic categories, it is widely believed that adherents of the categorical approach are and will be biologic in orientation. Similarly, since psychoanalytic, sociocultural, behavioral, and dimensional schools of psychiatry are predominantly individualistic, it is generally assumed that supporters of individualistic approach are and will be psychologic and sociocultural in orientation. These generalizations do not have

historic support. Many of the biologic physicians reviewed in this chapter have been individualistic in orientation. Some psychologic schools are categorical. In psychiatry, contemporary psychopharmacologists are moving away from an exclusive categorical approach as it becomes evident that medications such as the tricyclic antidepressants, lithium, and the antipsychotic agents each have value in treating several diagnostic groups. Imipramine, for instance, is an appropriate treatment for most affective disorders, some anxiety disorders, schizophrenic disorders with major affective components, and enuresis. In addition, several neurobiologic theories of certain aspects of mental illness now postulate a small number of neurochemical systems that must be in proper balance for the maintenance of mental health (45)—a concept not different in form from the humoral theories of ancient medicine. It appears that biologic psychiatry needs clinical categories for structure but then finds the limitations of a category or even dissolves the boundaries between categories.

Medicine and Psychiatry

Contemporary psychiatry is categorical *in emphasis*. The categorical nature of DSM-III-R, (despite its individualistic aspects) and the scientific events leading to its publication are having a significant and positive impact on education, research, and clinical care. Leston Havens, an astute observer of various schools of psychiatric thought, has referred to this as "Kraepelin's century"(25). Much of contemporary medicine is individualistic in emphasis. Support for this statement includes the development of primary care and family medicine specialities; the current interest in holistic medicine; the influence of the Weed Problem-Oriented Record, which addresses the patient's problems in addition to formal diagnoses (46); the use of clinical hypotheses from the social, psychodynamic, and behavioral areas to supplement knowledge about biologic diseases (47); the growing interest in illness behavior to understand the uniqueness of the individual (48, 49); the awareness by most clinicians that classical or "textbook cases" are statistical oddities; the many areas of medicine where functional or quantitative disabilities are often more important than categorical or qualitative distinctions (cardiac disability, stress, many problems of aging); the presence of general treatments for many medical conditions (rest, stress reduction, diet, exericse, aspirin, steroids, diuretics); and the interest in the maintenance of health and preventive medicine. It is not that medicine finds diagnosis unimportant. Medicine has the need to go beyond diagnosis (50) for its continued progress. New diagnostic methods, biologic discoveries, and psychosocial conceptualizations have supplemented old categories and rendered others obsolete. In the study of coronary artery diseases, for instance, greater knowledge of risk factors, sophisticated diagnostic techniques, and new surgical approaches require individualistic diagnostic formulations and treatment plans. With so much of medicine's past and present rooted in the individualistic approach to psychopathology, equating the categorical approach with psychiatry's "medical model" is both inaccurate and confusing. Medicine has been and should be both categorical and individualistic.

If the analysis above is correct, medicine and psychiatry are out of synchronization. Meyer made the same observation in 1926: "Dogmatic nosology . . . has become the rarest of all birds of late years in the general medicine of the day—but not as yet in psychiatry"(26). This asynchrony becomes a dilemma in clinical practice when the internist seeks a consultation to achieve a more comprehensive understanding of his patient and to receive advice as to how to manage particular behaviors and feelings in his patient—and sometimes in himself. A rigid categorical psychiatrist whose response is a categorical diagnosis understandably frustrates and disappoints the referring physician.

Contemporary Concepts of Disease

Early in this chapter I discussed the concept of disease or disorder. This point now needs further elaboration. In medicine, diseases are named after the symptom (migraine, nonspecific diarrhea); the physical sign (hypertension); the syndrome (rheumatoid arthritis, uclerative colitis); and the pathogenesis (thyrotoxicosis, porphyria). When we state that the etiology is known, we usually mean that one or several of many etiologic factors has been discovered. When we state that the pathogenesis is known, we usually mean that one or several links in the chain of events leading to the observed nosographic picture has been determined (2). Both medicine and psychiatry search for explanation by moving from symptoms and signs to syndrome, and from syndrome to etiology and pathogenesis. This is the model of Sydenham and Kraepelin.

Mental distress included under the rubic of psychiatric disorders is difficult to classify. Multiple explanatory models with their differing methods of clinical observations and a wide variety of treatments make it difficult to decide what sets of natural relationships should be circumscribed as diseases or disorders. Having done so, certain disorders will in all likelihood be more categorical than others. Engle and Davis (19, 51, 52) in a series of papers on medical diagnosis organize medical diseases into five categories according to the clarity of the phenomena. The first group includes some genetic abnormalities that result in predictable biochemical and anatomical manifestations. The second group includes the infectious diseases in which the necessary but not sufficient causes are known and in which the clinical picture shows many variations. The third group includes diagnoses that are almost entirely descriptive since little is known about etiology and pathogenesis. The fifth group includes the collagen diseases where etiology is unknown and clinical syndromes overlap and blend together.

Individualistic aspects of medical or psychiatric problems may be a manifestation of a multifactorial etiology in which pathogenic causal chains lead not to a final common pathway, as in some diseases, but to diffuse and protean symptoms or to symptoms in which a small number of important dimensions vary independently of one another.

A Perspective on DSM-III-R

Despite these problems in developing a satisfactory categorical approach for psychiatry, classification is important and DSM-III-R is necessary. It has enhanced clinical care, research, and intellectual debate. Its categories are necessary for further investigation. The historic perspective of this chapter suggests, however, that major parts of it will be superseded or modified in profound ways by new individualistic approaches from the biologic and psychologic sciences. These advances will, in turn, lead to a revised and more useful nosology including more valid categories.

For the present, this historic inquiry can help us be aware of the dangers inherent in each approach. Following the categorical approach there is the risk that the DSM-III-R will be used as a textbook rather than a diagnostic manual; that the categories will be used to explain or describe people rather than their disorders; that the categories will become reified rather than being understood as abstractions to be judged by their usefulness; that all categories will be assumed to be equally discrete and valid; that transitional forms of the category will be dismissed as nonrelevant or nonexistent; that alternate categories from other theoretical perspectives will be ignored; that the importance of an individualistic or dimensional approaches to some conditions will be ignored; and that categories will proliferate in an unproductive manner.

In following contemporary individualistic approaches, there is a risk that obvious diagnostic categories with clear therapeutic implications will be overlooked, that alternative individualistic theories will be ignored, and that the theories will lose their clinical base and become tortuous, abstract, and incomprehensible.

Followers of both approaches run the risk of forgetting that the major contributions of each approach to contemporary psychiatry are based predominantly on different patient populations—the categorical approach on the schizophrenias and the mood disorders, the individualistic approach on the personality disorders and nonsyndromal behaviors. Both groups run the further risk of becoming mired in emotional contempt for each other, thereby obscuring the truths each has to offer (3, 53).

SUMMARY AND CONCLUSIONS

This brief historic review suggests several points that may have clinical relevance, particularly to outpatient clinicians who attempt to assess and treat a heterogeneously patient population.

1. There has always been tension and debate in medicine and psychiatry as to whether categorical or individual approaches are most useful for understanding patients and for further scientific development in the field.
2. This is not a biologic versus psychologic debate, either in medicine or psychiatry.
3. The current use of the phrase "medical model" for the categorical approach is unfortunate since medicine both past and present has been deeply committed to individualistic approaches.
4. Both approaches have made great contributions to medicine and psychiatry to the degree that they have applied their approaches to the clinical areas to which they are best suited. Neither approach has had a monopoly on the use of the scientific method or clinical relevance.
5. Over the centuries, the debate between the two approaches has taken the form of a dialectic in which each approach has influenced the other in positive ways.
6. Although DSM-III-R is a categorical or Kraepelian approach, its multiaxial sys-

tem represents an important individualistic contribution.

7. There are serious clinical risks in becoming dogmatic adherents of either approach.

8. Our overriding task in understanding and developing psychiatric diagnosis and formulation is to be scientific and clinically relevant. This requires a spirit of open inquiry that encourages integrative efforts among biologic, psychologic, and sociocultural approaches on one hand and between categorical and individualistic approaches on the other (54–56).

References

1. 1. Sederer LI: *Inpatient Psychiatry: Diagnosis and Treatment,* ed 2. Baltimore, William & Wilkins, 1986.
2. Wulff H: *Rational Diagnosis and Treatment.* Oxford, London, Blackwell Scientific Publications, 1976.
3. Kendall RE: *The Role of Diagnosis in Psychiatry.* Oxford, London, Blackwell Scientific Publications, 1975.
4. Engelhardt HT Jr: The disease of masturbation: values and the concept of disease. *Bulletin of the History of Disease* 48:234–248, 1974.
5. Cartwright SA: Report on the diseases and physical peculiarities of the Negro race. *The New Orleans Medical and Surgical Journal* 7:707–709, 1851.
6. Achenbach TM: *Assessment and Taxonomy of Child and Adolescent Psychopathology.* Beverly Hills, CA, Sage Publications, 1985.
7. Spitzer RL, Williams JBW, Skodol AE: *International Perspectives on DSM-III.* Washington, DC, American Psychiatric Press, 1983.
8. Spitzer RL, Williams JBW, Skodol AE: DSM-III: the major achievements and an overview. *Am J Psychiatry* 137:151–164, 1980.
9. Klerman GL, Vaillant GE, Spitzer RL, et al: A debate on DSM-III. *Am J Psychiatry* 141:539–553, 1984.
10. Spitzer RL, Skeehy M, Endicott J: DSM-III: guiding principles. In Rakoff VM, Stancer HC, Kedward HB (eds): *Psychiatric Diagnosis.* New York, Brunner/Mazel, 1977, pp 1–14.
11. Guze SB: The validity and significance of the clinical diagnosis of hysteria (Briquet's Syndrome). *Am J Psychiatry* 132:138–141, 1975.
12. Kanfer FH, Saslow G: Behavioral analysis: an alternative to diagnostic classification. *Arch Gen Psychiatry* 12:529–538, 1965.
13. Eisenthal S: The sociocultural approach. In Lazare A (ed): *Outpatient Psychiatry: Diagnosis and Treatment.* Baltimore, Williams & Wilkins, 1979, pp 71–83.
14. Blank R, Blank G: *Ego Psychology: Theory and Practice.* New York, Columbia University Press, 1974.
15. Faber K. *Nosography in Modern Internal Medicine.* New York, Paul B. Hoeber, 1923.
16. Cohen H: *The Nature, Method and Purpose of Diagnosis.* Cambridge, England, Cambridge University Press, 1943.
17. Cohen H: The evolution of the concept of disease. *Proc R Soc Med* 48:155–160, 1953.
18. Temkin O: The scientific approach to disease: specific entity and individual sickness. In Crombie AC (ed): *Scientific Change.* New York, Basic Books, 1963, pp 629–647.
19. Engle RL: Medical diagnosis: past, present and future: II. Philosophical foundations and historical developments of our concepts of health, disease and diagnosis. *Arch Intern Med* 112:520–529, 1963.
20. Haggard HW: *The Doctor in History.* New Haven, CT, Yale University Press, 1934.
21. Sydenham T: Preface to the third edition of Observationes Medicae from the works of Thomas Sydenham, Volume I. In Caplan AL, Englehardt HT, McCartney JJ (eds): *Concepts of Health and Disease: Interndisciplinary Perspectives.* Reading, MA, Addison-Wesley, pp 145–155.
22. Taylor FK: *The Concepts of Illness, Disease and Morbus.* Cambridge, England, Cambridge University Press, 1979.
23. Entralgo PL: *Mind and Body. Psychosomatic Pathology: A Short History of the Evolution of Medical Thought.* London, Harvill, 1955.
24. Engelhardt HT Jr: The concepts of health and disease. In Engelhardt HT Jr, Spicker SF (eds): *Evaluation and Explanation in the Biomedical Sciences.* Dordrecht, Holland, Reidel Publishing, 1975, pp 125–141.
25. Havens LL: Twentieth-century psychiatry: a view from the sea. *Am J Psychiatry* 138:1279–1287, 1981.
26. Winters EE: *The Collected Papers of Adolf Meyer, Volume III.* Baltimore, John Hopkins University Press, 1951.
27. Winters EE: *The Collected Papers of Adolf Meyer, Volume II,* Baltimore, Johns Hopkins University Press, 1951.
28. Mora G: Adolf Meyer. In Kaplan HI, Freedman AM, Sadock JB (eds): *Comprehensive Textbook of Psychiatry/III.* Baltimore, Williams & Wilkins, 1980, pp 805–812.
29. Brill AA: Anticipations and correlations of the Freudian concepts from non-analytic sources. *Am J Psychiatry* 92:1127–1135, 1936.
30. Menninger K: *The Vital Balance: The Life Process in Mental Health and Illness.* New York, Viking Press, 1963.
31. Ferenczi S: Stages in the development of the sense of reality. In *Selected Papers of Sandor Ferenczi.* New York, Basic Books, 1913, vol. 1, pp 213–239.
32. Freud A: *The Concept of Developmental Lines. The Psychoanalytic Study of the Child.* New York, International Universities Press, 1963.
33. Abraham K: Psychoanalytical studies on character-formation. In *Selected Papers on Psychoanalysis.* London, Hogarth Press, 1927, pp 370–417.

34. Blank G, Blank R: *Ego Psychology II: Psychoanalytic Developmental Psychology*. New York, Columbia University Press, 1979.
35. Burstein B: A diagnostic framework. *International Review of Psychoanalysis* 5:2–31, 1978.
36. Gedo J, Goldberg A: *Models of the Mind*. Chicago, University of Chicago Press, 1973.
37. Lazare A: Hidden conceptual models in clinical psychiatry. *N Engl J Med* 288:345–351, 1973.
38. Tischler GL: Evaluation of DSM-III. In Kaplan HI Sadock BJ (eds): *Comprehensive Textbook of Psychiatry/IV*. Baltimore, Williams & Wilkins, 1985, pp 617–621.
39. Klerman GL: Diagnosis and Classification of Mental Disorders, Alcoholism, and Drug Abuse: The Contemporary American Scene. Unpublished manuscript.
40. Frances A: Categorical and dimensional systems and personality diagnosis: a comparison. *Compr Psychiatry* 23:516–527, 1982.
41. Lazare A, Klerman GL, Armor D: Oral, obsessive and hysterical personality patterns: replication of factor analysis in an independent sample. *J Psychiatr Res* 7:275–290, 1970.
42. Bellak L, Hurvich M, Gediman HK: *Ego Functions in Schizophrenics, Neurotics, and Normals*. New York, John Wiley & Sons, 1973.
43. Karasu TB, Skodol AE: VIth Axis for DSM-III: psychodynamic Evaluation. *Am J Psychiatry*, 137:607–610, 1980.
44. Eliot TS: *The Cocktail Party*. London, Faber and Faber, 1950.
45. Whybrow PC: *Mood Disorders: Toward a New Psychobiology*. New York, Plenum Press, 1984.
46. Weed LL: *Medical Records, Medical Education and Patient Care*. Cleveland, Press of Case Western Reserve University, 1969.
47. The Royal College of General Practitioners: *The Future of Practitioners: Learning and Technology*. London, Royal College of General Practitioners, 1972.
48. Mechanic D: The concept of illness behavior. *J Chron Dis* 15:189–194, 1962.
49. Eisenberg L: Interfaces between medicine and psychiatry. *Compr Psychiatry* 20:1–14, 1979.
50. McWhinney IR: Beyond Diagnosis. *N Engl J Med* 287:384–387, 1972.
51. Engle RL: Medical diagnosis: present, past and future. I. Present concepts of the meaning and limitations of medical diagnosis. *Arch Intern Med* 112:512–519, 1963.
52. Engle RL: Medical diagnosis: present, past and future. III. Diagnosis in the future, including a critique on the use of electronic computers as diagnostic aids to the physician. *Arch Intern Med* 112:530–543, 1963.
53. Jaspers K: *General Psychopathology*. Chicago, University of Chicago Press, 1963.
54. Engle GL: The need for a new medical model: a challenge for biomedicine. *Science* 196:129–136, 1977.
55. Engle GL: The clinical application of the biopsychosocial model. *Am J Psychiatry* 137:535–543, 1980.
56. McHugh Pr, Slavney PR: *The Perspectives of Psychiatry*. Baltimore, Johns Hopkins University Press, 1986.

9

Clinician/Patient Relations I:
Attending to the Patient's Perspective[a]

Aaron Lazare, M.D.
Sherman Eisenthal, Ph.D.

Responding to the needs of large numbers of patients who seek help in busy outpatient settings is a frustrating and fatiguing experience. Though patients are in considerable distress, many of them neither meet the traditional criteria for long-term psychotherapy nor fit the usual models for crisis intervention or brief psychotherapy. Psychodynamic formulations may be cumbersome, and official diagnostic categories have limited value for clinical intervention. The hypothesis testing approach (described in Chapter 7) using par-

[a] Adapted with permission from Lazare A, Cohen F, Jacobson AM, et al: The walk-in patient as a "customer": a key dimension in evaluation and treatment. *Am J Orthopsychiatry* 42:872–883, 1972 (Copyright 1972, the American Orthopsychiatric Association, Inc.); Lazare A, Eisenthal S: Patient requests in a walk-in clinic: replication of factor analysis in an independent sample. *J Nerv Ment Dis* 165:330–340, 1977 (Copyright 1977, the Williams & Wilkins Co.); and Lazare A, Eisenthal S, Wasserman L: The customer approach to patienthood: attending to patient requests in a walk-in clinic. *Arch Gen Psychiatry* 32:553–558, 1975 (Copyright 1975, the Archives of General Psychiatry and the American Medical Association).

tial formulations from four conceptual models enables the clinician to respond in a more comprehensive manner to a broad range of problems. Yet, it does not inevitably suggest the optimal clinical response.

All of the above approaches to diagnosis and treatment neglect the importance of eliciting and attending to the patient's perspective, a process that we have come to believe is an essential part of the initial interview. Our interest in the patient's perspective arose from a situation of crisis. We were assigned the dual responsibility of providing for (a) the clinical needs of over 300 patients a week who sought help at a walk-in clinic, and (b) the training needs of six first-year residents in psychiatry who were responsible for the care of these patients (each resident evaluated and treated walk-in patients for 2½ days each week throughout a 6-month rotation). Out of a sense of frustration over caring for patients and teaching residents in this setting, the senior author (A. L.) assisted by a college student (Frances Cohen) conducted brief interviews with several hundred patients who were waiting to be seen by the resident psychiatrist (1). The purpose of the interview was to determine what the patients were requesting from us or how they wanted us to intervene on their behalf to assist them in achieving their goals. We hoped that somehow this information would be of some clinical value. To our surprise we found that the elicitation of these requests not only provided important diagnostic information but also exerted a therapeutic influence on the interview itself.

As our attention on the patient's perspective expanded to include the clinician's perspective with the resultant conflict between patient and clinician, the research was named "A Negotiated Approach to Patienthood." This work has since been applied to other psychiatric settings and medical settings (2, 3).

We attempt to show in this chapter and the next how the conceptualizations and data of this research have been useful to us in our roles as clinicians, teachers, and administrators working in busy outpatient settings. This chapter describes the importance of hearing and responding to the patient's perspective. The next chapter describes clinician/patient conflict and the resolution of such conflict by negotiation.

PATIENT REQUESTS

The research began with a search for what patients in a walk-in clinic wanted from the clinicians who were there to serve them. It was our initial belief that by learning what patients requested, we would have a better idea as to how we might help. Our implicit assumption was that patients had requests in mind that they would share with clinicians under the proper conditions.

The Patient's Perspective

It soon became necessary to distinguish requests from other kinds of data that, together with requests, comprise what we term "the patient's perspective." This category of data encompasses (a) the definition of the problem including the complaint and the illness attribution ("I am depressed and anxious because of the unhappiness in my marriage."); (b) the goals of treatment ("I would like to feel like my old self so I can return to work."); and (c) the request or methods of treatment ("Would you give me pills?" or "Would you help me unload my painful feelings?" or "Would you have a talk with my wife?" or "Would you meet together with both of us?" or "Would you help me understand how I mess things up?" or "Would you testify at the divorce proceedings so I can get custody of the children?"). We soon learned that knowing the problem and the goal told us little about the nature of the request or the desired method of intervention. In other words, from the examples above, the clinician would be unable to predict which of the above six requests the depressed, anxious man would make in order to be able to return to work. This observation has important clinical implications, since most clinicians do elicit some aspect of the patient's understanding of the problem, as well as some goal(s) of treatment, but often fail to elicit the request, perhaps in the mistaken belief that the request is self-evident, not available, or irrelevant.

A Categorization of Patient Requests

To determine the range and definition of patient requests, we conducted brief interviews with several hundred patients who were waiting for their initial evaluation in the walk-in clinic. Most patients who came of their own volition were willing to state a request when the investigators asked the questions with enough persistence and compassion. It was then possible to compose definitions of what appeared to be 14 distinct requests in language that was both respectful and understandable to the patient while meaningful to the clinician. These categories, described below, were settled upon only after various members of the research team attempted to elicit the full range of requests from different patient samples in the clinic (1, 4, 5).

Administrative Request

The patient is seeking administrative or legal assistance from the clinic to help him or her with the current dilemma. The specific request may be to provide a disability evaluation, a draft deferment, a medical excuse to leave work, medical permission to return to work, permission to drive, admission to a hospital, or testimony in court. These powers are delegated by society to particular professionals or institutions.

Advice

The patient wants guidance about what to do in personal or social matters. He or she may already have formed an opinion, but now may want professional advice about the "right" thing, the "best" thing, or the "wisest" to do. The patient may want the advice in order to have the clinician share the responsibility for a decision about to be made.

Clarification

The patient wants help to put feelings, thoughts, or behaviors in some perspective. He or she does not want to be told what to do, but would rather take an active role in the therapeutic process. Often the patient wants the help in order to make a decision. He or she wants to understand and see the choices. The patient usually sees the problem as being acute and not a part of an ongoing neurotic pattern.

Community Triage

The patient is requesting information as to where in the community he or she can get the help that is needed. The clinic is seen as an available resource which has the necessary information.

Confession

The patient feels guilty about what he or she has said, thought, or done and hopes that by talking to the therapist he or she will feel better. Specifically, the patient wants to be forgiven. The patient hopes the clinician (authority figure) will see the misdeed as medical or psychological in origin and therefore not bad.

Control

The patient is feeling overwhelmed and out of control and may fear hurting him- or herself or someone else, or going crazy. This patient is saying, "Please take over. I can no longer manage."

Medical

The patient sees his or her problem as being physical in origin, like any other medical condition, as opposed to psychologic or situational in origin. The patient often refers to the problem as "nerves," or as a "nervous condition." The patient, accordingly, hopes for a medical kind of treatment such as pills, electroconvulsive therapy (ECT), hospitalization, or medical advice. He or she expects to take a passive role in the treatment.

Psychologic Expertise

The patient believes that the source of the problem is psychologic rather than physical or situational and is asking the professional to provide an explanation as to why the patient thinks, feels, or acts the way that he or she does. The patient anticipates playing a passive role in the interaction, contributing only that information which the expert requires.

Psychodynamic Insight

The patient perceives the problem as psychologic in origin, as evolving from his or her early development, and as having a repetitive quality. As a result, the patient is left feeling unhappy and unfulfilled, but not overwhelmed or out of control. The patient expects to take an active, collaborative role in talking about the roots of the problem and hopes that a better understanding of the problem will enable him or her to change.

Reality Contact

The patient feels that he or she is losing hold of reality and wants to talk to someone who is psychologically stable and "safe." The request is for the clinician to help the patient "check out" or "keep in touch with" reality.

Social Intervention

The patient sees the problem as residing primarily in the people or situations around him or her. Because the patient feels unequipped to effect the necessary change, the clinician is asked to intervene on the patient's behalf. The patient is asking not for the legal powers of the clinician, but for his or her social influence.

Succorance

The patient is feeling empty, alone, not cared for, deprived, or drained. He or she wants the clinician to care, to be involved, to be comforting, to be warm and giving so that the patient can feel replenished and warm inside. It is not so much the content of the interchange, that is requested as its affective quality of warmth and caring.

Ventilation

The patient would like to tell the clinician about various feelings and affect-laden experiences. The patient anticipates that getting it off his or her chest will be therapeutic. The patient feels like he or she is carrying around a burden which he or she would like to leave with the clinician. In contrast to the request for confession, the patient does not feel guilty and does not need or want forgiveness.

No Request

Patients who make no request are a heterogeneous group. They may have been referred without proper preparation; they may be psychotic; they may have problems, but are not seeking help at this time; they may want help, but are reluctant to state the problem; they may not need help; they may be in the wrong clinic.

These 14 requests have been measured by an 84-item Patient Request Form that was derived from patients' verbatim statements in clinical interviews. A factor analysis of the 84 items confirmed the relative mathematical independence of 13 of the 14 requests (4, 5).

THE CLINICAL VALUE OF ELICITING AND RESPONDING TO PATIENT REQUESTS

As we elicited patient requests, we became aware that gathering this data had considerable diagnostic value and a facilitative effect on the therapeutic flow of the interview. These two perspectives are illustrated in the following seven case histories (1, 6).

Case Histories

Case 1. A 40-year-old woman, whose chart referred to her condition as "chronic schizophrenic," was referred to the psychiatry clinic from the medical clinic, where she had stated her problem as "noise pollution." From her facial expression, her bizarre thought content, and the history of multiple-state hospitalizations, it seemed highly probable that the diagnosis was correct. It was also noted that she had been to our clinic several times. Each time she was referred back to her local mental health center. Now, much to our embarrassment, she came to our medical clinic. The diagnosis, the history, and the manner of presentation made the clinician feel helpless and angry. He knew she was ill and that he was expected to help. He believed he had nothing to offer.

After 15 minutes of a rambling, circuitous interview, the clinician asked in frustration how she hoped that he could help. She requested to be put "on a stronger pill." The patient was receiving chlordiazepoxide hydrochloride (Librium), but no antipsychotic medications. The clinician was immediately put at ease, since the request was reasonable. He no longer felt helpless. The clinician was then able to explore how the patient's daughter, now 13 years of age, was beginning to talk too much and too loudly. This situation seemed to coincide with the onset of the delusion about noise pollution. In addition to a change in medication, the patient was willing to accept the recommendation for casework to help her deal with the psychologic demands of her adolescent daughter.

The patient concluded by explaining that she was no longer accepting our referrals to her local mental health center because they hospitalized her before listening to her. She came to our medical clinic because she felt the psychiatry clinic, before today, had not listened to her either.

Case 2.   A 27-year-old man had the target complaint of "nerves . . . too much drinking." He communicated with considerable urgency his goal of discontinuing drinking and specifically requested pills to accomplish the goal. The clinician, who believed the request was reasonable but failed to share this belief with the patient, proceeded to inquire into other areas that might help explain the drinking. Tension in the interview mounted. Finally, the patient angrily responded, "My marriage is okay, my family is okay, everything is okay . . . Look, first, give me the pills, and then I'll sing." With the request clearly stated, the clinician assured the patient that he believed that pills were indicated and agreed to write a prescription at the end of the interview. The patient then proceeded to describe his marital difficulties that culminated in striking his wife. The loss of control was the decisive event that brought him to the clinic.

Case 3.   A 55-year-old hospital employee said that he was upset and depressed over his wife's recent hospitalization for a recurrent psychotic condition. The resident elicited symptoms of depression which he attempted to understand in terms of the patient's loneliness or guilt, or both, but was unable to elicit responses that would support this formulation. In response to the question "How did you wish we could help?" the patient replied, "I work here in the hospital kitchen and bring food up to the psychiatry ward. It's a nice clean place, and they treat the patients well. If you have space, would you call the state hospital and have her transferred? I would feel much better." The transfer was arranged, and the patient became asymptomatic.

Case 4.   A 42-year-old divorced woman came to the clinic and stated the following: "My house burned down 2 days ago. I need something for myself; I need pills for my nerves." The patient was given the opportunity to tell her story for the next 30 minutes. She seemed to use the time for ventilation, emotionally recounting in considerable detail the description of the fire. The clinician's supportive listening was a response to the first part of the patient's request for "something for myself." The clini-

cian could then respond to the second part of the request with, "I don't believe pills are necessary." The patient replied, "I agree with you. I'm feeling so much better already. Could you give me your name and phone number so I can call you and let you know how things work out?"

Case 5.   An unkempt 46-year-old chronic alcoholic man, smelling of alcohol but not acutely intoxicated, was guarded during the first few minutes of the interview as he tried to sense whether or not he would receive the unfriendly welcome often given the alcoholic patient. As he began to feel that the clinician was interested in finding out what was bothering him and what he wanted, he proceeded to tell his story. Born in Scotland, he had only one relative in this country, a sister living in Baltimore. The patient had lost contact with her when she was hospitalized 8 months ago. He could never muster the nerve to phone her for fear of learning of her death. His request of the clinician was for social intervention: "Would you phone her for me? Here is money for the call." The clinician made the call and successfully put him back in contact with his only relative. (An implicit request was for the clinician to be with the patient if he were to learn of his sister's death.) The patient then told the clinician that his visit today was triggered by his bringing his only companion into the hospital for cirrhosis.

As the clinician heard the story, he considered and ruled out the possibility that the patient was suffering from impending delirium tremens, Wernicke encephalopathy, or another condition that would have required some "negotiation" over necessary medical treatment.

Case 6.   A 56-year-old married male presented with a 5-month history of depressive symptoms following the death of his brother. The depressive syndrome was of the endogenous type. He appeared not to have experienced a normal grief for his brother.

Three weeks prior to his visit to the clinic, the patient had been treated by another psychiatrist, who had prescribed a low dosage of antidepressant medications. The patient was still able to work, and suicide was not a serious concern. He seemed to be still in control of his life situation.

From the above data, acquired during a 45

minute interview, it was not learned what the patient wanted the clinic to do. Several therapeutic approaches, nevertheless, seemed possible, including exploring and possibly renegotiating the patient's relationship with the former therapist, administering a higher dose of anti-depressant medication, and dealing psychotherapeutically with the unresolved grief. After a reasonable treatment program had been offered, which addressed itself to all three approaches, the patient announced that he came to the clinic to be admitted to the psychiatric ward of our hospital. By this time, the therapist was annoyed and pressed for time. He then hastily agreed that hospitalization was a reasonable disposition. Since the ward was filled, hospitalization elsewhere was arranged. The therapist failed to learn at the beginning of the interview that the patient had a specific administrative request. He therefore missed the opportunity to explore fully why the patient felt that hospitalization was necessary so that he could either agree with the patient or help him to deal with some possible irrational ideas about hospitalization and explore whether outpatient care could be provided (1).

Case 7 (from a medical clinic). A 47-year-old obese, married female presented to the medical clinic with low back pain 2 years in duration. The medical student, assuming that the patient wanted a cure for her symptom, obtained a complete history relevant to low back pain. Lab tests were negative. He was able to present to his supervisor an excellent differential diagnosis of the symptom, and his treatment was referral to a dietician for weight reduction. Her coming to the hospital from a considerable distance and the 2-year history should have made him suspicious that perhaps the patient wanted something else.

During a second interview, with an internist and psychiatrist serving as consultants, the history was focused on what the patient hoped that we could do. It was easily ascertained that the patient was not asking for a cure for low back pain. This symptom had not been of major concern to the patient until 2 weeks prior to the clinic visit at which time her sister had died at the same hospital of cancer that was metastatic to the spine. To complicate matters, 2 months before the visit the patient had been told by her family physician that she had "tumors of the womb," which was "nothing to worry about." Before her death, the sister had suggested to the patient that this hospital would tell her the cause of the back pain. The patient was requesting some basic diagnostic information: "Do I have cancer?" A dietician could not provide the answer (1).

Diagnostic Issues

Patients' statements of their request provide diagnostic information which enhances the efficiency and effectiveness of the clinical process. There are many clinical situations in which the patients' statement of what they want is exactly what the clinician believes that they need. Using the negotiated approach, the clinician gathers this information early in the interview and profits thereby from patients' ideas, a commonly ignored source of diagnostic data. In Case 1, the patient with schizophrenia wanted and needed stronger medication. This information may have emerged later in the interview. However, in a busy clinical setting, a patient with a history of frequent nonproductive visits may have been sent elsewhere before being adequately evaluated. In Case 2 the patient wanted and needed pills. In Case 3 the patient wanted and needed administrative assistance to obtain better care for his wife and to feel that he was doing all in his power to help her. If the request was not directly elicited, his needs would never have been known. In Case 4 the patient wanted and needed "something for myself." Had this part of the request not been elicited, the clinician might have administered or withheld medicines without being aware of a more important need. In Case 5 the patient wanted and needed someone to put him in contact with his sister and to be available for other supportive needs if it were learned that his sister was dead. Unless the patient felt comfortable enough to make the request, he would have left with his needs unmet. The clinician might have commented, "Just another alcoholic."

When the patient's request is clinically appropriate, learning the request can be very important in determining the precise clinical response. Take for example, the requests for *ventilation, confession,* and *reality contact* in three separate patients and assume that these requests represent valid clinical needs. An accurate diagnosis of the request/need will lead to three distinct clinical responses. For the patient who needs *ventilation,* the clinician can best help by taking the role of the interested listener. If the clinician breaks in to make interpretive comments, the patient is apt to tolerate the interruption, ignore the clinician's words, and go on with his or her story. For the patient who needs *confession,* the clinician can best help by an attitude and verbal response which puts the deed in a medical or psychologic perspective (when the guilt is neurotic) or which (when guilt is real) helps the patient bear the painful feelings. If the clinician were to assume the role of the interested listener (as for *ventilation*) the patient would take this response as confirmation of his or her guilt. For the patient who needs *reality contact,* it may be important for the clinician to actively share thoughts about what is real. Again, the role of the passive listener might aggravate the condition.

For the above examples, it can be seen that by distinguishing a wide variety of distinct requests or perceived treatment needs, the clinician can discard or go beyond the rubric of "supportive" and address specific patient needs with more precise clinical reponses. In the past, diagnosing the need for "supportive" help often elicited vague clinical responses that often turned out not to be supportive.

The request is of diagnostic value even when it seems clinically inappropriate and/or when it catches the clinician unawares. If these situations arise, it is likely that the clinician was on the wrong track in his understanding of the problem or the goal. This was the situation in Case 3, in which the hospital employee wanted the clinic to arrange for a transfer; in Case 6, in which the patient announced that he wanted to be admitted to a hospital; and in Case 7, in which the patient said she wanted to know if she had cancer. The interview would have been more efficient and more effective in these four situations if the request had been learned earlier.

The patient's response to the clinician's elicitation of the request may also have special diagnostic meaning when the patient is reluctant to or refuses to state what he wants (see "Resistance to Expressing Requests"). If the clinician pursues the matter, he or she will often learn important information about the personality of the patient. Patients have told us, for instance, that they are not worthy enough to ask for anything, that they are unwilling to commit themselves, that they will be obligated to give the clinician something in return, etc. Without these responses, exploration of significant psychologic issues may be delayed.

Process Issues

There is apt to be a great deal of wasted time and energy during an interview, in which the patient request is verbalized either late in the interview or not at all. Instead of speaking freely about the problem, the patient may be preoccupied, wondering whether the clinician is kind enough, respectful enough, wise enough, understanding enough, and flexible enough to hear the request. "When will the clinician be ready to hear?" "When will I have the guts to come right out with it?" The clinician, meanwhile, often unaware of these concerns, goes about the business of establishing diagnoses and making treatment recommendations, not understanding why the patient participates only reluctantly during the interview. On the other hand, when the patient has stated the request early in the interview and feels it has been supportively heard, he or she is apt to participate more freely and feel more satisfied at the end.

Sometimes the clinician unwittingly discourages the patient from stating the request. One may observe in this situation a sparring between the clinician and the patient. For example, the patient throws out a hint about the request: "I think I may need to be watched over for a time (alluding to a request for hospitalization)." The clinician then changes the subject without acknowledging the request. "Have you had any physical illness recently?" The patient responds with hostility: "I'm fed up with everything!"

Sometimes the patient, feeling that there is no opening, waits until the end of the interview before stating the request: "By the way, would you. . . ." The clinician now has new and essential data, but not enough time to evaluate or act on it. For example, a patient comes to a medical clinic allegedly for a general exam. As she is about to leave the office after the examination, she states the real request: "By the way, you don't think this is serious, do you?" Had the patient made the request earlier and had the clinician perceived the request as legitimate and important, the clinician could have explored the reasons for the patient's concern and learned what kind of explanation would be most appropriate.

In sum, by eliciting the request in an empathic manner, the clinician diminishes the patient's need to engage in evasive activities meant to test the clinician's flexibility, interest, and concern, conveys to the patient the collaborative nature of the interview, and changes the focus of the interview towards the task.

In many clinical situations, acknowledging the request or giving the patient what he or she asks for satisfies needs that must be met before a healthier request can be made. For instance, patients who first request control, reality contact, or succorance cannot be expected to progress to requests requiring their active collaboration, such as clarification, until the more basic requests are dealt with. In Case 2 satisfying the request for medication frees the patient to explore social or psychotherapeutic requests regarding the marriage. We refer to this process of shifting requests from sicker to healthier as progressive. Contrariwise, patients whose initial requests are rejected or not acknowledged may subsequently present with a sicker or regressive request. For example, if a request for social intervention is denied, the patient may request control or reality contact. The chronic alcoholic patient, Case 5, may have had such needs had his request to phone his sister been denied.

The elicitation of the patient request has, in many situations, an important impact on the clinician which, in turn, affects the entire course of the interview. In Case 1, for instance, the clinician's feeling changed from anger to compassion upon learning that there was something useful that he could do. Similarly, the clinician in Case 3, before hearing the request for assistance in transferring the patient's wife to a general hospital felt bewildered that neither biologic nor psychodynamic hypotheses explained the patient's presentation. In Case 5, the "incurable chronic alcoholic" became a human being in distress once his request had become known.

It is not uncommon for overworked clinicians, dealing with patient populations culturally different from their own, to believe that the patient wants radical changes in character and symptomatology that are hard to fulfill. The clinician, believing that the patient will expect these changes, then becomes angry at the patient for having such unreasonable demands. Having the patient state his or her request undercuts this series of projections, since what the patient wants is almost always more modest than what the clinician expected. Patients do not want to be different human beings. They want to feel better.

Social Class and Patient Requests

By defining a wide range of requests and encouraging clinical responses to them or negotiations over them, we believed the overlooked needs of the lower social classes would be better met. They were the patients, it was assumed, who wanted the supportive requests of ventilation, control, advice, and medical treatment, rather than the more "sophisticated" middle class requests of psychodynamic insight and clarification. This assumption has been used to explain why lower class applicants to psychiatric clinics were less readily accepted for psychotherapy, were more likely to be assigned to less experienced psychotherapists, were judged as being less socially improved upon termination from treatment, and were more apt to terminate prematurely. We were now saying to the clinician on the basis of our current concepts: "Take patients where they are. They may well know what they need. Even if you disagree, negotiations must start from the patient's perspective."

We subsequently examined the relationship between patient requests and social class (7). The major conclusion of this study was that patient requests are largely independent of social class. More specifically, patients from Classes I to IV did not differ from each other in the kinds of help (requests) they wanted from the clinic. Class V patients wanted more active help (e.g., social intervention, community triage, and administrative help) and more authoritarian information (e.g., psychologic expertise) than higher class patients, but just as much psychodynamic insight and clarification. The important findings, it seems to us, is that lower class patients want psychologic interventions much more than had previously been assumed and that middle and upper class patients want much more of the so-called "supportive" interventions than had been previously assumed. The implication of these findings is that patients of *all classes* have been shortchanged because of inaccurate preconceptions by mental health professionals of what each group needs or wants. In addition, the notion should now be dispelled that the inequities in care provided to lower class patients are a consequence of their having the "wrong" requests or expectations and that some requests are second class because of the groups of patients who make them.

THE EXPRESSION OF PATIENT REQUESTS

Elicitation of the Patient Request

Since the patient's statement of the request during the initial interview is a crit-

ical beginning of a negotiated approach, how the clinician elicits the request deserves special attention.

Sometimes the patient will state his or her request spontaneously at the beginning of the interview. When this does not occur, the patient request is best elicited after the clinician learns the patient's complaint and a meaningful part of the present illness. This preliminary interaction establishes the rapport necessary for the elicitation of the patient request. Eliciting the request at the very start of the interview before the patient has stated the problem increases the chances of placing the patient in the position of adversary rather than collaborator in the diagnostic and therapeutic process. "You asked me what I want. You do not even know what is wrong with me." Eliciting the request at the end of the interview deprives the clinician of the opportunity to negotiate or work with the request.

We have been most successful in eliciting the patient request by asking, "How do you hope (or wish) I (or the clinic) can help?" The question "What do you want?" and "What do you expect?" should be avoided, since they are more likely to be perceived as confrontations. The words "wish" or "hope," in contrast, give the patient permission to state requests that he or she does not necessarily expect will be granted. Even when the clinician finally asks the patient what he hopes for, the responses commonly are "I don't know. You are the therapist," or "I just want to feel better." In this kind of situation, the patient frequently has a rather specific request in mind that he or she is reluctant to state. The elicitation of the request then requires persistence, persuasion, and compassion. "You must have had some idea when you decided to come," or "it is important for me to know what your wishes are, even if I may not be able to fulfill them."

The initial statement of the request may be incomplete or stated in such general terms that it requires elaboration to achieve the specificity necessary for clinical utility. "You said you want me to help you understand things better. What in particular do you want to understand?'' or ''You thought you would feel better if I would fix up your family situation. How do you hope I can fix it up?'' When the request has finally been stated and elaborated, it is important that the clinician acknowledge having heard and understood the request. Otherwise, the patient may wonder whether the clinician heard the request, was offended by it, or didn't believe it worthy of a response.

The elicitation of the request undoubtedly depends on more than timing and phraseology for its effectiveness. Certainly, the clinician's attitude of interest and receptivity is crucial. We have observed, for instance, that the patient frequently hints at or alludes to the request, apparently waiting for some response from the clinician that will indicate that it is acceptable to continue or to become more specific.

As the interview proceeds, the clinician should listen for elaborations of or changes in the request resulting fron the developing relationship between clinician and patient. The patient thinks, ''Now that I have more trust in you, let me tell you what I really want,'' or ''Now that you have responded to my initial request, it occurs to me that there is something more important that I need.''

Research Findings

Moving from the clinical to the experimental, we felt that it was important to explore the assumption that serves as a basis for the clinical recommendation to elicit patient requests: that patients do come with requests, the expression of which depends on the sanctioning behavior of the clinician. In a series of studies (4, 5, 8, 9) we have shown that 99% of patients filling out a Patient Request Form (PRF) will state at least one request that they strongly endorse, whereas only 69% of patients will verbalize a specific request, using a structured preintake interview. In the natural setting of the clinical interview, we found the 63% of patients expressed

specific requests. This group breaks down into 37% of patients who spontaneously emitted a specific request and 26% of patients who verbalized a request after the clinician's elicitation. The importance of the clinician's behavior in eliciting the request was emphasized by the significant increase in patient's verbalizations of specific requests following a second elicitation inquiry.

These findings support the view that most patients (63 to 69%) are predisposed to express specific requests in an intake interview. It is not clear to what degree the remaining 31 to 37% of patients (*a*) have requests in mind, but have not had sufficient sanction from the clinician to express their requests and (*b*) do not have requests clearly formulated and need to have the experience of the clinical interaction to help them formulate exactly what they want. Similarly, one may ask whether the PRF, with its 99% endorsement, sanctions patients' expressing what they already have clearly formulated, or whether it functions like the clinical interaction which crystalizes for patients what had been a vague sense of what they wanted.

We attempted to identify which patients are most likely to express specific requests, since some patients do not state requests or state them in a nonspecific, general, or noncommittal form. The patients who tend to be specific can be characterized as (*a*) female, (*b*) coming to the clinic at their own instigation rather than at the suggestion of others, (*c*) prior patients to the clinic, and (*d*) having a complaint which is interpersonal or somatic, rather than one which is vague, general, or situational. These data suggest that clinicians may need to help certain identifiable patient groups in formulating and expressing their requests.

Resistance to Expressing Requests

Although verbalizing the patient request usually has considerable clinical value, there is an extraordinary amount of resistance on the part of clinicians in eliciting requests and of patients in expressing requests. It is as if there were a conspiracy between both parties, in which the patient agrees not to say what he or she wants and the clinician agrees not to ask. We have attempted to understand this resistance from the separate points of view of clinician and patient.

Clinicians describe several reasons why they neither elicit nor respond to patient requests. Some believe that by hearing the statement of the problem and the goal, they know the patient's request even though it has not been made explicit. For example, the clinician is apt to assume that an intelligent, insightful person who describes some apparent intrapsychic conflict wants psychotherapy. Other clinicians believe that patients either cannot verbalize what they want or that the verbalizations are conscious distortions of unconscious processes. For some, the issue of professional norms is at stake. It is feared that the patient will regard the clinician who elicits the patient's request as not professionally responsible. "You should know; you are the therapist." Another important issue has to do with authority. In these circumstances, the clinician may feel that asking the patient what he or she wants is tantamount to turning over the authority for treatment to the patient. We believe the most important issues which keep the clinician from finding out how the patient would like him or her to intervene are fears of impotence and helplessness. There is the concern in many of us that eliciting the request will open up a Pandora's box of unending, overwhelming, and depleting demands which the clinician would rather avoid.

We have observed three major reasons as to why patients find it difficult to tell the clinician what they want. The first has to do with their perception that it is the patients' role to state their problem, but not to evaluate how the help should be provided. Patients, nevertheless, reserve the right to take their business elsewhere if they are not satisfied. The second reason has to do with the patients' perception of the clinic or the clinician as the adversary who has the power to say no. As a result,

patients must hint at this request or present it in an indirect way which may maximize their chances of "winning." The third reason why patients find it difficult to say what they want has to do with a wide range of personality variables: (a) Some patients feel that making the request explicit diminishes the quality of the giving. "A caring person would know what I wanted without my asking." (This situation is similar to complimenting one's spouse's appearance only after he or she has requested it). (b) Some patients do not feel worthy enough to ask: "Who am I to ask for anything?" (c) Others feel humiliation and loss of pride if they have to ask for anything. (d) Some patients feel that stating their wish leads to too much intimacy or closeness, that they could become too open or exposed and therefore subject to criticism, ridicule, rejection, or even acceptance and other feared positive feelings. (e) Patients may be concerned that saying what they want is limiting by making it unlikely that they will get more. By keeping the request vague, it is possible to get more. (If you ask $150,000 for your house, no one will offer you $151,000). (f) Others are reluctant to state what they want because they will have then committed themselves and are not psychologically prepared to do so: "If I say what I want, you may take me seriously and hold me to what I say." (g) Some patients fear that if they verbalize their desires, the magnitude of their needs might embarrass them. (h) Some patients fear that by having their request granted, they would be forced to change their notion of the world as a mean, ungiving place. (j) Others fear that the clinician may yield to a request which may be clinically inappropriate. "He might do what I want and that might turn out to be a mistake." (k) Others may fear that the clinician, by saying yes to the request, will fail to set needed limits: "I needed him to say no!" (l) Finally, many patients perceive asking for what they want to be too aggressive an act.

The difficulty in stating what one wants, wishes, or hopes for is hardly limited to the clinician–patient relationship. It is deeply rooted in our culture. For example, in making wishes after blowing out the birthday candles or breaking the wishbone, we must keep wishes to ourselves if they are to have the best chance of coming true. In seeking out certain academic and industrial positions, one does not ask for the job. The chances for attaining the position are enhanced if someone else submits the applicant's name.

In sum, telling someone what you want from them is a most intimate and revealing communication.

SUMMARY

This chapter has reviewed clinical research on the value of attending the patient's perspective in the initial interview(s). Patient perspectives refer here to the patient's definition of the problem, goals of treatment, and requests or desired methods of treatment. Fourteen discrete request categories are described.

The elicitation of the patient's request (and perspective) is useful diagnostically by suggesting to the clinician with considerable specificity what the patient needs. In addition, the elicitation of the request enhances the process of the interview by (a) communicating to the patient the collaborative rather than adversarial nature of the interview, (b) satisfying some of the patient's needs so that he or she can be freed to make other requests, and (c) enhancing the morale of the clinician who now feels more effective and less intimidated by what he or she fears that the patient wants.

References

1. Lazare A, Cohen F, Jacobson AM, et al: The walk-in patient as a "customer": a key dimension in evaluation and treatment. *Am J Orthopsychiatry* 42:872–883, 1972.
2. Katon W, Kleinman AM: Doctor–patient negotiation and other social science strategies in patient care. In Eisenberg L, Kleinman AM (eds): *The Relevance of Social Science for Medicine*. Dordrecht, Holland, Reidel, 1981 pp 253–279.
3. Good M, Good B, Nassi AJ: Patient requests in primary health care settings: development and validation of a research instrument. *J Behav Med* 6:151–168, 1983.
4. Lazare A, Eisenthal S, Wasserman L, et al: Patient requests in a walk-in clinic. *Compr Psychiatry* 16:467–477, 1975.
5. Lazare A, Eisenthal S: Patient requests in a walk-in clinic: replication of factor analysis in an independent sample. *J Nerv Ment Dis* 165:330–340, 1977.
6. Lazare A, Eisenthal S, Wasserman L: The customer approach to patienthood: attending to patient requests in a walk-in clinic. *Arch Gen Psychiatry* 32:553–558, 1975.
7. Frank A, Eisenthal S, Lazare A: Are there social class differences in patients' treatment conceptions?: myths and facts. *Arch Gen Psychiatry* 35:1–69, 1978.
8. Eisenthal S, Lazare A: Specificity of patient requests in the initial interview. *Psychol Rep* 38:739–748, 1976.
9. Eisenthal S, Lazare A: Expression of patients' requests in the initial interview. *Psychol Rep* 40:131–138, 1977.

10

Clinician/Patient Relations II:
Conflict and Negotiation

Aaron Lazare, M.D.
Sherman Eisenthal, Ph.D.
Arlene Frank, Ph.D.

In the previous chapter, the patient's perspective was discussed, with particular emphasis on patient requests or preferred methods of intervention. Both the diagnostic and the therapeutic values of eliciting and responding to these requests were shown.

It soon became apparent, however, that conflict between the clinician and patient over their perspectives not only is a common ocurrence but also is often a central feature of the clinical process. Studies of such conflict in clinical practice deal with various aspects of the patient's perspective: expectations of treatment, (1–13) methods of treatment (14, 15), priorities or goals of treatment (15–22), and attitudes and behaviors of the clinician (23, 24). There is little discussion in these studies about how clinicians should respond to these conflicts. Most of this research was generated in response to the alarming number of patients who fail to comply with treatment recommendations (35), who comply but are dissatisfied with the treatment they receive (23), who terminate

treatment prematurely (1, 36), or who fail to show measurable therapeutic gains (37–39). It has been suggested by several investigators that a major cause of such instances of therapeutic failure is conflict between therapist and patient, particularly over their treatment conceptions (40).

In this chapter we attempt to conceptualize the types of conflict that occur between clinicians and patients in initial encounters of a general outpatient psychiatric practice and the variety of consensus-seeking strategies, particularly negotiation, that are used to resolve them. We believe, however, that this theoretical analysis can be applied to all clinical encounters between help seekers and help providers—not only in mental health but in medicine and its subspecialties.

Since the first publication of this chapter, there have in fact been numerous applications of the concept of negotiation to the medical encounter (41–45) and to psychoanalysis (46).

Social psychology and, to a lesser extent, medical sociology are the academic

137

disciplines that provide the language, the concepts, and the existing research on dyadic conflict and negotiation. By systematically applying these ideas to clinician–patient encounters, we hope to focus attention on an important but neglected dimension of patient care.

A CLASSIFICATION OF CONFLICT

Conflict between the clinician and patient may be classified as being over (a) the problem, (b) the goals of treatment, (c) the methods of treatment, (d) the conditions of treatment, and (e) the clinician–patient relationship. Knowledge of the type of conflict is essential to initiating the process of negotiation.

Conflicts over the Problem

In initial clinical encounters, patients and clinicians usually have divergent and incomplete views as to the nature of the problem, its causes, its seriousness, and, in the case of multiple problems, the treatment priorities. Typically, they differ in their experience with psychiatric problems, in their access to information about the meaning of symptoms (e.g., the patient's family and friends or mass media versus the clinician's colleagues and supervisors or professional journals), and in their belief systems, defenses, and coping mechanisms. The different life experiences of patient and clinician undoubtedly contribute to different conceptions of what is wrong, whether the problem is environmental, interpersonal, biologic, intrapsychic, or whether there is any problem at all.

For example, a patient may feel that the problem is anxiety, while the clinician may feel the problem is severe personality disorganization. The patient may not perceive his strange thoughts as a significant problem, whereas the clinician views the disturbed thought processes as a possible manifestation of schizophrenia and thus as a significant problem. Even if a patient and clinician agree on the nature of the problem, they may disagree as to its cause. For

example, a patient may attribute her memory problem to "emotional fatigue," while the clinician may attribute it to Alzheimer's disease. Similar differences may occur over the seriousness of the problem. For example, a patient may perceive his heart palpitations and shortness of breath as indicators of an impending heart attack and thus as being quite serious problems. For the clinician, these symptoms may signify anxiety, which is not necessarily a reason for serious concern.

Finally, in the case of multiple problems, patients and clinicians may have conflicting treatment priorities. For example, both patient and clinician may agree that the patient has two major problems that require attention: a chronic marital problem and an acute psychosis. The patient may first want to address her marital problem, which she may perceive as being more distressing as well as being the cause of the psychosis. The clinician may first want to deal with the psychosis, which he or she feels represents an insurmountable obstacle to any marital therapy.

Conflict over the problem can be much more complex than are the examples described above. Patients and clinicians at the beginning of psychotherapy, for instance, usually have somewhat divergent and incomplete views as to what is wrong. Part of the process of psychotherapy consists of an elaboration of the problem through clarifications, interpretations, and new historic data. It is hoped that in time, the clinician and patient approach a more comprehensive and congruent view of the problem (46).

Conflicts over the Goals of Treatment

Conflicts over the goals of treatment are common in clinical encounters but are seldom explicit (exceptions are behavior therapy and transactional analysis, in which explicit contracts are commonly set). For example, the patient may wish to find relief from intense anxiety, whereas the clinician wishes to assist the patient in achieving personality change. Most often these conflicts are unstated, subtle, and implicit. They may surface when there is a failure to agree over some method of treatment, such as hospitalization, or a condition of treatment, such as cost or time.

In our observation of the evaluation process, relatively few interviewers inquire intensively about the patient's goals. Differences in goals are thus likely to be overlooked or be unrecognized. One reason for this is the assumption by the clinician of congruence over treatment goals, namely, a return to health. The possibility of different subgoals and priorities is overlooked. Another reason is that the acknowledgment of conflicts and differences is unpleasant and, for that reason, is avoided.

Conflicts over goals may reflect divergent values. For example, in the case of manic–depressive illness, a conceivable conflict over goals (values) would be restitution and maintenance of the individual's best premorbid state (clinician's goal) versus return to a state of manic euphoria (patient's goal).

Conflict over the goals of treatment is likely to occur if the clinician has not resolved conflicts over the definition of the problem, especially over causal attributions. For example, the patient who believes the problem of outbursts of impulsive behavior is caused by excessive family control will set diminished family control as her primary goal, while the clinician who believes the problem is manic–depressive psychosis, a biologic illness, will set medical management of this illness as the primary goal.

Conflicts over Methods of Treatment

One of the most common types of conflicts that clinicians encounter is over the methods of treatment. Rare is the clinician who has not had to negotiate with a patient over the merits of medication versus psychotherapy, hospitalization versus outpatient treatment, or individual versus group psychotherapy. Since treatment disposition is of primary concern in the initial evaluation, it is not surprising that conflicts over methods arise so often. These conflicts arise for a number of reasons.

Often, the patient and clinician have failed to achieve a shared understanding of the problem. For example, a depressed patient may come to a clinician requesting psychotherapy. The clinician, after taking a history and conducting a mental status exam, may conclude that the most appropriate treatment is psychotherapy combined with medication. Although the explicit conflict is over the treatment method, the "real" or implicit conflict is over the nature of the problem. The clinician may have based his or her treatment recommendation on the belief that the patient's depression, characterized by frequent spontaneous recurrences with vegetative symptoms and a strong family history of depression, had a strong biologic component. The patient, on the other hand, may have requested psychotherapy because he believed that his depression was primarily the result of intrapsychic conflict and personal disappointment. Although patient and clinician agreed that the problem was "depression," neither elaborated his or her definition of depression. In this case, the conflict over the treatment might have been circumvented if they had achieved a shared understanding of the meaning and origin of the problem.

Even when a patient and clinician agree on the nature of the problem and the goals of treatment, they still may disagree on the methods of treatment. In these cases, the conflict may stem from several sources: (a) their preconceived notions about what is helpful; (b) their treatment preferences (e.g., the clinician, by virtue of his or her extensive experience and skill with groups, may prefer group psychotherapy as a treatment modality, while the patient may be uncomfortable in group situations and may prefer individual psychotherapy.); and (c) their unstated problems in the therapeutic relationship (E.g., a patient may object to a clinician's recommendation of hospitalization because the patient views it as avoidance of personal involvement, a personal rejection. The patient may feel that the clinician does not care enough about him or her personally to want to treat him or her or that the clinician questions the patient's ability to handle outpatient treatment. The clinician, in turn, may be recommending hospitalization because he or she is frustrated with the patient's many demands and wants to let go of the burden of caring for such a difficult patient).

The consequences of not resolving such conflicts are numerous and varied, as well as potentially serious. For example, the clinician may not accept the patient for treatment, or the patient may terminate the applicancy process. Even if the patient and clinician continue the applicancy process, they may encounter further relationship problems. The patient may initially comply with the clinician's treatment recommendation, only to later manifest his or her resentment toward the clinician for "forcing" a treatment method that the patient never really wanted. Finally, if the patient and clinician fail to reach a consensus over the methods of treatment, it is unlikely that they will be able to effectively negotiate the conditions of treatment.

Conflicts over the Conditions of Treatment

Among the most frequently observed explicit conflicts between clinician and patient are those over the condition of treatment. Conditions of treatment include where treatment should take place (a private office, a clinic, a waiting room, or at home), who should provide the treatment (a nurse, a social worker, a psychologist, a psychiatrist), how finances for the treatment should be arranged, and how frequently the treatment should take place. Resolution of conflicts over the conditions of treatment often rests on the clinician's perceptions of the patient's motivations and rights. A common rationalization of differences over time, place, or cost of treatment is the attribution by the clinician of a lack of motivation, resistance, or entitlement on the patient's part. It is our thesis that the patient's desires regarding the conditions of treatment should be taken seriously as a part of entering into a process of negotiating and resolving conflict. Otherwise an effective formation of a treatment alliance may be nipped in its formative stage.

Conflicts over the Relationship

Conflicts over the relationship (what the patient wants from the clinician and what the clinician wants from the patient) are of greatest consequence in the clinical interview. The patient's requirements of the clinician can be categorized around two basic dimensions—personal caring and technical competency. First, the patient wants to feel the clinician is sufficiently caring, respectful, and interested. The patient does not want to suffer humiliation or sacrifice self-esteem, honor, or principle. Conflicts over this dimension may arise when the clinician attempts to maintain a position of detachment despite the patient's desire for personal support. Second, the patient wants to believe the clinician is competent and expert—that he "knows his stuff." Conflict over this dimension may arise when the clinician's interview is brief, the diagnostic tests are few, and the explanation of the findings is meager. In this situation, although the evaluation and treatment plan may be adequate and accurate from the professional's point of view, the patient may question the clinician's competency and seek a more thorough examination.

A conflict over competence is often hinted at by the patient's questioning the clinician regarding his or her age, experience, or training. A conflict over personal caring may be suggested by the patient's complaining about another clinician's insensitivity. The degree to which the patient feels that both dimensions of the relationship are satisfied influences the quality and durability of the working relationship. In mental health encounters, the caring quality of the working relationship is perhaps more important than in other helping fields. For example, in surgery the patient may be willing to forego the need to be respected and cared for so long as he or she feels assured of the clinician's competency—"I have the best surgeon in the world. That's all that matters."

Let us now consider the clinician's requirements of the patient. At the least, the clinician may require that the patient not be physically violent, keep appointments, pay the fees, and be on time. The clinician may also desire that the patient be pleasant, intelligent, and psychologically minded and present an intellectually challenging problem. The fewer requirements the clinician has of the patient, the wider the range of patients the clinician will be able to help.

THE EXPRESSION OF CONFLICT

The clinical task of diagnosing and classifying conflict in the initial encounter requires that attention be paid to the ways in which conflict is experienced and expressed by the clinician and patient. We shall describe a threefold analysis of the expression and awareness of conflict. The first two aspects concern the expression of conflict—namely, implicit versus explicit conflict, and direct versus displaced conflict—while the third concerns the awareness of conflict, that is, conscious versus unconscious conflict.

Explicit Versus Implicit Conflict

A conflict is explicit when both parties verbalize divergent or opposing positions and is implicit when at least one party does not verbalize a divergent or opposing position that the other party has taken. Implicit conflicts, although unstated, are usually conscious and signify an effort to avoid confrontation, usually in favor of other, more indirect means of conflict resolution. For example, the patient may initially set a goal or request a method of treatment with which the clinician disagrees. The conflict is implicit if the clinician does not immediately verbalize his or her conflicting goals and methods. The clinician may be motivated by the concern that the ensuing confrontation might lead

to the patient's terminating the interview. Instead of making the conflict explicit, the clinician attempts to develop a relationship with the patient while inquiring into the patient's understanding of the problem, goals, and methods. The conflict may surface only indirectly by the tone and focus of questions and comments. If consensus is not achieved by the process, the clinician inevitably makes his or her conflicting position explicit by the end of the interview, for example, "I do not believe the medication you want is indicated for the problems you have described."

In practice, conflicts over the problems and conditions of treatment are apt to be explicit while conflicts over goals, methods, and the relationship are apt to be implicit. Conflicts over the problem are apt to be explicit since it is expected that the patient begins the interview by stating what is wrong and the clinician ultimately presents his or her belief about what is wrong. Since practical questions regarding the conditions of treatment inevitably arise, explicit conflict over the conditions of treatment are common in discussions of treatment planning. In contrast, conflicts over goals are apt to be implicit, since both the clinician and the patient often assume the goal is so obvious it does not need stating. The clinician always presents his or her proposed method of treatment, while the patient is often silent about an opposing view (see Chapter 9). Conflicts over the relationship are least likely to be explicit since they might be regarded as personal confrontations, insults, or statements that unnecessarily expose oneself: "I don't trust you," "You frighten me," "You are too aloof," "You are not smart enough," "You are too old," "You are too young."

Direct Versus Displaced Conflict

Clinicians need to be attuned to the fact that conflicts may be obscured not only by being implicit but also by being displaced from their original content or target. A patient may oppose, for example, a proposed treatment procedure when the real conflict is over the relationship with the provider of treatment. Thus, patients who complain about their medication may really be displacing conflicts over deficiencies in the expected relationship. Clinical sensitivity to disguised indirect communication is essential to the recognition and exploration of these conflicts. In addition, the clinician must work to develop a trusting relationship in order for the patient to be more open and direct, reducing the likelihood of displacement and increasing readiness to be direct.

Conscious Versus Unconscious Conflict

Under ideal conditions, negotiations can proceed in an orderly fashion when the conflicts are explicit, direct, and also conscious. Unfortunately, clinical experience leads us to believe that many significant conflicts may be unconscious or outside of awareness of either the patient or the clinician.

Conflicts in any of the areas subject to negotiation and consensus seeking (the nature of the problem, the relationship, the treatment method, the treatment conditions, and the goals of treatment) may be unconscious. In some cases, there will be awareness of interpersonal conflict, an awareness that a confrontation is taking place, without an understanding as to why. In other cases, one or both of the parties may be unaware of the impact of unconscious conflicts upon the nature of the transactions between them. Patients may respond negatively to a treatment plan, knowing they will not comply with the plan without knowing why and also without verbalizing this opposition to the clinician. Manifestly there is no conflict. This may be one of the reasons for the high rate of noncompliance over medications in general medical practice.

THE CLINICAL ENCOUNTER AS A NEGOTIATION

On the basis of the previous literature review (1–46), the above analysis of clinician–patient interactions, and our own clinical experience, we believe it is reasonable to conclude that conflict is present in the vast majority of clinical encounters. Conflict is particularly evident in the initial encounter in which the patient may have specific requests but may be quite uncertain as to what services are available or are deemed appropriate by the clinician. Later in treatment, after these differences in perspectives have been settled, conflicts are apt to be less frequent and less obvious.

Conflict between patient and clinician in the initial encounter has been generally regarded as deviant or counternormative behavior, that is, as uncharacteristic of normal clinician–patient interaction. Clinicians explain such conflict as a result of the patient's having the "wrong" expectations of treatment or inadequate motivation to change.

In our conception of clinician–patient encounters, we view conflict as normative—something to be expected, understood, even desired. It is a feature of normal interpersonal discourse in clinical and nonclinical settings, not the result, fault, or responsibility of either party. The resolution of such conflict, we contend, is an essential aspect of clinical practice, not an unexpected or unwanted dimension of the clinician–patient interaction.

Conflict between individuals or groups may be resolved by numerous methods, including a variety of legal procedures, the investment of power in a third party, violence or the threat of violence, or chance methods such as flipping a coin (47). *In clinical practice, we believe that an essential method of conflict resolution is negotiation (bargaining).* This is supplemented by various educative and persuasive techniques that some regard as conceptually distinct from the negotiation process.

According to social psychologists Rubin and Brown (47), negotiation (or bargaining) is "the process whereby two or more parties attempt to settle what each shall give and take, or perform and receive, in a transaction between them." They further characterize the negotiating relationship as having the following features: (a) At least two individuals or groups are involved; (b) the parties have a conflict of interest with respect to at least one issue; (c) the parties are at least temporarily engaged in a voluntary relationship; (d) the relationship is concerned with an exchange of specific resources or the resolution of intangible issues; and (e) the activity involves a sequential presentation of demands or proposals followed by concessions and counterproposals. Other authorities on negotiation and bargaining theory focus on specific aspects of the negotiation relationship. Young (48), for example, suggests that the applicability of a negotiation–bargaining approach rests on certain basic premises: First, the parties, lacking information essential to make decisions that would improve their outcome, need to coordinate their efforts through "interdependent decision making." Second, there must be the possibility for the parties involved to influence the expectations of the other party regarding the definition of the situation. Third, there must be the possibility of extensive communication between the parties involved. Finally, Deutsch (49) states, "The essential features of a bargaining situation exist when: (1) both parties perceive that there is a possibility of reaching an agreement in which each party would be better off, or no worse off, than if no agreement is reached; (2) both parties perceive that there is more than one such agreement which could be reached; and (3) each party perceives the other as having conflicting preferences or opposed interests with regard to the different agreements that might be reached."

The clinical encounter differs from other negotiation situations in one major way: The clinical encounter is not explicitly or usually defined as conflictual, requiring resolution by techniques such as negotiation. Several authors take exception to this position. Balint (50), a British psychoanalyst, describes the doctor–patient relationship as "always and invariably the result of a compromise between the patient's offers and demands and the doctor's responses to them." He goes on to discuss the doctor's attempts to "convert" the patient to his beliefs in the face of the pa-

tient's "chronic haggling." Scheff (51), a sociologist, describes both the medical and the psychiatric interview as a process of negotiation over "reality" in which the clinician can reject various patient "offers" until data, an attitude, or a theory of causality emerge consistent with the clinician's frame of reference. Finally, Levinson et al. (52) describe the optimal applicancy process in a psychiatric clinic as based on negotiations over the problems and methods of treatment.

To understand how clinical negotiations differ from situations such as economic bargaining, the distinction between distributive and integrative bargaining needs to be clarified. In *distributive bargaining* there is a competition for resources so that as one party wins or improves his or her position the other party loses or assumes an unfavorable position. In such a situation, the other party is the opponent, the relationship is competitive, and information exchange must be carefully managed. In *integrative bargaining* both parties have common motives, there is no competition for resources, the other party is identified as a partner or coparticipant, the relationship is cooperative, and information exchange is open. The focus is joint problem solving.

In clinical encounters, both clinician and patient usually attempt to define the situation as one of integrative bargaining, that what will fulfill one party as a clinician will simultaneously fulfill the other as a patient and that they both improve their situations simultaneously. ("If you give me this tranquilizer, you will be a good doctor, and I will get what I need for my nerves"; "If you accept this method of treatment, you will be fulfilled as a patient, and I will be an effective clinician.") Ideally, clinician and patient will appreciate their basic interdependence and need for cooperation regarding the definition of the problems, goals, methods, and conditions of treatment, so that consensus will be mutually rewarding and will not be seen as compromise, surrender, or giving in.

In practice, however, the clinical encounter commonly contains elements of both integrative and distributive bargaining. As described in the previous chapter, patients frequently view the clinician as an adversary.

STRATEGIES OF NEGOTIATIONS

The following strategies of negotiations were developed from observations of expert clinicians, from our own clinical experience, and from a review of the sociologic, social psychologic, and psychoanalytic literature. These strategies represent our initial attempt to conceptualize for pedagogic purposes what clinicians practice intuitively. It is evident that there is overlap among the categories and that a clinician is apt to use several of them simultaneously. The purpose of the negotiation is not only to have the patient accept that the clinician's definition of the problem, goals, and methods are "correct" (goals of traditional medicine), but to have the clinician accept the possibility that the patient's definitions of the problem, desired goals, and methods are appropriate. The negotiation strategies, in other words, will ideally lead to a situation of mutual influence in which the power of both parties is simultaneously enhanced, patients will receive what they believe they need, and the clinician will offer and have accepted that which he or she believes to be effective treatment. Despite the desirability for mutuality in the negotiation process, the clinician must take the initiative and assume the clinical responsibility, a role expectation held for the professional care provider. The clinician's leadership is required to legitimate the expression of differences and conflicts and thus to give this helping situation an added and unexpected meaning. He or she has the legitimate power to initiate the tone of the encounter as a mutual exchange of information in which differences can be resolved by negotiation.

We have divided the consensus-seeking and negotiation process into five major se-

quential stages, each of which has identifiable negotiating strategies associated with it. The first two stages, developing and sustaining an atmosphere for negotiation and establishing the nature of the conflict, are not strictly speaking negotiating strategies but rather are preconditions of negotiation. When the clinician attends to these two stages, consensus is usually attained and the majority of conflict situations are avoided. On the other hand, when there is an unfavorable atmosphere for negotiations and when the patient's perspective is not known to the clinician, the continuity of conflict is inevitable.

Developing and Sustaining an Atmosphere for Negotiation

Conflicts over the relationship from the patient's perspective may focus on the perception of inadequate respect and caring or lack of expertise on the part of the clinician. The clinician negotiates both these attributes throughout the course of the entire interview. If either of these relationship issues is inadequately attended to, negotiations over the problem, goals, methods, and conditions are unlikely to succeed.

Communicating Respect and Caring

The patient comes to the interview feeling vulnerable. He or she may be unable to cope psychologically; is often in a regressed state; fears the worst; has to ask for something; and may feel psychologically exposed and anticipate examination of his or her private thoughts. The patient may fear the clinician will criticize him or her for not coming sooner, for coming at all, or for attempting various self-help measures. The patient may fear the clinician will be unable or unwilling to hear his or her problem. Patients with this commonly held frame of mind are very susceptible to feeling judged, degraded, and humiliated, even with little basis in reality. Once in this state of mind, patients regard the clinician as a potential adversary. They are less apt to say what they want for fear of humiliation; they may lie and make threats; and they may listen for weakness in the clinician's position rather than try to understand it. In sum, these patients may regard the clinician not as a respectful, caring ally but as an adversary.

Given the vulnerabilities of patienthood with their untoward effects on clinical negotiations, the clinician must carefully maintain an attitude of respect, understanding, acceptance, openness, and authenticity, even in the face of a patient's rudeness and hostility. These attitudes must be communicated not only in direct clinician contact but also in the setting of the waiting room with secretaries and other personnel (54).

For clinicians to provide the necessary relationship supports for further negotiations, they must attend to their own needs for safety, creativity, emotional support, pride, and financial compensation. These needs, not to be taken lightly, are provided by the patient, the administrative structure in which the clinician works, peer and supervisory relationships, and a conceptual framework that puts meaning and interest into the clinical encounter.

Establishing Expertise

The clinician may be better able to exchange information and negotiate over the problem, goals, and methods if he or she is perceived by the patient as an expert. This may be effected in part by the reputation of the clinician, the reputation of the clinical setting, and the referring clinician's communications to the patient. The clinician may further the belief in his or her expertise by being thorough, being able to anticipate the patient's questions, and being able to educate the patient as to the nature of the illness. When the illness represents a constellation of symptoms, such as in depressive syndromes, the clinician's statement that the many symptoms represent a single problem commonly produces in the patient not only a sense of relief that there is only a single problem but a belief that the clinician is knowledgeable and expert. Clinicians must be careful in establishing their expert and authoritative status that they do not become authoritarian and

thereby diminish the patient's willingness to negotiate.

Establishing the Nature of the Conflict

A skilled negotiator strives to determine the other party's understanding of the problem, goals, methods, conditions, and relationship needs. In the clinician-patient relationship, partly as a result of culturally defined roles of both parties, the clinician is apt to assume that the patient does not know what he or she wants, that the patient has delegated these tasks to the clinician, that the patient's real needs are unconscious, or that it does not matter what the patient thinks about or wants. Patients may reinforce these assumptions by denying that they have any idea of what is happening or what they want from the clinician. They may say "You are the therapist. You tell me." In the vast majority of cases, the patient does have a belief as to what is the problem, what has caused the problem, how he or she would like to feel, and what he or she wants the clinician to do. There is a tendency on the part of patients to withhold this information because they think it is not their role, fear the clinician will ridicule or humiliate them, or regard the clinician as an adversary who has the power to withhold what they want and who therefore must be approached with caution (see Chapter 9).

Eliciting Definitions of the Problem, Goals, Methods, and Conditions of Treatment

The most effective way to elicit conflict is to first establish the proper atmosphere for negotiations. The sequence of inquiry should then be the problem, the goal, the method, and the conditions. In first eliciting the nature of the problem, clinicians are doing what is traditionally expected of them (finding out what is wrong). If one first elicits the goal or method before elaborating the problem, the patient may perceive one as uncaring, as evaluating the patient's suitability to available services, and as just wanting to make a disposition.

Conflicts over the problem are further elucidated by exploring the patient's illness attribution or theory as to what is the problem and its cause. This is difficult to do since the patient may anticipate that, at best, the clinician will not take his or her theories seriously and at worst will laugh at and ridicule them.

Role Reversal

Role reversal is a procedure in which one party verbalizes the viewpoint and feelings of the other in an accurate, warm, and authentic manner. The clinician's verbalization might include the patient's goals, the means of attaining these goals, the patient's rationale for having these goals met, and even the patient's arguments against accepting the doctor's recommendations. An example is "Let me see if I fully understand what you want. You feel you should not take medicine because if makes you feel like you have to depend on something or need a crutch and that you could even get dependent on them, almost like a narcotic." In role reversal, the clinician may ask the patient to describe what he or she (the clinician) has said. It has been established in a series of studies that role reversal "can be used effectively to increase the mutual understanding, interpersonal attraction, and perceived similarity of the parties involved in the conflict, as well as producing attitude change concerning the issue under negotiation and an increased probability of reaching an agreement" (55).

Verbalizing One's Intentions

When patients are unwilling or unable to state their goals and preferred methods, the clinician may verbalize his or her intention or provisional plan in order to elicit their reaction. Patients may then state what they want or emphatically reject the clinician's suggestion. By not being unequivocally committed to the proposal, the clinician can more easily negotiate a mutually acceptable solution. For example, the distraught and overwhelmed patient denies knowing how he would like to be helped. The clinician begins to outline a possible treatment program of outpatient care, only to be interrupted by the patient, who insists that only hospitalization can help. Negotiations then begin over the relative value of inpatient versus outpatient care.

General Negotiating Strategies

The following three negotiating and consensus-seeking strategies are commonly used by clinicians in dealing with either explicit or implicit conflicts.

Expanding the Clinician's Definition of the Problem

The clinician may need to go beyond official diagnostic categories and initial formulation to develop consensus with the patient over what is wrong. One attempt to expand one's understanding of the problem is through the expanded range of biologic, psychodynamic, sociocultural, and behavioral hypotheses described in Chapter 7. The clinician negotiates with the patient over a conceptualization of the problem that is mutually acceptable. To effect this negotiation the clinician needs to listen for the patient's language, cultural orientation, and theoretical orientation. The clinician also expands the definition of the problem for him- or herself and for the patient through the pursuit of more clinical data.

Clarification by Organizing the Issues and Priorities

The clinician may be unable to achieve consensus with the patient who is overwhelmed by the complexity of the problem, the goals, and the treatment. This difficulty can be overcome by organizing the issues. For instance, the clinician may say, "These problems have been with you for a long time and we will not deal with them at this time. There is an acute crisis that has led to the anxiety and this is what we have to work on now." In another example, the clinician may need to help the patient sort out the effects of the medicine versus the depressive symptoms so it can become clear what is wrong and what needs to be done.

Direct Education

In direct education, clinicians use their legitimate authority as experts to explain what is wrong, what should be done, and what methods should be used. This strategy is most likely to be effective when the clinician has attended to the relationship variables and is fully aware of the patient's perspective including the illness attribution. This approach may be successful because it responds to the desire of many patients to be taught by the expert. The educative strategy is apt to fail with patients who are too anxious to hear, too committed to their own beliefs to listen, or so dissatisfied with the relationship and the overbearing and condescending "lecture" they are receiving that they will not let themselves be influenced. The clinician cannot assume that consensus has been reached if the patient seems to acquiesce or does not object to the educational attempts. Educative attempts that fail on the initial encounter may succeed on subsequent encounters when the patient is less anxious, when the therapeutic relationship is stronger, and when the patient has had the opportunity to assimilate other knowledge about the illness.

Specific Negotiating Stategies

The negotiating strategies described below are used in specific clinical situations by particular clinicians.

Making a Concession

The clinician may make a concession (a classical element in all negotiations), that is, may grant the patient something that he or she wants, something that the clinician was not about to do or give. This may take the form of some assurance, a phone call to a relative, a pill, or time to think. The clinician conceives of these procedures as partially therapeutic or as neither therapeutic nor harmful. It is hoped that the concession will be followed by the patient's accepting and acting on the clinician's advice. The concession is more likely to be perceived as benevolent if the clinician is perceived to have done so willingly and

out of strength. The concession may be a response by the clinician to a preliminary need that should be met before the patient can consider the more central problem.

Providing a Sample Treatment

With a possible conflict over methods, the clinician may choose to provide the patient with a sample of treatment. This commonly occurs during the evaluation for psychotherapy in which the patient has a chance to experience the process of sharing intimate and painful feelings while the clinician provides clarifications and support. Patients reluctant to take medications because of feared side effects may benefit from the opportunity to sample the medication at low doses. In our walk-in clinic, patients had the chance to sample "group therapy" in short-term crisis groups.

Sharing Control

Some of the methods of treatment seem to some patients to be too intrusive or to render them too passive. On these grounds, they may refuse treatment. Sharing control (sometimes a form of concession) of the treatment may then be employed. This may be done (*a*) with medications for which the patient may be given the option to regulate the dosage within certain limits, (*b*) with frequency of visits, of (*c*) by setting a date for termination.

Analysis of Resistance by Confrontation and Clarification

Confrontation and clarification, derived from psychodynamic psychotherapy, may be useful when the patient disagrees with the clinician's recommendations for reasons not clearly conscious to the patient. In confrontation, the clinician directs the patient's attention to a piece of behavior evident to both parties. For instance, "You insisted on having an appointment at the earliest possible moment and you arrived one hour early. Now you tell me your problem is nothing to worry about and you want to stop all diagnostic procedures." The clinician could conclude with an empathic clarification: "You must be beside yourself with worry and wish you could forget the whole thing." A clarification is a restatement of the patient's communication, sometimes with changes and sometimes with particular emphasis. It is hoped that this restatement will sharpen the patient's awareness of his or her conscious thoughts. For example, a patient, after discussing her perceived inability to be of value to her growing children and to her parents, says, "I know I need your help but you have other patients who need you more." The clinician may respond empathically with, "You don't think you are worth being helped." Many patients will respond to this clarification with an immediate willingness to begin treatment.

Calling in a Third Party

In clinician–patient interactions, third parties are often helpful in resolving conflict. A family member or friend of the patient or another professional may be summoned under various conditions: (*a*) when the clinician enlists them as allies, as a source of support during the course of treatment, or when they are needed to help the patient evaluate and accept a difficult rercommendation (e.g., hospitalization); (*b*) when they are part of the problem and need to be involved in the treatment process; and (*c*) when they function as consultants to the clinician or to the patient.

End-State Negotiations

When the previous four sequential stages of consensus seeking and negotiation fail, the clinician needs to first review utilization of general and specific strategies and then consider special end-state strategies.

Acknowledging the Conflict and Requesting a Postponement

When negotiations reach an impasse, the clinician may acknowledge the conflict, delay further attempts at resolution, and continue to deal with other negotiable issues. The delay gives the clinician and patient the opportunity to review previously described tactics of negotiation, to consult with their constituencies (colleagues, friends, family), to further evaluate the quality and impact of

relationship conflicts, to allow previous humiliations to heal, and to continue to deal with other negotiable issues.

Compromise or Unilateral Concession

Both parties may compromise or one party may offer a unilateral concession when it is clear that consensus cannot be reached yet the end result is felt to be of value to the patient and professionally responsible to the clinician. Issues over which there may be compromise or unilateral concession are the frequency of psychotherapy visits, the dosage of medication, or the fee for treatment. In these situations the subsequent feelings of one or both parties (humiliation, defeat, loss of face, anger) need be attended to if the relationship necessary for future negotiations and treatment is to be maintained.

Reassessment

Before considering ending treatment, the clinician should give serious consideration to the possibility that he or she has misunderstood some aspect of the patient's perspective. Are the patient's goals and methods so unreasonable or is the patient telling the clinician something important that had previously not been clear? With psychotic patients in particular, the clinician may miss the symbolic nature of the patient's understanding of the problem. For example, the patient in Case Example 5 of Chapter 9 stated her problem was "noise pollution." This turned out to be a reasonable, although symbolic, statement of her problem when it was subsequently learned that she was feeling overwhelmed by her noisy adolescent daughter.

Threatening to End the Relationship

When all negotiation strategies fail and further compromise or unilateral concession would be professionally irresponsible, the clinician may have to explore with the patient the possibility of ending the relationship. Although this strategy involves high risk, it may be the only one that conveys to the patient and the clinician their mutually elective roles in the treatment.

The patient may then make a concession or terminate treatment. We have seen clinical situations in which the patients forced the clinician to terminate treatment because treatment was begun under duress. Only after termination could the patient reinstitute treatment and truly feel like a voluntary participant in a negotiated relationship. Some people who feel weak need to say no before they can say yes.

EVALUATION OF A NEGOTIATED APPROACH TO PATIENTHOOD

Five pieces of indirect evidence support the usefulness of the negotiated approach.

Referral Decisions

To the best of our knowledge, the clinic in which the research was carried out and its findings implemented is the only outpatient setting that has shown that the decision to refer a patient into the clinic system is made independent of diagnosis or social class (56). Previous studies have consistently shown that the upper classes and the healthier were preferentially referred to and accepted into the system. We believe this admission policy can be explained in part by the use of patient requests that are for the most part independent of social class and by the use of a negotiated approach that takes patients where they are, rather than where the clinician thinks they ought to be.

Patient Satisfaction

Evaluation of the initial interview in the clinic from the patient's perspective revealed that patients' satisfaction correlated better with indices of a negotiated approach than with symptom relief or a belief that their feelings and problems were understood. The indices of the negotiated approach include the patients' belief that the clinician helped them verbalize what it was that they wanted and the patients' belief that they participated in the treatment decision. These findings persisted even when the patients did not receive the treatment plan they requested (57).

Compliance with Referral

In a study of patients in a walk-in clinic who were referred within the institution for further treatment, it was found that those patients who gave higher ratings on measures of the negotiated approach were more likely to follow through with treatment recommendations. The specific aspects of negotiation most important to patients were their belief that (*a*) they participated in the disposition and (*b*) the clinician understood their request (35).

Training

We believe that the successful use of a walk-in clinic for training first-year residents in psychiatry can be accounted for, in part, by the availability of a conceptual framework (described in this and the previous chapter) that puts meaning and excitement into the clinical encounter. This setting provides the trainee with a unique opportunity to see large numbers of unscreened patients who present with a heterogeneous group of problems that do not easily lend themselves to official diagnostic categories or psychodynamic formulations. Without such an approach, we believe that frustration, fatigue, clinical uncertainty, and sense of helplessness would interfere with the treatment of these patients (58). Using the approach described in these chapters, even when the diagnosis in unclear, a request can be elicited, several clinical hypotheses can be considered, and the ensuing process and relationship can be understood as a negotiation. As a result, a sophisticated dialogue between trainee and supervisor can occur.

Applications to Other Settings

The negotiated approach as described in this chapter and Chapter 9 is being applied to the fields of primary care medicine, nursing, anesthesiology, and victimology. Clinicians and teachers in these settings are finding these concepts useful for clinical care, teaching, and research.

CRITICISM AND RESPONSE

The work described in this chapter and Chapter 9 has been subject to two major criticisms: (*a*) that it takes too much power away from clinicians and inappropriately gives it to patients and (*b*) that it inappropriately gives too much power to clinicians at the expense of patients. Critics who take the first position often believe that patients do not have requests or that patients assume the role of a shopper, taking what they please at a supermarket. Clinicians thereby dilute the most effective source of influence, their legitimate authority. They further fear that they will find themselves helpless and impotent as they open up a Pandora's box of unending, complex, insatiable demands. These beliefs and fears are unnecessary. Patients do have requests. The expression of requests does not bind clinicians to agree to fulfill them. They do make them more knowledgeable and encourage patients in turn to be influenced by them. The aim of negotiation is the maintenance of the highest professional standards, not their surrender. Finally, the expression of the request is usually a more modest statement of perceived needs than the clinician had anticipated.

Critics who take the second position argue that clinicians already have too much power over patients and that the tools provided by the negotiation paradigm, particularly the strategies of negotiation, put patients at an even greater disadvantage. We believe that the use of the negotiated approach—developing trust, establishing expertise, educating the patient, providing a sample treatment—is part of the clinician's job. If a clinician, for example, thinks lithium rather than electroconvulsive therapy is the treatment of choice, it is his or her task to make the best possible case for this belief and thereby to influence the patient. Should the clinician not attempt to develop trust, establish his or her expertise, or educate the patient? What is really at issue, we believe, is not the clinician's

skill at negotiating, but the possibility that he or she may influence patients to accept treatments not responsive to their needs or even deleterious to their well-being. The solution to these abuses is not to discourage the negotiation process, but to encourage patients to be more educated consumers and to support auditing of training programs and clinical practice. The negotiation process that is described and recommended in these chapters simultaneously enhances the power of both parties and leads to better clinical care.

A SUMMARY NOTE

After we had completed the previous sections of this chapter, a colleague called to our attention Adolph Meyer's thinking about negotiations in clinical psychiatry, as recollected and elaborated on by Wendell Muncie (59). What we have studied and described is so similar to Meyer's viewpoint that we quote Muncie's statement for our summary (the bracketed insertions are ours):

The most vivid memory I have of his [Adolph Meyer's] attitude to treatment does not appear in his collected works but derives from a statement made in staff meeting late in his tenure at the Phipps Psychiatric Clinic . . . It was substantially as follows: "The patient comes with his own view of his trouble [the patient's perspective]; the physician has another view [the clinician's perspective]. Treatment consists of the joint effort to bring about that approximation of those views which will be the most effective and the most satisfying in the situation." This struck me forcibly at the time, for it laid down what, I recognized, had been our established working method at the clinic, but which had never been so aptly stated.

This succinctly asserts a cardinal principle: Treatment is a matter of negotiation of viewpoints and attitudes. This discards immediately old authoritarian views of treatment and uses, instead, mutual education through the elaboration of the material of the history as well as the working relationships existing between patient and physician to enlarge the area of negotiation. This view of treatment to me appears so basic, so elemental, and so self-evident—like much of Meyer's wisdom—that one can hear oneself saying impatiently, "Yes, of course. Now how to negotiate?" (That is, "How about the techniques?"). Meyer was always interested in techniques, but he seems to have held the conviction that the great failures in psychiatry resulted more from a failure in basic attitudes [unresolved conflicts over the relationship] than from a failure in techniques [strategies]. Otherwise stated, if the basic attitudes were firmly established, every practitioner could be expected to develop, in time, those techniques commonly in good repute and to add his own variants depending on his own assets (and needs). Consequently, trainees under Meyer ended with the most diverse technical equipment, but all were touched to some extent by the simple basic elementals of treatment as noted above.

My observations over the years lead me to conclude that the concept of treatment as negotiation is basic for the best effort. I see this confirmed daily both in its observance and in its breach. Negotiation implies mutual respect and a willingness to give a sympathetic hearing to the other [eliciting the patient's perspective]. It is especially the obligation of the physician to rid himself of any sense of justification for coercion which might arise from superior knowledge and faith in techniques [methods]. It is a humbling thought that, in some ways, the patient always knows more of himself than we ever will. If we can help in a more useful assembling of this self-knowledge we will have served our purpose . . .

To be condemned are enthusiastic parochially tinged injunctions to therapy addressed to a patient in no wise prepared for such well-meant advice. Treatment starts and ends with what is possible, and tries constantly to enlarge the area of the possible through patient understanding of the problem and communication to the sufferer of this expanding view, with the need for encouraging a greater participation on his part in an expanded goal. As purveyors of a service to sufferers, we must recognize that the patient has the inalienable right to determine

the degree of his participation, and summary interference with his freedom of action in this regard can only be sanctioned when clear danger to himself or others is evident.[a]

References

1. Lorion RP: Patient and therapist variables in the treatment of low-income patients. *Psychol Bull* 81:344–354, 1974.
2. Overall B, Aronson H: Expectations of psychotherapy in patients of lower socio-economic class. *Am J Orthopsychiatry* 33:421–430, 1963.
3. Aronson H, Overall B: Treatment expectations of patients in two social classes. *Social Work* 11:35–42, 1966.
4. Williams H, Lipman RS, Uhlenhuth EH, et al: Some factors influencing the treatment expectations of anxious neurotic outpatients. *J Nerv Ment Dis* 145:208–220, 1967.
5. Heine RW, Trosman A: Initial expectations of the doctor-patient interaction as a factor in the continuance in psychotherapy. *Psychiatry* 23:275–278, 1960.
6. Borghi J: Premature termination of psychotherapy and patient-therapist expectations. *Am J Psychother* 22:460–473, 1968.
7. Garfield S, Wolper M: Expectations regarding psychotherapy. *J Nerve Ment Dis* 137:353–362, 1963.
8. Goin M, Yamamoto J, Silverman J: Therapy congruent with class-linked expectations. *Arch Gen Psychiatry* 13:133–137, 1965.
9. Goldstein AP: Therapist and client expectation of personality change in psychotherapy. *J Counsel Psychol* 3:180–184, 1960.
10. Goldstein AP: Participant expectancies in psychotherapy. *Psychiatry* 25:72–79, 1962.
11. Heitler JB: Preparatory techniques in initiating expressive psychotherapy with lower-class, unsophisticated patients. *Psycho Bull* 83:339–352, 1976.
12. Houts PS, MacIntosh S, Moos RH: Patient-therapist interdependence: cognitive and behavioral. *J Consult Clin Psychol* 33:40–45, 1969.
13. Levitt EE: Psychotherapy research and the expectation-reality discrepancy. *Psychother Theor Res Practice* 3:163–166, 1966.
14. Roop KL: The patient request: Therapist and patient perceptions. Unpublished master's thesis, Smith College for Social Work, 1973.
15. Hornstra RK, Lubin B, Lewis RV, et al: Worlds apart: patients and professionals. *Arch Gen Psychiatry* 27:553–557, 1972.
16. Hill JA: Therapist goals, patient aims, and patient satisfaction in psychotherapy. *J Clin Psychol* 25:455–459, 1969.
17. Orlinsky DE, Howard KI, Hill JA: The patient's concerns in psychotherapy. *J Clin Psychol* 26:104–111, 1970.
18. Polak P: Patterns of discord: Goals of patients, therapists and community members. *Arch Gen Psychiatry* 23:277–283, 1970.
19. Thompson A, Zimmerman R: Goals of counsel-

---

[a] From Muncie W: The psychobiological approach. In Arieti S (ed): *American Handbook of Psychiatry*. New York, Basic Books, 1959, vol 2, pp 1319–1320.

ing: Whose? When? *J Counsel Psychology* 16:121–125, 1969.

20. Wilson NC: The automated tri-informant goal-oriented progress note. *J Community Psychology* 1:302–306, 1973.
21. Wilson NC: The ATGON approach to program evaluation. Paper presented at the Annual Clinical-Community Workshop on Program Evaluation, Silver Spring, MD, 1974.
22. Gottlieb W, Stanley JH: Mutual goals and goal-setting in casework. *Social Casework* 98:471–477, 1967.
23. Strupp HH, Fox RE, Lessler K: *Patients View Their Psychotherapy*. Baltimore, Johns Hopkins University Press, 1969.
24. Mayer JE, Rosenblatt A: Clash in perspective between mental patients and staff. *Am J Orthopsychiatry* 44:432–441, 1974.
25. Orlinsky DE, Howard KI: The good therapy hour: experimental correlates of patients' and therapists' evaluations of therapy sessions. *Arch Gen Psychiatry* 16:621–632, 1967.
26. Polansky N, Kounin J: Clients' reactions to initial interview and field study. *Hum Relations* 9:237–264, 1956.
27. Kounin J, Polansky N, Biddle B, et al: Experimental studies of clients' reactions to initial interviews. *Hum Relations* 9:256–292, 1956.
28. Rogers CR, Gendlin ET, Kiesler DJ, et al (eds): *The Therapeutic Relationship and Its Impact: A Study of Psychotherapy with Schizophrenics*. Madison, University of Wisconsin Press, 1967.
29. Barrett-Lennard GT: Dimensions of therapeutic response as causal factors in therapeutic change. *Psychol Monogr* 70:42, 1962.
30. Farson RE: Introjection in the psychotherapeutic relationship. *J Counsel Psychol* 8:337–342, 1961.
31. Sapolsky A: Relationship between patient-doctor compatibility, mutual perception, and outcome of treatment. *J Abnorm Psychol* 70:70–76, 1965.
32. Feifel H, Eells J: Patients and therapists assess the same psychotherapy. *J Consult Psychol* 27:310–318, 1963.
33. Lorr M: Client perceptions of therapists: a study of the therapeutic relation. *J Consult Psychol* 29:146–149, 1965.
34. Strupp HH, Wallach J, Kogan M: Psychotherapy experience in retrospect: questionnaire survey of former patients and their therapists. *Psychol Monogr* 78:11, 1964.
35. Eisenthal S, Emery R, Lazare A, et al: Adherence and the negotiated approach to patienthood. *Arch Gen Psychiatry* 36:393–398, 1979.
36. Baekeland F, Lundwall L: Dropping out of treatment: a critical review. *Psychol Bull* 82:738–783, 1975.
37. Bergin AE, Suinn RM: Individual psychotherapy and behavior therapy. *Ann Rev Psychol* 26:509–556, 1975.
38. Brown JS, Kosterlitz N: Selection and treatment

of psychiatric outpatients. *Arch Gen Psychiatry* 11:425–438, 1964.

39. Erickson RC: Outcome studies in mental hospitals: a review. *Psychol Bull* 82:519–540, 1975.
40. Frank A, Eisenthal S, Lazare A: Are there social class differences in patients' treatment conceptions? Myths and facts. *Arch Gen Psychiatry* 35:61–69, 1977.
41. Bernarde MA, Mayerson EW: Patient:physician negotiation. *JAMA* 239:1413–1415, 1978.
42. Anderson TW, Helm DT: The physician–patient encounter: a process of reality negotiation. In Gartley Jaco E (ed): *Patients, Physicians, and Illness–A Sourcebook in Behavioral Science and Health*. New York, Free Press, 1979.
43. Heaton PB: Negotiation as an integral part of the physician's clinical reasoning. *J Fam Pract* 13:845–848, 1981.
44. Quill TE: Partnerships in patient care: A contractual approach. *Ann Intern Med* 98:228–234, 1983.
45. Schwartz CG, Kahne MJ: Medical help as negotiated achievement. *Psychiatry* 46:333–350, 1983.
46. Goldberg A: Psychoanalysis and negotiation. *Psychoanal Q* 56:109–128, 1987.
47. Rubin JZ, Brown BR: *The Social Psychology of Bargaining and Negotiation*. New York, Academic Press, 1975.
48. Young OR (ed): *Bargaining: Formal Theories of Negotiation*. Chicago, University of Illinois Press, 1975.
49. Deutsch M: *The Resolution of Conflict: Construction and Destructive Processes*. New Haven, Yale University Press, 1973.
50. Balint M: *The Doctor, His Patient, and the Illness*. New York, International Universities Press, 1957.
51. Scheff TJ: Negotiating reality: notes on power in the assessment of responsibility. *Social Problems* 16:3–17, 1968.
52. Levinson DJ, Merrifield J, Berg K: Becoming a patient. *Arch Gen Psychiatry* 17:385–406, 1967.
53. Walton R, McKersie RB: *A Behavioral Therapy of Labor Negotiations*. New York, McGraw-Hill, 1965.
54. Lazare A: Shame and humiliation in the medical encounter. *Arch Int Med* 147: 1653–1658, 1987.
55. Johnson DW: Role reversal: a summary and review of the research. *Int J Group Tensions* 1:318–334, 1971.
56. Lazare A, Eisenthal S, Frank A: Disposition decisions in a walk-in clinic: social and psychiatric variables. *Am J Orthopsychiatry* 46:503–509, 1976.
57. Eisenthal S, Lazare A: Evaluation of the initial interview in a walk-in clinic: the patient's perspective on a "customer approach." *J Nerv Ment Dis* 162:169–176, 1976.
58. Lazare A, Eisenberg L: Psychiatric residency training: an outpatient first-year program. *Semin Psychiatry* 2:201–210, 1970.
59. Muncie WS: The psychobiological aproach. In Arieti S (ed): *American Handbook of Psychiatry*, ed. 1. New York, Basic Books, 1959, pp 1317–1332.

11

Three Functions of the Clinical Interview

Aaron Lazare, M.D.

The purpose of this chapter is to propose a set of functions and objectives for the clinical interview and to describe the skills necessary to accomplish them. These functions, objectives, and skills are based on concepts presented in Chapters 2 through 10 in this book. They represent, in my opinion, what expert clinicians do in clinical practice. This chapter thus has both a summarizing and integrative function. (The reader who has not yet read the previous chapters is apt to find this material too condensed and difficult to comprehend.) I hope it has an additional value: as a guide for the teaching and conduct of the clinical interview.

The rationale for the organization of the interview into functions, objectives, and skills was first described by Bird et al. (1) in their proposals for teaching the medical interview. They argue that it is important from the perspective of educational principles to address separately the cognitive, affective, and behavioral domains of learning. They then relate the cognitive domain to the data-gathering skills of the interview, the affective domain to the emotional support skills of the interview, and the behavioral domain to the educational and motivational skills of the interview.

I would add to this rationale the broadening of the task of the interview to go beyond what many clinicians seem to regard as its unitary or central goal—making a formal diagnosis. I believe that teaching exercises, textbooks, and clinical practitioners do not sufficiently emphasize the importance of establishing more broadly based diagnoses, developing the therapeutic relationship, and implementing educational/treatment activities.

These three functions assure even greater importance in contemporary outpatient practice where so much may depend on the initial interview. It is a common occurrence, for instance, for the outpatient clinician to make an accurate *Diagnostic and Statistical Manual of Mental Disorders (Third Edition-Revised)* (DSM-III-R) diagnosis, only to have the patient not return for the follow-up visit because he or she did not feel adequately understood or cared for and did not believe he or she was offered an adequate explanation for the presenting problem or a reasonable plan for further diagnosis and treatment. In inpatient settings, in contrast, the single interview is apt to assume less importance because diagnostic, relational, and educational/treatment functions occur in the context of a treatment team, a therapeutic milieu, and a time frame of days to weeks or even longer.

It is proposed in this chapter that the clinical interview can be usefully organized

153

around three central functions: (*a*) determining the nature of the problem, (*b*) developing and maintaining a therapeutic relationship, and (*c*) communicating information and implementing a treatment plan (see Table 11.1). The second function proceeds simultaneously with the first and the third. The clinician, in other words, is always attending to the therapeutic relationship.

DETERMINING THE NATURE OF THE PROBLEM

In determining the nature of the problem, the clinician's objectives are to establish DSM-III-R multiaxial diagnoses, to formulate clinical hypotheses from at least four conceptual domains, and to learn other important aspects of the person's life story not included in the formal diagnoses or clinical hypotheses. Such diagnoses (used in the broadest sense) are simultaneously categorical, individualistic, and multidimensional.

The skills necessary to accomplish these objectives can be organized into five categories. First, the clinician must have a knowledge base of diseases, disorders, problems, and clinical hypotheses from multiple conceptual domains including the biologic/syndromal, psychodynamic, sociocultural, and behavioral domains. Second, the clinician must be able to elicit data for the above conceptual domains. This may be accomplished by encouraging patients to freely tell their stories, organizing the flow of the interview, characterizing the symptoms, performing the mental status examination, using associative anamnestic techniques, and conducting family interviews. Third, the clinician must be able to perceive verbal and nonverbal data from the above sources as well as from his or her subjective response to the patient. *Perceiving the data is not the same as eliciting it.* Fourth, the clinician must be able to use the knowledge base and the perceived data in order to entertain and validate or refute a wide range of clinical hypotheses. Fifth, the clinician must have an adequate therapeutic relationship (Function 2) in order

to elicit the data necessary for the execution of this diagnostic function of the clinical interview.

DEVELOPING AND MAINTAINING A THERAPEUTIC RELATIONSHIP

The clinician's objectives in developing and maintaining a therapeutic relationship include increasing the patient's willingness to provide diagnostic information, the general therapeutic effect of the relationship including the enhanced placebo effect, the patient's willingness to accept treatment or negotiate over treatment, patient satisfaction, and clinician satisfaction. The importance of clinician satisfaction and the skills necessary to achieve it is, in my opinion, a commonly overlooked aspect of the clinical exchange. The particular nature of the desired therapeutic relationship may vary according to the conceptual approach of the clinician and the nature of the patient's problems. For example, a biologically oriented clinician examining a patient with a presumed bipolar disorder may attempt to develop a therapeutic relationship quite different from a psychodynamically oriented clinician examining a high-functioning patient whose impairment is presumably the result of the unsatisfactory resolution of intrapsychic conflict.

The skills necessary to achieve these objectives are subtle, and they vary according to the categorical and individualistic aspects of the patient and the particular skills of the therapist. There are some general skills, however, that may be useful to list. First, the clinician needs to define the nature of the relationship. This may include the purpose and duration of the consultation and the nature of the financial arrangements. The relationship is further developed by allowing the patient to tell his or her story. The clinician, meanwhile, is hearing and supporting the patient's expression of painful feelings. The clinician's comments provide empathy, support, and reassurance when appropriate. The relationship is further strengthened by the clinician's providing meaning and coherence

Table 11.1   The Clinical Interview: Functions, Objectives, and Skills

Functions	Objectives	Skills
1. Determining the nature of the problem	1. *Diagnostic and Statistical Manual of Mental Disorders (Third Edition-Revised)* diagnoses	1. Knowledge base of diseases, disorders, problems, and clinical hypotheses from multiple conceptual domains: biologic/syndromal, sociocultural, psychodynamic, and behavioral.
	2. The formulation of clinical hypotheses from at least four conceptual domains.	2. Ability to elicit data for the above conceptual domains (encouraging the patient to tell his or her story, organizing the flow of the interview, the form of questions, the characterization of symptoms, the mental status examination).
	3. Learning other relevant aspects of the person's life story.	3. Ability to perceive data from multiple sources (history, mental status exam, physician's subjective response to patient, nonverbal cues).
		4. Hypothesis generation and testing.
		5. Developing a therapeutic relationship (see Function 2).
2. Developing and maintaining a therapeutic relationship	1. The patient's willingness to provide diagnostic information.	1. Defining the nature of the relationship.
	2. Relief of psychologic distress.	2. Allowing the patient to tell his or her story.
	3. Willingness to accept the treatment plan or negotiate over treatment.	3. Hearing and supporting the patient's expression of painful feelings.
	4. Patient satisfaction.	4. Appropriate and genuine interest, empathy, and cognitive understanding.
	5. Clinician satisfaction.	5. Attending to common patient concerns over embarrassment, shame, humiliation, and stigma.
		6. Elicitation of patient's perspective.
		7. Determining the nature of the problem (see Function 1).
		8. Communicating information and recommending treatment (see Function 3).
3. Communicating information and implementing a treatment plan	1. The patient's understanding of the nature of the illness.	1. Determining the nature of the problem (see Function 1).
	2. The patient's understanding of suggested diagnostic procedures.	2. Developing a therapeutic relationship (see Function 2).
	3. The patient's understanding of the treatment possibilities.	3. Establishing the differences in perspective between clinician and patient.
	4. Achievement of consensus between clinician and patient over the above (1–3).	4. Educational strategies.
	5. Achievement of informed consent.	5. Clinical negotiations for resolving conflict.
		6. Recommending treatment.

to a story that may seem confused to the patient. This communication of meaning may take the form of sharing with the patient possible explanations (taken from four conceptual frameworks) for his or her problems. The clinician should elicit at some point in the interview the patient's perspective, which would include the definition of the problem, the goals of treatment, and the desired methods for treatment. The empathic elicitation of this perspective is valuable in itself for the development of the relationship. The data gathered from this process is also necessary to implement the final function of the interview, communicating information and implementing a treatment plan. A skill, often the most important skill, in developing a therapeutic relationship is showing respect and attending to the patient's ubiquitous concerns over shame, embarrassment, and humiliation over the problem and/or over coming for help. Seeking a mental health consultation is commonly fraught with stigma despite the increased public enlightenment of the past few decades (2). Finally, the clinician's skill in determining the nature of the problem (Function 1) and communicating information and implementing a treatment plan (Function 3) can have a considerable bearing on the development of a therapeutic relationship.

COMMUNICATING INFORMATION AND RECOMMENDING TREATMENT

The clinician's objectives for this final function of the interview are to help the patient understand the nature of the illness and to suggest both diagnostic procedures and treatment possibilities, including methods of self-help. The achievement of some consensus between clinician and patient over some of these issues is desirable and necessary if the relationship is to continue. Treatment may involve a brief, intermittent, or long-term professional relationship requiring one or a combination of the psychotherapies, rehabilitation, medication, or hospitalization.

Achieving these goals requires the further objective of informed consent.

The skills required to accomplish these objectives include the successful accomplishment of the first two functions of the interview, developing and maintaining a therapeutic relationship and determining the nature of the problem. The clinician must also establish differences in perspective with the patient over the nature of the problem, the goals of treatment, the methods of treatment, and the relationship. These differences or conflicts are then dealt with by educational strategies or by clinical negotiations. Treatment plans and the patient's subsequent informed consent are thus the product of a negotiated consensus.

INTERVIEW STYLES

I have observed three prototypic styles in the conduct of the clinical interview. They are usually combined in some manner and rarely occur in pure form. In the first style the clinician actively and aggressively pursues the data for diagnosis. Although the goal is most often the establishment of the DSM-III-R diagnosis, this interview style is also used to establish behavioral, sociocultural, and even psychodynamic hypotheses, formulations, and diagnoses. In the second style, the clinician uses a nondirective technique, allowing the patient to determine the flow of the verbal material. The clinician may comment on key phrases to emphasize important themes and encourage associations. It is believed that this spontaneous flow of associations will provide crucial diagnostic information, primarily for psychodynamic inferences. In the third style, the clinician addresses the patient's theories about the cause of the problem, fears about the future, the experience of the illness, and hopes for treatment. All this is understood in the context of patient's life story. This style is most effective in establishing an empathic relationship.

The problem with the first two styles is that the clinician may gain the information he or she is seeking, but the patient may not return because he or she feels inadequately supported. The problem with the third interview style is that the patient may develop an effective working relationship with the patient but fail to elicit the information necessary for diagnosis and treatment.

I strongly believe that all three styles can and should be integrated for the most effective conduct of the interview. Elements of each style facilitate the use of the other styles. For instance, an effective inquiry into the relevant signs and symptoms helps convince the patient that the clinician is knowledgeable and therefore worthy of a growing therapeutic relationship. Similarly, the establishment of an empathic relationship by use of the third style makes it more likely that the patient will confide to the clinician important facts that otherwise would be too humiliating to reveal. How these three styles are integrated in a given interview depends on the skills of the clinician and the manner in which the patient presents him- or herself. It goes without question, however, that the skillful integration of all three interview styles is necessary to achieve the three functions and objectives of the clinical interview.

IMPLICATIONS FOR TRAINING

Early in this chapter, I commented briefly on the possible teaching value of this functional analysis of the clinical interview. Our initial efforts to use this model for teaching interviewing to medical students and psychiatric residents appear to be useful in three distinct ways. First, an explicit model of the interview provides clinicians with the opportunity to offer criticisms and suggest modification and revision to the proposed model. Second, demonstration interviews conducted by faculty or students can be critiqued according to how effective the interview skills have been applied and how well the interview objectives have been achieved. Third, in reducing the interview to a number of discreet skills, students can learn one or two at a time without being overwhelmed at the complexity of the entire task. For instance, the skills of eliciting data, perceiving data, hypothesis testing, eliciting the patient's perspective, and negotiating with the patient can be taught in separate exercises before integrating them into the clinical interview.

References

1. Bird J, Cohen-Cole SA, Mance R: The three-function model of medical interview. Unpublished manuscript, 1984.
2. Lazare A: Shame and humiliation in the medical encounter. *Arch Intern Med* 147:1653–1658, 1987.

Section II

Data for Assessment

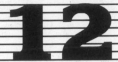

The Mental Status Examination

I. General Appearance and Behavior, Emotional State, Perception, Speech and Language, and Thinking

Theo C. Manschreck, M.D.
Martin B. Keller, M.D.

In this chapter and the next, we discuss a systematic approach to the observation of the patient. Such observation provides the data for determining the patient's clinical state. What features should the clinician examine? What findings may be discovered? Our approach is medical; we highlight observations relevant to medical (in the sense of biologic) hypotheses regarding psychopathology. The clinical state examination provides the fundamental picture of the patient. It is the guidepost for the remaining examinations and the basis on which all formulations ultimately rest. Our goal is to organize and define the wide range of specific facts necessary for a complete examination. If the chapter appears exhaustive and detailed, this merely reflects the complexity of the physical and emotional manifestations of psychpathology and the lack of simple laboratory tests for diagnosis. In the absence of easy and reliable means of ascertaining etiology, the diagnostic process will remain detailed and demanding of patience, skill, and knowledge.

GENERAL APPEARANCE AND BEHAVIOR

The assessment of general appearance and behavior forms the cornerstone of the mental status examination. Throughout the interview, the clinician has the opportunity to make many observations, to compare what the patient says with how he or she appears, and frequently to compensate for a limited history by investigating clues that may solve clinical puzzles. Dilated pupils, for instance, may suggest drug toxicity in a patient who is complaining of hallucinations.

Such observations may corroborate the patient's story. The depressed patient complains of anorexia and weight loss and displays hollow cheeks, temporal muscle wasting, and loosely fitting clothes. Other observations may contradict the patient's story. The patient's denial of delusional concerns may contrast sharply with his or her increased vigilance and poor eye contact. In those cases in which overt psychiatric disturbance is not apparent, careful and thorough descriptions may indicate personality or other disturbances. These and similar observations also provide the flavor and detail that give life to clinical description.

The clinician also learns the most global and crucial features of the patient's presentation. Does the patient appear well or ill? If ill, acutely or chronically so? Is the patient aware of surroundings and alert, or is the patient easily distracted? Furthermore, initial observations relating to the patient's self-awareness and orientation to surroundings are fundamental to the type of interview that the clinician performs. Confronted with a confused patient, the clinician will focus on an examination of higher intellectual functioning and a search for potential medical causes. For the patient demonstrating alertness and clarity of thinking, the clinician will be less concerned with such causes and will structure the interview accordingly. As these more global questions are answered, the clinician will make more specific kinds of observations.

The examination of general appearance and behavior also provides a basis for comparison with other observations in order to create a coherent picture of the clinical state. A patient complains of depressed mood and decreased interest in activities; examination discloses a lack of spontaneity. Further evaluation might reveal generalized slowness in the initiation and continuation of movement, findings consistent with the lack of spontaneity. The clinician looks for such consistencies in the clinical situation and if they are not to be found, carefully considers the meaning of their absence.

Level of Awareness and Appreciation of Surroundings

Although observations of general appearance and behavior occur throughout the interview, a useful starting point for assessing the clinical state is to estimate the patient's level of awareness. Most clinicians use the neurologic measuring stick of level of consciousness as the fundamental means for evaluating level of awareness. Cobb (1), a neuropsychiatrist, indicated the overlap of these two concepts, awareness and consciousness, and promoted the "neurologic" component of the assessment. We conceptualize disturbances of consciousness as falling on a continuum from normal and wakeful alertness to coma. Psychiatric examination deals primarily with the mild to moderate end of this continuum. Changes in consciousness can be subtle and often require an especially careful examination. They may be dreamlike, characterized by reduced sharpness, intensity, or clarity. We refer to such changes as *clouding of consciousness*, manifest as a mild global impairment of cognitive processes (e.g., thinking, attending, remembering, perceiving) in association with reduced awareness of the environment. Somewhat more severe changes of consciousness may be associated with intrusive abnormalities of perception (e.g., illusions and hallucinations) and affect as conceptualized in the syndrome of delirium.

The term *stupor* properly refers to a syndrome characterized by reduced or absent speech and spontaneous movement and apparent diminished response to external stimulation with the suggestion of impaired consciousness. However, the eyes are usually open and vigilant, able to follow visual stimuli, and, if closed, may resist opening by the examiner. Moreover, the patient may respond to external stimulation. After stupor has passed, the patient may be able to recall the experiences (2). *Catatonic stupor* refers to the retarded phase of catatonia when what appears to be stupor occurs with certain other features such as negativism, posturing, waxy flexibility, and anatomic obedience, among others. In general, simple stupor is a more serious condition that can progress to coma, whereas catatonic stupor is generally reversible and more benign.

There is, however, an additional arena of psychiatric concern—disturbances of awareness of self. Many psychiatric disorders, as well as medical and neurologic conditions, influence this form of awareness. The patient may lose awareness of ego boundaries or the continuity of identity over time. These disturbances shall be discussed separately and are often described as anomalies in the experience of self (3, 4).

Changes in consciousness and anomalies of experience of self should not be thought of as mutually exclusive. We distinguish between them for the purpose of theoretical clarity. However, they often occur together.

Disturbances of Alertness

Observations of alertness are made informally and formally throughout the interview. The patient's attentiveness, awareness of the environment, and comprehension of the interview serve as useful clues for determining the state or level of consciousness. Because most disturbances of alertness do not occur in isolation, associated difficulties in attention, perception, thinking, and memory frequently complicate the clinical picture. Evaluation of these functions may establish the degree of disturbed consciousness. Between coma (profound sleep or unconsciousness) and normal awareness (full, alert consciousness) there are several transitional states of reduced consciousness. Stupor and coma are the more profound disturbances, of course, and they usually call for neurologic consultation(5). When alertness is low or absent, the examination focuses on the de-

gree of reflexive response to sensory stimulation. In states of greater wakefulness, awareness is estimated by determining the frequency and intensity of stimulation response and the time required to react, the patient's capacity to maintain attention, and the quality of verbal responses and motor activity. In states in which awareness fluctuates, the discovery and characterization of orientation and periodic amnesia are important.

The clinical or formal tests of alertness include questions useful for evaluation of orientation. For example, does the patient know the time of day, date, place, name, etc.? These tests provide corroborating information for the clinical estimate of awareness.

Disturbances in the Experience of Self

Disturbances in the experience of self are not often discernible in the course of the evaluation. These experiences are subjective. They may be reported spontaneously, but generally the clinician should inquire to discover them. Drawing in part from Jaspers (6), we shall consider four areas (see Table 12.1) in which disturbances in the experience of self may occur.

The Experience of Reality of One's Self and the Environment. All events of consciousness are associated with a sense of conviction that one is real and that one's surroundings are real (7). Disturbances in this area are called *disturbances of incongruity.* To determine whether there is a disturbance of incongruity, the clinician should ask the following questions: Have

Table 12.1 Disturbances of Consciousness

Disturbances of alertness
  Normal wakefulness to coma; clouding of consciousness
Disturbances in the experience of self
  a. Alterations in the experience that one is real and that the environment is real (disturbances of incongruity)
  b. Alterations in the experience of continuity of identity with the passage of time (disturbances of discontinuity dissociative states)
  c. Alterations in the experience of unity of will and action (passivity experiences)
  d. Alterations in the experience of distinctiveness of self from surroundings (ego boundary disturbances)

---

you felt recently that things around you are not real, as if everything was being acted or an imitation? If so, for how long, and how intensely? Have you felt recently as if you were not real? If so, for how long, and how intensely?

In incongruity, the patient senses that the environment is altered from its normal conditions. The individual may be fully aware of self and actions as a unity, but may feel a lack of conviction in the reality of self or the environment. There are two basic abnormal findings in the sphere of incongruity. The first is *depersonalization*. Depersonalization represents a change in the awareness of self, in which the patient feels him- or herself to be unreal. This condition may be persistent or short lived (for hours or less), may be pleasant or unpleasant, and may vary in intensity. The second condition is *derealization*, which also represents a change in awareness of self (associated frequently with depersonalization); however, in this case the patient perceives

his or her surroundings as unreal, peculiar, or changed.

The Experience of Continuity of Identity with the Passage of Time.   One experiences oneself as persisting in time. Although life may bring different experiences, there is a quality of sameness that continues. Identity is not broken by periods of amnesia. Disturbances in this area are called *disturbances of discontinuity* of the experience of self. Disturbances of discontinuity are numerous and have been generally referred to as dissociative states (see Table 12.2). In assessing the continuity of the experience of self, the clinician is interested in learning several specific kinds of data. The clinician should note reports of memory loss and periods of wandering. Has the patient ever forgotten his or her own identity, or felt he or she was someone else? Also significant are episodes of behavior control loss resulting from drug use or small amounts of alcohol (*pathologic intoxication*).

Table 12.2 Dissociative States

Dissociation of affect	The patient becomes aware that feelings are disconnected from the rest of experience, giving the impression of a reduction of anxiety or a loss of tension in fairly stressful circumstances.
Dissociative trancelike states	Conditions characterized by a marked lack of response to the environment, often by immobility, and by total absorption of attention. They are also characterized by sudden onset, a duration from hours to days, a dazed appearance, and partial amnesia upon restoration of normal responsiveness.
Déjà vu experiences	An experience of estrangement in which there is an illusory sensation of familiarity with current experience.
Amnesia	A circumscribed or "patchy" loss of memory for events often occurs during a dissociative reaction. Patients are in a daze and unable to account for what is happening or has happened, or where they came from. They may in some cases forget their identity and name.
Multiple personality	In this condition there is an apparent coexistence of relatively distinct and autonomous personalities in the same individual; characteristically, there is amnesia for the operations of the alternate personality(ies). This condition is also associated with fugues (cf. below).
Automatic writing	An uncommon condition associated with dissociative trance states.
Fugue	The patient may suddenly leave a stressful situation and later may be in a daze, confused, and amnesic for his or her "flight." Occasionally, the patient demonstrates no self-concern or interest in his or her surroundings.
Frenzied or violent states of dissociative behavior	States in which there is sudden, abrupt onset of frenzied behavior for which there is amnesia. In other cultures, such states are so patterned that they are named specifically. Examples include *latah, running amok,* and *koro* (8). In Western culture, so-called pathologic intoxication is occasionally part of a dissociative reaction associated with a small amount of alcohol intake. Pathologic intoxication is usually abrupt in onset, is associated with impaired consciousness, and may last 1–36 hr following ingestion of alcohol. Frenzied, occasionally violent behavior may take place, clearly out of proportion to the amount of ingested alcohol.

Individuals may be aware of themselves and may note their individuality and initiation of activity, but may experience a detachment or change in the sense of identity over time. Amnesia for this change, once the patients feel restored to their original condition, is typical.

The Experience of Unity of Will and Actions. One normally experiences the control and power of one's body and its acts. One recognizes the discrepancies and intactness of one's identity. Disturbances in this domain (e.g., *passivity experiences*) are often severe and are considered in the section on disturbances of control of thinking.

The Experience of the Distinctiveness of Self Apart from Surroundings. This is a fundamental experience of self, requiring the ability to discriminate between self and environment; clinicians refer to this area of functioning with the concept *ego boundaries.* Disturbances of ego boundaries shall be considered in the discussion of disturbances of control of thinking (see page 184).

General Appearance

We have outlined the examination of general features of the patient. Though the actual process of examination may differ from the sequential order that we propose, the principle underlying our outline is that the clinician moves from observations of a more global nature to those that are more specific.

The patient's appearance provides considerable information. Initial observations reveal important global characteristics. The sex, race, and apparent age are noted. Each of these features may have a bearing on the type of psychiatric problem encountered and its impact. To the experienced clinician, these characteristics often suggest conditions for which the patient is at greater risk. Sexual development is estimated largely on the basis of secondary sexual characteristics (hair distribution, breasts, voice, etc.). Discrepancies between apparent and stated age suggest malingering or chronic illness. Maturation of features is considered in order to estimate the age of the patient. The patient's age

may be a critical clue to a variety of clinical judgments. Older depressed males tend to have a more serious risk for completed suicides, than, for instance, young women, who may have a greater risk for less serious or incomplete suicide attempts. Moreover, in the case of an elderly, confused patient, the clinician should investigate for probable neurologic or medical difficulties, instead of probing primarily for the unlikely onset of schizophrenic symptomatology.

A significant issue is the patient's apparent health or illness. Does the patient look ill? This judgment is based on a number of observations. Most pertinent are nutritional status, general color, alertness and self-awareness, body habitus, and attitude. If ill, what judgment can be made as to the length of illness?

Once these global assessments are made, the clinician searches for more specific clues about the nature of the difficulties facing the patient.

General Bodily Characteristics

The clinician observes the structure and proportions (body habitus) of the patient. It is not enough to note that a patient looks strange. The determinants of body habitus include heredity, hormones, nutrition, and the status of connective tissue. Abnormalities should alert the clinician to consider further investigations.

General examination should include an impression of height; skeletal proportions; circumference of head, chest, and abdomen; and symmetry. Except when the patient's familial background is in keeping with the patient's tallness or shortness, unusual stature may be the result of several factors. Excessively tall stature in the male may reflect a lack of androgens. Hypogonadism may be due to true eunuchism or Kleinfelter's syndrome, wherein the phenotype is male and the genotype XXY. Other causes of hypogonadism are less common. Excessive height may be a reflection of gigantism, which results from excessive growth hormone production prior to fusion of the epiphyses. A thin, asthenic, tall build is common in the not-so-rare-inherited disorder of connective tissue known as Marfan's syndrome. Long, spiderlike fingers and toes (arachnodactyly) and skeletal abnormalities of chest (pectus excavatum and pectus carinatum) and spine (scoliosis) are common in this syndrome.

In general, small stature (dwarfism) is a sympton of congenital or acquired disease. Pituitary dwarfism occurs because of growth hormone deficiency; a thin build with aging of the skin and relative preservation of youthful facies is characteristic. Turner's syndrome (ovarian dysgenesis) is a form of genetic dwarfism, wherein the patient possesses only the X chromosome. Webbed neck, a hairline low on the neck, a broad chest, narrow nails, and short fingers would alert the clinician to this possibility. The hypothyroid dwarf (cretinism) is uncommon in psychiatric clinics, but less profound deprivation of thyroid hormones at or around puberty may induce this state of reduced height; mental sluggishness; cool, dry skin; and puffy features. Other conditions leading to shortness in stature are less common in Western settings. These include nutritional deprivation or serious disease in childhood (e.g., chronic infections, such as tuberculosis, congenital heart disease, etc.).

Face, Ears, Head, and Neck

Examination of these features can provide information about general health (e.g., color and nutritional status), registration of affective responses (e.g., anger or laughter), and clues to specific disease entities (e.g., systemic lupus erythematosus). While cursory inspection of facial appearance may alert one to obvious abnormalities, careful evaluation of the individual features permits fuller appreciation of more subtle changes. Inspection of the facial components, the musculature, the forehead, nose, cheeks, mouth, and lips is necessary. Facial asymmetry may reflect muscular weakness. Lack of a dimple on one side, or a droop in the corner of the mouth, may signal partial or total facial nerve paralysis. Facial expression, both spontaneous and controlled, should be noted. Is the facial expression flat or animated? If lacking in animation, does the patient's face maintain a constant expression, a frown, sadness, etc., that suggests a powerful affective response not congruent with the thinking of the patient? Are the muscles of expression tightly contracted or relaxed? Lack of animation may indicate a depressive disorder, dullness, or parkinsonism. Certain facial appearances (facies) are considered classical for medical problems that may present psychiatrically. Among these are the syndromes of retardation, including Down's syndrome, in which the palpebral aperture is short and wide, having its highest point at the center of the lid. Others include the acneiform rash and moonlike facies of Cushing's syndrome, the staring facies of the hyperthyroid patient, and the puffy lids and dry skin of hypothyroidism. The puffy lid of nephrotic edema, urticaria, and insect bite should be differentiated from these disorders. In parkinsonian states, the face is characteristically immobile, the expression fixed and staring, the skin oily. There is little, if any, smile; the mouth is slightly open, and often there may be drooling. Though uncommon, it is useful to recognize the pattern of myasthenia gravis—gradual weakening of the musculature with the passage of the day and fatigue.

Darwin first commented on the imprinted quality of prolonged tension on the corrugator muscle that may appear on the forehead (the omega sign because the musculature resembles the Greek letter), a finding suggestive of depression. Maintenance of the forehead in a frown or expression of concentration may be a reflection of anxiety.

The nose may reveal many aspects of functioning. Asymmetry and the presence of dried or fresh blood indicate past or recent trauma. Rosacea, or reddening of the nose or cheeks, often characterizes the chronic alcoholic. A nose with a sunken bridge is classical for congenital syphilis. The reddened, butterfly-shaped rash that spreads symmetrically over the bridge of the nose may be a sign of systemic lupus.

The nose is large in acromegaly; in hypothyroidism it tends to broaden.

The cheeks are a common source of information about general health. Pallor can be noted, as well as wasting and dehydration (e.g., diabetes, depression, and severe diarrhea); rounded contours of the cheek may result from corticosteroid therapy.

The mouth and lips are useful for assessment of general color, particularly changes associated with cyanosis and jaundice; acneiform rash around the mouth, especially in nonadolescents, may be an early sign of bromide intoxication. The hygiene of the mouth may be an important clue to general health. Does the patient have a full set of teeth? If not, why not? What is the condition of the gums? Dryness may be associated with anxiety, anticholingeric poisoning, or psychotropic (with anticholingeric properties) drug treatment. Hypertrophy of the gums may be a reflection of chronic treatment with diphenylhydantoin (Dilantin). Tongue inspection may reveal hypoglossal nerve paralysis, hemiatrophy, or tremor (due to anxiety, thyroid disease, delirium tremens, general paresis of the insane or parkinsonism). It may also reveal early signs of tardive dyskinesia. A dry brown tongue suggests late stages of serious illness, for example, uremia. A magenta-colored, swollen tongue is found in riboflavin deficiency. Inflammation of the tongue and angular fissures may signal niacin deficiency.

The ears may reveal several abnormalities. The absence of well-defined lobes and fusion of ears to the face are common in mental retardation and some epileptic individuals. The ears are large in Down's syndrome.

The head and neck may give a clue to certain disorders. An immense head, with the appearance of sunken eyes, is characteristic of hydrocephalus. Generalized enlargement of the head may be the result of Paget's disease (osteitis deformans). Evidence of goiter or thyroid enlargement should be noted. Nodular irregularities in the head, neck, or face should orient the clinician to the possibility of primary or secondary tumor, or lymphadenopathy in Hodgkin's disease and acquired immune deficiency syndrome (AIDS).

Skin

In addition to the consideration of skin in the context of examination of the face and autonomic system, the following should be observed.

Skin color is influenced by pigmentation, blood (character and flow), and thickness of skin. Increased pigmentation from light to dark shades of brown is a classic indication of Addison's disease (adrenal insufficiency) and should be looked for on the elbows, on the hands, and in the mucous membranes of the mouth. The latter are not pigmented when changes in color are due to intestinal malabsorption, liver disease, and arsenic poisoning. Café au lait spots and neurofibromas are seen in von Recklinghausen's disease. Blood flow may be increased in sunburn and other forms of inflammatory response. Carbon monoxide poisoning may be suspected when patients appear to have a cherry red skin color. Changes in skin color to yellow may indicate jaundice or, rarely, carotenemia. Pallor is frequently due to anemia, unusual fright, or lack of pigmentation (albinism).

Texture of the skin may be altered by many influences. Heavy cigarette smoking may lead to "crows feet" at the corners of the eyes. Thyroid hormone in excess leads to moist, fine, smooth skin. In thyroid deficiency, the skin becomes dry, thickened, and scaly.

Skin turgor generally indicates the state of hydration. Dry, paperlike skin is seen in the dehydrated and elderly. Absence of axillary or body perspiration and sunken, soft eye globes suggest serious dehydration.

Rashes, of course, may be of great clinical importance. Of particular interest to the psychiatrist are the unusual rashes that develop secondary to drug overdose or susceptibility to drug reactions, the maculopapular rashes of secondary syphilis, the acneiform rash that develops with bromide intoxication, and the striae of Cushing's syndrome.

Hair and Nails

The character and distribution of hair are often altered by disease processes. Many serious illnesses lead to dryness and temporarily increased loss of hair. In hypothyroid states, the hair becomes thick and coarse and tends to fall out over the frontal region and, occasionally, from the outer aspects of the eyebrow. More complete loss of hair from the head and body generally is seen in anterior hypopituitary disease. Patchy loss of hair occurs in secondary syphilis and alopecia areata, a condition sometimes associated with "psychogenic" disturbances.

Increased hair (hirsuitism) in the female is worth noting, but is not necessarily a reflection of disease. For instance, slight degrees of increased hair over limbs, trunk, and in the moustache area are not pathognomonic for disease. Virilization should be considered, however, when the hair is more grossly distributed and requires shaving. Loss of hair from temporal areas in the female (under influences of testosterone) also suggests virilization rather than simple hirsutism.

The nails deserve attention. Short, irregular nails suggest excessive nail biting. Deficient grooming is often reflected in the nails. Brittle, pitted, or broken nails may indicate psoriasis, the aftermath of severe illness, or the presence of a malabsorption syndrome. The color of the nail bed itself may be a good indication of anemic changes. Clubbing of the nails is a nonspecific change associated with chronic conditions (such as pulmonary tuberculosis, chronic cyanosis, carcinoma of the lung, and subacute baterial endocarditis). Splinter hemorrhages may occur because of embolic phemonena in bacterial endocarditis and in various blood diseases.

Eyes

The eyes give the face much of its expression. Judgments about mood and character often derive from information revealed in the eyes. Pain, anxiety, fear, and even apathy are often expressed largely through them. Conditions with clear psychiatric relevance will be mentioned.

Observations of the orbit, the lids, the palpebral openings, pupils, conjunctivae, and sclerae are made. Exophthalmos (proptosis), if bilateral, suggests hyperthyroidism; if unilaterial, tumor or other retrorbital anomaly is suggested. Enopthalmos is a reflection of serious wasting diseases and dehydration. Certain congenital diseases lead to increased distance between the eyes (ocular hypertelorism, if greater than 40 mm between inner canthi). A puffy lower lid may indicate nephrosis or hypothyrodism. Ptosis refers to drooping of the lid and is indicative of myasthenia or any of a number of neurologic conditions that can interrupt nerve pathways to the lids. The stare of hyperthyroid disease results from the elevation of the upper lid, so that the white sclera becomes visible between the lid and the iris. Increased blinking may be due to a foreign object in the eye (e.g., contact lens) or excessive dryness of eye tissue—such as in atropine ingestion. A decrease in blinking is characteristic of parkinsonism and is observed in many schizophrenic patients.

The presence of vigilance should be distinguished from the stare of hyperthyroidism and should be evaluated with respect to degree of suspiciousness present. Vigilance may indicate fear or anxiety or may be a reflection of paranoid thinking.

The pupils should be equal in size. When greater than 5 mm, the pupil is described as dilated. Sympathetic discharge or interference with parasympathetic tone dilates the pupil. Thus intense anxiety, withdrawal from certain drugs such as narcotics and barbiturates, or intoxication with atropine preparations can lead to dilation. Constriction is due to parasympathetic discharge and is caused by intoxication with narcotics or interruption of sympathetic tone (e.g., Horner's syndrome with miosis, ptosis, and anhydrosis on the affected side). Conjunctival examination reveals color, vascularity, and hemorrhage. Anemia is evident with pale conjunctivae; infection and allergic disorders may be evident with inflammatory changes. In respiratory failure and polycythemia, a glistening appearance occurs. Hemorrhage may result from fracture of the skull or from blood diseases, as well as from local injury. The sclerae are yellow in jaundice. The cornea of arcus senilus reveals an opalescent ring on the periphery of the iris.

Dress and Grooming

Dress and grooming are fundamental features of normal functioning. They break down in a variety of ways, usually in response to fairly serious changes in mental state. Manner of dress and condition of clothing, as well as grooming, may reveal much about the patient's state of mind. The neatness of the obsessive patient's dress and grooming is well known. Exotic or unusual clothing may reflect individual or eccentric style, perhaps grandiosity in the patient with mood disturbance, the delusional thinking of psychosis, or the provocativeness of the attention seeker. Soiled, disheveled clothing suggests unusual poverty, severe depression, psychosis, or coarse brain disease, as well as other medical illness. Soiled face, hands, nails, and skin tend to increase suspicion of more serious disturbances.

Odors

Halitosis, bad breath, usually arises from dental conditions. In psychiatric settings, the clinician is particularly attuned to the smell of alcohol on the breath or person of the patient. Other odors include the unpleasant perspiratory odor of poor hygiene, the acetone odor of diabetes, or starvation acidosis. In some uremic patients, an odor of ammonia is recognizable on the breath. The sweet musty odor of liver disease is occasionally detected.

Autonomic Functions

The state of autonomic functioning may reflect the nonspecific influence of many psychiatric and medical conditions, as well as the more specific influence of pharmacologic and toxic intrusions. Anxiety, fear, the ingestion of caffeine, and cardiac disturbances are some of the many sources of marked changes in autonomic functions. The patient should be asked about "butterfly" sensations in the stomach, dizziness, dry mouth, giddiness, palpitations, circumoral and extremity tingling and numbness sensations, difficulty catching the breath, choking, unusual blushing, trembling, and sweating. For some of these disturbances (such as sweating, increased pulse rate, and respiration) the clinician can make direct observations to confirm the subjective report.

The pattern of occurrence of the above changes should also be noted. Do they occur spontaneously or in reaction to known stimuli? Are they accompanied by fear of dying? Their duration and frequency should be elicited as well as their association with any irrational fears (phobias) such as fear of spiders, snakes, or cockroaches (monophobias) or of open places, crowds, shopping centers, etc. (agoraphobia).

Motor Behavior[a]

Activity

In observing the patient, the clinician is looking for variations from normal motor behavior. Attention focuses on the degree of activity, the presence or lack of spontaneity, and special patterns or qualities.

In questioning the patient, the clinician tries to elicit the subjective experience associated with the motor behavior, because this information may provide clues regarding the nature of the particular motor problem. For example, two major disturbances of subjective experience associated with a variety of motor phenomena are (a) obsessional thinking that often leads to compulsive behavior, and (b) feelings of passivity (wherein patients experience their thoughts, feelings, and behavior as alien and not clearly under their control or influence) that are often associated with echolalia, perseveration, and other behaviors.

Obsessional thinking and feelings of

---

[a] See Chapter 24 for discussion of motor disturbances.

passivity are dealt with more fully in the discussion of disturbances of thinking.

Clinical evaluation of motor behavior initially focuses on the quantity and kind of activity the patient exhibits. Is behavior increased or decreased from normal? Stated differently, is the patient overactive or underactive? Motor activity falls along a continuum from motionlessness (akinesia) to frenzy. Once activity has been noted, the clinician observes whether it is slow or rapid, diffuse or more circumscribed and patterned in character. Does the behavior appear to be goal directed, spontaneous, adaptive, or purposeless? These features help to characterize more precisely the form of motor disturbance. The accompanying tables indicate the specific disturbances seen clinically with increased and decreased motor activity (see Tables 12.3 and 12.4).

In recent years, it has been routine to evaluate patients' involuntary movements prior to initiating antipsychotic treatment, as a means of monitoring potential motor effects in the course of such therapy. Two kinds of evaluations have been developed: the assessment of extrapyramidal movement disturbances (Table 12.5) and of "tardive dyskinesia" (Table 12.6).

Gait, Posture, and Station

Gait is influenced by the rhythm, rate, and character of the movements of walking. The examiner should observe the patient rising from the chair and walking, the pace of walking, and the character of turning around. One must be aware of the role of painful and restrictive conditions in the joints, muscles, and bones when evaluating the meaning of gait disturbance. Backward walking may accentuate abnormalities. Tandem walking (with heel to toe) helps demonstrate ataxia. Particular kinds of gait disturbance are described in Table 12.7.

The patient's posture should be observed and deviations noted. Postural reflexes are dependent on intact medullary functioning. Also influential are tonic neck reflexes, labyrinthine function, cerebellar function, and proprioceptive mechanisms.

Postural fixation is tested by having patients close their eyes and extend their fingers and arm in front of them. Arm and hand drifting are noted and may indicate weakness, tumor, hypotonia, or other abnormal movement. A positive Romberg test occurs when the patient, standing with eyes closed, experiences an actual loss of balance. A wide-based stance (station) may also be noted. Interference with the ability to stand may indicate vertigo (Table 12.7).

The Patient's Relationship and Attitude toward the Clinician[b]

An alliance with the patient is crucial for gathering optimal data in the interview. When lack of cooperation and an unfriendly attitude toward the examiner are present, the clinician should attempt to discover why.

Cooperation may be impaired because of confusion, dysphasia, suspicion, delirium, hostility, or irritability. For example, irritablity may be due to numerous conditions and often will not be attributable to the patient's personality. Among the potential causes for irritability are

1. Fatigue, which lowers thresholds for annoyances and strongly expressed responses;
2. Frustration;
3. Chronic illness, which weighs heavily on coping reserves of the patient;
4. Anxiety, the nonspecific sort associated with many psychiatric conditions and found often in schizophrenia;
5. Jaundice, perhaps because of metabolic disturbances affecting the central nervous system;
6. Diabetes, again probably related to the disturbances in metabolism and also the chronic nature of the disorder;
7. Central nervous system disturbances, such as dementia, delirium, head injury, and meningitis, in which irritability may be the only evidence in some phases of the illness;
8. Affective disorders.

---

[b] See Chapter 14 for discussion of psychodynamic features.

Table 12.3 Clinical Disturbances of Increased Motor Activity

Diffuse

Restlessness	A persistent or generalized increase in bodily movement.
Excitement	Prolonged bursts of energy, often chaotic and disorganized, frenzied in character.

Simple-patterned

Tremor	Involuntary, purposeless contractions of muscle groups which produce oscillating movements near a joint, or of the head. They may occur at rest, with arms extended (postural), resting, or with movement (intentional). Fine or coarse, regular or irregular, rapid or slow.
Stereotypic movements	Repeated performance of non-goal-directed behavior in a uniform manner, often with some remnant of purposive behavior in the movement. Repeated gestures or actions (sometimes thought to have symbolic significance), including continuous movement in and out of a chair, crossing oneself, and waving repeatedly in the air.
Spasms	Involuntary contractions of muscles or groups of muscles, sometimes associated with pain, embarrassment, and fear. Examples are habit spasm, spasms of swallowing or of the tongue, of the eyelids (blepharospasm) spasmodic torticollis, in which there are spasms of neck muscles, particularly the trapezius and sternocleidomastoid, which result in pulling of the head to one side.
Choreiform movements	Short, jerky movements that may affect the whole body. They may affect the periphery more than the trunk. They may be fine or coarse. Also, they may appear to be fragments of expression or gesture and are often disguised in this manner.
Athetoid movements	Spontaneous movements that are slow, writhing, and twisting (wormlike—hence, athetoid) involving generally distal muscles, but possibly proximal also, and bringing strange postures to the body, especially to the hands.
Dystonic movements	Defined as bearing similarity to athetoid movements, but usually involving large areas of the body musculature. Slowed, hypertonic, occasionally grotesque movements with maintenance of peculiar postures.
Myoclonic movements	Rapid contraction of either proximal or distal muscles, usually in a nonrhythmic fashion but sometimes with bilaterally symmetrical presentation. Usually spontaneous but can be elicited by auditory, visual, or tactile stimulation.
Perseverative movements	The involuntary continuation or recurrence of a movement more appropriate to a prior stimulus (e.g., request, command, etc.) the purpose of which is already served, in response to a succeeding stimulus. Perseverative movement may be noted by asking the patient to close the eyes, stick out the tongue or write for the examiner, as well as by close observation of interview behavior.
Impulsive movements	Sudden, apparently purposeless or involuntary acts, including screaming, biting, exhibition of genitals.
Carphologic movements	These including picking at bedclothes, skin, clothing in a purposeless manner.

Complex-patterned

Agitation	The subjective report of anguish, psychic tension, or anxiety of very unpleasant proportions *and* one or more of the following: pacing; fidgetiness; inability to sit still; wringing of the hands; pulling at skin, hair, or clothing; shouting or complaining in outbursts.
Akathisia	Motor restlessness, often subjectively experienced as centered in the lower extremities and accompanied by muscular or somatic tension, a feeling of having to move, and an intolerance of sitting still. In milder states, shuffling or tapping movements, shifting, rocking to and fro. In severer states, an inability to sit still at all and incessant movement.
Tics	Short, sudden, repetitive, jerky movements of small groups of muscles of face, neck, or upper trunk, often worsened by psychologic circumstances. Most commonly affecting the face, tics may be part of an unusual blink or distortion of the forehead, nose, or mouth. Swallowing, grunting, coughing, or shoulder movements may also be tics. More complex tics, such as compulsive touching of people or objects, may be very similar to mannerisms.
Tardive dyskinesia	Literally, this is a late disorder of motility. There are choreiform movements of the extremities, orofacial movements (such as flycatcher's tongue, unusual grimacing, snouting, etc.) and dystonic postures. Younger patients appear more affected in the extremities and trunk, while in older patients, there is a greater restriction to the oral region.

Table 12.3 *(Cont.)*

Mannerisms	These consist in an unusual variation in the performance of normal, goal-directed movement. Examples include unusual movements in greeting, shaking hands, or writing, strange uses of words, and unusual verbal expressions out of keeping with the situation. Stereotypies are often difficult to distinguish from mannerisms. The distinction that is often useful is that stereotypies generally do not have a direction or goal, nor do they form part of goal-directed behavior.

Table 12.4 Clinical Disturbances of Decreased Motor Activity

Diffuse

Retardation	Slowed in all activities, voluntary and vegetative, and often slowed in thinking and speech as well. Patients show little spontaneity, and goal-directed behavior is reported to be exhausting.
Poverty of movement	Reduction in the amount or quantity of motor activity, sometimes called hypokinesia.
Stupor	There may be almost no animation, spontaneous movement, or locomotion.

Patterned

Motor blocking (obstruction)	Episodic occurrence in which movement suddenly is reduced or halted in the midst of normal or increased activity. Later, the patient may be able to resume the movement. The patient may report the subjective experience of thought withdrawal or that the intended movement was forgotten following such episodes. Because of this disturbance, movement may appear stiff and awkward.
Cooperation	(a) *Mitmachen:* A variant of catalepsy (see under disturbances of posture) in which a displaced body part returns to its original position when released by the examiner. (b) *Mitgehen:* A more severe or extreme form of this disturbance in which the patient's body part continues to move in a given direction in response to light pressure.
Automatic obedience	The patient carries out all instruction, regardless of merit or propriety.
Negativism	A broad spectrum of motor behavior which is characterized by an apparently unmotivated failure to do what is suggested. This may lead to varying degrees of akinesia, or lack of movement. In its most severe form, it is also aptly described as stupor.
Ambitendency	This is considered a form of negativism, which consists in the patient making a series of tentative movements toward a goal which is not reached in response to a request to carry out a voluntary action. For example, the patient may walk toward the examiner in response to a request to come forward and then may halt halfway and return to the original starting position.
Parkinsonian movement	Characterized by lack of spontaneity, and associated with expressionless facies, fixed postures, and cog wheel rigidity of the limbs. A tremor at rest is often present.
Opposition (Gegenhalten)	Refers to the presence of muscular resistance to passive movement of the extremities.
Echopraxia	Patient imitates the simple behavior of the examiner or other patients, such as clapping or tapping the finger. In echolalia, speech is imitated.

Table 12.5 Simpson Neurological Rating Scale (9)

The examination should be conducted in a room where the patient can walk a sufficient distance to allow him/her to get into a natural rhythm, e.g., 15 paces.

   Each side of the body should be examined; if one side shows more pronounced pathology than the other, record more severe pathology.

   Cogwheel rigidity may be palpated when the examination is carried out for items 3, 4, 5, and 6. It is not rated separately and is merely another way to detect rigidity. It would indicate that a minimum score of 2 would be mandatory.

1.   GAIT: The patient is examined as he walks into the examining room—his gait, the swing of his arms, his general posture, all form the basis for an overall score for this item.
   1 = Normal
   2 = Mild diminution in swing while the patient is walking
   3 = Obvious diminution in swing suggesting shoulder rigidity
   4 = Stiff gait with little or no armswing noticeable
   5 = Rigid gait with arms slightly pronated; or stooped-shuffling gait with propulsion and repropulsion
   9 = Not ratable

2.   ARM DROPPING: The patient and the examiner both raise their arms to shoulder height and let them fall to their sides. In a normal subject, a stout slap is heard as the arms hit the sides. In the patient with extreme Parkinson's syndrome, the arms fall very slowly.
   1 = Normal, free fall with loud slap and rebound
   2 = Fall slowed slightly with less audible contact and little rebound
   3 = Fall slowed, no rebound
   4 = Marked slowing, no slap at all
   5 = Arms fall as though against resistance; as though through glue
   9 = Not ratable

3.   SHOULDER SHAKING: The subject's arms are bent at a right angle at the elbow and are taken one at a time by the examiner who grasps one hand and also clasps the other around the patient's elbow. The subject's upper arm is pushed to and fro and the humerus is externally rotated. The degree of resistance from normal to extreme rigidity is scored as detailed. The procedure is repeated with one hand palpating the shoulder cuff while rotation takes place.
   1 = Normal
   2 = Slight stiffness and resistance
   3 = Moderate stiffness and resistance
   4 = Marked rigidity and difficulty in passive movement
   5 = Extreme stiffness and rigidity with almost a frozen joint
   9 − Not ratable

4.   ELBOW RIGIDITY: The elbow joints are separately bent at right angles and passively extended and flexed, with the subject's biceps observed and simultaneously palpated. The resistance to this procedure is rated.
   1 = Normal
   2 = Slight stiffness and resistance
   3 = Moderate stiffness and resistance
   4 = Marked rigidity with difficulty in passive movement
   5 = Extreme stiffness and rigidity with almost a frozen joint
   9 = Not ratable

5.   WRIST RIGIDITY: The wrist is held in one hand and the fingers held by the examiner's other hand, with the wrist moved to extension, flexion and ulner and radial deviation or the extended wrist is allowed to fall under its own weight, or the arm can be grasped above the wrist and shaken to and fro. A "1" score would be a hand that extends easily, falls loosely, or flaps easily upwards and downwards.
   1 = Normal
   2 = Slight stiffness and resistance
   3 = Moderate stiffness and resistance
   4 = Marked rigidity with difficulty in passive movement
   5 = Extreme stiffness and rigidity with almost a frozen wrist
   9 = Not ratable

Table 12.5 (*Cont.*)

6.   HEAD ROTATION: The patient sits or stands and is told that you are going to move his head from side to side, that it will not hurt and that he should try and relax. (Questions about pain in the cervical area or difficulty in moving his head should be obtained to avoid causing any pain.) Clasp the patient's head between the two hands with the fingers on the back of the neck. Gently rotate the head in a circular motion 3 times and evaluate the muscular resistance to this movement.

        1 = Loose, no resistance
        2 = Slight resistance to movement although the time to rotate may be normal
        3 = Resistance is apparent and the time of rotation is shortened
        4 = Resistance is obvious and rotation is slowed
        5 = Head appears stiff and rotation is difficult to carry out
        9 = Not ratable

7.   GLABELLAR TAP: Subject is told to open eyes wide and not to blink. The glabellar region is tapped at a steady, rapid speed. Note number of times patient blinks in succession. Take care to stand behind the subject so that he does not observe the movement of the tapping finger. A full blink need not be observed; there may be contraction of the infraorbital muscle producing a twitch each time a stimulus is delivered. Vary speed of tapping to assure that muscle contraction is related to the tap.

        1 = 0–5 blinks
        2 = 6–10 blinks
        3 = 11–15 blinks
        4 = 16–20 blinks
        5 = 21 and more blinks
        9 = Not ratable

8.   TREMOR: Patient is observed walking into examining room and then is re-examined for this item with arms extended at right angles to the body and the fingers spread out as far as possible.

        1 = Normal
        2 = Mild finger tremor, obvious to sight and touch
        3 = Tremor of hand or arm occurring spasmodically
        4 = Persistent tremor of one or more limbs
        5 = Whole body tremor
        9 = Not ratable

9.   SALIVATION: Patient is observed while talking and then asked to open his mouth and elevate his tongue.

        1 = Normal
        2 = Excess salivation so that pooling takes place if mouth is open and tongue raised
        3 = Excess salivation is present and might occasionally result in difficulty in speaking
        4 = Speaking with difficulty because of excess salivation
        5 = Frank drooling
        9 = Not ratable

10.   AKATHISIA: Patient is observed for restlessness. If restlessness is noted, ask: "Do you feel restless or jittery inside; it is difficult to sit still?" Subjective response is not necessary for scoring but patient report can help make the assessment.

        1 = No restlessness reported or observed
        2 = Mild restlessness observed, e.g., occasional jiggling of the foot occurs when patient is seated
        3 = Moderate restlessness observed, e.g., on several occasions, jiggles foot, crosses and uncrosses legs or twists a part of the body
        4 = Restlessness is frequently observed, e.g., the foot or legs moving most of the time
        5 = Restlessness persistently observed, e.g., patient cannot sit still, may get up and walk
        9 = Not ratable

EMOTIONAL STATE

The observation, description, and characterization of the emotional state of the patient are difficult tasks, since both objective and subjective criteria play important roles. Objective observations of the face, general motor behavior, posture, gait, gestures, and responsiveness to the examiner should be considered. The occurrence of flushing, tears, perspiration, tachycardia, tremor, and changes in respiration or blood pressure call for special attention, since these manifestations may be present in excitement, fear, anxiety, depression, and a variety of medical disturbances.

Subjective observations are gained from

Table 12.6 Abnormal Involuntary Movement Scale (AIMS) (10)

INSTRUCTIONS:	Complete Examination Procedure before making ratings. MOVEMENT RATINGS: Rate highest severity observed. Rate movements that occur upon activation one *less* than those observed spontaneously.	CODE	0 = None 1 = Minimal 2 = Mild 3 = Moderate 4 = Severe		
FACIAL AND ORAL MOVEMENTS	1. Muscles of Facial Expression e.g., movements of forehead, eyebrows, periorbital area, cheeks; include frowning, blinking, smiling, grimacing				☐
	2. Lips and Perioral Area e.g., puckering, pouting, smacking				☐
	3. Jaw e.g., biting, clenching, chewing, mouth opening, lateral movement				☐
	4. Tongue Rate only increase in movement both in and out of mouth. NOT inability to sustain movement				☐
EXTREMITY MOVEMENTS:	5. Upper (*arms, wrists, hands, fingers*) Include choreic movements, (i.e., rapid, objectively purposeless, irregular, spontaneous), athetoid movements (i.e., slow, irregular, complex, serpentine). Do NOT include tremor (i.e., repetitive, regular, rhythmic)				☐
	6. Lower (*legs, knees, ankles, toes*) e.g., lateral knee movement, foot tapping, heel dropping, foot squirming, inversion and eversion of foot				☐
TRUNK MOVEMENTS:	7. Neck, shoulders, hips e.g., rocking, twisting, squirming, pelvic gyrations				☐
GLOBAL JUDGMENTS:	8. Severity of abnormal movements	None, normal Nominal Mild Moderate Severe	0 1 2 3 4		☐
	9. Incapacitation due to abnormal movements	None, normal Minimal Mild Moderate Severe	0 1 2 3 4		☐
	10. Patient's awareness of abnormal movements Rate only patient's report	No awareness Aware, no distress Aware, mild distress Aware, moderate distress Aware, severe distress	0 1 2 3 4		☐
DENTAL STATUS	11. Current problems with teeth and/or dentures	No Yes	0 1		☐
	12. Does patient usually wear dentures?	No Yes	0 1		☐

skillful questioning about experienced feelings. Care must be used to define carefully the nature of the patient's experience in his or her own words and not to suggest the interviewer's preconceived assessment.

The emotional state is evaluated with regard to mood and affect (see Table 12.8).

Assessment of self-esteem and suicide potential are dealt with in chapters 14 and 42, respectively.

Mood

Mood is a somewhat ambiguous term (11). It is often used interchangeably with the term *affect*, which adds confusion to clinical discourse. We choose, somewhat arbitrarily, to define mood as the more sustained and less flexible emotional state over a defined period of time. For our purposes, this time will be the length of the interview for objective observations

Table 12.6 (*Cont.*)

Examination Procedure

Either before or after completing the Examination Procedure observe the patient unobtrusively, at rest (e.g., in waiting room).

The chair to be used in this examination should be a hard, firm one without arms.

1. Ask patient whether there is anything in his/her mouth (i.e., gum, candy, etc.) and if there is, to remove it.
2. Ask patient about the *current* condition of his/her teeth. Ask patient if he/she wears dentures. Do teeth or dentures bother patient *now?*
3. Ask patient whether he/she notices any movements in mouth, face, hands, or feet. If yes, ask to describe and to what extent they *currently* bother patient or interfere with his/her activities
4. Have patient sit in chair with hands on knees, legs slightly apart, and feet flat on floor. (Look at entire body for movements while in this position).
5. Ask patient to sit with hands hanging unsupported. If male, between legs, if female and wearing a dress, hanging over knees. (Observe hands and other body areas.)
6. Ask patient to open mouth. (Observe tongue at rest within mouth.) Do this twice.
7. Ask patient to protrude tongue. (Observe abnormalities of tongue movement.) Do this twice.
*8. Ask patient to tap thumb, with each finger, as rapidly as possible for 10–15 seconds; separately with right hand, then with left hand. (Observe facial and leg movements.)
9. Flex and extend patient's left and right arms (one at a time). (Note any rigidity and rate on DOTES.)
10. Ask patient to stand up. (Observe in profile. Observe all body areas again, hips included.)
*11. Ask patient to extend both arms outstretched in front with palms down. (Observe trunk, legs, and mouth.)
*12. Have patient walk a few paces, turn, and walk back to chair. (Observe hands and gait.) Do this twice.

*Activated movements

and up to a week for subjective reports. Changes in mood are of course characteristic of depression and mania, but are also common in patients with a variety of disorders, including basal ganglia disease, cardiovascular disease, cerebral tumors, and head injury.

Subjective Report

The report of the patient on being asked how he or she feels provides the initial data. This question may be phrased in a variety of ways (e.g., "How are your spirits?" and "How are things going for you?"). We ask an open-ended question so that the patient's response can indicate the general way he or she feels. If the patient finds it difficult to respond to this general type of inquiry, the clinician can suggest more specific feelings to probe for the information (Does the patient feel happy? worried? blue? sad? anxious? frightened?).

A more careful description and characterization now become the goal. If the patient has been "blue," how intensely and with what associated behavior (crying, withdrawal, etc.)? The patient's own

words provide a unique report worth recording.

Objective Evaluation

The clinician then observes the patient's mood. Does the patient appear "blue"? When there are discrepancies between subjective reports and objective observations, the clinician should try to resolve them. For example, a vigilant and tremulous patient declares that he feels "fine." Is the patient merely not cooperating, suspicious and frightened, or too confused to respond? Often it is useful to ask patients to rate their mood. For instance, the clinician suggests that the patient estimate on a scale from 1 to 10, in which 1 represents the worst they have felt and 10 the best, where they would place themselves today. This estimate should corroborate the clinician's observation and the patient's verbal report and may enlighten the clinician concerning the severity of mood disturbances. Table 12.9, adapted from Preu (12), lists some of the descriptions of prevailing mood.

Table 12.7 Disturbances of Gait

Reeling or ataxic	The patient walks with a disorganized, staggering, lurching wavering walk.
Propulsive, festinating	This gait is characterized by neck and trunk rigidity, lack of associated (swinging) movements of the arms, and short shuffling steps (marché à petit pas) and the appearance of almost falling forward in line of movement.
Clownish	Walking is affected by grotesque movements caused by the involvement of purposeless involuntary acts.
Spastic	This gait has a quality of stickiness. The patient either swings the thigh or pushes the foot of the affected side along the floor
Bizarre or hysterical	A grotesque inconsistent unpatterned movement and accompanying postures may be used in walking.
Steppage	This gait is characterized by flaccid limbs, the thigh and leg being raised high to clear the ground. The gait may be uni- or bilateral and is often associated with foot drop.
Waddling	Wide-based feet, lordosis, and waddling motion centered in the pelvis.

Table 12.8 Assessment of Mood and Affect

Mood (during course of interview)
  Subjective report and rating from 1 to 10
  Objective or observed mood

Affect
  Subjective (awareness of affective experiences)
  Objective (types displayed)
    Overall qualities
      1. Range (full vs. constricted)
      2. Intensity (intense, flat, blunted)
      3. Changeability (stability vs. lability)
      4. Appropriateness to situation and content of thinking

Table 12.9 Descriptions of Mood (12)

1. Cheerful, silly, self-satisfied, boastful, grandiose, elated, exalted, ecstatic
2. Nostalgic, sensitive, sad, gloomy, pessimistic, depressed.
3. Worried, anxious, distressed, apprehensive, frightened, terrified, bewildered
4. Sarcastic, annoyed, irritable, angry, furious, enraged.
5. Cool, distant, aloof, disdainful, suspicious, defensive
6. Apathetic, indifferent, dull, affectless.

Affect

We use the term *affect* here to refer to more momentary emotional experiences than those described by "mood." Thus *affect* means the more immediate expressions and experiences of emotion that may occur in a variey of forms throughout the clinical interview. While patients may feel somewhat anxious in mood, they may be able to show joy, sadness, anger, frustration, and other affects during the examination. These latter observations are the focus of this part of the examination.

1. What the patient experiences when he or she appears frustrated, joyful, or sad is valuable information. Does the patient have a vocabulary to describe his or her emotional life? If so, how rich and detailed is it? These observations provide data regarding the patient's awareness of emotional experience.

2. The clinician notes the type of affects displayed. *Display* refers to the objective appreciation of affects (i.e., what the clinician sees) on the face and other features.

3. Having noted the types of affect, the clinician then assesses the overall qualities of the patient's affective experiences.

   a. Initially, one is interested in judging the range of affective behavior. Is there constriction to only a few related affective responses (e.g., only irritability, annoyance, anger) or is the range more full or variable?

   b. What is the intensity of these experiences and manifestations? Are they shallow, as in the fatuous affect of frontal lobe syndrome or dementia? If affective responses are virtually absent, the term *flattened affect* is used. The chronic anhedonia of schizophrenia is often described in this manner. If there is responsiveness, is it less than the situation merits? Blunting or decreased intensity may be seen in neurologic conditions in which lesions prevent the full expression of affective responses. It is also found in a number of other conditions, including depression. Affect may be very intense in depression, anxiety, and psychosis.

c. The clinician follows the changes from one affect to another. Are the transitions smooth or awkward? How rapidly are they made? Rapid changes in affect indicate liability of affect, a finding present in many organic disorders and occasionally in manic states.

d. The clinician assesses the appropriateness of the affect with respect to the situation and content of thinking. The appropriateness criterion probably has something to do with social propriety, but the key issue is the degree of congruency between affective display and thinking. Does the patient smile when discussing morbid information? Are tearfulness and despair evident when the patient discloses content to match these qualities? Clinically, patients with acute schizophrenic syndromes may present affects incongruent with thinking or situation. Bulbar palsies may perplex the clinician initially because of the rather intense and inappropriate displays of crying and laughter that characterize this condition. A catastrophic affective reaction may occur in response to questions that tax or challenge the patient especially in left hemispheric injuries and dementia.

PERCEPTION[c]

The assessment of perception calls for careful questioning of the patient, since there are few objective observations for this kind of disturbance. There are two fundamental categories of perceptual disturbance, *distortion* and *deception* (4). A distortion implies that there is a constant and real object as the basic stimulus for the perception but that for any of a variety of

---

[c] See Chapter 22 for discussion of perceptual disturbances.

reasons, the perception is altered. A deception implies that a new perception occurs that is usually not in response to an external stimulus.

Normal perception takes place through each of the sensory modalities and in the dimensions of time and space. In principle, there is the possibility for disturbance in each of these categories. The most significant problem in obtaining useful information about perceptual disturbances is determining their presence. Generally, patients find it easier to discuss and describe distortions than they do deceptions.

The information required by the clinician includes (a) the phenomenologic description of the perception; (b) the relation of the perception to external stimulation; (c) the environmental context of the perception (e.g., in light or in darkness, whether the surroundings are strange or familiar); (d) the relationship of the perception to affective state or thought content, especially delusions; (e) the subjective interpretation of the perception, e.g., its reality (is it real or imagined?); and (f) the attitude toward the hallucination (e.g., fear, enjoyment, a nonplussed response, etc.). The answers to these questions should alert the clinician to the nature of the disturbance and to possible causes.

Distortion

A perceptual distortion is due to a change in quality, intensity, or spatial form of a real experience. Distortions of temporal perception also occur. Tables 12.10 and 12.11 outline the visual and auditory distortions in perceptual disturbance.

Deceptions

There are two types of deception: *illusion* and *hallucination*. An illusion is a misinterpretation of stimuli arising from an external object, and a hallucination is a perception without adequate source of external stimulation.

Illusions

The patient adds features to the perception of a real object that it does not have.

Table 12.10 Visual Distortions

Changes in spatial form (dysmegalopsia)	This is the name for general type of disturbance in which there is a change in the spatial form of visual perception. Such distortions may create irregular mixtures of images in the visual field which may appear near, far, long, short, fat, or thin—all at the same time. There are two specific kinds of more uniform dysmegalopsia: *micropsia,* in which objects appear far away or smaller than they actually are, and *macropsia* in which objects appear nearer or larger than they actually are.
Changes in quality	Visual distortions may be manifest as changes in color. Terms such as xanthopsia (yellow), chloropsia (green), and erhythropsia (red) describe these experiences.
Changes in intensity	Certain features of visual images may appear more or less intense. Sometimes, colors appear more brilliant or pale, lines more or less distinct. Requesting that the patient close his or her eyes and apply a small amount of fingertip pressure to the globes of the eyes (taking caution, of course, to remove any contact lens) can often induce vivid patterns of colors in the eye, which the patient will report.

Shadows are seen, for instance, to be menacing figures threatening harm. Innocent gestures take on frightening significance for the patient. A creak in the stairs becomes the approach of some possibly sinister person. Voices are misheard. Occasionally, the attribution applied to these perceptions is difficult to distinguish from delusional and hallucinatory phenomena.

A particular and vivid kind of illusion is *pareidolia,* which results from a combination of imagination and impressive visual imagery. Patients, with little or no effort, and occasionally against their will, see lifelike pictures in the clouds, on the walls or carpeting, and in fires. The patient may be asked to look at the carpet or curtain in the examining office and describe what he or she sees to elicit this response.

The string test is a classic maneuver to elicit illusory visual phenomena. The clinician asks the patient if he or she can see anything between the partially separated hands of the examiner (the hands are held as if they are grasping the ends of a short string). The patient may describe both the presence and color, as well as other characteristics of the "string."

Hallucinations

Jaspers (6) defines hallucination as "a false perception, which is not a sensory distortion or misinterpretation and which occurs at the same time as real perceptions." This excludes dreams. There are other perceptual phenomena that must also be distinguished from hallucinations:

Imagery refers to experiences occurring in inner subjective space, which lack the substantial reality of perception. Fantasy, imaginative thinking, and daydreaming all fall into this category.

Pseudohallucination refers to phenomena that are vividly perceived (seen, heard, smelled, etc.); however, the patient is aware that they are not actual or true perceptions. The phenomenal experiences of hallucinogens may be of this character: "I see something but I know it's not real."

True hallucination, in contrast, refers to perceptions without adequate basis in objective space that carry the conviction of reality. *Negative hallucination* refers to failure to perceive things that are present.

Hallucinations may occur in each of the sensory modalities.

Vision (Visual Hallucinations). Visual hallucinations may be elementary such as light flashes, partly organized such as in patterns of various colors, or organized (complete), in which case the visual experience is of whole objects, people, scenes, etc. Often, visual hallucinations are associated with intense emotion, and frequently with fear. Special kinds are detailed in Table 12.12.

Appropriate questions that elicit or augment the description of visual hallucinatory experience include "Do you dream vividly?"; "Do you see visions in the daytime?"; and "Do you see flashes of light, patterns, figures, objects and so forth that others cannot see?"

Hearing (Auditory Hallucinations). Auditory hallucinations may also be elementary (unusual noises), partially orga-

Table 12.11 Auditory Distortions

Changes in spatial form	Some patients describe their experience of sound as if it arose from a distance. This is analogous to the visual experience of micropsia.
Changes in intensity	Patients complain of sound being too intense or almost inaudible (hyperacousis and hypoacousis). The experience of the former is often apparent in the inability to hear spoken conversation. The latter is described as unpleasant, distracting, and "nerve racking."

Table 12.12 Visual Hallucinations

Hallucinatory flashback	A drug related memory appears with particularly clear perception.
Visions	Some patients describe a vivid scene such as fire, religious experiences, etc.
Lilliputian hal lucination	Patients see little men and women; such a hallucination is often accompanied by an experience of enjoyment.
Autoscopy	This experience, often called *Doppelgänger*, occurs when patients see themselves and recognize that what they see are themselves.
Negative autoscopy	Occurs when patients look at a mirror but are unable to see themselves.
Mass hallucinations	Some patients report experiences of mass violence and brutality.
Extracampine hallucinations	Patients hallucinate outside the visual perceptual field. For instance, the patient sees an object in a house across the street or behind his head.
Hypnagogic hallucinations	The patient has hallucinatory experiences while falling asleep.
Hypnopompic hallucinations	The patient hallucinates while awakening.

nized (music), or completely organized (voices, also sometimes called *phonemes*). Typically, voices are perceived as either clear and distinct or vague; one or more voices may be heard; the voices may sound like normal ones or may be more spiritual, loud, or soft, etc. Voices may have potent impact or may not affect the patient's behavior at all. Usually, voices are abusive, but occasionally they are friendly, even comforting to the patient. They may berate, discuss, argue about, or converse with the patient. In true hallucinations, voices generally originate from outside the head; in pseudohallucinations, they may be more often described as in the mind of the patient. Specific kinds of auditory hallucinations are detailed in Table 12.13.

Questions that are often helpful in eliciting auditory hallucinations include "Do noises in your head, ears, or from the outside bother you?"; "Do you ever hear your own thinking, your own thoughts as if they were being spoken aloud?"; "Do you hear voices when no one else is around you who could be speaking? If so, whose voice? Is it clear? Abusive? Accusatory? A real voice, sound, or perhaps just your own thoughts?"; and "Can you stop the voices from occurring?"

Smell (Olfactory Hallucinations). Hallucinations of smell are often difficult to distinguish from delusional and illusory phenomena. Some patients may distinctly smell various unpleasant odors in the environment but may not be able to specify their origin. Others may feel that they are the source of an odor—usually unpleasant —from their body, perhaps from a tattooed area or a discolored spot on their skin. Most frequently, olfactory hallucinations occur with such noxious smells as gas, burning rubber, or ammonia.

Taste (Gustatory Hallucinations). Frequently, it is difficult to distinguish hallucinations of taste from secondary delusions or illusions, though they do occur.

Touch, Pain, and Vestibular Sensation Hallucinations. Patients may complain of tactile sensations, bugs crawling on the body (formication), and sexual sensations such as forced ejaculation or persistent feelings of coitus. Some patients may experience sensation from a previously amputated extremity, as if the extremity were still present, sensible and able to move (phantom limb). Patients may describe their flesh being twisted, torn, electrically

Table 12.13 Auditory Hallucinations

Command hallucinations	The patient is given instructions to carry out various tasks.
Audible thoughts (Gedankenlautwerden or echo de pensees)	The patient may report hearing his or her own thoughts being spoken aloud
Functional hallucinations	The patient reports a voice when the hum of a fluorescent bulb is present, but not when the light is off. Such hallucinations occur only in the presence of external noise.
Extracampine auditory hallucinations	The patient hears a voice from a distance well out of hearing range.
Voices arguing	The patient may hear two or more voices discussing or arguing, usually about the patient, who is referred to in the third person.
Voices commenting on the patient's actions	The content of the hallucination is a description of the patient's activities as they take place.

shocked, placed in a vise, etc. Some patients have sensations of sinking through the floor, of flying, or of falling from heights (kinesthetic hallucinations).

Perception of Time

Disturbances arising in sensory experience and the perception of space are relevant features to evaluate clinically. Less often considered are disturbances in the perception of time, which may also be informative. Temporal disorientation, which can be assessed formally by requesting that the patient tell the examiner the time of day, date, year, and season, is dependent on time perception and is usually associated with other impairments in higher intellectual functioning. An appreciation of the patient's subjective sense and estimation of the passage of time may suggest diagnostic possibilities in cases in which other cardinal symptoms and signs are not apparent. For instance, slowed time may be associated with depression; the rapid passage of time may be experienced in anxiety and mania. Disturbances in time perception are generally distortions, but because of the complex nature of this cognitive act, it is less useful to categorize the disturbance than simply to describe it.

Relevant questions include "Does time proceed slowly or quickly for you?"; "Does time ever seem to stand still?"; and "Do you experience periods of confusion or other changes when the distinction between past and present or present and future seems to blur?" The patient may be asked to estimate the passage of a minute or a shorter period, or to estimate the duration of the interview to the time of the question.

SPEECH AND LANGUAGE

Speech refers to the production of sounds (i.e., articulation and phonation) as a mode of communication. It is a motor function by which words, having been formulated, are converted into sound. Thus, it involves the lips, tongue, palate, vocal cords, and respiratory musculature. Language, on the other hand, refers to the comprehension and expression of meanings through the use of words. Hence, language functions include the proper use and construction of words. Generally, speech is the physical and language the symbolic form of verbal expression. Careful listening and the use of several simple tests are the keys to evaluating both speech and language.

Speech

As a clinician listens to the patient's speech, he or she should note and describe its spontaneity, volume, pitch, modality, slurring, intelligibility, and fluency. Are there accessory movements in the face and neck or emotional accompaniments to speaking, such as frustration or embarrassment? The rate of speaking should also be noted. Normal speech is generally spontaneous, of medium pitch and volume, and, because of normal hesitations or "uhs" and "ahs," may be far from fluent. The emotional expressions accompanying normal speech are appropriate to the content of what is being said. Prosody refers to the melody of speech, and dysprosody is a disturbance of the rhythm and rate of speech production. The latter is associated with Parkinson's disease, cerebellar disorders, and nondominant cortical lesions. Hoarseness should be noted and, if necessary, referral should be made for further evaluation. Keeping the voice at unusual levels of pitch (high or low) abuses the speech apparatus and may be associated with physical and/or psychiatric disorder. In aphonia, articulation is preserved and phonation is lost, and the patient speaks in a whisper. This disturbance may arise from vocal cord or laryngeal disease, but is most commonly not organic. Mutism, complete loss of speech in the conscious nonaphasic patient, is discussed in the evaluation of thinking. Disruptions in articulation, with audible or silent repetitions or prolongations of single words, sounds, or syllables, are the hallmarks of stuttering. If these disruptions are frequent and not readily controlled by the patient, more specific examination may be required, and a referral should be made to a speech pathologist.

Slurred speech should also be noted: It may be due to weakness of the articulatory muscles or to the rigidity and slowness of parkinsonism; or if characterized by unduly separated syllable formation; it may be due to cerebellar dysfunction. Explosive speech, sometimes associated with grimacing, may be seen as a severe accompaniment of slurring. This speech disturbance may be due to multiple sclerosis or conditions characterized by chorea and athetosis.

Language

Language assessment is relatively simple and should be routine in the psychiatric examination, particularly in acutely ill and older patients (in whom neurologic illness may masquerade as psychiatric complaints). Symbolic functions of verbal expression include the ability to comprehend, to repeat, to name, to read, and to write.

The patient's ability to comprehend is usually evident from the interview, but it is useful to ask the patient to perform a complex command such as touching the left ear with the right thumb. For repetition, ask the patient to repeat a phrase like "no ands, ifs, or buts." Then, to test naming ability, ask for the names of three objects, such as button, tie, and watch stem. Having the patient write a sentence and read still another completes the assessment.

Intact reading and writing functions generally rule out aphasia. Disturbances of these functions and of comprehension, repeating, or naming fall under the heading *aphasia* and are divided into two groups, *fluent* and *nonfluent*, depending on whether a specific disturbance in articulation (expression) characterizes speech. Nonfluent aphasia (Broca's aphasia) exhibits slow, slurred speech that is poorly articulated, is reduced in quantity, and in which short words such as conjunctions are omitted. The result is a telegraphlike production in which repetition is faulty, though single-word repetition may be performed without difficulty. Nevertheless, comprehension is usually intact.

Other aphasias are fluent and are distinguished by the pattern of disturbed functions discovered in the simple examination procedure outlined above. Table 12.14 provides guidance for specifying these disturbances. The presence of any of these patterns calls for neurologic consultation.

THINKING[d]

The examination of thinking can provide significant information regarding psychopathology and diagnosis. Obtaining this information, however, requires that adequate attention has already been directed at speech and language assessment. If the latter are intact, the evaluation of thinking can proceed. Many clinicians recognize disturbances of thinking quite frequently in their patients, but find it difficult to describe these disturbances clearly or explain

---

[d] See Chapter 21 for discussion of disturbances of thinking.

Table 12.14 Patterns of Aphasic Disturbance

Type of Aphasia	Fluency	Compre- hension	Repe- tition	Naming	Reading and Writing
Broca's	−	+	−[a]	+	−
Wernicke's	+	−	−	−	−
Anomic	+	+	+	−	+
Conduction	+	+	−	−	−
Global	−	−	−	−	−

+, ability present; −, ability absent.
[a] The repetition of single words may be intact.

their importance. Particularly troublesome are disturbances such as loosened associations (derailment), blocking, and flight of ideas. To counter these deficits, we propose a method of evaluation based on Fish (4) that, like all such schemes, is somewhat arbitrary, but carries two practical advantages: It is specific and it is clear.

The assumption underlying this scheme is that language is the vehicle of thought. That is, we must assume that language mirrors the process of thinking, or, put simply, that what we say is what we think. Obviously, language reflects only a part of thinking; there is a great deal of thinking that is not expressed spontaneously in language, and there may well be forms of thinking (such as problem solving and creative or imaginative thinking) that require little or no language at all. Thus a careful examination of thinking requires first that we listen closely to the patient and second that we question the patient to determine the subjective experience associated with his or her use of language. The latter helps to clarify our impressions of the "underlying processes."

Thinking is divided into four aspects: flow or stream, possession, content, and form.

Flow of Thinking (Also Called Stream or Progress of Thinking)

Flow of thinking has two characteristics: (a) the rate and (b) the train (or continuity) of thought.

Rate

Effective communication demands that we maintain a rate of language expression that can be comprehended. The range for this rate varies, but there are two kinds of extremes with which the clinician should be familiar.

In *slowed* or *inhibited thinking* (retarded thinking), the patient's language is reduced in rate. The patient frequently reports that ideas and mental images present themselves less frequently and that thought is slowed, sometimes to the point that neither ideas nor images enter consciousness. The range may be from mild slowing to complete slowing (that may be manifest as *mutism*).

In *rapid thinking*, the patient's language is increased in rate. The patient frequently reports that ideas come with unusual ease and speed and that the mind may be "racing." There is, of course, a range here as well; the rate may be described as a flight (almost always accompanied by pressured speech), wherein some semblance of understandability is retained and each thought has coherence. On the other hand, the connections between words and phrases may reflect the operation of chance factors such as rhymes, puns, or intense environmental stimulation, so that the product of thought becomes almost nonsensical. Further along this continuum, the patient may exhibit what can only be described as incoherence because thoughts come so rapidly that they are scarcely formulated into words.

Train or Continuity of Thinking

The train of thinking must be directed and consistent and stay on track if the patient is to make him- or herself understood. The following are examples of specific disturbances.

Circumstantiality. In circumstantiality the patient's thinking seems slow, overly detailed, and intricate; yet, somehow, by the most circuitous of routes, the goal is reached without the interviewer's intervention.

Tangentiality. In tangentiality the train of thought is disturbed by getting and remaining on a sidetrack. Consequently, the goal of thinking is not reached. On being questioned, the patient may report that he or she cannot recall what was being said or how the conversation started.

Thought Blocking.   In thought blocking the patient suddenly stops talking, without apparent cause, for seconds to minutes. When the patient begins again to speak, he or she often is on a completely different track and cannot remember what he or she was previously discussing. Occasionally, the patient may report a subjective experience of thought alienation. A similar disturbance in motor behavior, motor blocking, refers to the sudden interruption of movement without apparent cause.

Perseveration.   In perseveration the patient is unable to move from one track to the next and experiences an inability to free his or her thinking from verbal associations or previously spoken related ideas. Thus, language becomes repetitive of words, phrases, and questions, beyond the point of usefulness or relevance. This disturbance may have a counterpart in the motor sphere (motor perseveration), where the patient is unable to stop repeating an action or task after the appropriate stimulus for doing so has gone.

Control or Possession of Thinking

Control or possession of thinking means the subjective experience of self-determination operating in one's thinking and the sense that one's thoughts are one's own. There are two varieties of disturbances.

Obsessional Thinking.   Obsession refers to a type of experience in which the patient cannot be free of certain ideas, fears, images, or impulses that are recognized as senseless but that may be persistent and may dominate the content of consciousness. The essential feature is that these phenomena appear against the patient's will. Yet they are neither foreign nor outside the patient's control; they can be resisted. In short, the patient may describe being compelled to think his or her own thoughts. For the sake of clarity, we may distinguish several kinds of obses-

sional phenomena. Obsessional images are vivid images which occupy the patient's mind in an irresistible manner. Obsessional ideas are the content of ruminations about all manner of things, for instance, excessive and unnecessary worry, concern about irrelevancies, etc. Obsessional impulses may create a desire to touch, to count, to step on cracks, etc. An obsessional fear (phobia) is a baseless fear that the patient realizes dominates him or her without reason. According to standard usage, the term *compulsion* refers to action that may be mediated by obsessional images or thoughts.

Clinicians may recognize obsessional phenomena at work when patients engage in compulsive stereotyped movements (grimacing, coughing, gestures, clearing of the throat) or in more complex patterns such as arranging one's clothes repeatedly, washing hands over and over again, pacing over the same route in the waiting room, etc. Subjectively, the patients may complain of being preoccupied with obsessional phenomena or other worries well beyond an appropriate concern. Questions useful in eliciting these phenomena are listed in Table 12.15.

Table 12.15 Questions about Obsessional and Compulsive Behavior

1. Do you wash your hands more frequently than other people?
2. Are you frequently subject to doubts and decisions or troubles with your conscience?
3. Do you feel compelled to do things over and over again?
4. Do you recheck again and again to see if the doors are locked and the lights turned off when you leave your home?
5. Do you have to do things in the same way each time you do them?
6. Do you get bothered if someone rearranges your furniture or things in your office or room?
7. Are you beset with worries or thoughts that you cannot get rid of?
8. Do you have any special fears (animal, certain people, certain situations, such as crowds or high places, open or closed places, and sharp objects?)
9. Are these fears under your control? These acts?

Thought Alienation. Patients experiencing thought alienation (8, 11) describe thoughts as being under the control of an outside force or report that others are participating in their thinking to an extent that they no longer personally possess their thoughts. There are several varieties: thought insertion, in which patients feel that thoughts are not their own and that they are being inserted into the mind from outside; thought withdrawal, in which patients experience single thoughts or long trains of thought suddenly disappearing or being withdrawn from the mind and attribute this to a foreign influence; and thought broadcasting, in which patients feel that their thoughts are not confined to their mind but are escaping to be read out like a ticker tape or to be heard by others as they are thought.

Passivity Experiences. Passivity refers to a related kind of experience, in which patients feel they are the recipients not only of thoughts but also of imposed sensations, feelings, and impulses. As a result, they may no longer feel in control of their will, feelings, words, or actions. To help elicit disturbances of thought control, the clinician should ask whether the patient has felt forced to think, say, or do certain things; whether thoughts, feelings, or actions have been controlled by other people and how; whether the patient has felt that thoughts were not his or her own, that they were being broadcast, put aside, or removed from the head; and whether there is a meaning to these experiences.

Content of Thinking

The major concern regarding content of thinking is the presence of delusions, generally considered one of the most serious disturbances of thinking.

A delusion is a false, unshakable belief that is incommensurate with the patient's social and cultural background and cannot be influenced by reason or experience.

Patients may report delusions spontaneously, but usually specific questioning is required. Clues suggesting the presence of delusions include evasiveness, suspicion, or other indications of heightened sensitivity in the interview. Generally, a subtle, increasingly specific use of questions is the most appropriate interview strategy.

Delusions are classified according to the following characteristics.

Systematic Qualities

The patient may build a more or less logical and consistent understanding of a particular situation that is based entirely on one fundamental error, the deluded premise. For example, *paranoia* (now called delusional disorder) is the term used to describe a syndrome in which the logical nature of the system of belief is tight and coherent concerning persecution or threat, while evidence of other psychopathology is comparatively mild or absent.[e]

Type of Delusion

Delusions are generally classified according to their content, which appears to be dependent on social and cultural influences. Thus clinicians in the United States see more patients who consider the CIA or FBI to be on their track, for example, than patients who complain of witches and devils trying to do them harm. The latter manifestation might be more common among patients of the non-Western, nonindustrialized world. Various types of delusions are listed and described in Table 12.16.

The Patient's Response to Delusions

The clinician should note whether the patient is angry, quiet, unperturbed, or preoccupied in response to delusional content of thinking. Is there any suggestion of suicidal ideation, homicidal preoccupation, or an interest in carrying matters to Congress or the police? Another question that the clinician must ask is whether delusions arise from the apparent influence of depressed or heightened mood. For example, does the patient suffering from persecutory delusions view the persecution as justified because he or she is an evil and guilty person (mood-congruent delusions), or do

---

[e] See Chapter 39 for a discussion of delusional disorders.

Table 12.16 Types of Delusions

Delusions of persecution	Patients believe they are the victim of persecution by individuals, organizations, racial or ethnic groups. These delusions may take different forms: (*a*) *Delusions of self-reference* correctly identify the experience of patients who believe that people are talking about, slandering, or spying on them. (*b*) *Delusions of being poisoned or infected* are also in this category. (*c*) *Delusions of influence* that result logically from passivity experiences suggest to the patient a basis—witches, demons, hypnotism, atomic rays, etc.—for explaining them. (*d*) Delusions that strangers have taken the place of loved ones (capgras).
Delusions of jealousy	Delusions of marital or sexual infidelity. Such experiences may occur in patients who episodically interrogate and accuse spouses of illicit sexual activities.
Delusions of love	The patient believes that some person is in love with him or her, though they may not even have met. There may be an attempt to act on this belief through letter writing, appointment arrangements, and so forth.
Delusions of grandiosity or grandeur	The patient may believe in all degrees of self-importance and uniqueness, ranging from sainthood and historical greatness to relatedness to important figures, for example, "I am a good friend of the Kennedys."
Delusions of ill health (somatic delusions)	The patient believes he or she has some incurable malady, e.g., cancer or an infection. These are also called *hypochondriacal delusions,* and they are to be distinguished from preoccupation with or overawareness of normal visceral or peripheral sensation, hallucinations, misinterpretations, and real physical disease.
Delusions of guilt (self-depreciation)	Patients amplify mild self-reproach and criticism into a belief that they are a sinner and profligate. Delusions of guilt may give rise to delusions of persecution as the patients see a justifiable stance in the malevolence of others toward them.
Delusions of nihilism	Patients deny the existence of friends, family, the world, themselves, and their mind. They may even assert that they are dead.
Delusions of poverty	Patients believe that they are impoverished.

they have no relatedness to the patient's mood (mood-incongruent delusions)? Do delusions occur as a result of apprehension or impaired consciousness? Some questions that may help in eliciting delusional trends in the patient's thinking are listed in Table 12.17.

Form of Thinking

Form of thinking traditionally refers to several features. First of all, there is the logical character of thinking—do the patient's thoughts lead to conclusions in a manner that obeys the laws of deductive and inductive reasoning? Second, there is the feature of abstractability—is the patient able to conceptualize abstract thoughts and use them meaningfully? Third, there is the feature of coherence or connectedness of clauses, phrases, and sentences that provides the structure for the patient's utterances to be comprehensible. Fourth, there is the quality of associations, which if disturbed may reduce the coherence and com-

Table 12.17 Questions to Elicit Delusional Thinking

1. Have you felt that something was extremely wrong and that you could not put your finger on it? Did that bother you? How did you explain it?

2. Have you felt unusually well or in very good spirits? Has this resulted in any activities on your part? Do you have any special talents or abilities?

3. Do you feel that others might be responsible for your problems or the situation you are in?

4. Have you felt troubled about your marriage? Have you ever questioned the faithfulness of your wife or husband? How jealous have you felt?

5. Has anyone treated you badly or criticized you unfairly, annoyed you or bothered you in any way that was unusual?

6. Has anyone been paying particular attention to you, watching you, or talking about you?

7. Have you felt that people on radio or TV were talking about you in their reports? What is the basis for these unpleasant experiences? Why are they happening to you? Have they occurred before?

prehensibility of what is said. Are there intrusions (derailment, loosening of associations) in the train of expressed thought that decrease comprehensibility because their relatedness and possibly their relevance to what is being said appears tenuous? The relationship between intelligence and the first three of these features (logical character, abstractability, and coherence of thinking) is substantial as *they* require skill and ability in producing and editing thoughts. This is less true regarding the quality of associations, which appears to be governed by factors (e.g., arousal, semantic memory) relatively independent of intelligence.

Logic

The logic that the patient employs in thinking is difficult to evaluate. Normal individuals often make logical errors; however, instances of bizarre arguments or idiosyncratic inferences should be investigated. Most clinical judgments have the shortcoming of being vague and impressionistic. If the patient is illogical, the clinician should document examples.

Abstractability

Abstractability lies on a continuum with concreteness. According to Payne (14), concreteness is the inability to (*a*) formulate an abstract general principle from a group of particular items, or (*b*) recognize that a group of objects with some common characteristics can be grouped together under the same general category. This feature is generally evaluated by similarity tests and proverb interpretation. Concreteness is often referred to as a *negative formal thought disorder*. It is considered further in Chapter 21.

Coherence and Quality of Associations

The patient's thinking may show a variety of disturbances of these features, often termed *positive formal thought disorder*. Coherence refers to the internal relevancy and efficiency with which the patient's thinking is expressed. Coherence depends on several features of thinking; for example, the continuity or train of thinking must be intact for coherent thinking to be present. However, other sources of disturbance

may reduce the coherence of a patient's verbal production. For instance, the patient must achieve a certain high quality of associations (in terms of word choices, accepted uses of idioms, keeping to a theme, etc.). This latter quality is necessary, but not sufficient, to make language coherent. These two features, coherence and quality of associations, though logically separable, are frequently interdependent aspects of thinking. Generally, the greater the lack of coherence, the greater the likelihood that the quality of associations will be poor and vice versa. On the other hand, there may be cases in which lack of coherence of expressed thought does not indicate a marked disturbance of associations. However, almost any disturbance of association will detract from the coherence of thinking.

Other Features

There are other less common features of thinking that may be important in assessing psychopathology. Most of these features have limited clinical value, indicating only that abnormality is present. However, they may also be subtle, occur intermittently, and challenge the most disciplined ear to establish their presence. For example, the conclusion that a patient displays poverty of speech (reduced output) or that a patient exhibits impoverished thought (poverty of information conveyed, poverty of content of thinking) based on the quantity of factual or informative material produced rather than the mere amount of speech is singularly difficult, except in the most extreme cases. Andreasen (15) has proposed a rating scale (see Table 12.18) that calls for judgments on 21 features, including a global assessment. Nevertheless, the possible value of their use in monitoring treatment response, if not assisting in diagnosis, can be envisioned.

Each of these features is evaluated by listening to the patient. Except perhaps for abstractability, there is precious little to quantify in the evaluation of formal thinking; a clear description of what is observed remains the best source for judgments defining such disturbances in terms of psychopathology.

Table 12.18 Individual Items Rated on Andreasen's Thought, Language and Communication Assessment Scale

Poverty of speech	Word approximations
Poverty of content of speech	Circumstantiality
	Loss of goal
Pressure of speech	Perseveration
Distractible speech	Echolalia
Tangentiality	Blocking
Derailment	Stilted speech
Incoherence	Self-reference
Illogicality	Paraphrasia (phonemic)
Clanging	Paraphrasia (semantic)
Neologisms	

References

1. Cobb S: *Foundations of Neuropsychiatry.* Baltimore, Williams & Wilkins, 1948.
2. Lishman W: *Organic Psychiatry.* Oxford, Blackwell Scientific Publications, 1987.
3. Ey H: Disorders of consciousness in psychiatry. In Bruyn G, Vinken P (eds): *Handbook of Neurology.* New York, John Wiley & Sons, 1969, vol 3, pp 112–136.
4. Fish F: *Clinical Psychopathology.* Bristol, England, John Wright & Sons, 1985.
5. Plum F, Posner J: *Diagnosis of Stupor and Coma.* Philadelphia, F.A. Davis, 1972.
6. Jaspers K: *General Psychopathology* (trans 1963). Chicago, University of Chicago Press, 1923.
7. Reed G: *The Psychology of Anomalous Experience.* Boston, Houghton Mifflin, 1975.
8. Yap P: *Comparative Psychiatry.* Toronto, University of Toronto Press, 1974.
9. Simpson G, Angus JWS: A rating scale for extrapyramidal side effects. *Acta Psychiat Scand* 212: 11–19, 1970 (updated, 1986, National Institute of Mental Health).
10. National Institute of Mental Health: *Abnormal Involuntary Movement Scale (AIMS)* (US Public Health Service Publication No. MH-9-17). Washington, DC. U.S. Government Printing Office, 1974.
11. Ketai R: Affect, mood, emotion, and feeling: sematic considerations. *Am J Psychiatry* 132: 1215–1217, 1975.
12. Preu P: *Outline of a Psychiatric Case Study.* New York, Paul Hoeber, 1939.
13. Schneider K: *Clinical Psychopathology.* New York, Grune & Stratton, 1959.
14. Payne R: Cognitive abnormalities, in Eysenck H (ed): *Handbook of Abnormal Psychology.* San Diego, Robert Knapp, 1973, pp 420–483.
15. Andreasen N: Thought, language, and communicative disorders: clinical assessment, definition of terms, and evaluation of their reliability. *Arch Gen Psychiatry* 36:1315–1321, 1979.

13

The Mental Status Examination
II. Higher Intellectual Functioning

Martin B. Keller, M.D.
Theo C. Manschreck, M.D., M.P.H.

The clinical tests used by most clinicians to assess higher intellectual functioning were organized by Adolph Meyer in 1902 (1) and revised by George Kirby in 1921 (2). They have remained largely unchanged since that time. Most clinicians perform these tests by rote out of a desire to be "complete" and to make certain that organic syndromes have been ruled out, but they do so with little knowledge of the reliability or validity of these tests.

Evidence of reliability and validity will be reviewed for the tests commonly used for the higher intellectual functions. In addition, we shall discuss eight tests not commonly used that have a high degree of validity in distinguishing organic from functional syndromes.

The primary goal in assessing higher intellectual functioning is to alert clinicians to the possible presence of organic disease. Further investigation may then be necessary for definitive diagnosis and treatment. When a diagnosis or organic disease has already been established, assessment of higher intellectual functioning is often desirable for determining specific deficits and monitoring clinical

changes. The clinician can then formulate the plan of treatment, taking into account both the more immediate and long-term needs of the patient.

The structured nature of the clinical tests of the sensorium enables examiners to perform them with a high degree of reliability (3, 4). Unfortunately, this reliability has contributed to an overly optimistic view of the validity of these tests (5–7). Despite evidence to the contrary, most clinicians consider errors on these tests to be indications of cerebral damage and are reassured that the disorder is functional when the tests are performed without error. It is important to be aware that these tests may be normal in the presence of cerebral lesions or abnormal in individuals with no organic pathology.

Many of the higher intellectual functions are evaluated by the examiner without formal questioning through observation of how the patients follow and respond to history gathering and general questioning. However, major deficits may be masked in patients with a good vocabulary and skill in social interactions. For example, a hallmark of dementia is the preservation of social graces and conversational skills in the presence of gross deficits in one or several areas of higher intellectual functioning. This raises the controversial issue of when to recommend formal testing of higher intellectual functioning. Awareness that such deficits may go undetected unless the patient is thoroughly examined poses a particularly difficult dilemma for clinicians in an outpatient setting. The intrusive nature of these tests often makes clinicians reluctant to do them on patients who appear lucid. In practice, clinicians may go to extremes, abbreviating or ignoring systematic questioning or slavishly asking everything.

We recommend the following guidelines for the mental health clinician. The beginning clinician should do formal testing on all patients in order to learn the ranges of normal responses, gain experience in examining patients, develop a thorough and comprehensive approach, and minimize the chances of missing psychologic or somatic disease. As one becomes more experienced, it is possible to be less formal and "complete" in one's approach and still gain the relevant clinical data. For example, in those patients who do not present with symptoms consistent with organic syndromes and for whom the clinician has enough of an opportunity to observe an adequate range of normal intellectual functioning during the routine interview, it is reasonable to forego formal testing of higher intellectual functioning. In these instances, it is still necessary to consider organic disorders in the differential diagnosis.

Whenever there is suspicion of deficits in higher intellectual functioning based on historical data or other observations, formal and systematic testing should be performed.

Although these tests lend themselves to sequential performance, for certain patients it will be preferable to vary the format and integrate the questions throughout the interview to avoid undue irritation or fatigue for both the patient and the clinician.

STANDARD CLINICAL TESTS OF THE SENSORIUM

Memory

Memory refers to the ability to recall past experience. Memory has traditionally been divided into three functions: registration, retention, and recall. The actual process by which each of these stages occurs is still speculative, and the transition from one stage to another is not always easy to detect. The rationale for maintaining these distinctions is that memory deficits are often seen at one of these three stages, and deficits at a particular stage frequently form an important part of a specific clinical syndrome. Examples of such syndromes are the lack of registration in the presence of intact long-term memory following head trauma and the lack of retention in a patient who can register information, which may occur in Korsakoff's syndrome.

The standard clinical tests used to assess memory include the following:

1. Repetition of digits forwards and backwards, usually up to six forward and four backwards.
2. Repetition of objects after 2 minutes.
3. Repetition of a simple sentence such as "the Babcock sentence" (6), which states, "One thing a nation must have to be rich and great is a large, secure supply of wood."
4. Repetition of a logical memory story, such as the cowboy or donkey story, after 5 minutes: "The cowboy went to San Francisco with his dog which he left at a friend's while he left to buy a new suit of clothes. Dressed in his brand new suit, he came back to the dog, whistled to it, called it by name, and patted it. But the dog would have nothing to do with him in his new hat and coat, and gave him a mournful howl. Coaxing was of no avail, so the cowboy went away and put on his old suit, then the dog immediately showed its wild joy on seeing its master as the dog thought he ought to be."

5. Recall of recent and remote personal events and recent general events.

The clinical tests of memory are highly reliable (8), but their validity in establishing an organic diagnosis has not been demonstrated, since nonpathologic factors, such as intelligence and age, and states of functional pathology, such as anxiety and depression, may alter performance on tests of memory. A striking example of memory loss caused by functional pathology is depressive pseudodementia, a syndrome characterized by impairment in higher intellectual functioning, including diminished memory, in elderly depressed patients. This impairment remits after the depression improves.

Studies by Eysenck and Halstead (9) and by Zangwill (10) show that the results on most memory tests correlated with intelligence levels to such a degree that a "memory factor" could not be distinguished from intelligence. Such studies highlight the need for clinical tests that are less influenced by intelligence, although it may be that these functions are at some level not separable from each other. Crook, et al (11) found that standard digit span tests have limited validity for assessment of geriatric patients' memory ability. For verbal repetition of visually presented digits only, recall of 10 digits, far exceeding standard digit span length, differentiated memory-impaired aged persons from the normal elderly group.

Even if these tests are not valid as tests of memory per se, the question remains whether they are useful in differentiating organic illness from functional conditions. Shapiro et al. (12) found memory for remote personal events and memory for recent general events differentiated organic illness from functional conditions at a highly significant level. Hinton and Withers (8) found that recall of objects at 2 minutes and repetition of the Babcock sentence were significantly impaired in patients with organic brain syndrome.

In summary, the data suggest that repetition of digits forwards and backwards, repetition of a logical memory story, and recall of recent personal events should be eliminated as tests of either memory or organicity, and repetition of objects at intervals of up to 2 minutes and repetition of the Babcock sentence maybe useful tests of organicity, although they are less clearly tests of memory. Recall of remote personal events and recent general events appear to be the most useful tests of memory and the most useful tests for differentiating organic from functional illness.

Attention and Concentration

Attention and concentration refer to an individual's ability to focus selectively on stimuli in his or her environment. Clinically observable disorders of attention and concentration include inattentiveness to one's surroundings, inability to concentrate on a given task, distractibility, and increased attentiveness or vigilance.

Disorders of attention and concentration may be isolated to one area of functioning or may be more global. For example, inattentiveness to one's surroundings is seen selectively in the patient with unilateral visual agnosia and generally in the delirious or severely retarded patient. Inability to concentrate on given tasks may exist as the only abnormal finding in the area of attention in the early stages of a dementing illness or as part of a global disturbance in higher intellectual functioning often found in gross disorders of consciousness. Increased attentiveness ranges from normal inquisitiveness and curiosity to the hypervigilance seen in paranoid syndromes. It may be selective, as in catatonia, or global, as in paranoia. Distractibility may result from preoccupation, as is seen in obsessive or autistic thinking, but it may also be secondary to external stimulation as in manic states.

The following clinical tests are used to assess attention:

1. Subtraction of 7's starting from 100, or subtraction of 3's starting from 100.
2. Reversing the days of the week or the months of the year.

3. Spelling simple words such as "world" backwards.
4. Repeating a series of digits forwards and backwards.

These tests directly measure the individual's capacity to sustain effort on given tasks but do not formally test inattentiveness, increased attentiveness, or distractibility. Their high reliability has been demonstrated (8), but their validity in differentiating organic from other psychiatric disturbances is limited.

The Subtraction of Serial Sevens Test, originated by Kraepelin, is perhaps the most widely used of all the clinical tests of the sensorium. A number of studies seriously question its validity. Smith (13) found errorless performance in only 42% of 132 normal subjects. Twenty-four percent of subjects made between 3 and 12 errors, and three subjects abandoned the test completely. Milstein et al. (14) studied more than 300 patients with severe psychiatric disorders and compared them to a matched sample of nonhospitalized patients. They found little diagnostic specificity and no evidence that subtraction of serial sevens was useful in detection of organic brain disease among psychiatric patients. These studies lead to the conclusion that this widely used test has not demonstrated its value to detect organicity or specific psychiatric syndromes. Similarly, reversing the days of the week and repetition of digits forwards and backwards were not found to differentiate between organic and functional conditions, although performance was affected by intelligence, education, and age. There are no reports available for the test of spelling a simple word backwards.

In summary, the tests described above have little or no value in distinguishing organic from functional syndromes. When errors are made on these tests, decisions about further diagnostic investigation in a given patient should be made on the basis of the overall clinical situation. Moreover, as previously discussed, there are no clinical tests in current usage that assess inattentiveness to one's surroundings, increased attentiveness or vigilance, and distractibility. Observations concerning them should be made as part of the clinical examination of attention and concentration, because they represent an aspect of attention and concentration that may be disordered as part of a number of organic and functional psychiatric syndromes.

General Information

General information refers to fund of knowledge. It does not measure a specific function, such as language or memory, for which there are presumed to be more direct anatomic and physiologic correlates within the central nervous system. Rather, general information is felt to measure broadly a person's contact with the environment during the course of his or her lifetime and at the time of testing.

Of the routinely used clinical tests of the sensorium, tests of general information have been the least standardized. A representative selection of information from areas commonly asked includes asking the patient to

1. Name the last four presidents of the United States, starting with the current president.
2. Name the state governor, state senators, and city mayor.
3. Name four large cities in the United States.
4. Provide information concerning four widely known current events.
5. Describe what four famous people are known for, such as George Washington, Christopher Columbus, Albert Einstein, or William Shakespeare.

When given by examiners (8) using a standardized format, testing of general information had high test–retest reliability for a given individual, even when similar, but nonidentical, questions were used. Four studies have been reported which demonstrate that tests of general information are valuable experimentally in differentiating organic from functional illness.

Hopkins and Roth (15, 16) compared patients with senile psychosis, affective psychosis, and arteriosclerotic psychosis. They found a highly significant difference in the number of correct responses among the three groups. Senile psychotics averaged 20% correct responses, compared to 70% for those with untreated affective disorder. Shapiro et al. (12) found significant differences between patients with functional and organic disorders. Those with functional illness averaged 60% correct responses, compared to 40% for those with organic impairment. Hinton and Withers (8) found that although results correlated positively with intelligence level and were somewhat impaired by affective disorder, significant differentiation between patients with organic and functional syndromes was still possible.

The average percentage of correct responses is remarkably similar among the different studies, and the difference within each study is statistically significant in separating organic from functional groups. Despite this, the practical usefulness of these data is limited in that the percentage cutoffs found were for narrowly defined populations, thereby preventing generalization of these results to other populations.

In summary, tests of general information have been shown experimentally to distinguish between functional and organic disorders. However, standardization of specific questions between studies was poor, sample populations varied, and the range of differences in errors found are difficult to apply to clinical situations with any precision. With these qualifications in mind, such tests are valuable in alerting the clinician to organic illness, especially when one finds greater than 60% incorrect responses.

Calculation

The disorders of higher intellectual functioning that tests of calculation evaluate are generally covered by tests of attention, concentration, and intelligence. In addition, there is no literature concerning the reliability and validity of calculation tests. Although there does appear to be a wide range in ability to calculate without the aid of paper and pencil, there is no evidence that disturbances in calculation are useful diagnostically, except for the rare instances in which the ability to calculate is impaired out of proportion to other cognitive deficits. This occurs in the symptom of acalculia (or dyscalculia), which is one of the defining features of Gerstmann's sydrome, believed to be secondary to pathology of the dominant parietal lobe, and also includes agraphia, finger agnosia, and right–left confusion as clinical signs.

Tests of calculation include the following:

1. Simple addition, subtraction, division, and multiplication.
2. Computation in such tests as: (a) how many nickels there are in $1.35 and (b) the interest on $100 at 4% for 18 months.

Intelligence

Intelligence is defined differently by most clinicians and textbooks. One definition given by Linn (17) considers intelligence as the capacity to meet an unknown situation by improvising a novel adaptable response. He defines this capacity according to three factors: abstract intelligence, mechanical intelligence, and social intelligence.

It has been demonstrated that a person's intelligence may have a marked effect on how he or she performs on many tests of higher intellectual functioning and may be partially inseparable from memory, abstraction, general information, and calculation. Assessment of intelligence is therefore an important part of the mental status examination. There are no clinical tests that can be performed in several minutes that allow derivation of a precise intelligence measure. The patient's performance in school, occupational level and performance, vocabulary, and ability to use abstract ideas and symbols correlate well with intelligence (18) and, if they are fairly consistent with each other, usually allow for an adequate judgment of intelligence. Should gross discrepancies be found among these variables, specific psychologic testing (Wechsler Adult Intelligence Scale–Revised, Mill Hill, Raven Progressive Matrices) may be indicated.

Other situations that call for formal intelligence testing include suspected mental deficiency, progressive or potentially progressive dementia where baseline and follow-up measures allow for a monitoring of change, and vocational and rehabilitative evaluations.

Abstraction

Abstract thinking involves the patient's ability to make valid generalizations. However, responses to the formal tests of abstraction will often enable one to asses far more than the patient's range of concreteness and abstraction. The entire spectrum of formal disorders of thinking discussed in Chapters 12 and 21 may become evident from the patient's responses to these questions. To evaluate abstractions, the clinician asks the patient to

1. Describe the similarities between pairs of words, such as (a) dog and elephant, (b) apple and pear, and (c) plane and boat.
2. Give the meaning of a proverb such as (a) strike while the iron is hot, (b) people in glass houses shouldn't throw stones, and (c) a stitch in time saves nine.

A major drawback of these tests is that they have a very low interrater reliability. Andreasen et al. (19) showed a very wide range in judging levels of abstractions on proverb responses by members of the same academic psychiatry department.

Even if one improves interrater reliability, the validity of the information for diagnostic purposes will be quite limited for several reasons. Similarities and proverbs are greatly influenced by intelligence. In fact, they are both included as subtests on many of the standard psychometric exams from which intelligence quotients are derived, so that (perhaps more than any of the other tests of the sensorium) they directly measure intelligence. In addition, it has never been demonstrated that poor performance on these tests serves as an indicator of otherwise undetectable organic brain disease.

In summary, these tests have low interrater reliability, are easily affected by other cognitive impairments, and are dependent on intelligence. Their usefulness as differential indicators of organic brain disease has not yet been demonstrated. They may be of value in the assessment of functional psychiatric disorders, if the clinician goes beyond using them as measures of concreteness and abstraction and looks for bizarre or idiosyncratic responses as indicators of formal thought disorder.

Judgment

Judgment may be defined as the mental activity of comparing or evaluating alternatives within the framework of a given set of values for the purpose of deciding on a course of action. Accurate perception is necessary for good judgment, as is adequate recall to bring forth previously known information as a basis for comparison. It follows that in the presence of a gross disturbance of consciousness, orientation, memory, or attention and concentration, the prerequisites for making sound judgments will be lacking.

Evaluation of judgment has traditionally been included during testing of higher intellectual functioning by interpreting the patient's responses to standard hypothetical situations. The two most common questions are

1. What would you do if you were in a movie theatre and saw smoke coming from an empty section of the theatre?
2. What would you do if you found a stamped, sealed, addressed envelope in the street?

There is no evidence that responses to these questions will detect impaired higher intellectual functioning in the absence of disturbances on the other clinical tests of the sensorium. The types of judgments in which the clinician should be more interested may range from a patient's process of reasoning about daily or long-term life goals, to his or her capacity for homicidal or suicidal behavior, or his or her likelihood of acting on delusional beliefs or hallucinatory perceptions. Evaluation of such disturbances will be more properly done by exploring such areas with the patient during the interview than by asking the standard hypothetical questions of judgment.

Insight

Insight has an extremely wide range of meaning. It generally refers to one's ability to see and understand the connection between specific things or situations. At one extreme the term is used by clinicians solely to indicate a patient's ability to realize that he or she is suffering from an illness. At another extreme, it may refer to the patient's ability to comprehend various psychodynamic mechanisms that the patient and therapist determine have led to the formation of present-day feelings and attitudes.

No specific clinical tests have been devised to assess insight, yet this category has traditionally been included under the higher intellectual function section of the mental status examination.

Conditions that grossly alter consciousness, orientation, memory, and attention and concentration may greatly interfere with the patient's capacity for insight at a variety of levels. However, there is no evidence or any reason to suspect that assessment of insight is a useful indicator of organic illness or a specific aid in psychiatric differential diagnosis.

Summary of the Clinical Tests of the Sensorium

As was stated, the primary goal in assessing higher intellectual functioning is to alert clinicians to the presence of organic disease. Secondary goals include enabling the clinician to monitor changes in the patient's specific deficits in higher intellectual functioning.

Review of the literature on the standard clinical tests of the sensorium reveals that there have been very few research studies on their reliability and validity. The empirical data that are available show that such tests aid the clinician to only a limited degree in meeting the above-stated goals. Only several tests, such as recall of remote personal events and recent general events, repetition of objects at intervals up to 2 minutes, repetition of a simple sentence, and tests of general information, meet the primary goal of differentiating significantly between organic and functional illness, and even the clinical utility of these tests is limited by the difficulty in establishing cutoff levels for organicity. This results in part because the tests are not readily quantifiable. Lack of quantification also limits their capacity to monitor changes in the patient's clinical state, and therefore, none of these tests is very useful for this purpose in its present form. Eliciting specific areas of cognitive defects was shown to be accomplished validly by tests of memory, calculation, intelligence, and abstraction, although to a much lower degree than presumed by most clinicians.

Above all, the data documenting the reliability and validity of these tests are sparse, particularly when it is considered that the tests are performed so routinely by clinicians in the medical and mental health fields. Further attempts to replicate the findings that have been summarized here is strongly warranted.

SUPPLEMENTAL CLINICAL TESTS OF THE SENSORIUM

There are eight easily administered and readily quantifiable tests that address some of the deficiencies just described. These tests can be divided into three groups: (a) those that were designed specifically for the geriatric population; (b) those designed for use among medical and psychiatric patients; and (c) those that are similar to "neurologic examinations and standard

Table 13.1.   Reliability and Validity of Standard Tests of Higher Intellectual Functioning for Differentiating Organic from Functional Disorders[a]

Tests	Reliability	Validity
Memory		
Repetition of digits (forwards and backwards)	+ +	−
Repetition of objects		
2 minutes	+ +	+
5 minutes	+ +	−
Babcock Sentence	+ +	+
Logical memory story	+ +	−
Recent personal events	+ +	−
Remote personal events and recent general events	+ +	+ +
Attention and concentration		
Subtraction of serial	+	−
7's and 3's	+	
Reversing days of week or month	+ +	−
Spelling of words backwards	0	0
Repetition of digits	+ +	−
General information	+ +	+
Calculation	+ +	0
Intelligence	0	0
Clinical tests	No tests in usage	
Psychometric tests (WAIS, Raven, Mill Hill)	+ +	+ +
Abstractions	−	−
Judgment	0	0
Insight (clinical tests)	No tests in usage	

[a] 0 = no studies reported, + + = reliability or validity demonstrated to high degree on at least one research study, + = reliability or validity demonstrated to mild degree on at least one research study, − = unreliable or invalid on at least one research study.

psychometric examinations"(20) and applicable for use in the general population.

Supplemental Clinical Tests for Elderly Patients

The Mental Status Questionnaire (MSQ), the Short Portable Mental Status Questionnaire (SPMSQ), and the Set Test were designed to detect chronic organic disease and senile dementia among aged patients.

Mental Status Questionnaire

The MSQ was developed by Kahn et al. (21) and consists of 10 questions for differentiating confused from alert elderly patients. One point is given for each correct response.

Scores of 9 and 10 indicate alertness, scores between 6 and 8 indicate slight confusion, scores of 3 to 5 indicate moderate confusion, and scores of 0 to 2 suggest a severe confusional state. Brink et al. (22) found the MSQ performance in the low range among alert poorly educated immigrants, and therefore suggest adjustment of scores for poorly educated patients.

One version of the MSQ consists of the following 10 questions:

1. How old are you? (within 1 year)
2. When were you born? What year? (exact year)
3. What year is it now? (exact year)
4. What month is it now? (exact month)
5. What day of the week is it? (exact day)
6. What was the last meal you ate? (breakfast, lunch, or dinner)
7. What is the name of this place? (nursing home, name of facility)
8. Count backward from 10 to 0. (no errors)
9. (a) Who is the administrator of this facility? (if institutionalized)
   (b) Who is the governor of this state? (outpatients)
10. Who is the president of the United States? (22)

Research studies (20, 22) indicate that the MSQ is a reliable and valid measure of impairment in brain functioning. The MSQ accurately distinguishes alert patients from those who are confused and indicates the severity of the patient's confusional state.

Short Portable Mental Status Questionnaire

The SPMSQ, a derivate of the MSQ, also consists of 10 questions for detection of organic impairment. Pfeiffer (20, 23) devised the questionnaire in 1975 for use among geriatric outpatients. The SPMSQ reliably detects organic impairment and assesses the severity of organic disease. Future studies are needed to replicate the observed high validity and reliability of the MSQ and the SPMSQ.

Set Test

The Set Test was designed in 1972 by Isaacs and Kennie (20, 24) as a screening test to detect dementia among the elderly. The patient must name 10 items in each of four categories: (*a*) colors, (*b*) animals, (*c*) fruits, (*d*) towns. One point is given for each correct item and scoring is from 0 to 40.

The original study examined 199 patients aged 65 to 85. Patients were evaluated independently for dementia (25), affective disorder, and physical illness and were rated as to intelligence. The following results were obtained: A score of less than 15 corresponded closely to a clinical diagnosis of dementia; scores in the 15–24 range showed less association with dementia, and no one scoring over 25 was found to be demented.

On the basis of its initial clinical trial (25), the Set Test is a valid indicator of dementia in elderly patients. It is recommended as an excellent screening test for dementia in patients over 65. The data suggest that all patients who score less than 15 and most who score less than 25 be thoroughly evaluated medically. Again, further studies are needed to confirm the initial findings of this potentially valuable examination.

Examinations for Medical and Psychiatric Patients

Examinations found to be useful for a general population of medical and psychiatric patients include the Mini-Mental State Examination (MMSE) and the Cognitive Capacity Screening Test (CCSE).

Mini-Mental State Examination

The MMSE was designed and tested by Folstein and colleagues (4) as a practical method for grading the cognitive state of patients. It has a wide range of applicability, having been tested on a broad diagnostic spectrum of patients and with a population ranging in age from the twenties to the eighties.

The MMSE tests memory, attention, and orientation to assess higher intellectual functioning. The examination also tests visual and motor skills and linguistics. It requires 5–10 minutes to administer. There are 11 categories of questions requiring 30 responses. The examination is as follows:

Part 1

1. Ask the patient to name the year, season, date, day, and month. (5 points)
2. Ask the patient to name the state, country, town, hospital, and floor. (5 points)
3. Ask the patient to repeat three unrelated objects that you name for him. Have him repeat them right after you tell them to him and repeat them until he learns all three, if he has not learned them initially. (3 points)
4. Have the patient subtract 7 from 100, stopping after five subtractions. Or have him spell the word "world" backwards. (5 points)
5. Ask the patient to repeat the three objects that he had previously been told. (3 points)

Part 2

1. Show the patient a wristwatch and ask him what it is. Repeat this for a pencil. (2 points)

2. Ask the patient to repeat this phrase "No ifs, ands, or buts." (1 point)
3. Have the patient follow a three-point command, such as "Take a paper in your right hand, fold it in half, and put it on the floor." (3 points)
4. On a blank piece of paper, write the sentence "Close your eyes." Ask the patient to read it and do what it says. (1 point)
5. Give the patient a blank piece of paper and ask him to write a sentence. It must be written spontaneously. Score correctly if it contains a subject and a verb and is sensible. (1 point)
6. Ask the patient to copy a design which you have drawn for him on a piece of paper. (1 point)

Clinical trials (4, 20) have indicated that the MMSE is a valid and reliable test for differentiating organic and functional disorders as well as for distinguishing dementia from depression, schizophrenia, and neurotic disorders. The ability of the MMSE to monitor and document clinical changes in higher intellectual functioning has also been demonstrated in patients recovering from head trauma, delirium, and depression (20).

Although patients' intelligence influences performance on this test, it does not impede the examination's ability to detect organic disease. Anthony et al. (26) did find, however, that patients' age and educational background influenced performance on the MMSE.

Among a heterogeneous population of medical patients they found 100% specificity for detecting dementia and delirium among highly educated patients. However, there was low specificity for patients with a 7th-grade education or less. They also found the test more specific for patients under age 60 (26). Anthony et al. (26) conclude that earlier studies' selection bias resulted in observations of extremely high sensitivity and specificity of the instrument for detection of dementia and delirium.

On the basis of the MMSE's initial study, scores of 9 through 12 indicate a high like-lihood of dementia, and scores of 25 and above predominate for normal subjects and patients with neurosis, personality disorder, or functional disorder. Anthony et al. (26) used the more recently established cutoff score 23/24 (scores less than or equal to 23 indicate cognitive disturbance) as a detector of dementia or delirium, and suggest an adjustment of a 22/23 cutoff for testing a heterogeneous population.

Cognitive Capacity Screening Examination

The CCSE assesses short-term memory, orientation, and ability to calculate. Studies (27) have indicated that this examination has high validity and reliability for detecting organic syndromes.

Supplemental Neuropsychologic and Psychometric Examinations

The Face–Hand Test (FHT), the Bender Gestalt Visual Motor Test (BGVMT), and the Background Interference Procedure (BIP) version for the BGVMT are similar to neuropsychologic and psychometric tests (20).

Face–Hand Test

Fink and colleagues (28) first reported the FHT in 1952. The FHT is used to detect confusional states. It requires the patient's localization of the examiner's strokes on the cheek and back of hand as the patient holds his or her hands on knees with closed eyes. Repeated errors on this test imply the presence of organic illness. Cutoff scores on the FHT have not yet been established for differentiating confused and alert patients (20, 22). Nevertheless, clinical trials have indicated that it is a valid examination for detecting confusional states and intellectual deficits detrimental to brain functioning (22).

Bender Gestalt Visual Motor Test

The BGVMT was developed more than 30 years ago by Loretta Bender. Although quite popular with psychologists, it has been neglected by psychiatrists and neurologists. It consists of showing the patient nine figures on a card or a piece of paper and asking him or her to copy the design on another piece of paper.

The test requires that visual perception be grossly intact and that motor ability be sufficient to allow reproduction of the design by drawing. It is not affected by memory, and although performance is affected by age, education, and intelligence, its ability to discriminate organic illness is still highly significant when adjustment is made for these variables.

Brilliant and Gynther (29) found the BGVMT to be the best single measure of organicity when compared to several other psychometric tests (including the Benton Visual Retention Test and Graham-Kendall Memory for Designs Test). Using five copying errors as a cutoff point, the Bender Gestalt ruled out nonorganicity at 92% accuracy and detected organicity at 67% accuracy. Patients with acute and chronic brain disorders averaged 5.7 errors, patients with functional psychosis averaged 3 errors, and patients with personality disorders averaged 2 errors.

Shapiro et al. (12) reported that the BGVMT differentiated between patients with organic illness and functional illness at the highest level of significance (p = 0.001) when compared with each of the standard clinical tests of the sensorium described earlier.

Although further quantification of range of errors and cutoff criteria for the BGVMT would enhance its clinical value as an alerting measure of organicity, the results of these studies and others indicate that it differentiates organic conditions from functional conditions with a high degree of validity, perhaps higher than that of any other clinical test available. The authors strongly recommend it for testing the sensorium.

Background Interference Procedure

The BIP version for the BGVMT developed by Canter involves the standard copying procedure as well as copying the figures on paper with a background of distracting lines. A comparison of performance in the standard and interference conditions indicates the presence or absence of brain damage.

Reports by Canter (30) and Heaton et al. (31) provide supportive evidence of the BIP as one of the most effective screening tests for organicity. Despite these findings of high validity, when considering age, education, and ethnic background, Boake and Adams (32) conclude that the BIP has low validity.

SUMMARY OF TESTING OF HIGHER INTELLECTUAL FUNCTIONING

In summarizing the testing of higher intellectual functioning, it is important to re-emphasize that none of the standard tests, used alone or together, or any of the supplemental tests may be expected to provide a definitive diagnosis of an organic or functional state, let alone provide a definitive diagnosis of which specific syndrome is present. The standard tests may be an important part of the mental status examination, which may alert the clinician to organicity or to detect certain specific deficits in higher intellectual functioning. The supplemental tests appear to be useful both as general indicators of organicity and for monitoring changes in clinical state. Even if a series of clinical exams was devised that did not have the deficiencies found in each of these tests, they would at best provide only a more highly accurate means of generating specific hypotheses concerning differential diagnosis. The clinician must always take into account the entire mental status examination, history, and clinical situation when evaluating findings in any one particular sphere. This should be done prior to interpreting data and deciding whether to pursue physical examinations, laboratory studies, or referring the patient elsewhere. The differential diagnosis for each of the abnormalities found in the tests of higher intellectual functioning and the general mental status exam are covered in Chapter 23.

Finally, we again emphasize the often-ignored fact that a flawless performance on tests of cognition does not rule out organic disease, just as errors on these clinical tests may be found in a variety of functional psychiatric syndromes and in states of normality.

References

1. Meyer A: *Collected Papers*, vol 3. (Winters E, ed). vol. III. Baltimore, Johns Hopkins Press, 1951.
2. Kirby GH: *Guides for History-taking and Clinical Examination*. Albany, New York State Hospital Commission, 1921.
3. Withers E, Hinton J: Three forms of the clinical test of the sensorium and their reliability. *Br J Psychiatry* 119:18, 1971.
4. Folstein MF, Folstein SE, McHugh PR: Minimental state—a practical method for grading the cognitive state of patients for the clinician. *J Psychiatr Res* 12:189–198, 1976.
5. Hayman M: Two minute clinical test for measurement of intellectual impairment in psychiatric disorders. *Arch Neurol Psychiatry* 47:454–462, 1942.
6. Babcock M: An experiment in the measurement of mental deterioration. *Arch Psychol* 117:18, 1930.
7. Luria: *Higher Cortical Functions in Man*. New York, Basic Books, 1966.
8. Hinton J, Withers E: The usefulness of the clinical tests of the sensorium. *Br J Psychiatry* 119:9–18, 1971.
9. Eysenck HJ, Halstead H: The memory function, a functional study of fifteen clinical tests. *Am J Psychiatry* 102:174–180, 1945.
10. Zangwill MA: Clinical tests of memory impairment. *Proc R Soc Med* 36:576–580, 1943.
11. Crook T, Ferris S, McCarthy M: Utility of digit recall tasks for assessing memory in the aged. *J Consult Clin Psychol* 48:228–233, 1980.
12. Shapiro MB, Post F, Lofving B, et al: Memory function in psychiatric patients over sixty: some methodological and diagnostic implications. *J Ment Sci* 102:233–246, 1956.
13. Smith A: The serial sevens subtraction test. *Arch Neurol* 17:78–80, 1967.
14. Milstein V, Small J, Small I: The subtraction of serial sevens test in psychiatric patients. *Arch Gen Psychiatry* 26:439–441, 1972.
15. Hopkins B, Roth M: Psychological test performance in patients over sixty. I. *J Ment Sci* 99:439–450, 1953.
16. Roth M, Hopkins B: Psychological test performance in patients over sixty II. *J Ment Sci* 99:451–463, 1953.
17. Linn L: Clinical manifestations of psychiatric disorders. In Freedman AM, Kaplan HI, Sadock BJ (eds): *Comprehensive Textbook of Psychiatry* 2. Baltimore, Williams and Wilkins, 1975, vol 1, pp 783–825.
18. Preu P: *Outline of Psychiatric Case Study*. New York, Hoeber, 1939.
19. Andreasen NJC, Tsuang MT, Cantor A: The significance of thought disorder in diagnostic evaluations. *Compr Psychiatry* 15:27–34, 1974.
20. Keller MB, Manschreck TC: The bedside mental status examination—reliability and validity. *Compr Psychiatry* 22:500–511, 1981.
21. Kahn RL, Pollack M, Goldfarb AI: Factors related to individual differences in mental status of institutionalized aged. In Hoch PH, Zubin J (eds): *Psychopathology of Aging*. New York, Grune and Stratton, 1961, pp 104–113.
22. Brink TL, Capri D, DeNeeve V, et al: Senile confusion: limitations of assessment by the Face–Hand Test, Mental Status Questionnaire, and staff ratings. *J Am Geriat Soc* 26:380–82, 1978.
23. Pfeiffer E: A short portable mental status questionnaire for the assessment of organic brain deficits in elderly patients. *J Am Geriatr Soc* 23:433–441, 1975.
24. Isaacs B, Kennie A: The Set Test as an aid to the detection of dementia in old people. *Br J Psychiatry* 123:467–470, 1973.
25. Roth M: The natural history of mental disorder in old age. *J Ment Sci* 101:281–301, 1955.
26. Anthony JC, LeResche L, Niaz U, et al: Limits of the Mini-Mental State as a screening test for dementia and delirium among hospital patients. *Psychol Med* 12:397–408, 1982.
27. Jacobs JW, Bernhard MR, Delgrade A, et al: Screening for organic mental syndromes in the medically ill. *Ann Intern Med* 86:40–46, 1977.
28. Fink M, Green A, Bender MB: Face-Hand Test as a diagnostic sign of organic mental syndrome. *Neurology* 2:46, 1952.
29. Brilliant P, Gynther M: Relationships between performance on three tests of organicity and selected patient varables. *J Consult Psychol* 27:474–479, 1963.
30. Canter A: *The Canter Background Interference Procedure for the Bender-Gestalt Test: Manual for Administration, Scoring, and Interpretation*. Nashville, Counselor Recordings and Tests, 1976.
31. Heaton RK, Baade LE, Johnson KL: Neuropsychological test results associated with psychiatric disorders in adults. *Psychol Bull* 85:141–162, 1978.
32. Boake C, Adams RL: Clinical utility of the Background Interference Procedure for the Bender-Gestalt Test. *J Clin Psychol* 38:627–631, 1982.

14

The Mental Status Examination
III. Psychodynamic Dimensions[a]

Aaron Lazare, M.D.
Anne Alonso, Ph.D.

The mental status examination (MSE), originally named and described by Adolph Meyer in 1918 (1) and presented in contemporary form in the previous two chapters, is regarded as a basic tool for observing and recording parts of the psychiatric examination. It is the psychiatric equivalent of the physical examination in that it consists of data obtained primarily by direct observation of the patient, in contrast to data that are primarily historic in nature (2, 3).

The traditional MSE is particularly useful for the description and differentiation of those syndromes that have been studied and defined by the categoric (objective/descriptive, "medical") approach. For example, the MSE is essential in the assessment of major depression, bipolar disorders, schizophrenia, various organic mental conditions, and, to a lesser degree, the personality disorders (4–10).

We believe there are a wealth of clini-cally relevant observations that are not systematically observed or described in the MSE because they do not naturally emerge from the conceptual paradigm of the categoric model. Such observations may be relevant to psychodynamic, sociocultural, behavioral, existential, and other conceptual paradigms and would be applicable to all patients whether or not they meet the criteria for categoric diagnoses (11).

To facilitate the recording of psychodynamically relevant observations, this chapter attempts to develop a psychodynamic MSE. The observations contained herein represent our selections and descriptions of those styles, attitudes, and behaviors that we believe are related to psychodynamic inferences about conflict, ego strength, personality type, defensive strategy, self-concept, sexuality, aggression, superego, ego ideal, and the like. We have organized the clinical observations into a format similar to the traditional MSE so they can be easily incorporated into verbal presentations and written records of the traditional MSE (12–20).

---

[a] This chapter is adapted from "A Psychodynamic Mental Status Examination" by William A. Binstock, M.D., and Aaron Lazare, M.D., in the first edition of this book.

GENERAL APPEARANCE

There are manifestations of the patient's general appearance and behavior not usually described in the traditional mental status examination that are useful for assessing conflict, personality style, ego functioning, and other aspects of psychodynamic functioning, in addition to conveying an overall impression of the patient as a person. A suggested outline to record such observational data can be found in Table 14.1.

Mainly, we draw attention to particulars of dress, speech, locomotion, conversational style, and the like; we would add a strong caveat to avoid simplistic or formulaic inferences. Not all neat people are obsessive; not all emotionally intense patients are hysteric. The very essence of the psychodynamic method requires that we observe and record the here-and-now reality and then explore the less conscious meanings of these data on the basis of inferred unconscious dynamics of the patients.

The key to organizing these clues involves some judgment of normality and contextual appropriateness, and a curiosity about a patient's deviations from the norm—or for that matter, a too slavish conformity that blunts all orginality and personal taste.

Thus whether or not a patient is dressed in an age-appropriate manner, removes his or her coat, keeps on dark glasses, and sits very close to or very far from the the interviewer become signposts to begin building a diagnostic profile. These observations point toward a series of decision trees—they lead to inferences about the patient, and when the evidence begins to build in one direction or another, we can delve more deeply into the patient's inner life to rule in or rule out a diagnostic picture. For example, if a female patient is dressed in a jumble of bright clothing, is crying and wringing her hands, and is sitting close to the interviewer and interrupting often, we would want to know whether this collection of hysteric behaviors is indicative of a lifelong disorganization and lability, or whether she is responding understandably to the trauma of learning that her child has been abducted. In the latter case, we might find on further examination that she is showing us signals of the extreme chronic lability of an oral hysteric patient, but we might also learn that the current style is a regressive aberration in a competently organized person due to an acutely traumatic situation. In the latter case, calm composure would take on much more pathologic meaning than does her hysteria and anxiety.

The examiner's awareness of his or her internal state also aids in the psychodynamic assessment. The examiner may feel drained after listening to the seemingly reasonable discussion of stomach pains by a patient who will later prove insatiable in his demands for succor, or may feel pleasurably stimulated by a relatively healthy patient's sexual confusion. Attention to the reciprocal influence of each party to the interview on the other will be an important predictor of the alliance and the transference.

The way in which patients present their illness or themselves as people with problems convey not only their pain, but also what there is to be gained from the sick role in general and from their symptoms in particular. For example, it is necessary to assess whether it is the patient or only his or her social network that is suffering from the illness before a promising course of intervention can be planned. An apparent lack of distress over symptoms ("la belle indifference") hints at successful primary gain, which may include fulfillment of masochistic needs. Lack of distress over such severe manifestations as hallucinations or disabling psychogenic physical symptoms indicates chronicity, the acceptance of illness as a way of life. Such verbalizations as "This illness is driving my family crazy" provide more specific clues. (A woman who became depressed after her 21-year-old daughter moved away from home kept repeating "This illness of mine will be the death of my daughter.")

The patient's capacity to tolerate frustration, to delay gratification, is immediately manifest in the intiial interview. Performance on this continuum demonstrates ego strength rather directly. At one pole is the patient who "can't stand it another

Table 14.1.   Outline for a Psychodynamic Mental Status Examination

GENERAL APPEARANCE
1. Dress and grooming (neatness, fit, formality, color, appropriateness—to age, sex, occupation, occasion)
2. Posture and movement (arrival, gait, handshake, seating arrangements, distractibility, eye contact, body language, departure)
3. Blemishes, handicaps, and deformities
4. Characteristics of speech other than content (articulateness, tempo, tone, emphasis)
5. Sexuality (gender signals, asexuality or oversexualizing, security or confusion in sexual identity)
6. Aggression (inhibited, exaggerated, devious)
7. Superego and ego ideal (overall strategies for dealing with shame and guilt, consistent conscious ideals, use of models, rigid archaic morality, narcissistic entitlement to be an exception to the rules, infantile tolerance of blatant inconsistency in one's own rules, antisocial amorality)
8. Relationship with interviewer (passive, compliant, trusting, sexually and/or aggressively provocative, suspicious, competitive, demanding, obstinate, ingratiating)
9. Impact on interviewer (countertransference)
10. Relationship to Illness (primary and secondary gain)
11. Self-esteem (lowered in varying manners and degrees, maintained by compensatory grandiosity, i.e., the management of narcissism)
12. Tolerance for frustration (ability to delay gratification)
ASSOCIATIONS
1. General development of themes in the interview
2. Spontaneity of associations
3. Specific associative connections
4. Relationship of patient's words to clinician's words
5. Balance of primary process and secondary process organization (ratio of wishfully organized to conceptually organized thinking)
AFFECT AND MOOD
1. General range, expression and appropriateness of affect (including relationship to content)
2. General level of anxiety and ability to bear it
3. General level of depression and ability to bear it
4. Ability to express anger
5. Management of ambivalence of affect
6. Sadomasochism
7. Capacity for comfort and enjoyment
8. Ability to tolerate affective interchange
CONTENT
1. General content and recurrent theme
2. Style of content
3. Omissions, evasions, spontaneous denial, specific amnesias
4. Amnesia for childhood
5. Slips of speech or hearing
6. Words, phrases or metaphors with loaded meanings
7. Content highlighted by associated changes in affect, posture, loudness or pitch of voice, stuttering, or rhythm of speech
8. Inappropriately intimate or primary process (wishfully organized) content
9. Emphasized level of psychosexual and aggressive development (concept of a relationship)
INTELLECTUAL FUNCTIONS
1 Relationship between actual intellectual performance and inferred potential
2. Style of thinking (abstractness and concreteness, rigidity or flexibility, cognitive style, qualitative character typology)
3. Defensive strategy (characteristically prominent mechanisms of defense)
4. Psychological mindedness
5. Self-concept (clarity and quality)
6. Autonomous ego functions (conflict-free functioning, sublimations, interests, gifts, capacity to work effectively)
AUTOGNOSIS
1. Subjective responses of clinician
2. Evidence of therapeutic impasse

minute!''; at the other is the person who automatically assumes that doing his or her part in the clinical situation will lead to the desired result in due course of time. A capacity to delay can be understood in terms of the achievement of basic trust (in the nondestructiveness of one's own impulses and of one's relationships).

ASSOCIATIONS

One may apply to the clinical interview a psychodynamic analysis of associations. The general development of themes in the interview is important to note, particularly when the patient has the opportunity to provide some of the direction of the interview. There is usually a relatively small number of themes, which express the idiosyncratic concerns of this particular person at this specific moment in his or her life. The psychodynamic clinician, proceeding on the hypothesis that this simple consistency is determined by preconscious and unconscious processes, may hear patients' accounts of themselves and their dilemmas so clearly as to forget that the patients may not have heard it at all. Suppression suffices to keep different sections of the interview separated; only the material of the moment receives attention, so that even the persistent recurrence of a dominant theme can readily be kept from consciousness. In short, it is always vital to determine whether the patient hears the story that is coming across so clearly to the interviewer. The following example illustrates the emergency of a theme in the course of an interview: "My mother died when I was two. I've been married for two years and my wife is getting on my nerves. For two cents I'd leave her tomorrow."

The same considerations should be brought to bear on the discontinuities in the associations. On the psychodynamic assumption that all mental contents are connected, it can be expected that the missing link between seemingly disparate themes is there preconsciously or unconsciously. For example, aggressive themes followed by anxious or self-destructive associations may be evidence of conflict over

aggression. Complaints about the boss may be closely followed by talk of father or mother each time they occur. The subject of the presenting complaints may recur each time reference to the opposite sex is made (and also serve to prevent the completion of any story relating to this subject). Disruptions in the smooth flow of associations are evidences of the patient's areas of conflict.

Relatively healthy patients are in general able to present their stories in a relevant, goal-directed manner while responding appropriately to intermittent comments and questions from the clinician. The ability to pursue spontaneously one's conscious communicative goal is characteristic of ego strength. In the hysterical patient, the drama will easily unfold with little need for prompting. The lines of thought, however, are easily deflected by transient influences, and the general aim is toward being liked and cared for. Listening to a hysterical patient may leave an interviewer feeling somehow taken in: There was lots of talk and lots of energy, but surprisingly little factual information was communicated. The obsessional patient's associations are homogeneous and monotonous. There is little spontaneity, except perhaps at the beginning and at the end. After interviewing an obsessional patient, the clinician may find him- or herself with lots of information, but little information about the patient or about the relationship between the patient and the information. The schizoid patient, wary of commitment, may speak in a slow and halting manner similar to that of the depressed patient or in a boring, lifeless tone.

Specific associative connections may be obvious to the interviewer, as indicated above, even though the patient manages not to know about them consciously. In other cases, connections present as apparent disconnections—defensive disruption of the flow of associations may produce a gross gap or discontinuity. Such manifestations of active intrapsychic conflict present invaluble opportunities to the interviewer who pays attention to them. It is safe to infer that the disconnection was dictated by the need to avoid anxiety, and it is profitable to seek the missing material that had to be kept out of consciousness for this defensive purpose.

A psychologically minded patient may invite investigation of the point of discontinuity ("That's funny, I started to think about something else!"). Others may employ a glib cover-up that is also a clear signal to the alert listener ("Not to change the subject, but . . ."). Still others proceed in apparent unawareness of the awkward pause or jarring shift of direction. Tactful questioning at these points can be especially rewarding.

The relatively healthy patient is able to go on supported by a respectful show of interest on the part of the clinician. The hysterical patient may interrupt the associational flow by asking the clinician personal questions to engage his or her attention. The sociopathic patient may raise questions in order to discover the clincian's intentions, whereas the obsessional patient does it to control the conversation. General tendencies to direct the interview, seek direction, or control the flow are therefore revealing.

A rich response to the clinician's comments indicates an empathic interviewer, a psychologically minded patient, and the promise of a good alliance.

As thinking evolves in the course of individual development, its original wishful primary process organization in accordance with the quest for pleasure is supplemented by a conceptual secondary process organization in accordance with the dictates of external reality. Whereas the primary process is concrete and dominated by internal reality (especially the demands of the drives), the secondary process is abstract and takes cognizance not only of external reality, but also of the constraints of logic. Although extremes of one or the other type of organization are encountered (the wishful dream or daydream, the conceptual work of physical science), thought after infancy is always ruled by a compromise between the two competing types of organization. A characteristic balance of the two can be noted in a patient's spontaneous productions. Hysteric patients tend to lean toward wishful thinking beyond normal expectation ("I know you'll understand without my having to spell it out"), compulsive patients toward conceptual ("There are three more points I plan to cover, and then there will be 15 minutes left for you to explain to me what it means").

AFFECT AND MOOD

A healthy person has available a full range of appropriate affective responses and can express them in a well-modulated manner that greatly facilitates communication. Departures from this ideal characterize all temporary or long-term disturbances of optimal functioning. Hysterical personalities typically exhibit exaggerated, histrionic affects that strike the examiner as somehow not genuine. Obsessive patients, by contrast, are remarkably objective and even, appearing in this way, to be controlling anxiety and anger. Patients with schizoid personalities seem cut off from feelings. Paranoid and sociopathic types may appear (for different reasons) to be pleasant and cooperative at the start of the interview, only to become angry and antagonistic when they feel endangered (paranoid) or thwarted (sociopathic).

The presence of conflict may be reliably inferred (a) when antagonistic emotions occur simultaneously within the same context such as love and hate, pleasure and pain (a patient may smile while describing his "horror" at his father's near fatal surgery); (b) when the affective expression is out of proportion to the ideational content (a patient may weep or burst into a tirade while discussing an apparently neutral subject); (c) when the affect is inappropriate; and (d) when the predominant affects are all painful.

Anxiety and depression are unavoidable experiences; their absence is remarkable in a person seeking help with a problem. The healthy ability to tolerate them as circumscribed, ego-alien episodes is impaired in various personality styles.

A burden of chronic and diffuse free-floating anxiety invades and overwhelms all functioning in incipient psychoses or severe "borderline" conditions. This state may become apparent only as the investigation broadens beyond the area of the presenting complaint, revealing that there is *no* neutral area of the patient's life—*everything* generates anxiety.

An analogous burden of depression may, like the anxiety, appear at first a relatively appropriate situational response until the interviewer becomes aware that this is a characterlogic compromising of all the patient's functioning. Again, even severe depression may be an appropriate reaction to what is going on in the patient's life at the moment; it is by further investigation that the clinician learns that the depression is always, or usually, present.

The simple question as to whether the expression of anger is available to the patient is important in assessing the aggressive aspect of his or her life. (Anger is often, although not always, another of the painful affects, as are the moral anxieties of shame and guilt.) People's ways of concealing anger generally are more successful in deceiving themselves than in deceiving others. The obsessional individual whose speech becomes more and more measured and monotonous until its stilted formality is torturing the listener may herself experience the dehumanization of her discourse as a model of "rationality." The patient who sadistically teases the interviewer about some personal characteristic may believe himself to be lightening the atmosphere by "some good-natured kidding." The narcissistic patient who becomes offensively patronizing may experience herself as nobly generous in so enlightening and elevating her humble servant, the clinician. The hysteric patient who cuts off the interviewer's sentences with interruptions and jarring changes of subject may feel this intrusive, controlling behavior to be "enthusiasm." In these and similar cases, it will not be clear whether the patient is merely suppressing or is actually denying the evidence of anger that seems so obvious to the sensitive listener. Accordingly, the first order of business

may be a determination of whether or not the patient can admit being angry, annoyed, or irritated.

In assessing overall strength and maturity, the ego's management of ambivalence can be observed to range from alternating between love and hate toward the same object to a smooth integration and acceptance of mixed feelings. Opportunities to study this are prominent in initial interviews, which are so frequently precipitated by a loss of important relationships.

The healthiest patients seem to tolerate mixed feelings quite comfortably and to be able to decide and act on the dominant feeling. The sicker patient will tend to experience one or another side of his or her ambivalence, but not both simultaneously.

CONTENT

Specific observations of content are particularly useful in assessing personality, ego functioning, and areas of conflict.

Patients will usually convey areas of major concern by focusing on one or a few themes in the content they present spontaneously. There is a finite catalogue of themes that the clinician customarily hears: for example, loss, failure, separation, being intruded on or violated, fear of losing control and becoming destructive or sexually irresponsibile, fear of retaliation, fear of annihilation or engulfment, loneliness, and isolation.

Words, phrases, and metaphors with loaded meanings are of special interest. "You are saddled with me, and I am saddled with you." "It was a blinding observation." "I am starved for affection." Patients who "want to get things straightened out" may wish they could talk about their potency problems. Content referable to the body is reliably revealing: "I feel a hollow space in the pit of my stomach." "He is a pain in the neck." "My whole body feels like a raw nerve that is being tickled."

Ego weakness can be manifested through too open a presentation or too blatant a primary process organization of the content.

INTELLECTUAL FUNCTIONS

Intellectual functions, or more broadly, the patient's ways of knowing and not knowing, are revealing of his or her personality style. The more familiar topic of mechanisms of defense is included here because many of the defenses are cognitive maneuvers whereby the ego manages not to know what it knows.

The headline thinking of hysteric patients, conceptual objectivity of obsessional patients, glib plausibility of sociopathic patients, etc., provide excellent overview of character type (personality style). Alertness to mechanisms of defense yields some of the most precise and valuable technical inferences available to the psychodynamic clinician. What the investigator seeks is a short list of those mechanisms most prominently used. For example, isolation (supplemented perhaps by reaction formation) might dominate the picture in many interviews with patients of obsessional, schizoid, paranoid, or narcissistic character type; it would be of the greatest interest in such a case whether the other mechanism(s) noted in the dominant cluster are repression and/or suppression on the one hand, or projection and/or denial on the other.

A detailed listing of every mechanism of defense that can possibly be noted is an empty academic exercise; presumably, we all make some use of all of them. The absence of reality-respecting defenses (suppression, repression, rationalization, isolation, reaction formation, doing and undoing) is a more notable evidence of compromised functioning than the presence of reality-distorting ones (denial, projection, introjection). Insofar as the mechanisms can be ordered in an adaptive hierarchy, the prominence of one or another gives a rough cue to the relative health of character structure.

The inventory of predominant mechanisms of defense also complements qualitative judgments about style of thinking. Excessive use of suppression, repression, and denial will go with the vagueness of the lots-of-feeling-not-much-thinking type of mind. The very rational devotee of abstract purity and precision will rely inordinately on isolation, probably supplemented by reaction formation and undoing.

The role of introjection and identification in a patient's response to the interviewer can be revealing of major problems with the self. Someone who swallows whole the words of a clinician, accepting them wholesale without question as though they were marching orders or revealed truth, is demonstrating a deficiency in self-concept, a sense of self that is inadequate to support an autonomous role in the interchange. Another who picks up traits of the interviewer during the first session or so is obviously manifesting a diffuseness of his own identity, an uncertainty about who he is.

An assessment of psychologic mindedness is essential for planning further investigative and therapeutic efforts. This may be understood roughly as an openness to, or even a propensity for, the approach employed in the psychodynamic investigation. Unfortunately, such a conception can easily mislead one into accepting a patient's glib intellectual formulations as an expression of a genuine introspective approach. Psychologic mindedness entails a response to psychic pain that acknowledges its presence and proceeds to trace its origins internally. Psychodynamic formulations can be reified into external forces akin to possessing demons ("I know, I know, it's my father fixation"). When more than one interview is conducted, the clinician can readily note the opening up of additional areas from session to session. In contrast, a lack of psychologic mindedness can be grossly manifested in the closing of previously open areas.

The presence of spheres of conflict-free areas of functioning is an important component of ego strength. (For example, the patient whose difficulties in succeeding in love and career ambitions occupy much of her record may nevertheless have a basic capacity to get along with people and work effectively that is relatively unimpaired by her conflicts.) In clearly compromised egos, there may be important autonomous areas that are vital assets. A psychotic artist may be able to go on functioning as an artist to the envy of healthier peers. Gross failure in relationships may leave great verbal or mathematical abilities relatively unimpaired. Since diagnostic formulations always imply prognostic and therapeutic directions to the professional reader, it is essential to acknowledge in the record areas of functioning not compromised by illness.

AUTOGNOSIS

A final category of clinical observations that are useful for psychodynamic inferences comprises the clinician's observations of him- or herself in relationship to the patient. Such knowledge has been referred to by Messner as "autognosis," or diagnosis by the use of one's self (21). These observations include the clinician's total subjective response to the patient, including "awareness of perception, intuition, empathy, prejudices, emotions, fantasies, traits, skills, attitudes, motivations, and other internal events and processes of the clinician" (21). According to some theoreticians, this definition encompasses a greater range of subjective phenomena than does countertransference. Messner states that there are four major uses of autognosis. First, it is of value for the interpretation of clinical data for diagnosis and treatment. Second, it is useful for the diagnosis and resolution of therapeutic impasses. Third, it is useful in helping the clinician maintain optimal therapeutic activity. And finally, it is useful for personal growth.

In the appliction of subjective data for assessment, it is important to be aware that some of our subjective responses to patients are shared by a wide group of clinicians while others are quite idiosyncratic to the particular clinician. For instance, many clinicians feel, in the presence of many borderline patients, as if they are walking on eggs and that they may be verbally attacked as soon as they attempt to be helpful. A more idiosyncratic subjective response to borderline patients would be a sense of comfort and relaxation. For the sake of diagnosis, what is important is that a given clinician's responses, whether common or idiosyncratic, are reliable. In other words, the clinician can reliably assume that a particular subjective response in him- or herself suggests a particular diagnosis or the presence of a particular issue at a given point in the interview.

Just a few common subjective responses of clinicians that tend to have diagnostic value include the following feelings, wishes, and fantasies: the sense of fulfillment that one is helping another, a sense of mutuality, the desire to rescue the patient from insensitive or destructive family members, sexual excitement, the wish to have the patient move to another city or change clinicians, fear of the patient's physical or verbal violence, annoyance, boredom, humiliation, the desire to humiliate, the sense of being manipulated, and the sense of feeling emotionally drained and exhausted. It is probably the awareness and accurate use of these cues that constitute what we call hunches or intuition.

Some of these subjective responses, particularly when they are persistent, may be clues that there is a therapeutic impasse. Messner lists 16 such clues. These are

- an unreasoning distaste for the patient;
- becoming overemotional in regard to the patient's troubles;
- excessive fondness for the patient;
- sleepiness in the patient's presence;
- frequent lateness by the therapist;
- intense or frequent arguments with the patient;
- derogatory criticism of the patient;
- appearance of the patient in the clinician's dreams;
- forgetting material;
- persistence of thoughts of the patient in the clinician's fantasies;
- undue pessimism or optimism;
- thoughts of premature termination;
- active withdrawal;
- regression to orthodoxy;
- feelings of inadequacy;
- unusual handling of fees (21).

The awareness of these responses give clinicians the opportunity to explore both the patient's behaviors that provoke them as well as their own personal experiences, neurotic features, and maturational crises that lead to their vulnerability. Such an exploration allows clinicians to maintain optimal therapeutic activity with their patients as well as continue their own personal growth.

CONCLUSIONS

The psychodynamic MSE represents an initial attempt to organize and record psychodynamic interview observations. Our choice of outline, selection of suggested topics, and assignment of topics to one category or another leave much room for improvement by others. Some of the mainstays of psychodynamic psychiatry (such as the relationships of the patient to key figures, to work, and to play) have been ignored because these and other inferences are customarily drawn from the history and recorded with it.

There are three major problems with a psychodynamic MSE. The first is conceptual and has to do with the psychodynamic inferences or concepts to which the clinical observations are presumably related. Some of these concepts are characterized by imprecise, overlapping, and multiple definitions that approach at times the use of different languages (e.g., object relations theory versus drive and ego psychology). It is also uncertain whether psychodynamic clinicians agree in finding a particular concept useful. The second problem is empirical: How does one know that a particular observation is related to a psychodynamic inference? The third has to do with the necessarily subjective assessment of normality and appropriateness by the clinician. The examiner is hardly bias free, and what may be perceived as a "cold response" by an examiner from a Mediterranean ethnic background may seem very healthy to a more formal clinician from an emotionally restrained family. It is our hope that continued efforts at developing a psychodynamic MSE will focus much needed attention on these problems and lead to a more systematic and commonplace acceptance of its importance for the diagnosis and treatment of the psychiatric patient.

References

1. Meyer A: *The Collected Papers of Adolph Meyer* (Winters EE, ed). Baltimore, Johns Hopkins Press, 1951, vol. 3, pp 224–258.
2. Donnelly J, Rosenberg M, Fleeson, W: The evolution of the mental status—past and future. *Am J Psychiatry*, 126:997–1002, 1970.
3. Wertzel WD, Morgan DW, Guyden TE, et al. Toward a more efficient mental status examination. *Arch Gen Psychiatry* 28:215–218, 1973.
4. Redlich FC, Freedman DX: *The Theory and Practice of Psychiatry*. New York, Basic Books, 1966.
5. Whitehorn JC: Guide to interviewing and clinical personality study: *Arch Neurol* 52:197–216, 1944.
6. Sullivan HS: *The Psychiatric Interview*. New York, W. W. Norton & Co., 1954.
7. Stevenson I: The psychiatric interview (chap 9). The psychiatric examination (chap 10). In Arieti S (ed): *American Handbook of Psychiatry*. New York, Basic Books, 1959, vol 1, pp 197–214, 215–234.
8. Saul LJ: The psychoanalytic diagnostic interview. *Psychoanal Q*, 26:76–90, 1957.
9. Powdermaker F: The techniques of the initial interview and methods of teaching them. *Am J Psychiatry* 104:642–646, 1948.
10. Jacobson JG, Whittington HG: A study of of process in the evaluation interview. *Psychiatry*, 23:23–24, 1960.
11. Lazare A: Hidden conceptual models in clinical psychiatry. *N Engl J Med* 288:345–351, 1973.
12. Hendrickson WJ, Coffer RH Cross TN: The initial interview. *Arch Neurol* 71:24–30, 1954.
13. Gill MM, Newman R, Redlich FC: *The Initial Interview in Psychiatric Practice*. New York, International Universities Press, 1954.
14. Finesinger JB: Psychiatric interviewing: some principles and procedures in insight therapy. *Am J Psychiatry* 105:187–195, 1948.
15. *Reports in Psychotherapy: Initial Interviews* (No. 49). New York, Group for the Advancement of Psychiatry, 1961.
16. Langs R: *The Technique of Psychoanalytic Psychotherapy*. New York, Jason Aronson, 1973.
17. Tarachow S: The initial interview conference. *Hillsdale Hosp* 11:127–153, 1962.
18. MacKinnon RA, Michels R: *The Psychiatric Interview in Clinical Practice*. Philadelphia, W.B. Saunders, 1971.
19. Barish JI, Buchenholz B: A teaching technique for inferring psychodynamics. *Psychiatr Q* 34–103, 1960.
20. Deutsch F, Murphy WF: *The Clinical Interview* (vol 1). New York, International Universities Press, 1955.
21. Messner E: Autognosis: diagnosis by the use of the self. In Lazare A (ed): *Outpatient Psychiatry*. Baltimore, Williams & Wilkins, 1979, pp 231–237.

15

Use of the Laboratory in Outpatient Psychiatry

David Gitlin, M.D.
Aaron Lazare, M.D.

Since the publication of the first edition of this book in 1979, the importance of the laboratory in outpatient psychiatry has grown significantly. Whereas previously the laboratory was used primarily for the diagnosis of organic conditions, currently its use has expanded to include the monitoring of blood levels of therapeutic drugs and the determination of markers for some of the psychiatric disorders.

This chapter first discusses some definitions and general concepts relevant to laboratory testing, particularly in outpatient settings. The body of this chapter is then organized around five clinical functions of the laboratory: (a) testing for organic disease, (b) performing toxicology studies (c) testing organ functioning for patients receiving psychiatric medications (d) monitoring blood levels of psychiatric medications, and (e) diagnosing and monitoring psychiatric disorders.

DEFINITIONS AND GENERAL CONCEPTS

Sensitivity, Specificity, and Predictive Value

In order to interpret the significance of a given laboratory result, the clinician must be familiar with three statistical concepts: sensitivity, specificity, and predictive value. *Sensitivity* refers to the probability of the laboratory test's detecting the abnormality or establishing the diagnosis in those who suffer from the abnormality or the disease in question. If there were a laboratory test for schizophrenia, a sensitivity of 90% would mean that 90% of schizophrenic patients would test positive while 10% of schizophrenic patients would test negative and therefore be referred to as false negatives. *Specificity* refers to the probability of a negative test result for an individual who does not have the disease. In the hypothetical laboratory test for schizophrenia, a specificity of 90% means that 90% of patients who do not suffer from schizophrenia will have a negative test for schizophrenia while only 10% will be false positives; that is, they test positive but do not actually have the disease. *Predictive value* is the percentage of all positive results that are true positives. This, in turn is a function of sensitivity, specificity, and prevalence of the disease (1–4).

Problems Specific to Ambulatory Laboratory Testing

The attempt to develop standard guidelines for the use of laboratory testing in outpatient practice is complicated by the heterogeneity of ambulatory settings, ambulatory patients, and the clinicians who staff them. Of all outpatient settings, subspecialty clinics in teaching hospitals are most apt to use laboratory testing. This is because of the high percentage of clinicians who are psychiatrists, the nature of the clinical problems under investigation (affective disorders, eating disorders, etc.) the controlled flow of patients, and the interest in scholarly activities. Community mental health centers, in contrast, are less apt to use laboratory testing because of the small percentage of clinicians who are psychiatrists, the heterogeneity of the problems under investigation, the busy and uncontrolled flow of patients, and the financial constraints. In general, inpatient psychiatrists are more aggressive in ordering laboratory tests than their outpatient counterparts. This is because the disorders treated on inpatient settings are apt to be more serious and treatment resistant, and because the inpatient clinician has a relatively brief period of time for diagnosis and treatment.

Cost Versus Benefit in the Use of Laboratory Tests

For each laboratory test, the clinician must consider the cost to the patient versus the possible benefit of the test. The benefits may include increased probabililty that the diagnosis will be accurate, that treatment is being efficiently provided, that the patient's physical health is not being compromised by the treatment, and that the patient will perceive the clinician as careful, caring, and scientific. The costs include finances, inconvenience, the probability of the test's being inadequately performed, the confusion caused by false positive and false negative results, psychological trauma to the patient, and physical danger to the patient. The decision to perform a laboratory test, therefore, should be the result of a negotiated process leading to the informed consent of the patient and/ or his or her family.

TESTING FOR ORGANIC DISEASE

It is well established that physical morbidity and mortality are greater in psychiatric patients than in the general population. In Chapter 17 we review 19 studies of medical disease in various psychiatric populations including inpatient, outpatient, emergency room, community support programs, outpatient rehabilitation programs, and medical/neurologic services. These studies record the overall incidence of medical disease, the incidence of previously undiagnosed medical disease, and the incidence of medical disease causative of or contributory to the psychiatric presentation. It is sufficient to say for this chapter that the overall incidence of medical disease is significant but variable according to the nature of the clinical site and patients under study. These data lead to the inevitable conclusion that in the assessment of every psychiatric outpatient, the clinician must consider the hypothesis that an organic illness may be causing, contributing to, or coexisting with the psychiatric condition. This section describes the role of the laboratory in the diagnosis of organic illness.

Experts disagree over the appropriate use of the laboratory for the detection of organic disease in psychiatric outpatients. Some argue for comprehensive screening in all outpatients. Others argue for a diagnostic algorithm that provides various levels of assessment according to clinical findings. In other words, the clinician's decision to order laboratory tests should depend on clinical judgment, which in turn is based on the nature of the psychiatric history, the symptom picture, the medical history, a mental status examination, and a partial or complete physical examination. Clinicians vary considerably regarding the extent of the laboratory evaluation before making a referral to the appropriate medical specialist.

Complete Blood Count

The complete blood count (CBC) makes up the basic screening assessment of the cellular components of blood: red cells, white cells, and platelets. Red cells, essential for oxygen and carbon dioxide transportation, are assessed on the CBC by two measures—hemoglobin content and hematocrit (red cell volume in blood). White cells are necessary for major immune functions, and platelets are required for effective clotting. The differential analysis of specific white cell types is often helpful in the assessment of infections. (Other measurements of the CBC are not discussed here.)

Anemia, easily measured by decreased hematocrit, may cause a variety of neuropsychiatric symptoms such as fatigability, apathy, weakness, headaches, lightheadedness, numbness and tingling, lethargy, impaired concentration, anorexia, and decreased libido. (see Table 1) These symptoms may be confused with depressive and anxiety disorders.

Causes of anemia include acute or chronic blood loss, impaired red cell formation (from deficiencies of iron, folate, and B_{12}), and increased red cell destruction. Anemia of chronic disease is seen in malignancy, liver and renal failure, endocrine dysfunction, infection, and collagen–vascular disease. Deficiences in folate and B_{12}, as well as iron, are seen in alcoholics, drug abusers, and the chronic mentally ill. The psychiatric presentations of folate and B_{12} deficiencies may resemble organic brain syndrome with disturbances in awareness, thought, affect, and memory. Delay in diagnosis and treatment may make these conditions irreversible.

The most frequent cause of elevated white blood count is infection. This may be a critical test for the corroboration of infection, particularly in the elderly, where the fever response may be blunted. Significant increases in the band and neutrophil forms suggest bacterial infections, while increases in lymphocytes suggest viral infections. Infectious mononucleosis may show an increase in atypical lymphocyte forms. (Further localization of the infection, e.g., pulmonary, or urogenital, will suggest further laboratory testing.) Various forms of leukemia may cause a wide range of disturbances in the CBC from pancytopenia to significant elevations of white cells, red cells, and/or platelets.

Electrolytes

Many of the chemicals measured in the blood exist in ionized form (electrolytes), either as cations such as sodium and potassium or as anions such as chloride and bicarbonate. These and other electrolytes are involved in the functions of the body that require intracellular and extracellular exchange. The brain is especially sensitive to deviations in electrolyte concentrations, which may result in a variety of psychiatric manifestations.

Sodium, potassium, chloride, and bicarbonate represent the major electrolytes and are usually measured together as a separate "electrolyte screen." Calcium, magnesium, and phosphate can be ordered separately or may be ordered in blood chemistry analyses such as the sequential multichannel autoanalyzer (SMA)-16.

Sodium

Sodium, the major cation in the extracellular fluid, accounts for 90% of the total serum osmolality and is therefore critical to the maintenance of total body water. Concentration of sodium is controlled by a very efficient mechanism involving the hypothalamus, posterior pituitary, and the kidneys. Diseases affecting the kidneys or gastrointestinal and endocrine systems often lead to perturbations in sodium balance.

Hyponatremia may cause lethargy, confusion, stupor, coma, apathy, weakness, and irritability. Associated physical symptoms include anorexia, abdominal pain, headaches, muscle cramps and twitching, convulsions, nausea and vomiting. Hyponatremia may be caused by congestive heart failure, cirrhosis, nephrotic syndrome, renal failure, hypothyroidism, the various causes of volume depletion (diuretic abuse, adrenal insufficiency, severe vomiting, and diarrhea) and the syndrome of inappropriate antidiuretic hormone secretion (SIADH). Diuretic abuse and severe vomiting are commonly associated with eating-disordered patients; SIADH may be seen in patients with disorders of the central nervous system secondary to head injury, pulmonary disease, and various psychoactive drugs including carbamazepine, amitriptyline, narcotics, barbiturates, and acetominophen. Psychogenic polydipsia is a state of primary dilutional hyponatremia that occurs when the intake of water exceeds the kidney's ability to excrete. This condition, although rare, has been seen in psychotic patients and in Munchausen's disorder.

Hypernatremia may lead to confusion, lethargy, psychosis, stupor, weakness, and convulsions. Causes of hypernatremia include Cushing's syndrome, primary hyperaldosteronism, severe burns, diabetes mellitus, and diabetes insipidus. The latter may be seen in patients with head trauma, with neurosurgical procedures, and as a complication of lithium therapy. Hypernatremia also occurs in patients who have lack of access to water, e.g., postoperative, nursing home, institutionalized, and stroke patients.

Potassium

Potassium, the principal intracellular cation, plays a significant role in nerve conduction, skeletal and cardiac muscle function, and acid–base balance.

Hypokalemia may cause anxiety, depression, weakness, diarrhea, nausea, and vomiting. Associated decreased motor strength, hyporeflexia, paralysis, and cardiac arrhythmias or arrest can occur. Causes of hypokalemia include diuretic use, vomiting, hyperaldosteronism, Cushing's syndrome, steroid use, and metabolic alkalosis. Diuretic abuse and vomiting are commonly seen in patients suffering from somatoform and eating disorders.

Hyperkalemia may cause depression, weakness, and palpitations. The electrocardiogram may show bradycardia, heart block and arrhythmias. Causes of hyperkalemia include renal failure, adrenal insufficiency, diuretic abuse, hypoaldosteronism, metabolic acidosis, excessive potassium intake, and severe tissue trauma. Abuse of potassium-sparing diuretics is seen in patients suffering from somatoform and eating disorders.

Bicarbonate

Bicarbonate is one of several buffer systems involved in the regulation of pH through the removal of carbon dioxide, the most abundant acid substrate in the body. Control of the bicarbonate buffer system takes place in the lungs and kidneys. Primary decreases in barcarbonate lead to metabolic acidosis; increases, to metabolic alkalosis.

Metabolic acidosis may be associated with confusion, stupor, coma, fatigue, anorexia, and hyperventilation. Some causes of metabolic acidosis are renal failure, lactic acidosis, drug ingestions, diarrhea, and ketoacidosis (diabetic, starvation, or alcoholic). Acute and chronic alcoholism, usually in association with prolonged starvation and protracted vomiting, can lead to ketoacidosis. Drug ingestions commonly leading to acidosis include methanol, ethylene glycol, and alcohol.

Chloride

Chloride is the fourth ion measured in a basic electrolyte screen. Its concentration is interdependent with sodium concentration, with chloride ions basically following sodium in and out of cells. Chloride fluctuations are not directly related to any specific changes in mental status.

Blood Chemistries

There are various other chemicals in the intracellular and extracellular fluids, not in the ionized form, whose deviations from normal levels may result in psychiatric presentations. Among these are urea, glucose, and creatinine.

Urea

Urea, the end product of protein breakdown and the major nonprotein metabolized form of nitrogen, is formed in the liver and carried via the bloodstream to the kidneys to be excreted in the urine. The nitrogenous portion of the urea in the blood is measured as blood urea nitrogen (BUN). Since BUN is a gross measure of glomerular filtration rate, dysfunctions of the glomerulus may result in elevated BUN. Profound elevations in BUN are seen in uremia, although the BUN is not the actual toxin in this condition.

Degrees of renal insufficiency associated with elevated levels of BUN present with anorexia, apathy, confusion, stupor, drowsiness, lethargy, insomnia, restlessness, weakness, and decreased concentration. The most serious outcome of renal insufficiency is uremia, a type of encephalopathy resulting in altered sensorium. Associated physical symptoms include abdominal pain, easy bruisability, chest pain, hiccups, muscle cramps, myalgias, nausea and vomiting, nocturia, polyuria, and pruritis. Physical examination may reveal congestive heart failure, mental status changes, hypertension, pallor, purpura, dry and excoriated skin, myoclonus, and pericardial friction rub. The most common cause of a markedly elevated BUN is renal failure.

Calcium and Phosphorus

Calcium and phosphorus homeostasis is closely interrelated under the influence of the parathyroid glands, kidneys, and Vit D. Calcium plays a role in a variety of bodily functions including bone metabolism, hormone secretion, neurotransmitter release, muscle contraction, and enzyme activation and deactivation, and as an intracellular messenger. Calcium and phosphorus are both absorbed in the gastrointestinal tract and excreted via the kidneys, so diseases of these organ systems may also lead to impaired homeostasis.

Hypocalcemia may be associated with anxiety, paraesthesias, convulsions, dyspnea, twitching, neuromuscular irritability (carpopedal spasm, tetany), hyperventilation, and seizures. Some causes of hypocalcemia are primary and secondary hypoparathyroidism, malabsorption, osteomalacia, chronic renal failure, rickets and pancreatitis.

Hypercalcemia may be associated with lethargy, confusion, stupor, coma, apathy, depression, and psychosis. Associated physical symptoms include nausea, anorexia, constipation, vomiting, and weakness. Physical findings include proximal muscle weakness, hyporeflexia, band keratopathy, muscular atrophy, and pseudogout.

Causes of hypercalcemia include malignancies (especially breast), hyperparathyroidism, hyperthyroidism, Addison's disease, sarcoidosis and thiazide abuse. Reported symptoms range from mild personality disorders to severe psychiatric disturbances. Patients may experience multiple vague complaints that can be mistaken for psychosomatic illness or minor depression. In some patients, these may be the initial signs and symptoms of the condition.

Hyperphosphatemia may be associated with anorexia, dizziness, bone pain, and weakness. Physical findings include waddling gait and proximal muscle weakness. The most common cause is renal failure. Hypophosphatemia is occasionally associated with muscle weakness and respiratory failure.

Magnesium

Magnesium, like phosphorus, is intimately related to calcium and is necessary for proper calcium absorption from the gastrointestinal tract. It is also linked to neuromuscular transmission, hormone secretion, effective clotting, and numerous enzymatic processes. Hypomagesemia may be associated with fatigue, weakness, depression, organic brain syndrome, palpitations, growth failure, tremor, tetany, convulsions, and arrhythmias. Causes of hypomagnesemia are dietary deficiency, alcoholism, hyperaldosteronism, cirrhosis, malabsorption, and hypoparathyroidism. This condition is frequently encountered in the chronic alcoholic and may be at least partially responsibile for some of the long-term sequelae. Magnesium levels should be tested on patients presenting with alcoholism and disorders of cognition.

Glucose

Glucose is the major energy source in humans. Its metabolism is a result of a coordination of insulin, glucagon, and other hormones. Disregulation of the endocrine system, starvation, and liver disease may lead to disruptions in glucose metabolism.

Hypoglycemia may be associated with agitation, anxiety, lethargy, derealization, hallucinations (often visual), bizarre behavior, disorientation, stupor, and coma. Associated physical symptoms include palpitations, diaphoresis, shakiness, weakness, hunger, nausea, headaches, lightheadedness, paraesthesias, yawning, and syncope. On physical examination, there may be tachycardia, hyperventilation, confusion, tremor, trismus, convulsions and diaphoresis. Common causes of hypoglycemia are excess insulin (overdose, poor diabetic control, insulin-secreting tumors), alcoholism, liver failure, congestive heart failure, severe malnutrition, Addisonian crisis, and functional hypoglycemia. Functional or reactive hypoglycemia is a topic of heated debate among endocrinologists, many of whom doubt its existence. Since alcoholics account for greater than one-third of all exogenously induced episodes of hypoglycemia, it is important to distinguish hypoglycemia from alcohol intoxication in these patients. Hypoglycemia can also mimic other syndromes commonly seen in the alcoholic, such as alcoholic withdrawal, Wernicke-Korsakoff syndrome, hepatic encephalopathy, meningitis, subdural hematoma, and subarachnoid bleeding. Because of the serious and possibly irreversible effects of hypoglycemia, all patients presenting with alterations in sensorium require intravenous glucose once a serum glucose has been obtained. In alcoholics, thiamine should also be given to prevent acute Wernicke's encephalopathy which may be precipitated by the glucose load.

For patients presenting with symptoms of anxiety, the clinician may wish to consider functional (reactive) hypoglycemia in the differential diagnosis. This condition may be considered as causative of anxiety symptoms when a blood sugar of 45 mg/dl or less is obtained simultaneously with the symptoms. Confirmation of functional hypoglycemia is obtained by a 5-hour glucose tolerance test. In functional hypoglycemia, there is an exaggeration of the normal hypoglycemic portion of the test.

Creatinine

Creatinine, a by-product of muscle breakdown, is produced at a constant rate and excreted by the kidneys. Because it is completely removed by the glomerular complex and not resorbed in the tubules, it is a more specific and sensitive measure of glomerular filtration rate than the BUN.

Liver Function Testing

When liver disease occurs in psychiatric patients, the most common cause is substance abuse or hepatotoxic medications. Although alcohol is the obvious example, many psychotropic medications have the potential for hepatotoxicity including monoamine oxidase inhibitors, methyldopa, phenytoin, valproic acid, haloperidol, carbamazepine, chlorpromazine, and disulfuram. Early screening and continued assessment for possible liver disease can be accomplished by means of chemical analysis of selected enzymes and metabolic breakdown products in the hepatobiliary system. These include aspartate aminotransferase (AST), alanine aminotransferase (ALT), alkaline phosphatase, and total bilirubin. AST and ALT are also referred to as serum glutamic-oxaloacetic transaminase (SGOT) and serum glutamic-pyruvic transaminase (SGPT), respectively.

Aspartate Aminotransferase and Alanine Aminotransferase Both AST and ALT are hepatocellular enzymes that are very sensitive to disruptions in the integrity of the hepatocyte. Elevations may range from mild to moderate (cirrhosis, metastatic liver disease, pancreatitis) to severe (active hepatitis). ALT is a more specific indicator of intracellular liver disease than AST because the latter is present in significant concentrations in other tissues such as heart, muscle, and kidney.

Bilirubin Bilirubin, a breakdown product of hemoglobin, is eliminated from the body via conjugation within the hepatocyte with subsequent secretion into the bile. Processes that disrupt the hepatocyte or cause obstruction of the heptobiliary tree may lead to elevations in total bilirubin. These include alcoholic cirrhosis, hepatitis, cholestasis (secondary to drugs, portal hypertension), gallstones, and malignancy. Jaundince is the obvious physical sign of hyperbilirubinemia.

Alkaline Phosphatase Alkaline phosphatase, produced by many tissues including liver and excreted in the hepatobiliary tree, is the liver chemistry most sensitive to obstructions of this system. Pancreatic cancer, gallstone, and portal hypertension may all lead to elevations in alkaline phosphatase. Since pancreatic cancer may present with depression and other psychoneurotic features, the clinician should always be alert for signs and symptoms of obstruction in such patients and perform the appropriate laboratory tests. Alkaline phosphatase can be elevated, however, in the absence of liver disese, e.g., in Paget's disease and bony metatases.

Thyroid Function Tests

Hypothyroidism can present with symptoms of depression, general dulling of personality, delirium, and dementia. Hyperthyroidism can present as mania, depression, anxiety, schizophrenic-like psychosis, and delirium. Thyroid testing, therefore, is commonly performed for many of the above symptoms.

It is important to note that investigators have found perturbations in thyroid function tests at an increased rate in newly hospitalized psychiatric patients regardless of diagnosis (5). In the vast majority of cases, this perturbation resolves spontaneously in 7 to 10 days. It is unclear what relevance this may have to the outpatient evaluation of affective disorders with thyroid studies.

The laboratory tests of greatest ease and utility are measurements of serum thyroxine (T_4) and triiodothyronine resin uptake (T_3RU) (a technique for assessing availability of thyroid-binding globulin). When these are combined via a mathematical formula, the result, called the "free thyroxine index," is felt to be an effective test for screening thyroid function. When the free thyroxine indicates a hypothyroid state, a thyroid-stimulating hormone (TSH) level is useful in determining whether the problem lies in the thyroid gland (elevated TSH level) or the central nervous system (low or normal TSH level). When the free thyroxine is within the normal range, an elevated TSH level may indicate subclinical hypothyroidism.

The thyrotropin-releasing hormone (TRH) stimulation test may be useful in confirming a diagnosis of hypothyroidism when the plasma elevation of TSH is borderline. The usefulness of this test in the outpatient setting is unclear.

Testing for Syphilis

Neurosyphilis is rare since the advent of penicillin. Tests for syphilis use serology to detect the presence of *Treponema pallidum*, the causitive organism. The Venereal Disease Research Lab slide test (VDRL) is the most commonly used test, but can be plagued by false positive results in the range of 20%. If syphilis is suspected, a highly specific antibody test (such as flurescent treponemal antibody absorption test [FTA-ABS]) is used.

Human Immunodeficiency Virus Testing

Since the initial manifestations of acquired immune deficiency syndrome (AIDS) may be neuropsychiatric, the psychiatrist may be the first physician to see the infected patient. An increased index of suspicion should be raised if the patient is a member of a high-risk group such as homosexuals, intravenous drug users, hemophiliacs, and others who have had contact with blood-borne products. There are two major laboratory tests used to identify the human immunodeficiency virus, the presumed causative agent of AIDS. If the psychiatrist suspects that the patient is infected with AIDS or if a patient insists on being tested for AIDS, the psychiatrist should, after appropriate counseling, refer the patient to an internist or AIDS toxicity center.

Erythrocyte Sedimentation Rate

The erythrocyte sedimentation rate (sed rate) measures the speed at which red blood cells settle out of unclotted blood. The rate increases when red cells agglutinate, a process caused by numerous diseases that affect the cells. Among these are neoplasms, infections, collagen vascular disease, and various inflammatory dis-

eases. This test is neither very specific nor sensitive.

Urine Evaluation

Urine is a complex body fluid, the end product of metabolic reactions occurring in the body. Because it is so easily accessible, it can be useful in the assessment of some psychiatric illnesses.

Table 15.1   Psychiatric Symptoms Associated with Abnormal Laboratory Tests

Laboratory Tests	Normal Values	Symptoms with Elevated Levels	Symptoms with Decreased Levels
Hemocrit	Men: 40–52% Women: 36–42%		Fatigue, apathy, impaired cognition, decreased libido, anxiety
White blood count	4,300—10,300/mm^3	Depression	
Sodium	136–142 mmol/l	Lethargy, confusion, stupor, coma, apathy irritability, anorexia	
Potassium	3.5–5.3 mmol/l	Anxiety, depression, weakness	Depression, weakness
Bicarbonate	24–32 mmol/l		Confusion, stupor, coma, fatigue, anorexia
Chloride	97–110 mmol/l		
Calcium	8.5–10.5 mg/dl	Confusion, lethargy, stupor, coma, apathy, depression, psychosis, anorexia	Anorexia
Phosphate	2.5–4.5 mg/dl	Anorexia, weakness	Muscle weakness, respiratory failure
Magnesium	1.8–2.4 mg/dl		Fatigue, weakness, depression, delirium
Blood urea nitrogen	7—26 mg/dl	Anorexia, apathy, confusion, lethargy, stupor, coma, weakness, restlessness, poor concentration	
Glucose (testing)	65–105 mg/dl		Anxiety, lethargy, agitation, psychosis, confusion, stupor, coma
Creatine	0.6–1.2 mg/dl		
Liver function tests		Confusion, stupor, coma, delirium, dementia	
Aspartate aminotransferase (SGOT)	7–40 U/L		
Alanine aminotransferase (SGPT)	7–40 U/L		
Total bilirubin	0.5–1.2 mg/dl		
Alkaline phosphatase			
Thyroid function tests		Mania, psychosis, delirium	Depression, delirium, dementia
Thyroxine (T$_4$)	4.3–9.5 mg/dl		
Triiodothyronine resin uptake (T$_3$RU)	24–33%		
Free thyroxine index	4.4–9.4		
Thyroid-stimulating hormone (TSH)			
Thyrotropin-releasing hormone-stimulation test (TRH)			

Pregnancy Test

The placenta produces measurable amounts of human chorionic gonadotropic (HCG) as early as 14 days after conception. The common test is designed to detect the subunit β-HCG.

Urinalysis

The basic urinalysis is a means of detecting various properties of urine, including pH and specific gravity, as well as the presence of glucose, ketones, blood (red and white cells), and protein. The presence of these may indicate specific physiologic disruptions. Urinary symptoms such as dysuria and polyuria are indications for a urinalysis.

Porphyrins and Porphobilinogens

In healthy persons, insignificant amounts of porphyrin (a hemoglobin precursor) are excreted in the urine. However, in certain conditions such as porphyria, an inbred error of hemoglobin synthesis, levels are elevated.

Acute intermittent porphyria usually presents with abdominal pain followed by neurologic and psychiatric syptoms. The psychiatric presentation is often the initial one and may range from anxiety and depression to frank delirium, coma, and death. The acute but chronically intermittent symptoms may predispose to a histrionic presentation, and the diagnosis may be missed (7).

Neuropsychiatric manifestations are evaluated by qualitative assay of porphobilinogen in urine. The presence of porphobilinogen is pathognomonic for porphyria, and quantitative 24-hour levels may be 20- to 200-fold greater than normal levels (8). Patients with positive results require referral to a hematologist for full evaluation.

Urinary Metabolites

The evaluation of serotonin and norepinephorine metabolites in urine is currently being used in research on affective disorders and schizophrenia (see Chapters 3, 31, and 38).

In addition, evaluations of 24-hour urine assays for total metanephrines and vanillylmandelic acid, a catecholamine metabolite, may be useful in diagnosing pheochromocytoma, which can present with a variety of somatic symptoms associated with anxiety (see Chapter 18).

Myoglobin

Myoglobin is a breakdown product of muscle catabolism. In conditions of excessive muscle breakdown, such as neuroleptic malignant syndrome, myoglobin may be detectable in the urine. Its detection may be an ominous sign, sometimes indicating acute renal failure.

Electrocardiogram

The electrocardiogram (EKG) is a useful but generally nonspecific evaluation of cardiac status. Disturbances of rate, rhythm, and function may be apparent. An EKG may be helpful in patients with known cardiac history, smokers, patients over 40, and those presenting with symptoms of cardiac disease such as chest pain, palpitations, and syncope.

In patients with suspected arrhythmias, especially those in whom antidepressant therapy is considered, a continuous EKG reading may be obtained via a 24-hour Holter monitor. The EKG may also be useful in distinguishing the precordial distress of acute anxiety from arrhythmias. In addition it is also used as a baseline and monitoring test for patients being treated with cardiotoxic agents.

Chest Roentgenogram

In patients with a history of pulmonary disease, smoking, environmental exposures, or primary pulmonary symptoms (dyspnea, tachypnea, cough, wheezing), particularly with weight loss, a chest x-ray is recommended.

Neurologic Screening Tests
Electroencephalogram

The electroencephalogram (EEG) measures electrical activity of the brain. Abnormal EEGs have been noted in seizure disorders, toxic/metabolic derangements, CNS degenerative diseases, CNS inflammatory conditions, and with cerebrovascular lesions. Standard EEGs are being used by many clinicians to differentiate organic illnesses from functional illnesses, such as the assessment of dementia and delirium. Recent research suggests alterations in the EEG patterns of some schizophrenics, and extensive work has been done evaluating alterations of the EEG sleep patterns of patients with affective disorders. For example, a shortened rapid eye movement latency period may be a useful biologic marker for depression.

A recent and promising development in the use of the EEG, called brain electrical activity mapping (BEAM), uses a computer to transform EEG and evoked-potential data into multicolored maps of the brain. It is hoped that BEAM wil be useful in the investigation of various neurologic and psychiatric conditions without the radiation risk of positron emission and computerized tomographic scans. This technique is mainly used for research (2).

Computerized Tomographic Scan of the Head

Computerized tomography makes use of differences in tissue densities to identify structural abnormalities in the brain. Brain masses, abscesses, ventricular size and displacement, hemorrhage, swelling, and other changes can be detected. Possible indications for computerized tomographic scanning include dementias and movement disorders of unknown etiologies, initial presentations of psychosis, anorexia nervosa, prolonged catatonia, and initial presentation of affective disorders or personality changes after age 50 (9).

TOXICOLOGY STUDIES

The presentation of confusional states or other acute psychotic behaviors in previously healthy patients requires full evaluation for toxic agents. Besides the common presentation of alcohol intoxication, various other "street drugs" have been implicated in acute changes in mental status. Thus, an effective toxicology screen is quite useful to psychiatrists as well as to emergency room physicians. Their use, however, is fraught with problems of limited sensitivity and specificity, practicability and cost.

There are two commonly used methods in toxicology laboratory testing. The first are immunoassays, which use antibody–antigen reactions to detect drugs. The second are chromotography tests, which include thin-layer chromotography (TLC), high-performance liquid chromotography (HPLC), and gas chromotography usually used in combination with a mass spectrometry system (GC-MS). The standard toxicology screen used in most laboratories is the TLC. Its usefulness is limited, however, for several reasons. First, the sample often must be sent to a reference laboratory where results may not be available for 24 hours. Second, although its specificity is extremely high (95–99%), as are all the toxicology tests, it has poor sensitivity. Third, many commonly abused drugs, e.g., phencyclidine, marijuana, and tetra hydro cannabinol, and newer antidepressants may not be included in routine toxicology screens. Fourth, the assay needs to be done by a very experienced technician. Finally, TLC does not identify some drugs in low or even therapeutic ranges. Thus, some drugs that can cause neuropsychiatric symptoms at these doses may well be missed.

Immunoassays, as a rule, are more sensitive but less specific than TLC; that is they have less false negatives but cross-react with other substances and therefore have more false positives.

The GC-MS and HPLC tests use chromotography to separate compounds, followed by spectrometry to identify the fragments. These are the most sensitive and specific tests and are therefore recommended if available. However, they both require extensive sample preparation and are quite expensive.

The clinical circumstances are important in effectively utilizing these screens. Knowledge of common street drugs in the local area will often help direct the investigation. Identification of prescription drugs used by patients is also helpful. In general, the likelihood of a true positive assessment by toxicology screen is greatly enhanced by asking for specific agents.

Whereas a comprehensive drug evaluation includes screening for opiates, barbiturates, alcohol, amphetamines, benzodiazepines, methadone, phencyclidine, cocaine and cannabinoids, particular neuropsychiatric symptoms may suggest a more narrowed search. Psychotic patients with or without manic presentations should be tested for amphetamines, barbiturates, cocaine, alcohol, opiates, and phencyclidine. Depressed patients require tests for benzodiazepines, barbiturates, and alcohol.

The clinician should use the toxicology screen knowledgeably but with caution. Negative results do not mean the patient has not been abusing that drug. Low levels on a routine toxicology screen may not be detected. The drug may be quickly metabolized (e.g., cocaine), or the symptoms may represent drug withdrawal.

TESTING OF ORGAN FUNCTIONING FOR PATIENTS RECEIVING PSYCHIATRIC MEDICATIONS

All psychiatric medications have effects on organ systems outside of the central nervous system. Some of these effects may be serious or even fatal. Patients with known disorders of these organ systems as well as patients at increased risk for medical illness, such as the elderly, may require extensive evaluation of that organ system as well as consultation with a medical physician before proceeding with treatment. For women who have even a small chance of being pregnant, a pregnancy test should be obtained because of the possibility of teratogenicity. When monitoring of the status of a particular organ system is important, pretreatment as well as periodic monitoring may be indicated.

There are wide variations among authorities as to whether, and under what conditions, baseline testing and subsequent monitoring should be performed. We present, wherever possible, the consensus or the range of recommendations.

Lithium

The organ systems most seriously affected by lithium salts are renal, thyroid, and cardiac.

Renal

Potential renal effects include persistent polyuria and polydipsia, nephrogenic diabetes insipidus (inability to concentrate urine), increased sodium excretion, and permanent structural changes (10). Many clinicians suggest pretherapy renal studies including electrolytes, BUN/creatinine, and a 24-hour urine volume. Some recommend a 24-hour creatinine clearance as a more sensitive indicator of renal function than a single creatinine level. Others recommend a 12-hour dehydration test to assess baseline concentrating capacity as well as urinalysis. Tests conducted during maintenance therapy are essentially the same as the initial tests and are commonly carried out on a yearly basis. If testing suggests renal damage, more thorough renal evaluation is recommended.

Thyroid

Lithium inhibits several steps in the production of thyroxine by the thyroid gland. Approximately 30% of patients on lithium have elevated TSH levels, and 5% show signs of hypothyroidism. An initial assessment should include TSH levels and a free thyroxine index. These should be assessed on a regular basis. Some authors recommend TRH stimulation tests as a more sensitive indicator.

Cardiac

Although adverse cardiovascular reactions to lithium are unusual, they may include T-wave flattening or inversion on EKG, first-degree A-V block, sinus arrhythmias, increased premature ventricular contractions, congestive heart failure, and ventricular tachycardia, even with normal doses. Toxic effects include atrial fibrillation, and second- or third-degree A-V block. A baseline EKG is recommended with yearly follow-up.

Tricyclic Antidepressants

The major effects of tricyclic antidepressants (TCAs) that require laboratory monitoring are on the cardiovascular system. In addition, rare but potential agranulocytosis and hepatic effects should be considered for assessment.

Cardiovascular

Tricyclic antidepressants in therapeutic doses are generally safe and may even exert corrective effects on certain arrythmias. However, in excessive doses, especially in the elderly and in patients with certain kinds of cardiac disease TCAs may cause a variety of reactions, including postural hypotension, tachycardia, congestive heart failure, arrhythmias, and even sudden death. Changes in EKG at normal blood levels include Q-T prolongation, T-wave flattening or inversion, and tachycardia. Toxic levels may induce P-R and QRS widening, ST depression, A-V block, frequent PVCs, and interventricular conduction defects. A baseline EKG is commonly obtained, particularly in patients over age 40 or with a previous history of cardiac disease.

Hepatic

Tricyclic antidepressants may rarely cause a hypersensitivity reaction, leading to liver toxicity. Baseline and intermittent liver function tests are suggested by some authorities.

Hematologic

Tricyclic antidepressants rarely cause agranulocytosis. Some clinicians suggest baseline and maintenance CBCs.

Carbamazepine

Carbamazepine is structurally similar to the TCAs, and the same indications for laboratory monitoring should apply. How-

ever, an additional consideration for carbamazepine is the complication of aplastic anemia, as well as leukopenia, agranulocytosis and thrombocytopenia. Because these are potentially life-threatening complications, many clinicians recommend regular CBC, platelet, and reticulocyte counts. Testing may occur as frequently as weekly for the first 3 months of treatment and every 2 to 3 months thereafter.

Monoamine Oxidase Inhibitors

The monoamine oxidase inhibitors (MAOIs) can produce serious reactions, many of which resemble tricyclic effects. Severe hypertension, hyperthermia, and hypertonic reactions may also be observed.

Cardiovascular

At normal doses, MAOIs may produce orthostatic hypotension, tachycardia, and palpitations. Marked hypertension occasionally occurs at normal doses, but more commonly at high doses when combined with sympathomimetic agents, TCAs, or high-tyramine diets. Many other agents, including over-the-counter preparations, may lead to hypertensive states. The reader is referred to standard pharmacological resources for a complete list of food and drugs to be avoided. Guidelines for baseline and follow-up EKGs are similar to those for the TCAs.

Hepatic

Direct hepatotoxicity rarely occurs with MAOI. Some clinicians order routine baseline and maintenance liver function tests.

Antipsychotics

The organ systems affected by antipsychotic drugs that require laboratory evaluation are essentially the same as for TCAs, although the cardiac effects are less pronounced and the hepatic and hematologic effects more common. Baseline and maintenance EKG, CBC, and liver functions are recommended by some authorities.

Benzodiazepines

The benzodiazepines have not been noted to have any long-term adverse effects on any organ systems, although their potential for addiction and subsequent withdrawal is well known. There are no specific recommendations for baseline testing.

Disulfiram (Antabuse)

Disulfiram, a common treatment for chronic alcoholic patients, has a potential for serious liver toxicity and failure. All patients, on disulfuram should, therefore, have baseline liver functions tests, with a repeat assessment 10 to 14 days after initiation of therapy and every 3 to 6 months thereafter.

BLOOD LEVEL MONITORING OF PSYCHIATRIC MEDICATIONS

Plasma levels of psychotropic agents have two functions: to monitor toxicity and to maximize clinical response. The routine use for the latter function is an area of significant controversy in outpatient psychiatry. Of the major psychotropic agents, lithium and carbamazepine are the only ones for which there is general agreement that plasma level monitoring is essential in all patients. The use of plasma levels for maximizing clinical response for some of the TCAs clearly has value in many clinical situations. The value of plasma levels in other TCAs, MAOIs, neuroleptics, and benzodiazepines is controversial at best, and unsupported at worst. Before reviewing the various classes of medications, we shall review the general concepts of plasma levels and half-lives, toxicity, and technical problems in the interpretation of plasma levels.

General Concepts
Plasma Levels and Half-Lives

A plasma level reflects a quantity of free drug measurable at that point in time and is the function of absorption, metabolism, volume of distribution, and excretion. Of major interest in assessing plasma levels is the drug's half-life, which is the length of time needed to eliminate half the drug from the plasma. Drugs that are rapidly metabolized and excreted have short half-lives (1 to 4 hours), and drugs that are highly lipid soluble and thus only gradually released into the plasma have long half-lives (days). When a drug is in equilibrium between the intracellular and plasma compartments, it is said to be at a steady state, and it will essentially remain at that level as long as dosing requirements remain unchanged. Steady-state levels are obtained after a stable dosage has been taken for about five half-lives of that particular drug. Any level monitoring done prior to five half-lives may give false information regarding steady-state levels.

Toxicity

There is a level at which every drug becomes toxic to organs that accumulate it, usually the brain, liver, heart, and/or kidneys. Medications for which mean toxic levels are close to mean therapeutic levels, such as lithium and the tricyclic agents, are said to have a low therapeutic index. Medications in which the therapeutic range is far lower than its toxic range are said to have a high therapeutic index. With such medications, obtaining plasma levels to check for toxicity is usually unnecessary except for overdoses.

In certain populations, the absorption, metabolism, or excretion of drugs may be altered so as to produce toxic levels with usual therapeutic dosages. Geriatric patients may have higher levels than younger patients on the same dose of medications because of degenerative liver and renal disease. Patients with liver or renal disease may have significantly increased levels for the same reasons. Dehydration in patients treated with lithium may increase the risk of toxicity. Certain drug interactions may markedly increase the plasma level. For example, the addition of phenothiazines may raise the plasma level of a TCA.

The monitoring of plasma levels may help prevent toxicity. Systemic signs and symptoms of toxicity, especially of a cardiovascular nature, require plasma levels assessment. Also, the clinician must be aware that toxicity may mimic the underlying disorder. For example, toxic levels of nortriptyline frequently worsen depression while being misinterpreted as inadequate therapy. Finally, there may be a role for high-dose TCA in treatment-resistant depression, in which plasma level monitoring to prevent toxicity is recommended.

Technical Problems in the Interpretation of Plasma Levels

Problems in interpretation of the plasma levels may lead to incorrect conclusions and potentially serious consequences. Particular pitfalls are common and should be recognized and avoided.

In drugs with intermediate half-lives, including lithium, carbamazepine and TCAs, standard plasma levels should be drawn 10 to 14 hours after the last regular dosage. This is most easily done by drawing an early morning level, about 12 hours after patient's evening dose. Confusing levels may arise when the patient's blood is drawn outside the set time limits, or when the patient takes his or her morning dose prior to blood drawing. Patients should be carefully instructed on these points.

Errors in TCA levels may also occur as a result of incorrect collection systems. Numerous studies have demonstrated significantly elevated levels when specimens are collected in "vacutainer" systems. This can be avoided by use of tris-butoxethyl vacutainer tubes or the "Venoject" blood collection system.

The use of a dependable laboratory is critical. While lithium and carbamazepine levels are usually quite accurate, TCA levels may vary considerably depending on the method of laboratory determination. The physician who uses plasma levels should establish the reliability and efficiency of his or her laboratory.

Specific Medications

Lithium

Lithium has a very low therapeutic index. Its half-life is approximately 24 hours but can be much longer in geriatric patients or those with impaired renal function. Because of the seriousness of lithium toxicity, the suggested recommendation for plasma levels monitoring is approximately 2 to 3 days after each dosage change, particularly when initiating treatment. In outpatients lithium may be initiated more gradually and thus tested less often. A steady-state level may be obtained 5 to 7 days after stable dosage is reached. Once the patient is stable, level monitoring may be gradually decreased to every 3 to 4 months. Change in psychiatric presentation or symptoms suggestive of toxicity require plasma level assessment.

Tricyclic Antidepressants

Tricyclics have a low therapeutic index, as stated above. The mean half-life ranges from a low of approximately 16 hours for imipramine to a high of 80 hours for protriptyline (see Table 15.2). As a rule, the common tertiary amines (amitriptyline, imipramine, and doxepin) have 12 to 16 hours of half-life, and the common secondary amines (desipramine and nortriptyline) have at least 30-hour half-lives.

The importance of monitoring plasma levels of TCAs to maximize clinical response is a subject of considerable debate. At this time, only imipramine, nortriptyline, and, to a lesser extent, desipramine, appear to have consistent data supporting a relationship between plasma level measurements and clinical outcome. With nortriptyline, there appears to be a therapeutic window (a plasma level range of 50 to 150 ng/ml) outside of which a poor clinical response is likely to occur. Imipramine and desipramine have been shown to have linear or sigmoidal response curves with a therapeutic range but no drop-off in antidepressant response above this range. Investigations on the relationship between plasma level measurements and clinical outcome with amitriptyline offer contractory results. There are inadequate data on the other antidepressants.

Where plasma level measurements are related to clinical outcome, this test is useful for the following clinical situations: in patients who do not respond clinically to the usual oral doses, in patients who do respond clinically in order to determine whether they are slow metabolizers who may be on unnecessarily high doses, in high-risk patients who should be treated with the lowest possible effective dose, and where there is an urgency to reach therapeutic levels in the shortest possible time, such as with severely depressed patients.

The application of these results and recommendations to outpatient practice suffers from the following problem. Outpatient studies of the relationship of plasma levels to clinical response commonly show no clinical relationship. This is presumably the result of the vast majority of studies on TCAs involving inpatient populations, where the incidence of major or endogenous depression is higher than in outpatient populations. In this population, the clinical response to TCAs is better established. In outpatient studies the clinical population of depressed patients is presumably more heterogeneous (11, 12).

Carbamazepine

It is generally accepted that the maintenance of carbamazepine levels between 0.6 and 1.2 mg/ml is necessary in its use as an anticonvulsant. Most clinicians now believe that these plasma levels are also correlated with good clinical response in affective disorders. Initial half-lives can be lengthy (25 to 65 hours), but with chronic treatment half-lives usually decrease to at least 12 hours, since carbamazepine induces liver enzymes in its own breakdown. Therefore, initial doses may need to be increased to maintain the same therapeutic levels.

Monoamine Oxidase Inhibitors

While plasma level monitoring has not been shown to be useful with MAOIs, several studies have demonstrated that measurable activity of MAOIs has been correlated with response. That is, platelet inhibition greater than 80% correlates with clinical improvement. In patients who have poor responses, a low platelet inhibi-

tion may indicate need for an increase in dosage.

Antipsychotics

Over the past several years, much clinical research has attempted to identify a therapeutic range for antipsychotic drugs, in hopes of improving the efficacy of treatment. Some initial studies have shown a relationship between serum levels and therapeutic response, but most studies have failed to replicate this. No clear therapeutic range, therefore, exists for this class of drugs.

Measurement of levels may be useful in demonstrating compliance, which is a common issue in the treatment of schizophrenia. However, even several weeks of noncompliance may not be demonstrable because of lengthy half-lives of most antipsychotics.

Antipsychotics have a high therapeutic index, and therefore toxicity is of minimal concern beyond side effects, except with overdose. The relationship of plasma levels of antipsychotic agents to tardive dyskinesia and other neurologic sequelae has not been established. Currently, investigators are exploring this relationship.

Table 15.2   Half-Lives and Plasma Levels of Common Psychiatric Medications

Drug	Approx. Half-Life (hr)	Typical Plasma Levels
Antidepressants		
Imipramine	16	200–300 ng/ml
Amitriptyline	16	100–250 ng/ml
Doxepin	16	100–250 ng/ml
Desipramine	22	100–250 ng/ml
Nortriptyline	24	50–150 nl/ml
Protriptyline	126	100–250 ng/ml
Trazodone	5	800–1600 ng/ml
Lithium	22 ± 8	0.6–1.2 mEq/l
Carbamazepine	12–30	4–10 mg/l
Antipsychotics		
Chlorpromazine	5–16	100–600 ng/ml
Thioridazine	7–42	100–800 ng/ml
Fluphenazine	15–24	?
Perphenazine	8–21	?
Thiothixene	34	10–150 ng/ml
Haloperidol	13–36	2–260 ng/ml

Based on data from Baldessarini RJ: *Chemotherapy in Psychiatry.* Cambridge MA, Harvard University Press, 1985, pp 35, 97, 141.

DIAGNOSING AND MONITORING PSYCHIATRIC DISORDERS

During the past decade, there has been increasing hope that the laboratory would provide objective data for the diagnosis and monitoring of psychiatric disorders and for the selection of treatments. In this section we review laboratory tests from three areas of research that have been the topic of active discussion as holding future promise. The first is neuroendocrine research, the second is neurotransmitter research, and the third is visual brain imaging research. None of these tests currently have the proved value to be applied to routine outpatient practice.

Neuroendocrine Testing

Dexamethasone Suppression Test

Ever since Harvey Cushing described the high incidence of depressive features in patients with adrenal hyperfunction in 1932, researchers have investigated the connection between the hypothalamic–pituitary–adrenal axis and affective disorders. Cortisol secretion is suppressed in normal subjects when given dexamethasone, an exogenous steroid. In standard protocols of the dexamethasone suppression test (DST) patients are given either 1 or 2 mg of dexamethasone at 11:00 PM. Cortisol levels are assessed the next day at 4:00 PM and 11:00 PM (usually only 4:00 PM in outpatient practice). A normal response is suppression of cortisol, while an abnormal response is nonsuppression. Initial studies indicated a high rate of endogenous depression in patients with nonsuppression (90%), and a low rate of nonsuppression in patients without depression (10%). However, recent studies suggested the low sensitivity (30–70%) in depressed patients hampers the utility of the DST as a screening tool.

Many factors other than depression influence DST response. Nonsuppression has been noted in a variety of conditions including increased age, malnutrition, weight loss, dementia, mania, cerebrovascular accident, alcohol, withdrawal, and severe medical illness. Various drugs, including high-dose estrogens, barbiturates, TCAs, hypnotics, and anticonvulsants may cause nonsuppression (false positive), while high-dose benzodiazepine treatment may lead to false negative results.

Attempts have been made to find greater predictive value for the DST. It has been suggested that the test may be used to differentiate various subsets of depression (unipolar vs. bipolar, endogenous vs. exogenous, primary vs. secondary, psychotic vs. nonpsychotic), to predict responses to somatic therapy, and to monitor prognosis and long-term consequences. While many of the studies have shown statistically significant results, the low sensitivity renders the DST test inadequate as a screening or monitoring tool. There is however, good preliminary evidence that persistent DST nonsuppression in treated patients may indicate poorer long-term prognosis, with a significantly higher incidence of suicide, despite clinical improvement (1).

Thyrotropin-Releasing Hormone Stimulation Test

Thyrotropin-releasing hormone is secreted by the hypothalamus, stimulating the pituitary to release TSH, which in turn stimulates the production of T_3 and T_4 in the thyroid gland. As noted previously, affective disorders have been related to thyroid dysfunction. Many researchers believe that some depressed patients with normal thyroid function tests may have a subclinical hypothyroidism discernible by a TRH stimulation test. The test consists of a 0.5 mg infusion of TRH in the morning to a fasting, recumbent patient. Levels of TSH are taken prior to infusion and at intervals of 15 to 30 minutes after infusion up to 90 minutes. A positive test is defined as a change in TSH of less than 5–7 mIU/ml.

Research has demonstrated a positive test in 25 to 35% of depressed patients, but seldom in normal patients. When combined with DST results, predictive value is reportedly higher. Some investigators have also suggested its utility in separating unipolar from bipolar depression. However, blunted responses have been noted in alcoholism, mania, eating disorders, the elderly, and patients with renal failure. The low sensitivity and specificity of the TRH stimulation test thus limit its usefulness in outpatient settings.

Neurotransmitter Metabolites

Studies of metabolites of norepinephrine and serotonin have grown out of the research on TCA receptor binding. Initial studies indicated decreased levels of 3-methoxy-4-hydroxyphenylglycol (MHPG), the principal metabolite of norepinephrine, and 5-hydroxyindoleacetic acid (5-HIAA), the principal metabolite of serotonin, in depressed patients. Subsequent data, however, have been inconsistent, and no clinical differences in the subgroups, or correlations to treatment response, have been consistently demonstrated. There are some data that suggest a relationship between low central nervous system 5-HIAA levels and increased risk of suicide. The utility of these tests in clinical practice has not yet been demonstrated.

Visual Brain Imaging Techniques

Studies of brain metabolism have attempted to define reproducible differences in various psychiatric disorders compared with normal subjects. *Regional cerebral blood flow* uses radioactive xenon to study changes in certain cortical and subcortical areas. *Positron emission tomography* scanning makes use of cerebral glucose utilization during periods of specific brain activity. Although preliminary data from these techniques suggest specific abnormalities in schizophrenia, with both frontal cortex and subcortical changes, these data have been challenged by some. Both of these visual brain imaging techniques remain experimental in the evaluation of psychiatric illness. *Magnetic resonance imaging* is a relatively new imaging technique that provides high-resolution structural information about the brain as well as quantitative assessment of functional change. It holds considerable promise not only for research but as a diagnostic instrument.

CONCLUSIONS

The inclusion of sections on laboratory testing in textbooks is due in large part to the excitement over drug monitoring and the possibility of determining markers for mental disorders. It is an interesting paradox, therefore, that in our review of the use of the laboratory, the traditional use of the laboratory is far more important clinically than these newer uses of the laboratory. By traditional laboratory use, we refer to the assessment of medical illness in psychiatric patients, i.e., testing for organic disease, toxicology studies, and the use of the lab for baseline testing of organs affected by psychiatric medications. With hindsight, such material should have appeared in textbooks of psychiatry much sooner. The newer uses of the laboratory in clinical psychiatry, particularly drug monitoring, have value. But the importance of diagnostic markers is still a hope for the future.

The clinical decision as to the use of the laboratory presents a second paradox. The uninformed clinician may seriously underuse the laboratory as a result of lack of knowledge as to what testing has to offer. He or she may also overuse the laboratory by indiscriminately ordering tests. The informed clinician knows the use and the limitations of the laboratory and can perform a careful clinical assessment that will lead to its judicious use. In this sense the clinical challenge of the psychiatrist is similar to that of the medical physician.

References

1. Stahl SM, Kravitz KD: A critical review of the use of laboratory tests in psychiatric disorders. In Berger PA, Keith H, Brodie H (eds): *American Handbook of Psychiatry: Vol. 8. Biological Psychiatry.* New York, Basic Books, 1986, pp 1048–1084.
2. Mackinnon RA, Yudofsky SC: *The Psychiatric Evaluation in Clinical Practice.* Philadelphia, J.B. Lippincott, 1986.
3. Martin RL, Preskorn SH: Use of the laboratory in psychiatry. In Winokur G, Clayton PJ (eds): *The Medical Basis of Psychiatry.* Philadelphia, W.B. Saunders, 1986.
4. Pottash ALC, Gold MS, Exstein I: The use of the clinical laboratory. In Sederer LI (ed): *Inpatient*

Psychiatry: Diagnosis and Treatment. Baltimore, Williams & Wilkins, 1986.

5. Spratt DI, Pont A, Miller MB et al: Hyperthyroxinemia in patients with acute psychiatric disorders. *Am J Med* 63:41–48, 1982.
6. Kramlinger KG, Gharib H: Normal serum thyroxine values in patients with acute psychiatric illness. *Am J Med* 76:799–801, 1984.
7. Barkowsky H, Schady W: Neurologic manifestations of acute porphyria. *Seminars in Liver Disease* 2(2):108–124, 1982.
8. Bissell MD: Laboratory evaluation in porphyria. *Seminars in Liver Disease* 2(2):100–101, 1982.
9. Weinberger DR: Brain disease and psychiatric illness: when should a psychiatrist order a CAT scan? *Am J Psychiatry* 141:1521–1527, 1984.
10. Bennett DR (ed): Drugs used inaffective disorders. in *AMA Drug Evaluation*, ed. 5. Chicago, American Medical Association, 1983.
11. Task Force on the Use of Laboratory Tests in Psychiatry: Tricyclic antidepressants—blood level measurements and clinical outcome: an APA task force report. *Am J Psychiatry* 142:155–162, 1985.
12. Glassman AH, Schildkraut JJ, Cooper TB, et al: Tricyclic antidepressants: blood level measurements and clinical response, in Berger PA, Keith H, Brodie H (eds): *American Handbook of Psychiatry: Vol. 8. Biological Psychiatry.* New York, Basic Books, 1986, pp 373–385.

Suggested Readings

Baldessarini RJ: *Chemotherapy in Psychiatry.* Cambridge, MA, Harvard University Press, 1985.

Bassuk EL, Schoonover SC, Gelenberg AJ: *The Practitioner's Guide to Psychoactive Drugs,* New York, Plenum, 1983.

Daul SG: Plasma level monitoring of antipsychotic drugs—clinical utility. *Clinical Pharmacokinetics* 11:36–61, 1986.

Fischbach FT: *A Manual of Diagnostic Tests.* Philadelphia, J.B. Lippincott, 1980.

Freeman MC, Hoffman AR, Klausner RD, et al: *Medicine.* Philadelphia, J. B. Lippincott, 1981.

Giannini AS, Black HR, Goettsche RL: *Psychiatric, Psychogenic, and Somatopsychic Disorders Handbook.* Garden City, NY, Medical Examination Publishing, 1978.

Hall RCW: *Psychiatric Presentations of Medical Illness.* Jamaica, NY, Spectrum Publications, 1980.

Isselbacher KS, Adams RD, Braunwald E, et al: *Harrison's Principles of Internal Medicine,* ed. 9. New York, McGraw-Hill, 1980.

Kochar MS: *Textbook of General Medicine.* New York, John Wiley & Sons, 1983.

Schou M: *Lithium Treatment of Manic–Depressive Illness: A Practical Guide.* New York, Karger, 1980.

16

Psychologic Testing for Mental Disorders

William Vogel, Ph.D.

A HISTORICAL PERSPECTIVE

The role of the psychologist as a test examiner has changed dramatically since the 1940s. During the period immediately after World War II, psychologists who worked with patients in psychiatric treatment settings were primarily occupied with patient assessment by means of formal testing procedures. In many psychiatric inpatient settings and outpatient psychiatric units, all patients were routinely given a battery of psychologic tests as part of the intake procedure in order to obtain, as a psychiatrist colleague of mine put it, "an x-ray of the innermost recesses of the personality." During that period, many psychologists and other mental health workers had profound faith in the predictive power and the practical benefits of psychological test assessments. Psychologists were asked questions that only much later were understood to be inherently unanswerable, e.g., "What is this patient's potential for suicide?"

Starting in the 1960s, however, and continuing for some time into the 1970s, routine psychologic testing of patients became much less common. The consensus of opinion among psychologists came to be that routine assessment of patients by psychologic tests was not cost-effective in re-

gard to professional time, the financial cost to the patient, or the practical applicability of the results that were being obtained (1, 2). Further, the psychology testing movement came under severe scrutiny from the general public and the profession itself. Questions were raised as to whether the tests in widespread use incorporated cultural biases against women, minorities, and those with little education (3). Even more to the point, questions were raised as to the degree to which the tests were able to assess or predict the very behaviors they were specifically designed to assess or predict, e.g., academic performance (4, 5), job performance (6), or diagnoses and treatment outcome (1, 2).

By the mid-1970s, routine formal assessment by psychologic test procedures had become a rarity in most clinical settings, in part because of the issues discussed above and in part because psychologists had assumed much broader professional roles as psychotherapists, research scientists, industrial consultants, rehabilitative and educational specialists, etc.

Nevertheless, formal assessment of patients by clinical psychologic tests remained an important part of every well-trained psychologist's armamentarium. The testing came to be much more specific in purpose, as in questions of differential

227

diagnosis. In addition, new subspecialties of clinical testing evolved to deal with clinical problems in the areas of neuropsychologic impairment, forensic psychology, and rehabilitative medicine.

CURRENT USE OF PSYCHOLOGIC TESTS IN PSYCHIATRY

At present, psychologic tests are generally used to answer specific questions about specific patients that cannot be answered by clinical interview. Thus, patients might be referred for a differential diagnosis when that decision cannot be made on the basis of several interviews, for a forensic psychologic evaluation to determine competence as part of a pretrial evaluation, or for a clinical–educational evaluation to determine if a learning-disabled patient could benefit from a particular curriculum.

In making the referral, the psychologist and the referring agency must keep in mind the question of cost-effectiveness for the patient, as well as for the provider. Psychologic testing is expensive in terms of time and money. From the patient's point of view, a full battery of psychologic tests can cost between $500 and $1,000. That same amount of money could be used to pay for 10 to 20 treatment sessions. If the patient is an outpatient, and dependent on medical insurance, then under the terms of many insurance policies the psychologic testing alone might exhaust the patient's mental health outpatient insurance benefits for the year. Consequently, the decison to refer a patient for psychologic testing is not to be made lightly. As a practical matter, routine psychologic testing of adult psychiatric patients is far more common on inpatient services (where the costs are usually covered by the patients' hospitalization insurance) than on outpatient services.

CHARACTERISTICS OF PSYCHOLOGIC TESTS

The term *test* implies a standardized procedure, i.e., a procedure that is identical for all persons who are given the test. All examinees are presented with the same test material, with the same test instructions, and the answers are scored and interpreted according to the same pre-established criteria. The criteria are usually established by previous testing of a *standardization sample*, i.e., a large group of persons who share the same characteristics as the persons who are to be evaluated by the test.

In order to have usefulness, a test should be *reliable,* i.e., should yield stable results. *Test–retest reliability* involves giving examinees a test and then retesting them later in order to determine whether the text gives comparable results. A test–retest measure of reliability is appropriate to use when the characteristic to be assessed is presumed to be relatively stable over time, e.g., IQ score. It is not applicable when the variable to be assessed is known to be unstable and to fluctuate with time, e.g., assessment of depression in a group of acute psychiatric patients. *Interjudge reliability* of a test is appropriate to assess when the test involves the use of subjective judgment on the part of the test scorer. For example, on the Rorschach test, the psychologist employs systematic rules to score and interpret the test. It is essential that the rules be specific enough so that psychologists, trained in the use of the test, can be in agreement over the scores they obtain and the interpretations they make. Interjudge reliability provides an index as to the degree of such agreement.

Split-half reliability is a measure of the internal consistency of a test. For example, on the Wechsler Adult Intelligence Scale (WAIS), items within each subtest are presented to the subject in order of increasing difficulty. If within each subtest the items are divided into even- and odd-numbered items, the test results obtained with the even-number list should theoretically be identical with the results obtained with the odd-number list. Split-half reliability provides an index of the degree of such agreement.

The *validity* of a test is the extent to which the test measures what it purports to measure. How do we know, for example, that a test that we have labeled an "intelligence test" assesses "intelligent" behavior? The first step is to establish the test's *content validity,* i.e., the extent to which the test measures the full range of target behaviors.

Predictive validity and *concurrent validity* are measures of the degree to which the test relates to behavior; e.g., one would expect an intelligence test to predict (in the sense of relate to) academic performance, learning ability, occupational success, life achievement, etc. Similarly, scores on a test meant to select among candidates competing for promotion from a lower to a higher position in an organization should be related to job performance in the higher position. Challenges to such tests by women or members of minority groups are often made on the grounds of the test's poor predictive or poor concurrent validity, e.g., the tests do not measure or are not relevant to job performance.

Finally, *construct* validity is a measure of the degree to which the test measures a given trait. The construct validity of a test is established by determining how well it relates to other tests or measures that are accepted and established indicators of the behavior in question.

The relationship between reliability and validity is complex. Some of the most useful test devices in clinical psychology (e.g., the Rorschach Inkblot test and the Minnesota Multiphasic Personality Inventory [MMPI]) are, on the weight of the evidence, unquestionably valid for the clinical purposes for which they are generally employed. However, assessing the reliability of the devices can be highly complicated because of the fluctuating mental states of the acutely ill mentally patients who are most often given the tests.

STANDARD PSYCHIATRIC TEST BATTERY FOR ADULTS

Most psychologists do not use tests singly, but rather employ them in a battery. In testing adult psychiatric patients, there are several commonly employed tests: (*a*) the WAIS, (*b*) the Rorschach Inkblot test, (*c*) the Thematic/Apperception Test (TAT), (*d*) the Bender-Gestalt test; (*e*) figure drawings (in which the subject is asked to draw, free-hand, a person and also sometimes some common objects), (*f*) sentence completion tests, and (*g*) the MMPI.

In using such a battery, the psychologist typically employs each test as a kind of mini-experiment, testing the patient and formulating hypotheses from the test results. The psychologist then confirms or rejects these hypotheses and reformulates new ones while proceeding from test to test. Finally conclusions are reached that embody and are consistent with the results of all of the tests. For example, a psychologist might find that on the WAIS-Revised (WAIS-R), a patient has a high score on the Information subtest, but a relatively low score on the Comprehension subject (which assesses social judgment), a configuration that is common among obsessive–compulsive individuals. The psychologist would first test the hypothesis (of obsessive–compulsive neurosis) by determining if the patient showed other WAIS-R patterns associated with that diagnosis. If that were the case, the psychologist would determine if the patient showed a pervasive pattern of obsessive–compulsive "signs" on other tests, such as the Rorschach.

Should it be warranted on the basis of the results of the testing, the psychologist may decide to give additional tests or may recommend other diagnostic procedures to the referring clinician.

REFERRAL PROCESS

Psychologists most frequently test patients upon referral from psychiatrists. However, referrals may also come from other physicians, other psychologists, or other professionals (e.g., educators, lawyers). The referral process often presents problems to those professionals who are not thoroughly familiar with the nature of psychologic tests. Since most psychiatrists, other physicians, or psychologists request psychologic testing in only a very small proportion of their cases, those that are referred almost invariably present problems that are particularly puzzling or unique. Often the referral question that the psychologist receives is stated in very general terms (e.g., "Request psychometric tests"; "Request psychologic tests for differential diagnosis"; Request IQ testing") that are not useful to the psychologist, who is able to function optimally and be most helpful if the referral question is clearly stated in specific terms. It is best if the psychiatrist or other referral source consults with the psychologist before the formal referral is made in order to help delineate the specific nature of the puzzle the patient presents and determine whether or not psychologic testing is apt to be helpful in the solution of the particular problem.

It is also common for psychologists to receive referrals that raise questions they cannot answer. The largest category of such referrals comprise those that ask the psychologist to predict the patients' future behavior, e.g., "What is the patient's suicide potential?" (i.e., "Is this patient likely to attempt suicide?"); "What is this patient's potential for assaultive behavior?" (i.e.,"Is the patient likely to attack staff or other patients?"); "What is this student's academic potential?" (i.e., "Is this unstable but brilliant young man likely to flunk out of Harvard?"). In general, we psychologists are no better able to predict specific future behaviors of given individuals with our tests than clinicians are able to do using standard interview techniques. The assessment of patient behavior such as suicide and violence is best accomplished by reference to the patient's history and current mental status (see Chapters 29 and 42).

Questions we can reasonably attempt to answer are those that have to do with personality structure: psychopathology, intellectual skills, cognitive style, attitudes, motivation, socialization, interests, aptitudes, emotional life, etc. Using tests, a skilled psychologist should be able to obtain a broader and more complete picture of the patient in a shorter period of time than can be obtained from interview techniques alone.

Once the psychologist and the referral source have jointly determined that the patient should be tested, the referring person should explain to the patient why the referral is being made. Since most patients who are referred for psychological testing are apprehensive about the reason for the referral as well as the examination itself, this discussion should address the patient's anxieties as well as attempt to answer his or her questions. At this time the patient should be assured that the psychologist will set up a posttest meeting in order to discuss the test results with the patient.

PRETEST INTERVIEW

A psychologist should precede test examination of a patient by a careful examination of materials received from the referral source: the patient's mental status and medical, social, and psychiatric history, etc. Next, the psychologist should interview the patient in order to become familiar with the style and characteristics of the patient, so as to better conduct the examination. In addition, it is essential for a successful psychologic test examination that the patient should feel relatively comfortable and at ease with the examiner.

Once, when conducting a research program in a large state school for the mentally retarded, I had occasion to supervise the intelligence testing of a number of the retarded residents. I trained my assistants in my usual procedure, i.e., to hold a pretest session in order to establish rapport with the examinees. The intelligence scores that we subsequently obtained ranged from 10 to 25 points higher than those previously obtained at the school for the same residents. This was puzzling, especially since the usual finding for persons placed in large state institutions for the retarded at the time was for intelligence scores to *decrease* from 1 to 3 points with each year of continued institutionalization (7). Upon investigation, I found that the psychometricians in the school, who were under great pressure to test large numbers of people in a short time, had adopted the practice of beginning the psychologic testing upon meeting the resident, without scheduling any opportunity to establish rapport.

Another reason for the retest interview is to enable the psychologist to experience first hand those aspects of the patient's interview behavior that moved the clinician to make a psychologic referral in the first place.

KINDS OF PSYCHOLOGIC TESTS

Intelligence Tests

The intelligence test most frequently employed by psychologists is the (WAIS-R). The test consists of subtests, divided into Verbal (6 subtests) and Performance (5 subtests) tests. The rationale for this division was to permit assessment of both verbal (language) and nonverbal (cognitive–perceptual-motoric) intellectual aptitude. In fact, however, both Verbal and Performance subtests are mediated by language, although this is less the case for the latter. Wechsler meant each of the verbal tests to assess a particular cognitive function: Information, to assess fund of knowledge, and long-term memory; Comprehension, social judgment; Digits, attention, or short-term memory; Similarities, abstract reasoning; Arithmetic, concentration; Vocabulary, verbal fluency. However, factor analysis indicates that none of the subtests are factorially pure; i.e., none of them assess just a single cognitive function.

It is most important to recognize that psychologists, giving intelligence tests to adult psychiatric patients, are only rarely interested in the IQ score per se. Most often the psychologist is interested in assessing the pattern of intellectual performance in order to determine which functions are well or poorly developed, which are intact and which are impaired. Since most Americans have been in school at least until age 16, and have either been given intelligence tests or tests from which IQ can be esti-

mated, it is often possible to obtain past records for comparison with patients' current performance. Most often, psychologists will use the tests as a diagnostic device; e.g., schizophrenia, depression, obsessive–compulsive and hysterical neuroses, and brain injury are often reflected in intelligence test performance. For example, depressive patients tend to have relatively low scores on nonverbal com pared with verbal subtests; obsessive– compulsive patients tend to give pedantic and overelaborate vocabulary definitions; and schizophrenic patients, in comparison with other diagnostic groups, are often more likely to fail easy items but solve difficult ones.

The question of whether IQ tests are valid measures of intelligence for members of minority groups, women, and low socioeconomic status individuals does not arise in this context, since the psychologist is not primarily interested in comparing the patient to the general population. Rather, the psychologist is interested in the patterning of intellectual ability the person shows relative to that person's own general level of performance (e.g., whether the person shows a selective decrement in memory relative to functioning in other areas), and whether the person shows a change in intellectual performance over time (i.e., a current decrement as compared with the person's own test performance several years ago).

That being said, the question does at times arise as to how the patient's intellectual performance compares with that of the population at large. This comparison must always be made with the greatest caution. For example, I was once asked to examine a young man who had robbed a liquor store (where he was well known) with what was later found to be an unloaded handgun. He took several hundred dollars from the till, leaving several hundred additional dollars that, he said, he "didn't really need." The highly unusual circumstances of the robbery led to his being sent for observation to a state hospital where the psychiatrist referred him for psychometrics in order to rule out mental retardation. I found his IQ to be 64, within the range of mental retardation.

The question of mental retardation, in such a circumstance, is not an academic one. At the time, in the jurisdiction where the young man was arrested, he might, if found guilty, serve no more than 1 year in jail. However, if found "not guilty by reason of insanity" (for legal purposes in that jurisdiction, mental retardation was considered under the same rubric as insanity since both potentially impair one's capacity "to distinguish right from wrong") the man would be sent for an indefinite period to an institution for the criminally insane, until he was either "cured" or until he "no longer represented a danger to the community."

An examination of the test protocol indicated he performed well above the range of mental retardation in non-school-related areas, and within that range in school-related areas. His education was seriously deficient; he had completed less than six grades, all in a one-room schoolhouse in the rural southern United States in which all elementary grades were taught simultaneously. I concluded in my report, citing the facts above, that the man was not mentally retarded. He consequently stood trial as a "competent person."

This case illustrates an assumption that underlies all intelligence testing, i.e., that the persons tested have all had the same opportunity to gain the information and skills that are measured by the intelligence test as the persons who were represented in the test standardization sample did ("the assumption of equal opportunity"). If that assumption is wrong, the test is invalid.

Projective Tests

Projective tests are tests of personality in which the patient must interpret or structure ambiguous stimulus material. This material may be an inkblot, with the patient instructed to tell the examiner "what this might look like to you," or it may be a picture of several people, with the patient instructed to "make up a story" about the picture. The common element in all projective tests is that there is no "right answer" and that patients, in structuring the material, must draw on their own personalities; they must "project" their unique personality attributes into the task.

While the theory of projective testing may be very simply stated and its rationale may seem self-evident, there are, in fact, very complex theoretical issues involved that have to do with the relation of fantasy to behavior. If, for example, a person tells stories laden with achievement themes, or violent themes, may we infer that the person is achievement oriented in life, or that the patient is prone to violence? The evidence indicates no simple, one-to-one relationship between fantasy and behavior. Freud, in fact, argued that the relationship was inverse, that is, that fantasy was compensatory—a means of obtaining in imagination what could not be obtained behaviorally in life (8). There is some experimental evidence to support that view (9). Projective tests may reflect patients' cognitive styles, fantasies, motivations, and attitudes, but any predictive statements made about individual patient behavior on the basis of the patient's fantasy productions should be regarded as strictly inferential.

The best known of the projective tests is the Rorschach test. The test consists of 10 inkblots, all symmetrical, 5 of them colored and 5 of them achromatic. The patient's task is to "say what this might look like to you," and there is no further instruction. After the patient has been given the chance to respond to each of the blots, the examiner inquires, for each of the patients' responses, where in the blot the patient saw the percept (i.e., the location), and what made it look that way, i.e., the determinants. The determinants are the factors that influence patients to make a given response, e.g., color, shape, texture, shading, and apparent movement.

The patients' responses are scored according to any one of several theoretical systems. The basic elements that are scored are the location, determinants, and content (what the patient saw: a human, or animal, a landscape, a map, etc.). In classical Rorschach theory, the crucial factors in interpretation are the location and the determinants of the response, rather than the content. Some of the power of the test undoubtedly derives from the fact that the patient doesn't know what the examiner is looking for and generally assumes that it is the content of the response which is of primary interest to the examiner. Partly for that reason, it is extremely difficult for a naive patient (i.e., one not trained in the use of psychologic tests) to mislead a psychologist by giving manufactured rather than honest responses.

Another factor that makes it difficult for the patient to falsify the test results and mislead the psychologist is that in interpreting the test, the examiner takes *all* of the patient's behavior into account, not just the test responses themselves: the patient's style of approach, way of relating to the examiner, language, test-taking attitude, etc.

The Rorschach has been the subject of more research than any other projective test, and an impressive body of evidence confirms its usefulness as a personality assessment and diagnostic device (10, 11). The problem is that its proper use requires extensive supervised training and clinical experience, so that the usefulness of the test is unquestionably more a function of the skill of the examiner than of any qualities inherent in the test itself. The same criticism, in fact, may be made of all the projective tests.

The TAT (Thematic Apperception Test) consists of a series of 30 pictures, most of which are of one or more people. Usually, however, the clinician uses only 12 to 15 of the cards to examine any given patient, selecting the cards that are appropriate to the age and sex of the patient. The patient is instructed to tell who the person(s) in the card may be and then make up a story about the card, telling (*a*) what is happening, (*b*) what happened in the past to lead up to this, and (*c*) what might happen in the future. The patients' stories are individully interpreted in regard to content: the emotional, motivational, attitudinal, behav-

ioral, and cognitive characteristics of the protagonists, and the other characters in the stories; the nature of the social interactions among the characters; the structural aspects of the stories; etc. Through this analysis, the clinician hopes to be able to obtain a personality description that embodies the unique characteristics of the patient.

A number of scoring systems have been devised to quantitatively assess motivation from the subjects' TAT productions (e.g., need for achievement, need for affiliation, need for sex, need for power) but these motive-scoring systems have been employed in personality research, rather than in day-to-day clinical work.

Other commonly used projective tests include human figure drawing, in which the patient is asked to "draw a person," and then is given another sheet of paper and asked to "draw a person of the opposite sex." The clinician attempts to draw inferences from the tests about the patient's perceptions of "body image," or perceptions of self and of others. The patient's productions may also be analyzed structurally, in order to assess type and degree of psychopathology.

The sentence completion test has many different published versions. The patient is asked to fill in sentences such as "I feel very angry when ___" and "My sex life is ___." This test is used to assess the patients' attitudes and perceptions along a series of dimensions and to assess kind and degree of psychopathology.

Structured Psychologic Tests

The best known, best scientifically established, and most widely used structured clinical psychologic test is the MMPI (12–14). The test consists of 566 items to which the patient is instructed to answer "true" or "false" "as applied to you." The test can be scored quickly by hand, using templates, or can be scored by computer. The items are divided into clinical scales corresponding to clinical categories, e.g., "hypochondriasis," "depression," "hysteria," "psychopathic deviancy," "paranoia," "schizophrenia," and "hypomania," and also into "validity" scales. The validity scales consist of three scales designed to determine whether the person is attempting to project on unrealistically positive self-image (L scale); whether the patient is being guarded and defensive, but in a more subtle manner than would be suggested by on elevated L scale score (K scale); or whether the patient is yielding an invalid record by answering randomly or by attempting to present a bizarrely pathologic self-image, or perhaps simply because of failure to comprehend the items (F scale).

The various scales were all empirically validated, e.g., the items on the schizophrenia scale have been found to differentiate schizophrenic from normal individuals, whether or not the content of the item reflects behavior that clinicians ordinarily regard as reflecting a schizophrenic process. Thus, if the patient answers "true" to the item "During one period when I was a youngster I engaged in petty thievery," the item is scored in the pathologic direction on the schizophrenia scale, since that item has been found to reliably differentiate normal from schizophrenic persons in the studies that were done to establish and validate that scale.

The test is interpreted, first, by determining whether the test results are valid in terms of the examinee's performance on the validity sides; second, by determining which scales are abnormally elevated (i.e., which scales are in the range that statistically differentiates persons with psychiatric diagnoses from normal persons); and third, by determining the configuration of scores, or the patient's "MMPI code file" (i.e., on which scales the patient had the highest score, on which the second highest, etc.). Having made these determinations, the clinician may make a diagnosis and derive a personality description (a) on the basis of the clinician's own experience with the MMPI; (b) by reference to reviews of the scientific literature, which provides studies of diagnoses and personality characteristics associated with given MMPI codes; (c) by reference to an atlas of case histories of persons with given MMPI codes, or (d) by consulting any one of several computerized services that provide personality descriptions and "most probable diagnoses" for a given code profile. Many clinicians make use of all four sources, with any given case.

SPECIALIZED PSYCHOLOGIC TESTING FOR ADULT PSYCHIATRIC PATIENTS

Forensic Psychology

A forensic psychologist is a clinical psychologist who works in close collaboration with lawyers, judges, penologists and forensic medicine people, dealing with such legal questions as competence, criminal responsibility, etc. Judges have shown increasing acceptance of psychologists' testimony, probably because of the standardized, objective nature of the instruments psychologists employ to investigate questions regarding intellectual functioning (e.g., WAIS-R) and psychopathology (e.g., MMPI). Forensic psychologists almost invariably work with a forensic psychiatrist, and the two specialties operating as a team are often more effective in presenting case testimony than either would be working separately. Forensic psychologists differ from clinical psychologists less in the kinds of test instruments they employ than in the nature of the problems they investigate (clinical–legal as opposed to simply clinical) and the audience to whom they report (lawyers, judges, other legal system personnel, and jurors, as opposed to mental health professionals). The field of forensic psychology has experienced considerable growth during the past decade.

Neuropsychology

A neuropsychologist is a clinical psychologist who has additional training in clinical neurology and in the basic neurologic sciences (neurophysiology, neuroanatomy, etc.) and whose major interest is in the area of how brain abnormality affects psychologic function (15).

Clinical psychologists, as well as neuropsychologists, are trained to make a diagnosis of organic brain disorder from psychologic tests and to make a differential diagnosis between organic brain disorders and functional mental disorders. The clinical psychologist's first step must be to obtain results of the patient's premorbid intellectual performance from medical, educational, or military records, in order to compare current with previous level of intellecutal functioning and to ascertain the specific nature of the patient's disability. Failure to do so would greatly reduce the psychologist's ability to make any definitive statement about the consequences of the patient's brain injury.

Next, the clinical psychologist gives a standard battery of tests, generally including the WAIS-R, as well as other tests that are thought to be sensitive to the psychologic changes arising from organic mental dysfunction (e.g., Bender-Gestalt, Wechsler Memory Scale, Trail-Making Test), and analyzes the tests for the signs known to be associated with brain disease. For example, the WAIS-R is sensitive to impairments of memory, concentration, attention, abstraction ability, verbal language ability, perceptual motor functioning, social judgment, planning ability, and impulse control. The Bender-Gestalt, a test on which the patient copies geometric designs and also reproduces the designs from memory, is especially sensitive to organic brain dysfunction, particularly of the parietal lobes. The Wechsler Memory Scale is a test of various short- and long-term memory functions that was designed to provide a "memory quotient" score that, in a person with no memory impairment, would yield a number equivalent to the Wechsler "intelligence quotient" but which, in a memory-impaired person, would yield a lower score. The Trail-Making test is a screening device designed to differentiate brain-impaired from normal and from functionally psychopathologic persons.

The work of the neuropsychologist embraces all this and more. In the past, the neuropsychologist focused on attempts at localization of the site of the brain impairment. Today, however, it is recognized that similarly situated lesions can be associated with very different kinds of dysfunction in different individuals and that slight differences in lesion site can be associated with very different kinds of dysfunction across individuals. As a result, neuropsychologists focus on attempting to specify the nature of the psychologic dysfunction that results from brain lesions, rather than just on specification of the lesion site, for the purpose of designing treatment and rehabilitation programs (16, 17). The neuropsychologist, then, stands at the interface of psychology, psychiatry, and neurology.

Neuropsychologists usually employ standard screening tests (e.g., the Hunt-Minnesota and the Shipley Institute of Living Scale) and standard neuropsychologic test batteries (e.g., Halstead-Reitan, Smith's Neuropsychological Battery, and the Luria-Nebraska) that are designed to specify the nature of brain dysfunction. However, the neuropsychologist will almost invariably do extensive individual testing beyond the standard neuropsychologic battery, depending on the disability shown by a given patient. For example, patients with prominent dysfunctions of language will almost certainly be given additional tests, specifically designed to elucidate the specific nature of their disabilities (e.g., for aphasia, the Porch Index of Communicative Ability, the Eisenson, or the Minnesota Test of Aphasia, among others) (15). The eventual aim of the neuropsychologist is the development of individualized treatment programs designed to assess the speed of recovery and to plan the rehabilitation of the brain-injured patient (16, 17).

TEST REPORT

Psychologists tailor their report for the audience for whom it is intended. Consequently, it is vital that the psychologist know the use to which the report will be put. For example, a psychiatrist might request the report as part of an examination of the patient's legal competence, for purposes of differential diagnosis, as part of an examination because the patient is a student with adjustment difficulties who requires a special education program, or as an aid in psychotherapy. Thus, the eventual recipient of the report might be a judge and jury, a treatment team composed of many different kinds of health professionals, a school system, or the referring psychiatrist. A report meant for a courtroom should be written very differently from one meant for a treatment team; both will be written very differently from reports meant for educators or for psychiatrists.

It is important to recognize that psychologists typically expect their reports to be employed as a basis for dialogue leading to some intervention that will have impact on the patient's life. Consequently, the psychologist will commonly expect professional contact with the referring agency after the report has been completed and forwarded.

The psychologist should usually arrange to discuss the test results with the patient. Although some psychologists prepare a report for the patient, using lay language, most prefer to give the patient a verbal report first, since patients almost invariably have numerous questions about the testing that cannot be anticipated in a preprepared written report.

ABUSES OF PSYCHOLOGIC TESTING

Psychologic tests are subject to misuse and abuse, precisely because of their wide acceptance, and highly exaggerated conceptions of their predictive power on the part of the public. In no other country have psychologic tests gained the wide usage that they have in the United States for clinical, educational, and industrial purposes.

School teachers, for example, are highly influenced in their grading of students by their knowledge of the children's intelligence test scores, expecting, as do most nonpsychologists, that grades are largely a function of IQ. However, the correlation of intelligence tests with school grades is approximately 0.50 (5). In order to prevent

teachers (and parents) from being influenced in their attitudes toward children by what is known of a child's IQ score, some school systems have forbidden routine psychologic testing in the schools, testing a child only if there is medical–educational justification on a case-by-case basis. Consequently, it is important that psychiatrists who have ordered psychologic tests in children exercise the greatest care in informing parents and teachers of the test results. The information, when provided, should be in general rather than specific terms.

The same caution should be exercised when psychologists inform adult patients of the results of psychologic testing. Patients in an unstable or fragile mental state may have a tendency to attribute an unreasonable degree of power to the tests. Any comments they interpret as negative can therefore be detrimental to their self-esteem. In one case in which I was involved, a college student with excellent grades and recommendations was shaken in his determination to go on to graduate school because he decided "my IQ seems to me to be too low to allow for that."

SUMMARY

Properly used, psychologic testing is a valuable tool for any mental health clinician. The clinician should understand that on the one hand, it is not needed in the majority of cases, while on the other hand, it can be invaluable in cases that present a problem of differential diagnosis, cases in which there is a suspicion of organic involvement, and cases in which forensic questions are raised. In all cases, it is unwise to request psychologic testing and then consider the matter ended once the psychologic report is received. It is essential, if psychologic tests are to be used to full advantage, for the clinician and the testing psychologist to establish a close dialogue in regard to the case.

References

1. Meehl PE: *Clinical versus Statistical Prediction: A Theoretical Analysis and a Review of the Evidence.*

Minneapolis, University of Minnesota Press, 1954.

2. Meehl PE: Seer over sign: the first good example. *Journal of Experimental Research in Personality* 1:27–32, 1965.

3. Cleary TA, Humphreys LG, Kendrick SA, et al: Educational uses of tests with disadvantaged students. *Am Psychol* 30:15–41, 1975.

4. Sarason SB: Jewishness, blackness, and the nature–nurture controversy. *Am Psychol* 28:926–971, 1973.

5. Matarazzo D: *Wechsler's Measurement and Appraisal of Adult Intelligence*. Baltimore, Williams & Wilkins, 1972.

6. Anastasi A: *Psychological Testing*. New York, MacMillan, 1982

7. Vogel W, Kun KJ, Meshorer E: The cognitive development of mental retardates in response to conditions of environmental enrichment and environmental deprivation. *Journal of Consulting Psychology* 31:570–576, 1968.

8. Rapaport D: *Organization and Pathology of Thought*. New York, Columbia University Press, 1951.

9. Broverman DM, Jordan EJ Jr, Philips L: Achievement motivation in fantasy and behavior. *J Abnorm Soc Psychol* 60: 374–378, 1960.

10. Exner JE Jr: *The Rorschach: A Comprehensive System*. New York, John Wiley and Sons, 1974.

11. Exner JE Jr: *The Rorschach: A Comprehensive System: Volume 2. Current Research and Advanced Interpretations*. New York, John Wiley and Sons, 1978.

12. Dahlstrom WG, Welsh GS, Dahlstrom LE: *An MMPI Handbook: Volume I. Clinical Interpretation*. Minneapolis, University of Minnesota Press, 1975.

13. Dahlstrom WG, Dahlstrom LE: *Basic Readings on the MMPI: A New Selection on Personality Measurement*. Minneapolis, University of Minnesota Press, 1979.

14. Dahlstrom WG, Welsh GS, Dahlstrom LE: *An MMPI Handbook: Volume II. Research Developments and Applications*. Minneapolis, University of Minnesota Press, 1975.

15. Lezak MD: *Neuropsychological Assessment*, ed 2. New York, Oxford University Press 1983.

16. Miller E: *Recovery and Management of Neuropsychological Impairments*. Chicester, England, John Wiley and Sons, 1984.

17. Wedding D, Horton AM, Webster J (eds): *The Neuropsychology Handbook: Behavioral and Clinical Perspectives*. Springer, New York, 1986.

Section III

Differential Diagnosis of Psychiatric Presentations with Known Organic Causes

17

Medical Disorders in Psychiatric Populations

Aaron Lazare, M.D.

The importance of medical disorders in psychiatric patients, according to Bunce et al. (1), was first emphasized by Bonhoeffer (2) in 1912 and confirmed by Malzberg (3) in 1934 and Odegard (4) in 1952. They demonstrated that "both physical morbidity and mortality are greater in psychiatric patients than in the general population" (1). Phillips, in 1937, conducted the first of at least 19 studies of the incidence of medical diseases in a psychiatric population (5–23). In addition, there are at least six studies of medical populations in which misdiagnosed psychiatric disorders ultimately were found to have medical causes (24–30). The vast majority of the early studies on the incidence of organic disease were conducted on inpatient settings. The more recent studies have been conducted in outpatient settings including community support and rehabilitation programs. This is a reflection of the increased importance of outpatient settings in the overall provision of psychiatric care and of the importance of deinstitutionalization in particular.

In this chapter the aforementioned literature on medical disorders in psychiatric populations and misdiagnosed psychiatric patients in medical populations is reviewed. Problems in the medical evaluation of psychiatric patients are then described and some clinical principles for

the diagnosis of organic disease are presented.

STUDIES OF MEDICAL DISEASE IN PSYCHIATRIC POPULATIONS

Of the 19 studies that have attempted to determine the percentage of psychiatric patients who suffer from medical disease, many also report the percentage of patients whose medical disease caused or contributed to the psychiatric symptoms and the percentage of patients whose medical disease had been previously undiagnosed. The settings include eight inpatient units, six outpatient clinics, one brief stay observation unit, one day hospital, one emergency clinic, one community support program, and one outpatient rehabilitation program. Nine of the studies took place in England, seven in the United States, two in Canada, and one in Jamaica. The studies are summarized in Table 17.1, which represents a modification and update of similar tables by Koranyi (31) and La Bruzza (32).

These studies differ as to clinical setting, patient population, and methods of assessment for medical diagnosis. The data can be summarized as follows. On psychiatric inpatient services, 34% to 84% of patients

Table 17.1 Review of Studies Conducted to Determine Percentage of Psychiatric Patients with Medical Illness

Study	Year	Clinical Setting	No. of Patients Studied	Patients with Medical Disease		Patients with Medical Disease That Caused or Contributed to Psychiatric Condition		Patients with Medical Disease Previously Undiagnosed	
				No.	%	No.	%	No.	%
Phillips (5)	1937	Inpatient	164	137	84	74	45	—	
Marshall (6)	1949	Inpatient	175	77	44	39	22	—	
Herridge (7)	1960	Inpatient	209	103	49	54	26	—	
Eilenberg (8)	1961	Observation unit	1259	232	18	90	7	31	2
Davies (9)	1965	Outpatient	72	37	51	26	36	—	
Johnson (10)	1968	Inpatient	250	—		30	12	24	10
Maguire (11)	1968	Inpatient	200	67	34	—		33	17
Eastwood (12)	1970	Emergency clinic	100	40	40	—		16	16
Koranyi (13)	1972	Outpatient	100	49	49	10	10	35	35
Burke (14)	1972	Inpatient	202	86	43	—		—	
Burke (15)	1978	Day hospital	133	67	50	—		—	
Hall (16)	1978	Outpatient	658	—		60	9	—	
Hall (17)	1979	Inpatient	100	80	80	46	46	80	80
Koranyi (18)	1979	Outpatient	2090	902	43	622	29	417	20
Muecke (19)	1981	Outpatient	910	—		"A few"		185	20
Summers (20)	1981	Inpatient	75	31	41	14	19	21	65
Barnes (21)	1983	Outpatient	144	37	26	—		19	13
Farmer (22)	1987	Community support program	59	—		—		31	53
Roca (23)	1987	Outpatient rehabilitation program	42	39	93	—		18	43

were noted to have physical diseases. In these studies, the range of patients with physical disease previously undiagnosed was 10% to 80%. The range of patients whose physical disease caused or contributed to the psychiatric presentation was 12% to 46%. On the outpatient services, 26% to 51% of patients were noted to have physical disease, with 13% to 35% previously undiagnosed. The range of outpatients whose physical disease caused or contributed to the psychiatric presentation was from "a few" to 36%.

STUDIES OF MISDIAGNOSED PSYCHIATRIC DISEASE IN MEDICAL POPULATIONS

There are, to my knowledge, six systematic studies of patients in medical/neurologic settings who were given a psychiatric diagnosis to explain their physical findings (see Table 17.2). Comroe (25) studied pa-

tients who received various psychiatric diagnoses. In the remaining five studies, patients were diagnosed as having conversion symptoms or hysteria. The initial evaluations for nearly all of these patients were performed on medical, surgical, and neurologic inpatient services. Their subsequent care and follow-up were done predominantly in outpatient settings. The primary purpose of these studies was to determine the validity of the original psychiatric diagnoses. In these six studies, 13% to 30% of patients with psychiatric diagnoses were ultimately found to have organic disease to account for the symptoms on follow-up studies ranging from 6 months to 10 years. These studies offer some evidence that spontaneous improvement, improvement following amytal, or conversion patterns on the Minnesota Multiphasic Personality Inventory do not necessarily confirm the diagnosis of conversion rather than organic disease.

Table 17.2 Summary of Six Studies of Misdiagnosed Psychiatric Disease in Medical Populations

Study	Year	Setting	No. of Patients Studied	Average Length of Follow-up	Psychiatric Diagnosis	Patients With Organic Disease on Follow-up	
						No.	%
Comroe (25)	1946	Medical inpatient	100	8 months	Various psychiatric disorders	24	24
Gatfield (26)	1962	Neurologic and neurosurgic inpatient	37	2½–10 years	Conversion reaction	5	21
Slater (27)	1965	Medical and neurologic inpatient	73	7–11 years	Hysteria	22	30
Raskin (28)	1966	Neurologic inpatient and outpatient	50	6–12 months	Conversion reaction	7	14
Stefansson (29)	1976	Medical, surgical, and neurologic inpatient	64	3.3 years	Conversion reaction	8	13
Watson (30)	1979	Medical inpatient and outpatient	36	10 years	Conversion reaction	10	28

TYPES OF MEDICAL DISEASES IN PSYCHIATRIC PATIENTS

The most comprehensive reviews of the types of medical diseases found in psychiatric populations are presented in the outpatient studies of Hall et al. (16) and Koranyi (18). Koranyi, in a sample of 2090 patients, reports a total of 1298 medical diagnoses. (Some patients had more than one disease.) The frequency of disease types, without reference to their being causative of psychiatric symptoms, was as follows: cardiovascular 33%; central nervous system, 19%, endocrine, nutritional, and metabolic, 12%; gastrointestinal, 9%; respiratory system, 6%; genitourinary, 4%; hematopoietic, 4% neoplasm, 3%; infectious, 3%; adverse drug reaction, 3%; skin and subcutaneous tissue, 3%; and musculoskeletal and connective tissue, less than 1%. The author makes special note of the incidence of diabetes mellitus. There were 69 cases, 57 of which were diagnosed for the first time.

Hall, in a sample of 68 patients, lists 95 medical disorders believed to be causative of presenting psychiatric symptoms. The frequency of disease types was as follows: cardiovascular, 23%; endocrine, nutritional, metabolic, 22%, infectious, 15%; respiratory system, 13%; gastrointestinal, 9%; hematopoietic, 8%; central nervous

system, 5%; and neoplasm, 4%. From these two studies, it may be concluded that all the major disease types can present with psychiatric symptoms and the most frequently occurring types of medical diseases lead to the most frequent psychiatric presentations. The reader is referred to the specific articles for listings of the individual diseases.

PROBLEMS IN THE MEDICAL EVALUATION OF PSYCHIATRIC PATIENTS

The results presented above raise the immediate question as to why there is a disproportionate percentage of medical problems in psychiatric patients. The following explanations have been offered by the investigators of the studies reported above as well as by others.

1. Many of the patients who have been studied are from lower socioeconomic strata where there is often poor access to quality medical care.
2. Patients, because of their psychiatric condition, may be unable to seek proper medical care, tolerate long clinic waits, and adequately follow through on diagnostic testing.
3. Acutely and severely ill mental patients

are commonly offputting and tend to provoke negative feelings in the clinician (33, 34). They may be uncooperative and unmotivated to be examined; they may be aggressive, threatening, or generally unpleasant; they may be unclean and unkempt (35, 36); they may be unable to present a coherent or valid history; they may not communicate pain or physical discomfort that other patients are likely to experience and describe (37, 38). All these factors may contribute to incomplete and inadequate histories and physical examinations.

PROBLEMS OF MEDICAL EVALUATION IN OUTPATIENT SETTINGS

In addition to the general problems of medical evaluation for the mentally ill, the outpatient setting adds further complications:

1. The time available for examination may be limited.
2. The clinician is often unable to observe the natural history of the disorder.
3. The responsible clinician (psychiatrist, psychologist, social worker, psychiatric nurse) may lack the necessary diagnostic expertise, and there may not be easy access to consulting physicians.
4. Other clinicians are not apt to see the patient.
5. The common division of labor in community mental health centers and other outpatient facilities into "therapist" and "medication doctor" may fragment the collection of data necessary for establishing a medical diagnosis.
6. Laboratory facilities may not be easily accessible.

CLINICAL PRINCIPLES FOR THE DIAGNOSIS OF ORGANIC DISEASE

The following principles for the diagnosis of organic diseases in psychiatric populations have been described by the investigators and clinicians referred to above. I believe these principles would achieve consensus among the vast majority of practicing clinicians.

For every psychiatric outpatient, the clinician should consider the hypothesis that the psychiatric condition is caused or exacerbated by a medical illness concurrently with the psychiatric disturbance. Psychiatric patients, including outpatients, are at higher risk than the general population for medical disease; however, psychiatric inpatients are at 4 to 8 times greater risk for coexisting medical illness than psychiatric outpatients (39).

Patients even under the care of medical physicians may present to psychiatric inpatient or outpatient settings with medical diseases that are causative or coexistent with the psychiatric presentation (16–18). Hall et al. found that previous treatment with a medical physician correlated poorly with a diagnosis of physical illness. They offer three possible explanations: First, most patients had not been examined by that physician during the previous year. Second, the examinations tended to be incomplete. And third, at the time of the psychiatric evaluation the medical symptom picture was often incomplete (39).

Referral to a medical physician for "medical clearance" does not ensure an adequate medical work-up. The medical evaluation is more apt to be effective if the psychiatrist informs the medical physician what he or she is looking for, orders appropriate lab tests in advance, and discusses with the medical physician the clinical and laboratory findings.

Disturbances in memory, sensorium, and orientation are highly discriminative of a primary medical/neurologic disorder. These symptoms, however, may occur in the so-called functional disorders such as major depression, mania, and schizophrenia.

Visual hallucinations, distortions, and illusions are particularly suggestive of an underlying medical/neurologic disorder.

The more acute the onset of psychotic behavior, the more likely the condition is organic in etiology. Schizophrenia or manic–depressive psychosis does not develop over the course of several days.

The presence of an apparent precipitating event should not lead to the automatic conclusion that the disorder is functional. Precipitating events are sometimes too easily found.

Normal functioning of higher intellectual processes occurs in a wide variety of medical conditions that present with psychiatric symptoms. Secondary mania caused by brain tumor and depression caused by cancer of the pancreas are two examples. Normal intellectual functioning, therefore, never rules out the possibility of medical causes of psychiatric symptoms.

A significant percentage of patients who receive the label of "hysteria," particularly on inpatient medical settings, will eventually receive an organic diagnosis for the condition (24).

Patients who present psychiatric symptoms for the first time in their life after age 40 are more likely to have a causative medical illness than younger patients.

Elderly patients who present with psychiatric symptoms have a greater chance of having causative or contributory medical conditions than younger patients with the same presenting symptoms.

For patients with a known medical condition, there is a significant chance that the psychiatric presentation is a result of a decompensation of the disease or a complication of the treatment.

In situations in which a nonpsychiatrist mental health professional and a psychiatrist (medical "back-up") share the clinical responsibility for a patient, there is reasonable risk that neither party is apt to learn the whole clinical picture. In such situations, both parties need to be particularly aware that the medical responsibilities are properly attended to.

CONCLUSIONS

A difficult but unanswered question is the specific nature of the medical evaluation for psychiatric outpatients. Some argue for routine physical examination and comprehensive laboratory screening for all outpatients. Others believe that such a practice is impractical given the low rate of positive findings with clinical significance (40). They argue, instead, for a diagnostic algorithm that "proceeds from the simple and inexpensive to the costly and dangerous" (40–42). In other words, the clinician's decision to pursue a further medical inquiry should depend on his or her index of suspicion of medical illness, which in turn depends on the presenting symptom, the medical history, the mental status examination, the patient's current level of medical care, and other factors that determine that patient's risk for medical illness. The resolution of this controversy will require further studies using a wide variety of outpatient clinical settings and patient populations.

Chapter 15 discusses the use of laboratory testing in outpatient practice. Chapters 18 through 30 provide more precise guidelines for the medical evaluation of specific psychiatric presentations.

References

1. Bunce DF, Jones LR, Badger LW, et al: Medical illness in psychiatric patients: barriers to diagnosis and treatment. *South Med J* 75:941–944, 1982.
2. Bonhoeffer K: Die Psychosen im Gefolge von akuten Infektionen Allgemeiner Krankungen. In Aschaffenburg GL (ed): *Handbuch der Psychiatrie.* Leipzig, Germany, Deuticke, 1912, vol 3, pp 1–60.
3. Malzberg B: *Mortality Among Patients with Mental Disease.* Utica, NY, New York State Hospital Press, 1934.
4. Odegard O: The excess mortality of the insane. *Acta Psychiatr Neurol Scand* 27:353–367, 1952.
5. Phillips RJ: Physical disorder in 164 consecutive admissions to a mental hospital. *Postgrad Med* 54(2):78–84, 1973.
6. Marshall HES: Incidence of physical disorders among psychiatric in-patients. *Br Med J* 2:468–470, 1949.
7. Herridge CF: Physical disorders in psychiatric illness. *Lancet* 2:949–951, 1960.
8. Eilenberg MD, Whatmore PB: Physical disease and psychiatric emergencies. *Compr Psychiatry* 2:358–363, 1961.
9. Davies DW: Physical illness in psychiatric outpatients. *Br J Psychiatry* 111:27–33, 1965.
10. Johnson DAW: The evaluation of routine physical examination in psychiatric cases. *Practitioner* 200:686–691, 1968.
11. Maguire GP: Granville-Grossman KL: Physical illness in psychiatric patients. *Br J Psychiatry* 115:1365–1369, 1968.
12. Eastwood MR, Mindham RHS, Tennent TG: The physical status of psychiatric emergencies. *Br J Psychiatry* 116:545–550, 1970.
13. Koranyi EK: Physical health and illness in a psy-

chiatric outpatient department population. *Can Psychiatr Assoc J* 17(Suppl):109–116, 1972.

14. Burke AW: Physical illness in psychiatric hospital patients in Jamaica. *Br J Psychiatry* 121:321–322, 1972.
15. Burke AW: Physical disorder among day hospital patients. *Br J Psychiatry* 133:22–27, 1978.
16. Hall RC, Gardner ER, Stickney SK et al: Physical illness manifesting as psychiatric disease. *Arch Gen Psychiatry* 37:989–995, 1980.
17. Hall RCW, Gardner ER, Stickney SK, et al: Physical illness manifesting as psychiatric disease: II. Analysis of a state hospital inpatient population. *Arch Gen Psychiatry* 37:989–995, 1980.
18. Koranyi EK: Morbidity and rate of undiagnosed physical illnesses in a psychiatric clinic population. *Arch Gen Psychiatry* 36:414–419, 1979.
19. Muecke LN, Krueger DW: Physical findings in a psychiatric outpatient clinic. *Am J Psychiatry* 138:1241–1242, 1981.
20. Summers WK, Munoz RA, Read MR, et al: The psychiatric physical examination—Part II: Findings in unselected psychiatric patients. *J Clin Psychiatry* 42:99–102, 1981.
21. Barnes RF, Mason JC, Greer C, et al: Medical illness in chronic psychiatric outpatients. *Gen Hosp Psychiatry* 5:191–195, 1983.
22. Farmer S: Medical problems of chronic patients in a community support program. *Hosp Community Psychiatry* 38:745–749, 1987.
23. Roca RP, Breakey WR, Fischer PJ: Medical care of chronic psychiatric outpatients. *Hosp Community Psychiatry* 38:741–745, 1987.
24. Lazare A: Current concepts in psychiatry: conversion symptoms. *N Engl J Med* 305:745–748, 1981.
25. Comroe BI: Follow-up study of 100 patients diagnosed as "neurosis." *J Nerv Ment Dis* 83:679–684, 1936.
26. Gatfield PD, Guze SB: Prognosis and differential diagnosis of conversion reactions: a follow-up study. *Dis Nerv Syst* 23:623–631, 1962.
27. Slater ETO, Glithero E: A follow-up of patients diagnosed as suffering from "hysteria." *J Psychosom Res* 9:9–13, 1965.
28. Raskin M, Talbott JA, Meyerson AT: Diagnosed conversion reactions: predictive value of psychiatric criteria. *JAMA* 197:530–534, 1966.
29. Stefansson JG, Messina JA, Meyerowitz S: Hysterical neurosis, conversion type: clinical and epidemiological considerations. *Acta Psychiatr Scand* 53:119–138, 1976.
30. Watson CG, Buranen C: The frequency and identification of false positive conversion reactions. *J Nerv Ment Dis* 167:243–247, 1979.
31. Koranyi EK: Somatic illness in psychiatric patients. *Psychosomatics* 21:887–891, 1980.
32. La Bruzza AL: Physical illness presenting as psychiatric disorder: guidelines for differential diagnosis. *Journal of Operational Psychiatry* 12:24–31, 1981.
33. Groves JE: Taking care of the hateful patient. *N Engl J Med* 298:883–887, 1978.
34. Goodwin JM, Goodwin JS, Kellner R: Psychiatric symptoms in disliked medical patients. *JAMA* 241:1117–1120, 1979.
35. Kampmeier RH: Diagnosis and treatment of physical disease in the medically ill. *Ann Intern Med* 86:637–645, 1977.
36. Hoffman RS, Koran LM: Detecting physical illness in patients with mental disorders. *Psychosomatics* 25:654–660, 1984.
37. Talbott JA, Linn L: Reactions to schizophrenics to life-threatening disease. *Psychiatr Q* 50:218–227, 1978.
38. Marchand WE: Occurrence of painless myocardial infarction in psychotic patients. *N Engl J Med* 253:51–55, 1955.
39. Hall RCW, Beresford TP, Gardner ER, et al: The medical care of psychiatric patients. *Hosp Community Psychiatry* 33:25–34, 1982.
40. Horvath TB: The psychological presentations of somatic disorders. In Berger PA, Brodie KH (eds): *American Handbook of Psychiatry*, ed 2. New York, Basic Books, 1986, vol 8, pp 899–943.
41. Hendrie HL: Brain disorders: clinical diagnosis and management. *Psychiatr Clin North Am* 1:3–19 1978.
42. Fauman MA: The emergency psychiatric evaluation of organic mental disorders. *Psychiatr Clin North Am* 6:233–257, 1983.

18

Anxiety

Ted Lawlor, M.D.
Aaron Lazare, M.D.

Anxiety is one of the most common conditions for which patients seek psychiatric or medical help. Such patients generally present with a combination of psychologic and somatic experiences. The psychologic experiences include fear, dread, foreboding, impending doom, and panic, while the somatic manifestations include diaphoresis, tremulousness, tachycardia, lightheadedness, and butterflies in the stomach. Tables 18.1 and 18.2 provide an extensive list of these psychologic and somatic experiences. It is not known why some patients have certain symptom constellations rather than others.

The presenting complaints for anxiety conditions are varied and include "anxiety," "nerves," fear of "losing my mind," feeling "wired all the time," feeling like "I'm having a nervous breakdown," feeling "afraid all of the time." Even in the presence of these complaints, the true manifestations of anxiety can be determined only by an inquiry into the presence of the signs and symptoms listed in Tables 18.1 and 18.2. A patient complaining of "nerves," for instance, may be referring to feelings of depression or angry outbursts, not anxiety.

Given the vast array of somatic manifestations, it is easy to understand why so many patients suffering from anxiety

Table 18.1 Somatic Manifestations of Anxiety

Cardiovascular distress (elevated blood pressure, increased pulse, palpitations)
Chest pain or discomfort
Choking
Dizziness, lightheadedness, or unsteady feelings
Dry mouth
Faintness
Gastrointestinal distress (butterflies, pain, cramps, nausea, vomiting, diarrhea, loss of appetite, increased appetite)
Headache
Motor tension (trembling, twitching, shaking, fine tremor of extremities, feeling shaky, muscle tension, aches or soreness, restlessness, easy fatigability)
Respiratory distress (rapid breathing, shortness of breath, smothering sensations)
Numbness or tingling sensations (paresthesias)
Pupillary dilatation
Sexual dysfunction
Sleep difficulties (insomnia)
Tendon reflexes, brisk and increased
Tinnitus
Urinary distress (frequency, hesitancy, urgency)
Vasomotor distress (coldness of extremities, chills, flushing, pallor, sweating)
Vertigo
Vision, blurred

present intially to their medical physicians. They may come with the medical emergency of a feared myocardial infarction or stroke, or they may come after reading a popular magazine about anxiety symptoms resulting from mitral valve prolapse or hypoglycemia.

Table 18.2   Psychologic Manifestations
of Anxiety

Aggressiveness
Anxiety
Apprehension
Concentration impairment
Dread
Depersonalization or derealization
Edginess
Fear of dying
Fear of going crazy or losing one's mind
Fear of losing control
Feeling of impending doom
Feeling keyed up or "wired"
Feeling scared
Fright
Impulsiveness
Inability to concentrate
Irritability
Nervousness
Panic
Restlessness
Suicidal ideation
Tension
Terror
Uneasiness
Uptight feeling

The initial task of the clinician, after determining that the patient has clinical manifestations of anxiety, is to establish the categorical diagnosis. This is no easy task since anxiety can be a manifestation of a normal conditon, one of the anxiety disorders, one of the other functional psychiatric disorders, or the organic anxiety syndrome. This chapter first reviews the differential diagnosis of anxiety and then suggests clinical guidelines for the approach to the patient. Major emphasis is placed on the organic anxiety syndrome. (Chapter 34 reviews the anxiety disorders.)

CLASSIFICATION OF CONDITIONS CHARACTERIZED BY ANXIETY

We propose four major categories of conditions in which symptoms of anxiety are prominent: normal states, psychiatric syndromes (excluding anxiety disorders), anxiety disorders, and the organic anxiety syndrome.

Normal States

Normal anxiety refers to those symptomatic anxiety responses that are logical, understandable, time limited, and perhaps adaptive to the stressful situation. Examples are the anxiety of a soldier about to parachute from a plane, a student about to take an examination, or a pedestrian who witnesses or barely escapes an accident. Pathologic anxiety may be defined by its impairment of function or performance, by its persistence in time, by its persistence away from the stressful situation, and by its association with known psychiatric syndromes. The treatment of normal anxiety is education and reassurance.

Psychiatric Syndromes (Excluding Anxiety Disorders)

Anxiety symptoms, even appearing as the syndrome of panic attacks, may occur in the context of many of the major psychiatric disorders. When this occurs, anxiety is considered secondary to the primary disorder, and treatment is directed at the primary disorder. The most common syndromes in which anxiety occur are schizophrenia, bipolar disorder, depressive disorders, other psychotic disorders, the adjustment disorders, and the somatoform disorders, particularly somatization disorder and hypochondriasis. In schizophrenia, manic disorders, and depression, the anxiety may precede by days the full-blown syndrome of the predominant disorder. Once the full-blown syndrome is in evidence, the anxiety is apt to go unnoticed by the clinician, who becomes more concerned with delusions, hallucinations, or depressive symptoms. With the somatoform disorders, there may be acute symptoms of anxiety superimposed on the chronic syndrome that can be discerned from history. The key to establishing the diagnosis when the presenting symptom is anxiety is the awareness of the possibility that another major syndrome is causative. With this mind-set, the clinician will actively pursue other confirmatory signs and symptoms of the syndromes and even use time—perhaps days—to observe the emergence of confirmatory data. There is no evidence that the presence of anxiety as part of the major syndrome alters the treatment or course of the syndrome.

Anxiety Disorders

The anxiety disorders include all the so-called functional states of pathologic anxiety with the exception of the disorders listed above. Known organic causes of anxiety (described below) are also excluded. The anxiety disorders, described in detail in Chapter 34, include the following seven categories according to the *Diagnostic and Statistical Manual of Mental Disorders (Third Edition-Revised)* (DSM-III-R): panic disorder, agoraphobia without history of panic disorder, social phobia, simple phobia, obsessive–compulsive disorder, post-traumatic stress disorder, and generalized anxiety disorder.

Organic Anxiety Syndrome

The organic anxiety syndrome, now an official diagnostic category of DSM-III-R under the broader category of organic mental disorders is defined or diagnosed by three criteria: (*a*) prominent, recurrent, panic attacks or generalized anxiety; (*b*) evidence from the history, physical examination, or laboratory tests of a specific organic factor (or factors) judged to be etiologically related to the disturbance; and (*c*) not occurring exclusively during the course of delirium. In our experience, the organic anxiety syndrome represents a small minority of the cases that present with anxiety.

CAUSES OF ORGANIC ANXIETY SYNDROME

Before the clinician can make a diagnosis of normal anxiety, one of the anxiety disorders, or one of the other functional disorders characterized by anxiety, careful consideration must be given to the possibility that the condition has an organic etiology. Table 18.3, based on a composite of several sources (1–8), presents an extensive but incomplete list of organic causes of anxiety symptoms. We shall review only those conditions that are more common, that are difficult to diagnoses, or that patients are apt to discuss.

Cardiovascular/Pulmonary Disease

A variety of cardiovascular/pulmonary conditions may present as anxiety. Myocardial infarction commonly presents with chest pain, shortness of breath, sensation of choking, diaphoresis, and the fear of impending death. Electrocardiogram (ECG) and cardiac enzymes establish the diagnosis with certainty. The chest pain, palpitations, and shortness of breath of angina pectoris can be difficult to distinguish from the symptoms of anxiety, particularly when the ECG stress test is normal. Pain described as squeezing or pressure is more apt to be associated with coronary artery disease, while pain described as stabbing or throbbing is more likely to be associated with anxiety (9). Paroxysmal atrial tachycardia may be confused with anxiety. The pulse of an anxiety attack may be normal but is not apt to exceed 120, whereas the pulse of paroxysmal atrial tachycardia often exceeds 200. Twenty-four-hour ECG monitoring may be necessary to record the period of the symptomatology in question. Distinguishing functional anxiety from the cardiac conditions described above is difficult since patients commonly have anxiety secondary to the cardiac condition. Although patients with panic disorder have a higher risk of mitral valve prolapse than is found in the general population, a causal relationship between the two has not been established. Hypoxia, which may be caused by a variety of conditions such as emphysema, atelectasis, and asthma, commonly presents as anxiety.

Endocrine and Metabolic Disease

Hypoglycemia

Hypoglycemia is a final common physiologic state that can cause symptoms of

Table 18.3 Medical Disorders Presenting with Anxiety Symptoms

---

Dietary, drug-induced, and toxic conditions
  Caffeinism (and other xanthine derivatives)
  Monosodium glutamate
  Sympathomimetic agents
    (amphetamine, ephedrine, cocaine, etc)
  Hallucinogens
  Anticholinergics
  Antipsychotics (akathisia)
  Tricyclic antidepressants
  Monoamine oxidase inhibitors
  Amylnitrite
  Withdrawal syndromes
    (alcohol, sedative-hypnotics)
  Insulin
  Thyroid medication
  Corticosteroids
  Mercury
  Arsenic
  Phosphorus
  Organophosphates
  Carbon disulfide
  Benzene
  Lactic acid

Cardiovascular
  Angina pectoris
  Myocardial infarction
  Congestive heart failure
  Paroxysmal atrial tachycardia
  Other arrhythmias
  Mitral valve prolapse
  Hyperdynamic β-adrenergic state
  Hypovolemia

Hematologic
  Anemia

Pulmonary
  Acute asthma
  Chronic obstructive pulmonary disease
  Pneumonia
  Pneumothorax
  Pulmonary edema
  Pulmonary embolus

Endocrinologic/metabolic
  Hyperadrenalism (Cushing's syndrome)
  Hypocalcemia (hypoparathyroidism and
    other causes)
  Hypokalemia
  Hypoglycemia
  Hyponatremia
  Hyperthyroidism
  Thyroiditis
  Addison's disease
  Hypopituitarism
  Metabolic acidosis (diabetic and other causes)
  Menopausal symptoms
  Carcinoid syndrome
  Pheochromocytoma
  Acute intermittent porphyria
  Malnutrition, vitamin deficiency (B_{12},
    pellagra)

Neurologic
  Partial complex seizures
  Grand mal epilepsy
  Transient ischemic attacks
  Cerebrovascular insufficiency
  Subarachnoid hemorrhage
  Migraine
  Multiple sclerosis
  Tumors
  Encephalopathies
  Cerebral trauma and postconcussion
    syndrome
  Vertigo
  Myasthenia gravis
  Wilson's disease
  Tremors
  Degenerative diseases

Infectious Disease
  Febrile illness and chronic infection
  Infectious mononucleosis
  Posthepatitis syndrome
  Meningitis

---

anxiety as well as other psychologic behavioral manifestations such as psychosis. Hypoglycemia can result from excess doses of insulin or oral antidiabetic agents with inadequate carbohydrate intake, with early diabetes, with insulin-secreting islet tumors of the pancreas, following large carbohydrate loads, during fasting, following subtotal gastrectomy, with cirrhosis, with Addison's disease, and with hypopituitarism (5, 7). It is generally believed that the public's concern for the possibility of functional hypoglycemia is exaggerated. Most of these patients after careful medical work-up are found to have one of the functional anxiety disorders. A glucose tolerance test is required to document the presence of hypoglycemia (blood level of 45 mg/dl or less). The only certain method of determining whether anxiety is caused by hypoglycemia is to measure the blood glucose at the time of the anxiety symptoms.

Thyroid Disease

Hyperthyroidism is apt to present as generalized anxiety with feelings of jitteriness associated with weight loss and heat intolerance. Panic attacks are uncommon.

Hypoparathyroidism

Hypoparathyroidism, usually the result of thyroid surgery, leads to hypocalcemia, which in turn may cause symptoms of anxiety as well as other psychiatric symptoms such as depression and irritability. The scar of thyroid surgery should raise the clinician's index of suspicion. Low calcium blood levels are diagnostic.

Pheochromocytoma

Pheochromocytoma, a rarely occurring tumor that secrets high levels of catecholamines continuously or intermittently, is apt to present as episodic panic attacks. The classical presentation includes headache, excessive sweating, and palpitations. High blood pressure, pallor followed by flushing, and nervousness are also common symptoms. The diagnosis is made by elevated urinary levels of vanillylmandelic acid, a catecholamine metabolite.

CLINICAL APPROACH TO THE PATIENT

The foundation for the clinical assessment of anxiety is a careful history elicited in the context of a broad knowledge of the differential diagnosis. A single transient anxiety episode following a significant trauma suggests normal anxiety. The anxiety disorders usually have characteristic histories, but the diagnosis can be made only in the absence of other psychiatric syndromes and organic anxiety disorders. The diagnosis of other psychiatric syndromes, particularly as they present early in their course, may be suspected by age of onset, family history, and previous psychiatric history. A first episode of anxiety at age 50, for instance, is more likely to represent the beginning of a mood disorder than an anxiety disorder. In general the clinician should suspect an organic disorder if the patient is older than 40 years at the onset of symptoms, if the patient has a negative family history for anxiety disorders, or if the patient is unable to identify an event with significant psychologic meaning related to the onset of symptoms (8).

In pursuing the organic differential diagnosis of anxiety, the clinician should inquire of all known medical illnesses and family histories of medical illness (which may be genetically transmitted). At the same time he or she should inquire of medications the patient may be taking for the disease as well as any other prescription or over-the-counter or illicit medication. The clinician should also inquire about any other unusual dietary habits such as excessive caffeine ingestion. Recent discontinuation of medication and alcohol can be equally important. The time of the anxiety attack should alert the clinician to the possibility of hypoglycemia. The location of the somatic focus should alert the clinician to a further set of decision points. Chest pain, for instance, may lead the clinician to order the appropriate diagnostic tests for coronary insufficiency and myocardial infarction. Headache, dizziness, faintness, and/or tremor may alert the clinician to the possibility of neurologic disease. Knowledge of the symptoms of hyperthyroidism, hypothyroidism, and pheochromocytoma helps the clinician consider these possibilities and order the appropriate tests.

The nature of the history and the mental status examination will determine whether the clinician should perform a physical examination and in how much detail, what laboratory tests should be ordered, and whether and when a specialist needs to be consulted.

References

1. Rosenbaum JF: Anxiety. In Lazare A (ed): *Outpatient Psychiatry*. Baltimore, Williams & Wilkins, 1979, pp 252–257.
2. Hall RCW: Anxiety. In Hall RCW (ed): *Psychiatric Presentations of Medical Illness*. Jamaica, NY, Spectrum Publications, 1980, pp 13–35.
3. Jefferson JW, Marshall JR: *Neuropsychiatric Features of Medical Disorders*. New York, Plenum Press, 1981.
4. Cummings JL: *Clinical Neuropsychiatry*. New York, Grune and Stratton, 1985.
5. McNeil GN: Anxiety. In Soreff SM, McNeil SM (eds): *Handbook of Differential Diagnosis*. Littleton, MA, PSG Publishing, 1986, pp 1–56.
6. Van Valkenburg CV: Anxiety symptoms. In Winokur G, Clayton PJ: *The Medical Basis of Psychiatry*. Philadelphia, PA, WB Saunders, 1986, pp 400–413.
7. Horvath TB: The psychological presentations of somatic disorders. In Berger PA, Brodie KH (eds): *American Handbook of Psychiatry, ed 2*. New York, Basic Books, 1986, vol 8, pp 900–943.
8. Mackenzie TB, Popkin MK: Organic anxiety syndrome. *Am J Psychiatry* 140:342–344, 1983.
9. Levine OL: Chest pain: prophet of doom or nagging neurosis? *Acta Med Scand (Suppl)* 644:11–13, 1981.

19

Depression

Paul J. Barreira, M.D.

The complaint of depression is one of the most common reasons why people seek psychiatric treatment (1). Although the majority of these patients suffer from minor psychologic distress, grief, or affective disorders, a significant proportion may be suffering from an organic affective syndrome; that is, the depressive symptoms are caused by medications or a medical disorder. Several studies indicate that medical disorders present in approximately 45% of psychiatric outpatients and are the sole cause of psychiatric symptoms in 9% of the cases (see Chapter 17). Hall's findings suggest that depression is the second most common psychiatric symptom whose etiology is ultimately determined to be organic (2). If an organic affective syndrome goes unrecognized, and treatment of a functional affective disorder is initiated, valuable time may be wasted, a reversible condition may go untreated, and the patient may be subject to unnecessary treatments with their associated risks. Therefore, an initial diagnostic evaluation of depressive symptoms should include the assessment of possible organic etiologies.

Many organic conditions can be detected by a careful history and review of systems. Others will require physical examination and laboratory tests. Once identified, the organic condition may be a sufficient cause and explanation for the clinical presenta-

tion. In other cases, the medical condition may aggravate or complicate a preexisting depression.

DRUGS ASSOCIATED WITH DEPRESSION

Drugs are the main cause of organic depressive states, and drug-induced depressions are being reported with increasing frequency (3). Usually a careful medical history will identify possible offending agents. Recent evidence suggests that drug-induced depressions occur more often in patients with a positive family history for affective disorder, in those with a personal history of depression, or in the elderly. One should attempt to establish a temporal relationship between the initiation of medication and development of symptoms. Although the depressive symptoms usually appear within days or weeks after the introduction of medication, symptoms may not appear for several months. A trial period off medication should help to establish the role of medication. Besides the many drugs that have been reported to cause depression, the clinician should consider that any drug might be a contributing factor, especially in a predisposed individual. The actual incidence of drug-induced depression is difficult to define, in part because the definition of depression is broad and lacks the specificity of other symptoms such as mania. Also it is easy to mistake drug-induced psychomotor slowness and sedation for a depressive syndrome. Table 19.1 lists the most common agents associated with depressive symptoms.

Antihypertensive drugs including reserpine, methyldopa, and propranolol have been frequently implicated in the etiology of depressive symptoms. In most instances, the development of depressive symptoms is not dose dependent. Propranolol is an exception, with higher doses more commonly associated with depression. Mood change is insidious and accompanied by changes in sleep patterns, fatigue, and decreased libido. Hyponatremia, a frequent electrolyte abnormality of antihypertensive drugs, may also cause a depressive picture.

Sedative hypnotic agents, especially the benzodiazepines, can cause depression. The development of depression with these drugs is related to dose and length of time on the drug. Patients complain of fatigue and poor concentration. Occasionally the patient may have signs of chronic sedative intoxication such as nystagmus.

Whenever a patient presents with depression and alteration in behavior, one must consider the role of alcohol. Alcoholism is a major health problem and can mimic many other disorders. Eliciting an accurate history of alcohol intake is not as straightforward as reviewing medications, since denial plays such a dominant role in alcoholism. If one suspects that alcohol is contributing to the depression, discussions with family members can be helpful (see Chapter 36).

Elderly patients are at higher risk for developing depression with any drug. In part, this is due to increased exposure to medications. Also, older patients seem more vulnerable to the potential depressive effects of medications. Many drugs, like digitalis and antiinflammatory agents, which are commonly prescribed in the geriatric population, may cause depression at normal doses.

Many other medications have been reported to cause depressive symptoms; oral contraceptives and other steroid agents are examples. Like for the previously described medications, the onset of depressive symptoms is insidious and patients often fail to associate the medication with the depression. Since the incidence of depressive symptoms caused by medications is not known, the burden rests with the clinician to identify possible offending agents and evaluate their role in the clinical presentation.

MEDICAL DISORDERS ASSOCIATED WITH DEPRESSION

Medical disorders that are associated with depression include endocrine, meta-

Table 19.1   Drugs Associated with Depression

Analgesics/anti-inflammatory agents	*Antiparkinsonian agents*
Ibuprofen	*Cytotoxic agents*
Indomethacin	
Opiates	*Hormones*
Pentazocine	Andrenocorticotropic hormone
Phenacetin	Corticosteroids
Phenylbutazone	Estrogen
	Oral contraceptives
Anticonvulsants	
	Immunosuppressive agents
Antihistamines	
	Psychotropic medications
Antihypertensive agents	Barbiturates
Clonidine	Neuroleptics
Guanethidine	Benzodiazepines
Hydralazine	
Methyldopa	*Miscellaneous*
Propranolol	Alcohol
Reserpine	Amphetamine withdrawal
	Baclofen
Antimicrobials	Caffeine
Ampicillin	Cimetidine
Cycloserine	Digitalis
Dapsone	Disulfiram
Griseofulvin	Fenfluramine
Isoniazid	Halothane
Metronidazole	LSD (lysergic acid diethylamide)
Nalidixic acid	Methysergide
Nitrofurantoin	Metrizamide
Procaine penicillin	Phenylephrine
Streptomycin	Procainamide
Sulfonamides	
Tetracycline	
Trimethoprim-sulfamethoxazole	

bolic, infectious, and other disorders (4) (see Table 19.2). In many instances, mental status changes precede physical signs or symptoms of the medical disorder. Endocrine disorders tend to cause global changes in personality including behavior, mood, and cognition rather than

Table 19.2   Medical Disorders Associated with Depression

Collagen–vascular	Metabolic
Giant cell arteritis	Acidosis
Periarteritis nodosa	Alkalosis
Rheumatoid arthritis	Hyperkalemia
Systemic lupus	Hypocalcemia
erythematosus	Hypokalemia
	Hypomagnesemia
Endocrine	Hyponatremia
Acromegaly	Uremia
Diabetes mellitus	
Hyperadrenalism	*Neoplasm*
Hyperparathyroidism	Intercranial
Hyperthyroidism	Leukemia
Hypoadrenalism	Lymphoma
Hypoglycemia	Oat cell carcinoma
Hypoparathyroidism	Pancreatic
Hypopituitarism	
Hypothyroidism	*Neurologic*
Menopause	Alzheimer's disease
Postpartum	Chronic subdural
	hematoma
Gastrointestinal	Huntington's disease
Cirrhosis	Multiple sclerosis
Inflammatory bowel	Organic brain
disease	syndrome
Pancreatitis	Parkinson's disease
Whipple's disease	Head trauma
	Stroke
Hypovitaminosis	
Ascorbic acid	*Miscellaneous*
Folate	Amyloidosis
Iron	Gout
Niacin	Psoriasis
Pernicious anemia	Sarcoidosis
Pyridoxine	Wilson's disease
Thiamine	
Infectious	
Brucelleosis	
Encephalitis	
Hepatitis	
Infectious	
mononucleosis	
Influenza	
Malaria	
Pneumonia	
Syphillis	
Tuberculosis	

physical signs or symptoms (e.g., goiter). Furthermore, the changes may be so insidious and subtle that the individual adapts to them over time, which leads the clinician to feel that the alteration is a result of psychologic rather than organic causes. Endocrine disturbances may cause an exacerbation in a preexisting psychiatric disorder (e.g., affective disorder). Treatment of the endocrine disturbance usually results in remission of symptoms. Thyroid dysfunction is the most common of the endocrine disorders to cause depression. Either an excess or a deficiency of the hormone results in changes in mood or behavior. Usually, the hyperthyroid patient appears to have an anxiety state or agitated depression, while the hypothyroid patient has a retarded depression. Hyperthyroidism causes an increase in the metabolic rate with symptoms of sensitivity to heat, tremor, sweating, increased pulse, and (later) exophthalmus. Hypothyroidism is associated with hoarseness of voice, pale skin, slow pulse, sensitivity to cold, fatigue, and edema. Diseases of other endocrine glands can cause depression, but less commonly.

Depressive symptoms are common in many neurologic disorders. The most difficult to assess is the group of chronic, degenerative disorders that early in the illness may not show clear organic symptoms other than subtle changes in memory and other cognitive functions. Included in this category are Alzheimer's disease, Parkinson's disease, and Pick's disease (see Table 19.2). At times it is difficult to distinguish the cognitive impairment due to major depression, so-called pseudodementia, from a dementing illness. Age of onset, history of affective illness, or response to treatment may help to make the diagnosis (see Chapter 23). Many other medical illnesses including infections and tumors have been reported to present initially with depressive symptoms. The list of potential organic causes is extensive.

Fortunately, most patients who present with depressive symptoms suffer from a functional depressive disorder and will respond to standard psychologic and pharmacologic treatments. If the clinician is careful to evaluate for possible organic etiologies of depression in the initial evaluation, the most common causes, drugs and medical conditions, should be identified without needless and costly laboratory tests. When a previously diagnosed depressive disorder does not respond to conventional treatment, a more comprehensive investigation is warranted.

References

1. Koranyi EK: Morbidity and rate of undiagnosed physical illnesses in a psychiatric clinic population. *Arch Gen Psychiatry* 36:414–419, 1979.
2. Hall RCW, Popkin MK, De Vaul R, et al: Physical illness presenting as psychiatric disease. *Arch Gen Psychiatry* 37:989–995, 1980.
3. Katerndahl DA: Nonpsychiatric disorders associated with depression. *J Fam Pract* 13:619–24, 1981.
4. Fava GA: Diagnosis and treatment of depression in the medically ill. *Prog Neuro-Psychopharmacol Biol Psychiatry* 610:1–9, 1986.
5. Hall RCW (ed): *Psychiatric Presentations of Medical Illness: Somatotropic Disorders.* New York, Spectrum Publications, 1980.

20

Manic Behavior

Ann Ohm Massion, M.D.
Sheldon Benjamin, M.D.

He proclaimed that he was the younger son of the Virgin Mary. He planted twigs into the soil of the gardens around the clinic believing they would flourish as little Maupassants. He would howl like a dog and lick the walls of his cell. He deliberately practiced retention, saying his urine was "all diamonds . . . all jewels . . ." (1)

Maupassant's manic behavior was typical of the expansive form of general paresis of the insane. In the 10 years before his death in 1893 at age 43, Guy de Maupassant had become an unbelievably prolific writer. At the same time he had become irritable, insomnic, restless, grandiose, somewhat paranoid, and prone to lavish spending and pressured speech (2). The form of neurosyphilis that affected Guy de Maupassant was perhaps the most common organic cause of mania at the turn of the century.

For over 70 years psychiatrists have known that mania can be organically induced (3–5). Karl Bonhoeffer noted in 1909 that psychiatric symptoms could predominate in organic illness whether directly or indirectly involving the brain. He felt, however, that exogenous manic psychoses were unrelated to manic–depressive mania (4, 6). In 1916, Eugen Bleuler defined the "organic psychosyndrome" as a set of behavioral symptoms of diffuse cerebral damage, including emotional liability and impairment of impulse control, memory, judgment, attention, and discrimination (5). In the wake of the 1918 influenza epidemic, his son, Manfred Bleuler, recognized the postencephalitic syndromes, with their disturbed impulse control, drives, and mood, but preserved intellect, as "focal psychosyndromes" (7). He emphasized that that same manic syndrome could be found in a variety of different diseases such as general paresis of the insane (a form of neurosyphilis), Huntington's disease, brain tumors, and cerebral arteriosclerosis (8).

Since the reexamination of the subject of organically induced mania by Krauthammer and Klerman in 1978 (9), a large body of literature describing "secondary manias" has developed. This chapter reviews that literature and suggests a framework for evaluating the patient presenting with manic behavior of unknown etiology.

256

DEFINITION AND DIAGNOSTIC CRITERIA

The early distinction of primary versus secondary affective disorder defined secondary affective disorder as one occurring after a previous psychiatric illness other than a primary affective disorder (10). However, in 1978, Krauthammer and Klerman (9) commented that mania following other psychopathology was not only rare but a "rather empty classification." They proposed that "secondary mania," a term introduced by Klerman and Barrett (11), be defined in keeping with medical terminology as a manic syndrome secondary to medical and/or pharmacologic antecedents. Excluded were manic syndromes coexisting with delirium, dementia, or confusional states, as well as those occurring with a previous history of manic–depressive or other affective disorder (9). This is consistent with the usage of the term '"secondary" in other fields of medicine, analogous to the difference between essential (primary) hypertension and hypertension secondary to known medical causes such as renal artery stenosis.

The syndrome defined by Krauthammer and Klerman differs from the *Diagnostic and Statistical Manual of Mental Disorders (Third Edition)* (DSM-III) organic affective syndrome, manic type (Table 20.1) in two ways: (*a*) Krauthammer and Klerman exclude the diagnosis if there is a prior history of affective disorder, and (*b*) they observe that psychotic symptoms of either mood-congruent or mood-incongruent type can occur. The DSM-III-Revised (DSM-III-R) subsumes secondary mania under the category of organic mood syndrome, allowing manic, depressed, or mixed forms. Symptoms of delirium can be present as long as the mood disturbance does not occur exclusively during the delirious phrase. Thus DSM-III-R allows more leeway in establishing the diagnosis of organic mood syndrome (Table 20.2).

Jamieson and Wells (12) proposed that the manic symptoms should be coterminous with the appearance of the somatic disorder. This presents some difficulty in

Table 20.1   DSM-III Criteria for Organic Affective Syndrome[a]

A) The predominant disturbance is a disturbance in mood, with at least two of the associated symptoms listed in criterion B for manic or major depressive episode.[b]

B) No clouding of consciousness, as in delirium; no significant loss of intellectual abilities, as in dementia; no predominant delusions or hallucinations, as in organic delusional syndrom or organic hallucinosis.

C) Evidence, from the history, physical examination, or laboratory test, of a specific organic factor that is judged to be etiologically related to the disturbance.

[a] Reprinted with permission from *Diagnostic and Statistical Manual of Mental Disorders (Third Edition)*. Washington, DC, American Psychiatric Association, 1987. Copyright 1987 American Psychiatric Association.
[b] Symptoms included in criterion B for manic episode are 1) increase in activity (either socially, at work, or sexually) or physical restlessness, 2) more talkative than usual or pressure to keep talking, 3) flight of ideas or subjective experience that thoughts are racing, 4) inflated self esteem (grandiosity, which may be delusional), 5) decreased need for sleep, 6) distractibility, i.e., attention too easily drawn to unimportant or irrelevant external stimuli, 7) excessive involvement in activities that have a high potential for painful consequences which is not recognized, e.g., buying sprees, sexual indiscretions, foolish business investments, reckless driving.

Table 20.2   DSM-III-R Criteria for Organic Mood Syndrome[a]

A) Prominent and persistent depressed, elevated, or expansive mood.

B) There is evidence from the history, physical examination, or laboratory tests of a specific organic factor [or factors] judged to be etiologically related to the disturbance.

C) Not occurring exclusively during the course of delirium.

Specify: manic, depressed, or mixed.

[a] Reprinted with permission from *Diagnostic and Statistical Manual of Mental Disorders (Third Edition-Revised)*. Washington, DC, American Psychiatric Association, 1987. Copyright 1987 American Psychiatric Association.

view of evidence that the onset of the manic syndrome and other psychotic syndromes may be significantly delayed after the onset of the underlying disorder [up to 6 years in one report of 20 cases of posttraumatic mania (13); up to 11 years after a vascular cerebral lesion such as stroke or hemorrhage (14, 15); and over 10 years in a series of 317 posttraumatic psychoses, including 47 affective psychoses of which 3 were manic (16)].

In our experience, the criteria defined by Krauthammer and Klerman seem more useful, with the caveat that manic behavior at times can present with disorientation or confusion but the predominant disturbance clearly is one of mood.

APPROACH TO THE PATIENT

For every patient with new-onset manic behavior, the clinician should first decide if there is evidence of a primary affective disorder. The workup should include medical and psychiatric history, medication review, physical examination, toxicology screen, thyroid studies, syphilis serology, and routine chemistries. In addition to screening for prior personal or family history of affective disorder, the clinician must consider diagnoses that can be confused with mania (e.g., agitated delirium) and other psychiatric disorders that can include maniclike behavior (e.g., schizoaffective disorder) before considering the diagnosis of secondary mania.

Agitated delirium, which can occur in almost any acute medical illness under the right circumstances, is a condition in which the predominant disturbance is fluctuating attention and level of arousal, during which the symptoms typically wax and wane. The onset is fairly rapid and the duration usually brief, though chronic delirium states can also occur. In organic delusional syndromes, delusions predominate in the presence of a specific organic factor judged to be etiologically related. In organic hallucinosis, persistent or recurrent hallucinations are the predominant feature. Although dementia should also be ruled out (see Chapter 23), some dementing illnesses may first present as secondary manias (Table 20.3)

A rare syndrome that may occur in the context of mania, but can also be caused by a host of other psychiatric organic conditions, is catatonic excitement. Signs include extreme overactivity; loud pressured speech reflecting delusions and hallucinations, often with an idiosyncratic psychotic content; severe rage attacks; and streams of repetitive psychotic mannerisms and gestures. Moments of deep guilt can lead to self-mutilation. Restraint can exacerbate the condition and increase the risk to the patient of dehydration, hyperthermia, and sudden death. Neuroleptics, which can cause hypothalamic side effects, can complicate the course by masking the hyperthermia.

Other psychiatric disorders that can include manic symptomatology at some time during their course are cyclothymic disorder and schizoaffective disorder. Cyclothymia is characterized by periods of depression and hypomania, of insufficient severity and duration to meet the criteria for a major depressive or manic episode. The patient is never without hypomanic or depressive symptoms for greater than 2 months at a time during at least a 2-year period. There are no associated psychotic features, such as delusions, hallucinations, or loosening of associations. The condition should not be initiated or maintained by a specific organic factor such as repeated intoxication.

Schizoaffective disorder refers to a heterogeneous group of disorders consisting of mixtures of schizophrenic and affective symptoms. This diagnosis has been used when the clinician is unable to differentiate between affective disorder and either schizophreniform disorder or schizophrenia. Researchers who have begun to investigate this group more closely describe two subtypes—a primarily affective type and a primarily schizophrenic type. The former group, which may represent a lithium-responsive bipolar variant, lacks premorbid schizoid features and has mood-incongruent psychotic features only during the predominant mood disturbance. The latter group has premorbid schizoid features or has schizophrenia-like psychotic symptoms that persist for at least a week after the affective symptoms remit (17). According to the DSM-III-R criteria for schizoaffective disorder, at least 2 weeks of psychotic symptoms in the absence of mood disorder are required during an episode.

The question of primary versus secondary mania arises when a patient without personal or family history of affective disorder, frequently an older patient, presents with new onset of mania. Table 20.3, compiled from a large number of case reports, illustrates the panoply of disorders that can present as secondary mania (see Cummings for another comprehensive review [18]). Several cases are identified in which the mania described did not fulfill one of the Krauthammer and Klerman criteria. In some other case reports, though the patients did show manic behavior, insufficient historical data were given to determine whether or not all criteria were satisfied. The category headings in Table 20.3 were chosen to illustrate a common approach to differential diagnosis. The clinician can cover most of the diagnostic possibilities for a given symptom by systematically considering whether conditions in any of these categories could be causative.

In eliciting the patient's history, clinicians often overlook past head injury, seizures, or central nervous system (CNS) infection when evaluating possible secondary mania. History of stroke, tumor, substance abuse, or peculiar drug effects is of potential significance. A history of learning disorder or cognitive disability could become important if a question of congenital right hemisphere syndrome is being entertained (128). A thorough search for repetitive stereotypic behaviors associated with a change in state of consciousness should be included to evaluate the possibility of complex partial seizure phenomena. In addition to the routine laboratory evaluation, head computed tomographic scan and electroencephalogram should be performed on any middle-aged or elderly patient with new-onset mania and no personal or family history of affective illness. The neurologic examination and cognitive status examination dictate what areas should be focused on in these studies.

Apart from seeking obvious focal neurologic findings, it is important to conduct a detailed mental status examination. If confusion (disorientation, fluctuating level of alertness) dominates the clinical picture, an agitated delirium rather than a true secondary mania may be present. During the mental status examination, the clinician should focus on right hemisphere, deep midline and frontal function. The mental status exam may be notable for signs of right hemisphere dysfunction: hemi-inattention, hemi-neglect (of any sensory modality), or denial of deficit (anosognosia) or of its significance (anosodiaphoria); constructional apraxia; impaired visuospatial memory, map localization, and direction sense; motor impersistence; or motor or sensory emotional aprosodia (129). Because of the tendency toward denial of deficits, it may be necessary to interview other family members to obtain an accurate history (interestingly, this is often the case in primary mania as well). There may be signs of deep midline hemispheric dysfunction: movement disorders, neurovegetative signs, temporolimbic epilepsy. Orbitofrontal pathology, giving rise to euphoria, disinhibition, affective liability, difficulty maintaining and shifting set, and impaired goal-oriented behavior (impulsivity), may be difficult to distinguish on mental status exam from manic behavior. In fact, some cases described in the past as frontal lobe syndromes might also be described as secondary mania today.

The observation that a patient's mania is responsive to lithium therapy does not aid in the differentiation of primary from secondary mania since there have been numerous reports of lithium-responsive secondary manias (19, 34, 79–81). Antidepressant-induced mania is generally regarded as evidence of an underlying primary affective disorder, not secondary mania. Although primary and secondary mania often look identical, some secondary manias appear to be phenomenologically different from classic or primary mania. For instance, in a recent review of 20 cases of posttraumatic mania, irritability was a presenting symptom in 85%, compared with euphoria in only 15% (13).

On the other hand, primary mania may look organic and present as a manic pseudodementia (130, 131). Though the re-

Table 20.3   Reported Causes of Secondary Mania

Neoplasm
  Midbrain (19)
  Diencephalic (20–23)
  Suprasellar (24)
  Frontal lobe
    Bilateral (25, 26)
    Right (25)
    Left (27)
  Right frontoparietal (28)
  Intraventricular (29)
    (Right lateral ventricle)
  Left subtemporal (30)
  Right temporoparietal (25)
  Right temporal (25)
  Pituitary (25)

Vascular
  Right hemisphere stroke
    R temporoparietal infarct
      (15)
    R temporooccipital infarct
      (25)
    R temporal hematoma (14)
    R internal carotid occlusion
      (31)
    R middle cerebral infarction
      (32)
    R thalamic infarct (33)
    R thalamocapsular infarct (25)
    R thalamocapsular
      hemorrhage (25)
  Left hemisphere stroke
    L frontal infarct (25)
    L middle cerebral artery
      occlusion (34)
    L middle cerebral artery
      aneurysm (32)
  Brainstem stroke (31)
      (R midbrain, L cerebellar)
  *Right frontal arteriovenous
    malformation* (35)

Inflammatory
  Systemic lupus (36)
  Multiple sclerosis (37–39)

Infection
  Neurosyphilis (40–44)
  Herpes encephalitis (6)
  Postencephalitic parkinsonism
    (40, 45–47)
  Cryptococcal meningitis (48)
  Infectious mononucleosis (49)[a]
  Influenza A (50)[a]
  Q fever (51)
  Acquired immune deficiency
    syndrome (52, 53)

Degenerative
  Pick's disease (54)
  Parkinson's disease (55)
  Wilson's disease (56)
  Huntington's disease (57)

Metabolic/Endocrine
  Hypocalcemia (58, 59)
  B12 deficiency (60–63)
  Pellagra (64)[a]
  Dialysis encephalopathy (65)
  Hepatic encephalopathy
    (66–70)
  Grave's Disease (60, 71, 72)
  Klein-Levin syndrome (73)
  Premenstrual syndrome (74)[a]
  Postpartum mania (75, 76)
  Carcinoid (77)[c]
  Barotrauma (78)

Posttraumatic
  Head trauma (13, 16, 25, 79,
    80)
  Postsurgical
  R temporal (81)
  R hemispherectomy (82)
  Hypothalamic (23)

Seizure Disorders
  Temporal lobe epilepsy
    Interictal psychosis (83)

Toxic
  Drug-induced
    Antidepressants[b]
      Tricyclics (84, 85)
      Trazodone (86)
      Fluoxetine (87, 88)
      Tomoxetine (89)
      Bupropion (90)
      Monoamine oxidase inhibi-
        tors/Isoniazid (91, 92)

Anxiolytics
  Alprazolam (93)
Dopamine agonists
  Bromocriptine (92, 94, 95)
  L-Dopa (92, 96–98)
Dopamine antagonists
  Metaclopramide (92, 99)
Adrenergic agents
  Yohimbine (100)
Decongestants/bronchodilators
  (101)
Psychostimulants
  Amphetamine (9, 92)
  Pemoline (102)[c]
Antihypertensives
  Propranolol (92)
  Clonidine (103)[d]
  Hydralazine (104)
  Captopril (105, 106)[a]
Anticholinergics (107)
Antiarrhythmics
  Propafenone (108)
    (related to Bupropion)
Central muscle relaxants
  Baclofen (92, 109–111)
  Cyclobenzaprine (92, 112)
Nonsteroidal anti-inflammatories
  Tolmetin (113)[a]
Antiparasitic agents
  Niridazole (92)
Antineoplastics
  Procarbazine (114)
  Cyclosporin A (92, 115)
Histamine H2 receptor blocker
  Cimetidine (116)
Hallucinogens
  LSD (117)
  PCP (118)
Hormonal agents
  Corticosteroids (119, 120)[e]
  Thyroxin (92)

Metals
  Manganese (121, 122)
  Copper (56)
  Vanadium (123)
  Bromide (124, 125)

Myelographic contrast
  Metrizamide (126)

Congenital
  Multiple lentigines
    syndrome (127)[a]

[a] May not fulfill one of the Krauthammer and Klerman criteria.
[b] Not true secondary mania (see text).
[c] Prior family history of mania but no personal history.
[d] Mania followed abrupt withdrawal of drug.
[e] Dose-dependent effect (115).

ported cases of this disorder occurred in the context of either a family or a personal history of bipolar disorder, the diagnoses became clear only after the patients were successfully treated with lithium.

TREATMENT

Though the central tenet in treatment of secondary mania is to treat the underlying disorder, successful therapy with antimanic agents has been well described, even if the primary underlying disorder is not treatment responsive (12). Despite the observation that patients with CNS disorders may be more susceptibile to lithium neurotoxicity even at therapeutic levels (132, 133), lithium is often effective in this population. If the patient's symptoms are lithium resistant or if lithium is not tolerated, carbamazepine is frequently effective. Apart from being a second-choice antimanic agent for the above situations, there is mounting evidence that carbamazepine alone or in combination with lithium may be the treatment of choice for certain subsets of bipolar patients. This has been alleged in cases of secondary mania (32, 82, 134). In one study of 130 manic patients, two factors, mixed mania and presence of a second neuropsychiatric illness, correlated with lithium resistance. Mixed mania was found to be highly correlated with CNS dysfunction of any form. Many of these patients responded to anticonvulsants (usually carbamazepine) or combination lithium/carbamazepine therapy (135). If the temporal lobe syndrome is present (see chapter 30) with or without seizures, carbamazepine has been found to be effective (136). DeGreef et al. have suggested that atrophy on computed tomographic scans (indicated by lateral ventricular enlargement) generally is a sign of poor treatment outcome in bipolar patients (137).

POSSIBLE MECHANISMS

As Krauthammer and Klerman pointed out, the very existence of secondary mania, with its multitude of causes, casts doubt on any unitary single-agent hypothesis of the etiology of mania (9). Mania may represent a common pathway for expression of altered brain function due to a variety of mechanisms. We shall therefore summarize several lines of evidence linked to development of the vegetative symptoms, motoric excitement, and expansive mood that compose manic behavior.

Deep midline structures of the limbic system, basal ganglia, diencephalon, and midbrain are involved in the regulation of emotions and vegetative functions. The hypothalamus, which regulates appetite, sleep, and libido, is implicated in the production of the vegetative symptoms of mania. Many tumors reported to cause secondary mania have been in the region of the 3rd ventricle, especially on the right (33). It is also known that lesions of the medial hypothalamus in animals produce tremendous irritability (138).

Frontal lobe syndromes include symptoms seen in manic behavior, such as irritability, euphoria, grandiosity, and hyperactivity. The grandiose form of general paresis of the insane (neurosyphilis), a classic example of secondary mania, is interesting in that treponemal concentration in the frontal lobes was often a postmortem finding. In a recent study, analysis of CT lesion location in 12 patients with mania following focal brain lesions revealed that the affected area in 10 of 12 cases involved or was functionally connected to the frontal lobes. Of these, 9 cases involved the right hemisphere, 7 exclusively (25).

On the basis of experience with braindamaged individuals, epileptics, and specifically lesioned animals, it is fairly well established that the limbic system is related to the emotions. Not surprisingly, mania is among the postencephalitic psychiatric phenomena of herpes encephalitis (which has a predilection for temporolimbic areas) and of encephalitis lethargica (which was associated with lesions of the limbic system and striatum). Euphoria and elation are among the interictal behavioral changes attributed to temporolimbic epileptics (see Chapter 30). Interictal manic psychosis also occurs. Both of these conditions have been reported to be more frequently associated with right than left hemisphere epileptic foci (139, 140).

It has been proposed that the limbic system is responsible for generating extremes of emotional display, while the right hemisphere in concert with the limbic system appears to play a role in understanding and generating the more graded aspects of emotion (129). Both irritative and destructive lesions of the right hemisphere have been associated with development of mania. Mania has been reported to occur with right hemisphere tumors and strokes (Table 20.3). Cummings and Mendez reviewed 24 cases of mania secondary to focal cerebrovascular lesions and found that the majority involved diencephalic lesions and were lateralized to the right side (33). Whether the crucial factor is loss of a right hemisphere function or the resulting unopposed expression of an adjacent or left hemisphere function is yet unclear (140). Mood elevation occurs during Wada tests (intracarotid barbiturate injection for preneurosurgery determination of language dominance) of the right hemisphere (141) and after right hemispherectomy (82). Euphoric indifference occurred in roughly three times as many right than left hemisphere strokes in a cohort of 80 patients with each type (142). Motoric hyperactivity follows right more than left hemisphere injury in the rat (143). In addition, right hemisphere lesioned rats show depletion of biogenic amines whereas left hemisphere lesioned rats show no change (143, 144).

In the first controlled study of manic behavior following focal brain lesions, Starkstein et al. reported finding that (*a*) focal lesions tended to involve the limbic system more so on the right, and (*b*) ventricular brain ratios were greater than those for normal controls, lesion controls, and bipolar controls (145). However, half of their secondary mania subjects had a prior history of depression and one quarter had a family history of affective disorder. Secondary mania subjects with a positive family history had significantly less atrophy than those without such a history.

On the basis of earlier animal work, a literature review, and the above findings, Starkstein et al. proposed that the necessary conditions for developing secondary mania might be preexisting atrophy of anterior subcortical areas due to either perinatal insult or genetic vulnerability, plus a later asymmetric biogenic amine response to a right-sided lesion of either limbic or limbic-connected structures (25, 145).

The entire range of neurotransmitter-active agents (norepinephrine, serotonin, Y-aminobutyric acid, acetylcholine, and dopamine) have resulted in manic syndromes (Table 20.3). The fact that both tricyclic antidepressants that selectively inhibit serotonin reuptake (fluoxetine) and those that selectively inhibit norepinephrine reuptake (tomoxetine) can precipitate mania lends further support to the hypothesis that multiple neurotransmitter systems are involved. Although studies of the endogenous opioid system in mania have been inconclusive, it has been shown in experimental animals that stimulation of enkephalin-rich midline nuclei (in diencephalon and midbrain) can cause a mania-like mood elevation. In a classic paradigm, experimental animals with in-dwelling electrodes in "reward-oriented," enkephalin-rich, deep midline nuclei chose repeated self-stimulation of these areas (146). In one report, a persistent pseudomanic euphoria (with confusional state) developed in a patient being treated with intrathecal β-endorphin (147).

Some interesting data on the calcium/calcitonin system in bipolar disorder have emerged in recent years. Serum calcium has been found to increase concomitant with decrease in cerebrospinal fluid calcium in rapid-cycling patients entering the manic phase. Calcitonin has been shown to have antimanic effects. There is evidence that lithium increases serum calcitonin and that antidepressants tend to decrease cerebrospinal fluid calcitonin (58). Calcium channel blockers have also been shown to have some antimanic effects (148).

Clearly, the etiologies of mania are diverse. Studies of patients with bipolar disorder point to its heterogeneity. Patients without a family history of affective disorder appear to be more likely to have EEG abnormalities (149), neuropsychologic deficits (135), and larger ventricular brain ratios on CT scan (145), and are more lithium resistant (135). Further study of such "acquired manias" may eventually lead to a better understanding of the genesis of manic behavior.

SUMMARY

In summary, secondary mania should be considered in any patient without family history or prior personal history of affective disorder who develops new-onset manic behavior in late life. Such patients merit a thorough neuropsychiatric and laboratory evaluation for possible etiologic factors. Although treatment of any discovered underlying condition is the mainstay of therapy, these patients often respond to antimanic regimens. In some patients, carbamazepine or a combination of lithium/carbamazepine therapy may be the treatment of choice.

References

1. Critchley M: Five illustrious neuroluetics. In Critchley M (ed): *The Divine Banquet of the Brain.* New York, Raven Press, 1980, pp 203–217.
2. Ignotus P: *The Paradox of Maupassant.* New York, Funk and Wagnalls, 1966.
3. Kraepelin E: *Manic-Depressive Insanity and Paranoia.* Edinburgh, E&S Livingstone, 1921.
4. Bonhoeffer K: Exogenous psychoses (1909). In Hirsch SR, Shepherd M (eds): *Themes and Variations in European Psychiatry.* Charlottesville, University Press of Virginia, 1974, pp 46–52.
5. Bleuler E: *Textbook of Psychiatry.* New York, Arno Press, 1976 (Reprint from 1916).
6. Koehler K, Guth W: The mimicking of mania in "benign" herpes simplex encephalitis. *Biol Psychiatry* 14:405–411, 1979.
7. Lipowski ZJ: Organic mental disorders: their history and classification with special reference to DSM-III. In Miller NE, Cohen GD (eds): *Clinical Aspects of Alzheimer's Disease and Senile Dementia.* New York, Raven Press, 1981, pp 37–45.
8. Bleuler M: Psychiatry of cerebral diseases. *Br Med J* 2:1233–1238, 1951.
9. Krauthammer C, Klerman GL: Secondary mania. *Arch Gen Psychiatry* 35:1333–1339, 1978.
10. Robins E, Guze SB: Classification of affective disorders: the primary–secondary, the endogenous–reactive, and the neurotic–psychotic concepts. In Williams TA, Katz MM, Shield J ASA (Eds): *Recent Advances in the Psychobiology of the Depressive Illnesses* (DHEW Publication No. HSM 70-9053) Washington, DC, Department of Health, Education and Welfare, 1972, pp 289–293.
11. Klerman GL, Barrett JE: The affective disorders: clinical and epidemiological aspects. In Gershon S, Shopsin B (eds): *Lithium, Its Role in Psychiatric Research and Treatment.* New York, Plenum Press, 1973, pp 201–236.
12. Jamieson RC, Wells CE: Manic psychosis in a patient with multiple metastatic brain tumors. *J Clin Psychiatry* 40:280–282, 1979.
13. Shukla S, Cook BL, Mukherjee S, et al: Mania following head trauma. *Am J Psychiatry* 144:93–96, 1987.
14. Cohen MR, Niska RW: Localized right cerebral hemisphere dysfunction and recurrent mania. *Am J Psychiatry* 137:847–848, 1980.
15. Levin DN, Finklestein S: Delayed psychosis after right temporoparietal stroke or trauma: relation to epilepsy. *Neurology* 32:267–273, 1982.
16. Achte KA, Hillbom E, Aalberg V: Psychoses following war brain injuries. *Acta Psychiatr Scand* 45:1–18, 1969.
17. Levinson DF, Levitt MEM: Schizoaffective mania reconsidered. *Am J Psychiatry* 144:415–425, 1987.
18. Cummings JL: Organic psychoses *Psychiatr Clin North Am* 9:293–311, 1986.
19. Oyewumi LK, LaPierre YD: Efficacy of lithium in treating mood disorder occurring after brain stem injury. *Am J Psychiatry* 138:110–112, 1981.
20. Stern K, Dancey TE: Glioma of the diencephalon in a manic patient. *Am J Psychiatry* 98:716–719, 1942.
21. Greenberg DB, Brown GL: Mania resulting from brain stem tumor. *J Nerv Ment Dis* 173:434–436, 1985.
22. Malamud N: Psychiatric disorder with intracranial tumors of limbic system. *Arch Neurol* 17:113–123, 1967.
23. Alpers BJ: Relation of the hypothalamus to disorders of personality. *Arch Neurol Psychiatry* 38:291–303, 1937.
24. Guttman E, Hermann K: Ueber psychische Storungen bei Hirnstammerkrankungen und das Automatosesyndrom. *Ztschr f d ges Neur u Psychiat* 140:439–472, 1932.
25. Starkstein SE, Boston JD, Robinson RG: Mechanisms of mania after brain injury. *J Nerv Ment Dis* 176:87–100, 1988.
26. Ackerly S: Instinctive, emotional, and mental changes following prefrontal lobe extirpation. *Am J Psychiatry* 92:717–729, 1937.
27. Robinson BW: Limbic influences on human speech. *Ann NY Acad Sci* 280:761–771, 1976.
28. Oppler W: Manic psychosis in a case of parasag-

ittal meningioma. *Arch Neurol Psychiatry* 64:417–430, 1950.

29. Binder RL: Neurologically silent brain tumors in psychiatric hospital admissions: three cases and a review. *J Clin Psychiatry* 44:94–97, 1983.
30. Bourgeois M, Campagne A: Maniaco-dépressive et syndrome de Garcin. *Annales Médico-Psychologiques, Paris* 125(Suppl. 2):451–460, 1967.
31. Van Der Lugt PJM, DeVisser AP: Two patients with a vital expansive syndrome following a cerebrovascular accident. *Psychiat Neurol Neurochir* 70:349–359, 1967.
32. Jampala VC, Abrams R: Mania secondary to left and right hemisphere damage. *Am J Psychiatry* 140:1197–1199, 1983.
33. Cummings JL, Mendez MF: Secondary mania with focal cerebrovascular lesions. *Am J Psychiatry* 141:1084–1087, 1984.
34. Herlihy CE Jr, Herlihy CE: Lithium and organic brain syndrome. *J Clin Psychiatry* 40:455, 1979.
35. Gross RA, Herridge P: A maniclike illness associated with right frontal arteriovenous malformation. *J Clin Psychiatry* 49:119–120, 1988.
36. Feinglass EJ, Arnett FC, Dorsch CA, et al: Neuropsychiatric manifestations of systemic lupus erythematosus: diagnosis, clinical spectrum and relationship to other features of the disease. *Medicine* 55:323–339, 1976.
37. Kwentus JA, Hart RP, Calabrese V, et al: Mania as a symptom of multiple sclerosis. *Psychosomatics* 27:729–731, 1986.
38. Mapelli G, Ramelli E: Manic syndrome associated with multiple sclerosis: secondary mania? *Acta Psychiatr Belg* 81:337–349, 1981.
39. Surridge D: An investigation into some psychiatric aspects of multiple sclerosis. *Br J Psychiatry* 115:749–764, 1969.
40. Lishman WA. *Organic Psychiatry.* Oxford, Blackwell Scientific Publications, 1978.
41. Mapelli G, Bellelli T. Secondary mania. *Arch Gen Psychiatry* 39:743, 1982.
42. Binder RL, Dickman WA: Psychiatric manifestations of neurosyphilis in middle-aged patients. *Am J Psychiatry* 137:741–742, 1980.
43. Cummings JL, Benson DF: *Dementia: A Clinical Approach.* Boston: Butterworth, 1983.
44. Ravi SD, Roach FL, O'Rourke CJ: Neurosyphilis and late onset mental changes in the elderly. *J Clin Psychiatry* 45:484, 1984.
45. Weisert KN, Hendrie HC: Secondary mania? A case report. *Am J Psychiatry* 134:929–930, 1977.
46. Fairweather DS: Psychiatric aspects of the postencephalitic syndrome. *J Ment Sci* 93:201–254, 1947.
47. Holt WL: Epidemic encephalitis. *Arch Neurol Psychiatr* 38:1135–1144, 1937.
48. Thienhaus OJ, Khosla N: Meningeal cryptococcosis misdiagnosed as a manic episode. *Am J Psychiatry* 141:1459–1460, 1984.
49. Goldney RD, Temme PB: Case report: manic depressive psychosis following infectious mononucleosis. *J Clin Psychiatry* 41:322–323, 1980.
50. Steinberg D, Hirsch SR, Marston SD, et al: Influenza infection causing manic psychosis. *Br J Psychiatry* 120:531–535, 1972.
51. Schwartz RB: Manic psychosis in connection with Q fever. *Br J Psychiatry* 124:140–143, 1974.
52. Kermani E, Drob S, Alpert M: Organic brain syndrome in three cases of acquired immune deficiency syndrome. *Compr Psychiatry* 25:294–297, 1984.
53. Perry S, Jacobsen P: Neuropsychiatric manifestations of AIDS-spectrum disorders. *Hosp Community Psychiatry* 37:135–142, 1986.
54. Neumann MA: Pick's disease. *J Neuropath Exp Neurol* 8:255–282, 1949.
55. Schwab RS, Fabing HD, Prichard JS: Psychiatric symptoms and syndromes in Parkinson's disease. *Am J Psychiatry* 107:901, 1951.
56. Pandey RS, Screenivas KN, Patil NM, et al: Dopamine-beta-hydroxylase inhibition in a patient with Wilson's disease and manic symptoms. *Am J Psychiatry* 138:1628–1629, 1981.
57. Folstein SE, Franz ML, Jensen BA, et al: Conduct disorder and affective disorder among the offspring of patients with Huntington's disease. *Psychol Med* 13:45–52, 1983.
58. Carman JS, Wyatt ES, Smith W, et al: Calcium and calcitonin in bipolar affective disorder. In Post RM, Ballenger JC (eds): *Neurobiology of Mood Disorders.* Baltimore, Williams & Wilkins, 1984, pp 340–355.
59. Groat RD, Mackenzie TB: The appearance of mania following intravenous calcium replacement. *J Nerv Ment Dis* 168:562–563, 1980.
60. Lassen E, Ewald H: Acute organic psychosis caused by thyrotoxicosis and vitamin B_{12} deficiency: a case report. *J Clin Psychiatry* 46:106–107, 1985.
61. Zucker DK, Livingston RL, Nakra R, et al: B_{12} deficiency and psychiatric disorders: case report and literature review. *Biol Psychiatry* 16(2):197–205, 1981.
62. Evans DL, Edelsohn GA, Golden RN. Organic psychosis without anemia or spinal cord symptoms in patients with vitamin B_{12} deficiency. *Am J Psychiatry* 140:218–221, 1983.
63. Goggans FC. A case of mania secondary to vitamin B_{12} deficiency. *Am J Psychiatry* 141:300–301, 1984.
64. Spivak JL, Jackson DL. Pellagra: an analysis of 18 patients and a review of the literature. *Johns Hopkins Med J* 140:295–309, 1977.
65. Jack RA, Rivers-Bulkeley NT, Rabin PL. Secondary mania as a presentation of progressive dialysis encephalopathy. *J Nerv Ment Dis* 171:193–195, 1983.
66. Read AE, Sherlock S, Laidlaw J, et al: The neuropsychiatric syndromes associated with chronic liver disease and an extensive portal–systemic collateral circulation. *Q J Med* 141:135–150, 1967.
67. Adams RD, Foley JM: The neurological disorder associated with liver disease. In Merritt HH, Hare CC (eds): *Metabolic and Toxic Diseases of the Nervous System.* Baltimore, Williams & Wilkins, 1953.

68. Havens LL, Child CG: Recurrent psychosis associated with liver disease and elevated blood ammonia. *N Engl J Med* 252:756–759, 1955.

69. Summerskill WHJ, Davidson EA, Sherlock S, et al: the neuropsychiatric syndrome associated with hepatic cirrhosis and an extensive portal collateral circulation. *Q J Med* 25:245–266, 1956.

70. Sherlock S, Summerskill WHJ, White LP, et al: Portal-systemic encephalopathy. *Lancet* 2:453–457, 1954.

71. Villani S, Weitzel WD: Secondary mania. *Arch Gen Psychiatry* 36:1031, 1979.

72. Young LD: Organic affective disorder associated with thyrotoxicosis. *Psychosomatics* 25:490–492, 1984.

73. Jeffries JJ, Lefebvre A: Depression and mania associated with Kleine-Levin-Critchley syndrome. *Can Psychiatr Assoc J* 18:439–444, 1973.

74. Williams EY, Weekes LR: Premenstrual tension associated with psychotic states. *J Nerv Ment Dis* 116:321, 1952.

75. Kadrmas A, Winokur G, Crowe R: Postpartum mania. *Br J Psychiatry* 135:551–554, 1979.

76. Brockington IF, Cernik KF, Schofield EM, et al: Puerperal psychosis. *Arch Gen Psychiatry* 38:829–833, 1981.

77. Lehmann J: Mental disturbances followed by stupor in a patient with carcinoidosis. *Acta Psychiatr Scand* 42:153, 1966.

78. Stoudemire A, Miller J, Schmitt F, et al: Development of an organic affective syndrome during a hyperbaric diving experiment. *Am J Psychiatry* 141:1251–1254, 1984.

79. Sinanan K: Mania as a sequel to a road traffic accident. *Br J Psychiatry* 144:330–331, 1984.

80. Cohn CK, Wright JR III, DeVaul RA: Post head trauma syndrome in an adolescent treated with lithium carbonate—case report. *Dis Nerv Syst* 38:630–631, 1977.

81. Rosenbaum AH, Barry MJ. Positive therapeutic response to lithium secondary to organic brain syndrome. *Am J Psychiatry* 132:1072–1073, 1975.

82. Forrest DV. Bipolar illness after right hemispherectomy. *Arch Gen Psychiatry* 39:817–819, 1982.

83. Flor-Henry P: Psychosis and temporal lobe epilepsy. *Epilepsia* 10:363–395, 1969.

84. Dilsaver SC, Greden JF: Antidepressant withdrawal phenomena. *Biol Psychiatry* 19:237–257, 1984.

85. Pickar D, Cowdry RW, Zis AP, et al: Mania and hypomania during antidepressant pharmacotherapy: clinical and research implications. In Post RM, Ballenger JC (eds): *Neurobiology of Mood Disorders.* Baltimore, Williams & Wilkins, 1984, pp 836–845.

86. Warren M, Bick PA: Two case reports of trazodone-induced mania. *Am J Psychiatry* 141:103–104, 1984.

87. Chouinard G, Steiner W: A case of mania induced by high-dose fluoxetine treatment. *Am J Psychiatry* 143:686, 1986.

88. Settle EC, Settle GP: A case of mania associated with fluoxetine. *Am J Psychiatry* 141:280–281, 1984.

89. Steinberg S, Chouinard G: A case of mania associated with tomoxetine. *Am J Psychiatry* 142:1517–1518, 1985.

90. Shopsin B: Bupropion: a new clinical profile in the psychobiology of depression. *J Clin Psychiatry* 44:140–142, 1983.

91. Rothschild AJ: Mania after withdrawal of isocarboxazid. *J Clin Psychopharmacol* 5:339–341, 1985.

92. Abramowicz M (ed): Drugs that cause psychiatric symptoms. *Med Letter Drug Ther* 28:81–86, 1986.

93. France RD, Krishnan KRR. Alprazolam-induced manic reaction. *Am J Psychiatry* 141:1127–1128, 1984.

94. Vlissides DN, Gill D, Castelow J: Bromocriptine-induced mania? *Br Med J* I:510, 1978.

95. Brook NM, Cookson IB: Bromocriptine-induced mania? *Br Med J* I:790, 1978.

96. Harsch HH, Miller M, Young LD. Induction of mania by L-dopa in a nonbipolar patient. *J Clin Psychopharmacol* 5:338–339, 1985.

97. Ryback RS, Schwab RS: Manic response to levodopa therapy. *N Engl J Med* 285:788–789, 1971.

98. Lin JT-Y, Ziegler DK: Psychiatric symptoms with initiation of carbidopa-levodopa treatment. *Neurology* 26:699–700, 1976.

99. Ritchie KS, Preskorn SH: Mania induced by metoclopramide: case report. *J Clin Psychiatry* 45:180–181, 1984.

100. Price LH, Charney DS, Heninger GR: Three cases of manic symptoms following yohimbine administration. *Am J Psychiatry* 141:1267–1268, 1984.

101. Waters BGH, LaPierre YD. Secondary mania associated with sympathomimetic drug use. *Am J Psychiatry* 138:837–838, 1981.

102. Sternbach H: Pemoline-induced mania. *Biol Psychiatry* 16:987–989, 1981.

103. Tollefson GD: Hyperadrenergic hypomania consequent to the abrupt cessation of clonidine. *J Clin Psychopharmacol* 1:93–95, 1981.

104. Paykel ES, Fleminger R, Watson JP. Psychiatric side effects of antihypertensive drugs other than reserpine. *J Clin Psychopharmacol* 2:14–39, 1982.

105. Zubenko GS, Nixon RA: Mood-elevating effects of captopril in depressed patients. *Am J Psychiatry* 141:110–111, 1984.

106. McMahon T: Bipolar affective symptoms associated with use of captopril and abrupt withdrawal of pargyline and propranolol. *Am J Psychiatry* 142:759–760, 1985.

107. Coid J, Strang J: Mania secondary to procyclidine. ('Kemadrin') abuse. *Br J Psychiatry* 141:81–84, 1982.

108. Jack RA: A case of mania secondary to propafenone. *J Clin Psychiatry* 46:104–105, 1985.

109. Arnold ES, Rudd SM, Kirschner H: Manic psychosis following rapid withdrawal from baclofen. *Am J Psychiatry* 137:1466–1467, 1980.

110. Kirubakaran V, Mayfield D, Rengachary S: Dyskinesia and psychosis in a patient following ba-

clofen withdrawal. *Am J Psychiatry* 141:692–693, 1984.

111. Wolf ME, Almy G, Toll M, et al: Mania associated with the use of baclofen. *Biol Psychiatry* 17:757–759, 1982.

112. Harsch HH. Mania in two patients following cyclobenzaprine. *Psychosomatics* 25:791–793, 1984.

113. Sotsky SM, Tossell JW: Tolmetin induction of mania. *Psychosomatics* 25:626–628, 1984.

114. Carney MWP, Ravindran A, Lewis DS. Manic psychosis associated with procarbazine. *Br Med J* 284:82–83, 1982.

115. Wamboldt FW, Weiler SJ, Kalin NH. Cyclosporin-associated mania. *Biol Psychiatry* 19:1161–1162, 1984.

116. Hubain PP, Subolski J, Mendlewicz J. Cimetidine-induced mania. *Neuropsychobiology* 8:223, 1982.

117. Horowitz HA. The use of lithium in treatment of drug-induced psychotic reactions. *Dis Nerv Syst* 36:159–163, 1975.

118. Pearlson GD: Psychiatric and medical syndromes associated with phencyclidine (PCP) abuse. *Johns Hopkins Med J* 148:25–33, 1981.

119. Ling MHM, Perry PJ, Tsuang MT. Side effects of corticosteroid therapy. *Arch Gen Psychiatry* 38:471–477, 1981.

120. Boston Collaborative Drug Surveillance Program: Acute adverse reactions to prednisone in relation to dosage. *Clin Pharmacol and Ther* 13:694–698, 1972.

121. Schuler P, Oyanguren H, Maturana V, et al: Manganese poisoning. *Industrial Medicine and Surgery* 167–173, April, 1957.

122. Penalver R: Manganese poisoning. *Industrial Medicine and Surgery* 1–7, January 1955.

123. Yung CY: A synopsis on metals in medicine and psychiatry. *Pharmacol Biochem Behav* 21(Suppl 1):41–47, 1984.

124. Sayed AJ: Mania and bromism: a case report and a look to the future. *Am J Psychiatry* 133:228–229, 1976.

125. Carney MWP. Five cases of bromism. *Lancet* 2:523–524, 1971.

126. Kwentus JA, Silverman JJ, Sprague M: Manic syndrome after metrizamide myelography. *Am J Psychiatry* 141:700–702, 1984.

127. Loyd DW, Tsuang MT, Benge JW: A study of a family with Leopard syndrome. *J Clin Psychiatry* 43:114–116, 1982.

128. Weintraub S, Mesulam M: Developmental learning disabilities of the right hemisphere. *Arch Neurol* 40:463–468, 1983.

129. Ross ED. Modulation of affect and nonverbal communication by the right hemisphere. In Mesulam M-M: *Principles of Behavioral Neurology*. Philadelphia, F.A. Davis, 1985, pp 239–257.

130. Koenigsberg HW: Manic pseudodementia: case report. *J Clin Psychiatry* 45:132–134, 1984.

131. Thase ME, Reynolds CF: Manic pseudodementia. *Psychosomatics* 25:258–260, 1984.

132. Himmelhoch JM, Neil JF, May SJ, et al: Age, dementia, dyskinesias and lithium response. *Am J Psychiatry* 137:941–945, 1980.

133. Rifkin A, Quitkin F, Klein DF: Organic brain syndrome during lithium carbonate treatment. *Compr Psychiatry* 14:251–254, 1973.

134. Folks DG, King D, Dowdy SB, et al: Carbamazepine treatment of selected affectively disordered inpatients. *Am J Psychiatry* 139:115–117, 1982.

135. Himmelhoch JM, Garfinkel ME: Sources of lithium resistance in mixed mania. *Psychopharmacol Bull* 22:613–620, 1986.

136. Blumer D, Heilbronn M, Himmelhoch J: Indications for carbamazepine in mental illness. In: Proceedings of the 139th Annual Meeting of the American Psychiatric Association. Washington DC, American Psychiatric Association, 1986.

137. DeGreef G, Mukherjee S, Bilder RM: CT scan findings in bipolar patients. Presented at Symposium 33, ''Neuropsychiatry of Bipolar Disorders,'' Annual Meeting of the American Psychiatric Association, Chicago, 1987.

138. Kandel ER, Schwartz JH (eds): *Principles of Neural Science*, ed 2. New York, Elsevier, 1985.

139. Bear DM: Hemispheric specialization and the neurology of emotion. *Arch Neurol* 40:195–202, 1983.

140. Flor-Henry P: *Cerebral Basis of Psychopathology*. Boston, John Wright, 1983.

141. Sackheim HA, Greenberg MS, Weiman AL, et al: Hemispheric asymmetry in the expression of positive and negative emotions. *Arch Neurol* 39:210–218, 1982.

142. Gainotti G: Emotional behavior and hemispheric side of the lesion. *Cortex* 8:41–55, 1972.

143. Robinson RG: Differential behavioral and biochemical effects of right and left hemispheric cerebral infarction in the rat. *Science* 205:707–710, 1979.

144. Robinson RG, Coyle JT: The differential effect of right versus left hemispheric cerebral infarction on catecholamines and behavior in the rat. *Brain Res* 188:63–78, 1980.

145. Starkstein SE, Pearlson GD, Boston J, et al: Mania after brain injury. *Arch Neurol* 44:1069–1073, 1987.

146. Olds J: Self-stimulation of the brain. *Science* 127:315–324, 1958.

147. Pickar D, Dubois M, Cohen MR: Behavioral change in a cancer patient following intrathecal beta-endorphin administration. *Am J Psychiatry* 141:103–104, 1984.

148. Dubovsky SL: Calcium antagonists: a new class of psychiatric drugs? *Psychiatr Ann* 16:724–728, 1986.

149. Cook BL, Shukla S, Hoff AL: EEG abnormalities in bipolar affective disorder. *J Affect Disord* 11:147–149, 1986.

21

Disturbances of Thinking

Theo C. Manschreck, M.D.
Martin B. Keller, M.D.

A careful interview together with additional information from family and friends usually provides adequate data to assess the possibility of a disturbance in thinking. Occasionally, because of the patient's lack of cooperation or the brevity of the evaluation, the clinician may need to reserve judgment regarding thinking disturbance until further evaluation is possible. Another problem interfering with assessment is the fact that many disturbances occur intermittently and may not be present during the interview. Despite these limitations, the assessment of thinking may disclose abnormalities that contribute important data to comprehensive diagnosis.

The approach to differential diagnosis of thinking should be as follows. First, knowing the four features of thinking to observe—flow (or stream), possession (or control), content, and form—the clinician can systematically judge their intactness (1). Second, as the clinician becomes aware of abnormalities, he or she needs to describe them precisely. Third, by evaluating additional information (e.g., history, laboratory, and other observations), the clinician can organize the search to pin down the possible source for these abnormalities.

In this chapter, discussion of differential diagnosis will cover disturbances related to each of the four features of thinking. Then we suggest a clinical approach to thinking disturbance that emphasizes certain simplifying principles and organizes the evaluation efficiently.

See chapter 12 for a description of disturbances of thinking in the mental status examination.

DISTURBANCES IN THE FLOW OF THOUGHT (STREAM OR PROGRESS)

See Table 21.1 for a list of disturbances in flow of thought.

Rate Disturbances

Slowed or inhibited thinking occurs in retarded depression so regularly that many clinicians mistakenly consider it to be diagnostic. Slowed thinking may be due to anxiety or preoccupation, even in depressed patients. Not to be forgotten is a variety of brain disorders, including frontal and postconcussive syndromes, as well as delirium, in which slowed thinking occurs as a prominent feature. In these cases the appropriate diagnosis derives from consideration of additional features.

Mutism strongly suggests organic sources (e.g., akinetic mutism, presenile

Table 21.1 Disturbances in the Flow of Thought

Rate disturbances	
Slowed or inhibited thinking	Occurs in retarded depression. Changes in rate may also be due to the influence of anxiety and preoccupation or a variety of brain disorders including prefrontal and postconcussive syndromes as well as delirium.
Mutism	Strongly suggests organic sources (e.g., akinetic mutism, presenile dementia, subdural hematoma) that should be carefully ruled out. Mutism is often present in patients who are severely depressed or catatonic.
Rapid thinking	Occasionally a normal occurrence, but typical of excited states in psychiatry. May be associated with dissociative disturbances, catatonia, and morbid elation. Certain causes are exogenous: tricyclic, antihistaminic, and anticholinergic toxic states: marijuana, barbiturate, or other sedative–hypnotic toxicity; and intoxication and central nervous system stimulants. In the case of anxiety and hypomanic states, may be accompanied by *pressured speech. Flight of ideas* may also be present in manic states.
Disturbances of the train or continuity of thinking	
Circumstantiality	Frequently encountered in elderly patients experiencing changes in intellectual ability, in patients suffering from brain damage, in obsessional patients, and in central nervous system disturbances that induce mild intellectual deficits.
Tangentiality	Seen most often in schizophrenia, but may occur as an isolated disturbance of thinking in patients suffering from severe short-term memory losses (e.g., Korsakoff's syndrome). Also seen in patients suffering from a variety of intellectual disturbances, including dementia.
Thought blocking	Sign of schizophrenic illness. May also occur in anxious or tired normals.
Perseveration	Seen in adolescence, schizophrenia, and obsessional disorder. It is increased by fatigue, tension, and anxiety. As a persistent symptom, it may be a reliable sign of brain disease (delirium and dementia, closed head injury, carbon monoxide poisoning, and alcohol and sedative–hypnotic drug intoxication).

dementia, and subdural hematoma) that should be carefully ruled out. Mutism is present occasionally in patients who are severely depressed or suffering from catatonic disturbances. However, such a finding is unusual in these disorders without simultaneous occurrence of stupor. In recent years there have been reports of phenothiazine toxicity inducing a state of mutism. "Hysterical aphonia" may be distinguished from organically caused mutism by the patient's ability to cough. In more difficult cases sodium amobarbitol interview and electroencephalography may be helpful in establishing the diagnosis. The former may strongly suggest a psychogenic mutism, if the patient is able to speak under the influence of the drug; the latter may disclose changes consistent with specific disease.

Rapid thinking occasionally occurs with no specific import. Yet, dissociative disturbances, catatonia, and morbid elation should be considered. Classically, rapid thinking occurs in anxiety and hypomanic states accompanied by *pressured speech. Flight of ideas* is the term typically used to describe rapid thinking in manic states. Yet without other symptoms or signs of mania, flight of ideas may be difficult to interpret. It may occur in anxious or excited schizophrenia patients.

Certain causes of rapid thinking are exogenous. These include tricyclic, antihistaminic, and anticholinergic toxic states; marijuana, barbiturate, or other sedative–hypnotic toxicity; and intoxication with central nervous system stimulants. Careful history, evaluation of vital signs, occasionally a therapeutic trial (as, for example, in anticholinergic toxicity, where challenge with appropriate doses of physostigmine may be indicated), and complete mental status examination generally disclose the source of rapid thinking disturbances.

Disturbances of the Train or Continuity of Thinking

Circumstantiality is most frequently encountered in elderly patients experiencing changes in intellectual ability and in the brain damaged. For instance, in epileptic patients, pedantic, overly detailed speech may serve to compensate for mild disturbances in conceptualization and efficiency of thought production. By the same token, circumstantiality is often seen in central nervous system disturbances that induce mild intellectual deficits. Obsessional patients may exhibit circumstantial thinking when they are literally unable to come to the point.

Tangentiality is classically observed in schizophrenia. In such cases, other features of thought disturbance are usually evident. However, tangentiality may occur as an isolated disturbance of thinking in patients suffering from severe short-term memory losses, as in chronic alcoholism (e.g., Korsakoff's syndrome), affecting thalamic and mammillary body functioning. Tangentiality is also seen in patients suffering from a variety of intellectual disturbances, including dementia.

Thought blocking is a particularly striking sign of schizophrenic illness. However, there is a tendency to identify as thought blocking the hesitations, pauses, and losses of train of thought that occur in anxious or tired normals and in patients with other conditions, such as petit mal epilepsy.

Perseveration in thinking may be present in normals (particularly in adolescence) and in psychiatric conditions (such as schizophrenia and obsessional disorder). It is increased by fatigue, tension, and anxiety. If persistent and regularly present, it may be considered a reliable sign of brain disease, including the manifold varieties of delirium and dementia, but especially closed head injury, carbon monoxide poisoning, alcohol and sedative–hypnotic drug association, liver disease, and electrolyte disturbances. Focal disturbances and the frontal lobe and a high percentage of aphasic disorders have associated perseverative disturbances of thinking (2).

CONTROL OR POSSESSION OF THINKING

See Table 21.2 for a list of disturbances in control or possession of thinking.

Obsessional thinking occurs in normal children and adults, where it may be aggravated and sustained by intense anxiety. Nevertheless, obsessional thinking commonly occurs in psychopathologic conditions such as schizophrenia, depression, and phobic and anxiety states. These cases are usually distinguished on the basis of the prominence of their more cardinal symptoms so that diagnosis is not difficult. If obsessional thinking is the most prominent feature of psychopathology, the patient may be suffering from an obsessional disorder. Organic sources for obsessional thinking should not be overlooked. Classically, encephalitis has been associated with obsessional states; however, other potential sources include dementia, posttraumatic states, postencephalitic states, and hypothyroidism.

Thought alienation and passivity experiences typically occur in schizophrenia. Schneider (3) observed that similar experiences may be seen in cases with generalized brain disease as well. Infrequently, depression, manic states, and personality disorder may occur with these symptoms. Currently, this kind of disturbance is frequently associated with hallucinogenic intoxication or other drug and alcohol states.

Table 21.2 Control of Possession of Thinking

Obsessional thinking	A normal feature of child and adult function that may be aggravated and sustained by intense anxiety. Also occurs in obsessional disorder, schizophrenia, depression, and phobic and anxiety states. Possible organic sources include encephalitis lethargica, dementia, post-traumatic states, postencephalitic states, and hypothyroidism.
Thought alienation and passivity experiences	Typically occurring in schizophrenia but may also be seen in cases with generalized brain disease. Depression, manic states, and personality disorder may occur with these symptoms.

CONTENT OF THINKING DISTURBANCES OR DELUSIONS

See Table 21.3 for a list of types of delusions.

Delusions are divided into various types, such as delusions of persecution, jealousy, and love, according to the content of the delusion. Generally, delusions can and do appear in virtually all varieties of disorder—both classical psychiatric disorders and traditional medical and neurologic disease—that have psychotic manifestations (4). The clinician may gather significant information relevant to diagnosis by recognizing the type and setting of delusions encountered.

Among the useful hints:

1. *Try to discover the relationship between the delusion and the patient's mood.* Is the patient with a delusion of persecution being arbitrarily singled out for punishment or other unusual treatment, or is there a kind of extreme justice being exacted for past sins, wickedness, or indiscretions? Similarly, with delusions of grandeur, does the heightened sense of importance attached to this delusion parallel or seem to flow from an unusually high tide of cheerfulness, elation, euphoria, or boundless energy? Does the delusion in these circumstances appear to be an "understandable" development of mood? If so, affective disorder may be present.
2. *Try to determine the relationship between delusions and level of awareness.* In many medical conditions, the acute occurrence of delusions is frequently associated with disturbances in orientation, or clouding of consciousness. Generally, schizophrenia and affective disorders exhibit delusions in clear consciousness.
3. *Try to determine the relationship between delusions and activities planned in response to them.* Certain delusions, particularly jealousy, for instance, have been associated repeatedly with premeditated acts of revenge, including murder. Generally, when delusions form the major and perhaps only symptom in a clinical presentation, the patient may be more organized and capable of acting on such thoughts. Hence, inquiry about plans for acting on delusional concerns may disclose the patient most dangerous to himself or others.

The lack of a specific relationship between particular disorders and particular delusions has several consequences for the clinician. First, a delusion is evidence more of *severe* psychopathology than of *specific* psychopathology. Second, discovery of a delusion requires a thorough investigation of medical, neurologic, and psychiatric possibilities for understanding the clinical presentation. Third, even the most cherished clinical psychiatric maxims about delusions must be considered suspect. These include the following: (*a*) Delusions of grandeur indicate mania and manic–depressive disorder. Such delusions, though they occur in manic states, occur in schizophrenic disorder and a multitude of organic conditions as well, e.g., steroid psychoses, hallucinogenic intoxications, and frontal lobe syndromes. (*b*) Delusions of persecution indicate schizophrenia. Often they do, but persecution is also typical of psychotic depression, even mania, delusional disorders and a number of organic disorders. (*c*) Somatic delusions indicate schizophrenia. Somatic delusions are known to occur in schizophrenia. Their occurrence in psychotic depression is also well documented. Furthermore, they routinely appear in dementia, other chronic brain disease, drug-induced psychoses, and also in delusional disorders.

For those types of delusion that have not

Table 21.3   Delusion Types[a]

Persecution	Poverty
Love (erotomania)	Guilt
Jealousy	Nihilism
Ill health (somatic defect)	Reference
Grandeur	Influence
	Imposture

[a] See Chapter 12 for a discussion of types of delusion.

been mentioned in this general discussion, the same principles apply. Namely, all delusions are nonspecific. Hence, they may occur in a variety of psychiatric and neurologic or medical conditions. Differential diagnosis must be based on other features.

Certain bizarre or impossible delusions are predominantly associated with schizophrenia. These include delusions of influence and delusional perceptions. Occasionally, brain disease, both focal and general, may result in this kind of delusion. The most likely brain diseases in this domain are the epileptic disorders, particularly temporal lobe disease. Nevertheless, because there is a variety of disturbances that can cause delusions; the clinician must be careful to assess neurologic findings thoroughly in all cases of delusion (3, 5).

FORMAL DISTURBANCES OF THINKING (FORMAL THOUGHT DISORDER)

See Table 21.4 for a list of formal disturbances of thinking.

Traditionally, formal thought disturbance was considered an essential finding for the diagnosis of schizophrenia (5, 6). Furthermore, it has generally been accorded the status of pathognomonicity in schizophrenia. It is now known that we must temper our enthusiasm for these clinical teachings. Other psychiatric and medical disorders may result in formal thinking disturbance (7, 8).

Logical errors in thinking occur regularly in normals regardless of educational background. They are more frequently seen in states of fatigue or tenison. Mentally retarded, delirious, and demented patients may be unable to present thoughts logically. In schizophrenia, what appears to be poor logic may be more the result of highly unusual or bizarre inferences when thinking is examined more closely (9). Often, such strange thoughts are based on premises that reflect idiosyncratic insights or associations, and the conclusions the patient draws from the premises may be quite logical. The difficulty arises, of course, as to how to determine what the premises are. This determination, perhaps more than any other aspect of evaluation in thinking, can disclose crucial clues (such as delusions or unusual perceptual experiences) regarding the nature of the patient's cognitive disturbances. In short, knowing what the premises are in many cases may be more helpful than recognizing that the patient's logic seems to be aberrant.

The *ability to abstract* is often impaired in psychiatric patients, yet the portent of such a finding is difficult to estimate. Intelligence appears to influence this ability greatly. Goldstein (10), who pioneered investigations using the abstract–concrete dimension of thinking, founded his ideas on careful observations of brain-injured patients. As might be expected, patients with deficits in intellectual functioning, particularly patients with dementia, mental retardation, and prefrontal syndromes, commonly exhibit concrete thinking. In schizophrenia, concrete thinking has been put forward as a cardinal feature. Yet, in observations of schizophrenia,

Table 21.4 Formal Disturbances of Thinking (Formal Thought Disorder)

Logical errors	Occurring regularly in normals, aggravated by states of fatigue and tension. Mentally retarded, delirious, and demented patients may be unable to present thoughts logically. In schizophrenia, logical errors may be more the result of highly unusual or bizarre inferences.
Incoherence	Difficult to evaluate because disturbances in coherence lead to disruption in the comprehensibility of thinking. If the disturbance is in associations (e.g., derailment), the diagnostic possibilities should include aphasic disorders, schizophrenia, manic–depressive disorder, and drug intoxication. May occur as a severe manifestation of schizophrenia, manic–depressive illness, mental retardation, dementia, delirium, aphasic disorders, and a host of other organic conditions. Other contributing features include impoverished thinking and neologisms.

concrete responses may be inconsistently present.

Coherence is a sophisticated feature of thinking and is often difficult to evaluate, partly because disturbances in coherence lead to disruption in the comprehensibility of thinking. If a disturbance in coherence is minimally or moderately severe, then the clinician should assess the *continuity of thinking* (compare above discussion) and the *quality of the patient's associations*, both of which influence coherence (11). This assessment will generally help in sorting out alternative diagnostic possibilities, among which must be those discussed above in the section on disturbances in continuity. If the disturbance is in associations, then the diagnostic possibilities should include aphasic disorders, particularly the fluent aphasias, schizophrenia, manic–depressive disorder, and drug intoxication (12). An important differential point is that incomprehensible thoughts occur involuntarily in these disorders. The self-aware patient may be able to tell the clinician that what is intended to be said and what is said are different. Frustration may be an accompanying emotional feature in these conditions.

Occasionally, individuals who are tired or anxious may converse incomprehensibly. However, such incomprehensibility is transient. If the disturbance is severe enough, then thoughts may become *incoherent*, and the clinician's task is doubly difficult because incoherence is so nonspecific that other features of the patient's condition must guide the differential diagnostic process. Incoherence may occur as a severe manifestation of schizophrenia, manic–depressive illness, mental retardation, dementia, delirium, aphasic disorders, and a host of other organic conditions.

CLINICAL APPROACH

To assess thinking disturbance, the clinician must listen with a disciplined ear to the patient's spontaneous verbal productions and inquire about the patient's subjective experience regarding flow, continuity, control, and form of thinking. Disciplined listening implies knowledge of the disturbances discussed above and the skill to discuss and record them in the case record.

The clinician should avoid the temptation to use clinical maxims rather than comprehensive evaluation as a foundation for differential diagnosis. Circumstantiality does not mean schizophrenia, delusions of persecution occur routinely in a variety of organic and psychiatric disturbances, and rapid thinking does not necessarily mean manic–depressive disorder.

Finally, the clinician should integrate findings in the area of thinking within the total picture of the patient's history, examinations, and laboratory data. While it is true that thinking disturbances have little pathognomonic value, they should be consistent with the formulation that the clinician develops. Inconsistencies suggest mistaken or forgotten diagnostic possibilities. This limitation imposes heightened responsibility on the clinician to evaluate the patient thoroughly.

References

1. Fish F: Disorders of thought and speech. In: *Clinical Psychopathology*. Bristol, England, John Wright, 1974, pp 33–57.
2. Allison R: Perseveration as a sign of diffuse and focal brain damage. I and II. *Br Med J* 2:1027–1032, 1035–1101, 1966.
3. Schneider K: *Clinical Psychopathology*. New York, Grune & Stratton, 1959.
4. Manschreck T, Petri M: The paranoid syndrome. *Lancet* 2:251–253,1978.
5. Slater E, Roth M: *Clinical Psychiatry*. Baltimore, Williams & Wilkins, 1969.
6. Bleuler E: *Dementia Praecox or the Group of Schizophrenias*. New York, International Universities Press, 1950.
7. Ianzito B, Cadoret R, Pugh D: Thought disorder in depression. *Am J Psychiatry* 131:703–707, 1974.
8. Lipowski ZJ: Delirium, clouding of consciousness, and confusion. *J Nerv Ment Dis* 145:227–255, 1967.
9. Maher B: The language of schizophrenia: A review and interpretation. *Br J Psychiatry* 120:3–17, 1972.
10. Goldstein K: *Language and Language Disturbances*. New York, Grune & Stratton, 1948.
11. Maher B: A tentative theory of schizophrenic ut-

terance. *Progress in Experimental Personality in Research* 12:1–52, 1983.

12. Benson DF: Disorders of verbal expression. In Benson DF, Blumer D (eds): *Psychiatric Aspects of Neurologic Disease*. New York, Grune & Stratton, 1975, pp 121–135.

22

Perceptual Disturbances

Theo C. Manschreck, M.D.
Martin B. Keller, M.D.

Perceptual disturbances occur in each of the sensory modalities and may interfere with the patient's appreciation of spatial and temporal relationships. The clinician determines whether the patient's perception is abnormally altered and, if so, assesses the form (i.e., distortion or deception), content, and circumstances in which the perception occurs. These characteristics help orient differential diagnosis. This determination may be straightforward or difficult, depending on the patient's ability to communicate such experiences. Herein lies a fundamental limitation of the assessment of perceptual disturbance. To repeat an important distinction: A *distortion* implies that there is a constant and real object as the basic stimulus for a particular perception but the perception is altered. A *deception*, on the other hand, implies a new perception that may not be in response to an external stimulus. There are two types of deception: *illusion* and *hallucination*. The former is a misinterpretation of stimuli arising from an object, and the latter is a perception without adequate source of external stimulation.

See Chapter 12, pp 177–180, for mental status observations of perceptual disturbances.

DISTORTIONS

Changes in Size or Spatial Form

Changes in size, when objects appear either smaller or farther away (*micropsia*), or larger and nearer than they actually are (*macropsia*), occur as a result of retinal disease, disturbances of convergence and accommodation, or brain disease (particularly lesions of the temporal lobe). In psychiatry, the most common sources of these changes are drug ingestions (which often affect peripheral visual mechanisms) and disease of the temporal lobe. In the latter, there may be an association of dysmegalopsia (a distortion of space) with an epileptic discharge (1). Patients with peripheral visual disease may recognize perceptual disturbances and complain about them as representing visual problems. When the visual experience is intimately tied to central nervous system disease, however, the patient may attribute any changes to unusual powers operating upon him or her. Here careful history and neurologic examination offer the best means to disclose the source of perceptual distortion.

Changes in Quality

Changes in quality are most frequently noted in visual perception. Certain drugs can bring about changes in the color of perception (e.g., digitalis). Fish (1) noted that santonin, an antihelminthic drug, could produce yellow or violet vision. This is not a typical psychiatric complaint, and a thorough search for toxic substances is the best guide to proper diagnosis if such cases occur in clinical psychiatric practice.

Changes in Intensity

The intensity of sensations may be either increased (*hyperesthesia*) or decreased (*hypoesthesia*). Such changes may affect the whole range of sensory experience, often involving several sensory modalities simultaneously. They may result from intense emotional experiences or changes in the physiologic threshold for experiencing a particular sensation. Psychiatric disturbances are associated with both mechanisms. For example, in tense and anxious patients, certain sounds may occur with such intensity that the patients complain they cannot sleep or concentrate; patients with delirium may have difficulty hearing or seeing accurately because of heightened thresholds for auditory and visual perception. The clinician may gloss over perceptual changes in intensity because they lack the bizarre or dramatic qualities of certain hallucinations. This is a mistake, because perceptual changes in intensity reliably indicate that alterations in emotional experience or physiology have occurred. For example, distortions of visual, spatial, auditory, and somatic perception are among the earliest symptoms in schizophrenia (2).

DECEPTIONS

Illusions

The occurrence and nature of illusions— misinterpretations of stimuli arising from an external object—depend on how intact the perceptual apparatus is and the setting in which perceptions take place. The potential (risk) for developing illusory experiences increases when vision or hearing is altered (due to age or disease, for instance) or when the patient is isolated, withdrawn, or in a dark place. Hence, it is not surprising to find such misinterpretations occurring in the evening and nighttime hours among the older, more ill, and socially isolated individuals. However, illusory experiences may be caused by other conditions, for example, severe fever, independent of risk factors such as age.

The clinician must keep in mind that illusory experiences occur in a variety of diseases and that certain factors increase the risk of their incidence. Illusory experiences occur most frequently in disorders which alter normal consciousness; delirium, both mild and severe, is a common source. Of particular importance to clinicians then are the broad range of alcohol, drug, febrile, and metabolic states, the symptoms of which may include illusions. *Pareidolia* refers to a particular illusion which may be elicited by having a patient passively attend to clouds or to carpeting. These patients often report in response to such stimulation that they see complex figures or patterns, even movement. These experiences have been a common finding for years among patients who have a history of ingesting hallucinogenic drugs. It is unclear why this phenomenon occurs long after discontinuation of drug use.

Hallucinations

Some forms of hallucination occur in individuals who are not mentally ill (3). The significance of such experiences is unclear; the term *pseudohallucination* has been applied to indicate that the subject usually recognizes them as unreal perceptions (4). Children occasionally describe clear images of persons as imaginary playmates. During some healing and religious activities, individuals may experience visions, and others hallucinatory states. Grieving persons may see or hear the deceased. Hypnogogic (while falling asleep) and hypnopompic (while awaking) hallucinations are among such experiences, although the former have been associated with narcolepsy. Life-threatening stress or prolonged periods without sleep, sensory stimulation, or adequate food and water have produced hallucinatory experiences in otherwise normal subjects.

Visual Hallucinations

Traditionally, clinicians have been taught that *visual hallucinations* indicate brain disorder. Indeed, visual phenomena, including hallucinations, frequently accompany states of delirium and many diseases, and this maxim is useful. It may also be helpful to specify the phenomenology of the hallucinatory experience as a clue to diagnosis.

For example, in delirium, the hallucinations (accompanied by fear) are often of small animals or insects and are characterized by color, richness of detail, and movement. Frequently such hallucinations are also transient. Alcohol withdrawal can be one of the most frequent causes of such hallucinations that occur as part of delirium tremems. Patients who report hallucinatory scenes or visions (often of a religious nature and associated with highly charged emotions, such as anger, joy, or sadness) should be investigated for temporal lobe disease or evidence of cortical lesions (especially occipital and temporoparietal areas). Convulsive disorders and migraine may be associated with hallucinations as well as some cases of dementia and other brain diseases. Visual hallucinations occurring primarily at night probably indicate brain disorder; visual hallucinations occurring in the absence of other psychopathology almost always indicate drug intoxication or physical illness (for example, metabolic disorders, chemical toxicities, autoimmune disorders, acquired immune deficiency disorders). With drugs, other unformed visual phenomena may precede the occurrence of hallucinations, causing changes in size, color, shape, and movement. And, following repeated drug ingestions, some persons experience flashbacks, often months after abstinence, which are seemingly spontaneous recurrences of illusions and visual hallucinations, similar to those experienced during drug intoxication. Other drugs known to cause visual hallucinations include digoxin, beta-blocking agents (such as propranolol), benztropine, trihexiphenidyl, atropine, and other anticholinergic drugs (which may cause Lilliputian hallucinations). The wise clinician will add to this list as new drugs are introduced and older drugs manifest their full range of effects.

Schizophrenic patients, of course, may experience visual hallucinations. In a series of 50 schizophrenics studied by Small et al. (5), approximately 30% of the patients had experienced visual hallucinations. In a study by Bowman and Raymond (6) of 2500 cases, visual hallucinations were almost always accompanied by other significant perceptual disturbances in schizophrenia, most frequently in the auditory but also in the tactile, olfactory, and gustatory modalities (7). Hence, isolated visual hallucinations occurring in schizophrenia are unusual. The content of visual hallucinations in schizophrenia has been examined in two studies. These studies have shown that principal family members and other persons who are well known to the patient figure prominently in their visual hallucinatory experiences (5, 8).

One particular and unusual kind of visual hallucination is the *autoscopic hallucination*, in which patients experience seeing themselves vividly and unmistakably as an image in front of themselves, despite the absence of a mirror. This kind of hallucination tends to occur when patients are drowsy and anxious. It carries a sense of belief that the image is a physical and intimate part of the patient. Autoscopic hallucinations are strongly associated with epilepsy. However, migraine, encephalitis, focal disease of the brain, and post-traumatic disorders have also been reported with autoscopic phenomena. Lhermitte (9) emphasized the importance of suspecting medical disease in all cases with "apparition of the double," as autoscopic hallucinations are often called (10).

Auditory Hallucinations

Auditory hallucinations may be evidence of schizophrenia. Small et al. (5) found that 66% of schizophrenic patients had evidence of auditory hallucinations. The majority of these hallucinations appeared to the patients to originate from family members or friends and concerned family matters, accusations, and threats. One-third of those experiencing auditory hallucinations were afraid, most were indifferent, and only a small group derived comfort from these experiences.

Chronic auditory hallucinosis, a rare condition related to alcohol (and chloral hydrate) abuse, may occur after withdrawal and while the patient is no longer drinking. It is also known that auditory hallucinosis may accompany acute alcohol withdrawal. Auditory hallucinations frequently occur with temporal lobe disorders, amphetamine and cocaine psychoses (11), and the influence of other drugs (3). *Synesthetic hallucinations* arise when an individual, perhaps under the influence of hallucinogenic drugs, experiences auditory hallucinations in response to bright lights or loud noises. Progressive bilateral hearing loss has also been associated with the occurrence of auditory hallucinations.

Auditory hallucinations in schizophrenia appear to have particular characteristics which may distinguish them from other abnormal auditory phenomena. Schneider (12) asserted that certain types of auditory hallucination were diagnostic of schizophrenia if coarse brain disease were not present. These included (*a*) hearing one's own thoughts (*Gedankenlautwerden*), (*b*) hearing conversing voices arguing or referring to the patient in the third person, and (*c*) hearing hallucinatory voices maintain a running commentary on one's behavior. Mellor (13) has corroborated the usefulness of Schneider's ideas on hallucinations, while Carpenter et al.

(14) have noted limitations to calling them pathognomonic. On the basis of his research, Sedman (15, 16) restricted diagnostic significance to those auditory hallucinations which he called "true hallucinations," i.e., those in which the patient feels the voices are alien and that some external agency is responsible for their occurrence. Sedman thus excluded voices of conscience, imagery, or other kinds of auditory experience from the true hallucination category. As the criteria for calling certain auditory hallucinations pathognomonic for schizophrenia become increasingly refined, the clinical significance of auditory hallucinations that do not meet such criteria becomes difficult to determine, for all too often the vague reports that patients give concerning hallucinations fall short of meeting any particular set of descriptive criteria. In such cases, there are certain general guidelines to fall back on that are derived from clinical experience and clinical studies (17). First, auditory hallucinations occur, like other kinds of hallucinations, in a wide variety of disorders; and, second, the value of auditory hallucinations in differential diagnosis is that they alert the clinician to a range of psychiatric and medical disorders and not to one diagnostic category.

Olfactory, Gustatory, Somatic, Tactile, and Other Hallucinations

The occurrence of olfactory, gustatory, somatic, and/or tactile hallucinations should arouse suspicions of organic illness. Temporal lobe disorder is a common cause, but other brain diseases affecting smell and taste centers can result in deceptions in olfactory and gustatory modalities. Tactile hallucinations (e.g., formication) may occur in cocaine and amphetamine intoxications (11).

Somatic hallucinations have frequently been described in schizophrenia, but they also occur in many other psychiatric conditions. Schizophrenic patients frequently complain of simple bodily sensation hallucinations, for example, being touched, rubbed, cut, etc. (5). Sometimes a physical illness may contribute to the hallucinatory content (18). For example, a patient with asthma may complain of butterflies moving within his or her chest. Also, schizophrenic patients frequently have passivity experiences that may take the form of such bodily sensations; these patients may complain of hallucinatory feelings of pain, "electricity," or sexual excitement that they attribute to external forces. In addition, Lunn (19) has described coenaesthetic hallucinations, in which the whole body or parts of it feel distorted or changed in some bizarre way. Lukianowicz (20) reported on this type of unusual disturbance in 50 patients, 23 of whom were schizophrenic. Interestingly, bizarre somatic hallucinations that can form the basis of delusions were not uncommon in other psychoses and in organic brain syndromes. Furthermore, as with visual hallucinations, it is unusual for somatic hallucinations to be an isolated symptom in schizophrenia (7).

Negative hallucinations are infrequent, but suggest various dissociative conditions when they occur. The phantom limb is a good example of kinesthetic hallucination, in that it may involve the false perception of motion in an amputated extremity.

CONCLUSION

The clinical evaluation of perceptual disturbance is complicated. The fundamental limitation is the fact that patients may be unable to give more than a vague account of the nature of their experiences. Thus, establishing whether a patient is hallucinating may itself be difficult. Of course, the better the description the patient offers regarding psychopathologic experience, the more helpful that information can be in differential diagnosis. Nevertheless, even with excellent clinical descriptive data, differential diagnosis, particularly in assessing deceptions (hallucinations and illusions) may be problematic. Hallucinations, for instance, occur widely and nonspecifically in psychiatric and medical conditions. Their presence certainly indicates that something is wrong but does not usually indicate what it is. Hence, hallucinations may have special value in monitor-

ing improvement or deterioration in the clinical state. Clinical studies have also shown that certain kinds of hallucinations seem to occur regularly in temporal lobe disease and schizophrenic disorders (21). Furthermore, it is unusual to see schizophrenic patients with visual, but not auditory, hallucinations. However, there are enough exceptions to underscore the limits of these principles. Perhaps the most useful maxim for the clinician to keep in mind is that similar perceptual abnormalities occur in a variety of disorders, and, as in so many other clinical situations, establishing the diagnosis requires a careful assessment of all available information. Premature diagnostic decisions based on the discovery of certain prominent or unusual perceptual disturbances should be avoided.

References

1. Fish F: *Clinical Psychopathology*. Bristol, England, John Wright, 1974.
2. Chapman J: The early symptoms of schizophrenia. *Br J Psychiatry* 112:225–251, 1966.
3. Asaad G, Shapiro B: Hallucinations: theoretical and clinical overview. *Am J Psychiatry* 143:1088–1097, 1986.
4. Taylor FK: On pseudo-hallucinations. *Psychol Med* 11:265–271, 1981.
5. Small I, Small J, Andersen J: Clinical characteristics of hallucinations of schizophrenia. *Dis Nerv Syst* 27:349–353, 1966.
6. Bowman KM, Raymond AF: A statistical study of hallucinations in the manic–depressive psychoses. *Am J Psychiatry* 88:299–309, 1931.
7. Frieske DA, Wilson WP: Formal qualities of hallucinations: A comparative study of the visual hallucinations in patients with schizophrenic, organic and affective psychoses. In Hoch PH, Zubin J (eds): *Psychopathology of Schizophrenia*, New York, Grune & Stratton, 1966, pp 49–62.
8. Higashi H, Koshika K: On the comparative study of hallucinations in the schizophrenias and organic psychoses. *Bull Osaka Med Sch* 12 (Suppl):155–161, 1967.
9. Lhermitte J: Visual hallucinations of the self. *Br Med J* 1:431–434, 1951.
10. Lukianowicz N: Autoscopic phenomena. *Arch Neurol Psychiatry* 80:199–220, 1958.
11. Manschreck T, Laughery J, Weisstein C, et. al: Characteristics of freebase cocaine psychosis. *Yale J Biol Med* 61:112–115, 1988
12. Schneider K: *Clinical Psychopathology*. New York, Grune & Stratton, 1959.
13. Mellor C: First-rank symptoms of schizophrenia. *Br J Psychiatry* 117;15–23, 1970.

14. Carpenter WT, Strauss JS, Muleh S: Are first rank symptoms pathognomonic for schizophrenia? *Arch Gen Psychiatry* 28:847–852, 1973.

15. Sedman G: "Inner voices": phenomenological and clinical aspects. *Br J Psychiatry* 112:485–490, 1966.

16. Sedman G: A comparative study of pseudo-hallucinations, imagery, and true hallucinations. *Br J Psychiatry* 112:9–17, 1966.

17. Goodwin DW, Alderson P, Rosenthal R: Clinical significance of hallucinations in psychiatric disorders. *Arch Gen Psychiatry* 24:76–80, 1971.

18. Southard EH: On the somatic sources of somatic delusions. *J Abnorm Psychol* 7:326–339, 1912.

19. Lunn V: Body hallucinations. *Acta Psychiatr Scand* 41:387–399, 1965.

20. Lukianowicz N: "Body image" disturbance in psychiatric disorders. *Br J Psychiatry* 113:31–47, 1967.

21. American Psychiatric Association: *Diagnostic and Statistical Manual of Mental Disorders (Third Edition-Revised)*. Washington, DC, American Psychiatric Association, 1987.

23

Disturbances of Higher Intellectual Functioning

Gary S. Moak, M.D.

Disturbances of higher intellectual functioning include impairments of cognitive functions such as orientation, selective attention, language, memory, information processing, calculation, abstract reasoning, praxis, and visuospatial skills. Cognitive impairment is among the cardinal signs of all psychiatric disorders and is commonly seen in many psychiatric settings (1). In outpatient practice, the principle goal in assessing cognitive function is to evaluate the diagnostic, functional, and therapeutic significance of disturbances of higher intellectual function.

This chapter focuses on general aspects of the clinical methods necessary for cognitive assessment. Techniques for gathering and interpreting clinical data are discussed further in Chapters 12 through 16 and in the other chapters on the differential diagnosis of psychiatric presentation with known organic causes. This chapter shall first discuss the importance of viewing disturbances of higher intellectual functioning as cardinal features of all psychiatric disorders. It will then focus on three psychiatric syndromes in which acquired disturbances of higher intellectual functioning are the predominant part of the presentation at some stage of the disorder.

COGNITIVE IMPAIRMENT IN ORGANIC AND "FUNCTIONAL" DISORDERS

A common convention in medicine has been to separate pathology into organic and functional categories. This has been true in psychiatry, where the routine assessment of higher intellectual functioning as part of the mental status examination is thought of as screening for organicity. Unfortunately, the differential diagnosis of organic and the so-called functional disorders on the basis of cognitive impairment is simplistic and clinically unreliable. In fact, in practice this distinction often cannot be made.

Many primary psychiatric disorders increasingly are being understood in terms of cerebral dysfunction (2). Acutely or chronically psychotic patients with mania, schizophrenia, or depression may appear to be demented or delirious (1, 3, 4). Such states of pseudodelirium or pseudodementia may simply reflect the more global behavioral disorganization experienced by psychotic patients. Psychotic illness often disrupts attention, tracking, and memory as much as organic mental disorders do (1). Moreover, severe anxiety adversely affects cognitive performance. Recent research has also identified more specific, localizing patterns of neuropsychologic deficits associated with primary psychiatric disorders (5). In fact, cerebral physiology can become sufficiently disorganized in patients with major depression that lateralized hard neurologic signs have been observed as concomitants of depressive episodes. These neurologic signs disappear with effective antidepressant treatment (6). Whether the cognitive impairment seen in functional disorders is an epiphenomenon or a manifestation of focal, reversible cerebral dysfunction is not resolved. Notwithstanding this uncertainty, the predictive value of signs of cognitive impairment in diagnosing organic mental disorders should not be overestimated.

Patients with localized or diffuse organic brain pathology manifest behavioral signs which may be misinterpreted as functional in origin. This is especially true in the outpatient setting, where signs of cognitive impairment are often subtle. Motor impersistence associated with right hemisphere damage can be misinterpreted as uncooperativeness (7). Patients with dysprosodia, also associated with right brain pathology may manifest affective signs and symptoms resembling those seen in functional mood disorders. The dysprosodias are disturbances of emotional communication which are emotional analogues of the aphasias (8). The formal thought disorder of schizophrenia may be difficult to distinguish from the language disorder of aphasia (9). Furthermore, patients with frontal lobe pathology (e.g., Pick's disease) may present with behavioral symptoms which initially are much more prominent than are the signs of higher intellectual dysfunction (10).

The psychiatric presentation of patients with organic mental disorders is complicated further by these patients' psychologic reaction to their deficits. Most patients experience clinically significant emotional distress in reaction to intellectual dysfunction or the associated personal and social disruption (11). This is commonly true of patients with amnestic syndromes or early dementing illnesses or in the prodromal or recovery phases of delirium. Depending on premorbid personality and narcissistic investment in cognitive abilities, such patients may develop symptoms of difficulty in coping with the mental changes they are experiencing.

Thus, more often than not, the task of psychiatric assessment involves evaluating syndromes with mixtures of behavioral and cognitive signs and symptoms. The goal is to describe accurately and reliably disturbances of higher intellectual functioning in the context of disturbances of other dimensions of behavior which then define clinical neuropsychiatric syndromes. A careful description of the clinical syndrome can then lead to an appropriate list of differential diagnoses. In this way, the diagnostic significance of disturbances of higher intellectual functioning can meaningfully be assessed so that accurate diagnosis is not delayed.

Adhering to a syndromal approach to diagnosis provides a framework for interpreting the meaning of signs of disturbance in higher intellectual functioning. Level of education and premorbid intelligence must be considered as possible confounding variables when interpreting the significance of apparent deficits of cognitive performance. Motivation to participate in testing must also be taken into consideration. Psychiatric patients are often poorly motivated to perform cognitive tasks and may appear falsely impaired. Furthermore, the frankly uncooperative patient presents an additional challenge. Fewer reliable conclusions can be drawn about the intellectual functioning of an uncooperative patient. A common mistake is to assume that patients who are mute or uncooperative or who only respond nonverbally are severely cognitively impaired. This may not necessarily be the case. In such cases, inferences must be made from other aspects of the mental status examination.

Another common mistake is failure to recognize cognitive impairment or appreciate its significance in the presence of more predominant psychiatric symptoms.

For example, when patients with presenile dementia of the Alzheimer type present with depressive symptoms, the correct diagnosis can be overlooked while vigorous attempts are made to treat what appears to be an episode of major depression (12). Notwithstanding the importance of treating depressive symptoms in demented patients, this oversight is problematic. Delay in the diagnosis of delirium or treatable dementia can be catastrophic. Moreover, delay in the recognition of a progressive, nonarrestable dementing illness also may potentially adversely affect outcome by delaying initiation of appropriate interventions such as psychotherapy, family therapy, involvement of community resources, and legal counseling, or possibly by exposing the patient unnecessarily to incorrect pharmacotherapy.

Effective treatment of syndromes with mixed behavioral and cognitive symptoms requires ongoing reassessment of cognitive status. Since it is often not possible initially to distinguish between organic and functional illnesses, the diagnosis may have to be modified as treatment progresses. Moreover, serial assessment of higher intellectual functioning is essential to sort out the therapeutic or adverse effects of treatment from changes in the mental state related to progression of an illness or changes in the patient's personal life. One common scenario illustrates this dilemma. Electroconvulsive therapy (ECT) often is indicated for the treatment of elderly depressed patients with mixed affective and cognitive symptoms. As the course of treatment progresses and depressive symptoms resolve, it is necessary to carefully assess the significance of persistent cognitive symptoms. Do they represent still-to-be-treated symptoms of depression, an underlying dementing disorder, or an ECT-induced amnestic or confusional syndrome? Appropriate decisions to continue or stop therapy depend on being able to resolve these syndromes clinically.

It is also crucial to pay attention to psychodynamic aspects of the mental status of patients with disturbances of higher intellectual functioning. The behavioral morbidity associated with cognitive impairment can be understood much better when its meaning is appreciated in the context of individual and family dynamics. Moreover, several diagnoses of disturbed intellectual functioning depend on a more extensive knowledge of the patient's life circumstances and intrapsychic functioning. In hysterical pseudomentia, complaints of difficulty with memory, concentration, or other cognitive tasks occur as conversion symptoms. The cognitive symptoms have a symbolic meaning and may be associated with secondary gains. In Ganser's syndrome (factitious disorder with psychological symptoms; 13), the patient voluntarily produces a disturbance of higher intellectual functioning in order to assume the patient role. This disorder is often known as the "syndrome of approximate answers," because of the patient's tendency to give near-miss responses during cognitive assessment. Such patients often appear worse while being observed and may be suggestible in the range of symptoms which they will endorse. They typically exhibit severe personality disorders and often have histories of substance abuse. Finally, cognitive impairment can be seen in malingering, in which there is some external goal to the symptom which can be recognized given sufficient knowledge of the patient's life circumstances. An example would be a person who attempts to obtain benefits on the basis of a cognitive disability. One of the hallmarks of malingering is inconsistent performance on batteries of tests of neuropsychologic functioning (11).

Thus, most psychiatric disorders are best thought of as complex syndromes with varying disturbances in the behavioral dimensions of emotionality, thinking, movement, modulation, and information processing. It is essential to carefully assess higher intellectual functioning as part of the diagnostic evaluation and treatment of all psychiatric disorders. Moreover, since the differentiation of functional and organic disorders often cannot be made on the basis of cognitive signs, the significance of disturbances of higher intellectual functioning, or apparent absence of such, must be interpreted in a syndromal context with a prospective approach to diagnosis.

AMNESIA

Patients with disturbances of memory illustrate many of the clinical issues discussed above. Symptoms of memory disturbance are seen in a wide range of psychopathologic syndromes of organic or functional etiology in outpatient practice. In functional psychiatric disorders, short-term memory may be nonspecifically affected by poor motivation or inattention. Certain dissociative disorders produce psychogenic memory loss which can be clinically dramatic. Memory disturbances are also commonly seen in organic mental disorders. Amnesia refers to a relatively circumscribed disturbance of the higher intellectual function of memory. In dementia and delirium (see below) symptoms of amnesia present as components of more global syndromes of cognitive impairment.

An amnestic syndrome per se represents a specific impairment of the neurophychologic function of memory. According to the *Diagnostic and Statistical Manual of Mental Disorders* (*Third Edition-Revised*) (DSM-III-R), a diagnosis of amnestic syndrome requires the presence of deficits in short- and long-term memory in the absence of a clouding of consciousness (13). The impairment of short-term memory, known as anterograde amnesia, refers to the inability to learn new material. The disturbance of long-term memory, or retrograde amnesia, refers to difficulty remembering previously learned material. Typically, remote memory is preserved better than recent memory. Immediate recall is intact in amnestic syndromes. A specific organic factor causing the syndrome is presumed to exist. If the amnestic syndrome is severe, associated disorientation and confabulation may occur (14, 15). The various types of amnestic syndromes are listed in Table 23.1.

Patients with amnestic syndrome may experience a wide range of symptoms, including disorientation, perplexity, apathy,

Table 23.1   Disturbances of Memory

Amnestic syndromes
  Alcohol amnestic syndrome (Korsakoff's Psychosis)
  Posttraumatic amnesia
  Poststroke amnesia
  Anoxic amnesia
  Postinfectious amnesia
  Herpes or other limbic encephalidities
  Postelectroconvulsive therapy amnesia
  Transient global amnesia
Drug-induced amnesia
  Alcohol
  Benzodiazepines
Syndromes of global impairment
  Dementia
  Delirium
Functional disorders
  Psychogenic amnesia
  Psychogenic fugue
  All psychiatric disorders capable of disrupting attention and memory
Benign senescent forgetfulness

depression, agitation, and delusions. Such symptoms may reflect a number of possible psychopathologic processes. There may be an associated organic delusional syndrome, organic hallucinosis, or organic affective syndrome. Psychiatric symptoms may reflect the patient's emotional reaction to the loss of memory function. Behavioral disturbances also may arise from the patients' misinterpretation of their circumstances due to their inability to remember and integrate new information. Such behavioral symptoms may be sufficiently dramatic and unexpected that the memory disturbance can go unrecognized, leading to incorrect diagnosis and management (16).

The amnestic syndrome is a distinct neuropsychologic entity which must be distinguished from other forms of memory disturbance (Table 23.1). In psychogenic amnesia, the patient experiences a sudden inability to recall important or psychodynamically significant personal information. This may include knowledge of personal identity. The sudden loss of memory is often preceded by a psychologic stress. In psychogenic fugue there is amnesia for a period of time. During the period for which the patient is amnestic, there may be wandering away (14).

One entity commonly seen in outpatient settings which deserves mention is benign senescent forgetfulness. This age-related memory disturbance is characterized by difficulty recalling details of events without amnesia for the actual experiences. The problem is one of retrieval of information rather than storage, since the details may be remembered at a later time (17). Although this disturbance of memory function is not fully understood, it should be considered a normal, age-related change in higher intellectual functioning. People who experience this sometimes report considerable fear that they have Alzheimer's disease. Such anxiety usually responds to reassurance supported by a thorough clinical evauation.

DELIRIUM

Delirium is a term which still is used inconsistently in the medical literature. It traditionally is defined as an acute, reversible organic brain syndrome. This is problematic since the etiology of delirium may not be fully reversible and the onset may not be well demarcated. Many authors differentiate the subdued form of the delirium syndrome with terms such as "toxic psychosis," "beclouded state," "metabolic or toxic encephalopathy," or "acute confusional state" (18); the term *delirium* is reserved for agitated, hyperactive confusional states. This distinction introduces needless confusion. Lipowski has provided a helpful definition of delirium as "a psychiatric syndrome characterized by a transient disorganization of a wide range of cognitive functions due to widespread derangement of cerebral metabolism, with fluctuation over a day and worse at night in the dark" (19). This definition seems more useful since it defines delirium as a syndrome with heterogeneous etiologies and behavioral manifestations and a common pathophysiologic process.

According to DSM-III-R, delirium is a clouded state of consciousness manifested by difficulty sustaining selective attention, sensory misperception, and thought disor-

der with abrupt onset (13). The hallmark of delirium is a fluctuating level of attention or consciousness. There usually is a sleep–wake disturbance, and it may be associated with alterations of psychomotor activity, illusions or hallucinations, and varying degrees of global cognitive impairment (Table 23.2). In contrast, in uncomplicated dementia there is widespread disturbance of higher intellectual functioning without alteration of consciousness.

The fluctuating or altered attention in delirium is manifested by distractability, poor concentration and tracking, and impersistence. The patient may be either hyper- or hypoalert, with associated alterations in activity. In the hyperactive variant, the patients appear vigilant and hyperresponsive and manifest increased sympathetic tone. Delirium tremens is the prototype hyperactive delirium. The constellation of psychotic symptoms, agitation, vigilance, and behavioral response to hallucinations may present a syndrome resembling mania or schizophrenia. The hypoactive variant manifests as decreased alertness, inattention, sluggish responsiveness, and bewilderment. This presentation can be mistaken for dementia or depression.

Depending on the etiology and the course of the disorder, delirium may present in the outpatient setting, where its presence may be subtle. The onset of delirium is generally rapid (hours to days) but it may not be demarcated clearly. During the prodromal phase, patients may experience anxiety, difficulty concentrating and thinking clearly, restlessness, irritability, and fatigue. Mildly delirious patients may be alarmed or embarrassed by their difficulty controlling their own thinking. Such patients may attempt to conceal cognitive deficits by evading questions (19). The evaluation of such patients poses a diagnostic challenge in outpatient psychiatric or general medical practice.

Recovery from delirium may occur over days to months. The outcome is variable and may include complete recovery, transitional confusional states, psychosis, progression to dementia, or death (19).

Table 23.2   Diagnostic Criteria for Delirium

A. Reduced ability to maintain attention to external stimuli (e.g., questions must be repeated because attention wanders) and to appropriately shift attention to new external stimuli (e.g., perseverates answer to a previous question).
B. Disorganized thinking, as indicated by rambling, irrelevant, or incoherent speech.
C. At least two of the following:
    (1) reduced level of consciousness, e.g., difficulty keeping awake during examination
    (2) perceptual disturbances: misinterpretations, illusions, or hallucinations
    (3) disturbance of sleep-wake cycle with insomnia or daytime sleepiness
    (4) increased or decreased psychomotor activity
    (5) disorientation to time, place, or person
    (6) memory impairment, elg., inability to learn new material, such as the names of several unrelated objects after five minutes, or to remember past events, such as history of current episode of illness
D. Clinical features develop over a short period of time (usually hours to days) and tend to fluctuate over the course of a day.
E. Either (1) or (2):
    (1) evidence from the history, physical examination, or laboratory tests of a specific organic factor (or factors) judged to be etiologically related to the disturbance
    (2) in the absence of such evidence, an etiologic organic factor can be presumed if the disturbance cannot be accounted for by any nonorganic mental disorder, e.g., manic episode accounting for agitation and sleep disturbance

Reprinted with permission from American Psychiatric Association: *Diagnostic and Statistical Manual of Mental Disorders* (*Third Edition-Revised*). Washington, DC, American Psychiatric Association, 1987. Copyright 1987 American Psychiatric Association.

Psychiatrists often have a central role in the outpatient follow-up of delirious patients. Even the completely recovered patient may experience anxiety or depression related to the experience of delirium. This may require psychiatric intervention. When delirium is diagnosed, a thorough workup must be initiated to identify the specific etiology (Table 23.3). The approach to clinical evaulation is discussed below.

DEMENTIA

Dementia is a syndrome of acquired cognitive impairment of sufficient severity to interfere with normal social or occupational functioning. The cognitive impairment generally involves a wide range of disturbances of higher intellectual functioning, but dementia may present with more focal deficits, in the areas of language or memory for example. The mental state is more stable in dementia and there is no clouding of consciousness as in delirium. Dementia may be complicated by delirium or other behavioral disturbances such as delusions, depression, agitation, insomnia, or

wandering. Dementia is not a specific disorder but a syndrome. According to DSM-III-R, a specific etiology is presumed to exist if one is not clinically evident (13) (Table 23.4). For specific diagnoses of dementia such as primary degenerative dementia of the Alzheimer type, multiinfarct dementia, or dementia associated with alcoholism, there are additional diagnostic criteria. It is worth noting that although one of the criteria for primary degenerative dementia of the Alzheimer type is a uniformly progressive course, some research has shown that the rate of progression of the senile onset form may vary during the course of the disorder (20) (Table 23.5).

There are two clinical constructs of some controversy in the dementia literature which shall be discussed because of their conceptual importance in the differential diagnosis of dementiform presentations in psychiatry. These are pseudodementia and subcortical dementia.

Pseudodementia

Much attention has been paid in the literature to the often difficult differential di-

Table 23.3   Causes of Delirium

Intoxication
  Alcohol
  Organic compounds
  Drugs—anticholinergics, sedative–hypnotics,
    opiates, anticonvulsants
  Heavy metals
  Carbon monoxide
Withdrawal states
  Alcohol—delirium tremens
  Sedative–hypnotics
Metabolic encephalopathies
  Hepatic
  Hypoxic
  Hypoglycemia
  Endocrinopathies
  Electrolyte imbalances
  Dehydration
Infections
  Systemic
  Central nervous system
    meningitis or encephalitis
Seizure disorders
Trauma
Cerebrovascular disease
  Stroke
  Subarachnoid hemorrhage
  Subdural hematoma
Intracranial mass lesions

agnosis of dementia and depression. The concept of depressive pseudodementia has been used effectively to draw attention to the fact that some patients who appear to be demented may have a diagnosable depressive illness. The poor cognitive performance of such patients may be more symptomatic of depression, which must not be overlooked since treatment often will be helpful. Unfortunately, the pseudodementia construct as discussed in the literature is heterogeneous and has not been validated adequately.

Classically, patients with depressive pseudodementia present with complaints out of proportion to the degree of functional impairment. They report severe dysmnesia but exhibit little interest in attempting cognitive tasks, typically answering most questions with "I don't know." Cognitive impairment is more evident on tasks which demand effort (1). The truly demented, nondepressed patient attempts to arrive at the correct answer or actively evades the question. The history may re-

veal that depressive symptoms antedated the cognitive impairment, which then developed with a subacute time course.

The concept of pseudodementia, although useful, can be misleading: It implies that depression can manifest as dementia in the absence of dysphoric symptoms, which is rarely the case. The concept has more meaning when applied to patients who present with mixed depressive and cognitive symptoms. Most have a depressive disorder complicating an underlying dementia (22). In such patients, "pseudodementia" may appropriately refer to the component of cognitive impairment that improves with treatment. There has been a tendency to overestimate the prevalence of dementia that resolves entirely with treatment of depression. More often than not, depressive symptoms improve but some cognitive impairment remains (23).

Subcortical Dementia

Another controversy in behavioral neurology has to do with the classification of dementias into cortical and subcortical clinical types (24). Classically, dementia is conceptualized as a dysfunction of the cerebral cortex. According to this scheme, the early hallmarks of the cortical dementias—Alzheimer's disease being the prototype—are aphasia, agnosia, and apraxia; speech, motor functioning, and personality remain intact until the advanced stages. Subcortical dementia refers to dementia associated with dysfunction of subcortical structures such as the basal ganglia and thalamus. This syndrome has been applied to the dementia seen in patients with Parkinson's disease, progressive supranuclear palsy, Huntington's disease, etc. These patients often are apathetic or depressed, have a movement disorder, and exhibit hypophonic or dysarthric speech. Their cognition is described as "dilapidated": They are forgetful, and their thinking is bradyphrenic or sluggish (25, 26). They are not truly amnestic in that their forgetfulness appears to be related to difficulty retrieving stored information and cognitive inefficiency.

Table 23.4   Diagnostic Criteria for Dementia

A. Demonstrable evidence of impairment in short- and long-term memory. Impairment in short-term memory (inability to learn new information) may be indicated by inability to remember three objects after five minutes. Long-term memory impairment (inability to remember information that was known in the past) may be indicated by inability to remember past personal information (e.g., what happened yesterday, birthplace, occupation) or facts of common knowledge (e.g., past Presidents, well-known dates).

B. At least one of the following:
   (1) impairment in abstract thinking, as indicated by inability to find similarities and differences between related words, difficulty in defining words and concepts, and other similar tasks
   (2) impaired judgment, as indicated by inability to make reasonable plans to deal with interpersonal, family, and job-related problems and issues
   (3) other disturbances of higher cortical function, such as aphasia (disorder of language), apraxia (inability to carry out motor activities despite intact comprehension and motor function), agnosia (failure to recognize or identify objects despite intact sensory function), and "constructional difficulty" (e.g., inability to copy three-dimensional figures, assemble blocks, or arrange sticks in specific designs)
   (4) personality change, i.e., alteration or accentuation of premorbid traits

C. The disturbance in A and B significantly interferes with work or usual social activities or relationships with others.

D. Not occurring exclusively during the course of delirium.

E. Either (1) or (2):
   (1) there is evidence from the history, physical examination, or laboratory tests of a specific organic factor (or factors) judged to be etiologically related to the disturbance
   (2) in the absence of such evidence, an etiologic organic factor can be presumed if the disturbance cannot be accounted for by any nonorganic mental disorder, e.g., major depression accounting for cognitive impairment

Criteria for severity of dementia:

Mild: Although work or social activities are significantly impaired, the capacity for independent living remains, with adequate personal hygiene and relatively intact judgment.

Moderate: Independent living is hazardous, and some degree of supervision is necessary.

Severe: Activities of daily living are so impaired that continual supervision is required, e.g., unable to maintain minimal personal hygiene; largely incoherent or mute.

Reprinted with permission from American Psychiatric Association: *Diagnostic and Statistical Manual of Mental Disorders* (*Third Edition-Revised*). Washington, DC, American Psychiatric Association, 1987. Copyright 1987 American Psychiatric Association.

When formally tested such patients usually do not have aphasia, apraxia, or agnosia (27).

Despite the active debate over the construct validity of subcortical dementia, the concept is of heuristic value. It draws attention to the heterogeneity of the dementia syndrome and the different neuroanatomical loci which may serve as substrates for cognitive functioning. It also highlights the fact that dementia often involves disturbances in other dimensions of behavior (movement, motivation, and emotionality) in addition to higher intellectual functioning. From the description of subcortical dementia, it is clear that this syndrome overlaps significantly with the pseudodementia syndrome (4). Although the validity of both constructs is controversial, they draw attention to the conceptual problem underlying the difficult differen-

tial diagnosis of depression and dementia in patients who present with widespread cognitive impairment, functional incapacity, and depressive symptoms.

Dementia may present in a number of ways in the outpatient setting. While patients themselves often are aware of early cognitive deficits, it is the family members who usually initiate referral. At time of presentation, family members commonly report symptoms of memory disturbance which has been of several months to a few years duration. Families appear to be quite tolerant of mild cognitive deficits. More often referral appears to be precipitated by behavioral symptoms which the family is not able to manage or tolerate. These include depression, anxiety, agitation, hostility, aggressiveness, delusions, wandering, or personality change. A retrospective history of forgetfulness, confusion,

Table 23.5   Etiologies of Dementia

Cortical dementias
  Primary degenerative dementia of the Alzheimer
    type
  Pick's disease
Subcortical dementias of extrapyramidal disorders
  Parkinson's disease
  Progressive supranuclear palsy
  Huntington's disease
  Hallervorden-Spatz syndrome
  Spinocerebellar degenerations
Vascular dementias (cortical, subcortical, or both) or
    multiinfarct dementia
  Lacunar state
  Cortical strokes
  Binswanger's disease
Infectious
  Central nervous system syphilis
  Viral
  Jakob-Creutzfeldt disease
  AIDS (21)
  Progressive multifocal leukoencephalopathy
  Subacute sclerosing panencephalitis
Chronic fungal meningitis
Paraneoplastic encephalomyelitis
Metabolic
  Chronic hypoxia and anoxia
  Sleep apnea
  Chronic renal failure
  Dialysis dementia
  Hepatic failure
  Recurrent hypoglycemia
  Electrolyte disturbances
  Cushing's syndrome
  Addison's disease
  Hypothyroidism
  Apathetic hyperthyroidism
Vitamin deficiencies
  Thiamine—B_1
  Cyanocobalamin—B_{12}
  Folate
  Niacin
Toxic
  Metals
  Industrial compounds
  Drugs
  Alcohol
Normal-pressure hydrocephalus
Trauma
  Subdural hematoma
  Dementia pugilistica

Behavioral symptoms may develop as psychobiologic concomitants of the neuropathologic process causing dementia. Alternatively, they may be precipitated by "revealing events" which overwhelm the patient's limited behavioral reserve, leading to decompensation from a previously precarious equilibrium (28). Such revealing events include acute medical illness, hospitalization or change to other unfamiliar environments, and loss of a spouse or other close family member. Again, many patients may develop regressed behavior, anxiety, or depression in reaction to their awareness of deficits or loss of independence. It is essential to understand these processes and be able to identify them in order to arrive at a correct diagnosis and treatment plan.

There are a number of other presentations of nonreversible disturbances of higher intellectual functioning which need to be differentiated from dementia (Table 23.6). First, patients with infarction of the left parietotemporal cortex may develop a constellation of receptive aphasia and other cognitive deficits that mimics the presentation of Alzheimer's disease (29). Second, patients with amnestic disorders or benign senescent forgetfulness must be distinguished from those with early dementing illnesses. Finally, measurable cognitive impairment in the absence of diagnosable dementia can be found in a significant percentage of elderly community populations, as was demonstrated by Folstein et al. (30). The meaning of such cognitive impairment is unclear. Some of these patients may have been screened during the preclinical stages of a dementing illness. On the other hand, some people with cognitive impairment experience no concomitant social or occupational con-

getting lost, or mismanaging finances is then obtained. Such patients may have been started already on one or more psychotropic drugs by another physician. This can complicate the differential diagnosis since the current state may reflect any combination of partially treated symptoms and cognitive side effects of medication.

Table 23.6   Nonreversible disturbances of Higher Intellectual Functioning Which Are Not Dementia

Receptive aphasia
Amnestic syndromes
Benign senescent forgetfulness (17)
Cognitive deficit without diagnosis (30)

sequences and should not be identified as cases.

CLINICAL APPROACH TO DIFFERENTIAL DIAGNOSIS

The problematic nature of the traditional organic versus functional classification of psychiatric disorders has already been pointed out: In the presence of mixed cognitive and behavioral symptoms, this distinction often cannot be made. Two basic principles of differential diagnosis should be observed. The first is that assessment should be guided by a syndromal approach. The second is that assessment should be ongoing or prospective; this is discussed below.

In the psychiatric assessment of syndromes with disturbances of higher intellectual functioning, the importance of speaking with family members and other close people or caretakers cannot be overemphasized. As in all other areas of medicine, the diagnosis depends most on the history. Cognitively impaired patients may be unable to relate a meaningful history. On the other hand, they may provide a very cogent-sounding history which omits, denies, evades, or distorts problems. Corroborating history as to symptoms, onset, past history, and course is essential. By speaking with as many informants as are available, the interviewer can begin to assess whether the presenting complaint is the problem of the patient or the caregivers, and the extent to which the behavioral (and cognitive) symptoms are caused or exacerbated by environmental or interpersonal stress. Data provided by informants can then be compared with inferences based on the history related by the patient and the mental status examination findings. In assessing cognitively impaired patients, as much attention may need to be paid to interpersonal and psychodynamic aspects as to the neurobiologic evaluation (31) (see Chapter 14).

The history must include a description of the onset and course. Did the behavioral symptoms antedate or follow the onset of cognitive symptoms? Were there other symptoms which coincided, such as "spells," focal neurologic deficits, automatisms, or shortness of breath? Was the onset related to a medical illness, prescription change, or use of illicit drugs or alcohol? Has the course been steady, progressive, or stepwise, or has there been fluctuation? A clinical sleep history from the patient and the bed partner may be necessary (32). Sleep apnea may present with daytime cognitive impairment (33).

The mental status examination must include careful attention to documenting higher intellectual functioning using a consistent technique that can be reproduced serially during follow-up evaluation and treatment. When clinically significant cognitive impairment is suspected, validated instruments such as the Mini Mental State Exam may be used to quantitate the severity of the impairment (34). This easy-to-use instrument is well suited for longitudinal surveillance in outpatient practice. The physical examination should include a careful search for signs of drug intoxication, abuse, and withdrawal or dependence. The neurologic examination should include testing for the presence of frontal lobe release reflexes (35).

Since most, if not all, systemic illnesses can produce psychiatric symptoms, and few if any psychiatric symptoms cannot be caused by systemic disease, the basic diagnostic testing should screen functions in the major organ systems (Table 23.7). Computerized tomography (CT scan) and the electroencephalogram (EEG) are standard components of the diagnostic batteries for delirium and dementia. When these disorders present with unknown etiology, a CT scan is indicated (36). An EEG may be useful in the assessment of delirium and dementia in at least two ways that a CT scan is not. First, the background frequency of the waking EEG can be correlated with the patient's mental state: If the patient clinically is severely impaired and the EEG is relatively normal, the patient may have pseudodementia; if the patient presents with an early or mild dementia syndrome and the EEG is very abnormal (i.e., slow), this may indicate a reversible

Table 23.7   Diagnostic Tests for Delirium and Dementia

	SCREENING TESTS
Heart	—Electrocardiogram, chest x-ray
Lungs	—Chest x-ray (PPD)
Urinary system	—Blood urea nitrogen, creatinine, urinalysis (urine culture and sensitivity)
Hematologic	—Complete blood count with differential count, platelets, B_{12}, folic acid (iron, total iron binding capacity)
Metabolic/endocrine	—Electrolytes, glucose, calcium, phosphate, T_4, resin T_3 uptake, thyroid-stimulating hormone, liver function tests
Central nervous system	Electroencephalogram, computerized tomography
	SUPPLEMENTAL TESTS IF INDICATED
Serology	—Venereal Disease Research Laboratories test, rapid plasma-reagin, automated reagin test, fluorescent treponemal antibody-absorption
Drug levels	—Anticonvulsants, tricyclic antidepressants, digoxin, drugs of abuse, lithium
Central nervous system	—Sleep studies, cerebrospinal fluid, magnetic resonance imaging

or arrestable encephalopathy. Second, the EEG can also help identify disturbances of higher intellectual functioning related to seizure disorders (37). While many of the indications for an EEG in psychiatry are also indications for hospitalization, the EEG should not be forgotten as part of the outpatient workup of psychiatric presentations of disorders with disturbance of higher intellectual functioning.

Neuropsychologic testing is often helpful in the outpatient evaluation of disturbances of higher intellectual functioning (11). Neuropsychologic data may aid in differential diagnosis by identifying the pattern of cognitive deficits more precisely. The findings may be useful in guiding management issues such as the need to obtain guardianship or restrict driving privileges. Test results also can be used to document disability and are valuable for longitudinal surveillance of changes in cognitive status. One caveat regarding neuropsychologic testing has to do with the common tendency to overestimate their diagnostic value: Diagnoses cannot be made on the basis of neuropsychologic test results, especially in the presence of mixed cognitive and behavioral symptoms.

A number of other brain-imaging techniques deserve mention because of their potential to increase our understanding of cerebral dysfunction in neuropsychiatric disorders. Such techniques include regional cerebral blood flow, positron emission tomography, brain electrical activity mapping, and magnetic resonance imaging (MRI). With the exception of MRI, these imaging methods are largely research techniques (38). MRI increasingly is being used clinically in a number of centers to supplement CT imaging, but its utility in outpatient psychiatry is unclear.

SUMMARY

Varying degrees of disturbance of higher intellectual functioning are seen in most if not all psychiatric disorders. Patients with "functional" psychiatric disorders such as schizophrenia, mania, or major depression, may manifest significant cognitive impairment. On the other hand, patients with organic brain syndromes causing widespread cognitive deficits, such as delirium and dementia, may present with clinical pictures predominated by psychiatric symptoms. It is often difficult or impossible to distinguish "functional" from organic disorders at all, let alone on the basis of disturbances in higher intellectual functioning. Under these circumstances, assessment must be guided by a syndromal approach. This approach depends on assessment of the psychodynamic and psychosocial aspects of a presentation in addition to the neurobiologic features. This is especially critical in the outpatient setting where cognitive dysfunction and psychopathology are reciprocally affected by the patient's environment.

References

1. Tariot PN, Weingartner H: A psychobiologic analysis of cognitive failures. *Arch Gen Psychiatry* 43:1183–1188, 1986.
2. Flor-Henry P: *Cerebral Basis of Psychopathology.* Boston, John Wright PSG, 1983.
3. Thase ME, Reynolds CF: Manic pseudodementia. *Psychosomatics* 25:256–260, 1984.
4. Caine ED: Pseudodementia. *Arch Gen Psychiatry* 38:1359–1364, 1981.
5. Flor-Henry P: Neuropsychological studies in patients with psychiatric disorders. In Heilman KM, Satz P (eds): *Neuropsychology of Human Emotion.* New York, Guilford Press, 1983, pp 193–220.
6. Freeman RL, Galaburda AM, Cabal RD: The neurology of depression: cognitive and behavioral deficits with focal findings in depression and resolution after electroconvulsive therapy. *Arch Neurol* 42:289–291, 1985.
7. Rosse RB, Ciolino CP: Motor impersistence mistaken for uncooperativeness in a patient with right-brain damage. *Psychosomatics* 27:532–534, 1986.
8. Ross ED: The aprosodias. *Arch Neurol* 38:561–569, 1981.
9. Faber R, Abrams R, Taylor M, et al: Comparison of schizophrenic patients with formal thought disorder and neurologically impaired patients with aphasia. *Am J Psychiatry* 140:1348–1351, 1983.
10. Mesulam MM: Frontal cortex and behavior (editorial). *Ann Neurol* 19:320–325, 1986.
11. Lezak MD: *Neuropsychological Assessment,* ed. 2. New York, Oxford University Press, 1983.
12. Liston EH: Diagnostic delay in presenile dementia. *J Clin Psychiatry* 39:599–603, 1978.
13. *Diagnostic and Statistical Manual of Mental Disorders (Third Edition-Revised).* Washington, DC, American Psychiatric Association, 1987.
14. Kopelman MD: Amnesia: organic and psychogenic. *Br J Psychiatry* 150:428–442, 1987.
15. Benson DF, Blumer D: Amnesia: a clinical approach to memory. In Benson DF, Blumer D (eds): *Psychiatric Aspects of Neurologic Disease.* New York, Grune and Stratton, 1982, vol 2, pp 251–278.
16. Signoret JL: Memory and amnesias. In Mesulam MM (ed): *Principles of Behavioral Neurology.* Philadelphia, F.A. Davis Company, 1985, pp 169–192.
17. Kral VA: Senescent forgetfulness: benign and malignant. *Can Med Assoc J* 86:257–260, 1962.
18. Lipowski ZJ: Transient cognitive disorders (delirium, acute confusional states) in the elderly. *Am J Psychiatry* 140:1426–1436, 1983.
19. Lipowski ZJ: *Delirium.* Springfield, IL, Charles C Thomas, 1980.
20. Dastoor DP, Cole MG: The course of Alzheimer's disease: an uncontrolled longitudinal study. *Journal of Clinical Experimental Gerontology* 7:289–299, 1985–1986.
21. Navia BA, Jordan BD, Price RW: The AIDS dementia complex: I. Clinical features. *Ann Neurol* 19:517–524, 1986.
22. Reifler BV, Larson E, Hanley R: Coexistence of cognitive impairment and depression in geriatric outpatients. *Am J Psychiatry* 139:623–626, 1982.
23. Reifler BV: Mixed cognitive–affective disturbances in the elderly: a new classification. *J Clin Psychiatry* 47:354–356, 1986.
24. Mayeux R, Stern Y, Rosen J, et al: Is "subcortical dementia" a recognizable clinical entity? *Ann Neurol* 14:278–283, 1983.
25. Benson DF: Subcortical dementia: a clinical approach. In Mayeau R, Rosen WG (eds): *The Dementias.* New York, Raven Press, 1983, pp 185–194.
26. Cummings JL: Subcortical dementia: neuropsychology, neuropsychiatry, and pathophysiology. *Br J Psychiatry* 149:682–697, 1987.
27. Huber SJ, Paulson GW: The concept of subcortical dementia. *Am J Psychiatry* 142:1312–1317, 1985.
28. Drachman DA, Long RR: Neurologic evaluation of the elderly patient. In Albert ML (ed): *Clinical Neurology of Aging.* New York, Oxford University Press, 1984, pp 97–113.
29. Cummings JL, Benson DF: *Dementia: A Clinical Approach.* Boston, Butterworth, 1983.
30. Folstein M, Anthony JC, Parhad I, et al: The meaning of cognitive impairment in the elderly. *J Am Geriatr Soc* 33:228–235, 1985.
31. MacKinnon RA, Michels R: *The Clinical Interview in Clinical Practice.* Philadelphia, Saunders, 1971.
32. Kales A, Soldatos CR, Kales JD: Taking a sleep history. *Am Fam Physician* 22:101–107, 1980.
33. Reynolds CF, Kupfer DJ, Taska LS, et al: Sleep apnea in Alzheimer's dementia: correlation with mental deterioration. *J Clin Psychiatry* 46:257–261, 1985.
34. Folstein MF, Folstein SE, McHugh PR: Mini-Mental State—practical method for grading the cognitive state of patients for the clinician. *J Psychiatr Res* 12:189–198, 1975.
35. Granacher RP: The neurologic examination in geriatric psychiatry. *Psychosomatics* 22:1981.
36. Weinberger DR: Brain disease and psychiatric illness: when should a psychiatrist order a CAT scan? *Am J Psychiatry* 141:1521–1527, 1984.
37. Weiner RD: EEG in organic brain syndrome. In Hughes JR, Wilson WP (eds): *EEG and Evoked Potential in Psychiatry and Behavioral Neurology.* Boston, Butterworth, 1983, pp 1–24.
38. Brown RP, Kneeland B: Visual imaging in psychiatry. *Hosp Community Psychiatry* 36:489–496, 1985.

24

Disturbed Motor Behavior

Theo C. Manschreck, M.D.

CLINICAL APPROACH

When confronted with abnormal movement, the clinician should observe whether it represents increased or decreased activity and whether it is diffuse or patterned. These divisions are naturally somewhat arbitrary and serve only as guideposts to further investigation. Neurologic examination is virtually essential in assessing motor disturbances in order to provide the fullest information for differential diagnosis. Anatomic localization may then be possible. When the motor disturbance has been described and classified, diagnostic possibilities based on knowledge of motor phenomena will be evident.

There are several useful points to remember in assessing motor behavior. First, no motor abnormality should be ignored simply because prominent symptoms are present that suggest specific psychiatric disorder. Neurologic disease may, of course, occur with such disorders. Second, it is striking that motor disturbances lack pathognomonic import. They may be the consequence of numerous disorders. Hence, the clinician will find more possibilities, not fewer, to account for the clinical presentation when recognizing the presence of motor disturbances. Third, heightened suspicion, nevertheless, should be held for those common conditions known to disturb general be-

havior as well as motor behavior, e.g., certain drugs, alcohol, delirium, dementia, schizophrenia, mania, and depression. Fourth, careful medical and psychiatric history, either from the patient or another informant can be useful in sorting out many of these possibilities. Extensive laboratory testing may be necessary, e.g., toxic screens, serology, electroencephalogram, serial mental status examinations, and computerized tomography. Fifth, the more acute the development of symptoms, the more likely it is that the cause is organic. Sixth, even more chronic conditions should not be diagnosed as psychologic disorders unless the entire clinical picture has a convincing coherence and other possibilities have been excluded. Seventh, it is essential to rule out treatable and/or identifiable causes before deciding that motor disturbances are part of schizophrenic, depressive, or other disorders. Finally, virtually none of the motor disturbances to be discussed occurs in the absence of other major symptoms and signs. Hence, consideration of the entire clinical picture is necessary to avoid serious mistakes.

In discussing differential diagnosis of disturbed motor behavior, the clinician's task may be simplified by classifying the abnormalities as disturbances of increased and decreased activity. In this chapter, each of these categories shall be further divided into diffuse and patterned movement disorders. Disturbances of posture, gait, and station (stance) are then considered. The reader may wish to refer to Chapter 12, pp 168–173, to review the descriptive features of the motor behavior disturbances to be discussed here.

DISTURBANCES OF INCREASED ACTIVITY

Diffuse Types of Disturbance

Restlessness is a common finding among psychiatric patients. It may be a manifestation of tension or anxiety, but it may also signal other potentially serious conditions, including early delirium, encephalitis, presenile dementia, meningitis, hypoparathyroidism, hyperthyroidism, pheochromocytoma, lead and lithium toxicity, xanthine (caffeine, theophylline, theobromine, and aminophylline), and other central nervous system (CNS) stimulant toxicity (1).

Excitement has been associated with psychopathologic conditions including dissociative states, catatonic states, and states of elation. Most of the conditions which lead to restlessness may also result in excitement which represents a more serious and extreme form of movement disturbance. Excitement also occurs in tricyclic, antihistaminic, and atropine toxicity, barbiturate and other sedative–hypnotic toxicity, marijuana toxicity, and certain encephalopathies (particularly Wernicke's).

For a list of diffuse types of disturbance, see Table 24.1.

"Simple" Patterned Disturbances

Tremors are among the most common motor disturbances encountered in psychiatric evaluations. Although tremors are associated with anxiety states, fatigue, and other psychiatric conditions, they should be carefully assessed before it is decided that psychologic disturbance accounts for their presence (1).

Resting tremors tend to diminish or disappear with volitional activity. Hence, while the interview is proceeding, the in-

Table 24.1 Diffuse Patterns of Increased Activity

Disturbance	Possible Causes
Restlessness	Common nonspecific psychiatric complaint, psychotropic drug effect, delirium, encephalitis, meningitis, presenile dementia, central nervous system stimulant toxicity, lead toxicity, phenochromocytoma, hyperthyroidism, hypoparathyroidism (or hypocalcemic states)
Excitement	Dissociative, catatonic, and manic states and most of the conditions associated with restlessness; also tricyclic, antihistaminic, atropine, barbiturate, sedative–hypnotic, and marijuana toxicity; encephalopathy

terviewer should observe particularly the hands, head, and feet. Phenothiazines, carbon monoxide and manganese poisoning, and parkinsonism may be their source. Resting tremors are also common in metabolic encephalopathies. In Wilson's disease, in addition to a resting tremor, a "wing-beating tremor" may be observed.

Requesting that the patient extend the arms increases the tone of the musculature and may elicit *postural tremors*. Postural tremors tend to be either fine and rapid or coarse and slow. A fine, rapid tremor occurs in hyperthyroid states, fatigue, excitement, anxiety states, hypoglycemia, uremia, epinephrine, cocaine, amphetamine intoxication, and lead or mercury poisoning.

General paresis has a fine rapid tremor often associated with tremor of the tongue, eyelids, and lips. Barbiturates, bromides, glutethimide, nicotine, and monoamine oxidase inhibitors are also associated with fine rapid tremors. On the other hand, a coarse tremor frequently characterizes alcohol and related compound withdrawal (also hypnotic sedative drugs, e.g., chloral hydrate) and may be a prominent additional feature (cf. resting tremor above) in Wilson's disease. Familial tremor is a coarse tremor with onset in adolescence and preponderance in males. Benign essential tremor does not appear to be genetically transmitted and occurs in older individuals.

Certain *intentional* (*action*) *tremors* may appear when patients must make goal-directed movements, as in the finger–nose–finger test of cerebellar testing. As the goal is approached, the tremor increases in amplitude. These tremors are characteristic of cerebellar disease and may be seen in multiple sclerosis, Friedrich's ataxia, and severe alcoholism.

Certain tremors may be present at rest, with postural extension, and with movement. Among these are the coarse tremor of lithium toxicity and the coarse tremor known as senile tremor that occurs late in life and is usually accompanied by a nodding or rotatory tremor of the head. Senile tremor may in fact be a variant of familial tremor, which occurs in younger individuals.

Stereotypic movements have been classically linked with the catatonic subtype in schizophrenia. However, they are also seen in other schizophrenic subtypes and in CNS stimulant (e.g., amphetamine, cocaine, or related compounds) intoxication.

Spasmodic movements have traditionally been considered psychogenic. However, spasmodic torticollis, for instance, appears to be a distinct neurologic disturbance, probably of basal ganglia origin, which involves spasms of the neck muscles (the sternocleidomastoids and trapezeii, in particular), which pull the head toward the same side and twist the face in the opposite direction. Other spasmodic movements such as blepharospasm have been associated with CNS syphilis and antipsychotic drug treatment. Habit spasms such as unusual coughing, clearing of the throat, and swallowing are generally considered normal, but may fluctuate in severity in relationship to psychologic factors (2).

Choreiform movements generally indicate medical illness. Huntington's chorea may present with psychiatric symptoms (such as mood disturbance, intellectual impairment, and/or psychotic features) and only later may manifest the chronic motor signs classically associated with it. Reduced magnesium in the body, resulting from various conditions including chronic alcoholic disease, diabetes (acidosis), and diuretic treatment, may result in choreiform movements. Wilson's disease and other liver abnormalities, Sydenham's rheumatic chorea, and mercury toxicity may exhibit similar motor disturbances. Hyperthyroidism, neurosyphilis, lupus erythematosus, and reserpine and antipsychotic drug toxicity (e.g., tardive dyskinesia) are other conditions in which chorea may be seen.

Athetoid movements may also be seen in patients who suffer from hypomagnesemia. Antihistamine, lithium, and phenothiazine toxicity are somewhat uncommon, but are potential causes of athetoid movements. The clinician should consider basal ganglia disease, subacute combined degeneration, tabes dorsalis, and the recovery phase of hemiplegia in the differential diagnosis of athetoid conditions. Phenylketonuria and amaurotic familial idiocy (particularly Kufs and Spielmeyer-Vogt diseases) may have athetoid movements as a prominent feature (1). Athetoid movements are rare if they occur at all as part of schizophrenic disorders.

Myoclonic movements are associated with a number of cortical neuron diseases. In psychiatric patients such movements should alert the clinician to consider epileptic disorder, inclusion body encephalitis, Alzheimer's disease, Wilson's disease, and Jakob-Creutzfeldt's disease. Phenothiazine and other antipsychotic drug toxicity is also associated with such movements.

Perseverative movements may occur in normal, emotionally disturbed, and brain-damaged individuals. The incidence of perseverative movements is high in children; it tends to level off in adolescence, stabilize in adulthood, and rise again in old age. Like many other motor signs, they may be increased by tension, anxiety, and fatigue. Where pronounced and more or less constantly present day to day, perseverative movements are reliable indicators of disturbed brain function. They occur in schizophrenia, but are rarely encountered in pronounced forms in states of depression and anxiety. Among brain disturbances, perseverative movements may occur in delirium, carbon monoxide intoxication, as an early sign of dementing illness (e.g., Alzheimer's and Pick's diseases), and with severe closed-head injury. Perseverative movements may also be an early sign of cardiovascular failure, internal hemorrhage, alcohol and drug intoxication, electrolyte disturbance, hypoglycemia, and hepatic encephalopathy. Focal brain diseases, particularly of the frontal lobes, and a variety of aphasic disturbances have associated perseverative movement disorders (3).

Impulsive movements generally occur in individuals with brain disturbances, particularly with deteriorating intellectual abilities. Delirious and demented states are frequently associated with impulsive movements, but mania, drug and alcohol intoxication, and even agitated depressive states should be considered.

Carphologic movements are common manifestations of confusion, as seen in delirium and dementia. In many patients these movements should alert the clinician to the possibility of anticholinergic intoxication. However, they may also occur in anxiety states, amphetamine intoxication, hallucinogen intoxication, and Korsakoff's syndrome. Less commonly, they are seen in schizophrenia.

For a list of simple patterned disturbances, see Table 24.2.

Complex Patterned Disturbances

Akathisia is a frequent manifestation of antipsychotic drug administration. It generally occurs after an initial period of treatment of 1 to 2 weeks or even later. The severity is reflected in the amount of move-

Table 24.2 "Simple" Patterns of Increased Activity

Disturbance	Possible Causes
Resting tremor	Parkinsonism, carbon monoxide poison, manganese poison, Wilson's disease, metabolic encephalopathies, phenothiazines
Postural tremor Fine, rapid	Thyrotoxicosis, fatigue, hypoglycemia, excitement and anxiety states, general paresis, epinephrine, amphetamine, cocaine, lead, mercury poisoning, barbiturates, bromides, glutethimide, nicotine, monoamine oxidase inhibitors
Coarse, slow	Wilson's disease, alcohol withdrawal, familial or benign essential tremor
Intentional tremor	Multiple sclerosis, Friedrich's ataxia, severe alcoholism, lithium toxicity, senile tremor
Stereotypic movements	Catatonic syndrome in schizophrenia, amphetamine and cocaine intoxication
Spasmodic movements	Traditionally considered psychogenic; basal ganglia disturbance, central nervous system syphilis; antipsychotic treatment
Choreiform movements	Huntington's chorea, reduced level of magnesium (chronic alcohol disease, diabetes, diuretic treatment), Wilson's disease, Syndenham's rheumatic chorea, mercury toxicity, lupus erythematosus, hyperparathyroidism, hyperthyroidism, neurosyphilis, reserpine and phenothiazine toxicity
Athetoid movements	Hypomagnesemia, antihistamine toxicity, lithium and phenothiazine toxicity, basal ganglia disease, tabes dorsalis, phenylketonuria, amaurotic familial idiocy, recovery phase of hemiplegia
Myoclonic movements	Cortical neuron disease, epileptic disorder, inclusion body encephalitis, Creutzfeldt-Jakob's disease, antipsychotic and lithium toxicity
Perseverative movements	Delirium, carbon monoxide intoxication, Alzheimer's and Pick's diseases, severe closed-head injury, cardiovascular failure, internal hemorrhage, alcohol and drug intoxication, electrolyte disturbance, hypoglycemia, hepatic encephalopathy, focal brain disease
Impulsive movements	Delirium and dementia, mania, drug and alcohol intoxication, agitated depressive states
Carphologic movements	Delirium and dementia, anticholinergic intoxication, anxiety states, amphetamine intoxication, hallucinogen intoxication, Korsakoff's syndrome

ment and the patient's inability to remain at rest (4).

Agitation is commonly encountered in depressive states. Nevertheless, agitation may complicate the treatment of depression or endogenous anxiety states when MAO inhibitors are administered. Less common but potentially dangerous sources of agitation include hypoglycemia, congestive heart failure, and hypertensive encephalopathy. Hallucinogenic drugs may also induce agitation. Treatment with piperazine phenothiazines, butyrophenones, and thioxanthenes are also linked to agitation as an early sign of CNS excitation.

The etiology of *tics* is not well understood. They seem to increase with intense emotion and have frequently been regarded as psychogenic. It must be remembered, however, that facial nerve damage is associated with the development of tics. Further differential considerations in tic evaluation include dystonic musculorum deformans. Disorders which cause athetosis have also been implicated in the development of tics. Gilles de la Tourette disorder, an uncommon syndrome involving motor and verbal tics, should be considered, particularly in adolescents and in patients treated with antipsychotic drugs.

Dystonic movements frequently occur early in the course of antipsychotic treatment, usually within the first week. Acute dystonias may occur in association with sweating, pallor, or even fever, as well as with oculogyric crises, opisthotonus, and grimacing. The tongue, neck, mouth, and shoulders are the usual sites for such disturbance. These symptoms are often mistaken for hysteria, tetanus, and muscle injury in psychiatric practice. Congenital and familial dystonic diseases should be considered in those cases involving unusually large areas of bodily musculature and occurring as a chronic disturbance, particularly when the dystonias appear unresponsive to appropriate medical treatment (4). Wilson's disease, extrapyramidal disease, and Huntington's chorea may also show dystonic movement disturbances.

Tardive dyskinesia has been repeatedly linked to chronic antipsychotic drug treatment and to changes in treatment regimen, e.g., introduction of new agents in a chronic treatment. The essential prevalence rate is 10 to 15%. Those older than 50 are at greater risk than younger patients. Early recognition of this syndrome and prompt discontinuation of antipsychotic drugs when appropriate may reduce the occurrence of this disorder (5). Patients with senile dementia, severe depression, and CNS damage have also exhibited spontaneous dyskinesias with features similar to those of tardive dyskinesia. Antipsychotic treatment history may help distinguish such cases.

Mannerisms may be difficult to assess precisely because they are often part of normal motor behavior. Their association with schizophrenia has been a classic teaching since Kraepelin. Nevertheless, normal individuals, particularly in adolescence, may show manneristic behaviors, and patients with diffuse neurologic disturbance (e.g., dementia and delirium) may also show this behavior. Though striking when observed, there is nothing pathognomonic about mannerisms; they should be considered in the light of a comprehensive evaluation of the patient.

For a list of complex patterned disturbances, see Table 24.3.

DISTURBANCES OF DECREASED ACTIVITY

Diffuse Decreased Activity

Retarded movement occurs classically in severe depression. General slowing of movement is also seen in parkinsonism, cerebellar disease, and related neurologic conditions. For example, delirium and dementia may exhibit retarded movement.

Poverty of movement (hypokinesia) is associated with catatonic and depressive states. Muscle disease, including myotonia and myasthenia gravis, may also cause poverty of movement. Other possible sources for this disorder include cerebellar disease and parkinsonism, as well as delirium and dementia.

Table 24.3   Complex Patterns of Increased Activity

Disturbance	Possible Causes
Akathisia	Frequent side effect of antipsychotic drugs
Agitation	Depressive states, hypoglycemia, hypertensive encephalopathy, hallucinogenic drugs, antipsychotic drugs, cardiac disease
Tics	Frequently regarded as psychogenic, facial nerve damage, dystonia musculorum deformans, Gilles de la Tourette disorder
Dystonic movements	Antipsychotic medication, Wilson's disease, extrapyramidal disease, Huntington's chorea, tetanus
Tardive dyskinesia	Chronic antipsychotic drug treatment, senile dementia, central nervous system damage
Mannerisms	Schizophrenic disorders; may be present in adolescents and in other patients with diffuse neurologic disturbance

Severe muscular *rigidity* may be the consequence of antipsychotic drug treatment. If accompanied by fever, both the extrapyramidal symptoms (e.g., muscular rigidity) and the fever need to be addressed vigorously, since they may be somewhat independent features, in a condition with potentially poor prognosis. This constellation (including autonomic instability, fever, and stupor) has been called the "neuroleptic malignant syndrome." Levinson and Simpson, however, prefer to emphasize the heterogeneous causes of these features (6).

Stupor has traditionally been associated with severe states of depression and catatonic schizophrenia (7). These stuporous conditions are less common now in clinical practice. However, at times, they must be differentiated from stuporous conditions due to severe delirium and disturbances of consciousness (8). In depression, stuporous patients may appear almost frozen in inactivity. In schizophrenia, stupor is one among other catatonic features; including negativism, posturing, echopraxia, and related phenomena. There may be a degree

of reduced activity associated with suspicion, withdrawal, a glistening alertness in the eyes, (related to paranoid concerns or hallucinatory activity), and unexpected ability to move the eyes; the patient's posture may have symbolic connections to his or her delusions.

Table 24.4 presents the range of possible causes in a follow-up diagnostic study of 100 cases of stupor (9). It should be noted that stupor may form part of the neuroleptic malignant syndrome, a condition described after Joyston-Bechal's report on causes of stupor.

For a list of diffuse decreased-activity disturbances, see Table 24.5.

Patterned Disturbances of Decreased Activity

Motor blocking is characteristic of schizophrenia, particularly its catatonic forms. Its differential diagnosis, therefore, requires close scrutiny of those conditions which may mimic schizophrenia, particularly temporal lobe epilepsy.

Cooperation in its mild form, *Mitmachen*, and its more extreme version, *Mitgehen*, is a feature of schizophrenia, particularly catatonic schizophrenia. Similar guidelines for diagnosis hold.

Automatic obedience occurs most frequently in catatonic forms of schizophrenia. However, it is found occasionally in dementia.

Negativism suggests schizophrenia, particularly catatonia. However, it is incorrectly used to refer to hostility, inability to

Table 24.4   Causes of Stupor in 100 Cases[a]

All Cases		Organic Cases	
Schizophrenic disorder	31	Dementia	7
Depression	25	Confusional state	4
Organic diseases	20	Intracranial tumor	3
"Neurosis/hysteria"	10	Neurosyphilis	3
Unknown	14	Postencephalitic disorder	2
Total	100	Postepileptic	1
		Total	20

[a] Adapted from Joyston-Bechal (9).

Table 24.5   Diffuse Patterns of Decreased Activity

Disturbance	Possible Causes
Retarded movement	Severe depression, parkinsonism, cerebellar disease and related neurologic conditions, delirium, and dementia
Poverty of movement (hypokinesia)	Catatonia, depression, muscle disease (myotonia and myasthenia gravis), parkinsonism, cerebellar disease, delirium, dementia, stupor
Rigidity	Muscular response to antipsychotic drug treatment, lethal catatonia
Stupor	Catatonia, depression, neurologic disturbances of consciousness, antipsychotic-induced extrapyramidal symptoms with fever

cooperate, and motivated refusal. Hence, depressed psychotic patients who display apprehension and avoidance would be incorrectly labeled negativistic regarding motor behavior. Other potential sources of negativistic behaviors include mental retardation and dementia (2, 7).

Ambitendency is generally considered a variety of negativism and occurs in similar conditions.

Parkinsonian movements, of course, refer to those movements which are characteristic in parkinsonian states. In psychiatric practice, parkinsonian movements are associated with antipsychotic drug treatment. Manganese toxicity from industrial exposure may induce parkinsonian movements, and lithium treatment has been associated with such movements. Other

sources to consider are degenerative disease, infectious diseases, vascular disorders, metabolic conditions, and certain neurologic disorders, such as normal-pressure hydrocephalus.

Echopraxia may occur in schizophrenia, but it is also associated with dementia, transcortical aphasia, mental retardation, delirium, fatigue, and inattentiveness in normals, and with temporal lobe epilepsy (10).

Opposition (*Gegenhalten*) is a classic sign of frontoparietal disease. It is frequently associated with catatonic schizophrenia and thus calls for the same general approach to differential diagnosis that other so-called pathognomonic signs of schizophrenia require.

For a list of patterned decreased-activity disturbances, see Table 24.6.

DISTURBANCES OF POSTURE, GAIT, AND STATION

For a list of posture, gait, and station disturbances, see Table 24.7.

Drooping shoulders and inerect posture suggest fear, sadness, depression, old age, and debilitating disease. Stooped posture is typical of parkinsonian states and makes the patient appear to move forward in the line of movement. The maintenance of a postural position (*postural persistence* or *catalepsy*) indicates a catatonic state (see Table 24.8). Catatonia is mentioned here because of its diagnostic importance and the fact that many motor features are associated with it. This syndrome has a variety of motor and verbal manifestations. It

Table 24.6   Patterned Disturbances of Decreased Activity

Disturbance	Possible Causes
Motor blocking	Schizophrenia (see causes of catatonia), epilepsy
Cooperation	Schizophrenia (catatonia)
Automatic obedience	Schizophrenia (catatonia), dementia
Negativism	Schizophrenia (see causes of catatonia), mental retardation, dementia
Ambitendency	A variety of negativism; hence it may be part of catatonia and occurs in similar conditions
Parkinsonian movements	Antipsychotic drugs, manganese toxicity
Echopraxia	Schizophrenic disorders, dementia, transcortical aphasia, mental retardation, delirium, fatigue, inattentiveness in normals, temporal lobe epilepsy
Opposition (Gegenhalten)	Frontoparietal disease, schizophrenia (catatonia)

Table 24.7 Disturbances of Posture, Gait, and Station

Disturbance	Possible Causes
Stooped posture	Parkinsonism, debilitating disease, old age, depression, fear, sadness
Bizarre posture	Arthritis, kyphosis (Paget's disease, osteoporosis, acromegaly), ankylosing spondylitis, extrapyramidal syndromes, hysteria
Reeling or ataxic gait	Cerebellar disturbance, posterior column disease, vestibular disorder
Propulsive or festinating gait	Parkinsonian states
Spastic gait	Hemiplegia
Clownish gait	Huntington's chorea
Grotesque gait	Hysterical disorder and disturbances involving bilateral cerebral disease
Steppage gait	Popliteal nerve damage or damage to the roots of L5 and S1
Waddling gait	Muscular dystrophy
Positive Romberg test	Posterior column disease (tabes dorsalis), cerebellar disturbance, acute and chronic alcoholism
Vertigo	Acute labyrinthine disease or structural lesions affecting the vestibular pathways

Table 24.8 Manifestations of Catatonia

Excitement	Other Manifestations	Stupor
Violence	Stereotypies	Catalepsy (postural persistence)
Exhaustion	Mannerisms	Rigidity
	Echopraxia/echolalia	Negativistic motor behavior
		Last-minute responses
		Mutism

can be present in very mild forms or dramatically dominate the clinical picture. Catatonic features do not arise only from schizophrenic disorders (see Tables 24.9 and 24.10) (10–13). These and other postural abnormalities are closely related to the variety of disturbances discussed above in the section on disturbances of motor activity.

Arthritis, if severe, may lead to bizarre postures and difficulty standing. Diseases of bones and joints may cause characteristic postures. For instance, kyphosis occurs in Paget's disease, osteoporosis, and acromegaly and leads to a stooped appearance. Ankylosing spondylitis patients stand with rigid backs and sometimes with the head apparently flexed on the chest. Other abnormal postures may be the result of loss of muscle tone and movement control. They may occur in extrapyramidal syndromes and hysteria. In the latter, postures are generally unusual and unexplainable on a physiologic or anatomic basis. A general awkwardness or clumsiness of movement is frequently observed in schizophrenic disorders and often is asso-

Table 24.9 Differential Diagnosis of Catatonia[a]

Psychiatric Disorders	Neurologic Disorders
Affective disorders	Epileptic disorders
Schizophrenic disorders	Encephalopathy
Dissociative disturbances	Frontal lobe disease
Reactive psychoses	Basal ganglia disease
	Limbic system disorder
	Temporal lobe disorder
	Diencephalon disorder
	Narcolepsy
	Head injury
	Intracranial hemorrhage
	Subdural hematoma
	Cerebral cortex infarction

Drug-Related Disorders	Metabolic Disorders
Amphetamine	Diabetic ketoacidosis
Acetylsalicylic acid	Heptatic encephalopathy
Disulfiram	Hyperparathyroidism
Glutethimide withdrawal	Porphyria
Cortisone	Systemic lupus
Antipsychotics	erythematosus
Alcohol	Glomerulonephritis
Illuminating gas	Homocystinuria
Mescaline	Pellagra
Phencyclidine	
Organic fluorides	

[a] Adapted from Gelenberg (12) and Stoudemire (13).

Table 24.10   Causes of Catatonia in 55 Cases[a]

Cause	%
Mania (n = 34)	62
Endogenous depression (n = 5)	9
Schizophrenic disorder (n = 4)	7
Course brain disease, including epilepsy, toxic psychosis, encephalitis, alcoholic degeneration, drug-induced psychosis (n = 9)	16
Reactive psychosis (n = 3)	5

[a] Data from Abrams and Taylor (11).

ciated with repetitive movements, such as stereotypies (14).

Reeling or *ataxic gait* disturbance suggests cerebellar disturbance (as in alcoholic cerebellar degeneration and alcohol intoxication), posterior column disease, and vertibular disorder (as in acute vestibular labyrinthitis). If the disturbance is cerebellar in origin, the patient may compensate by walking with the feet placed widely apart. If the origin is posterior column disease, as in tabes dorsalis, the gait usually worsens when the eyes are closed.

Propulsive or *festinating gait* is seen in parkinsonian states. A *spastic gait* is typical of hemiplegia. A *clownish gait* is characteristic of Huntington's chorea. A *grotesque gait* is associated with hysterical disorder but may also be seen in disturbances involving bilateral cerebral disease. *Steppage gait* is usually due to popliteal nerve damage or damage to the roots of L5 and S1 and may be unilateral or bilateral (tumors of the cauda equina and advanced polyneuropathies). In peripheral neuropathies, steppage gait is usually associated with pain and hyperesthesias of the foot. *Waddling gait* is typical of muscular dystrophy. Much of the differential concerning disturbances of station is covered above. A *posi-*

tive Romberg test suggests posterior column disease and, specifically, tabes dorsalis. A wide-based stance suggests cerebellar disturbance due to intrinsic disease or the toxic effects of acute and chronic alcoholism. *Vertigo* may be due to acute labyrinthine disease or to structural lesions affecting the vestibular pathways.

References

1. Walker S: *Psychiatric Signs and Symptoms due to Medical Problems.* Springfield, IL, Charles C Thomas, 1967.
2. Fish F: Motor disorder. In Hamilton M (ed): *Clinical Psychopathology.* Bristol, England, John Wright, 1985, pp 91–114.
3. Allison AS: Perseveration as a sign of diffuse and focal brain disease. I and II. *Br Med J* 2:1027–1032, 1035–1101, 1966.
4. Marsden CD, Tarsy D, Baldessarini R: Spontaneous and drug-induced movement disorders in psychotic patients. In Benson DF, Blumer D (eds): *Psychiatric Aspects of Neurologic Disease.* New York, Grune & Stratton, 1975, pp 219–266.
5. Tarsy D, Baldessarini RJ: Tardive dyskinesia. *Am Rev Med* 35:605–623, 1984.
6. Levinson D, Simpson G: Neuroleptic-induced extrapyramidal symptoms with fever. *Arch Gen Psychiatry* 43:839–848, 1986.
7. Kraepelin E: *Dementia Praecox and Paraphrenia.* Edinburgh, E and S Livingstone, 1919.
8. Lishman WA: *Organic Psychiatry,* ed 2. Oxford, England, Blackwell Publications, 1987.
9. Joyston-Bechal MP: The clinical features and outcome of stupor. *Br J Psychiatry* 112:967–981, 1966.
10. Stengel E: A clinical and psychological study of echo reactions. *Journal of Mental Science* 93:598–612, 1947.
11. Abrams R, Taylor M: Catatonia. A prospective clinical study. *Arch Gen Psychiatry* 33:579–581, 1976.
12. Gelenberg A: The catatonic syndrome. *Lancet* 1:1339–1341, 1976.
13. Stoudemire A: The differential diagnosis of catatonic states. *Psychosomatics* 23:245–252, 1982.
14. Manschreck T: Motor abnormalities in schizophrenic disorders. In Nasrallah H, Weinberger D (eds): *The Neurology of Schizophrenia.* Amsterdam, Elsevier, 1986, pp 65–96.

25

Pain

Anthony Bouckoms, M.D.

Psychiatrists, like other physicians who work in ambulatory clinical care, commonly encounter patients with the complaint of pain. When pain is the primary presentation, the patient has usually been referred by a physician who has decided that the pain is psychologic in nature—meaning insufficient physical pathology to explain the suffering. When patients are self-referred, the pain complaint is more often part of a psychiatric syndrome. In either situation, the psychiatrist has the responsibility for a systematic assessment of the pain complaint to determine the contributions of organic and psychologic factors.

The complaint of pain always represents a physical and psychiatric phenomenon (1). Pain means physical tissue damage in the mind of the sufferer (malingering or factitious illness excepted). The association of pain with tissue damage is necessary for survival. Pain triggers basic reflexes necessary for survival: withdrawal, stress analgesia, vocalization, orientation to the stimulus, and sympathetic activation. These basic pain reflexes help protect the organism from further damage, underscoring the biologic necessity for the association between pain and tissue damage. Pain is also always in the mind. Patients who insist that their pain is not in their mind wish to deny the existence of their central nervous system (CNS). Pain is always in the mind; otherwise one would not know that one was in pain. Accordingly, a good definition of pain is the perception of nociception, where nociception is the irritation of specialized pain receptors in skin, joints, muscle, or viscera. Perception is a CNS-mediated psychologic phenomenon and hence so is pain. The mind perceives the sum of what the brainstem reticular activating system directs it toward, and what the thalamus filters through, either into the limbic system for an emotional response or into the cortex for a cognitive response. Pain, therefore, always represents a complex combination of physical and psychologic features requiring the most critical differential review of psychopathology and neuropathology (2). The purpose of this chapter is to describe how the psychiatrist might define and critically review the neuropathology and psychopathology of a patient presenting with pain and emotional suffering.

The task of differential diagnosis of pain complaints requires the following eight skills, in accordance with which this chapter is organized.

1. Knowledge of the basic types of pain and putative mechanisms.
2. The ability to accurately describe and understand the nature of altered sensitivity to painful stimuli.
3. Knowledge of the diagnostic implica-

tions of the sensory description of pain.
4. Recognition of the typical features of central pain disorders.
5. Familiarity with the association between pain and psychiatric problems, particularly the psychologic, statistical, and diagnostic obstacles that make diagnosis problematic.
6. The principal psychiatric diagnoses found in pain patients.
7. Knowledge of the standard psychiatric examination of the somatizing patient, as well as the interview style and diagnostic tools that make the process possible, easier, and more accurate.
8. Painful physical disorders that may mimic psychiatric pathology.

PAIN TYPES

There are five main pain types: nociceptive (peripheral), central (neuropathic or deafferentation), visceral, referred, and psychogenic. A psychiatrist should be particularly familiar with the nociceptive, central, and psychogenic types. They are common and their features may overlap. A summary description of these pain types, their sensory description, and their mechanism is presented in Table 25.1. The sensory description of the different pain types varies greatly and is most important in the differential diagnosis. Classically, nociceptive or peripheral pain due to tissue trauma presents with an aching sharp pain much like a toothache. In comparison, pain resulting from a central mechanism presents as a vague, shifting discomfort with exquisite hypersensitivity, even to nonpainful stimulus. Therefore, the first task is the ability to accurately describe and understand the nature of altered sensitivity to painful stimuli.

ALTERED SENSITIVITY TO PAIN

The complaint of altered sensitivity to pain is commonly heard by the psychiatrist. The patient may impute physical or psychologic factors for this altered sensitivity. Rarely, patients will tell the physician that their current fear or past experience makes the reactive emotional component of the pain a greater burden for them than most. Usually the comment will be intended to convey the opposite; emphasizing the robust strength of body and psyche, if it weren't for the pain. The patient wants to impress the doctor that the new painful sensitivity is entirely physical—not the result of some psychologic deficit. Accurate diagnosis at this psychosomatic interface requires that the psychiatrist recognize physical states of the CNS that result in altered sensitivity to touch, thermal, and pain stimuli (3). Numbness and analgesia are but two extremes of the alterations in sensory thresholds and response to stimuli that can occur. There are normal variations in sensation, such as paresthesia (a not unpleasant abnormal sensation either spontaneous or evoked, e.g., "pins and needles") and dysaesthesia (an unpleasant abnormal sensation either spontaneous or evoked, as might be felt if you fall asleep on your arm).

Increased sensitivity to touch, thermal, or painful stimuli, (defined as hyperaesthesia), is usually pathologic and requires critical analysis to decide if there is a disorder of sensation mediated by the sensory system or a global complaint of suffering suggestive of a primary psychiatric problem. This differential diagnosis is a major part of the psychiatrist's consultation. Three questions must be answered

Table 25.1   Pain Types

Type	Sensory Description	Mechanism
Nociceptive (peripheral)	Aching, sharp	Tissue damage
Central (neuropathic)	Dysaesthesia, allodynia, hyperaesthesia	Disinhibition of central nervous system
Visceral	Deep colicky pressure	Distension of viscera
Referred	Sensitive skin/muscles	Convergence of afferents
Psychogenic	Diffuse, intense, variable	Psychiatric illness

for a positive diagnosis of sensory pathology.

First, what is the threshold to light touch and painful stimuli? Lowered threshold to stimuli implies CNS pathology, assuming one excludes acute pain where inflammation or acute tissue injury is present. Two kinds of hyperaesthesia may accompany a lowered sensory threshold: allodynia and hyperalgesia. Hyperaesthesia may be accompanied by hyperalgesia if the stimulus and response are in the same modality, allodynia if the stimulus and response are in different modalities, or hyperpathia if there is summation of response to the original stimulus. A raised threshold to stimulation is a frequent finding in patients with neuralgic pain. Partial nerve injury is the usual antecedent to such a neuralgic pain syndrome. The raised threshold is always associated with increased sensitivity to some sensory stimulus (hyperaesthesia). Increased response with a raised threshold produces the syndrome of hyperpathia. It can be identified by faulty identification of the kind, intensity, and localization of the stimulus, delay, and then summation of the pain even after the stimulus has been removed, producing an explosive, distressing after-sensation. If the threshold is raised but the response decreased, then hypoalgesia exists. This decreased pain response to a stimulus that produces pain requires (by definition) that the stimulus and response are in the same mode.

Second, is the response to touch, temperature, and pain increased or decreased? In all cases of hyperaesthesia except for hypoalgesia, the response to stimulation is increased. The kind of stimulus and associated response and any alteration in threshold will determine the kind of hyperaesthesia present, as described above.

Third, are the sensory stimulus and response in the same mode? In other words, does light touch elicit pain (altered mode of response), or is a normally painful sharp pinprick required to elicit pain? Consider a common example found in trigeminal neuralgia where a slight whiff of cold air may elicit severe hyperaesthesia. This is a change in modality from a thermal stimulus to pain.

IMPLICATIONS OF THE SENSORY DESCRIPTION OF PAIN

The psychiatrist armed with a detailed description of sensory features of the pain complaint is at the very least able to precisely denote changes in the patient's state. In patients suffering from chronic pain, this classification system allows a precise prospective study of an evolving neurogenic disorder to be more assiduously tracked. Similarly, an inconsistently described sensory metaphor for psychic angst can be identified. Much more use can be made of the information on threshold, response, and stimulus–mode correlation. For example, the implications of the stimulus–response modality suggest that wide dynamic range cells in the CNS are involved in the pain if the modalities are different or that nociceptive specific cells in the traditional spinothalamic pathway are the putative mechanism if the modality is the same. Consider if allodynia is present, where light touch elicits pain. This cannot be due to nociceptive specific cells as are found mainly in the spinothalamic pathway. There must have been some convergence or facilitation of neurons not usually found in the acute pain response. The multimodality wide-dynamic-range neurons found in the CNS may have been recruited. Whatever the exact mechanism, it involves the CNS and changes the treatment considerations to include things that alter aberrant neuronal firing, e.g., anticonvulsants, anaesthetic membrane stabilizing agents, and monoaminergic medicines (4).

Another clinical value of the psychiatrist's knowing precisely the sensory pain features is that it allows useful collaboration between treating physicians. The psychiatrist and neurologist can now speak the same language, avoiding the tendency to assign some difficult problems to each other's specialty. Patients with chronic pain often get caught in this multitreater merry-go-round, a setup for alienation and despair when they are least able to cope. If these problems are avoided, then appropriate collaboration between psychiatrist and neurologist in the use of psychotropic agents, anticonvulsants, and assessment of suffering are possible. A final advantage of the psychiatrist's sensory knowledge is to speedily identify sensory descriptions that are not consistent with neurophysiologic functioning of the sensory system. Examples of such inconsistencies are a lowered threshold and a lowered response to stimulation, allodynia with a raised sensory threshold, hyperalgesia without hyperaesthesia, or hyperpathia without hyperaesthesia.

CENTRAL PAIN SYNDROMES

Afferent pain information is usually thought of as moving from the peripheral nerve to specialized nociceptive-specific cells in the dorsal horn and then passing rostrally in the neospinothalamic tract to more nociceptive-specific cells in the lateral thalamus and then cortex. However, this textbook pathway for the conveyance of afferent information is quite incomplete, certainly with regard to understanding the mechanisms of chronic central pain states and why they are so difficult to treat. Pain is also conveyed rostrally through the paleospinothalamic tract and the dorsal columns, and diffusely through the brainstem reticular activating system, thalamus, and limbic system (5). Wide-dynamic-range cells that respond to many nonnoxious stimuli may also be involved. This CNS component of pain means that pain can be perceived even without an obvious nociceptive stimulus. This kind of pain is called central or sometimes neuropathic or deafferentation pain. It is estimated that centrally mediated pain problems occur in 50% of chronic pain states. Neurophysiologists have established that nerve damage can result in changes in the receptive fields and recruitment of neurons at multiple levels in the nervous system from the dorsal horn to the brainstem to the thalamus and cortex. This diffuse spreading of electrical ac-

tivity results in a kind of partial seizure for pain. Understanding that these mechanisms may be present is very important to diagnosing this clinical syndrome and administering appropriate treatment (6). The clinical features of central pain syndromes are outlined in Table 25.2. The changes in sensory threshold and hypersensitivity which are classical for central pain states have been described in the previous section. The multiple features of this syndrome indicate that CNS pain is not a single well-defined phenomenon. Peripheral nociceptive pain associated with tissue damage may trigger a central pain exacerbation. There may also be a referred component to the pain because of convergent sensory afferents or sympathetic fibers proximal to the peripheral site of perceived pain. The sympathetic nervous system may become involved and present with a syndrome of reflex sympathetic dystrophy. The treatment of these central pain states has been previously reviewed in other publications (4).

THE ASSOCIATION OF PAIN WITH PSYCHIATRIC PROBLEMS

Pain is a common presenting complaint of affective, psychotic, stress-related, and somatoform disorder patients (7, 8). Pain in the head, neck, chest, abdomen, back, and extremities is very common in these psychiatric disorders, often affecting many bodily parts with a diffuse vague presentation. Merskey and Boyd (9) found that 38% of those complaining of pain in a se-

Table 25.2   Features of Central Pain Syndromes

Delay in onset of pain after injury—days to months
Gradual onset of uncomfortable dysaesthesia
Unprovoked lightninglike attacks of pain
Change in sensory threshold—typically light touch is painful
Lack of efficacy of narcotics
Efficacy of anticonvulsants, e.g., clonazepam
Diffuse and variable distribution of pain
Trigger points (variable) elicit pain
Verbal description difficult and variable—often "burning, sensitive"

ries of general medical patients had a psychiatric disorder. Usually the pain was not accompanied by an organic disease. In those patients with an emotional disorder, 74% complained of pain. The conclusion was that pain is apt to occur in conjunction with psychologic problems as often as with physical disorders. In a later study Merskey (10) reviewed 13 studies reporting the frequency of pain in 7542 patients in a variety of medical clinics. On average 50% had pain without a relevant physical lesion but with psychiatric illness. Bridges and Goldberg (11) reported on 497 illness inceptions in general practice and diagnosed them according to the physical diagnosis and *Diagnostic and Statistical Manual of Mental Disorders* (*Third Edition*) (DSM-III) psychiatric criteria. They found that 33% of these illness inceptions were of a primary psychiatric illness. Thirty-two percent of the DSM-III disorders presented with a purely somatic presentation, while a further 24% had mixed physical and somatic complaints (11).

Further erudition of the association of psychiatric disorders with pain is complicated by three problems, statistical, diagnostic, and psychologic. The statistical problem involves sample selection, base rate variation, and differences in researchers' application of diagnostic criteria, which significantly affect prevalence reports and reliability statistics. For example, Sherman's (12) study of 5000 American veteran amputees found that 78% of them reported significant phantom pain, yet only 54% of these victims discussed pain with their physicians. A random population sample of 500 patients studied by Crook (13) to determine the prevalence of pain complaints and contact with medical resources found that 16% of the individuals had experienced chronic pain problems, and 75% of these people had contacted their family physicians at least once for pain problems. This population sample of people with persistent pain used health services, both physicians and hospital care, more frequently than did those with only temporary pain.

Low base rates may further complicate statistical assessment of diagnostic reliability and validity. For example, somatoform disorders are said to occur in 3.5% of the population in the sample described in DSM-III. The kappa statistic for measuring diagnostic agreement between diagnosticians is 0.42 for somatoform disorders. This kappa statistic measures the proportion of observed agreements compared to agreement that could be reached by chance alone. Kappa may be inappropriately low, with low base rates giving smaller values as the base rate gets smaller (14). Therefore, on the one hand the low kappa may be erroneously low because of the small number of cases available in most studies, or it may reflect the real problem of making fine distinctions in homogeneous populations.

The threshold of diagnostic criteria used also affects the frequency of psychiatric disorder identified. The literature has figures ranging from 5% to 100% of pain patients exhibiting psychiatric disorder. The problem of diagnostic threshold criteria is demonstrated in a tertiary neurosurgery pain population where depression as defined by depressive symptoms was present in 60% of intractable pain patients, but major depression as defined by DSM-III was present in only 24% (15).

The second problem in understanding the association between psychiatric disorders and pain is diagnostic in nature. Pain and psychopathology have an extremely complex and tenuous relationship. For example, trigeminal neuralgia, which can be an excruciatingly severe pain, is associated with a psychiatric diagnosis in only 5% of cases. Milder cases of pain with less obvious distress, as might be seen in mild headache or work-related back pain, are frequently associated with a psychiatric disorder and disability. The matter is further complicated by the chicken-and-egg argument. Sternback and Timmermans showed that neuroticism associated with chronic pain is often the result of the pain, since it may be reversible when the pain is reduced or abolished surgically (16). An important example of the multivariate relationship between pain and psychopathology is provided in the work of Sigvardsson et al. (17). They compared 859 adopted women with nonadopted controls who were matched individually for social and demographic variables. Using the criterion of two or more sick-leave days per year, a somatization syndrome could be identified with brief, non-medically-substantiated periods of disability. The chief complaints were neck and headache, backache, and abdominal pain. This somatization syndrome was consistently associated with psychiatric impairment. These somatizers accounted for 36% of all cases of psychiatric disability and 48% of all sick-leave occasions in adopted women. Examination of the genetic and environmental antecedents of the backgrounds of these somatizers showed a high frequency of alcoholism and antisocial behavior, similar to the findings in families of patients with somatization and antisocial disorders. The implication is that somatoform disorders are much more common (36%) than is usually recognized by most physicians. This highlights problems of diagnostic criteria in somatoform disorders, their differential from affective and Axis II disorders, and the temporal effect on data as genotype evolves to phenotype.

The third problem is the denial and avoidance found in many chronic pain patients. A straightforward psychiatric screening interview often leads to no clear psychiatric diagnosis even in the most wary and seasoned clinician. One potent reason for this difficulty is that denial is one of the most common indices of psychopathology found in chronic pain patients. This denial extends from denial of current affect, particularly anger, to denial of earlier life traumatic events. Psychologic trauma causing covert emotional conflicts (which are denied by the patient) were found to be the commonest single kind of psychopathology in one chronic pain sample referred to a tertiary neurosurgery service. At 54% this was more common than any DSM-III psychiatric disorder (15). The problem for the clinician then is that a common index of psychopathology in pain is denied and covert and therefore missed

unless it is specifically assessed. This obfuscation of accurate diagnosis of affect in somatic patients has recently been reiterated by Stoudmire et al., who showed that even in patients referred to a psychosomatic unit the true diagnosis of affective disorders tripled from admission to discharge when the patient was better known (18).

PSYCHIATRIC DIAGNOSIS IN PAIN PATIENTS

A good introduction to the psychiatric diagnosis of physical complaints and irrational anxiety about physical illness can be found in the Appendix of DSM-III-Revised (DSM-III-R;19). This decision tree outlines differential diagnostic points in the somatoform category of illnesses. However, psychiatric diagnoses associated with pain occur in a wide range of DSM-III-R diagnoses, listed in Table 25.3.

The commonest major DSM-III-R psychiatric diagnosis found in pain patients is major depression. Twenty-four percent of 63 pain patients with organic causes for their pain had major depression in Bouckoms et al.'s (15). This figure is remarkably consistent in similar published studies that have used DSM-III or Research Diagnostic Criteria. It is consistent that about one-

Table 25.3 Psychiatric Diagnosis Associated with Pain

Major affective disorder
Anxiety disorders
Somatoform disorders
Somatization
Conversion
Psychogenic pain
Hypochondriasis
Atypical somatoform
Psychosis
Affective
Schizophrenic
Organic
Malingering
Factitious disorder
Psychologic factors affecting physical condition
Post-traumatic, stress-related chronic pain syndrome
Personality disorders

quarter of chronic pain patients will have a major depression. Many more have psychologic factors affecting their physical condition, minor depression, depressed mood, or adjustment disorders. The effects of criterion threshold and sampling are so variable with these diagnoses that the prevalence figures vary greatly between 5 and 100%. Outcome of pain in these "minor" diagnoses would be most telling as to their significance. Unfortunately, no studies have been done in this regard. Somatoform disorder is not too common in chronic pain patients, being found in approximately 5%. The problems with this group of diagnoses are many, some having been mentioned in the section on the psychiatric exam. Somatization syndrome is difficult to reach threshold on because of the necessity for having 12 different physical symptoms that have been attended to or treated in the context of chronic sickness occurring before age 30. Furthermore, the very tendency of somatizers to attribute pain to somatic causes, even when there is doubt about the etiology, obliges the assiduous clinician to default some likely candidates for this somatization diagnosis. Establishing the other somatoform diagnoses of conversion and psychogenic pain disorder is problematic not only because of difficulty reaching diagnostic criteria, but because of the vagueness in the diagnostic criteria. These two diagnoses require that psychologic factors be shown to be etiologic in the pain. The criteria given for this etiologic component are that the pain is temporally associated with a psychologic event or that there is some clear avoidance or secondary gain because of the pain. It is a rare case where one of these factors is unequivocally causative of the pain. On the other hand, an advocate for these diagnoses might see these psychologic factors present in most chronic pain patients. This problem probably explains why the degree of agreement between expert clinicians for the somatoform disorders is poor (kappa < .5). Psychotic people may have pain as their calling card to doctors. Schizophrenia, depressive psychosis, monosymptomatic delusions, and organic psychoses may all present with pain. Depressive psychosis is the commonest type of psychosis and the easiest to recognize because of the depressive symptoms. The other kinds of psychoses are quite rare, particularly for the psychiatrist since most patients with these do not go to psychiatrists. It is the nonpsychiatrist who most likely will see these delusional patients. Other psychiatric diagnoses that may be seen with pain include malingering, factitious disorder, and post-traumatic stress syndrome. These are all rare psychiatric syndromes associated with pain and shall not be discussed further. It is also important to remember that many chronic pain patients have no psychiatric diagnosis of any kind. Consider trigeminal neuralgia, which is a very severe pain and can be quite disabling. The prevalence of psychiatric dysfunction in these patients is 5%, less than one might expect in an average population of sick people. Bouckoms et al.'s series of chronic pain patients, a sample biased because of intractability and chronic suffering, have no psychiatric diagnosis in 36%. Chronic pain, even with severe suffering, is not a form of psychopathology.

PSYCHIATRIC EXAMINATION OF THE CHRONIC PAIN PATIENT

Examining the patient who is in chronic pain requires knowledge of the normal "psychopathology" of the long-suffering pain patient, particular resistances found in pain patients with psychologic problems, and knowledge of selected techniques for the clarification of areas of putative psychopathology (20).

The psychologic perception of pain always carries with it some kind of psychologic reaction. This may range from feelings of hopelessness, angry accusations of others' incompetence, or stalwart denial and long suffering to ward off the fear of asking for help. Normal suffering is not a homogeneous phenomenon; rather, it is determined by many things in the patient's current and past life. Nevertheless, there are common features of "normal suffering" that should be recognized as such, and not necessarily indicative of psychopathology. These normal attributes may still be extremely upsetting to the patient and the physician, making them difficult and important to recognize as within the realm of normal coping. Patients may demonstrate any of four common features of normal psychologic coping with pain: SOUR—angry, bitter feelings; SWEET—endearing to others, unduly self-effacing and passive; STRONG—intense affect and need as manifest through episodes of anxiety, depression, anger, and demands; and WEAK—low self-esteem, counterdependent bravado.

Psychologic coping becomes maladaptive when narcissistic injury is prominent. The pained self-esteem will then elicit a narcissistic reaction the degree of which is determined by the severity of the injury and the person's character structure. Intense fluctuating affect, denial and avoidance, efforts for psychologic recompensation, and projection of problems to external causes are all common features seen in chronic pain. The psychiatrist seeing such a patient will almost inevitably be subject to these reactions, particularly if they are conflictual for the patient. The chances are good that this will be the case in patients whom a psychiatrist is asked to see. A caricature of these features has been given the nominative classification, "pain-prone person" (21). This is defined as someone with long-standing pain and depression, characterized by guilt and long suffering which the pain serves to expiate. Strong but unfulfilled aggressive drives and equally strong yearnings for dependence are satisfied in part by the pain. Denial of problems in the face of many long-standing difficulties, both in the patient and the family, is characteristic.

The psychiatrist's general approach to the pain patient should be to initially allow the patient to talk about his or her pain or any aspects of the suffering associated with it. The goal is not to threaten the patient with an inquisition into psychologic weakness or threatening interpersonal problems, but instead to allow the patient to relate his or her own history in a straightforward manner so that the pain, psychologic losses and life changes, and fluctuations in treatment response can be correlated. That is, a classical objective descriptive medical history taking is likely to be much more productive than an anamnestic psychologic approach (22).

Certain diagnostic tools have proved to be of particular value in the delineation of psychopathology associated with chronic pain. These tools are the interview itself, bedside pencil-and-paper tests, the Minnesota Multiphasic Personality Inventory (MMPI), limbic evaluation, and the developmental history.

The Interview

The clinical interview must involve a strategy which evaluates the feelings and behavior observed during the information-gathering process as well as the facts of the emotional and physical state of the patient. The subtle psychologic problems and their presentation, which are not recognizable as bona fide psychiatric illnesses, at least initially, require a special kind of skill. The central concept to keep in mind is that fluctuations of mood and cooperation frequently encountered in the clinical interview of the intractable pain patient are symptomatic of a damaged self-esteem—a narcissistic injury. The techniques for interviewing narcissistically injured pain patients are designed to establish a diagnostic working relationship with these patients, while increasing their emotional experience of themselves and increasing their capacity for insight. This allows an accurate medical history to be elicited, avoids mistrust between doctor and patient, and allows a more effective treatment plan to be administered (23). The general guidelines are as follows:

1. Listen to the pain story. This provides an initial degree of catharsis, avoids mistrust, and provides a valuable impression of the patient's cognitive style and interpersonal relationships.

2. Focus the interview. Once the pain story has been told the interviewer should actively reflect back to the patient interesting points of content. Empathic statements, counterprojective statements, the maintenance of neutrality, and avoidance of misplaced sympathy are the hallmarks of the interview. These interventions also label the patient's distorted idealized view of caregivers and imply that the person must assume some responsibility for treatment. Labeling overt and covert roles assigned by the patient to the doctor are important early interventions to uncover and make explicit distorted beliefs about the people involved. The longer one waits to confront these distortions, the less effective any intervention will be.

3. Encourage the expression of affect. Aside from diagnostic need to understand the degree of depression, anger, and anxiety, it is also often helpful to the patients to be able to label exactly what their suffering feelings are. Avoidance of strong affect with too much support does not bypass psychologic problems, but rather may actually increase conflicted feelings over withholding, control, and a frail sense of self.

Bedside Diagnostic Aids

A detailed drawing of the pain with its distribution and character marked is one of the simplest and helpful diagnostic tests both neurologically and psychologically. Patients can draw their pain in their own time, pay attention to detail, and avoid the frequently cited problem of "I don't know how to describe it." A second useful aid is a visual analog scale, a simple 10-cm line with "severe pain" marked at one end and "no pain" at the other. Patients use this as a simple scale which they can mark as often as the physician requires. During diagnostic testing it may be every few minutes, or for routine follow-up it may be only daily. During periods of investigation and acute treatment, three times a day is a helpful minimum. This simple test is inexpensive, reliable, and extremely sensitive to slight changes in pain. More sophisticated elaborations of these tests can be found in instruments more typically used in research settings. The McGill-Melzack Pain Questionnaire is the foremost example of this (24).

The Minnesota Multiphasic Personality Inventory

Repression of hostility, denial of affect, difficulty in expressing feelings, and long-standing covert psychologic problems are often associated with chronic pain problems. The value of the MMPI in assessing these traits suggests that it could be useful in assessing the chronic pain patient. Psychologists, however, have been critical of the use of the MMPI for the study of an individual patient. They are cautious about the extrapolation of population data to single findings or scales in one individual. Even so, certain aspects of the MMPI may be useful for the assessment of individual chronic pain patients. Holmes et al.'s study (25) of the MMPIs of 31 chronic pain patients is particularly valuable because it compares this pain group with a control group of nonpain patients who were physically ill and had emotional problems. Holmes et al. found that hysteria, psychopathic deviate, and paranoia were the three MMPI scales showing consistently elevated subtle versus obvious scores in the chronic pain population. Subtle scores were considered to be significantly different from obvious scores on the MMPI when there was a difference of 7 or more points between them. Subtle items provide a more accurate index of psychopathology and less susceptibility to faking or the effects of personality style than the obvious items. Supplementary evidence of these denied feelings as being valid and relatively specific to the chronic pain population was shown with the finding that the MMPI covert hostility scale was elevated significantly more often than the overt hostility scale in the chronic pain population. This was not true in the control group.

This pervasive denial of feelings defined by the MMPI was validated by its association with interview-derived ratings of covert psychologic conflict in the person's past. The MMPI scales of resentment, aggression, and repression were elevated in chronic pain patients but not significantly more than in the other physically sick people with emotional distress, making these scales less useful diagnostically.

Confounding the generalizability of these findings is disagreement regarding the specificity of subtle MMPI scales. Jackson has stated that obvious nonsubtle scales were the more relevant and predictive of a particular trait (26). Burkhart et al. have written that normal subjects with higher intelligence had approximately equal or more subtle than obvious scores while those of lesser intelligence had higher obvious than subtle scores (27). However, these questions are not so problematic in these chronic pain patients where faking good and denial of problems are just what we want to examine. It has been shown that subtle scores increase and obvious scores decrease when subjects are instructed to intentionally fake good on the MMPI, and thus deny the presence of problems. Burkhart et al. stated (27) that given their inherent resistance to faking, subtle items may be especially useful in the clinical testing situation. Additional studies have further evaluated the merit of obvious and subtle scales within the various clinical scales of the MMPI and have shown that there is support for the predictive validity of subtle items. Holmes et al. also found that the typical psychoneurotic inverted V was quite rare in pain patients (p < .002). Instead the conversion V was significantly more common in chronic pain patients, being found in twice as many of these patients as control (p < .05).

In summary, it is suggested that the MMPI is useful for the detection of denial in chronic pain patients. Evaluation of this denial and affect can be readily ascertained and used by the practicing clinician by pursuit of specific items on the MMPI that strongly indicate denial and are not often found in other psychiatrically–medically ill patients. The specific items are as follows:

1. Higher subtle than obvious scores on the hysteria, psychopathic deviate, and paranoia scales. Hypochondriasis and depression may also be elevated but less often have the subtle greater than obvious scoring.
2. The configuration of the conversion V is more often found in chronic pain patients than the psychoneurotic inverted V. The latter is more often found in other types of emotionally distressed patients with physical illness.
3. The covert hostility scale is frequently elevated significantly more than the overt hostility scale.

It is recommended that if none of these three criteria are found on the MMPI, then hidden psychopathology is an unlikely cause for the pain complaint. However, caution should be exercised in that the MMPI alone should never be used to make a definitive diagnosis, but rather it should be used as an exploratory or confirmatory test.

Limbic Evaluation

The psychosomatic physician might well live by the aphorism "The limbic system never lies" (28). Limbic response denotes the person's instinctive reflex emotional response, either to the content or the interpersonal situation during the examination. The instantaneous smile, abrupt downward gaze of the eyes, instant denial, or strident avoidance of the question are all examples of emotional reflexive or limbic behavior at work. These are emotional reactions that are not highly intellectualized or planned according to what the person might think is appropriate, but rather are swift gut-level reactions that are not under conscious cortical control. These reactions are most telling about the emotional valance of a subject under discussion, the presence of conflict if the limbic reaction is at odds with the verbal reaction, and the detection of less than straightforward problems in the pain behavior of the patient. The majority of this limbic evaluation consists of careful assessment of the subtleties of the emotional response during the routine interview. The limbic evaluation can be supplemented with the following:

1. Hold up a clenched fist and ask the person, "What would you do with one of these?" Excessive denial of affect, particularly anger, will be indicated with the statement that they don't know what you mean. Angry but basically psychologically sound persons will smile broadly and designate two or three people they would like to express their anger at.

2. Label contradictory limbic responses and verbal responses in order to see whether the patient can integrate these divergent pieces of his or her own emotional life. Significant emotional pathology and conflict will be indicated by the person's inability to integrate these feelings often expressed through denial or avoidance of acknowledging that there is a problem. A healthier person with reactive rather than primary psychopathology will carefully consider the information and offer some response, indicating an ability to consider mixed emotional feelings.

Psychologic Developmental History

Pain behavior with maladaptive affective response and increasingly angry and dejected affective response is often a reflection of long-standing, unmet interpersonal needs. The question is whether such a response is simply an acute reaction to a novel and painful situation, in which case it should be expected to resolve spontaneously in the near future, or whether it is a reflection of more long-standing interpersonal difficulties that need a specialist's help. The assessment of the early psychologic developmental history can determine if early emotional deprivation and interpersonal problems have occurred. A detailed family background history with particular emphasis on loss, separations, and the quality of adequate parental care is important. Sources of emotional nuturance, conflictual or discrepant parental behavior, subtle emotional and physical deprivation should all be assessed as indicators of early psychologic developmental problems (15).

PAINFUL PHYSICAL DISORDERS MIMICKING PSYCHIATRIC DISORDERS

Psychiatric diagnosis should never be made by exclusion. Patients presenting with somatic complaints without obvious physical cause were often loosely assigned the label of hysterical or conversion. Such impressionistic labeling led to diagnostic errors in about 50% of cases. Reed (29) in a follow-up study of 15 cases of "hysterical pain" found that 6 had developed clear organic pathology explaining their pain, and only 2 others had recovered as might be expected in patients with truly hysterical symptoms. However, in addition to assiduous pursuit of a definitive psychiatric diagnosis, the possibility of other disease-mimicking psychopathology should always be kept in mind. Syphilis and multiple sclerosis are the two great mimics, presenting with multisystem, vague, and varying symptoms in the early stages. Other diseases that should be included in a differential of unusual pain cases would include hidden tumors, porphyria triggered by barbiturate use, sickle cell anemia, systemic lupus and other connective tissue autoimmune diseases, subcortical dementia, and partial complex seizures. Less common physical problems are drug withdrawal states, pheochromocytoma, Cushing's syndrome, carcinoid mital valve prolapse, and tuberculosis. Not dismissing the possibility of some hidden organic disease is the psychiatrist's responsibility as well as the primary physician's.

CONCLUSION

Americans consume 18 million tons of aspirin per year and lost 550 million work days per year because of pain (30). Pain is clearly a common costly and catastrophic problem. The majority of these personal and financial costs are incurred by a minority of people, who just never seem to improve. Social problems account for a portion of this problem, but psychiatric disease and unusual sensory descriptions of pain that confuse professionals and patients alike account for some of the intransigence. Depression, somatoform disorders, and covert psychologic problems are the major psychiatric problems. Depression alone is one of the major factors associated with a poor prognosis. No one in the series of pain patients seen by this author who sustained complete improvement had depression on initial evaluation. Smith has shown that a patient with somatization disorder costs nine times the national average in health care costs. Stoudemire has shown that the true prevalence of affective disorders in somatizing patients is one-third higher than initial prevalence unit. I have found that up to one-half of chronic pain patients may have central or neuropathic pain syndromes. If assiduous differential psychiatric and neurologic diagnosis can be pursued, then chronic pain patients may be diagnosed by positive diagnostic criteria, not by exclusion. This is helpful not only from an educational/research point of view but also as a prerequisite to the assignment of appropriate treatment for specific pain problems.

References

1. Loeser J: Components of chronic pain. Presented at a symposium on chronic back pain, University of Massachusetts, Worcester, 1980.
2. Cassem NH: Pain. In Rubenstein E, Federman DD (eds): *Scientific American Medicine. Current Topics in Medicine, Subsection II*. New York, Scientific American, 1983, 1–14.
3. Merskey H: Pain terms. *Pain* 6:249–252, 1979; Merskey H: A supplementary note. *Pain* 14:205–206, 1982.
4. Maciewicz R, Bouckoms A, Martin J: Drug therapy of neuropathic pain. *Clin J Pain* 1:39–49, 1985.
5. Melzack R, Loeser JD: Phantom body pain in paraplegics: evidence for a central "pattern generating mechanism" for pain. *Pain* 4:195–210, 1978.
6. Kruger L, Liebeskind J: *Advances in Pain Research and Therapy: Vol. 6. Neural Mechanisms of Pain*. New York, Raven Press, 1984.
7. Wilson DR, Widmer RD, Cadoset RJ: Somatic symptoms. A major feature of depression in a family practice. *J Affect Dis* 5:199–207, 1983.
8. Lipowski ZJ: Somatization: a borderland between medicine and psychiatry. *Can Med Assoc J* 135:609–614, 1986.
9. Merskey H, Boyd D: Emotional adjustment and chronic pain. *Pain* 5:173–178, 1978.
10. Merskey H: The role of the psychiatrist in the investigation and treatment of pain. In Bonica J (ed): *Pain*. New York, Raven Press, 1980, pp 249–259.
11. Bridges KW, Goldberg DP: Somatic presentation of DSM-III psychiatric disorders in primary care. *J Psychosom Res* 29:563–570, 1985.
12. Sherman RA, Sherman CJ, Parker L: Chronic phantom and stump pain among American veteran: results of a survey. *Pain* 18:83–96, 1984.
13. Crook J, Rideout E, Browne G: The prevalence of pain complaints in a general population. *Pain* 18:299–314, 1984.
14. Spitznagel EL, Helzer JE: A proposed solution to the base rate problem in the K statistic. *Arch Gen Psychiatry* 42:725–728, 1985.
15. Bouckoms AJ, Litman RE, Baer L: Denial in the depressive and pain-prone disorders of chronic pain. In Fields HL, et al. (eds): *Advances in Pain Research and Therapy*. New York, Raven Press, 1985, pp 879–888.
16. Sternbach RA, Timmermans G: Personality changes associated with reduction of pain. *Pain* 1:177–191, 1975.
17. Sigvardsson S, von Knorring AL, Bohman M, et al: An adoption stud of somatoform disorders: I. The relationship of somatization to psychiatric disability. *Arch Gen Psychiatry* 41:853–862, 1984.
18. Stoudmire A, Kahn M, Trig Brown J, et al: Masked depression in a combined medical–psychiatric unit. *Psychosomatics* 26:221–228, 1985.
19. *Diagnostic and Statistical Manual for Mental Disorders (Third Edition-Revised)*. Washington, DC, American Psychiatric Association, 1987.
20. Cassem NH: Functional somatic symptoms and somatoform disorders. In Hackett TP, Cassem NH (eds): *Massachusetts General Hospital Handbook of Psychiatry*. Littleton, MA, PSG Publishing Company, 1987, pp 42–68.
21. Blumer D, Heilbronn M: Chronic pain as a variant of depressive disease. *J Nerv Ment Dis* 170:381–389, 1982.
22. Hackett TP, Bouckoms AJ: The pain patient: evaluation and treatment. In Hackett TP, Cassem NH (eds): *Massachusetts General Hospital Handbook of Psychiatry*. Littleton, MA, PSG Publishing Company, 1987, pp. 42–68.
23. Bouckoms AJ, Litman RE: Chronic pain patients: clues in the clinical interview. *Psychiatr Med* 4:1–7, 1987.

24. Melzack R: *Pain Measurement and Assessment*. New York, Raven Press, 1983.
25. Holmes VF, Rafuls WA, Bouckoms AJ, et al: Covert psychopathology in chronic pain. *Clin J Pain* 2:79–85, 1986.
26. Jackson D: The dynamics of structured personality tests: 1971. *Psychol Rev* 78:229–248, 1971.
27. Burkhart B, Gunther M, Fromuth M: The relative predictive validity of subtle vs. obvious items on the MMPI depression scale. *J Clin Psychol* 35:748–751, 1980.
28. Murray GB: Limbic music. In Hackett TP, Cassem NH (eds): *Massachusetts General Hospital Handbook of Psychiatry*. Littleton, MA, PSG Publishing Company, 1987, pp 116–125.
29. Reed JL: Hysteria. In Silverstone T, Barraclough B (eds): *Contemporary Psychiatry*. Ashford, Canton, England, Headley Bros., 1976, pp 141–149.
30. Louis Harris and Associates: *Nuprin Pain Report*. New York, New York, Louis Harris and Associates, 1985.

26

Sexual Dysfunction

Mai-Lan Rogoff, M.D.

Complaints of sexual dysfunction, particularly of loss of sexual interest or of chronic erectile dysfunction, are often seen in patients coming to outpatient services. These may be primarily psychogenic in origin or may have a more complex combined organic/psychologic etiology. Since the normal sexual response cycle involves a spinal reflex arc requiring intact vascular, nervous, and hormonal systems which is then cortically perceived and modified, it is not surprising that a multitude of neuromedical and psychiatric disorders as well as drugs may also cause sexual symptoms.

CLASSIFICATION OF SEXUAL DYSFUNCTIONS

Kaplan has suggested dividing the sexual response cycle into three phases: desire, arousal, and orgasm (Tables 26.1–26.4) (1). Disorders of the sexual response cycle termed "psychosexual dysfunctions" in the *Diagnostic and Statistical Manual of Mental Disorders* (*Third Edition*) (DSM-III; 2) have been classifed in DSM-III-Revised (DSM-III-R; 3) into three phases plus two sexual pain disorders (dyspareunia and vaginismus). The disorders of desire are hypoactive sexual desire disorder, or loss of sexual interest, and sexual aversion disorder, in which there is aversion and/or avoidance of genital sexual con-

Table 26.1   Illnesses Causing Desire-Phase Disorders

General debility and/or pain
  Chronic obstructive pulmonary disease
  Degenerative diseases
  Infections
  Malignancies
  Endocrine (nonspecific; also specific effects [see below])
  Renal (also via low zinc levels)
Psychologic depression
Endocrine
  Lowered androgen levels
    Liver diseases
    Alcoholism
    Feminising tumors
    Primary gonadal abnormalities
      Klinefelters' syndrome
      Testicular agenesis
      Orchitis
    Hypothalamic–pituitary abnormalities
      Pituitary infarction or tumor
      Kallman's syndrome
      Prader-Willi syndrome
    Hypothyroidism
Central nervous system disorders, particularly of temporal or frontal lobe
  Vascular
  Tumor
  Infection
  Ideopathic epilepsy

tact with a partner. The disorders of arousal are female sexual arousal disorder, manifested by difficulty with lubrication and swelling accompanied by lack of a subjective sense of sexual excitement in women, and male erectile disorder, characterized by

314

Table 26.2 Drugs Which May Cause Desire-Phase Disorders

Antihypertensives
  Adrenergic blockers: aldomet
  Thiazide diuretics (acetazolamide)
  Beta-blockers: propranolol, nadolol, atenolol
Psychotropics
  Benzodiazepines (may also help through
    relaxation)
  Heterocyclic antidepressants
  Neuroleptics
  Lithium
Central nervous system depressants
  Narcotics
  Barbiturate abuse
  Alcohol abuse, especially chronic
Others
  Cimetidine
  Clofibrate
  Digoxin
  Fenfluramine

Table 26.3 Illnesses Causing Arousal/Orgasm Disorders

Vascular (arousal)
• Leriche's syndrome (large vessel blockade)
• Thrombosis
• Trauma
• Systemic vascular disorders (microvascular
  blockade)
    Arteriosclerosis
    Leukemia
    Sickle cell disease
Peripheral nervous system (arousal or orgasm)
• Diabetes mellitus (acts primarily by nervous and
  vascular effects rather than primary endocrine
  effect)
• Alcoholic neuropathy
• Primary autonomic nerve degeneration (Shy-
  Drager syndrome)
• Surgical disruption of L4 sympathetic ganglion
  or sacral nervous output
    Aneurysm repair, aortic surgery
    Back fusion
    Lumbar sympathectomy
    Abdominal or pelvic surgery interrupting nervi
      erigentes
    Retroperitoneal node dissection
Spinal cord (arousal or ogasm)
• Multiple sclerosis
• Tabes (Lues)
• Amotrophic lateral sclerosis
• Syringomyelia
• Myelitis
• Herniated disc
• Stenosis of lumbar canal
Central nervous system (mainly arousal)
• Temporal lobe epilepsy
• Chromophobe adenoma (pituitary tumor) via
  pressure
Endocrine (arousal, more effect on libido)
• Hypothalamic lesions
• Low testosterone/high prolactin
Severe renal disease (arousal)
Dyspareunia and/or vaginismus
• Irritation of vagina
    Chemical
    Infections
    Post-trauma (accident, surgical)
• Pelvic pathology
    Pelvic inflammatory disease
    Endometriosis
    Ovarian pathology
• Peyronie's syndrome (mechanical obstruction
  or pain)
Failure of ejaculation despite orgasm
• Diabetes mellitus
• Gonadal hormone insufficiency
• Bilateral ganglionectomy
• Extensive rectal operations
• Incompetence of bladder neck
• Peripheral neuropathy

difficulty initiating or sustaining an erection together with lack of sexual excitement in men. Men tend to call this state "impotence," and the persistence of this term probably reflects its accuracy in expressing the psychologic reaction to erectile dysfunction. The major disorders of the orgasm phase are inhibited male and female orgasm. Premature ejaculation and the specific ejaculatory disorders, such as retrograde ejaculation, also occur during this phase. Vaginismus, or involuntary contraction of the muscles surrounding the outer third of the vagina, and dyspareunia, or pain on intercourse, are classified separately because they may occur as part of inhibited sexual desire, during arousal, or during orgasm.

With the exception of certain disorders of ejaculation, it is rare that the cause of sexual dysfunction can be clearly classified into organic or psychologic categories. More often, underlying compromise of neurologic, endocrine, or vascular systems is complicated by the patient's anxiety about both the sexual dysfunction and the meaning of organic causes to the patient. This is particularly true in illnesses such as diabetes mellitus, in which the occurrence of sexual symptoms may represent the first in a series of feared microvascular complications. The symptom picture of sexual

Table 26.4   Drugs Which May Cause Arousal, Orgasm/Ejaculation Disorders

Anticholinergic gastrointestinal preparations (arousal disorders; also decrease volume of ejaculate)
   Banthine
   Probanthine
   Atropine
   Scopolamine
Antihypertensives
   Arousal disorders
      Diuretics (thiazides, spironolactones)
      Norepinephrine depleters (guanethidine, bretylium)
      Beta-blockers (propranolol, nadolol, atenolol)
   Arousal disorders, retarded ejaculation
      Adrenergic blockers (methyldopa)
      Ganglionic blockers (quaternary ammonium compounds)
   Absence of ejaculate despite orgasm
      Phenoxybenzamine
      Reserpine
      Guanethidine
      Methyldopa
Heterocyclic antidepressants
   Arousal disorders
   Ejaculation disorders (retarded, painful)
   Anorgasmia, delayed or "weak" orgasm
Monoamine oxidase inhibitors
   Delayed orgasm
   Retarded ejaculation
   Absence of ejaculate despite orgasm
Neuroleptics
   Arousal disorders
   Retarded ejaculation
   Premature ejaculation
   Retrograde ejaculation
   Priapism
   Absence of ejaculate despite orgasm
High-dose sedative–hypnotics
   Delayed orgasm
   Retarded ejaculation
Stimulants (high doses)
   Delayed organism
   Retarded ejaculation
Other drugs causing arousal disorders
   Antabuse (also causes retarded ejaculation)
   Cimetidine
   Clofibrate
   Digoxin
   Lithium

dysfunction seen by the evaluating physician usually results from a synergistic combination of an organic base and psychogenic intensification. Although psychologic factors play a prominent role in human sexuality, it is important to look for underlying organic causes of sexual dysfunction for several reasons: (*a*) The underlying cause may be directly treatable (as in hormonal deficiencies) or may suggest other organic therapy (such as a penile prosthetic implant for intractable microvascular problems), (*b*) the sexual complaint may be the first presenting symptom of a more serious illness (as in pituitary adenomas), and (*c*) the direction of psychotherapy may need to be reoriented. When organic illness plays a significant role, restoration of function may become less the goal than helping the patient to accept the organic aspect of the dysfunction and decrease the psychogenic contribution of anxiety. The knowledge that failure to regain full function does not represent a failure of "will" on the part of the patient, may actually be therapeutic.

Organic causes of sexual dysfunction may be classified into factors primarily affecting desire and those primarily affecting performance, with a secondary effect on desire. Effects on arousal and orgasm, however, often develop into disorders of desire as a result of the anticipation of performance problems. Disorders of desire may also effectively result in disorders of arousal and orgasm if the patient attempts sexual activity despite the absence of desire. By the time patients present requesting therapy, problems have often become persistent, and it may be difficult to differentiate whether in fact the disorder started as one of desire or later in the sexual response cycle. The answer may be significant in the consideration of organic factors and in the orientation of psychotherapy. Questions such as "When did you or your partner first become concerned?" and "What did you notice at that time?" may help. Determining whether sexual dissatisfaction originally concerned frequency of intercourse or whether the actual episodes of coitus were problematic may also help.

In considering organic causes of sexual dysfunction, two problems stand out. One is that the actual frequency of disorders caused by various drugs and illnesses usually is not known; the other is that most studies of pharmacologic and hormonal causes of sexual dysfunction have been carried out in men rather than women. Reports of sexual dysfunction are often anecdotal, particularly for drug effects. In considering antidepressants, for example, the number of people for whom decreased depression results in improved sexual function probably outweighs the known cases of sexual dysfunction induced by these drugs. Imipramine has even been successfully used to treat ejaculatory dysfunction following surgical disruption of pelvic nerves (4). The conclusion should not be drawn, therefore, that use of particular drugs or the presence of illness will inevitably lead to sexual dysfunction.

With regard to the problem of gender, the hypothesis based on the work of Masters and Johnson and others is that parallel pathways and mechanisms are active in women and men. Regardless of whether this is physiologically true, the effects of illness and drugs in women appear to be less specific than in men. The reason is unclear. Women may be less aware of early difficulties in lubrication than men are of difficulties in achieving or maintaining erection. Secondary psychologic consequences (e.g., fear of failure, performance pressure, anxiety, fear of humiliation) might then be less severe in women, rendering the progression of arousal disorders slower in women than in men. It may also be that women are able to have a satisfactory sexual experience with a greater amount of psychologic compromise than is possible for men, again because of the mechanical difficulties inherent in sustaining an erection. And finally, women may be able to enjoy the less genitally focused aspects of lovemaking more than men, who tend to look toward orgasm and ejaculation as a necessary part of sexual response. Women would then continue to report that sex was "satisfactory" in situations in which men might not.

In this chapter, causes of disorders are classified by the phase in which they tend to occur. Male and female disorders are not differentiated because of inadequate information. Sexual effects of illnesses or drugs, however, are generally less predictably deleterious in women than in men.

NEUROANATOMICAL BASIS OF SEXUAL BEHAVIOR

The normal sexual response cycle has major spinal reflex and vascular, endocrine, and cortical components. Disturbance of any of these functions, as well as disturbance of local genital anatomy or muscular response, will disturb sexual response.

On a subcortical level, genital innervation is both sensory and autonomic. Direct sensory innervation is via the pudendal nerve and its branches, the dorsal nerve of the clitoris, and the analogous dorsal nerve of the penis. Erection in men and presumably vaginal lubrication and engorgement in women are mediated by sacral parasympathetics arising in S2, 3, and 4. Psychogenic erection in men is thought to be mediated by T12–L1 and is sympathetically innervated (5). Orgasm in men consists of two phases: emission and expulsion. Emission is rapidly followed by formation of a pressure chamber in the posterior urethra, both processes being controlled by the hypogastric nerve, which is sympathetically innervated. Expulsion, which is accompanied by contractions of the striated bulbocavernosus and ischiocavernosus muscles in both men and women, is under control of the pudendal nerve. Both sympathetic and parasympathetic autonomic pathways are therefore involved in male sexual response. Since the female orgasm involves only the expulsive phase, parasympathetic pathways appear to be more involved than sympathetic in female sexual response.

Orgasm, however, is more than a spinal reflex arc. It is a subjective sensation, cortically perceived. The powerful, learned component of human sexuality which may suppress or enhance the spinal reflex arc probably involves frontal and associative cortex, as well as more central brain structures in the limbic system. The usual electroencephalographic pattern during orgasm consists of hippocampal theta and general cortical arousal. Ablation of temporal lobes in animals leads to hypersexuality (6), and there is general agreement that destructive lesions, such as tumor, may mimic the Kluver-Bucy syndrome in humans (7). Stimulatory lesions of temporal lobe in humans have also been described as leading to hypersexual behavior in a few cases (8–11). Contemporary work, however, seems to support the position that temporal lobe and other epilepsies are most often associated with decreased sexual activity (12–14). In the hypothalamus, the preoptic nuclei and connections to septum and hippocampus are particularly involved in sexual response. This suggests that variations in the monoamine neurotransmitters may have some direct effects on sexuality, although precise mechanisms have yet to be developed. L-dopa, for example, induces hypersexuality in about 10% of patients (15). This may be a result of improvement in Parkinson's disease, with increased motility in addition to any direct sexual effect of monoamine systems.

HORMONAL BASIS OF SEXUAL BEHAVIOR

Hormonally, the degree of sex drive appears to be androgen dependent in both males and females. Castration of adult male animals results in decreased ejaculation, which develops over time into decreased mounting. The effect can be reversed by administration of testosterone (16). Hypogonadal men often describe lack of sexual interest (17). Unsuspected low testosterone levels or high prolactin levels have been found to be associated with impotence; reversal of the erectile dysfunction occurs after testosterone or bromcriptine administration (18). Subsequent work strongly suggests that testosterone replacement influences libido but not erectile performance, unless the erectile dysfunction is secondary to loss of sexual interest (19, 20).

The evidence for the role of androgens in libido is not as direct in women as in men. Waxenberg et al. found that ovariectomy did not change the intensity of the sexual desire in women, but women who underwent both ovariectomy and adrenalectomy (adrenals are the primary source of female androgen) lost their libido (21).

Although some workers (5) have not found supporting evidence for a role for testosterone in female libido, other work supports the contention that androgen appears to drive female libido. A common clinical observation is that women receiving androgens for control of breast malignancies often report increased libido. There has also been a report (22) that women who had a higher level of androgen at the midpoint of their menstrual cycle tended to have more intercourse throughout the cycle than did those women with a lower level. Shader and Elkins have suggested that androgens may "prime the circuit" for dopamine and serotonin effects (23).

INCREASED SEXUAL ACTIVITY AND INTEREST

The search for substances which would act as aphrodisiacs may be almost as old as human sexuality, although increased sexual activity may also present as a complaint if it is "driven" or is accompanied by antisocial behavior. The appeal of some substances sold as aphrodisiacs appears to have been their scarcity or association with the strength and prowess of the animal from which they were extracted (e.g., rhinoceros horn). Others, such as Spanish Fly (Cantharides), are genitourinary tract irritants which may produce bladder irritation, urinary frequency, and priapism. Vasodilators such as yohimbine, a parasympathetic indole alkaloid with adrenergic blocking activity, and amyl nitrite, an antianginal drug, have also been used as aphrodisiacs. Yohimbine has been used in various aphrodisiac combinations, and some sexual effect has been shown for it in animals (24), although no definitive evidence of its effectiveness in humans has been demonstrated. Amyl nitrite ("poppers") may produce the sensation of prolonged orgasm through transient cerebral ischemia rather than actual prolonged sexual response (25).

Among street drugs, the primary drug currently being used for sexual effect is cocaine, which, together with the older stimulants, is said to increase sexual excitement. Stimulants have been associated with compulsive or driven sexual activity, including some of the paraphilias, such as public masturbation. Some street drugs which had been promoted as aphrodisiacs, such as methaqualone, have subsequently been shown to be associated with sexual dysfunctions. Others, such as marijuana and the hallucinogens have been reported both to enhance and diminish sexual response. Since much of the data has been gathered from drug abusers, the relative contribution of the drug versus the lifestyle is difficult to determine (26).

Compulsive, driven sexual activity and priapism have been reported as side effects of phenothiazines (27, 28), usually considered to be drugs with a risk of decreasing sexual activity. Varga et al. have even described a Kluver-Bucy-like syndrome induced by neuroleptics and relieved by antiparkinsonian drugs in two patients, marked by hypersexuality (29).

Probably the only reliable "aphrodisiacs" are those drugs which relieve syndromes associated with sexual dysfunction. These include the antidepressants, which may on occasion also be associated with sexual dysfunction; testosterone and bromcriptine in cases of hypogonadism or hyperprolactinemia; and vasoactive drugs which produce erection when injected directly into the corpora cavernosa by the patient and are used in the treatment of erectile dysfunction. During initiation of treatment with cyclazocine (an opiate antagonist) male addicts showed increased sexual interest and frequent erections, probably as a result of decreasing opiate activity (7). As previously mentioned, L-dopa may also be associated with increased sexual activity in a few patients.

DECREASED LIBIDO

Illnesses which result in fatigue, general debility, difficulty in breathing, or pain will be associated with loss of sexual interest. Similarly, any catastrophic illness or major surgery may result in decreased sexual interest because of associated anxiety and depression. Psychologic depression is com-monly associated with decreased libido which is considered one of the "biologic signs" of depression; Beck reported that 60% of the patients with moderate–severe depression had loss of libido (30). Illness which disrupts the hypothalamic–pituitary–gonadal axis will result in decreased sexual interest, as will hypothyroidism. Illness which results primarily in disruption of events later in the sexual response cycle may also have secondary effects on libido.

With the exception of chronic abuse of central nervous system depressants such as alcohol or narcotics, drugs such as the antihypertensives tend to have primary effects on arousal and orgasmic phases rather than on sexual interest. Antihypertensives, both alpha- and beta-blockers, have also been reported to decrease libido. The effect of anxiolytics is unclear: Theoretically they should help in disorders characterized by inhibition anxiety (1). When compared with testosterone, greater improvement has been shown in the testosterone group, but similar effects have not been seen with testosterone versus placebo, raising the possibility that benzodiazepines may act as other central nervous system depressants do to inhibit sexual interest (31). Thioridazine has also been reported to have a specific antilibido effect useful in treatment of sexual offenders, but these reports are unsubstantiated (23).

DISORDERS OF AROUSAL

Illnesses causing disorders of arousal act by disrupting the normal peripheral, autonomic, or vascular response; by causing pain on coitus or arousal; or by causing mechanical obstruction to coitus. Some illnesses act by disrupting more than one mechanism. Severe renal disease may result in erectile dysfunction via peripheral neuropathy and by lowering zinc levels (33). The mechanisms of illnesses causing arousal dysfunctions include most of the processes of pathophysiology: infectious, autoimmune, tumor, trauma, arteriosclerotic, and idiopathic. The frequency with which dysfunctions will be observed varies with the cause, reaction to the illness, and by sex. In diabetes, for example, a 30 to 60% prevalence of erectile dysfunction in men has been described (5), while both orgasmic difficulties (33) and no sexual effects (34) have been described for diabetic women. In addition, some men recover function despite the continued presence of peripheral neuropathy (35). This variability argues for consideration of cases individually, with educated concerns but without prior assumptions.

Most of the drugs which have sexual effects do so by their effect on autonomic nervous system, primarily an anticholinergic effect, or by causing alpha or beta blockade (35). Some drugs, such as the H^2-receptor antagonist cimetidine act as antiandrogens or raise serum prolactin. The mechanisms of action of other drugs, such as diuretics, in causing sexual dysfunctions are less clear.

DISORDERS OF ORGASM

The primary disorder of the orgasm phase is delayed or inhibited orgasm. In cord injury involving upper motor neurons, ejaculation is particularly vulnerable. Usually sexual function is impaired first in cord injury, then micturition and finally defecation. Cord injury may result from trauma or other processes which compromise neurologic function, such as illness or compression. Ejaculation is also particularly sensitive to drug effects on autonomic nervous system. Since both sympathetic and parasympathetic nervous systems are involved in ejaculation, drugs which disrupt either system may have sexual consequences. The delaying effect of some drugs on orgasm has been used in treatment of premature ejaculation (37). Chronic abuse of stimulants may slow orgasm through exhaustion of catecholamines and possibly through an amphetamine metabolite (p-hydroxy-norephedrine) which may act as a false neurotransmitter for peripheral adrenergic neurons (26).

In addition to delay or absence of orgasm, men may also develop ejaculatory pain or orgasm without ejaculation (aspermia, sometimes through retrograde ejaculation). Ejaculatory pain presents as a cramplike pain in the perineum or shaft of the penis and is caused by painful involuntary spasm of cremasteric or perineal muscles. It may last from a few seconds to a few days. The urologic examination is usually normal between spasms, and the cause is unclear. Orgasm without ejaculation is produced by a variety of drugs and should be differentiated from lack of orgasm/
ejaculation through history taking. Among the neuroleptics, thioridazine accounts for most of the cases reported in the literature (for unclear reasons), with about 100 reported cases and an unknown actual incidence (23). Less common disorders of the orgasm phase include orgasmic headaches (cephalalgia), particularly in patients with hypertension; cataplexy, which may be seen on orgasm in narcolepsy; and "female ejaculation," which may represent stress incontinence but is felt to represent the secretory products of a "female prostate" by one group of workers (38).

CONCLUSION

Human sexuality is a topic in which the duality between psyche and soma fades and the interaction of mind and body comes into evidence. Although only a minor portion of our lives is spent actually engaging in sexual intimacy, our sexuality goes far beyond genital activity and has profound implications for our sense of well-being and self. Multiple physical and mental systems must perform for normal sexuality to occur. The intense pleasure of sexual activity is cortically perceived; depends on a complex interaction of physical systems which are easily interfered with by illness, surgery, or medications; and is facilitated or inhibited by thoughts and feelings. A careful search for organic causes of sexual dysfunction together with an understanding that even with an organic underpinning, most sexual dysfunction has crucial psychogenic components, is most helpful to the patient.

References

1. Kaplan H: *The New Sex Therapy.* New York, Brunner-Mazel, 1974.
2. American Psychiatric Association: *Diagnostic and Statistical Manual of Mental Disorders (Third Edition).* Washington, DC, American Psychiatric Association, 1980.
3. American Psychiatric Association: *Diagnostic and Statistical Manual of Mental Disorders (Third Edition-Revised).* Washington, DC, American Psychiatric Association, 1987.
4. Nijman JM, Jager S, Boer PW, et al: The treatment of ejaculation disorders after retroperitoneal lymph node dissection. *Cancer* 50:2967–2971, 1982.
5. Schiavi R, Schreiner-Engel P: Physiological aspects of sexual function and dysfunction. *Psychiatr Clin North Am* 3:81–95, 1980.
6. Kluver H, Bucy PC: Preliminary analysis of functions of the temporal lobes in monkeys. *Arch Neurol Psychiatry* 42:979–1000, 1939.
7. Karczmar AG: Drugs, transmitters and hormones, and mating behavior. In Ban TA, Freyhan FA (eds): *Drug Treatment of Sexual Dysfunction.* Basel, Karger, 1980, pp 1–76.
8. Mitchell W, Falconer MA, Hill D: Epilepsy wtih fetishism relieved by temporal lobectomy. *Lancet* 2:626–630, 1954.
9. Epstein AW: Relationship to fetishism and transvestism to brain and particularly to temporal lobe dysfunction. *J Nerv Ment Dis* 133:247–253, 1961.
10. Rosenblum JA: Human sexuality and the cerebral cortex. *Dis Nerv Syst* 35:268–274, 1974.
11. Andy OJ: Hypersexuality and limbic system seizures. *Pavlov J Biol Sci* 12:187–228, 1977.
12. Bear D: Interictal behavior changes in patients with temporal lobe epilepsy. In Hales RE, Frances AJ (eds): *American Psychiatric Association Annual Review.* Washington, APA Press, 1985, vol 4, pp 190–210.
13. Fenwick PB, Toone BK, Wheeler MJ, et al: Sexual behaviour in a center for epilepsy. *Acta Neurol Scand* 71:428–435, 1985.
14. Herzog AG, Seibel MM, Schomer DL, et al: Reproductive endocrine disorders in men with partial seizures of temporal lobe origin. *Arch Neurol* 43:347–350, 1986.
15. Sathananthan O, Angrist BM, Gershon S: Response threshold to L-Dopa in psychiatric patients. *Biol Psychiatry* 7:139–146, 1973.
16. Resko JA, Phoenix CH: Sexual behavior and testosterone concentrations in the plasma of the rhesus monkey before and after castration. *Endocrinology* 91:499–503, 1972.
17. Raboch J, Mellon J: Hypogonadotropic eunuchoids and Klinefelter's: sexual development and activity. In Dorner G, Kawakami M (eds): *Hormones and Brain Development.* Amsterdam, Elsevier/North Holland, 1978, pp 381–389.
18. Spark RF: Impotence is not always psychogenic: newer insights into hypothalamic–pituitary–gonadal dysfunction. *JAMA* 243:750–755, 1980.
19. Bancroft J: Hormones and human sexual behavior. *J Sex Marital Ther* 10:3–21, 1984.
20. O'Carroll R, Bancroft J: Testosterone therapy for low sexual interest and erectile dysfunction in men: A controlled study. *Br J Psychiatry* 145:146–151, 1984.
21. Waxenburg SE, Finkbeiner JA, Drellich MG, et al: The role of hormones in human behavior: II. Changes in sexual behavior in relation to vaginal smears of breast cancer patients after oophorotomy and adrenalectomy. *Psychosom Med* 22:435–442, 1960.
22. Persky H, Dreisbach L, Miller WR, et al: The relation of plasma androgen levels to sexual behaviors and attitudes of women. *Psychosom Med* 44:305–319, 1982.
23. Shader RI, Elkins R: The effects of antianxiety and antipsychotic drugs on sexual behavior. In Ban TA, Freyhan FA (eds): *Drug Treatment of Sexual Dysfunction.* Basel, Karger, 1980, pp 91–110.
24. Clark JT, Smith ER, Davidson JM: Enhancement of sexual motivation in male rats by yohimbine. *Science* 225:847–849, 1984.
25. Kaplan H: *Disorders of Desire.* New York, Brunner-Mazel, 1979.
26. Petrie WM: Sexual effects of antidepressants and psychomotor stimulant drugs. In Ban TA, Freyhan FA (eds): *Drug Treatment of Sexual Dysfunction.* Basel, Karger, 1980, pp 77–90.
27. Lovett Doust JW, Huska L: Amines and aphrodisiacs in chronic schizophrenia. *J Nerv Ment Dis* 155:261–264, 1972.
28. Gottlieb JI, Lustberg T: Phenothiazine induced priapism: a case report. *Am J Psychiatry* 134:1445–1446, 1977.
29. Varga E, Haher JE, Simpson GM: Neuroleptic-induced Kluver-Bucy syndrome. *Biol Psychiatry* 10:65–68, 1975.
30. Beck AT: *Depression: Causes and Treatment.* Philadelphia, University of Pennsylvania Press, 1967.
31. Mathews A: Progress in the treatment of female sexual dysfunction. *J Psychosom Res* 27:165–173, 1983.
32. Mahajan SK, Prasad AS, Rabbani P, et al: Zinc deficiency: a reversible complication of uremia. *Am J Clin Nutr* 36:1177–1183, 1982.
33. Kolodny RC: Sexual dysfunction in diabetic females. *Diabetes* 20:557–559, 1971.
34. Ellenberg M: Sexual aspects of the female diabetic. *Mount Sinai J Med* 44:495–500, 1977.
35. Jensen SB: Sexual dysfunction in insulin-treated diabetics: a six-year follow-up study of 101 patients. *Arch Sex Behav* 15:271–283, 1986.
36. Story N: Sexual dysfunction resulting from drug side effects. *J Sex Res* 10:132–149, 1974.
37. Eaton H: Clomipramine (Anafranil) in the treatment of premature ejaculation. *J Int Med Res* 1:432–434, 1973.
38. Perry JD: G Spot co-author replies to Hoch and Alzate (letter). *J Sex Marital Ther* 10:142–144, 1984.

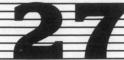

Disturbances of Sleep and Arousal

Milton K. Erman, M.D.

The psychiatrist is likely to hear complaints of disturbed sleep from patients whether in inpatient or outpatient settings. Although it might be understandable to respond by prescribing medication appropriate for the complaint—sedatives for the insomniac, stimulants for the hypersomniac—it cannot be emphasized too strongly that in this area, as in any medical or psychiatric subspecialty, effective treatment is based on accurate diagnosis. Furthermore, it is often important in assessing the significance of a patient's symptomatic complaint to determine whether features seen are characteristic of major sleep disorders, such as narcolepsy, sleep apnea, etc.

In this chapter, I do not attempt to provide a comprehensive introduction to sleep, but some basic information about sleep physiology is appropriate. Contrary to older concepts of sleep as a static state of low arousability and relative inactivity of the central nervous system (the "sleeping brain"), current wisdom suggests that sleep is a dynamic, highly organized compendium of physiologic processes. On the basis of scoring criteria derived from electrophysiologic research (1), sleep can be divided into two separate and distinct states: rapid eye movement (REM) sleep

and non-rapid eye movement (NREM) sleep. These states are defined by characteristic patterns of cortical electrical activity as measured by the electroencephalogram (EEG), by eye movement patterns as defined on the electrooculogram (EOG) channel, and by muscle tone and activity as measured by the electromyogram (EMG). Other channels of the polygraph may record the electrocardiogram (ECG), respiratory effort and airflow, blood oxygen and/or CO_2 levels, presence of leg or body movements, presence or absence of penile tumescence, or other physiologic parameters of interest to the clinician or researcher.

Through use of these standard parameters REM sleep, with its low-voltage EEG, actively inhibited EMG, and striking phasic events (REMs, muscle twitches, and erections) is easily differentiated from the NREM state. Non-rapid eye movement sleep is further divided into Stages 1 through 4; Stages 3 and 4 are characterized by the presence of abundant synchronized slow-wave EEG activity. The presence of this delta-wave EEG activity provides an alternative name—delta sleep—for this sleep, which is often experienced as being the "deepest" or most restful type of sleep. It is often extremely difficult to arouse individuals from delta sleep, and this is the type of sleep replenished with the greatest vigor after sleep deprivation.

There is no evidence to prove conclusively what functions these two major sleep states, REM and NREM, serve in human development and homeostasis, although there has been considerable speculation over the years. The ontogenetic hypothesis (2) suggests that REM sleep, which is seen in high concentration at birth and diminishes as a percentage of total sleep time through the crucial early childhood years, plays a role in stimulating development in the central nervous system (CNS). Recent research supports this hypothesis (3).

In adults, REM sleep is associated with increases in cerebral blood flow and glucose metabolism relative to levels in the NREM state. These findings, suggesting increased cerebral activity in REM compared with NREM sleep, have lead to suggestions that REM sleep may serve a role in CNS homeostasis and memory storage. The role of NREM sleep is less clear, although increases in the amount of delta sleep after vigorous exercise (4) have lead to suggestions that repair or maintenance body functions may occur in the NREM state.

Despite a lack of certainty with regard to the specific physiologic needs served by the type and amount of sleep that we obtain, it is now clear that a certain minimal amount of sleep is required for normal function and, indeed, to sustain life. Elegant animal experiments performed at the University of Chicago (5) have shown that in rats, total sleep deprivation will lead to death or a moribund state associated with pathologically inactive EEG activity. All animals showed ataxis, disturbances of metabolism and temperature regulation, hair loss and other changes in their coats, and swelling of the paws. The research design ensured that these changes were not associated with increased physical activity, since rats forced by a yoked design to endure equal levels of physical activity but allowed to sleep did not show these changes. In humans, a disorder called fatal familial insomnia (6), associated with an essentially complete loss of the ability to sleep, has also been described.

This chapter is organized according to the four distinct groups of sleep disorders using the "Diagnostic Classification of Sleep and Arousal Disorders" of the Association of Sleep Disorders Centers (ASDC) (7). These are as follows:

1. Disorders of initiating and maintaining sleep (DIMS)—the insomnias;
2. Disorders of excessive somnolence (DOES)—the hypersomnias;
3. Disorders of the sleep–wake schedule; and
4. Parasomnias

For a partial listing of disturbances of sleep, see Table 27.1.

DISORDERS OF INITIATING AND MAINTAINING SLEEP (THE INSOMNIAS)

Insomnia is the sleep complaint most prevalent in the general population (8), as well as among psychiatric patients (9). It must be emphasized that insomnia is a symptom and a subjective complaint, not an illness. As in any medical specialty area, including psychiatry, treating a symptomatic complaint without first having established a diagnosis is poor and dangerous medical practice.

Insomnia can be defined as the inability to sleep properly, including difficulty falling asleep, awakening too early, or feeling unrefreshed after a full night's sleep. How frequently is insomnia severe enough that it is reported as a complaint by patients? Studies show that insomnia is reported more frequently by women than by men and by older individuals more frequently than by younger ones (10). Reviews of studies measuring the prevalence of sleep complaints in the general population suggest that about one-third of Americans over the age of 18 perceive themselves as having had trouble sleeping within a given year (11).

The absolute number of prescriptions for hypnotic medications has been used as an-

Table 27.1   Disturbances of Sleep (Partial Listing)

Disorders of initiating and maintaining sleep (insomnias)
  Psychophysiologic
    Transient
    Persistent
  Associated with psychiatric disturbances
  Associated with use of drugs and alcohol
  Associated with sleep-related myoclonus and
    restless legs
  Associated with sleep-related respiratory
    impairment
  Associated with other medical, toxic, and
    environmental conditions
    Somatic pain
    Endocrine disorders
    Cardiac disease
    Gastrointestinal disease
    Dermatologic problems
    Pregnancy
    Infectious disease
Disorders of excessive somnolence (hypersomnias)
  Narcolepsy
  Associated with sleep-induced respiratory
    impairment (sleep apnea)
  Associated with sleep-related myoclonus
  Psychophysiological
  Associated with use of drugs and alcohol
  Associated with psychiatric disorders
  Associated with other toxic, environmental, or
    medical conditions
    Hypothyroidism
    Hypoglycemia
    Central nervous system (CNS) mass
      lesions
    Generalized or CNS infection
    Electrolyte disturbances
  Kleine-Levin syndrome
Disorders of the sleep–wake schedule
  Jet lag
  Frequently changing sleep–wake schedule
  Delayed sleep phase syndrome
Parasomnias
  Sleepwalking (somnambulism)
  Sleep terror (night terror)
  Dream anxiety attacks (nightmares)
  Sleep-related enuresis

---

other measure of the prevalence of insomnia complaints. These data have also been raised as a consideration in discussions regading the extent to which these medications are used appropriately in the treatment of insomnia complaints. Although 25.6 million prescriptions were written for sleeping pills in 1977, this large number in fact reflects a decline from the 41.7 million prescriptions written in 1971

(11). There has been a sharp decline in the number of prescriptions for barbiturate and barbiturate-like compounds, with a shift to the much safer benzodiazepine agents, and there have been suggestions that these drugs are now being prescribed more appropriately in the treatment of insomnia (12).

Causes

The capacity to make a specific diagnosis using formal, validated diagnostic criteria is an important and necessary step in determining appropriate treatment for any medical disorder. The stimulus for the development of a formal sleep nosology was frustration derived from the inability of sleep practitioners to describe and define specific sleep disorders in a fashion which facilitated standardized diagnosis and treatment (13). The ASDC diagnostic classification (7) allows the identification of a number of common and specific causes of insomnia.

Psychophysiologic Insomnia

The transient psychophysiologic insomnias are the most common sleep disorder seen in general medical and psychiatric patient populations. The transient form of this disorder may be the consequence of any acute stress or, including family or school pressures, interpersonal conflicts, or development of a medical illness. Indeed, hospitalization, with all of its attendant changes in routine, sleep schedule, and sleep environment, as well as the anxiety associated with admission to the hospital, may well be the ideal model for this type of insomnia.

The persistent form of this disturbance is seen in association with the development of negative conditioning to sleep and the sleep environment. Patients become more anxious as bedtime approaches and will often "try too hard" to fall asleep, increasing their level of arousal and anxiety and further diminishing their ability to fall asleep. They are afraid to get up from bed for fear of "really waking up," and become more frustrated as they lie in bed, awake, establishing the negative associations between the bed, the bedroom, and the inability to sleep.

Psychiatric Disturbances

Clearly, psychiatric patients are very much at risk for experiencing insomnia. Very specific changes in sleep physiology have been described in major psychiatric disorders, most particularly in association with depression. Specific findings seen in depression include sleep continuity disturbances, diminished slow-wave sleep, an abbreviated first NREM sleep period leading to the early appearance of the first REM sleep period, and altered intranight distribution of REM sleep, with increased REM time and activity in the first half of the night (14).

From a clinical perspective, sleep changes have also served as a hallmark of severe or endogenous depression. Both early morning awakening and delayed sleep onset are typical complaints in serious depressions. Although most depressed patients report decreased sleep time a smaller number report increased sleep time and daytime sleepiness. These hypersomniac complaints tend to be seen most often in the depressed phase of bipolar affective disorder (15).

The sleep disturbance in mania is also well described (16), with marked decreases in total sleep time and time in bed. Manic patients, however, often deny or are unaware that such changes have occurred. As part of the general psychiatric history, and particularly where mania (or depression) are suspected, it may be helpful to ask a spouse, family member, or roommate about changes in the patient's sleeping habits. Although the manic patient may feel quite well with 4 or 5 hours of sleep per night for long periods of time, those who must endure his or her hyperactivity are aware of the change in sleep patterns and typically are eager to report it, hoping for some relief.

Acute schizophrenia is also associated with a sleep disturbance, with delayed sleep onset, decreased total sleep time, and increased time awake after sleep onset (17).

Although considerable interest has been expressed for many years about the possibility that schizophrenic hallucinations might be associated with abnormalities in REM sleep, no specific findings reflecting this have been described. There also appear to be no specific sleep changes associated with chronic schizophrenia.

Drug and Alcohol Use

An important cause of insomnia complaints is chronic hypnotic drug use, as first described by Kales et al. (18). They demonstrated that patients on chronic drug regimens for periods of time ranging from months to years found that their sleep disturbances were exacerbated by their medication, but if they were abruptly stopped, the resulting withdrawal syndrome made sleep even more difficult. In a similar fashion, withdrawal from alcohol or from antianxiety agents may also lead to insomnia.

This disturbance is far more likely to be seen with the older barbiturate and barbiturate-like drugs than with newer benzodiazepine compounds. However, a drug-rebound insomnia may be seen with short and ultra-short half-life benzodiazepine agents, especially when used in high doses and/or for long periods of time on a nightly basis (19).

Another, perhaps obvious cause of insomnia can be stimulant use or abuse. Illicit stimulant drug use can obviously lead to a disturbance of this sort, as can excessive ingestion of tea, coffee, or caffeine-containing over-the-counter stimulants. Legal restrictions and changes in medical practice have limited the extent to which stimulant compounds are now prescribed, but excessive use or abuse of these agents may obviously also lead to excessive stimulation and insomnia complaints.

Sleep-Related Myoclonus

A relatively common cause of insomnia is the presence of arousing leg or body movements in sleep. This phenomenon, known as nocturnal myoclonus, periodic movements in sleep, or periodic leg movements, is most prevalent in older populations. Although many individuals with this disturbance may be asymptomatic, it accounts for 10 to 15% of patients presenting with complaints of chronic insomnia to sleep disorders centers (20). In this condition, patients demonstrate pronounced, simultaneous, repetitive jerks in one or both legs. Despite the presence of many such movements patients may be unaware of their presence. The formal diagnosis is made in the sleep laboratory on the basis of characteristic EMG patterns, usually associated with EEG arousal patterns. However, a report from a spouse or bed partner that he or she is kicked repeatedly at night is helpful in suggesting the diagnosis.

A related cause of insomnia is restless legs syndrome. This is a severe, hard-to-describe dysesthesia that is felt deep within the lower extremities. It is often associated with muscle twitches or jerks. It typically occurs when the patient has been at rest for a period of time and leads to an irresistible desire to move the legs. It has been estimated that a least one-third of patients with restless leg syndrome report a family history, and an autosomal dominant mode of transmission has been suggested (21). It is frequently reported by patients with nocturnal myoclonus, and as many as 90% of restless legs patients will demonstrate myoclonus when studied polysomnographically. Patients sometimes are so embarrassed by these bizarre symptoms that they do not report them.

Sleep Apnea

Sleep apnea may also be a cause of insomnia complaints, although it is far more likely to be associated with complaints of excessive sleepiness. The three categories of sleep apnea—central, peripheral, and mixed—are well described in the medical literature and have become much more widely appreciated by physicians in recent years. In those cases where patients experience insomnia secondary to sleep apnea (perhaps 1 to 5% of all insomniacs), the disturbance is most often of the central type (22). Central apnea is characterized by the transient absence of respiratory muscle activity during sleep. As with all apneas, the breathing interruption must last at least 10 seconds to be considered of clinical significance. These patients rarely are aware of the apnea. In many cases loud snoring is a chronic problem, and this and an abnormal breathing pattern may frequently be confirmed by a bed partner. The diagnosis can be made with certainty only with an all-night sleep recording.

Medical Conditions

Complaints of DIMS can develop as a result of various types of medical problems. Somatic pain or physical discomfort will lead to arousals as a consequence of disturbances such as arthritis, trauma, surgery, metastatic malignancy, peptic ulcer, pruritis, nocturia or polyuria, or rectal urgency. Cardiac symptoms such as angina pectoris, orthopnea, or paroxysmal nocturnal dyspnea may lead to disturbed sleep on the basis of anxiety as well as physical discomfort. Primary pulmonary disorders such as chronic obstructive pulmonary disease, cystic fibrosis, and hypoventilation secondary to polio, paralysis, or scoliosis will often lead to drops in oxygenation, arousal, and disturbed sleep. Other organic causes include endocrine disorders such as hyperthyroidism and hypoglycemia, gastroesophageal reflux, and renal disease.

Treatment

Although treatment approaches for the insomnia disturbances are determined on the basis of their specific etiologies, some common approaches can be suggested. Patients should be advised to avoid ingestion of caffeine in any form and should decrease or completely stop alcohol consumption, especially in the evening or at bedtime. Incorporation of a regular exercise routine may be helpful, as may training in biofeedback, relaxation, meditation, or self-hypnosis. Establishing regular bedtimes and awakening times will help to diminish the tendency for the insomniac to spend too much time in bed "trying to sleep," a pattern which lowers sleep efficiency and leads to increased frustration and insomniac complaints.

Various treatment approaches for the psychophysiologic insomnias have been suggested. For the transient or situational insomnias, if the initiating or inciting stress can be removed, the insomnia will likely disappear. If this is not possible, it is helpful for the involved clinician to take a supportive stance, emphasizing the acute and usually self-limited nature of the problem. Support by family members and friends should be encouraged.

A general approach to persistent psychophysiologic insomnias is derived from behavioral psychology. Therapeutic strategies may include such tactics as regularizing the daily schedule, including bedtime; not spending time in bed if sleep remains elusive; not going to bed until tired; not remaining in bed if unable to sleep; and not using the bed or bedroom for non-sleep activities such as reading, eating, and watching television (23).

Another behaviorally derived approach is that of sleep restriction therapy (24). This technique is based on the belief that excessive time spent in bed trying to maximize sleep time is an important factor in the development and perpetuation of insomnia. By limiting time spent in bed to the number of minutes that the patient feels he is actually sleeping, more highly efficient sleep is produced. Sleep is consolidated, and sleep patterns become more regular and predictable. Total time in bed is allowed to increase as the patient demonstrates the ability to continue to sleep in an efficient and consolidated fashion.

The treatment of the various major psychiatric disturbances is discussed elsewhere in this volume. As a general rule, successful treatment, with resolution of the target psychiatric symptoms, typically is associated with the disappearance of the related sleep disturbance. When this is not the case, the possibility of an independent sleep disturbance should be considered.

Treatment of drug withdrawal insomnia and withdrawal states from alcohol or sedative drugs necessitates cautious, gradual reduction in dose. This may need to be performed over a period of from weeks to months, and consideration should be given to the possibility of inpatient detoxification in severe cases. The clinician must be aware of possible hazards, including potentially fatal convulsions, and the patient should be educated about these dangers and urged to comply with the withdrawal regimen. The physical hazards of withdrawal from stimulants are not so great, though the psychologic and interpersonal effects of "crashing" from an amphetamine or cocaine high can be quite devastating.

Nocturnal myoclonus and restless legs syndrome pose treatment problems. Their causation is not understood, making treatment difficult on any rational basis. Reports of successful treatment are frequently based on individual cases or small case series. Various medications have been tried in treatment without outstanding results. These agents have included opiates, L-dopa, sedatives, and anticonvulsants such as carbamazepine or clonazepam. The sleep disruption associated with myoclonus may be diminished by use of hypnotic medications such as temazepam, which presumably decrease the tendency to awaken with each jerk.

Sleep apnea poses another therapeutic problem. There is at present no specific treatment for the central type of sleep apnea, the type most frequently associated with insomnia. Treatments with various agents such as tricyclic antidepressants, medroxyprogesterone, naloxone, and bronchodilators have been reported in small case series without evidence of spectacular results. Acetazolamide may provide greater benefit for at least some patients (25). Sedatives are generally contraindicated.

The treatment approach for the various medical causes of insomnia is, whenever possible, to attempt to treat the underlying medical problem. When insomnia is due to somatic pain, analgesics may help with sleep by their inherent sedating qualities, as well as by diminishing the noxious stimuli which tend to awaken the patient or keep him awake.

When medications are needed, some guidelines may be helpful. Medications used in the treatment of sleep disorders are listed in Table 27.2. Barbiturates and barbiturate-like drugs (e.g., ethchlorvynol, glutethimide) are rarely, if ever, indicated for use in outpatient psychiatric treatment. The dangers of these drugs are discussed at length elsewhere (26), but a brief discussion here is appropriate. The barbiturates have historically been the drugs most commonly used to commit suicide, and their low therapeutic index also makes accidental overdose common. This is especially true in combination with other sedatives or alcohol. As many as 5000 people died in the United States in 1975 from barbiturate overdoses (27). The popularity of these agents for abuse and recreational use is well known, as is the risk of habituation with frequent use and the potential severe risks associated with their withdrawal syndromes.

The chloral derivatives are relatively inexpensive and are reported to be fairly safe with regard to overdosage. Gastric irritation is frequently reported by patients using these agents, and tolerance to their use develops rapidly with regular use. These drugs affect anticoagulant levels by displacing protein-bound drug and increasing the concentration of the active free drug, thereby potentiating its clinical effect. There is little to suggest that chloral hydrate is preferable to available benzodiazepines on grounds of safety or efficacy.

Various antihistamines are prescribed as sleeping aids, and these compounds frequently compose the active ingredient in over-the-counter sleeping pills. They are relatively inexpensive but may lead to respiratory depression and are abused by some patients. In addition, if used to excess, their anticholinergic properties can lead to serious side effects.

The tricyclic antidepressants are often prescribed for use as sleeping aids, typically in lower doses than those used for treatment of depression. The sedating properties of these agents are felt to be secondary to their antihistaminic effects. The anticholinergic properties of these

Table 27.2 Generic and Trade Names of Medications Used to Treat Sleep Disorders

Generic	Trade
Acetazolamide	Diamox
Carbamazepine	Tegretol
Chlorazepate dipotassium	Tranxene
Chlordiazepoxide	Librium
Clonazepam	Klonopin
Diazepam	Valium
Ethchlorvynol	Placidyl
Flurazepam	Dalmane
Glutethimide	Doriden
Lorazepam	Ativan
Medroxyprogesterone	Provera
Naloxone	Narcan
Oxazepam	Serax
Prazepam	Centrax
Triazolam	Halcion

agents may lead to problems with side effects even in low doses, generating complaints of dry mouth, constipation, and blurring of vision. Orthostatic hypotension may develop with these agents, and overdosage, whether intentional or accidental, may be lethal.

The benzodiazepines are remarkably safe and effective agents for the treatment of anxiety and insomnia complaints (28) and are the category of hypnotic medications appropriate for use for virtually all patients. Three benzodiazepine compounds are currently marketed as hypnotic agents in the United States: flurazepam, with a long half-life of 40 to 150 hours; temazepam, with an intermediate half-life of 10 to 20 hours; and triazolam, with an ultra-short half-life of 1.5 to 5 hours. The long and intermediate half-life agents may produce unwanted daytime sedation on the basis of prolonged therapeutic effects, particularly at high doses and with prolonged use. The short half-life agent triazolam does not seem to lead to these types of problems but may generate rebound insomnia complaints, especially when used at high dosage levels for prolonged periods of time. Whenever possible, use of these agents should be restricted to brief periods at the lowest possible dosage levels or on an infrequent and intermittent basis as needed.

Potential problems associated with use of the benzodiazepines include their potential for abuse, their relatively high cost, and the possibility of physiologic addiction. These drugs should be avoided or used with caution in patients with prior histories of alcoholism or of addiction to or abuse of other drugs. The risk of withdrawal convulsions with these agents does exist, particularly if they have been used in high doses for prolonged periods of time or if they are discontinued abruptly without a gradual period of withdrawal.

DISORDERS OF EXCESSIVE SOMNOLENCE (HYPERSOMNIAS)

Causes

Narcolepsy

Narcolepsy has been the best known hypersomnia disorder and for many years has been considered to be the most prevalent cause of complaints of excessive daytime sleepiness. Although it is now clear that sleep apnea is a more common cause of hypersomnia complaints, narcolepsy remains an important disorder of particular interest in understanding the etiology of specific sleep disorders. This is particularly so since there is strong evidence suggesting a hereditary basis for this disorder, and recent research raises the possibility that autoimmune factors may play a role in its development.

Narcolepsy typically presents with the complaint of irresistible sleep attacks of short duration. Frequently, but not always, these attacks are accompanied by cataplexy (partial or complete loss of muscle tone), sleep paralysis (usually at the transition between wakefulness and sleep), and hypnagogic phenomena (usually auditory or visual hallucinations). A hallmark of narcolepsy is evidence of dysregulation of control of REM sleep, often manifested in these patients as an immediate REM sleep onset at the start of the night, contrasted with the normal NREM sleep onset. Excessive sleepiness during the daytime is demonstrated by increased tendencies to fall asleep quickly when the opportunity for sleep is present, with a marked predisposition for the immediate appearance of REM sleep in daytime naps as well.

Sleep Apnea

Sleep apnea of the mixed and obstructive types may lead to excessive daytime drowsiness. In almost all cases loud snoring is a chronic problem, and this and an abnormal breathing pattern may frequently be confirmed by a bed partner. It should be considered whenever loud snoring or apparent respiratory pauses are seen in association with excessive daytime somnolence. It is seen predominantly in men over the age of 50, but children and young adults may also present with significant apnea disturbances, particularly in association with tonsillar hypertrophy, micrognathia, or other craniofacial or oropharyngeal abnormalities which tend to occlude the oropharyngeal outlet. Women who present with significant apnea are likely to be obese or postmenopausal. Although the majority of these patients are overweight, they do not necessarily demonstrate the classic Pickwickian body habitus with extreme or morbid obesity.

Various types of symptoms and disturbances are caused by sleep apnea. They include automatic behavior while asleep, morning headaches, abnormal motor activity during sleep, nocturnal enuresis, and high blood pressure. Patients often report changes in emotional regulation, with complaints of marked irritability and of anxiety and depression. Memory and attention span are often described as being diminished, and work performance, particularly in sedentary settings, is impaired. Libido and sexual function are often reported to be diminished. Beyond these subjective reports of altered mental function due to sleep apnea, objective decrements in cognitive function, attention, and memory have been described in these patients (30).

For sleep apnea patients in particular, sedative agents with respiratory depressant effects should be scrupulously avoided. Patients with obstructive sleep apnea who are given hypnotics with respiratory suppressing properties or who ingest large amounts of alcohol may experience exacerbation of their apnea or potentially dangerous impairment of breathing.

Sleep apnea may also lead to the development of right-sided heart failure (cor pulmonale) (31). These cardiac complications are associated more closely with the obstructive apnea and do not appear to be a consequence of the central type.

Nocturnal Myoclonus

The phenomenology of myoclonus is discussed in the section on insomnia. Excessive sleepiness may be a consequence of this disorder as well. This is most likely to be the case if sleep is interrupted by partial arousals associated with these events, rather than leading to frank awakenings which lead to the perception of insomnia.

Toxic, Environmental, and Medical Causes

Neurologic disturbances, including encephalitis, subdural hematoma, and brain tumor, may lead to a decreased level of activity and awareness that may be confused with hypersomnia. Stupor may also be seen with generalized infection or metabolic abnormalities such as hypoglycemia, hypothyroidism, electrolyte disturbances, or ketosis.

Kleine-Levin Syndrome

Kleine-Levin syndrome is a rare periodic hypersomnia disturbance characterized by periods of bizarre, withdrawn behavior and increased sleep tendency. Episodes of sleep may last for from one day to several weeks. When awakened or aroused, patients are restless and irritable, and often demonstrate compulsive, hyperphagic eating behavior. It is seen most often in adolescent and young adult males, who are amnestic for much of what occurs during their hypersomniac episodes. The bizarre nature of this syndrome often leads to the impression that this must be a primary psychiatric disorder. The etiology of this disorder is not known, but appears clearly to be organic in nature.

Treatment

Treatment of each disorder is specific and must be based on accurate diagnosis. Although stimulant medications may lead to transient improvements in most cases, side effects, loss of efficacy and residual deficits are likely to ensue.

The treatment of narcolepsy is complicated. Amphetamines and methylphenidate have been used in the past, but tolerance tends to develop, and patients frequently complain of side effects. Pemoline, a less tightly regulated stimulant compound, is of benefit in many cases. Tricyclic antidepressants are often useful for the control of accessory symptoms of narcolepsy such as cataplexy, sleep paralysis, and hypnogogic hallucinations. Protriptyline, the most stimulating tricyclic compound available for use, is often used in treatment, although anticholinergic side effects often limit doses which can be prescribed. Gamma-hydroxybutyrate, a compound not yet available in this country except under research protocols, has been effective in the treatment of the cataplexy component of the narcolepsy syndrome. A combination of tricyclic antidepressants and stimulants may provide safe and effective treatment.

Several highly effective treatments for obstructive sleep apnea are now available. Continuous positive airway pressure ventilation has been available as a treatment for this disorder for over 6 years with generally excellent results (32). This treatment uses a tightly fitting nasal mask which transmits pressurized air through the nose, functioning as a "pneumatic splint" to keep the airway patent during sleep. The cognitive and performance decrements associated with apnea appear to improve with treatment (33) although it is not clear whether this improvement reflects a partial or full resolution of symptoms.

A number of surgical procedures have been used in the treatment of this disorder. To date, no single surgical approach has provided predictably successful treatment for serious apnea. When specific craniofacial abnormalities are present and appear to play a major role in the onto-genesis of apnea, procedures such as com-bined mandibular and maxillary advance-ment may be appropriate and of benefit.

In extreme cases tracheostomy, at one time the only effective treatment for this disorder, may still be required. When a permanent tracheostomy is required, the tracheostomy can be opened at night, pre-venting the apneic episodes, and closed during the day, allowing normal speech and respiration. Results are dramatic, with rapid clearance of many clinical complaints.

When morbid obesity is present massive weight loss may be helpful, although this is rarely accomplished and, by itself, may not fully ameliorate the apnea tendency.

DISORDERS OF THE SLEEP–WAKE CYCLE

Sleep schedule disorders include jet lag, a consequence of rapid shifts across mul-tiple time zones; shift work; frequently changing sleep and waking schedules; and other more persistent biologic rhythm dis-orders. One of these, delayed sleep phase syndrome, is often seen in young individ-uals who report the inability to fall asleep or awaken at desired conventional times. They are able to fall asleep easily at de-layed sleep times (e.g., 2:00 to 4:00 AM) and feel well if allowed to obtain a full night's sleep through the mid-morning. Circadian rhythm disturbances can lead to com-plaints of insomnia or hypersomnia, and are often seen in medical house officers, nurses, airline flight personnel, policemen, firemen, and others with variable work schedules or irregular bed times.

PARASOMNIAS

Causes

Parasomnias are disorders that occur during sleep or during partial arousals from sleep. Many, but not all, are associ-ated with specific sleep stages. Linkage with specific sleep stages determines the timing of stage-associated events, since deep NREM sleep is most prevalent in the early hours of the night and REM sleep is most concentrated toward morning.

Somnambulism

Somnambulism is a relatively common problem, estimated to have a prevalence in children of 6 to 15%. There is evidence that it is familial (34). It was thought in the past to be associated with dreaming, but is now recognized as a NREM phenomenon, es-pecially associated with delta sleep (Stages 3 and 4), when dreams are rare. Somnam-bulists show low levels of awareness, re-activity, and motor skills and are amnestic on awakening for events that have oc-curred.

Sleep Terrors

Sleep or night terrors are also largely a disturbance of Stages 3 and 4 of NREM sleep. They are states of partial arousal from sleep, with extreme levels of auto-nomic discharge, vocalization, and poor awareness of or responsiveness to the en-vironment. Patients are usually amnestic for events the next morning. Sleep terrors occur far more frequently in children than in adults and typically occur during the early hours of sleep. In children, sleep ter-rors are rarely indicative of psychologic disturbance, though they are more likely to be present in periods of stress or sleep deprivation. When seen in adults, psycho-pathology is more common.

Dream Anxiety Attacks (Nightmares)

In contrast with sleep terrors, night-mares tend to occur toward morning when dreams are longer and more active. Those experiencing nightmares are usually easily aroused, can report fairly detailed dream content, and have full awareness of the event and recall for it the next morning. These dreams are often recurrent, with similar content night after night.

Sleep-Related Enuresis

Primary enuresis is now considered to be a sleep disturbance and may not be re-flective of underlying psychopathology. Primary enuresis (no consistent dry periods ever) is quite different from the secondary type (relapse after at least one period of several months of dryness), which is more likely to be seen in association with emotional disturbance.

Treatment

Conservative treatment is usually indicated for all of the parasomnic disorders. The most important consideration in somnambulism is protecting the patient. This is done by locking doors and windows, removing potentially dangerous objects, or even having the patient sleep on the first floor. Somnambulism typically stops by age 15, and children usually outgrow it without developing any significant psychopathology.

Children also usually outgrow sleep terrors without harmful effects. However, when treatment is indicated for either somnambulism or sleep terrors, both of which appear to result from a partial-arousal from NREM sleep, diazepam or alprazolam may be helpful, perhaps as a result of suppressing Stage 4 of NREM sleep (35).

Nightmares are of greatest concern when they are recurrent, disrupt sleep, or contain elements which are distressing or anxiety provoking for the patient. Psychotherapeutic exploration of the sources of anxiety is helpful in these patients; when symptoms are extreme, antidepressant agents which suppress REM sleep may diminish the frequency and intensity of these disturbances.

Primary enuresis is usually outgrown. If it persists, or if secondary enuresis develops, the child's parents should be counseled to avoid overreaction which may induce guilt and anxiety in the child and make the enuresis worse. A structured behavioral approach with a wetness sensitivity pad and loud bell can be very successful (36). Antidepressant medications have been used in treatment. Relapse rates tend to be high when the drug is withdrawn, and safety concerns are always present when tricyclic agents are used in any age group.

THE SLEEP DISORDERS CENTER

It is neither appropriate nor advisable for every patient with sleep complaints to be sent for a sleep disorders evaluation, or for every patient sent to a sleep center to undergo polysomnographic evaluation. Medical practitioners who are interested in these problems can acquire sufficient knowledge to manage most sleep complaints without the need for formal laboratory studies.

At the same time, it should be emphasized that important objective data are obtained from polysomnographic evaluation, and this information is of benefit in understanding the origins of and establishing a treatment plan for any sleep disorder. These studies are of particular benefit in differentiating between narcolepsy and sleep apnea and in assessing the severity of either of these disorders when treatment plans must be made. They are also invaluable in uncovering organic causes of insomnia or hypersomnia, such as nocturnal myoclonus or sleep apnea, which might otherwise be missed, generating erroneous hypotheses about the psychogenic cause of these sleep complaints.

References

1. Rechtschaffen A, Kales A: *A Manual of Standardized Terminology, Techniques and Scoring System for Sleep Stages of Human Subjects.* Bethesda, MD, National Institute of Neurological Diseases and Blindness, 1968.
2. Roffwarg H, Muzio J, Dement W: Ontogenetic development of the human sleep–dream cycle. *Science* 152:604–619, 1966.
3. Oksenberg A, Marks G, Farber J, et al: REM sleep deprivation in kittens: behavioral and pharmacological approaches. *Sleep Research* 16:532, 1987.
4. Griffin S, Trinder J: Physical fitness, exercise, and human sleep. *Psychophysiology* 15:447–450, 1978.
5. Rechtshaffen A, Gilliland M, Bergmann B, et al: Physiological correlates of prolonged sleep deprivation in rats. *Science* 221:182–184, 1983.
6. Lugaresi E, Medori R, Baruzzi A, et al: Fatal familial insomnia and dysautonomia with selective degeneration of thalamic nuclei. *N Engl J Med* 315:997–1003, 1986.
7. Sleep Disorders Classification Committee, Association of Sleep Disorders Centers: Diagnostic classification of sleep and arousal disorders. *Sleep* 2:5–137, 1979.

8. Mellinger G, Balter M, Uhlenhuth E: Insomnia and its treatment. *Arch Gen Psychiatry* 42:222–232, 1985.

9. Berlin R, Litovitz G, Diaz M, et al: Sleep disorders on a psychiatric consultation service. *Am J Psychiatry* 141:582–584, 1984.

10. Hammond E: Some preliminary findings on physical complaints from a prospective study of 1,000,064 men and women. *Am J Public Health* 54:11–22, 1964.

11. Solomon F, White C, Parron D, et al: Sleeping pills, insomnia and medical practice. *N Engl J Med* 300:803–808, 1979.

12. Treating insomnia. *Lancet* 2:253, 1985.

13. Roffwarg H, Erman M: Evaluation and diagnosis of the sleep disorders. In Hale R, Francis A (eds): *Psychiatry Update: American Psychiatric Association Annual Review*. Washington, DC, American Psychiatric Press, 1985, vol 4, pp 294–328.

14. Reynolds C, Kupfer D: Sleep research in affective illness: state of the art circa 1987. *Sleep* 10:199–215, 1987.

15. Reynolds C, Shipley J: Sleep in depressive disorders. In Hale R, Francis A (eds): *Psychiatry Update: American Psychiatric Association Annual Review*. Washington, DC, American Psychiatric Press, 1985, vol 4, 341–351.

16. Hartmann E: Longitudinal studies of sleep and dream patterns in manic–depressive patients. *Arch Gen Psychiatry* 19:312–329, 1968.

17. Kupfer D, Wyatt R, Scott J, et al: Sleep disturbances in acute schizophrenic patients. *Am J Psychiatry* 126:1213–1223, 1970.

18. Kales A, Bixler E, Tan T, et al: Chronic hypnotic drug use. *JAMA* 227:513–517, 1974.

19. Kales A, Scharf M, Kales J: Rebound insomnia: a new clinical syndrome. *Science* 201:1039–1041, 1978.

20. Coleman R: Diagnosis, treatment and follow-up of about 8,000 sleep/wake disorder patients. In Guilleminault W, Lugaresi E (eds): *Sleep/Wake Disorders: Natural History, Epidemiology, and Long-Term Evolution*. New York, Raven Press, 1983, pp 87–97.

21. Boghen D, Peyronna J: Myoclonus in familial restless leg syndrome. *Arch Neurol* 33:1241–1245, 1976.

22. Guilleminault W, Dement W: Sleep apnea syndromes and related sleep disorders. In Williams R, Karacan I (eds): *Sleep Disorders: Diagnosis and Treatment*. New York, John Wiley & Sons, 1978–9, pp 9–28.

23. Bootzin R, Nicassio P: Behavioral treatments for insomnia. In Hersen M, Eissler R, Miller P (eds): *Progress in Behavior Modification*. New York, Academic Press, 1978, vol 6, pp 1–45.

24. Spielman A, Saskin P, Thorpy M: Treatment of chronic insomnia by restriction of time in bed. *Sleep* 10:45–56, 1987.

25. White D, Zwillich C, Pickett C, et al: Central sleep apnea: improvement with acetazolamide therapy. *Arch Intern Med* 142:1816–1819, 1982.

26. Cohen S: The barbiturates: has their time gone? *Drug Abuse and Alcoholism Newsletter* 6:5, 1977.

27. Cooper J: *Sedative Hypnotic Drugs: Risks and Benefits*. Washington, DC, National Institute of Drug Abuse, 1977.

28. Greenblatt D, Shader R: The clinical choice of sedative hypnotics. *Ann Intern Med* 77:91–100, 1972.

29. Langdon N, Welsh K, Van Dam M, et al: Genetic factors in narcolepsy. *Lancet* 2:1178–1180, 1984.

30. Findley L, Barth J, Powers D, et al: Cognitive impairment in patients with obstructive sleep apnea and associated hypoxemia. *Chest* 90:686–690, 1986.

31. Schroeder J, Motta J, Guilleminault W: Hemodynamic studies in sleep apnea. In Guilleminault W, Dement W (eds): *Sleep Apnea Syndromes*. New York, Alan R. Liss, 1978, pp 196–210.

32. Lombard R, Zwillich C: Medical therapy of obstructive sleep apnea. *Med Clin North Am* 69:1317–1335, 1985.

33. Watson R, Greenberg G, Deptula D: Neuropsychological performance following treatment of sleep apnea. *Sleep Research* 16:456, 1987.

34. Bakwin H: Sleepwalking in twins. *Lancet* 2:446–447, 1970.

35. Cameron O, Thyer B: Treatment of pavor nocturnus with alprazolam. *J Clin Psychiatry* 46:504, 1985.

36. Scharf M: *Waking Up Dry: How to End Bedwetting Forever*. Cincinnati, OH, Writer's Digest Books, 1986.

28

Disturbances of Eating and Body Weight

Linda Zamvil, M.D.
William E. Falk, M.D.

Disturbances of eating and body weight encompass a broad range of medical and psychiatric problems and require an accurate diagnosis in order to plan appropriate treatment. In this chapter we shall discuss approaches to the problems, differential diagnoses, and initial management goals.

Patients do not usually come for psychiatric help with a chief complaint of weight or appetite disturbance. More commonly, they are referred by internists or family physicians who believe the weight disturbance is a result of a psychiatric disorder, or they are self-referred because of "depression" or "anxiety." Even when a patient is referred by an internist, the clinician should assess the completeness of the medical workup. Specifically, do the history, physical examination, and laboratory data rule out remediable medical illnesses?

Whether the problem is excess or insufficient weight, certain basic questions should be answered in the evaluation, as outlined in Table 28.1. Of prime importance is listening to the patient's perception of the problem, which permits an initial view of defensive and adaptive styles, provides a vocabulary for the problem that is acceptable to the patient, and may suggest important clues to etiology.

Table 28.1 Important Points to Review with a Patient Who Has an Eating or Weight Disturbance

1. Client's perception of problem—Is there a disturbance in body weight?
2. Onset—childhood versus adult
3. Course—exacerbations and remissions
4. Diet/activity history
5. Medical history, including history of drugs and alcohol (used or abused)
6. Review of systems, looking particularly for precipitating or aggravating medical problems
7. Family history of weight disturbance, genetic abnormalities, and illnesses associated with weight disturbances
8. Psychiatric history and mental status examination

Keep in mind that psychiatric and medical illnesses can coexist, or one can result from the other. For example, the psychiatric symptoms of depression can be a manifestation of hypothyroidism, while the medical symptoms of diarrhea and bowel complaints may result from severe anxiety states.

INCREASE IN BODY WEIGHT AND APPETITE

Obesity is defined as an increase in body fat above statistical norms for a given

334

height and body build. It is perhaps the most common medical problem encountered in clinical practice. Although significant increases in mortality occur among those patients who are 15 to 20% overweight, (1) massively obese patients (sometimes greater than 100% overweight) regularly suffer severe medical, psychologic, and social consequences. Statistical tables, which specify norms in body weight according to height and body build, and triceps skinfold thickness measurements are useful methods of determining the presence of obesity, while body mass index or BMI (weight divided by height squared) has the best correlation with body fat (2). However, no single method of determination is entirely reliable, and Stunkard's dictum that if a patient looks fat, he is fat will usually serve in the outpatient psychiatry setting (1). If the patient and clinican agree that obesity is a problem, then the etiology may be investigated and plans for treatment discussed. Sometimes there is disagreement between the patient and clinician whether the weight is a problem. A careful evaluation of the patient's concern or lack of concern and thoughtful negotiation can often resolve the conflict.

The most common cause of obesity is when caloric intake exceeds expenditure. If purely medical causes are ruled out (see Table 28.2), obtain a complete history (Table 28.1) and dietary and activity data (Table 28.3).

Obesity is related to the regulation of body weight, primarily body fat. The notion that body weight is regulated and, in normal weight persons, relatively constant is called the "set point" theory (3). According to this theory, obesity may be triggered by an elevation in set point and a resultant inability to regulate weight voluntarily. Although the cause or causes of set point elevation are not well understood, it usually commences in childhood, thus making the prevention and treatment of childhood obesity extremely important. An additional factor is gender, since obesity is more prevalent among women and an inverse relationship exists between the level

Table 28.2   Causes of Increased Body Weight

Simple obesity
  Hyperplastic
  Hypertrophic
  Hypertrophic–hyperplastic
Endocrine dysfunction
  Cushing's disease
  Hypothyroidism
  Insulinoma
Lesion of ventromedial hypothalamus
  Tumor
  Infection
  Trauma
  Kleine-Levin syndrome
Genetic
  Prader-Willi syndrome
  Morgagni-Stewart-Morel syndrome
  Stein-Levinthal syndrome
  Familial?
Medication
  Oral contraceptives
  Exogenous steroids
  Insulin
  Oral hypoglycemic agents
  Major tranquilizers
  Antidepressants
  Lithium carbonate
  Phenytoin
  Reserpine
  Cyproheptadine
  Cannabis
  Alcohol excess
  Discontinuation of anorexic drug
  Cessation of cigarettes
Psychiatric–social
  Binge eating syndrome
  Night eating syndrome
  Depression
  Dealing with feelings of
    Inadequacy
    Dependency
    Anxiety
    Fear of intimacy
    Fear of aggressive impulses
  Coping with
    Masochistic traits
    Obsessions
    Delusions
  Symbolic obesity

of fatness in adult females and levels of education, income, and occupation (4).

An increase in body weight is not synonymous with an increase in body fat, since increased fluid or muscle mass can also account for weight gain. The clinican must distinguish among these possibilities by history and physical exam. Treatment would obviously be different if, for exam-

Table 28.3   Dietary and Activity History

Diet
  What is eaten?
  How much?
  How often?
  When and where?
  With whom?
  Associated activities (e.g., reading, watching television)?
  Eating related to altered emotional states?
  Past attempts at dieting and results?
Activity
  Present and past athletic history
  Type of job—active, sedentary, involved with food?
  Living conditions?
  Active versus sedentary life-style (e.g., does patient prefer stairs or elevator?)

ple, edema appeared to be the major cause of weight gain.

Complications of obesity are numerous. Hypertension is three times more prevalent in overweight individuals than nonoverweight individuals (5). Pulmonary infections and insufficiency (the extreme being the Pickwickian syndrome) are hazards, particularly in the massively obese. Endocrine complications include diabetes, hyperlipidemias, increased glucocorticoid production, hirsutism, amenorrhea, and infertility (6). In addition, there exists an increased risk of gall-bladder problems, kidney stone, certain cancers, skin infections, arthritis of weight-bearing joints, and varicosities. Given these complications, it is not surprising that excess weight is associated with a shortened life span.

Sometimes only sensitive inquiry reveals the extent of the psychosocial complications of obesity. How does obesity affect self-image, body image, the handling of intrapsychic conflicts, interpersonal relations, activities of daily living, and job performance? In this era of cost containment, the price of obesity's medical and social consequences is high.

General Classification

Recent literature suggests that "simple" obesity can be divided into two types: hyperplastic and hypertrophic. The former re-

fers to an absolute increase in adipose cell (adipocyte) number occurring in childhood that continues throughout life. The latter refers to an increase in the size, but not number, of adipocytes and occurs in adulthood. Pertinent to this distinction is the finding that a majority of obese children become obese adults and are clinically more refractory to treatment than are patients with adult-onset obesity. The childhood-onset obese may have five times as many fat cells, and some suffer from combined hypertrophic–hyperplastic obesity.

Terms such as "hyperplastic" obesity, "hypertrophic" obesity, "exogenous" obesity, and "obesity of undetermined origin" all denote a weight disturbance without a specific medical cause and represent the vast majority of case presentations. When a medical cause is suspected, further examination and laboratory data may confirm a diagnosis and, at worst, minimize the patient's feeling of guilt about his or her problem. The medical complications of obesity, when discovered, may add impetus to an obese dieter's resolve. In some cases, treating the secondary complications may assist in the overall management of the obese patient by decreasing morbidity and providing positive reinforcement for continued weight loss.

Endocrine Disorder

Hormonal dysfunction is always considered in the differential diagnosis of obesity. Although rare, endocrinopathies are usually treatable. One example of a treatable disorder is Cushing's disease, with signs that include truncal obesity, "moon-facies," a fatty "buffalo-hump" at the junction of neck and back, and violaceous striae on the abdomen. Aside from the body fat distribution, which is central in location, elevated serum cortisol and urine free corticoids will distinguish this syndrome from simple obesity, as will nonsuppression on the dexamethasone suppression test.

Another example is hypothyroidism, in which obesity occurs in slightly less than half of the cases. When symptoms of weight gain are associated with lethargy, constipation, cold intolerance, slow pulse, coarse hair, raspy voice, slow return phase of deep tendon reflexes, and a goiter, hypothyroidism is the likely diagnosis. Abnormalities or thyroid function studies such as thyroid-stimulating hormone (TSH), T_4, and resin T_3 uptake would confirm the diagnosis.

Rare disorders producing an excess of insulin, as in an insulinoma, are also associated with obesity. If postprandial symptoms of low blood sugar are obtained by history, a glucose tolerance test, including a 5-hour postprandial blood sugar, may assist in the diagnosis, but again, more sophisticated testing may be required (7). More often, patients complain of "hypoglycemia" as a cause of weight gain when there is no medical evidence to support their concern.

Hypothalamic—Genetic Causes

In the hypothalamic region of the brain, neuropeptides regulate appetite. A combination of the raphe (serotonergic) nuclei tract and the ventral adrenergic bundle appear to be responsible for mediating the satiety effects of the ventromedial hypothalamus. Conversely, dopaminergic nigrostriatal tracts are associated with the lateral hypothalamic feeding center. To further add to the system's complexity, opioid receptors appear to modulate appetite with β-endorphins being responsible for enhanced feeding in experimental animals (8). Naloxone and naltrexone, opiate antagonists, have been noted to reduce feeding, but as yet they have not been shown to be significantly effective in reducing food intake and inducing body weight loss in humans (9).

Hypothalamic causes of obesity are exceedingly rare, but lesions of the satiety center of the ventromedial hypothalamus by tumor, trauma, or inflammation can lead to excessive eating behavior (10). Kleine-Levin syndrome (periodic hypersomnia and hyperphagia) represents such a presentation.

Genetic causes of obesity due to hypothalamic dysfunction are very uncommon.

Mental retardation and other findings may accompany the obesity as in the Prader-Willi (11) and Morgagni-Stewart-Morel (hyperostosis frontalis) syndromes. On less firm ground is the possibility that certain forms of obesity may be familial. Nature and nurture remain difficult to separate.

Metabolic Disorder

Impaired cellular thermogenesis, specifically involving the sodium–potassium pump, may play a role in the development of obesity, but this remains a highly controversial area. Some investigators suggest that the energy cost of pumping sodium out of the cell may be lower in obese individuals, thus making more energy available for fat synthesis (12). Others have found no difference between obese and thin subjects (13) or have even found a higher energy requirement in the obese (14).

Weight Gain Caused by Medications

Medications can effect an increase in body weight by causing enhanced appetite, fluid retention, fat deposition, or a combination of these factors. Oral contraceptives, exogenous steroids, or inappropriately high insulin dosages are examples of hormonal agents that can contribute to obesity. Sulfonylureas, oral hypoglycemic agents, can also result in increased fat production by stimulating insulin release from the pancreas. Major tranquilizers, antidepressants, and lithium carbonate may cause increases in appetite and body fluid, while phenytoin (Dilantin) and reserpine more rarely can result in such increases. Cyproheptadine (Periactin) reportedly can lead to obesity in some children. The chronic use of cannabis may lead to increased appetite and weight, and chronic alcohol abuse may increase body fat and fluid. Discontinuation of anorexic medication or the recent cessation of cigarette smoking may also result in some weight gain.

Psychiatric Origins

The vast majority of cases of obesity are simply due to an excess of calories ingested over those expended. However, of these patients some may present with a psychiatric problem that contributes to the weight disturbance. For example, Stunkard described two patterns of eating behavior present in some obese patients, bulimia and the night eating syndrome (1). Bulimia (15), or binge eating, occurs in approximately 5% of obese individuals. However, it is seen more often in normal-weight individuals or those with anorexia nervosa (see Chapter 33). The bulimic individual's awareness of this abnormal eating pattern results in self-deprecating thoughts and depressed mood. Like bulimia, the night eating syndrome is found almost entirely in women and may be an atypical form of depression. It is characterized by morning anorexia, evening hyperphagia, and nocturnal insomnia.

Excessive eating is also seen in some clinically depressed and grieving patients, for whom certain foods seem to act as an antidepressant. Wurtman (16, 17) described a population of obese individuals who craved carbohydrates and speculated that they consumed high-carbohydrate snacks for their psychopharmacologic effect. She noted that carbohydrates stimulate the synthesis and release of brain serotonin and theorized that an antidepressant effect results. Wurtman has demonstrated that the administration of d,1-fenfluramine (which stimulates serotonin release) significantly reduces carbohydrate consumption in these patients (16, 17).

Further evidence for the association between carbohydrates and mood is seen in seasonal affective disorder, in which an increase in carbohydrate consumption occurs during depressive episodes and decreases during periods of euthymia (17). Interestingly, among non-carbohydrate-craving obese patients, consumption of a high-carbohydrate meal results in feelings of depression and fatigue (18).

Abnormal patterns of eating behavior can be precipitated by stress. On a psychologic level, obese patients may confuse hunger with other dysphoric affects and use eating behavior as a means of coping with these feelings, such as occurs with grieving. Ingestion of food can be used as a means of dealing with feelings of inadequacy, dependency, anxiety, fear of intimacy, or fear of aggressive impulses. Overeating can also be seen as a means of coping with masochistic traits, obsessions, or delusions. The clinician should also look for a disturbance in body image, for even if a weight disturbance is corrected, the body image disturbance may persist. Finally, obesity may have social or cultural determinants which reinforce positively the patient's obese status. For example, an individual may view obesity as symbolic of success or power. Excessive eating and obesity can be observed in a wide range of psychiatric disorders, which emphasizes the need for a complete history and mental status examination.

Management

After establishing a correct diagnosis and assessing physical, social, and psychologic sequelae of the weight disturbance, the clinician negotiates a treatment plan with the patient. When they are discovered, primary medical or pharmacologic contributors to the problem should be corrected. In the vast majority of cases, without such specific causes, the obesity should be considered a long-term problem for which life-long changes in eating behavior are necessary. The initial weeks of treatment may show a rapid weight loss (due to fluid loss) that will not be sustained in subsequent weeks. If a treatment alliance is established, reasonable goals have been set, and continued support has been offered, the stage is set for planning long-term treatment. While psychotherapy and psychoanalysis have been found to have a favorable impact on body image (19), behavior modification techniques, combined with dieting and exercise, appear to be most promising (20).

Stunkard outlined four major steps of behavior modification, each requiring a high degree of patient involvement (21). First, the patient describes the behavior to be controlled using daily records of amount, time, and circumstances of eating behavior. Second, the patient is guided in modifying and controlling the uncovered stimuli which appear to govern his or her eating behavior. For example, the patient may be encouraged to eat in one place at specific times with a distinctive table setting and without distractions. Third, techniques to control the act of eating are instituted, such as counting mouthfuls of food, being aware of chewing the food, or pausing every couple of minutes. Finally, prompt reinforcement of behavior that delays and controls eating should be encouraged, particularly in group settings such as TOPS (Take Off Pounds Sensibly) and Weight Watchers. While the assistance of a dietician in planning palatable menus can be invaluable, anorexic medication has no proved long-term benefit (22). Exercise alone is an inefficient way to lose calories, but can be helpful in an overall treatment regimen by decreasing caloric intake and by improving self-image (20). Surgical procedures should be considered only for the severely obese (greater than 100% overweight), but in this patient population it is the most successful form of treatment. A relatively new procedure, gastric stapling, holds particular promise (3).

DECREASE IN BODY WEIGHT AND APPETITE

As with weight gain, an evaluation of weight loss requires a careful history, physical exam, and pertinent laboratory data. Although weight loss may be viewed positively by many patients, an unexplained loss of 10 pounds or more is clinically significant. In the absence of deliberate dieting it is highly likely that a serious medical or psychiatric illness is the cause. If the weight loss is greater than 25% of ideal body weight, the importance is magnified, for if the loss continues, it is potentially life threatening.

A first step in determining the cause of weight loss is to separate general medical or pharmacologic etiologies from psychiatric causes. One should also consider the possibility that medical and psychiatric conditions coexist. Evaluation begins with a careful history, covering areas such as substance abuse, family illnesses, travel, dietary habits, sexual relations, and review of systems (e.g., fever, sweats, heat intolerance, symptoms referable to the gastrointestinal tract). The clinician should also listen to the patient's perception of the difficulty, elicit a careful psychiatric history, and perform a mental status examination.

The dysfunction of almost any physiologic system of the body may result in decrease in appetite and/or weight loss. Some representative entities are discussed below and outlined in Table 28.4.

Occult Malignancies

As is well known, cancer may initially present as an unexplained weight loss, with or without anorexia. Particular attention to this possibility should be made when the patient is middle-aged or older. In both men and women lung and gastrointestinal tumors should be suspected, while in women, focus should also be on breast and gynecologic pathology. History of pain, a mass, or unusual bleeding may assist in diagnosis. An alteration in food preferences may be noticed at times. For example, some cancer patients describe a revulsion to protein and a craving for carbohydrate-rich foods.

Chronic Infections

Pulmonary or disseminated tuberculosis, pyelonephritis, and other chronic bacterial, fungal, parasitic, and viral disorders may present with weight loss as a prominent symptom. Weight loss of 10 to 15% of body weight in individuals with human immune deficiency virus positivity may represent the first clinical sign of AIDS (acquired immune deficiency syndrome)-related complex or AIDS. This disease is found not only among homosexual males and intravenous drug abusers but also

Table 28.4   Causes of Decreased Body Weight

Occult malignancy
  Bowel
  Lung
  Breast
  Gynecologic
Chronic infection
  Bacterial
  Fungal
  Parasitic
  Viral (hepatitis, acquired immune deficiency syndrome)
Renal or liver disease
  Infection
  Toxic exposure
  Congenital defects
Endocrine dysfunction
  Hyperthyroidism
  Adrenal insufficiency
  Pituitary insufficiency
  Diabetes insipidus
  Diabetes mellitus
Gastrointestinal dysfunction
  Decreased intake
  Decreased absorption
  Increased fluid and food loss
Lesions of lateral hypothalamus
  Tumor
  Trauma
  Infection
Medications
  Thyroid hormone preparations
  Diuretics
  Laxatives
  Stimulants (amphetamines, cocaine, and related compounds)
  Digitalis preparations
  Antihypertensive agents
  Alcohol abuse
  Narcotic drug abuse
  Medications that decrease taste acuity
Psychiatric
  Depression
  Chronic anxiety states
  Schizophrenia
  Food phobia
  Conversion hysteria
  Obsessive–compulsive neurosis
  Anorexia nervosa
  Bulimia

among heterosexuals, particularly women. Systems review, blood transfusion history, travel history, social and sexual histories will assist in determining appropriate laboratory studies.

Renal and Liver Diseases

Diseases of the kidney and liver systems unrelated to infection may also present with weight loss. Signs of liver or kidney failure, a history of toxic substance exposure (e.g., alcohol or carbontetrachloride for the liver, certain antibiotics or phenacetin for the kidney), or family histories of diseases like polycystic kidney should be sought.

Endocrine Dysfunction

Hyperthyroidism, pituitary–adrenal insufficiency, diabetes mellitus, and diabetes insipidus may have weight loss as major signs. Although thyrotoxicosis may be unmistakable, with its cardinal signs of tachycardia, increased deep tendon reflexes, and exophthalmos, milder forms of the disease can be ruled out only by thyroid function studies. Hypotension, lassitude, nausea, vomiting, and, more rarely, hypothermia are the symptoms of adrenal insufficiency or Addison's disease. Pituitary insufficiency results from hemorrhage or infarction of the pituitary (Sheehan's syndrome), occurring postpartum. Symptoms include amenorrhea, vaginal atrophy, muscular weakness, and an initial weight gain followed by progressive cachexia. Diabetes insipidus and diabetes mellitus may have weight loss as part of their clinical picture, with polydipsia and polyuria being prominent signs. Also, diseases resulting in hypercalcemia or hypokalemia may have increased urinary output and weight loss as symptoms. In their severe forms, most of these disorders require immediate hospitalization and specialized medical care. It is important to reemphasize that many endocrine and metabolic disturbances may present with psychiatric symptoms such as agitation, depression, and confusion. Correct diagnosis obviously is necessary in order to initiate appropriate treatment (11).

Gastrointestinal Dysfunction

Many disorders of the gastrointestinal tract can result in poor nutritional balance and weight loss. This can occur as a result of decreased intake, decreased absorption, or increased food and fluid loss. Partial bowel obstruction, secondary to stricture, mass, or herniation, could lead to decreased intake. Diseases of the pancreas and liver could cause diminished absorption, as can malabsorption, sprue-like syndromes, regional enteritis, and severe food allergies. Any disease, whether infectious or structural, causing persistent diarrhea or vomiting will result in weight loss (23).

Lesions of Lateral Hypothalamus

Lesions of the brain's "feeding center," such as an invasive tumor, may account for decreased interest in food and resultant weight loss.

Drug-Induced Weight Loss

Medication history should include not only prescribed medications but also over-the-counter, "social," or illicit drugs. Excessive doses of thyroid hormone (including desiccated thyroid, thyroglobulin, sodium levothyroxine, sodium liothyronine, and liotrix) cause symptoms identical to hyperthyroidism. Diuretics such as ethacrynic acid, furosemide, thiazides, and others may cause gastrointestinal upset and anorexia, in addition to fluid loss. Laxatives, particularly cathartics like castor oil or magnesium citrate, and chronic enema usage may result in poor gastrointestinal absorption and weight loss. Stimulant agents, such as amphetamines and methylphenidate, probably decrease appetite by acting on the hypothalamus. Not only would chronic abuse lead to considerable weight loss in some individuals, it can also cause significant central nervous system effects. Newer synthetic agents which are reputed to have less central effects have been marketed as anorexics. These include fenfluramine, phentermine, phenylpropanolamine, phenmetrazine, and others. Digitalis preparations, some antihypertensive drugs, and phenformin, an agent used in adult-onset diabetes, have also been associated with weight loss. Many pharmacologic agents, such as cancer chemotherapy drugs, can have nausea and vomiting as significant side effects. Chronic alcoholism,

cocaine abuse or narcotic drug usage may cause both decreased taste acuity and decreased interest in food. A number of drugs including griseofulvin, penicillamine, clofibrate, and lincomycin, may cause unpleasant taste sensation with diminished food intake.

Psychiatric Origins

Numerous psychiatric illnesses cause weight loss. Despite a "classic" psychiatric presentation, however, a case may still be caused by a medical illness with associated psychiatric symtoms. Therefore, a high index of suspicion about the presence of medical illness should be maintained.

Depression is the most common cause of weight loss, since lack of interest in food may be a major symptom accompanying sleep disturbance, lack of energy, low self-esteem, and depressive mood. Chronic anxiety states may also present with considerable weight loss due to decreased appetite and increased metabolism. More rarely, schizophrenia with delusions of being poisoned, food phobias, conversion hysteria, or obsessive–compulsive disorder could also result in diminished weight. Anorexia nervosa is perhaps the most dramatic cause of weight loss due to psychiatric illness (see Chapter 33). Differential diagnosis of anorexia nervosa includes other psychiatric illnesses, as noted above, plus pituitary insufficiency and various malabsorption syndromes. A distinction from Sheehan's syndrome can usually be made on the basis of history, as well as normal plasma cortisol and adrenocorticotropic hormone levels. With malabsorption syndromes, anemia and hypoproteinemia are often present, but are rare in anorexia nervosa (15).

Initial Management

After a diagnosis has been established, a series of questions must still be answered. Is the underlying illness serious enough to require immediate hospitalization? Are there emergency measures to be taken? If the problem can be handled as an outpatient, is referral to a specialist required? If the primary disorder is psychiatric, is the patient a danger to him- or herself or others? Examples of medical problems requiring in-hospital management were mentioned above. Anorexia nervosa, a potentially fatal disease, may require immediate hospitalization if the patient's body weight is considerably less than 75% of normal, particularly if this is associated with a rapid pulse, suggesting hypovolemic shock. A depressed patient with marked psychomotor changes associated with weight loss may require hospitalization in order to provide sufficient nutrition.

CONCLUSION

Disturbances of eating and body weight require careful evaluation, which may seem beyond the capabilities of inexperienced clinicians. However, when the problem is approached in a logical and thoughtful manner, appropriate diagnosis and effective management will result.

References

1. Stunkard AJ: Obesity. In Kaplan HL, Sadock BJ (eds): *Comprehensive Textbook of Psychiatry IV*. Baltimore, Williams and Wilkins, 1985, pp 1133–1142.
2. Bray GA: Obesity: definition, diagnosis and disadvantages. *Med J Aust* (Special suppl) 142:S2–S8, 1985.
3. Stunkard AJ, Stinnett JL, Smoller JW: Psychological and social aspects of the surgical treatment of obesity. *Am J Psychiatry* 143:417–429, 1986.
4. Paige DM, Owen G: Obesity. In Paige DM (ed): *Manual of Clinical Nutrition*. Pleasantville, NJ, C. V. Mosby, 1985, pp 38.1–38.28.
5. National Institute of Health Consensus Development Conference: Health implications of obesity. *Ann Intern Med* 103:147–151, 1985.
6. Harlass FE, Plymate SR, Fariss BL, et al: Weight loss is associated with correction of gonadotropin and sex steroid abnormalities in the obese anovulatory female. *Fertil Steril* 42:649–651, 1984.
7. Olefsky JM: Obesity. In Braunwald E, Isselbacher KJ, Petersdorf RJ, et al. (eds): *Harrison's Principles of Internal Medicine*, ed 11. New York, McGraw-Hill, 1987, pp 1671–1676.
8. Bray GA: Autonomic and endocrine factors in the regulation of food intake. *Brain Res Bull* 14:505–510, 1985.
9. Morley JE, Levine AS: Neuropeptides and appetite regulation. *Med J Aust* (Special suppl) 142:S11–S13, 1985.
10. Maggio CA, Presta E, Bracco EF, et al: Naltrexone and human eating behavior: a dose-ranging inpatient trail in moderately obese men. *Brain Res Bull* 14:657–661, 1985.
11. Foster DW: Gain and loss in weight. In Braunwald E, Isselbacher KJ, Petersdorf RJ, et al. (eds): *Harrison's Principles of Internal Medicine*, ed 11. New York, McGraw-Hill, 1987.
12. DeLuise M, Blackburn GL, Flier JS: Red-cell sodium–potassium pump in human obesity. *N Engl J Med* 303:1017–1022, 1980.
13. Beutler E, Kuhl W, Sacks P: Sodium-potassium-ATPase activity is influenced by ethnic origin and not by obesity. *N Engl J Med* 309:756–760, 1983.
14. Mir MA, Charalambous BM, Morgan K, et al: Erythrocyte sodium-potassium ATPase and sodium transport in obesity. *N Engl J Med* 305 (21):1264–1268, 1981.
15. American Psychiatric Association: *Diagnostic and Statistical Manual of Mental Disorders (Third Edition)*. Washington, DC, American Psychiatric Association, 1980, pp 69–71.
16. Wurtman JJ: Neurotransmitter control of carbohydrate consumption. *Ann NY Acad Sci* 145–151, 1986.
17. Wurtman JJ: *Carbohydrate Cravings: A Disorder of Food Intake and Mood*. Cambridge, MA, Massachusetts Institute of Technology, in press.
18. Lieberman HR, Wurtman JJ, Chew B: Changes in mood after carbohydrate consumption among obese individuals. *Am J Clin Nutr* 44:772–778, 1986.
19. Rand CSW, Stunkard AJ: Obesity and psychoanalysis: treatment and four-year follow-up. *Am J Psychiatry* 140:1140–1144, 1983.
20. Blundell JE: Behavior modification and exercise in the treatment of obesity. *Postgrad Med J* 60:37–49, 1984.
21. Stunkard AJ: Behavioral management of obesity. *Med J Aust* (Special suppl) 142:S13–S20, 1985.
22. Galloway S, Farquar DL, Munro JF, et al: The current status of antiobesity drugs. *Postgrad Med J* 60 (Suppl 3): 19–26, 1984.
23. Isselbacher KJ: Anorexia, nausea and vomiting. In Braunwald E, Isselbacher KJ, Petersdorf RJ et al. (eds): *Harrisons's Principles of Internal Medicine*, ed 11. New York, McGraw-Hill, 1987, pp 173–175.

29

Violent and Aggressive Behavior

Linda Gay Peterson, M.D.
Bruce Bongar, Ph.D.
Steven K. Hoge, M.D.

Aggressive and violent behavior both frightens and fascinates the professional no less than the layperson. For the professional, the fear of physical harm and the potential for lengthy involvement in legal proceedings often encountered in working with violent patients may discourage the outpatient clinician from seeing such patients. However, the possibility of finding a correctable etiology for such behavior is a potent reason to engage in the evaluation of these cases. The reluctance of clinicians to become involved in evaluating violent patients is demonstrated in survey data showing that of psychiatrists in Boston in the 1970s less than half were involved in assessing and treating violent patients (1). This is of note since even in private hospital settings at least 3% of patients have recently manifested assaultive behavior toward other persons (2), and in some settings the rate may be as high as 60% (3).

Furthermore, not only do many patients present in emergency settings because of violent acts, but also in most jurisdictions the standard for civil commitment requires that a person be mentally ill and "dangerous." Also, an increasing number of state courts have found that mental health professionals have a duty to protect third parties from their patient's violence. Therefore, it is important that clinicians become familiar with the assessment of potentially violent patients as well as the management and associated legal responsibilities. This chapter strictly focuses on assessment (for comprehensive discussion of management and legal responsibilities, see Monahan's monograph on this subject [4]).

Before discussing the details of assessment, it is first necessary to effect working definitions of violent and agressive behavior. In this chapter *violence* is used to refer to

acts characterized by the application of or overt threat of force which is likely to result in injury to people. This use of the term includes, but is not restricted to, such criminal acts as homicide, mayhem, aggravated assault, forcible rape, battery, robbery, arson, and extortion. Criminal behaviors not likely to result in injury to people, such as noncoercive thefts or vandalism, are excluded, as are business practices which, although injurious to people, do not involve the application of force. (5)

Aggressive behavior is more difficult to define and has broader parameters, since it can be both verbal and physical, person or object directed, or even nondirectional. Because of this variability, rating scales for evaluating aggressive behavior which categorize aggressive behavior by type and level of intensity have been developed. One example of such a scale is the Overt Aggression Scale developed by Yudofsky et al (6). Other rating scales include the Buss Durkee Hostility Inventory (7), a self-rating scale for aggressive behavior. General behavioral rating scales can also be used, such as the Nurses' Observation Scale for Inpatient Evaluation (for nurses to rate behavioral observations) (8) and the Brief Psychiatric Rating Scale, which is used by trained observers to rate psychopathologic behavior in psychiatric inpatients (9).

Although rapid assessment is important in some settings, especially in emergency settings where self-protection for the clinician may be as critical as differential diagnosis, a more in-depth approach shall be taken here (10-16).

Violent behavior is a complex and multidetermined phenomenon (17, 18); no single model has been able to explain or fully inform violence. Therefore, the four conceptual models presented in Chapter 2 are used here to describe a comprehensive clinical approach to assessing and understanding violent and aggressive behavior. Table 29.1 provides a summary of those factors found to be associated with aggressive and violent behavior in each dimension.

SOCIOCULTURAL FACTORS

Social factors have been demonstrated to be strongly linked to violence, particularly violent crimes. Socioeconomic status as well as job and home instability have been linked to the commission of such crimes (19-21). In a similar fashion, these crimes have been found to be far more

Table 29.1   Factors Associated with Violent Behavior

Sociocultural
Job instability
Home instability
Urban setting
Low socioeconomic status
Biologic
Male sex
Youth
Low IQ
Illness
Alcohol abuse
Substance abuse
Medical
Delirium
Neoplasm, cerebral
Head trauma
Psychodynamic
Narcissistic injury
Paranoia
Cognitive distortions
Behavioral
Modeling
Frustration

common among urban populations than among rural populations (4). It seems reasonable to infer that the stressors attendant to urban living and low socioeconomic status predispose the individual to violent behavior.

As Wolfgang has noted, "Serious crimes within the family are most commonly related to subcultural values that, at best, do not much inhibit physical responses or, at least, condone and encourage them" (20, 22). In fact, spouses and other family members are the most frequent targets of assault among psychiatric outpatients (22). Men are more likely than women, and young men more likely than old, to be assaultive. Sex role expectations may contribute to this difference. In relation to violent behavior, the issue of role expectations even within different regions of our own country has been argued in several recent studies (23, 24).

There is also the factor of race. For psychiatric outpatients, Tardiff noted no statistical difference in rates of violence between racial groups (2). This lack of significance does not hold for the general population, where there is a higher rate of violent crimes among Blacks.

PSYCHODYNAMIC FORMULATIONS

In the psychodynamic approach to the differential diagnosis of violent patients, the clinician's own countertransference is helpful in understanding the basis of the violent behavior (25). The clinician must be aware of his or her own rational and irrational response to violence (10). Both denial and overreaction may interfere with successful evaluation. The patients who arouse feelings in the clinician of being taken advantage or of being "conned" frequently are personality disordered, whereas those patients with severely impaired reality testing generally evoke a more uneasy anxious reaction. The organic patient typically elicits a more sympathetic, but cautious caretaking response.

Often the clinician may come to understand the particular relationships, as seen through the transference, which elicit aggressive reactions on the part of an individual. Some theorists have hypothesized the presence of super ego lacunae as being responsible for the violence seen in psychopathy (26-28). These individuals are often perceived as cold, emotionally distant, aloof, and without regard for others. Aggression has also been conceptualized as an instinctual drive of equal stature with the libidinal drive, and it may well be that the interplay between these two drives together shape much of the unconscious life. Abnormalities in the integration of these two drives in a meaningful way has been posited as the underlying structural deficit of borderline personality disorder (29, 30).

Many clinicians have noted the frequent historic finding of a narcissistic injury preceding a violent act. Under this conceptualization the initial humiliation and subsequent narcissistic injury leave the individual feeling shamed and vulnerable. The consequent feelings of rage which emerge as a result of this experience leads to a violent act. The latter serves a defensive function reassuring the individual that he or she is not vulnerable (31).

Patients suffering from paranoid disorders, ranging from paranoid personality disorders to paranoid schizophrenia, have also been noted clinically to be more violent than other patients. Core psychodynamic difficulties in these patients include the placement of the locus of responsibility outside the individual and an exquisite sensitivity to shame. These patients seek to correct the stressors in their life by retaliating against those whom they perceive as being the cause of their problem.

Cognitive distortions may also play an important role in the dynamics of violence. Some patients may come to perceive situations in a way particularly prone to creating a violent interchange. For example, it has been noted by those conducting research into sexual offenders that many of these people share the belief that women enjoy and actually seek out rape (32). Also, individuals may perceive affronts and insults where none objectively exist. In this group of patients the shared psychopathology is a defect of reality testing.

BEHAVIORAL CONCEPTS

In the behavioral understanding of violence, two main themes emerge: the frustration–aggression theory and the social learning theory (33). Frustration–aggression theory, developed in the 1930s, hypothesizes that aggressive behavior is the result of frustration in achieving goals. The relevance of this model to clinical assessment is that frustration may be a chronic rather than acute phenomenon and that frustration of different types may be cumulative. This is useful in understanding aggression seen among young children, where multiple familial disruptions leading to loss of normal nurturance appears common (34).

Social learning theory hypothesizes that aggressive behavior is acquired through imitation as well as through direct experience (18). This model may be used in understanding the presence of violent behavior in patients who were brutalized as children. The recurrent theme of multigenerational child abuse and violent lifestyles may be related to learning of cultural scripts, along with other factors yet to be discusssed (e.g., biologic factors) (35).

An additional factor in violent behavior is the strong association of male sex and violence. Although there may be some biologic underpinning for this related to testosterone and its effect on the brain, there are also clearly issues of expected sex role behaviors. Males have been found to exhibit far more aggressive and violent behavior in a variety of contexts, both clinical and criminal. This finding has been consistent across many cultures. This may be secondary to sex role expectations. However, the consistency of this finding suggests that a more biologic factor underlies male violence. Causality remains elusive and equivocal. Studies investigating the association between plasma testosterone levels and violent behavior and sexual crimes have failed to find a consistent correlation (36-38).

Investigations of violence in both clinical and forensic settings have also consistently found youth to be associated with violence. The peak ages for the occurrence of violent crimes and violent behaviors seems to be between 18 and 25 (4, 39). The existence of subcultural values among the young may encourage such behavior, but the consistent findings suggest the possibility that a biologic factor may underlie violence in youth.

BIOLOGIC/SYNDROMAL CONSIDERATIONS

Disturbances of the mind and body may underly some instances of violent and aggressive behavior. This is probably even more so in the clinical setting. The factors in this category can be broken down further for analysis and include: (a) genetic factors, (b) neurotransmitter correlations, (c) the effects of exogenous mind-altering substances, (d) psychiatric disorders, and (e) medical disorders.

Genetic Factors

Much research has been conducted in search of genetic factors that contribute to violent and criminal behavior. While there is some evidence that property crimes have a familial and possibly genetic basis, there has not been any association of violent crimes or violence of a genetic nature that has stood up to critical investigation. For a time there was a great deal of attention focused on male with XYY chromosome abnormalities. However, more conclusive research has indicated that these individuals are no more violence prone than the general population (40).

Neurotransmitter Studies

A strong association between low cerebrospinal fluid serotonin and a history of violent behavior have been found by Brown (41). This finding has been replicated by other investigators and extended to include a correlation with self-directed aggression as well, e.g., violent suicide attempts (42). At this time the clinical relevance of this finding is limited.

Substance Use

Clearly alcohol and other central nervous system depressants have a disinhibiting effect on aggressive behavior, which results in much of the socialized violence in our society (e.g., barroom brawls). The clinician should always suspect alcohol use in relation to domestic violence or other aggressive acts. Fifty percent of all violent crimes and 50% of all domestic violence are alcohol associated (43). More than one-half the patients seen in one study of violence in a general hospital emergency room had consumed alcohol before their aggressive actions occurred (44). Twenty-five percent of psychiatric patients involved in violence are alcohol intoxicated (45-47).

Other substances contribute to violence in different ways. Central nervous system stimulants such as cocaine, amphetamines, phencyclidine, and even prescription agents such as theophylline increase arousal and therefore the likelihood of aggressive acts. Hallucinogens, such as lysergic acid diethylamide dimethyltryptamine and mescaline less often lead to violence, except in rare cases. Heroin, other narcotics, cocaine and other street drugs of abuse lead to violence. Histories of drug use or histories suspiciously laden with drug-related behaviors suggest the need for spot urine screens and active confrontation, since patients will rarely admit to active drug use.

These disorders can be distinguished in the process of obtaining the clinical history and doing a careful mental status examination. The presence of a diagnosis of substance abuse disorder should not, however, preclude careful assessment of possible underlying medical disorders as well, since patients with substance abuse problems are also likely candidates for head injury and secondary metabolic disturbances. Distinguishing characteristics of these disorders include whether the violent behavior is well organized and goal directed or poorly organized and randomly directed toward the environment. Goal-directed behavior is more characteristic of personality disordered individuals, whereas episodic outbursts, not related to substance use, are more suggestive of episodic dyscontrol, explosive personality, or seizure-related aggressiveness.

Other Psychiatric Disorders

The psychiatric diagnoses other than substance abuse most frequently associated with violence are (a) antisocial personality disorder, (b) episodic dyscontrol syndrome, (c) explosive personality disorder, and (d) paranoid schizophrenia. Other diagnoses which must be considered include borderline personality disorder; histrionic personality disorder; organic brain syndromes; and other psychotic disorders besides paranoid schizophrenia, particularly mania.

Medical Disorders

Nonpsychiatric medial disorders will require more in-depth physical examination, laboratory studies, and electroencephalographic and radiologic studies. The importance of medical evaluation of violent patients is underscored by the fact that 20% of all violent patients seen in psychi-

atric outpatient settings were found to have organic mental disorders (48). Organic conditions encountered in outpatient settings include the following: toxic, including substance use; metabolic; infectious; neoplastic; degenerative; traumatic; cardiovascular; connective tissue disorders and other systemic disorders; and, less commonly, even delerium and dementia.

Toxic conditions other than substance abuse disorders include lead poisoning, intoxications from inadvertent inhalation of fumes, especially hydrocarbons (e.g., carpet laying), and even use of home remedies by elderly patients. Toxicologic screening assistance is necessary from poison control centers or other sources to ascertain the most appropriate assessment battery available.

Metabolic abnormalities presenting with behavior change in an outpatient setting are most likely to be insidious in nature, such as hypo- or hyperthyroidism, Cushing's syndrome, and hypo- and hyperparathyroidism. New aggressive behavior could also reflect more immediate changes in a preexisting medical condition. One example might be violent behavior by an elderly patient on a hypotensive regimen, which has caused low potassium levels and an ensuing organic brain syndrome; another example is a patient recently placed on carbidopa–levodopa (Sinemet) for parkinsonism. Thus, careful attention to medications and concomitant medical illness is indicated in assessing the violent patient, along with basic laboratory evaluation which will often give clues to more elusive disorders requiring more elaborate evaluation, e.g., anemia and hypercholesterolemia in the lethargic, irritable patient, which suggests an evaluation for hypothyroidism.

Infectious processes can be acute or chronic. Acute processes will often be accompanied by fever, malaise, headache, and other symptoms of acute illness. More chronic processes such as cytomegalovirus infection in an immune-compromised patient or toxoplasmosis may be accompanied by other neurologic signs and symptoms. Neoplastic conditions include brain tumors, especially (*a*) slow-growing tumors (meningiomas) which produce gradual personality deterioration with gradual loss of appropriate inhibition of primitive behaviors and (*b*) tumors that produce hormones which affect behavior, e.g., oat cell or ovarian carcinoma, which may produce adrenocorticotropin-hormone-like substances. A computerized axial tomographic scan and careful physical examination will assist in determination of these conditions.

Hypoxia from poor cardiac output and hypertensive encephalopathy are examples of cardiovascular conditions which may cause behavioral effects resulting in aggressive or violent behavior. A common example is agitated aggressive behavior following a cardiac arrest. Connective tissue and systemic disturbances such as lupus erythematosus may cause cerebritis with concomitant behavioral aberrations. An abnormal electroencephalogram and elevated sedimentation rate, along with a positive antinuclear antibody, are suggestive of connective tissue disease.

Degenerative disorders are of several types, including congenital self-mutilating disorders such as Lesch-Nyhan syndrome and congenital absence of pain sensibility such as Reilly O'Day syndrome. These two disorders may cause violent behavior at any time as the result of the primary syndrome. Other degenerative disorders producing complex, partial, or grand mal seizures cause seizure-related violence. Both ictal and interictal periods can be associated with violent or aggressive behavior. In the ictal and postictal period following grand mal seizures, nondirected agitated aggressive behavior is uncommon, but this is the most frequent association between aggressive behavior and seizure disorders. "Aggressive behavior has been extensively reported in association with temporal lobe epilepsy. In fact, it would be difficult to cite either from case reports or a literature review another medical or neurologic illness in which aggressive behavior is described so regularly" (49).

Although electroencephalography is helpful in positively identifying a seizure disorder, negative results, unless done with sophisticated 24-hour telemetry and special transphenoidal leads, do not necessarily rule out an epileptic condition. Referral of patients for in-depth neurologic assessment is indicated where temporal lobe epilepsy is suspected.

Traumatic conditions resulting in violent behavior are mostly posttraumatic epileptic disorders or subdural hematomas. Therefore, a history of recent trauma is important in assessing new aggressive behavior or changes in aggressive behavior, since antisocial personalities and substance abusers are likely to have violent histories. Changes in patterns of aggression may suggest the need to rule out effects of recent trauma. (For further information on assessing the contribution of medical illnesses to violent behavior, see Lishman's *Biological Psychiatry* [50].)

CONCLUSIONS

Violent behavior is a multidetermined and complex phenomenon requiring a multilayered, multidisciplinary approach to assessment. Assessment is the first step in the management and treatment of these disorders. No single unidimensional understanding will suffice in developing a comprehensive approach to evaluation of this complex behavioral phenomenon.

The clinical interview, with adjunctive aids previously discussed, is important in testing the relevance of the contribution of each of these approaches to the final assessment. Even then, the clinician will often have to adjust his or her thinking on the spot, on the basis of additional historical, observational, or laboratory information obtained in the course of treatment. The comprehensive assessment of violent and aggressive behavior is a continuing and dynamic task that the practicing clinician needs to include in day-to-day practice, no less than in emergency settings.

References

1. Tardiff K: A survey of psychiatrists in Boston and their work with violent patients. *Am J Psychiatry* 131:1008–1011, 1974.

2. Tardiff K, Konigsberg HW: Assaultive behavior among psychiatry outpatients. *Am J Psychiatry* 142:960–963, 1985.

3. Mungus D: An empirical analysis of specific syndromes of violent behavior. *J Nerv Ment Dis* 171:354–361, 1983.

4. Monahan J: *The Clinical Prediction of Violent Behavior.* (NIMH DHHS Pub # (ADM) 81–921) Washington, DC, U.S. Department of Health and Human Services, 1981.

5. Megargee E: The prediction of dangerous behavior. *Criminal Justice and Behavior* 3:3–21, 1976.

6. Yudovsky SC, Silver JM, Jackson W, et al: The Overt Aggression Scale for the objective rating of verbal and physical aggression. *Am J Psychiatry* 143:35–39, 1986.

7. Buss AH, Durkee A: An inventory for assessing different kinds of hostility. *J Consult Psychol* 21:343–349, 1957.

8. Honigfeld G, Gillis RD, Klett CJ: Nurses' Observation Scale for Inpatient Evaluation: a new scale for measuring improvement in chronic schizophrenia. *J Clin Psychol* 21:65–71, 1965.

9. Overall JE, Gorham DR: The Brief Psychiatric Rating Scale. *Psychol Rep* 10:799–812, 1962.

10. Rada RT: The violent patient: rapid assessment and management. *Psychosomatics* 22:101–109, 1981.

11. Wood KA, Khuri R: Violence—the E.R. patient. In Turner JT (ed): *Violence in the Medical Care Setting: A Survival Guide.* Rockville, MD, Aspen Publications, 1984, pp 57–84.

12. Lion JR, Reid WH: *Assaults Within Psychiatric Facilities.* New York, Grune and Stratton, 1983.

13. Tardiff K: The violent patient. In Guggenheim FG, Weiner MF (eds): *The Manual of Psychiatric Consultation and Emergency Care.* New York, Jason Arnson, 1984, pp 15–22.

14. Skodol AE: Emergency management of potentially violent patients. In Bassuk EL, Birk AW (eds): *Emergency Psychiatry: Concepts, Methods, and Practices.* New York, Plenum Press, 1984, pp 83–96.

15. Slaby AJ, Tancredi LR: *Handbook of Psychiatric Emergencies.* Garden City, NY, Medical Examination, 1981.

16. Bassuk EL, Birk AW: *Emergency Psychiatry: Concepts, Methods, and Practices.* New York, Plenum Press, 1984.

17. Shiared MH: Clinical pharmacology of Aggressive behavior. *Clin Neuropharmacol* 7:173, 1974.

18. Roberts TK, Mock LAT, Johnstone EE: Psychological aspects of the etiology of violence. In Hays JR, Roberts TK, Solway KS (eds): *Violence and the Violent Individual.* New York, SP Medical and Scientific Books, 1981, pp 9–34.

19. Pritchard D: Stable predictors of recidivism. *Journal Supplement Abstract Service* 7:72, 1977.

20. Wolfgang M, Figlio R, Sellen T: *Delinquency in a Birth Cohort.* Chicago, University of Chicago Press, 1972.

21. Cook P: The correctional carrot: better jobs for parolees. *Policy Analysis* 1:11–54, 1975.

22. Wolfgang ME: Sociocultural overview of criminal violence. In Hays JR, Roberts TK, Solway KS (eds): *Violence and the Violent Individual.* New York, SP Medical and Scientific Books, 1981, pp 97–115.

23. Allen NH: Suicide statistics. In Hatton CL, McBride-Balente S (eds): *Suicide: Assessment and Intervention,* ed 2. Norwalk, CT, Appleton-Century-Crofts, 1984, p 17–32.

24. Peterson LG, Bongar B, Netowski M: Regional use of violent suicidal methods. *Am J Emerg Med,* in press.

25. Lion JR, Pasternak SA: Countertransference reactions to the violent patients. *Am J Psychiatry* 130:207–210, 1973.

26. Kozol H, Boucher RJ, Garofalo RF: The diagnosis and treatment of dangerousness. *Crime and Delinquency* 18:371–392, 1972.

27. Hare RD: Psychopathy and violence. In Hays JR, Roberts TK, Solway KS (eds): *Violence and the Violent Individual.* New York, SP Medical and Scientific Books, 1981, p 53–74.

28. Cleckley H: *The Mask of Sanity,* ed 5. St. Louis, MO, Mosby, 1976.

29. Wollheim R: *Sigmund Freud.* New York, Cambridge University Press, 1971.

30. Fancher RE: *Psychoanalytic Psychology: The Development of Freud's Thought.* New York, WW Norton, 1973.

31. Lewis HB: Personal communication, May 16, 1983.

32. Abel GG, Becker JV, Skinner LJ: Behavioral approaches to treatment of the violent sexual offender. In Roth L (ed): *Clinical Treatment of the Violent Person* (DHHS Pub No. (ADM) 85–1425). Washington, DC, U.S. Department of Health and Human Services, 1985.

33. Megargee EI: The psychology of violence: a critical review of theories of violence in crimes of violence (staff report to the National Commission on the Causes and Prevention of Violence). Washington, DC, U.S. Government Printing Office, 1969.

34. Lewis DO, Shanik SS, Grant M, et al: Homicidally aggressive young children: neuropsychiatric and experiential correlates, *Am J Psychiatry* 140:148–153, 1983.

35. Justice B, Justice R: Treatment of child abusing families. In Hays JR, Roberts TK, Solway KS (eds): *Violence and the Violent Individual.* New York, SP Medical and Scientific Books, 1981, pp 375–390.

36. Krevz LE, Rose Rm: Assessment of aggressive behavior and plasma testosterone in a young criminal population. *Psychosom Med* 34:321–332, 1972.

37. Meyer-Bahlberg HFL, Boon DA, Sharma M, et al: Aggressiveness and testosterone measures in man. *Psychosom Med* 36:269–274, 1974.

38. Rada RT, Laws DR, Kellner R: Plasma testosterone levels in the rapist. *Psychosom Med* 38:257–268, 1976.

39. Zimring F: Background paper. In *Confronting*

Youth Crime: Report of the Twentieth Century Fund Task Force on Sentencing Policy Toward Young Offenders. New York, Holmes and Meier, 1978.

40. Shiavi RC, Theilgaard A, Owen DR, et al: Sex chromosome anomalies, hormones, and aggressivity. *Arch Gen Psychiatry,* 41:93–99, 1984.

41. Brown GL, Goodwin FK, Bunney WE: Human aggression and suicide: their relationship to neuropsychiatric diagnoses and serotonin metabolism. In Ho BT, Schoolar JC, Usdin E (eds): *Serotonin in Biological Psychiatry.* New York, Raven Press, 1982, pp 287–307.

42. Asberg M. Bertillson L, Martensson B: CSF monoamine metabolites, depression and suicide. *Adv Biochem Psychopharmacol* 39:87–97, 1984.

43. Coleman KH, Weinman M: Conjugal violence: a comparative study in a psychiatric setting. In Hays JR, Roberts TK, Soloway KS (eds): *Violence and the Violent Individual.* New York: SP Medical and Scientific Books, 1981, pp 231–242.

44. Piency D: Violence in the medical care setting. In Turner JT (ed): *Violence in the Medical Care Setting: A Survival Guide.* Rockville, MD, Aspen Publications, 1984, pp 123–151.

45. Bach-y-Rita G, Lion JR, Clinment CR: Episodic dyscontrol: a study of 130 violent patients. *Am J Psychiatry* 127:1473–1478, 1971.

46. Bach-y-Rita G, Veno A: Habitual violence: a profile of 62 men. *Am J Psychiatry* 134:1015–1017, 1974.

47. Lion JR, Bach-y-Rita G, Ervin FR: Violent patients in the E.R. *Am J Psychiatry* 125:1706–1711, 1969.

48. Cummings JL: *Clinical Neuropsychiatry.* Orlando, FL, Grune & Stratton, 1985.

49. Devinsky A, Bear D: Varieties of aggressive behavior in temporal lobe epilepsy. *Am J Psychiatry* 141:651–655, 1984.

50. Lishman WA: *Organic Psychiatry.* Oxford, England, Blackwell Scientific Publications, 1978.

30

Organic Personality Syndromes

David M. Bear, M.D.

Organic personality syndromes are alterations in behavior caused by structural, chemical, or electrophysiologic alterations in the nervous system detectable by current diagnostic methods (1). While overzealous advocates of the biologic approach may suggest that all psychiatric disorders will eventually be shown to have an organic basis, this is mistaken logic (2). Persons with normal brains may be taught appropriate or inappropriate responses, and functional factors operating on structurally normal nervous systems account for many forms of maladaptive behavior (3). Therefore, clinicians will always be obliged to consider both organic (biologic) and functional (psychodynamic, behavioral, or sociocultural) hypotheses to account for the behavior of their patients.

Just as the distinction between organic versus functional causes cannot be willed away by biologic reductionism, it is not resolved by uncritical holism which suggests that behavior invariably involves interaction of biologic and environmental factors. It is clear that neurologic lesions in phylogenetically ancient areas of the nervous system can produce behavior unaccounted for by prior personality or environmental stresses (4). In practice, the degree of interaction between organic and functional factors in a particular situation becomes evident only after the location of the organic lesion and the resultant level of emotional discontrol are determined.

Unfortunately, the legitimate and necessary diagnostic distinction between organic and functional behavioral symptoms is often difficult to make. This is especially true of the organic personality syndromes, which by definition, lack the obvious cognition deterioration of delirium or dementia, grossly psychotic features, prominent affective symptoms, or hallucinations (1).

However, several principles help to organize the initially heterogenous clinical presentation of organic illnesses. Lesions selectively affecting emotions and behavior are most frequently located within areas of the human brain specialized for control of biologic drives such as aggression, flight, sexual reproduction, and feeding. Neurons regulating these drives are typically clustered and interspersed between specific sensory neurons, which inform them of stimuli relevant to drives, and effector neurons, which command endocrine, autonomic, extrapyramidal, or pyramidal responses preparatory to drive consummation.

During the course of primate evolution,

351

multiple levels of neurologic organization, initially adapted for the morphology and life-style of specific phyletic stages, have developed. The human nervous system may be viewed as a type of fossil record, with structures appearing earliest in phylogeny forming first in the developing brain and eventually assuming caudal and medial positions. Phylogenetically newer structures, which form and mature later in embryogenesis, take up progressively more rostral and lateral orientations. While the exact number, origin, and boundaries of these levels will always be speculative, the generalizations above can be applied to three gross levels of organization: the brainstem, limbic lobe, and cortical mantle (Fig. 30.1).

The spatiotemporal correlation schematized in Figure 30.1 forms the basis of a functional hierarchy among neuronal circuits. Areas more rostral and lateral— newer—normally control the function of those caudal and medial to these; higher levels rely on processing performed at lower levels, bringing into the process of emotional control successively subtler analyses of the environment, more versatile pathways of expression, and increasingly complex principles of decision making regarding the appropriateness and orchestration of responses.

Because of the ubiquitous survival value of the biologic drives, aggregates of neurons controlling feeding, reproduction, fight, and flight are represented at each of

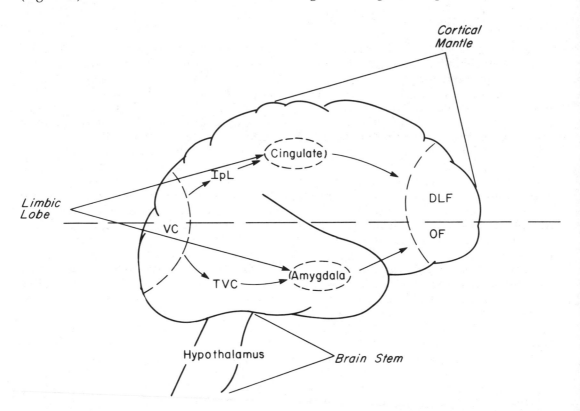

Figure 30.1.   Within the human brain, three ascending levels of organization may be readily distinguished: the brainstem (thalamus and hypothalamus, midbrain, pons, and medulla), the limbic lobe (amygdala, hippocampus, cingulate gyrus, and septal complex), and the cortical mantle (gray matter of occipital, parietal, temporal, and frontal lobes). *Arrows* indicate sequential processing of information within each of two major pathways which relate sensory perception (vision, for example) to motivation (limbic structures) and motor behavior (frontal lobe). VC = primary and association visual cortex; TVC = temporal visual cortex; IPL = inferior parietal lobule; DLF = dorsolateral frontal cortex; OF = orbital frontal cortex.

these levels. The functions of these structures, and the characteristic signs of their dysfunction, are consequences of distinctive forms of sensory information arriving to a particular center, the output channels addressed by each structure, and, most important, the contrasting principles of functional integration incorporated in their connections.

This anatomical view of emotional processing serves to organize and clarify the diversity of organic personality syndromes. To illustrate its clinical application, I shall compare and contrast behavioral alterations resulting from organic lesions to emotion-controlling centers at representative levels of the nervous system: within the brainstem, the hypothalamus; within the limbic lobe, the temporal pole amygdala and the inferior parietal lobule-cingulate; and within the cortical mantle, the prefrontal granular cortex (Fig. 30.1). The clinical examples illustrate two additional factors: hemispheric specialization for emotional control and the combinatorial effects of lesions to multiple structures.

HYPOTHALAMIC BEHAVIORAL SYNDROMES

Input to the hypothalamus is focused on the internal milieu, that is, the oral cavity, visceral organs such as heart or stomach, and osmotic and hormonal composition of the blood stream. Direct outputs are to the autonomic nervous system, pituitary gland controlling neuroendocrine responses, and midbrain and spinal centers which coordinate stereotypic motor movements.

In controlling biologic drives such as eating or aggression, hypothalamic nuclei appear to be organized into antagonistic excitatory and inhibitory regions, a form of push–pull control. For example, stimulation of lateral hypothalamic areas initiates feeding or precipitates preparation for attack ("sham rage") in many animal species, stimulation of ventromedial areas terminates feeding and initiates defensive posturing, chemical destruction or anatomical lesioning of the lateral hypothala-

mus leads to appetite loss and passivity, and ventromedial lesions produce obesity and aggressiveness (4).

Specific neurotransmitters infused into the hyothalamus elicit characteristic drive responses. For example, hypothalamic instillation of acetylcholine elicits predatory aggression in docile rats or cats and cholinergic blockers prevent attack in naturally predatory animals (5, 6).

In humans, hypothalamic lesions have produced behavioral effects consistent with observations in animals. The behavioral changes tend to be quantitative—too much or too little hunger, anger, or sexual desire independent of the stimuli which elicit these responses. Unlearned stereotypic behaviors such as biting or scratching often distinguish hypothalamic lesions. Other signs of dysfunction in the hypothalamus and adjacent brainstem are disruptions of homeostasis—deficits in thermoregulation, circadian hormonal rhythms, autonomic balance, or regulation of the sleep–wake cycle (4).

Examples

A previously normal young woman became bulimic and increasingly aggressive, indiscriminately scratching all those who approached. She developed a fever and lost the normal diurnal variation in serum cortisol. Autopsy revealed a vascular neoplasm of the ventromedial hypothalamus (7).

An adolescent man developed profound anorexia nervosa. His disgust for food, loss of interest in dating, and temper outbursts were initially attributed to the stress of terminal illness in a parent. Over the course of 6 months, he began to sleep excessively, complained of feeling cold, and passed large quantities of dilute urine. A computerized tomographic (CT) scan subsequently revealed invasion of the lateral hypothalamus by tumor (thought to be a pineal germinoma). Radiation therapy preserved his life, and with endocrine replacement, behavioral changes were ameliorated (4).

A child, who had suffered intrauterine

toxoplasmosis, engaged in vicious biting attacks; he had bitten off the ear lobe of one victim. He denied the intention to bite, warning that he could not control this behavior. During multiple pharmacologic trails, his attacks were uniquely suppressed by cholinergic antagonists (4). By contrast, exogenous chemicals increasing the availability of central acetylcholine, such as cholinesterase inhibitors, have precipitated simultaneous aggression in cat and humans (8) and possibly contributed to a homicide (6).

BEHAVIOR CHANGES FOLLOWING TEMPOROLIMBIC LESIONS

The amygdala is a complex of nuclei within the anterior medial temporal lobe which, like other limbic structures, has an extensively documented role in the control of aggression, feeding, and sexuality. In contrast to the hypothalamus, the lateral amygdala receives many afferents from neocortical sensory areas reporting on the external milieu via the visual, auditory, and tactile systems. Major input to and output from the medial amygdala reaches the hypothalamus via the ventral amygdalofugal pathway and the stria terminalis.

Converging evidence from neuroanatomy, physiologic psychology, and neurophysiology has implicated the amygdala in a central emotional process: the formation and retrieval of associations between stimuli in the outside world and appropriate biologic drives (9). Thus the visual discrimination of a food object, sexual partner, or enemy depends on amygdalar connections between the temporal visual cortex and the hypothalamus (10). This function of sensory–emotional association may be likened to the Freudian concept of cathexis, in which, through experience, a particular object takes on emotional valence (10).

Destruction of the anterior temporal lobe and amygdala would be expected to disrupt the association of familiar stimuli with their drive-related (emotional) associations. Following bilateral anterior temporal lobectomy, Rhesus monkeys lose both fear and aggressive responses to human caretakers; they copulate indiscriminately and mouth metal junk objects or feces as readily as monkey chow (11). An analogous syndrome of sensory–emotional dissociation has developed in humans following bilateral temporal lobe surgery or trauma, temporolimbic degeneration as in Pick's or Alzheimer's disease, or following medial temporal encephalitides (limbic encephalitis, herpes simplex encephalitis) (12,13).

Example

A middle-aged school teacher developed headache, neck pain, difficulty concentrating, and fever. During her hospitalization, a lumbar puncture documented lymphocytosis, a CT scan revealed bilateral lucencies of the temporal lobes, and a herpes simplex titer was diagnostically elevated.

Following resolution of the acute illness, her personality was drastically altered. She recognized her children but showed them no emotional response. She masturbated frequently, often in the presence of strangers. She attempted to mouth and swallow foreign objects, such as magazines and pieces of her suitcase. Much of the time her behavior was apathetic. Like other patients with extensive medial temporal lobe damage affecting the hippocampus, she was impaired in learning new facts or recalling recent events but had preserved long-term memory (4).

Fortunately, the Kluver-Bucy syndrome in humans is rare, usually associated with additional neurologic symptoms. However, a much more prevalent and subtle group of illnesses affect the temporolimbic structures. Epilepsy involving the temporal lobe, the most common seizure disorder in adulthood, may develop for many reasons: congenital malformation, birth complication, scarring from febrile convulsions in childhood or head trauma. In most cases, the structural injury to the brain is clinically silent, so that the majority of patients have normal neurologic examinations (14).

In contrast to removal or destruction of neurons, temporal lobe epilepsy represents a discharging lesion in which damaged neurons of the epileptic focus rapidly fire action potentials outside the usual physiologic controls. If repeated seizure discharges reach the amygdala via multiple convergent pathways from sensory association cortices, they may have the progressive and lasting effect of lowering the threshold for conduction of normal signals through the amygdala ("kindling"; 15). This process would be predicted to alter and generally increase the number and intensity of emotional associations (11).

The study, prevention, and treatment of behavioral changes in temporal lobe epilepsy constitute potentially one of the most important enterprises in neuropsychiatry. However, several points should be clarified to prevent basic misunderstanding. First, it is clear that during the majority of characteristic complex partial seizures, patients do not act on strong emotions like rage. Typically, the limbic functions of emotional association and memory formation are blocked rather than activated during the ictus, as reflected in the older terms "absence," "automatism," and "psychoparesis" (14). Behavioral changes described below are persistent rather than episodic features of personality which develop after months or years of epilepsy; they are observed during the interictal period.

Second, while temporolimbic structures may be directly implicated by history, aura, or specialized electrophysiologic monitoring in some patients, neither the location of the initial structural lesion, the seizure type experienced by the patient, nor the scalp-derived electroencephalogram (EEG) excludes secondary amygdala abnormality in additional individuals. Thus altered limbic physiology may lead to interictal behavioral changes in patients whose epilepsy ostensibly began in a nonlimbic site.

Third, the proposal of altered sensory–emotional associations suggests, and much clinical research confirms, a distinctive cluster of interictal behavior changes in many patients with temporal lobe epilepsy (14). This view does not imply that the behavioral changes are unique to temporal lobe epilepsy. In fact, much of the interest in temporal lobe epilepsy as a model illness rests on the possibility that other processes activating limbic circuits may produce similar behavioral symptoms, so that parallel aspects of currently obscure psychiatric conditions would be illuminated by the study of behavior in temporal lobe epilepsy. While the clustered behavioral changes of temporal lobe epilepsy have a distinctive quality, classic descriptions have emphasized "schizophrenialike" features (16) and frequent depressive symptoms (17).

Recent efforts have focused on the description and documentation of an interictal behavior syndrome in temporal lobe epilepsy (18, 19). The following examples illustrate features of these syndromes: alterations in sexual behavior and aggression, deepened religious or philosophic feelings reflected in extensive writing (hypergraphia), attention to and elaboration of detail, and an inappropriate sense of familiarity and interpersonal closeness (enhanced social cohesion) (14).

Additional observations suggest that the product of emotional associations may differ in right- versus left-sided temporal lobe epilepsy. Schizophrenia-like features or changes in ideation have been associated with left temporal lobe foci, and overt emotional or affective symptoms with right temporal lobe foci. Patients with right temporal lobe foci appear to minimize socially undesirable features of behavior such as aggression or polymorphous sexuality; in extreme cases, their behavior is seen as ego alien, resulting from an alternative personality (20).

Examples

A 36-year-old man suffered febrile convulsions in childhood, later developing complex partial seizures with an aura of fear, rotation of his head to the left, and lip smacking. The EEG revealed a right temporal lobe spike focus. Working as a professional writer, the patient was criticized by his editor for endless recitation of seemingly extraneous detail. For his first appointment with a new physician, he brought a 20-page essay summarizing sexual experiences in childhood. He emphasized a lack of interest in sexual matters, preferring "platonic relationships" with both men and women throughout high school. In college, he was ridiculed for ignorance of sexual anatomy or dating experience. Denying previous erotic sensations, he nonetheless began to consummate multiple relationships with men and women. For some months, he entertained a sexual and deeply emotional relationship with a woman 40 years his elder. Subsequently, he began cross-dressing followed by masturbation in front of a mirror. His mannerisms and vocal habits became effeminate, and he eventually developed a homosexual preference (14).

A 40-year-old man had experienced high fevers in childhood. In his 20s, he developed recurrent attacks of flushing, tachycardia, and diaphoresis. Extensive medical examinations revealed bilateral temporal lobe spike discharges and an enlarged temporal horn of the left lateral ventricle. Approximately 18 months after the onset of his autonomic spells, his military records documented the onset of multiple forms of aggression. Intensely self-critical, he once furiously punched a door, injuring knuckles of his right hand. He was imprisoned for multiple fights with fellow servicemen; believing that he had been treated unfairly, he destroyed the plumbing fixtures within his cell. When the military court refused to hear his explanation, he threatened to murder the magistrate.

After neurologic examination led to release from prison, he successfully controlled his temper for many years, developing religious and philosophic views which precluded violence. Nonetheless, when questioned about his temper, the patient responded, "I have more of a problem with anger than anyone I have ever met in my life." He then emphasized a constant conflict between angry feelings, which were elicited by a sense of injustice, and a strict moral conviction that he should never attack a person. His moral and religious convictions led him to voluntarily change and clean bed pans on a hospital ward and to write extensively about the clash of good and evil in the modern world (21).

A 42-year-old man suffered complex partial seizures initiated by an abdominal aura, followed by clonic movements of the right side of his body. Multiple EEGs showed spike and wave discharge from the left temporal lobe. He underwent a left temporal lobectomy; pathologic examination revealed a mesial temporal hamartoma. Though seizure frequency was markedly reduced, he has remained psychotic. His delusions relate anal stimulation to sexual arousal and seizure prevention. He is a frequent letter writer, usually sending one letter per week to his physician. The communications are remarkable for third-person self-references and excessive inclusion of identifying details, such as date, time, social security number, telephone, and post office box numbers. Often he follows the arabic numeral with its spelling. He has filed litigation against employers, the owner of a restaurant in which he experienced a seizure, his landlord, former physicians, and the Post Office for failure to deliver his many letters (14).

A 23-year-old woman had experienced déjà vu sensations and losses of consciousness since age 14; after age 20, she began to experience generalized clonic–tonic convulsions. Her EEG revealed bilateral abnormalities, with spikes thought to originate in the right temporal lobe. The patient described herself as aggressive and outspoken. She wrote poetry and long letters and kept a diary filled with philosophic speculation. At age 17, she experienced a change from heterosexual to homosexual preference. At about age 15, she had experienced the first of several prolonged dissociative experiences. At this time, she found herself in another city answering to a male name, and she was unaware of events during a 3-week period.

Subsequently, she underwent repeated psychiatric hospitalizations for dissociative experiences. The patient's roommate was able to describe two distinct personalities which emerged during dissociative episodes: One was masculinized, angry, tough, and threatening; the other was a "childlike little girl," sweet, shy, cooperative, and withdrawn. In separate incidents, the aggressive personality had beaten a man to unconsciousness, held a psychotherapist hostage at knife point, and telephoned a death threat to her physician (20).

PARIETO–LIMBIC LESIONS OF THE RIGHT HEMISPHERE

Pathways from sensory association cortices through the temporal lobe and amygdala, extending into orbital frontal cortex, represent a major connecting system relating perception and motivation to the initiation of behavior. In parallel to this temporo–limbo–frontal (ventral) route is a dorsal, parieto–limbo–frontal pathway, as indicated in Figure 30.1. For primates, vision has become the predominant sensory modality for exploring the world; the anatomy and physiology of visual limbic pathways are best understood, so that clues to the function of this second polymodal sensory–limbic system may be derived from its visual connections.

Much recent evidence suggests that the parietal visual system is concerned with spatial properties—the "where" of vision rather than the "what." The parieto–cingulo–frontal pathway appears critical for noticing and locating biologically important stimuli, especially in peripheral space. Its connections allow two important functions: (a) orientation and arousal mediated by the midbrain reticular formation, median raphe, and locus ceruleus; and (b) the initiation of tracking head and eye movements by frontal cortex. Several principles distinguish functions of the dorsal from the ventral visual limbic system: (a) simultaneous or parallel scanning of large sectors of peripheral space versus concentration on foveal vision; (b) extraction of

global spatial information rather than analytic object recognition; (c) surveillance for a broad class of motivationally relevant events rather than association to a particular stimulus; and (d) initiation of activating or orienting responses rather than production of coordinated motor or consummatory behaviors (22).

These generalizations are derived largely from experiments on monkeys, but a group of additional observations are based on clinical literature. These findings indicate extensive hemispheric asymmetries in both anatomy and function involving the parieto–limbic circuits. In brief, the dominant left hemisphere in most individuals contains a larger volume of architectonically distinctive cortex (Tpt) which, at the junction of parietal and temporal association systems, may mediate the extensive crossed-sensory associations critical for language. By contrast, the right hemisphere possesses a larger parieto–visual association area (PEG) which may confer superior spatial surveillance and attentional functions, compromised in the left hemisphere by language specialization (22).

These facts may partially account for the remarkable behavioral syndromes resulting from damage to the dorsal right hemisphere in humans. Symptoms include persistent neglect and misconstruction of extra personal space; slowed reactions and blunted autonomic responses to stimuli presented to the patient's left or right; failure to read emotional messages conveyed through vocal intonation (prosody) or facial expression of others; denial or minimization of deficits, which often extends beyond the patient's immediate illness to prior injuries, pressing financial or personal problems, and catastrophic events (22).

Example

A middle-age man sustained a severe contusion and hemorrhage within the right hemisphere when he was struck by an automobile at a traffic intersection. Neurosurgic treatment required the evacuation of extensive areas of his right parietal lobe.

The patient initially minimized his dense left hemiparesis and hemianopia, emphasizing cheerfully that he was "handicapable rather than handicapped." Years after the injury, he continues to walk into objects on his left. He is strikingly unconcerned about his wife's progressive loss of vision and the couple's deteriorating finances. Despite the obvious distress it provokes in his wife and caretakers, he engages in continual inappropriate punning and joking. He speaks in an apparently emotionless, unmodulated voice (motor aprosodia). Underestimating his physical limitations, he attempted to climb stairs on one occasion and suffered a serious fall (4).

Other observations have suggested that congenital abnormalities of the parietal association cortex in the right hemisphere, in some sense the mirror image of dyslexia resulting from dysmorphogenesis of the left temporo–parietal junction, may result in crippled social communications, awkwardness in interpersonal relationships, and deficits in spatial construction (22, 23).

BEHAVIOR FOLLOWING FRONTAL LOBE LESIONS

The frontal lobe is the major cortical meeting place for interoceptive–hypothalamic input, highly analyzed exteroceptive information from sensory association cortices, and, as suggested by Figure 30.1, the eventual destination of ventral and dorsal sensory–limbic pathways which inform it of emotionally relevant stimuli. Frontal cortex is also the major control center in the primate brain, regulating the older extrapyramidal system via extensive connections with the caudate nucleus and containing the cells of origin of the newer pyramidal system, through which we execute complex learned movements, speak, and write.

The mixed sensory, limbic, and motor capacities consolidated within the vastly expanded human frontal lobe provide the basis for its most critical function: constructing a course of action which, in the light of the current environment and past experience, will optimally satisfy long-range emotional goals. The best summary of the multifaceted operations of the frontal cortex is "judgment."

Characteristic lapses in judgment which follow frontal lobe lesions reveal components of the complex, underlying processes. Behavioral changes include failure to notice and be motivated by emotionally relevant stimuli, leading to apathy or abulia (especially with lesions to dorsal frontal cortex); transient, reflexive emotional outbursts without consideration of consequences (especially with ventral, orbital frontal lesions); neglect of social rules regarding the timing and expression of biologic drives such as elimination, sexual desire, or aggression; and absence of long-range behavioral planning or personal strategy. This seemingly paradoxical mixture of behaviors has been aptly termed "irritable euphoric apathy" (2, 24).

Example

Phineas Gage was a polite and conscientious railroad worker whose frontal lobes were pierced by a crowbar following a dynamite explosion. Although he was able to walk away from the accident, retaining his memory and ability to speak, his personality was profoundly affected: "The equilibrium or balance, between his intellectual faculties and animal propensities seems to have been destroyed. He is fitful, irreverent, indulgent at times in the grossest profanity, manifesting but little deference for his fellows, impatient of restraint or advice when it conflicts with his desires, at times pertinaciously obstinate yet capricious and vacillating, devising many plans of operation, which are no sooner arranged than they are abandoned in turn for others appearing more feasible. A child in his intellectual capacity and manifestations, he has the animal passions of a strong man"(4).

A middle-aged nurse and mother of two abruptly lost interest in work and home life. Previously, she had suffered episodes of blurred vision, right-sided weakness, and clumsiness. After the behavioral changes, a CT scan revealed an extensive demyelinating plaque of multiple sclerosis within the right frontal lobe. During a typical day, the patient was awakened by her morning alarm but did not arise or dress for work. She spent hours lying passively in bed, inattentive to the needs of her family. She was often incontinent of urine, but showed no embarrassment when bed clothes were changed. She generally was apathetic, expressing little spontaneous affection for her mother or children. By contrast, when food was presented, she ate it wolfishly. Irritated by the cries of her young son, she abruptly burned him with cigarette butts on several occasions. Moments later, she denied anger but was unconcerned about the consequences of her actions.

BEHAVIORAL EFFECTS OF COMBINED LESIONS

The disparate behavioral changes associated with the hypothalamus, temporal-pole-amygdala, parieto–limbic cortex of the right hemisphere or frontal lobe are best appreciated by considering focal lesions to each area. However, many circumstances can produce damage to multiple neural levels. An unfortunately frequent setting for combined lesions is head trauma, which may result in contusion to the orbital frontal cortex as well as posttraumatic temporolimbic epilepsy. The resulting changes in behavior may be severe and distinctive, reflecting complementary features of the individual syndromes. Thus emotions may be experienced frequently and intensely in association with the temporolimbic epileptic focus while loss of judgment concerning consequences of action, related to orbital frontal damage, further impairs behavioral control.

Example

Following a limb fracture, a young man sustained severe closed head injury when the ambulance in which he was riding collided with an automobile. Over a period of months he became, according to his devout parents, "a religious fanatic" who was rejected by the Jehovah's Witness movement as overzealous. He kept a voluminous diary of religious writings, punctuated by angry diatribes against former girlfriends whom he described as agents of Satan. He was hospitalized after attempting to murder his parents. Examination documented epileptic spiking in the left amygdala and structural damage to both frontal lobes (6).

IMPLICATIONS

In this overview of the organic personality syndromes, I have stressed an essential consideration: clinical recognition of these syndromes, which will lead to prompt medical–neurologic diagnosis and, where possible, reversal of the underlying cause. In situations such as benign pituitary tumors, encephalitis, meningiomas affecting temporal or frontal lobes, normal-pressure hydrocephalus or resectable epileptic foci, definitive treatment is possible. The efforts to localize neurobehavioral syndromes may take on special importance as methods of transplanting and regrowing particular neural circuits reach fruition during this decade.

However, it should be obvious that human beings cannot be reduced to the operation of specific neuronal circuits. For most patients, neuropsychiatric assessment is a necessary step in the crafting of a realistic, multidimensional program of therapy based on the individual's spared as well as impaired capacities. In the future, the organic personality syndromes may cast a light on the neurology of emotional processing which will illuminate the darker corners of psychiatry.

References

1. American Psychiatric Association: *Diagnostic and Statistical Manual of Mental Disorders (Third Edition).* Washington, DC, American Psychiatric Association, 1980.
2. Geschwind N: The borderland of neurology and psychiatry: some common misconceptions. In Benson F, Blumer D (eds): *Psychiatric Aspects of Neurologic Disease.* New York, Grune and Stratton, 1975, vol 1, pp 1–8.

3. Bear D, Freeman R, Greenberg M: Alterations in personality associated with neurologic illnesses. In Michels R (ed): *Psychiatry*. Philadelphia, J. P. Lippincott, 1985, Chapter 28.

4. Bear D, Fulop M: The neurology of emotion. In Hobson A (ed): *Behavioral Biology in Medicine*. Norwalk, CT, Kimmich Press, 1988.

5. Smith DE, King MD, Hoebel BG: Lateral hypothalamic control of killing: evidence for a cholinoceptive mechanism. *Science* 167:900–901, 1970.

6. Weiger, W, Bear D: The neuropsychiatry of aggression. *J Psychiatr Res* 22:85–98, 1988.

7. Reeves AG, Plum F: Hyperphagia, rage and dementia accompanying a ventromedial hypothalamic neoplasm. *Arch Neurol* 20:616–624, 1969.

8. Bear D, Rosenbaum J, Norman R: Aggression in cat and man precipitated by cholinesterase inhibitor. *Psychosomatics* 26: 535–536, 1986.

9. Geschwind N: Disconnexion syndrome in animals and man. *Brain* 88:237–294, 1965.

10. Bear DM: Temporal lobe epilepsy—a syndrome of sensory limbic hyperconnection. *Cortex* 15:357–384, 1979.

11. Kluver H, Bucy PC: Preliminary analysis of functions of the temporal lobes in monkeys. *Arch Neurol Psychiatry* 42:979–1000, 1939.

12. Marlowe WB, Mancall EL, Thomas JJ: Complete Kluver-Bucy syndrome in man. *Cortex* 11:53–59, 1975.

13. Terzian H, Dalle Ore G: Syndrome of Kluver and Bucy reproduced in man by bilateral removal of temporal lobes. *Neurology* 5:373–380, 1955.

14. Bear D, Freeman R, Greenberg M: Psychiatric aspects of temporal lobe epilepsy. In Hales R, Frances A (eds): *Psychiatry Update: American Psychiatric Association Annual Review*. Washington, DC, American Psychiatric Press, 1985, vol 4, pp 190–210.

15. Goddard GV, McIntyre D, Leech C: A permanent change in brain function resulting from daily electrical stimulation. *Exp Neurol* 25:295–330, 1969.

16. Slater E, Beard AW: Schizophrenia-like psychoses of epilepsy. *Br J Psychiatry* 109:95–150, 1963.

17. Mendez MF, Cummings JL, Benson DF: Depression and epilepsy. *Arch Neurol* 43:766–770, 1986.

18. Waxman SG, Geschwind N: Hypergraphia in temporal lobe epilepsy. *Neurology* 24:629–636, 1974.

19. Bear DM, Fedio P: Quantitative analysis of interictal behavior in temporal lobe epilepsy. *Arch Neurol* 34:454–467, 1977.

20. Schenk L, Bear DM: Multiple personalities and dissociative responses in temporal lobe epilepsy. *Am J Psychiatry* 138:1311–1316, 1981.

21. Devinsky O, Bear D: Varieties of aggressive behavior in temporal lobe epilepsy. *Am J Psychiatry* 141:651–656, 1984.

22. Bear DM: Hemispheric specialization and the neurology of emotion. *Arch Neurol* 40:195–202, 1983.

23. Weintraub S, Mesulam MM: Developmental learning disabilities of the right hemisphere. *Arch Neurol* 40:463–468, 1983.

24. Blumer D, Benson DF: Personality changes with frontal and temporal lobe lesions. In Benson DF, Blumer D (eds): *Psychiatric Aspects of Neurologic Diseases*. New York, Grune & Stratton, 1975, pp 151–170.

Section IV

Selected Problems in Outpatient Practice

31

Mood Disorders

Paul J. Barreira, M.D.
Aaron Lazare, M.D.

Disorders of mood, especially depression, are among the most common problems that individuals bring to psychiatrists, medical physicians, psychologists, psychiatric social workers, psychiatric nurses, and other mental health professionals. It is also one of the most common conditions that individuals cope with and endure without seeking professional help. For example, only one-third of patients suffering from current depressive episodes (or within the past 6 months) seek treatment for the condition, and only half of those who seek treatment receive help from a mental health professional (1).

People with mood disorders experience a high degree of suffering. They endure intense personal feelings of anguish; they have a high suicide rate; they are heavy users of medical services; they often have associated problems with alcohol and substance abuse; their family and friends are often profoundly affected by the disorder; and their suffering often becomes chronic. Yet, mood disorders are often treatable, usually with profound or at least moderate success. These facts underline the need for careful diagnosis and vigorous treatment of patients with mood disorders (2).

The emphasis of this chapter is on the diagnosis and clinical care of patients with mood disorders in outpatient settings. We will use "mood disorder," following the *Diagnostic and Statistical Manual of Mental Disorders (Third Edition-Revised)* (DSM-III-R, to refer to that group of disorders characterized by disturbances in mood, accompanied by a full or partial manic or depressive syndrome in which the symptom cluster is not due to any other physical or mental disorder. This includes the diagnostic categories of major depression, dysthymia, bipolar disorder, and cyclothymia (3) (see Table 31.1).

Before embarking on a discussion of the mood disorders, it is useful to acknowledge the following point of view about the heterogeneity of causation and clinical manifestations of mood disorders. According to

Table 31.1 DSM-III-R Classification of Mood Disorders

Depressive disorders
Major depression
  Single episode
  Recurrent
Dysthymia (or depressive neurosis)
Depressive disorder NOS (not otherwise specified)
Bipolar disorders
Bipolar disorder
  Mixed
  Manic
  Depressed
Cyclothymia
Bipolar disorder NOS

Akiskal (2), the mood disorders, like many medical disorders, can be usefully conceptualized as

the final common pathway of various somatic and psychological processes. This means that putative etiologic factors can independently cause an affective syndrome, or that, more commonly, many such factors interact to produce the final common clinical picture. From this perspective, clinical variations can be conceived as resulting from genetic heterogeneity and differences in biological stressors and personality and social forces.

This perspective is helpful in making sense of the complex literature on mood disorders. For instance, in considering the multiple hypothesized etiologies and various treatments for mood disorders, the reader should consider that many or all are correct or useful for a given subpopulation of patients with the disorder.

TERMINOLOGY AND NOSOLOGIC CONCEPTS

Terminology in mood disorders has been a source of considerable confusion. This is a result of the lay use of the word "depression," the historical evolution of various etiologic and nosologic concepts about mood disorders, and the hetergeneity of phenomena subsumed under the rubric "mood disorders."

The Term "Depression"

The common and ambiguous use of the term "depression" makes it essential to review and clarify its various meanings. First, "depression" may be used simply to refer to a transient dysphoric *affect* which the person equates with sadness or feeling blue and which is not associated with psychopathology. Second, the term may be used to refer to a dysphoric *mood* which has a more lasting quality and which may be associated with a variety of psychiatric and medical disorders. The quality of the

mood is thought to be qualitatively different from normal sadness. Third, "depression" may be used to refer to a syndrome or a constellation of signs and symptoms which include depressed mood, insomnia, weight loss, loss of interest in surroundings, and suicidal ideation. And finally, the term may be used to refer to a nosologic entity (a disorder, a disease, an illness, or a diagnostic category).

Depression as a Nosologic Entity

When professionals refer to patients as having major depression (or bipolar disorder) in a diagnostic, nosologic, or disease sense, what is meant besides the fact that the DSM-III-R criteria have been met? Depression in this sense means that acknowledged experts, based on empirical data, believe that it is useful for clinical and research purposes to circumscribe a particular set of signs and symptoms (taking into account certain exclusion criteria) into a distinct category. This designation separates patients with these criteria from those with other criteria which are designated by other categorical diagnoses. Such a designation represents our best attempt at this time to develop a homogeneous sample which then gives clinicians and researchers greater power to predict etiologic mechanisms, natural history, and treatment response. Even as we learn that the etiology of the nosologic entity (i.e., major depression) is multifactorial, its recognition continues to be useful if conceived of as a final common pathway of various psychologic and biologic processes. For example, the diagnosis still has considerable predictive value about these patients' perception of the world and themselves, about suicidal ideation, and about treatment response. In other words, to say that a patient has the diagnosis of major depression places him or her in a category of patients whose members are apt to share certain common features. At the same time, clinicians should be aware of enormous differences among patients who share the same diagnostic category. There are two explanations for these differences. First, the diagnostic category consists of several subgroups that have not yet been distinguished. Second, each person suffering from depression is unique when one takes into account all the biologic, psychologic, and social patterns and events that antedate and postdate the affective episode (see Chapter 8).

The concept of depression as a disorder or a disease can be further clarified by an analogy to hypertension (sustained elevation of blood pressure). In both conditions, the transient, situational *symptom* of depression and elevation of blood pressure do not constitute the *disease* or disorder of depression or hypertension, although these may be signs of early onset. In both conditions, there is no clear boundary between normal and abnormal ranges, although severe cases of each are unmistakable. In both conditions, severity can lead to death. Both conditions afflict from 10% to 20% of the population with varying degrees of severity. In both conditions, a minority of cases are caused by known medical conditions, while the majority of cases are of unknown etiology, referred to as functional or primary depression and essential hypertension. In both conditions, a variety of pharmacologic and nonpharmacologic treatments may be useful (e.g., verbal therapies and antidepressants for depression; and exercise, meditation, low-salt diet, weight reduction, and antihypertensive medication for hypertension). In both conditions, there is a small but significant group of treatment-resistant cases. For both conditions, there is the expectation that an increased knowledge of etiology and pathogenesis will lead to more useful nosologic entities. Most importantly, however, both conditions have proved to be useful diagnostic categories because, regardless of etiology and pathogenesis, they provide valuable information about course and treatment.

Primary Versus Secondary Affective Syndromes

Primary depressions arise independent of and are not preceded by or associated with other psychiatric and medical syndromes, whereas secondary depression chronologically follow other psychiatric or medical conditions. Secondary mania is known to follow medical conditions but rarely if ever follows other psychiatric conditions.

Patients with depression secondary to other psychiatric disorders, in contrast to patients with primary depression, more often report suicide attempts and are less apt to be delusional. These patients are not as likely as primary depressives to respond to antidepressants or electroconvulsive therapy and are less likely to recover. Patients with depression secondary to medical illness, in contrast to primary depressives, are likely to be older, less likely to have a family history of affective disorder, less likely to have a prior depressive episode, less likely to consider suicide or take one's life by suicide, and less likely to respond to antidepressant medications (4). The primary/secondary distinction has not yet been recognized in the official diagnostic categories.

Unipolar Versus Bipolar Depression

"Unipolar" refers to the disorders of patients characterized by one or more depressive episodes. (Unipolar manic conditions are rare.) "Bipolar" refers to the disorders of patients characterized by at least one manic episode. Of all the dichotomies listed in this section, the unipolar versus bipolar has proved to be the most useful in distinguishing clinical categories. Genetic, biochemical, and pharmacologic evidence supports this distinction. This distinction is reflected in the DSM-III-R classification. The material in the body of this chapter is based on this distinction.

Historic Terms and Dichotomies

There are several terms, many of them dichotomous, that are part of the history of our knowledge of affective disorders (5). Their use commonly leads to clinical and conceptual confusion.

Reactive/Neurotic Versus Endogenous Depression

It had been thought that the depressions could be usefully divided into those that were caused by external, psychosocial events (reactive or neurotic) and those that were caused by internal, genetic, or biologic causes (endogenous). It was further believed that these two types of depressions could be distinguished by their respective symptom patterns. Endogenous features were believed to be those now referred to by DSM-III-R as the melancholic type. It is currently believed that there is no relationship between the presence or absence of a precipitating event and the symptom picture.

Neurotic Versus Psychotic Depression

In the past, psychotic depression referred to a diagnostic category characterized by severe depression, depression with "endogenous features," or depression with psychotic symptoms of delusions and/or hallucinations. Currently, "psychotic" is not regarded as a nosologic entity but as an adjective modifier for major depression or bipolar disorder based on the presence of delusions and/or hallucinations (5).

Involutional Depression

Depressions that occurred for the first time during the involutional period were thought to have distinctive characteristics and therefore constituted a useful nosologic entity. It is currently believed that such depressions do not have unique clinical characteristics, so the term is not useful.

Agitated/Anxious Versus Retarded Depression

The agitated/anxious versus retarded dichotomy was once thought to have nosologic value. Currently, these terms represent modifiers to describe symptoms of mood disorders.

DEPRESSIVE DISORDERS (UNIPOLAR DEPRESSION)

Definition

Depressive disorders, according to DSM-III-R, are mood disorders characterized by one or more periods of depression

without a history of manic or hypomanic episodes. (This corresponds to the term "unipolar depression.") The two kinds of depressive disorders are major depression, in which there are one or more major episodes of depression (see Table 31.2), and dysthymia, in which the criteria for major depression are not met but the illness has a duration of at least 2 years (see Table 31.3). The DSM-III-R diagnoses of major depression and dysthymia correspond to *International Classification of Diseases–Ninth Edition* (ICD-9) diagnoses of major depressive disorder, reactive depressive psychosis, and neurotic depression (3).

Etiology
Psychosocial Causation

Psychosocial theories and hypotheses include psychodynamic approaches, personality factors, life events and environmental stress, learned helplessness, and cognitive theories.

The major contributors to the psychodynamic theories of depression are S. Freud, Abraham, Rado, Gero, E. Bibring, Bowlby, and Jacobson (6). There is no uniform psychodynamic approach because the theories of depression have evolved over the decades along with the evolving psychodynamic approaches (see Chapter 4). Another reason for the lack of uniformity in psychodynamic approaches is that various authors often refer to different clinical populations. Many contemporary pschotherapists regard Bibring's (7) contribution as the clearest and most useful of the psychodynamic approaches to depression. He states that depression is an affective state characterized by loss of self-esteem which can be lowered as a result of a variety of psychologic conditions. Bibring's contribution was to broaden the concept of self-esteem and relegate guilt and anger turned on the self as among the many dynamics in the etiology of depression.

It has long been postulated that certain personality disorders predispose patients to depression. Using DSM-III categories, there is comorbidity between depressive

Table 31.2   DSM-III-R Diagnostic Criteria for Major Depressive Episode[a, b]

A. At least five of the following symptoms have been present during the same 2-week period and represent a change from previous functioning; at least one of the symptoms is either (1) depressed mood or (2) loss of interest or pleasure. (Do not include symptoms that are clearly due to a physical condition, mood-incongruent delusions or hallucinations, incoherence, or marked loosening of associations.)
   (1) depressed mood (or can be irritable mood in children and adolescents) most of the day, nearly every day, as indicated by either subjective account or observation by others
   (2) markedly diminished interest or pleasure in all, or almost all, activities most of the day, nearly every day (as indicated by either subjective account or observation by others of apathy most of the time)
   (3) significant weight loss or weight gain when not dieting (e.g., more than 5% of body weight in a month), or decrease or increase in appetite nearly every day (in children, consider failure to make expected weight gains)
   (4) insomnia or hypersomnia nearly every day
   (5) psychomotor agitation or retardation nearly every day (observable by others, not merely subjective feelings of restlessness or being slowed down)
   (6) fatigue or loss of energy nearly every day
   (7) feelings of worthlessness or excessive or inappropriate guilt (which may be delusional) nearly every day (not merely self-reproach or guilt about being sick)
   (8) diminished ability to think or concentrate, or indecisiveness, nearly every day (by either subjective account or as observed by others)
   (9) recurrent thoughts of death (not just fear of dying), recurrent suicidal ideation without a specific plan, or a suicide attempt or a specific plan for committing suicide
B. (1) It cannot be established that an organic factor initiated and maintained the disturbance.
   (2) The disturbance is not a normal reaction to the death of a loved one (uncomplicated bereavement). *Note:* Morbid preoccupation with worthlessness, suicidal ideation, marked functional impairment or psychomotor retardation, or prolonged duration suggest bereavement complicated by major depression.
C. At no time during the disturbance have there been delusions or hallucinations for as long as 2 weeks in the absence of prominent mood symptoms (i.e., before the mood symptoms developed or after they have remitted).
D. Not superimposed on schizophrenia, schizophreniform disorder, delusional disorder, or psychotic disorder NOS.

Major depressive episode codes: fifth-digit code numbers and critiera for severity of current state of bipolar disorder, depressed, or major depression:
   1-*Mild:* Few, if any, symptoms in excess of those required to make the diagnosis, *and* symptoms result in only minor impairment in occupational functioning or in usual social activities or relationships with others.
   2-*Moderate:* Symptoms or functional impairment between "mild" and "severe."
   3-*Severe, without psychotic features:* Several symptoms in excess of those required to make the diagnosis, *and* symptoms markedly interfere with occupational functioning or with usual social activities or relationships with others.
   4-*With psychotic features:* Delusions or hallucinations. If possible, **specify** whether the psychotic features are *mood congruent* or *mood incongruent.*
   Mood-congruent psychotic features: Delusions or hallucinations whose content is entirely consistent with the typical depressive themes of personal inadequacy, guilt, disease, death, nihilism, or deserved punishment.
   Mood-incongruent psychotic features: Delusions or hallucinations whose content does *not* involve typical depressive themes of personal inadequacy, guilt, disease, death, nihilism, or deserved punishment. Included here are such symptoms as persecutory delusions (not directly related to depressive themes), thought insertion, thought broadcasting, and delusions of control.
   5-*In partial remission:* Intermediate between "in full remission" and "mild," *and* no previous dysthymia. (If major depressive episode was superimposed on dysthymia, the diagnosis of dysthymia alone is given once the full criteria for a major depressive episode are no longer met.)
   6-*In full remission:* During the past 6 months, no significant signs or symptoms of the disturbance.
   0-*Unspecified.*
Specify chronic if current episode has lasted 2 consecutive years without a period of 2 months or longer during which there were no significant depressive symptoms.
Specify if current episode is *melancholic type.*

---

[a] A "major depression syndrome" is defined as criterion A.
[b] Reproduced with permission from American Psychiatric Association: *Diagnosis and Statistical Manual of Mental Disorders (Third Edition–Revised).* Washington, DC, American Psychiatric Association, 1987.

Table 31.3.   Diagnostic Criteria for Dysthymia[a]

A. Depressed mood (or can be irritable mood in children and adolescents) for most of the day, more days than not, as indicated by either subjective account or observation by others, for at least 2 years (1 year for children and adolescents).
B. Presence, while depressed, of at least two of the following:
   (1) poor appetite or overeating
   (2) insomnia or hypersomnia
   (3) low energy or fatigue
   (4) low self-esteem
   (5) poor concentration or difficulty making decisions
   (6) feelings of hopelessness
C. During a 2-year period (1 year for children and adolescents) of the disturbance, never without the symptoms in A for more than 2 months at a time.
D. No evidence of an unequivocal major depressive episode during the first 2 years (1 year for children and adolescents) of the disturbance.
   Note: There may have been a previous major depressive episode, provided there was a full remission (no significant signs or symptoms for 6 months) before development of the dysthymia. In addition, after these 2 years (1 year in children or adolescents) of dysthymia, there may be superimposed episodes of major depression, in which case both diagnoses are given.
E. Has never had a manic episode or an unequivocal hypomanic episode.
F. Not superimposed on a chronic psychotic disorder, such as schizophrenia or delusional disorder.
G. It cannot be established that an organic factor initiated and maintained the disturbance, e.g., prolonged administration of an antihypertensive medication.
Specify primary or secondary type:
   Primary type: The mood disturbance is not related to a preexisting, chronic, nonmood, Axis I or Axis III disorder, e.g., anorexia nervosa, somatization disorder, a psychoactive substance dependence disorder, an anxiety disorder, or rheumatoid arthritis.
   Secondary type: The mood disturbance is apparently related to a preexisting, chronic, nonmood Axis I or Axis III disorder.
Specify early onset or late onset:
   Early onset: onset of the disturbance before age 21.
   Late onset: onset of the disturbance at age 21 or later.

[a] Reproduced with permission from American Psychiatric Association: *Diagnostic and Statistical Manual of Mental Disorders, Third Edition–Revised.* Washington, DC, American Psychiatric Association, 1987.

disorders and borderline, histrionic, dependent, and avoidant personality disorders (8). There are a variety of explanations for comorbidity (see Chapter 35). Personality disorders do not necessarily predispose patients to mood disorders. A major problem of studies of personality and depression is that reports of personality traits during the depression do not necessarily represent premorbid traits.

Many clinicians believe that life events play a major role in causing mood disorders. Although there is evidence to support this belief, reearch data have not yet answered the following objections: stressful events might be caused by the depression and identified in retrospect by the patient as an explanation of the depression; stressful life events are nonspecific and therefore may precede other psychiat-

ric illnesses; and the association may be coincidental (9).

Cognitive theories of depression postulate that depressive mood and behavior are caused by pathologic cognitive states (10). The two most prominent cognitive theories are Beck's cognitive–behavioral theory of dysfunctional attitudes (11) and Seligman's model of learned helplessness (12). Beck postulates that depression results from the activation of specific cognitive distortions which relate to how people evaluate themselves and relate to others. The theory of learned helplessness developed from studies in which animals showed depressive behaviors after being exposed to experimental situations which were out of their control. These new behaviors were termed "learned helplessness." These findings were reformulated as a model for human depression (13). Based on this theory, behavioral approaches attempt to teach the patient a sense of control and mastery of the environment.

Neurobiologic Causation

There is strong evidence for genetic causation of some of the unipolar depressions, based on rates of illness in relatives and twin studies. Genetic issues that remain unsettled are (a) the genetic relationship between unipolar and bipolar illness, (b) evidence for heterogeneity of depression, based on illness patterns in families and clinical characteristics of patients, (c) mode of inheritance, (d) linkage with genetic marker traits, and (e) biologic risk factors (14). The genetic contribution for unipolar disorders is considerably less than that for bipolar disorders.

There are several promising biochemical hypotheses about the pathophysiology of mood disorders. The following is a brief review of the major hypotheses.

The biogenic amine hypothesis proposes that depression is a result of a deficit in the available norepinephrine, serotonin, or indole amine available to postsynaptic receptors. This theory was supported by the observation that drugs such as reserpine that deplete brain amines cause depression. According to this hypothesis, monoamine oxidase inhibitors (MAOIs) decrease the breakdown of monoamines, while tricyclic antidepressants prevent reuptake of the monoamines. A second theory suggests that there is diminished receptor functioning in depressed states and that the therapeutic effects of some antidepressants are mediated through their changes in receptor sensitivity. A third hypothesis relates to neuroendocrine functioning resulting from the regulation of the hypothalamo–pituitary–adrenal axis by biogenic amine neurotransmitters.

There is a growing consensus that none of the above theories alone can explain all of the biologic abnormalities in depression. Older hypotheses will have to be extended and integrated with newer ones before they can better explain specific affective disorders. The reader is referred to more comprehensive reviews of the biology of depressive disorders (15–18).

Epidemiology and Risk Factors

Reports of the prevalence and incidence of depressive disorders vary according to the population under study and the definition of the disorder, which varies according to the nomenclature and research criteria most widely accepted at the time of the study. Epidemiologic data are reported as point prevalence, morbid risk or lifetime risk, annual incidence, and risk factor. *Point prevalence* refers to the proportion of people in the population who have the disorder at a given point in time. *Morbid risk* refers to the lifetime risk of an individual having a first episode of the disorder. *Incidence* is the number of new cases in the population throughout a period of time, usually 1 year. *Risk factor* refers to any factor that increases the chances of the person developing the disorder (19).

In more recent studies in industrialized nations, the point prevalence is 3.2 per 100 males and 4.5 to 9.3 per 100 females. The incidence of depressive disorders is 82 to 201 new cases per 100,000 men per year and 247 to 7,800 new cases per 100,000 women per year. The lifetime expectancy rate is 8% to 12% for men and 20% to 26% for women. Boyd and Weissman (19) summarized the risk factors as being female and between the ages of 35 and 45. In addition,

having a family history of depression or alcoholism; having childhood experiences in a disruptive, hostile and generally negative environment in the home; having had recent negative life events, particularly exits; lacking an intimate confiding relationship; having had a baby in the preceding six months.

Clinical Picture

With major depression, the symptoms may reach a peak in 1 to 6 weeks, but patients tend not to come for treatment until 3 to 5 months after the onset, when they realize they are having difficulty coping. Patients will describe their mood as sad, blue, despondent, low, or miserable. They will say, if they are articulate, that this mood is qualitatively different from their normal state of sadness. There may be a history of spontaneous crying often triggered by empathic comments of the interviewer. Alternatively, the patient may present with physical symptoms and complain of loss of pleasure or interest or anxiety. According to Hamilton (20), the most common symptoms in depressive illness are depressed mood, loss of interest, anxiety, difficulty falling asleep, loss of appetite, lack of energy, fatigability, and suicidal thoughts. Other symptoms often associated with depression include diurnal variation, constipation, decreased libido, and ruminations of guilt.

The DSM-III-R defines a major depressive episode as having five of nine criteria present during the same 2-week period: depressed mood, diminished interest, significant weight loss or gain, insomnia or hypersomnia, fatigue or loss of energy, feelings of worthlessness or guilt, diminished ability to think or concentrate, and recurrent thoughts of death. Psychotic features, if present, are noted to be mood congruent or mood incongruent. Congruency refers to the consistency of the content with depressive themes such as inadequacy, guilt, and disease. The major depressive episode is thought to be of the melancholic type if it meets five of nine criteria formerly associated with drug-responsive or endogenous depression. See Chapter 15 for the use of laboratory findings in the diagnosis of depression.

Clinical Course

Until the past 5 to 10 years, psychiatrists thought that most patients suffering from depressive disorders recovered from their acute episodes and returned to their previous level of well-being. Recent studies performed at university medical centers have cast serious doubt on these assumptions. (The generalizability of these studies, which are described below, to the general population are limited due to the sampling of the depressed populations under study.)

Depressive disorder can occur anytime in a person's life, with the peak ages for men and women being between 20 and 40 years of age, with a median age of 37 years. Of all patients with depressive disorders, almost 20% become ill in their teens, and more than 90% have had an episode before they reach 65. Ten to fifteen percent of patients with apparent depressive disorders will eventually experience a manic or hypomanic disorder and be reclassified as bipolar. Ten to twenty percent of patients who have an episode of major depression will go on to have a course characterized by long-term chronicity. At 6-month follow-up, 65% will have recovered; at 12-month follow-up, 76% are likely to have recovered; at 18-month follow-up, 78% are likely to have recovered; and at 5-year follow-up, 90% are likely to have recovered. Others studies report that 15% to 20% of patients treated for depression experience incomplete recovery and show fluctuation and chronic symptoms, often for years. This means the patient's chances for recovery decrease the longer the depression continues. The chances of recovery are enhanced by the acute onset of symptoms, by the absence of dysthymia, and by the presence of primary depression. Depression secondary to alcoholism in particular predicts a more chronic course (21–24).

Relapse or recurrence will occur in 50% to 85% of patients after the first depressive episode, with a mean number of lifetime episodes of five to six. The highest rate of relapse occurs during the first few months of recovery, with decreasing probability of relapse with the passage of time. An increased rate of relapse is related to greater numbers of previous depressive episodes, older age, and depression secondary to nonaffective psychiatric disorder. During the well interval between depressive episodes, a high proportion of patients have some psychosocial impairment and some residual symptoms. The lifetime rate of suicide, which accounts for almost all the excess mortality in depressive disorders, is 15% (24).

The term "double depression" refers to the clinical condition in which a major depressive episode is superimposed on a dysthymic disorder which preceded the major depression by at least 2 years. Patients with double depression are more apt to return to their premorbid dysthymic state than depressed patients without dysthymia are able to return to a symptom-free condition. At the same time, patients with double depression who recover from major depression are more prone to relapse than patients who do not have an underlying depression.

Dysthymia

The above discussion of double depression calls attention to the need to clarify the nosologic entity of dysthymia (see Table 31.3). Dysthymia was first introduced in DSM-III as a mild, chronic, subsyndromal level of depression on a spectrum with the more florid and acute manifestations of affective disorders. Even this nosologic entity is believed by several investigators to include several heterogeneous populations including patients with lifelong depressions which resemble personality disorders in terms of onset and time course, patients with chronic depressions which follow failure of complete remission of major depression, and patients with chronic depression which follows medical conditions or with demoralization following stress. The definition of dysthymia remains in flux (DSM-III versus DSM-III-R versus proposals for DSM-IV), and this entity is currently an area of increasing investigation (25–27).

Comorbidity

Patients who suffer from depressive disorders commonly suffer from a variety of other coexisting disorders. The diagnosis of the additional disorders is important because the presence of one may predispose the patient to the other and the combination of the disorders may have a synergistic effect, leading to more serious implications than would have been the case with one disorder alone. Furthermore, it is not uncommon for the clinician to diagnose one disorder and ignore the second. The disorders most commonly associated with the depressive disorders are alcohol abuse, anorexia nervosa, bulimia nervosa, and anxiety disorders (24).

Differential Diagnosis

Uncomplicated Bereavement

Uncomplicated bereavement is regarded as a normal reaction to the death of a loved one. The reaction may include a full depressive syndrome. The reaction rarely occurs after the first 2 to 3 months. A "morbid preoccupation with worthlessness, suicidal ideation, marked functional impairment, psychomotor retardation, or prolonged duration suggests that bereavement is complicated by major depressive disorder" (3, 28) (see Chapter 32).

Adjustment Disorder with Depressed Mood

Adjustment disorder with depressed mood requires a maladaptive reaction to an identifiable stressor and persists no longer than 6 months. This condition may not be distinguishable from the early stages of some depressive disorders.

Organic Mood Syndrome with Depression

Various medical illnesses and medications may produce a picture of depressive disorder. See Chapter 19 for further discussion and a list of medical conditions.

Dementia

A significant percentage of elderly patients with depressive disorders suffer from reversible cognitive impairment referred to as "pseudodementia." This may be a difficult condition to distinguish from Alzheimer's disease or other dementias. In pseudodementia, there is a relatively abrupt onset of memory disturbance, the memory disturbance follows the mood disorder, the patient is distressed over the memory impairment, and there is often a family history of mood disorder. In patients with true dementia, the onset of memory disturbance is apt to be more gradual, it precedes the mood disorder and shallow emotionality leads to less distress over the memory disturbance. The response to treatment for depression may be the best diagnostic test.

Schizoaffective Disorder

Schizoaffective disorder, a confusing and controversial nosologic entity in psychiatry, is distinguished from major depression with psychotic features by having a 2-week period during the episode in which there is an absence of prominent mood symptoms.

Treatment

A variety of psychosocial and somatic treatments are very effective in the treatment of most mood disorders. The psychosocial treatments include (*a*) short- and long-term traditional psychodynamic psychotherapies; (*b*) short-term interpersonal, cognitive, and behavioral therapies; and (*c*) couple, family, and group therapies. The somatic treatments include antidepressant agents, lithium salts, antipsychotic agents, and electroconvulsive agents. Hospitalization may be necessary for some as an additional aspect of treatment. In clinical practice, the treatment, combination of treatments, and sequencing of treatments are determined, whenever possible, by their proven efficacy for the particular clinical presentation. In many clinical situations, however, the particular skills and experience of clinician as well as some trial-and-error strategies are commonly employed.

Psychosocial Treatments

The following psychosocial treatments have been studied and used primarily for patients suffering from unipolar depressions of mild to moderate severity. Patients who are delusional, hallucinated, suicidal, or bipolar or who meet the criteria for melancholia are unlikely to respond to the psychosocial treatments alone.

The traditional psychodynamic psycho-therapies (see Chapter 4), both short- and long-term, are perhaps the most commonly used psychotherapies for the treatment of the mild to moderate unipolar depressions. Because of the difficulty in standardizing such treatments, there is little evidence as to their efficacy. Antidepressant agents are commonly used simultaneously.

During the past decade, several standardized short-term therapies have been developed which have proved to be of value for the treatment of the mild to moderate depressions. These include interpersonal therapy, cognitive–behavioral therapy, and several specific behavioral therapies including self-control therapy, social skills training, and psychoeducational treatment. These treatments are discussed in greater detail in Chapter 45. Marital, family, and group therapy have also been found to be useful in the treatment of depression, sometimes in combination with antidepressant agents. With all the psychosocial treatments, there is strong evidence that one of the most important variables is the quality of the therapeutic relationship. Current research attempts to assess the effects of these therapies on the natural history of the disorder, compare the standardized therapies, determine subpopulations most responsive to particular treatments, and determine the effectiveness of combinations of treatments.

Somatic Treatments

The most common somatic treatment for unipolar depression is antidepressant drug therapy. Two main classes of antidepressant agents are used. The first group are the heterocyclic antidepressants (HCAs), which increase biogenic amines at the synaptic junction by preventing reuptake of these amines. The second group are the MAOIs, which prevent the degradation of amines by destroying the enzyme responsible for amine breakdown.

Heterocyclic antidepressants are the most commonly used agents in the treatment of depression. For the most part, all the HCAs demonstrate the same therapeutic efficacy, although some patients will respond better to one medication than to another. They are most effective in patients who have melancholic symptoms such as loss of interest in almost all activities, psychomotor retardation, significant appetite and weight loss, early morning awakening, a distinct quality of depressed mood, episodicity with normal functioning between episodes, and a family history of depression. Such cases have a response rate of 90% compared with an overall response rate of 60% to 75%. In addition, they have proved useful in a subgroup of patients with dysthymia. It is important to note that therapeutic response to antidepressant drugs is delayed after the initiation of treatment. Although a change in sleep pattern commonly occurs almost immediately after initiating treatment, changes in mood take longer. While some improvement in mood is observed in the first weeks of treatment, a return to normal mood may take more that 4 weeks.

Side effects are common with these agents and often cause problems with patients' compliance with medication. Common side effects include dry mouth, inability to urinate, constipation, blurred vision, and lowered blood pressure. Often hypotension causes patients to fall and suffer fractures. This is a frequent problem with elderly patients. Some agents cause more potent side effects than others. A new antidepressant, fluoxetine, is a pure serotonin agonist which is reported to have no anticholinergic side effects.

Until recently, MAOIs have not been the first-choice agent for treatment of depression. Recent studies, however, indicate that these agents are as effective as the HCAs in treating depression. The possibility of serious side effects still causes MAOIs to be a second-choice agent. If patients are exposed to tyramine in their diet, severe headaches, hypertension, and death can result. Less severe but more common side effects include lower blood pressure and fatigue.

Electroconvulsive treatment (ECT) is useful in outpatient settings for drug-resistant patients and the elderly in whom the side effects of antidepressant agents may be too dangerous. There are broader uses of ECT in the treatment of depressive disorders on inpatient services. For psychotic depressions, ECT is the most effective treatment.

There are a group of depressed patients referred to as treatment refractory, drug resistant, or treatment failures. This group may account for 10% to 30% of patients seeking treatment. Some of these patients respond to the combination of an HCA or MAOI with lithium, thyroid, neuroleptics, or methylphenidate. HCAs and MAOIs are sometimes combined in treatment-resistant cases. Psychotic depressions are best treated with a combination of a neuroleptic plus an antidepressant.

General psychiatrists commonly refer many of the so-called treatment resistant patients (29) to subspecialists in psychopharmacology or to psychopharmacology clinics which specialize in the treatment of these patients.

BIPOLAR DISORDERS

Definition and Classification

Bipolar disorders, according to DSM-III-R, are mood disorders whose essential feature is the presence of one or more manic or hypomanic episodes. The three kinds of bipolar disorders are (*a*) bipolar disorder in which there are one or more manic episodes, (*b*) cyclothymia in which there are numerous hypomanic episodes and numerous periods with depressive symptoms, and (*c*) bipolar disorder not otherwise specified (bipolar NOS). See Tables 31.4 and 31.5 for diagnostic criteria for manic episode and cyclothymia. Bipolar NOS includes a clinical condition referred to as bipolar II which is characterized by brief hypomanic episodes and episodes of major depression. Current evidence suggests that these patients are more closely related to other bipolar patients than to unipolar depressed patients, but that they may have enough distinguishing characteristics to warrant a separate nosologic category.

Table 31.4   DSM-III-R Diagnostic Criteria for Manic Episode[a, b]

A. A distinct period of abnormally and persistently elevated, expansive, or irritable mood.
B. During the period of mood disturbance, at least three of the following symptoms have persisted (four if the mood is only irritable) and have been present to a significant degree:
   (1) inflated self-esteem or grandiosity
   (2) decreased need for sleep, e.g., feels rested after only three hours of sleep
   (3) more talkative than usual or pressure to keep talking
   (4) flight of ideas or subjective experience that thoughts are racing
   (5) distractibility, i.e., attention too easily drawn to unimportant or irrelevant external stimuli
   (6) increase in goal-directed activity (either socially, at work or school, or sexually) or psychomotor agitation
   (7) excessive involvement in pleasurable activities which have a high potential for painful consequences, e.g., the person engages in unrestrained buying sprees, sexual indiscretions, or foolish business investments
C. Mood disturbance sufficiently severe to cause marked impairment in occupational functioning or in usual social activities or relationships with others or to necessitate hospitalization to prevent harm to self or others.
D. At no time during the disturbance have there been delusions or hallucinations for as long as 2 weeks in the absence of prominent mood symptoms (i.e., before the mood symptoms developed or after they have remitted).
E. Not superimposed on schizophrenia, schizophreniform disorder, delusional disorder, or psychotic disorder NOS.
F. It cannot be established that an organic factor initiated and maintained the disturbance. **Note:** Somatic antidepressant treatment (e.g., drugs, ECT) that apparently precipitates a mood disturbance should not be considered an etiologic organic factor.
Manic episode codes: fifth-digit code numbers and criteria for severity of current state of bipolar disorder, manic or mixed:
   1-Mild: Meets minimum symptom criteria for a manic episode (or almost meets symptom criteria if there has been a previous manic episode).
   2-Moderate: Extreme increase in activity or impairment in judgment.
   3-Severe, without psychotic features: Almost continual supervision required in order to prevent physical harm to self or others.
   4-With psychotic features: Delusions, hallucinations, or catatonic symptoms. If possible, **specify** whether the psychotic features are *mood congruent* or *mood incongruent.*
   Mood-congruent psychotic features: Delusions or hallucinations whose content is entirely consistent with the typical manic themes of inflated worth, power, knowledge, identity, or special relationship to a deity or famous person.
   Mood-incongruent psychotic features: Either (*a*) or (*b*):
   (*a*) Delusions or hallucinations whose content does *not* involve the typical manic themes of inflated worth, power, knowledge, identity, or special relationship to a deity or famous person. Included are such symptoms as persecutory delusions (not directly related to grandiose ideas or themes), thought insertion, and delusions of being controlled.
   (*b*) Catatonic symptoms, e.g., stupor, mutism, negativism, posturing.
   5-In partial remission: Full criteria were previously, but are not currently, met; some signs or symptoms of the disturbance have persisted.
   6-In full remission: Full criteria were previously met, but there have been no significant signs or symptoms of the disturbance for at least 6 months.
   0-Unspecified.

[a] A "manic syndrome" is defined as including criteria A, B, and C. A "hypomanic syndrome" is defined as including criteria A and B, but not C, i.e., no marked impairment.
[b] Reprinted with permission from American Psychiatric Association: *Diagnostic and Statistical Manual of Mental Disorders* (*Third Edition-Revised*). Washington, DC, American Psychiatric Association, 1987.

Etiology

The importance of genetic factors in the transmission of bipolar disorders is indisputable. This is the conclusion from twin studies, adoption studies, and family studies of patients with bipolar disorder. Concordance rates for bipolar disorders are 68% for monozygotic twins and 23% for same-sex dizygotic twins. According to family studies, a bipolar patient is apt to have a 52% chance of having a parent with an affective disorder and a 63% chance of-having an affective illness in a parent or an extended family member (30).

There have been multiple biochemical approaches to the search for mediating mechanisms in bipolar disease. Goodwin and Jamison (31) have categorized studies on biologic parameters into six classes: (*a*) electrolytes, (*b*) membrane transport, (*c*) peptides, (*d*) neuroendocrine output and response, (*e*) neurotransmitter receptors, and (*f*) neurotransmitters, their metabolites, and related enzymes. For the most part, these abnormalities are not specific to bipolar disease. The reader is referred to several reviews of the biochemical theories of bipolar disorders (31, 32).

Epidemiology and Risk Factors

The lifetime risk of bipolar disorder for both sexes ranges from 0.6% to 0.9% in industrialized nations. The incidence of new cases per 100,000 per year is 9 to 15.2 for men and 7.4 to 32 for women. The rates of bipolar disorders are generally believed to be the same for men and women. These patients probably occur more frequently in the upper socioeconomic classes. The modal age of onset is 30, but up to 20% of new cases may occur after age 50, while 20% occur by age 20. The greatest risk for the disorder is having a family history of bipolar disorder. There is no relationship between incidence of bipolar disorders and race, religion, marital status, or urban/rural status (19).

Clinical Picture

The essential features of a manic episode are well known and generally easily identified. In the outpatient setting, the challenge is the recognition of the early signs of bipolar illness and the ability to distinguish these symptoms from normal variations in mood.

The early changes associated with a manic mood swing are subtle. Patients appear well. Indeed they may feel energetic, productive, and self-reliant. Since this may be reflected in their behavior, friends and relatives provide confirmatory data. Moreover, the generally positive, optimistic, festive, and energetic mood is contagious, causing others around the patient to feel good. Unless a history of previous mood swings is known, it is not possible to diagnose with certainty an early or pathologic mood swing. In fact, many individuals have been known to function quite well with these minor mood swings and never or only later in life develop a clear manic episode. Nevertheless, even with these minor swings, both the patient and family identify these times as distinct periods that have clear beginnings and endings. Families often accommodate themselves to these periods.

If the mood swing progresses, patients become more expansive in mood and disinhibited and embarrass others by ignoring social protocol. They are easily distracted and may show a flight of ideas, rapid digression from one idea to another, and pressure of speech. At this point they may see themselves as powerful and important beyond reason. They exercise poor judgment, usually manifested in buying sprees, poor business decisions, and sexual promiscuity. A sleep disturbance almost invariably accompanies these changes, characterized by a decreased need for sleep without loss of energy or feelings of fatigue. The typical accelerated pace of thinking as well as motor activity occurs during this time. Sexual interest and often sexual behavior increases (33, 34).

In later stages of mania, the euphoric mood may be replaced by irritability and anger; humor is replaced by a contentious, threatening manner. In addition to grandiose ideas or delusions, patients may develop psychotic features of delusions and hallucinations.

Since the 1800s, psychiatrists have observed the seasonal nature in the occurrence of untreated bipolar affective disorders, with mania occurring in the spring and summer and depression occurring in the fall and winter. Recently, a number of investigators have identified the following features of what is now referred to as seasonal affective disorder. Patients are usually women with onset of bipolar illness in the second or third decades of life. Depression tends to occur in October or November, and mania, in the spring and summer. The depressive episode is characterized by hypersomnia, anergia, carbohydrate craving, and weight gain in addition to other common depressive symtoms. First-degree relatives suffer from nonseasonal unipolar and bipolar disorders (35).

Clinical Course

The bipolar disorders are a recurring, episodic illness. Studies indicate that 85% to 90% of patients who present with a manic episode will experience multiple recurrences of major depressive and manic episodes. Despite its favorable outcome compared with that of schizophrenia, a significant number of bipolar patients remain symptomatic. Winokur et al. (36) reported that in a 2-year follow-up of 28 patients, 29% never achieved more than a partial remission and 11% were chronically ill. Predictors of slow recovery rate in bipolar patients include endogenous features, severity of depressive symptoms, psychotic features, psychomotor retardation, suicidal tendencies, anxiety, and alcoholism. For those patients who initially present as depressive disorders but eventually have a manic episode, an average of two to four depressive episodes over 6.4 years occur before the first manic episode. Change to bipolarity is associated with young age, hypersomnic and retarded phenomenology, psychotic depression, postpartum episodes, a family history of bipolarity, and pharmacologic hypomania.

Differential Diagnosis

Schizophrenia

The symptom picture of schizophrenia and mania is often difficult to distinguish, since between 20% and 50% of bipolar cases have hallucinations, delusions, and Schneiderian first-rank symptoms. A manic episode is more apt to be acute (except for the depressive prodrome) and associated with a good premorbid adjustment, previous history of mood disorder, current disturbance in mood, and family history of bipolar disorder. Schizophrenia is more apt to be associated with poor premorbid adjustment, absence of previous history of mood disorder, and negative family history for mood disorder. A catatonic presentation is statistically more apt to be a manifestation of bipolar illness than schizophrenia.

There is a growing consensus that patients with manic and schizophrenic symptoms referred to as "schizoaffective mania" should be regarded as bipolar disorders because of their common features of acute onset of episodes, sex ratios, and high rates of affective illness in relatives.

Organic Mood Syndromes

There are numerous medical conditions which can present a symptom picture identical with mania. These fall into the categories of medications, neurologic, endocrine, and infectious. A high index of suspicion on all clinical presentations of mania is important. Of particular concern are patients over the age of 50 who are having their first affective episode, patients with an identified medical illness known to cause mania, and patients on medications which are known to cause mania. (See Chapter 25 for a detailed clinical approach to the organic differential diagnosis of mania.)

Personality Disorders or Substance Abuse

Antisocial behavior and/or substance abuse may present with behaviors that may be confused with bipolar disorder. A stable premorbid adjustment, change in behavior, depressive or manic symptoms, and family history support the diagnosis of bipolar disorder.

Treatment

A common task of the outpatient clinician after establishing the diagnosis of manic episode is to arrange for hospitalization, particularly when the symptoms are socially disruptive and psychotic. Even with mild to moderate symptoms, the clinician must consider the possibility of a

Table 31.5   DSM-III-R Diagnostic Criteria for Cyclothymia[a]

A. For at least 2 years (1 year for children and adolescents), presence of numerous hypomanic episodes (all of the criteria for a manic episode, except criterion C that indicates marked impairment) and numerous periods with depressed mood or loss of interest or pleasure that did not meet criterion A of major depressive episode.
B. During a 2-year period (1 year in children and adolescents) of the disturbance, never without hypomanic or depressive symptoms for more than 2 months at a time.
C. No clear evidence of a major depressive episode or manic episode during the first 2 years of the disturbance (or 1 year in children and adolescents).
   Note: After this minimum period of cyclothymia, there may be superimposed manic or major depressive episodes, in which case the additional diagnosis of bipolar disorder or bipolar disorder NOS should be given.
D. Not superimposed on a chronic psychotic disorder, such as schizophrenia or delusional disorder.
E. It cannot be established that an organic factor initiated and maintained the disturbance, e.g., repeated intoxication from drugs or alcohol.

[a] Reprinted with permission from the American Psychiatric Association: *Diagnostic and Statistical Manual of Mental Disorders (Third Edition-Revised)*. Washington, DC, American Psychiatric Association, 1987.

rapid exacerbation of symptoms. Hospitalizing the patient requires persuasive skills, a good working relationship with the family, and, sometimes, commitment proceedings. Pharmacologic treatment for the acute episode is a neuroleptic–lithium combination, an antiparkinsonian drug, and, when this combination fails, ECT. Treatment with lithium alone is possible in milder cases without gross hyperactivity and psychotic features. Carbamazepine is used in place of lithium in patients who are unresponsive to lithium and in whom lithium is unsafe because of undue side effects, renal impairment, certain neurologic conditions, and pregnancy. Bipolar patients who present with depression should be treated with lithium or a combination of lithium and tricyclics or MAOIs.

The outpatient clinician has the responsibility to continue lithium treatment, to monitor the side effects of the medication, and to decide with the patient about the merits of indefinite maintenance. After the second or third episode, maintenance treatment is indicated for most patients. The following factors argue for earlier maintenance: male sex, onset after age 30, a first episode of mania rather than depression, sudden onset of the manic episode, onset unrelated to external events, and poor family and social support system. Together, these factors contribute to more frequent episodes that are unlikely to be treated rapidly (38, 39).

Noncompliance with medications is a common problem in patients with bipolar disorder. These patients complain of side effects of the medications, the loss of energy, feeling "flat," and decreased creativity. They miss certain aspects of what they perceive as the illness, such as feeling "high." These complaints are further complicated by manic behavior, such as testing of limits, flattery, shifting responsibility for action to others, exploiting others' weaknesses, and provoking anger.

Jamison and others have described the importance of psychotherapeutic issues in the clinical management of patients suffering from bipolar disorders (40–42).

Cyclothymia

Cyclothymic disorder (Table 31.5) is characterized by mood swings that are less severe and of shorter duration than those of bipolar disorder. Cyclothymia presents in the late teens and early 20's. Adolescence and early adulthood is often marked by disruptive relationships with family and friends and poor performance in school and work. Since the cycles occur in an irregular fashion with abrupt and unpredictable mood changes, the clinician may mistakenly conclude that the patient is suffering from a personality disorder. Individuals suffering from cyclothymia frequently abuse alcohol and drugs; have a history of multiple geographic moves; experience tempestuous and unstable relationships; and have an erratic job history.

Treatment with lithium is effective in approximately 60% of cyclothymic patients. Antidepressants should be used cautiously to treat the depressive cycle because of the possibility of inducing a hypomanic or manic episode.

THE CLINICAL INTERVIEW IN OUTPATIENT SETTINGS

Determining the Nature of the Problem

There are several problems of clinical diagnosis and assessment in patients suffering from mood disorders. Many of these problems have special relevance to outpatient settings. The first has to do with the difficulty in diagnosis resulting from the presentation in the early stages of the illness, mild to moderate symptomatology, atypical aspects of the clinical picture, or the patient's stoicism in not complaining about symptoms. We have seen patients with diagnosable mood disorders who have had symptoms for over a decade without ever seeking consultation. In one case, the internist providing medical care was quite surprised at the diagnosis of major depression because the patient had never appeared depressed and had never complained of depressive symptoms. Yet the patient had a long and continuous history of depressed mood, insomnia, fatigue, feelings of worthlessness, and suicidal ideation. Many patients present with atypical forms of mood disorders. In some, the somatic manifestations may predominate, even overshadowing the expression of depressed affect. These patients are more apt to be seen in primary care medical settings than in the offices of mental health professionals. Other depressed patients present themselves not with feelings of depression but with feelings of frustration, anger, helplessness, boredom, loss of interest or pleasure, disturbed interpersonal relationships, problems at work, and the loss of meaning in life. Couples therapists commonly observe that one member of the couple has a diagnosable mood disorder that plays a major role in the marital difficulty. Often, patients present with mild symptomatology that resolves spontaneously or with brief supportive therapy. The diagnosis may be adjustment disorder or normal bereavement. It is not until the patient returns months or years later that the diagnosis of mood disorder becomes clear.

A second problem in the diagnosis and assessment of mood disorders is the presence of concomitant problems which distract the clinician from eliciting and listening for the clinical signs and symptoms of depression. These include alcoholism, drug abuse, eating disorders, mental retardation, personality disorders, marital conflict, medical illness, and aging.

A third and very serious problem in the assessment of patients with mood disorders are clinicians who ideologically oppose nosologic entities such as major depression and dysthymic disorder. These clinicians see the nosologic approach as pigeonholing patients, labeling them as having a disease, or conceding that biologic treatments are inevitable. They prefer to view patients from an individualistic approach, attending to aspects of personality, details of the precipitating events and reactions to stress to describe each patient as a unique individual. This approach, while of considerable value, ignores the added and often necessary value of the diagnostic category for prognosis and treatment.

A related problem to the above are clinicians who see the patient as suffering only from a mood disorder, to the exclusion of the unique individual problems. Such a limited assessment results in an inadequate understanding of the patient, limited treatment options, and, often, the patient's seeking another clinician.

A fifth problem is the assessment of whether the depression is the cause of the patient's maladaptive behaviors or whether the maladaptive behaviors are causing the depression. We have seen different clinical situations in which one or the other explanation predominates. Common examples of the former are those dysthymic patients whose apparently self-defeating behaviors fail to respond to psychotherapy but respond to antidepressant medications. Here the maladaptive behaviors would be seen not as causing the depression but as a manifestation or result of depression. Common clinical situations in which maladaptive behaviors appear as causal factors in depression are the personality disorders where the pathologic behaviors create interpersonal situations which are self-defeating and isolating.

For all patients who are depressed, it is important for the clinician to initiate an inquiry as to the degree of suicidal potential. It may be helpful to let the patient know that it is common for depressed patients to have suicidal thoughts. Beginning clinicians commonly have the unfounded fear that an inquiry of suicidal intentions will be detrimental to the therapeutic relationship or will give the patient the idea of suicide that he or she did not entertain until that time. We believe that asking difficult but important questions of this nature strengthens the therapeutic alliance.

For the problems in establishing the nature of the problem, there are two parts to the solution. First, the clinician should consider the hypothesis for all patients that there is a mood disorder, despite the patient's appearance and presenting complaints. This is particularly important in patients with medical illness, personality disorders, the aged, the mentally retarded, the drug abuser, and the alcoholic. Second, the clinician must provide a comprehensive, individualistic evaluation for patients with mood disorder and not assume that the assessment is adequate because a DSM-III-R diagnosis has been established. For both parts of the solution, the clinician may need to evaluate the patient for an extended period of time and/or may need to obtain confirmatory data from the patient's family.

Developing and Maintaining a Therapeutic Relationship

With the depressed patient, it is essential that the clinician communicate a genuine sense of appreciation of the uniqueness of the patient's distress. This can be done by listening to the patient's story, attempting to understand the meaning of the events antecedent to the depression, eliciting the patient's current depressive behaviors, discussing suicidal thoughts, and communicating an appreciation for the impact of the symptoms on the patient's life. In collecting this data, the clinician maintains a calm and supportive attitude, even if the situation requires firm and direct action, such as hospitalization. The clinician attempts to convey a sense of hope, reduce guilt, and provide a plan that indicates that something can be done to help the patient. Such hope is facilitated by the clinician's communication that the patient's depression is something that he or she has observed in other patients who are depressed. At the same time, premature statements of understanding may seem patronizing and ingenuine to the patient. Focusing primarily on the depressive syndrome to the virtual exclusion of the patient's life story will leave the patient feeling not understood and unwilling to go on with the evaluation and treatment. The relationship may be strengthened by the clinician's educating the patient about the causes and symptoms of depression. For certain patients, attending to their feelings of shame and humiliation over their incapacity can be quite important. For patients whose thinking and judgment have been impaired as a result of the depression, the clinician may need to be more active in the interview and more authoritative in explaining what is wrong and what needs to be done. As with the problem of assessment, it may be necessary to develop a relationship over several interviews before the patient gains enough trust to follow certain treatment recommendations.

Patients experiencing hypomania or manic episodes are notorious for their difficulty in forming a therapeutic relationship. They often present with a sense of entitlement, an intolerance of others' opinions, and a denial that anything is wrong. Paranoid ideation, when present, further complicates the situation. Bipolar patients often come for consultation only at the insistence of a relative, and it is only through the leverage provided by this relationship that assessment and treatment can be conducted. For many patients with bipolar disorder, hospitalization is necssary for the establishment of the relationship.

Communicating Information and Implementing a Treatment Plan

Many patients find it useful to learn from the clinician about the syndromal nature of their disorder. This informs them that they have one, not several, disorders and that this represents a recognizable pattern with which the clinician is familiar. The syndromal definition of the disorder can lead to the naming of the disorder: "depression," "bipolar disorder," or "manic depressive disease." Some patients find the naming and description of the disorder a relief. They may also want to think of the etiology in biologic terms, thereby medicalizing the problem. To them this helps remove the stigma. Others regard the medicalizing of the disorder to be stigmatizing and prefer to think of the problem as part of a complicated life story, an understandable psychologic response to life stress.

The major problem with a patient's particular attribution is its possible influence on which treatments a patient thinks are acceptable. Assuming that medications and psychologic treatments are helpful and complementary to a significant percentage of patients, treatment negotiations become complicated when medically minded patients view psychologic understanding as meaningless and when psychologically minded patients view medications as unhelpful, harmful, and even shameful. In our experience, psychologically minded patients who need and resist medications often accept the treatment recommendations when they feel that the clinician understands the psychologic nature of their problem and the psychologic resistance to taking medications. Medically minded patients often make use of psychologic interventions so long as

they do not have to admit to their importance.

The communication of information to the patient with bipolar disorder may require more specificity than that required for the patient with depressive disorder. Jamison (42) suggests a series of specific points that the clinician needs to communicate, such as (a) that the illness is serious but treatable; (b) if the illness is left untreated, the risk of recurrence is high; (c) lithium is effective, but has a time delay; (d) certain side effects are temporary, and others are apt to be permanent; (e) temporary setbacks are common; and (f) alcohol is apt to complicate the condition.

References

1. Weissman MM, Merikangas KR, Boyd JH: Epidemiology of affective disorders. In Michels R, Cavenar JO, Brodie HK, et al (eds): *Psychiatry*, vol 1. Philadelphia, JB Lippincott, 1968, chap 60, pp. 1–14.
2. Akiskal HS: The clinical management of affective disorders. In Michels R, Cavenar JO, Brodie HK, et al (eds): *Psychiatry*, vol 1. Philadelphia, JB Lippincott, 1986, chap 61, pp. 1–27.
3. American Psychiatric Association: *Diagnostic and Statistical Manual of Mental Disorders (Third Edition-Revised)*. Washington, DC, American Psychiatric Association, 1987.
4. Coryell W: Secondary depression. In Michels R, Cavenar JO, Brodie HK, et al (eds): *Psychiatry*, vol 1. Philadelphia, JB Lippincott 1988, chap 66, pp. 1–9.
5. Lehmann HE: Affective disorders: clinical features. In Kaplan HI, Sadock BJ (eds): *Comprehensive Textbook of Psychiatry/IV*, vol 1. Baltimore, Williams & Wilkins, 1985, pp 786–810.
6. Mendelson M: Psychodynamics of depression. In Paykel ES (ed): *Handbook of Affective Disorders*. New York, Guilford Press, 1982, pp 162–174.
7. Bibring E: The mechanism of depression. In Greenacre P (ed): *Affective Disorders*. New York, International Universities Press, 1953, pp 14–47.
8. Docherty JP, Fiester SJ, Shea T: Syndrome diagnosis and personality disorders. In Frances AJ, Hales RE (eds): *The American Psychiatric Association Annual Review*, vol 5. Washington, DC, American Psychiatric Association, 1986, pp 315–355.
9. Paykel ES: Life events and early environment. In Paykel ES (ed): *Handbook of Affective Disorders*. New York, Guilford Press, 1982, pp 146–161.
10. Hirschfeld RMA, Goodwin FK: Mood disorders. In Talbott JA, Hales RE, Yudofsky SC (eds): *Textbook of Psychiatry*. Washington, DC, American Psychiatric Press, 1988, pp 403–441.
11. Beck AT, Rush AJ, Shaw BF, et al: *Cognitive The-*

ory of Depression. New York, Guilford Press, 1979.

12. Seligman MEP: Helplessness: On Depression, Development, and Death. San Francisco, Freeman, 1975.

13. Abramson LY, Seligman MEP, Teasdale JD: Learned helplessness in humans: critique and reformulation. J Abnorm Psychol 87:49–75, 1978.

14. Goldin LR, Gershon ES: The genetic epidemiology of major depressive illness. In Frances AJ, Hales RE (eds): Review of Psychiatry, vol 7. Washington, DC, American Psychiatric Press, 1988, pp 149–168.

15. Hughes CW, Preskorn SH, Adams RN, Kent A: Neurobiological etiology of schizophrenia and affective disorders. In Michels R, Cavenar JO, Brodie HK, et al (eds): Psychiatry, vol 1. Philadelphia, JB Lippincott, 1986, chap 64, pp. 1–16.

16. Ballenger J: Biological aspects of depression: implications for clinical practice. In Frances AJ, Hales RE (eds): Review of Psychiatry, vol 7. Washington, DC, American Psychiatric Press, 1988, pp 169–187.

17. Lingjaerde O: The biochemistry of depression. Acta Psychiatr Scand 302 (suppl): 36–51, 1983.

18. Meltzer HY, Bunney WE, Coyle J, et al (eds): Psychopharmacology, the Third Generation of Progress. New York, Raven Press, 1987.

19. Boyd JH, Weissman MM: Epidemiology. In Paykel ES (ed): Handbook of Affective Disorders. New York, Guilford Press, 1982, pp 109–125.

20. Hamilton M: Symptoms and assessment of depression. In Paykel ES (ed): Handbook of Affective Disorders. New York, Guilford Press, 1982, pp 3–11.

21. Keller MB, Shapiro RW, Lavori PW, et al: Relapse in major depression disorder. Arch Gen Psychiatry 39:911–915, 1982.

22. Keller MB, Shapiro RW, Lavori PW, et al: Recovery in major depressive disorder. Arch Gen Psychiatry 39:905–910, 1982.

23. Keller MB, Lavori PW, Endicott J, et al: Double depression: two-year follow-up. Am J Psychiatry 140:689–694, 1983.

24. Keller MB: Diagnostic issues and clinical course of unipolar illness. In Frances AJ, Hales RE (eds): Review of American Psychiatry, vol 7. Washington, DC, American Psychiatric Press, 1988, p 188–212.

25. Akiskal HS, King D, Rosenthal RL, et al: Chronic depressions: part 1. Clinical and familial characteristics in 137 probands. J Affective Disord 3:297–315, 1981.

26. Akiskal HS: Subaffective diorders: dysthymic, cyclothymic, and bipolar II disorders in the 'borderline' realm. Psychiatr Clin North Am 4:25–46, 1981

27. Akiskal HS. Dysthymic disorder psychopathology of proposed chronic depressive subtypes. Am J Psychiatry 140:11–20, 1983.

28. Van Eerdewegh M, Clayton PJ: Bereavement. In Michels R, Cavenar JO, Brodie HK, et al (eds): Psychiatry, vol 1. Philadelphia, JB Lippincott 1986, chap 67, pp 1–11.

29. Prien, RF: Somatic treatment of unipolar depressive disorder. In Frances AJ, Hales RE (eds): Review of Psychiatry, vol 7. Washington, DC, American Psychiatric Press, 1988, pp 213–234.

30. Rice, JP, McGuffin P: Genetic etiology of schizophrenia and affective disorders. In Michels R, Cavenar JO, Brodie HK, et al (eds): Psychiatry, vol 1. Philadelphia, JB Lippincott, 1986, chap 62, pp 1–24.

31. Goodwin FK, Jamison, KR: Manic-Depressive Illness. New York, Oxford University Press, in press.

32. Potter WZ, Rudorfer MV, Goodwin FK: Biological findings in bipolar disorders. In Hales RE, Frances AJ (eds): The American Psychiatric Association Annual Review, vol 6. Washington, DC, American Psychiatric Press, 1987, pp 32–60.

33. Keller MB: Differential diagnosis, natural course, and epidemiology of bipolar disorders. In Hales RE, Frances AJ (eds): The American Psychiatric Association Annual Review, vol 6. Washington, DC, American Psychiatric Press, 1987, pp 10–31.

34. Clayton PJ: Bipolar illness. In Winokur G, Clayton P (eds): The Medical Basis of Psychiatry. Philadelphia, WB Saunders, 1986, pp 39–59.

35. Rosenthal NE, Sack DA, Gillin JC, et al: Seasonal affective disorders: a description of the syndrome and preliminary findings with eight therapists. Arch Gen Psychiatry 41:72–80, 1984.

36. Winokur G, Clayton PJ, Reich T: Manic Depressive Illness. St Louis, CV Mosby, 1969.

37. Akiskal HS, Khani MK, Scott-Strauss A: Cyclothymic temperamental disorders. Psychiatr Clin North Am 2:527–554, 1979.

38. Goodwin FK, Roy-Byrne P: Treatment of bipolar disorders. In Hales RE, Frances AJ (eds): The American Psychiatric Association Annual Review, vol 6. Washington, DC, American Psychiatric Press, 1987, pp 81–107.

39. Post RM, Uhde TW: Clinical approaches to treatment-resistant bipolar illness. In Hales RE, Frances AJ (eds): The American Psychiatric Association Annual Review, vol 6. Washington, DC, American Psychiatric Press, 1987, vol 6, pp 125–150.

40. Jamison KR, Goodwin FK: Psychotherapeutic treatment of manic-depressive patients on lithium. In Greenhill M, Gralnick A (eds): The Interrelationship of Psychotherapy and Psychopharmacology. New York, Macmillan, 1983.

41. Jamison KR, Akiskal HS: Medication compliance in patients with manic-depressive illness. Psychiatr Clin North Am 6:175–192, 1983.

42. Jamison KR: Psychotherapeutic issues and suicide prevention in the treatment of bipolar disorders. In Hales RE, Frances AJ (eds): The American Psychiatric Association Annual Review, vol 6. Washington, DC, American Psychiatric Press, 1987, pp 108–124.

32

Bereavement and Unresolved Grief

Aaron Lazare, M.D.

Outpatient clinicians frequently see patients with bereavement reactions (the responses to the loss of important persons) for two fundamental reasons. First, bereavement reactions are psychologically distressful conditions that are common occurrences in the general population. Second, the social institutions of family and religion that provided the support for the bereavement reactions throughout the centuries have waned in their importance to individuals in Western culture, particularly during the last half of this century.

Patients with bereavement reactions come to the attention of outpatient clinicians under several circumstances. The patient may come for evaluation during the bereavement process; a medical practitioner may seek consultation about a bereaved patient that he or she is currently treating; a patient may come for treatment for a problem that ultimately turns out to be related to a bereavement reaction that occurred years before; or the bereaved or a friend or relative of the bereaved may approach the clinician informally or on a social basis for some "advice" about the course of the bereavement process.

Because the bereavement process is so universal and predictable, it is considered normal in its uncomplicated state and has been included under a "V" code in the *Diagnostic and Statistical Manual of Mental Disorders* (*Third Edition-Revised*) (DSM-III-R) (1). Complications of bereavement are commonly thought to lead to diagnosable disorders of mood. I believe they can contribute to or complicate other diagnosable psychiatric conditions as well as psychopathology that does not meet the criteria for DSM-III-R diagnoses.

This chapter is divided into two parts. The first part reviews the current state of knowledge about normal bereavement including the depression of normal bereavement. This is essential knowledge for the outpatient mental health clinician and medical practitioner who are commonly called on to provide professional advice to patients and referring sources. The second part presents a clinical approach to conditions of unresolved grief.

BEREAVEMENT

The Epidemiology of Bereavement

The 1-year incidence rates of bereavement in the general population are estimated to range from 5% to 9% (2, 3). The wide range is a result of the various samples under study and the nature of the relationship of the loss under question. Frost and Clayton (4) report a 6% one-year incidence of bereavement in first-degree relatives in a population with an average age of 61. The death of a parent is reported to occur in 5% of the population annually. There are currently 12 million widows and widowers in the United States with a female-to-male ratio of 5 to 1 (3).

The Relationship of Bereavement to Health

Despite the methodologic complexities and limitations of studies on mortality following bereavement, results of several studies suggest that some people are at increased risk for death (3). In particular, there is a significant increase in the mortality of widowers between the ages of 55 and 74. The risk is greatest during the first year of bereavement and up to 6 years for those who do not remarry. For widows, there is no risk during the first year. Some studies show an increase in risk during the second year (2). Causes of increased death for men are infectious disease, accidents, suicides, and cardiovascular disease. Causes of increased death for women are cardiovascular disease and cirrhosis of the liver.

During the first year of bereavement, there are an increased number of medical visits for those who are already ill. Most studies in the United States show no change in physician visits or hospitalizations. Most studies do show an increase in alcohol consumption, cigarette smoking, and tranquilizer or hypnotic use. There are many reports and suggestions that bereavement leads to exacerbation of preexisting medical conditions such as cardiovascular disease, hyperthyroidism, and many others. There are little systematic data which confirm or refute this hypothesis (3).

Several studies have shown that suicide rates are higher for the widowed than for the married. Most of the suicides occurred during the first 4 years following the death, particularly during the first year. Widowed males over 60 are particularly vulnerable.

Psychological Reactions to Bereavement

Before considering the problem of unresolved grief, clinicians must be familiar with the course of uncomplicated or normal bereavement. This enables them to better identify various manifestations of pathologic grief and to be familiar with the psychologic processes that inevitably emerge in its successful treatment.

The descriptions by Lindemann (5), Parkes (6), Raphael (7), Marris (8), and Kubler-Ross (9) of the response to loss are in basic agreement with each other and correspond to the observations of most clinicians. According to these authors, the first phase, referred to as "numbness" or "impact," may last from a few hours to 2 weeks. The response to learning of the loss is shock and disbelief: "Impossible." "You are joking." "I don't believe it." Immediately thereafter, there may be outbursts of tearfulness and restlessness alternating with numbness, blunted affect, or frozen withdrawal. With the full realization of loss, the bereaved, as described by Lindemann, experiences a syndrome of somatic distress, characterized by feelings of tightness in the throat, choking with shortness of breath, the need for sighing, an empty feeling in the abdomen, lack of muscular power, and intense tension or mental pain. This somatic distress, precipitated by mention of the deceased, occurs in waves lasting from 20 minutes to 1 hour. The bereaved becomes intensely preoccupied with the deceased. "I am completely occupied by him." "I am so full of him." "I am obsessed by thoughts of her." "I wish I could get my mind off of her." At the same time, the bereaved may take on symptoms, mannerisms, habits, or personality traits of the deceased. "Sometimes when I am speaking, I do not know whether it is he or me." The bereaved yearns and pines for the deceased, walks about restlessly as if searching for him, sees people whom, for an instant, are mistaken for the deceased, and sometimes calls out the deceased's name. He or she may express irritability, anger, bitterness, resentment, and rage over the loss. These feelings may be directed toward the deceased or toward the family and friends in close proximity. There is often an attempt to focus blame and responsibility, particularly on him- or herself. "How could this have happened?" "Why didn't I insist that he see the doctor?" "I should have known." "I should not have let her drive by herself." The preoccupation with the deceased and the psychologic and somatic distress is so great that the bereaved is unable to concentrate or maintain the usual patterns of behavior. There is no zest. Every task seems a major effort. Time drags. Life seems to have no meaning.

As the bereavement process continues, the bereaved review a variety of memories associated with the deceased and their relationship to him or her. Bereaved individuals discuss these memories in considerable detail and, stimulated by the repeated inquiries of visitors, review them again and again. Eventually, they regain interest in the outside world and are able to reinvest in new relationships.

Uncomplicated grief, as described above, is said to last for less than 6 months. It is felt to be minimally disruptive to normal functioning so that the bereaved stays home from work for only a few days to 2 weeks, rarely attempts suicide, and rarely seeks psychiatric assistance. The impact of the loss, however, may last for many years in a less severe form.

The Depression of Bereavement

Despite the commonly held belief that people return to normal within 6 months of the loss, there is a persistence of depressive symptomatology in a significant number of people well after this period of time. The incidence, the nature, and the course of these depressions have been described in a series of carefully designed studies by Clayton et al. (10–13). This group studied 109 widows and widowers 1 and 13 months after the death of their spouses. By means of structured interview, they attempted to clarify the natural history of depression in the bereaved. The criteria for the diagnosis of depression were based on the Feighner et al. (14) research criteria, which include feeling depressed, sad, despondent, discouraged, blue, and low plus four of the following eight symptoms: "(1) loss of appetite or weight loss; (2) sleep difficulties including hypersomnia; (3) fatigue; (4) agitation or retardation (feeling restless); (5) loss of interest; (6) difficulty in concentrating; (7) feelings of guilt; and (8) wishing to be dead or thoughts of suicide. This cluster had to be present at the time of the interview." Using these criteria, 35% of the bereaved population were depressed at 1 month and 17% at 1 year. Thirteen percent were depressed for the entire year and 45% were depressed at some time during the year.

The depressed group, in contrast to those who were not depressed, were less apt to have attended church before the death, more apt to experience a severe reaction on the anniversary of the spouse's death, and less apt to be living with their families at the time of the last research interview (12–13 months after the death).

Since a significant percentage of bereaved people have depressive symptomatology similar to that of patients who suffer from primary affective disorder, the important question arises as to whether these two groups are the same. Bornstein et al. (13) have found that in contrast to those with primary affective disorders, the depressed bereaved are less apt to have first-degree relatives with primary depression, are less apt to have first-degree relatives with alcoholism or heavy drinking, are not more commonly women than men, and are not more commonly those with a previous treatment history of depression. In addition, the depressed bereaved rarely if ever experience the depressive symptom of retardation and are less apt to be suicidal or attempt suicide, see a psychiatrist, experience the fear of losing their mind, or require psychiatric hospitalization.

The clinical significance of these studies is threefold: First, these studies establish prospectively in a random population of bereaved the incidence and course of depressive signs and symptoms. Second, they describe some of the social factors associated with depression in the bereaved. Third, they distinguish the depression of bereavement from primary affective disorders.

Biologic / Psychodynamic / Sociocultural Aspects of Bereavement

The Biology of Bereavement

Little is known about the biology of the grieving process even though clinical observations of grieving and the morbidity of grieving suggest that cardiovascular, endocrine, and immune systems are involved. Two areas of active research on the bereavement process during the past several years are the study of the hypothalamus–pituitary–adrenal axis by use of the dexamethasone suppression test (DST) and the study of the immune response. In the three DST studies to date (15–17), it appears that those bereaved who meet the criteria for depression have normal adrenocortical responses suggesting that the depression of bereavement is (at least on this dimension) a different biologic entity than unipolar depression. Studies on the immune response suggests that there is some lymphocyte suppression in the bereaved (18–20).

Psychodynamic Perspectives on Bereavement

From observations on normal grief, Freud (21), Abraham (22), Bowlby (23, 24), Fenichel (25), Loewald (26), Siggins (27), and others have made the following psychodynamic inferences which prove useful in understanding the bereavement process.

The bereavement process in many ways prolongs in the mind the existence of the deceased until that loss can be gradually accepted. This process prevents the person from being overwhelmed by the kind of panic seen in a small child who has been abandoned by his or her mother. To accomplish this task, bereaved adults, at first, flatly deny that the death occurred. Then they search for the lost person, call

for her, cry, and express resentment in hopes that she will return as she always did in the past. When the reality of permanent separation is acknowledged, a remarkable psychologic event occurs. Whereas the bereaved may have consciously thought of their mother every few days, they now think of her con-stantly. The deceased is their obsession, is in them, is part of them, and is at times indistinguishable from them. (This is the process of introjection.) "My love object is not gone, for now I carry it within myself and can never lose it." By this mechanism the deceased is kept alive, but at a terrible price. The bereaved feel consumed, taken over, not themselves, unable to function. The ego must now begin to give up the lost object piecemeal through the review over a period of weeks and months of hundreds of separate memories and situations of expectancies. This prolonged mourning, characterized by "introjecting the relationship with the lost object, and then loosening each tie to the now internalized object" (27), prevents the flooding of feeling. In the process, "the relationship to the lost person is not abandoned but the libidinal ties are so modified" (27) that a new relationship is established based on vital and satisfying identifications.

Sociocultural Perspectives on Bereavement

There are many features of contemporary Western society that may negatively affect the recovery from bereavement. These include "the decline of kinship and religion, the nuclearization and high mobility of the family, a diminished sense of community, and the disengagement of the elderly" (28). All these factors diminish what has been referred to as social support. Kaplan et al. (29) include in the concept of support, supportive religious and social rituals, supportive values and beliefs which comfort individuals and families, norms that provide meaning, social networks, the supply and availability of nurturant others, the ability to seek and receive support, the availability of supportive others who facilitate emotional release, and the structural supports of the community and work.

There is a significant social morbidity of bereavement, particularly in widows, which has been described by Maddison and Raphael (30), Parkes (6), and Lopata (31, 32). Many widows are isolated, spend much time alone, and experience a loss of contact or change in relationship with old friends. They may be regarded as a "minority group facing discrimination, poverty, and exclusion from full participation in society. They are seen as handicapped in that they lack a mate, much of the discrimination against them being based on the fact that they are visibly different in any situation requiring a male escort. Their loneliness is often exploited, and they may be dealt with unfairly in business affairs. They also tend to be avoided because their grief and their loneliness are threatening to others, who are made anxious by such emotions" (30). This social morbidity is lessened to the degree that the widow has achieved psychologic independence and an identity separate from her husband during her married life.

The diminished social stimulation may, in itself, account for some depressive manifestations of the postbereavement period. In addition, the absent or diminished social support system deprives the person of the necessary conditions for the process of mourning.

Interventions for Uncomplicated Grief

The treatment of uncomplicated grief consists of support for expression of the various affects of grief, including sadness, anger, anxiety, hopelessness, helplessness, and despair, and facilitation of the mourning process, including review of the positive and negative aspects of the lost relationship. This treatment is elaborated in the remainder of this chapter. Raphael recently studied the lowering postbereavement morbidity in the recently bereaved. She found a significant lowering of morbidity in a high-risk intervention group as compared to a control group (33). Many

bereaved express satisfaction from the help they receive from various support groups. The value of these groups has not been documented by research.

UNRESOLVED GRIEF

Unresolved or pathologic grief refers to the clinical processes and conditions which follow the loss, usually through death, of a significant person and is characterized by (*a*) inhibition, suppression, or absence of the grief process; (*b*) exaggeration or distortion of certain symptoms or behaviors which normally occur with grief; or (*c*) the prolongation of normal grieving. Any one of these three dimensions may occur singly or simultaneously in any combination.

Many clinicians, particularly those of psychodynamic persuasion, find the concept of unresolved grief invaluable in their clinical practice. They seem to understand its theoretical basis and believe they can successfully apply the principles of treatment to a large number of suffering patients. Other clinicians and investigators find the concept of unresolved grief to be so vague and elusive that they question whether there is such a condition or whether the concept can be meaningfully applied in clinical practice. This confusion and elusiveness, I believe, is a result of there being no clearly observable syndrome of unresolved grief similar to most of the DSM-III-R categories. This is because the failure of satisfactory resolution of grief is more a process than a clearly observable behavioral constellation, and it affects individuals in unique ways according to other aspects of their psychologic functioning. In other words, it more effectively lends itself to individualistic than to categorical formulations (see Chapter 8).

The material presented in this section represents a synthesis of the work of S. Freud (21), H. Deutsch (34), Lindemann (5), Bowlby (23, 24), Parkes (6), Raphael (7), Volkan (35), and Klerman and Weissman (36) together with my own clinical observations and inferences. The content has been organized in such a way to help readers to test the value of the ideas in their own clinical practices and research facilities.

Causes of Grief Other Than Death

At the outset, it is worth extending the concept of bereavement and unresolved grief, for clinical purposes, to include losses other than death. In *Mourning and Melancholia*, Freud (21) described mourning as following the loss of some abstraction which has taken the place of a loved person, such as love of one's country, liberty, or an ideal. Clinicians also describe mourning resulting from separations, aging in loved ones, the loss of one's children's dependence, change in neighborhood, change in body image resulting from surgery (mastectomy, amputation), aging (loss of teeth, hair, beauty), and even finishing a good book. Grayson (37) has described grief reactions during psychotherapy in response to the relinquishing of unfulfilled aspirations, missed experiences, infantile wishes, and youth and dreams of youth. When this grief work occurs years after the event, it may be regarded as an unresolved or delayed grief.

My experience is similar to Grayson's— grieving is an important aspect of relinquishing neurotic behavior in psychotherapy. One patient told me in anger: "You robbed me of my gods. I must give up hope of getting back my childhood. I had a dream of being in a war, fighting for my life. . . . Now I'm left holding the bag. There is nothing any longer to cling to." Another patient reported how as a result of therapy she was losing her pathologic attachment to her depressed mother as well as losing her own lifelong depression. "I can't get depressed any longer. It makes me feel sad, lonely, and frightened." A third patient said how pleased he was that he could relinquish the neurotic belief that success would be punished by withdrawal of parental love and succorance. Remaining a small boy had sustained his feeling of security. His smile turned to tears as he said, "This calls for a celebration. How about a funeral?"

Social Causes of Unresolved Grief

Unresolved grief may result from a variety of social and psychologic factors which interfere with the patient's ability to complete the process of mourning. By such social factors it is meant the physical or psychologic unavailability of an adequate social support system which most individuals need for mourning. Psychologic factors would be aspects of the patient's personality or psychologic resources for coping which interfere with the completion of mourning. Although there is often some admixture of social and psychologic factors, one commonly sees relatively pure groups: patients who suffer unresolved grief because of personality factors even though there is a good social support system and patients who are psychologically healthy but fail to complete their grieving because of inadequate social supports.

In the proposed classification of the causes of unresolved grief (see Table 32.1, considerable weight is given to social factors, particularly the unwillingness or inability of physically available social supports to acknowledge and help the individual deal with the loss. This is consistent with the findings of Maddison et al. (30) that widows who become symptomatic or depressed perceive the environment as "overtly or covertly opposed to their free expression of emotions, particularly those of grief and anger." A further rationale for this classification is my clinical impression that patients who are unable to resolve

Table 32.1 Causes of Unresolved Grief

Social factors
  1. Social negation of the loss
  2. The socially unspeakable loss
  3. Social isolation
  4. The social role of the strong one
  5. Uncertainty over the loss
Psychologic factors
  1. Guilt and ambivalence
  2. The loss as an extension of self (narcissistic loss)
  3. Reawakening an old loss
  4. Overwhelmed by multiple loss
  5. Inadequate ego development
  6. Idiosyncratic resistance to mourning

their grief because of these social factors, in the absence of serious personality disturbances, represent a large and somewhat homogeneous group who respond to a specific treatment program which is easy to implement.

Social Negation of the Loss

Although members of a person's social network are usually supportive following the death of a parent, grandparent, sibling, or child, they may not offer support following other losses which they do not define as a loss. Common examples of such losses are abortions and miscarriages, following which friends and relatives suggest "Just forget it ever happened" (abortion) or "Just get pregnant again and then you will forget it" (miscarriage). What may never be dealt with is intense guilt over the decision to abort, rage followed by guilt toward the miscarried fetus who the mother believed almost killed her, and the loss of the patient's frustrated dreams—having the perfect child who would be fulfilled (and would fulfill the mother) in childhood, academic life, marriage, and career. I have treated patients who, following abortions or miscarriages, suffer anniversary reactions, displace their conflicted feelings onto the next born child, or search for their dead child in the faces of all children who were born the same year the fetus died.

The death of certain relationships may represent powerful losses to a person, but not elicit the necessary social support. Such relationships include divorced spouses, in-laws of divorced spouses, friends, parents of friends, household help, and pets.

In 1975 my wife and I were one of many couples who were awaiting the arrival of Amerasian Vietnamese children whom we were planning to adopt. All of us had been in communication with these children for 6 months to 2 years through the exchange of photographs and letters. The death of many of these children in a plane crash led to acute grief reactions in all the parents with whom I was acquainted.

My wife and I learned of the crash at 6:30 A.M. and spent the rest of the morning with another equally anxious couple awaiting word as to whether our children that we were about to adopt from Allambie Orphanage in Saigon were on the ill-fated plane. Our anxiety turned to acute grief at 2:30 P.M. when we received word that all of the older children on the plane from Allambie had died. My wife and I went home to stare at the photographs of our two boys, reread all of our correspondence, review our hopes and dreams, blame ourselves for not completing the paper work sooner, and weep. Some friends and relatives phoned, visited, and brought food. Others had no appreciation that the deaths of children we never met could represent a loss. They would say, "If you want to adopt children, I am sure there are plenty more in this world. Why are you so upset over these two?" This would be an example of social negation of a loss, similar in some ways to the conditions surrounding a miscarriage.

At 10:30 P.M. on the day of the plane crash, my wife and I were informed that our boys had been held from that flight and were therefore the only two survivors from Allambie. During the subsequent years, we have learned that the idealized fantasies of our grief bore little resemblance to the two real boys (now young men) who are our sons, one of whom is now a U.S. Marine and one of whom is serving in the U.S. Army.

The Socially Unspeakable Loss

There are losses which the bereaved and those around acknowledge as losses but feel are not socially appropriate to discuss. These include the death of an illicit lover (homosexual or heterosexual), death caused by the bereaved either intentionally or accidentally, death by suicide, or giving up a child for adoption. Such losses leave the bereaved feeling embarrassed, shamed, or humiliated.

With the loss of an illicit lover, the person most available for help, the spouse, is not available for support. Others may feel the bereaved deserves punishment and does not warrant any kindness. When the bereaved feels responsible or is believed to be responsible for the loss (the driver of the car in which the fatal accident occurred, the person who held the gun that accidentally fired, the mother who didn't see the child wander into the street, the mother who murdered her infant), the important people in the patient's life may fear (or wish) that they will inflict further injury by the usual inquiry, "How did it happen? Tell me about it."

I had the experience of treating a 54-year-old female whose 24-year-old daughter died from an overdose of morphine. The deceased was an attractive, intelligent, well-educated, and apparently psychologically healthy person who had no previous history of drug abuse. It was never determined whether the death was a suicide, the result of foul play, or an experiment in getting high. In the weeks following the death, no one felt comfortable asking the bereaved mother the usual questions such as when, where, and how it happened. The patient failed to grieve but developed depressive symptoms for the first time in her life. One month after the death, she made a serious suicide attempt and after a brief hospitalization was referred to me. In this therapy, which occurred weekly for 10 weeks, she experienced a typical grief reaction and terminated following the resolution of her depressive symptoms. Therapy consisted of encouraging the patient to tell her story and express emotions surrounding the loss of her daughter. During the 9 years following treatment, there has been no recurrence of depressive symptoms.

Social Isolation

Patients may be socially isolated because of their psychologic difficulty in getting close to people or because important people are unavailable for support. The latter situation has occurred on a national level as a result of such developments as (a) social mobility leaving many people geographically distant from loved ones, (b) the breakdown of the extended family, (c) the diminished importance of religious institutions with subsequent loss of their social resources, and (d) the decline in impor-

tance of the family physician. As a result, many people do not have the opportunity to get the social support necessary for grief work. Some of these people, realizing their need, present to psychiatric or medical clinics during the period of acute grief with complaints of depression or various somatic ills. Their symptoms are typical for grief—but they feel they must assume the sick role to elicit the necessary social response. The most tragic situation of social isolation occurs when the entire social support system is lost through death—the death of a person's only friend or entire family.

The Social Role of the Strong One

Optimally, the bereaved is permitted to temporarily relinquish some of the usual responsibilities of working, making financial arrangements, entertaining, cleaning house, or cooking. Neighbors and relatives bring food, while siblings or other relatives make funeral arrangements. Freed from these tasks, the individual is allowed and encouraged to be "weak," to mourn. Many of the social situations previously described leading to the absence of social support force the individual to continue his or her tasks, make the funeral arrangements, and provide psychologic support for his or her children. The bereaved is designated as the strong one who must ignore his or her own wounds and help others mourn.

Sometimes those who might provide support may insist that a bereaved person remain "strong" either because of a cultural attitude that one should always maintain a stiff upper lip or because they believe that someone in a particular role (army officer, operating-room nurse, priest, psychotherapist) should not cry or "be weak."

Uncertainty Over the Loss

In situations where there is uncertainty over the loss, those who have the opportunity to help the bereaved (as well as the bereaved themselves) are unwilling to acknowledge the loss. Such situations occur when the deceased had been kidnapped or listed as missing in action years before.

When the bereaved makes the psychologic decision that death has occurred, who will be there to help? Similarly, grief may be complicated when the "deceased" is kept alive in an intensive care unit. The acknowledgment of death by the bereaved and by those who support him or her may thus be weeks or months apart. This dilemma of uncertainty over the loss may explain some of the difficulties a spouse may have in coming to terms with a divorce. "Maybe we can get together again. Maybe she will change. There still is some possibility. I have not lost her yet." The major issue, however, which complicates grief resolution over divorce, in my opinion, is the loss of self-esteem, humiliation, and subsequent rage on the part of the person who feels betrayed.

Psychologic Factors in Unresolved Grief

Guilt and Ambivalence

The bereaved may be unable to grieve because of the enormous guilt they anticipate experiencing should the mourning process proceed. This concern over guilt occurs most commonly in patients with harsh superegos (often having many obsessional personality features) whose feelings toward the deceased are markedly ambivalent. Along with their positive feelings for the deceased is an intense hate coupled with the superego injunction "Thou shalt not hate." These mourners feel guilty because they wished the death or are relieved by the death. This ambivalence is illustrated by a man who hated his mother so intensely that he insisted an autopsy be performed despite the obvious cause of death and he urged that the body be placed in the coffin unclothed. One year later his internist referred him for psychiatric treatment when he refused to take medication for severe hypertension. Symptoms and behaviors of unresolved grief (described in the next section) were apparent in the initial interview. I ultimately concluded that his refusal to accept treatment for hypertension represented a punishment for his destructive impulses.

Guilt may result not only from ambivalent feelings but also from a responsibility patients felt they ignored, for example, not driving carefully, failing to anticipate a suicide, not watching a child go into the road or the ocean.

The Loss as an Extension of Self (Narcissistic Loss)

There may be difficulty in mourning when the person who is lost is perceived as an extension of the patient. A man who lost a son to whom he had such a relationship described his "empire" being shattered. One woman referred to her dead mother as "half of myself." Another young woman who lost a daughter who promised to be everything the patient was not felt that the death left "a gaping hole, as if something was torn out by the roots." She later explained why she had to suppress the grief response: "If I believe that she is dead, then I am dead." In psychoanalytic terminology, this may be regarded as a narcissistic loss, an "injury at a point of developmentally determined vulnerability" (38). This is in contrast to the loss of a separate, libidinally cathected object. (Undoubtedly, there are elements of narcissistic attachments in all love relationships.) Patients who suffer such a loss of self may feel they can never be the same again. "I will get over this, but I will be a different person."

Reawakening an Old Loss

Some individuals are unable to grieve a current loss because of a previous unresolved grief. It is as if acknowledging the current loss, even an apparently minor one, will reawaken all of the conflicts surrounding the previous one. These dynamics are illustrated by the case of a 54-year-old mother of one child who developed her first depressive syndrome shortly after her 22-year-old daughter moved to an apartment four blocks from the mother's home. From further historical investigation together with the associational material, the following picture emerged. The patient at age 30 failed to grieve the death of her own mother. Within 1 year, she married and gave birth to a child whom she named after her mother. The patient would not take her baby home from the hospital for 3 weeks for fear that she would drop her. It became clear that as a result of the patient's failure to grieve, the daughter was made the displaced recipient of the patient's ambivalent attachment to her own mother. When the daughter moved, feelings surrounding her mother's death were reawakened. The patient's symptoms became an angry attack on her daughter: "This illness of mine is so terrible, it will be the death of my poor daughter."

Overwhelmed by Multiple Loss

Many individuals with multiple loss have difficulty grieving. They seem too exhausted to muster the energy for the work of mourning. One patient lost eight close relatives within a few years. She had not finished grieving for one person when someone else died. (Her situation was complicated by her current condition of social isolation. Those who could have supported her grieving were now dead.) A second patient with multiple losses suffered five miscarriages due to a uterine disorder. (Her situation was complicated by the social negation of the loss.) In therapy, the patient grieved the loss of each fetus. She had had for each a name and a set of hopes and dreams.

Inadequate Ego Development

There are a group of patients (see Chapter 4) who have not achieved an adequate integration of basic ego functions necessary to experience the process of mourning. Such patients may respond to the loss of a significant other or any separation with serious ego repression. They may experience depression, anxiety, explosive rage, despair, or a hopelessness which is defended against by primitive mechanisms often leading to psychotic behavior. Masterson (39) suggests that the ego's achievement of object constancy is essential to the ability to mourn. (Object constancy, according to Masterson, refers to the "capacity to maintain object relatedness irrespective of frustration or satisfac-

tion and is associated with and perhaps dependent on the capacity to evoke a stable consistent memory image or mental representation of the mother whether she is there or not" [39]). "If one cannot evoke mental images of the lost object, how can one resolve all the painful feelings caused by this loss to form new object relations? If one cannot mourn, he becomes fatally vulnerable to object loss" (39). In a similar vein, Zetzel (40) suggests that only through developmental achievements of the early years does the ego develop the capacity for a "mature passive acceptance of the inevitable . . . a prerequisite to the remobilization of available adaptive resources at all times."

Idiosyncratic Resistances to Mourning

There are many resistances to mourning which may ultimately lead to unresolved grief. This is often more a fear of the mourning process itself than a fear of acknowledging the loss. (a) Some people feel shame when they experience themselves as weak or being seen by others as weak. The yearning and the sadness of mourning is a surrender, an injury to their self-esteem. (b) Others are concerned that their mourning will hurt those who are available and want to help. "I don't want to upset you, doctor." (c) Another common resistance stems from the patient's fear that he or she will lose control and never regain it, specifically as it relates to the outpouring of tears and emotions. One patient related, "I am afraid I will cry and cry and never stop. I will cry in the streets. I'll cry all over the entire world. And then I will drown in my tears. And then I will be a pariah." In this situation, there is the fear of damaging and being damaged by mourning. (d) Some people feel guilty as a result of the satisfying feeling of grieving.

The Diagnosis of Unresolved Grief

Diagnosing unresolved grief is a complicated task. Many clinicians, in the belief that much of living is losing while none of us fully grieve what is lost, see unresolved grief in all clinical situations. Other clinicians, observing that the vast majority of the bereaved resume functioning without the need of psychiatric help, believe unresolved or pathologic grief to be rare clinical occurrences.

From a clinician's perspective, I have formulated tentative diagnostic criteria based, in part, on response to treatment (see Table 32.2). More specifically, when one or a combination of the following symptoms or behaviors occurs after a death and continues beyond the usual period of bereavement (6 months to 1 year), I consider the diagnosis of unresolved grief. The greater the number of symptoms and behaviors, the greater the likelihood of unresolved grief. The criteria are the following:

1. A depressive syndrome of varying degrees of severity beginning with the death and lasting over 1 year. Usually these symptoms are so mild that the person does not seek psychiatric help for them.
2. A history of delayed or prolonged grief.
3. Symptoms of guilt, self-reproach, panic attacks, and somatic expressions of fear such as choking sensations and breathing attacks.
4. Somatic symptoms representing identification with the death person, often the symptoms of the terminal illness.
5. Physical distress under the upper half of the sternum, accompanied by expressions such as "There is something stuck inside" or "I feel there is a demon inside of me."
6. Searching behavior. Patients may describe moving from city to city without awareness of what they are looking for. One patient, a city dweller who had lost his mother, became obsessed with the idea of owning a farm, "searching for mother earth."
7. Recurrence of depressive symptoms and searching behavior on specific dates, such as anniversaries of the death, birthdays of the deceased, achieving the age of the deceased, and holidays, especially Christmas.
8. A feeling that the death occurred yesterday, even though the loss took place months or years ago.
9. Unwillingness to move the material possessions of the deceased. The patient often keeps the room of the deceased intact and refuses to give away or move the clothes of the deceased.
10. Change in relationships following the death. There is often change in social relationships, especially toward those who seem to be replacing the dead

Table 32.2   Symptoms and Behaviors of Unresolved Grief

1. A depressive syndrome of varying degree of severity beginning with the death.
2. A history of delayed or prolonged grief.
3. Symptoms of guilt, self-reproach, panic attacks, and somatic expressions of fear such as choking sensations and breathing attacks.
4. Somatic symptoms representing identification with the dead person, often the symptoms of the terminal illness.
5. Physical distress under the upper half of the sternum accompanied by expressions such as "There is something stuck inside" or "I feel there is a demon inside of me."
6. Searching behavior.
7. Recurrence of depressive symptoms and searching behavior on specific dates, such as anniversaries of the death, birthdays of the deceased, and holidays, especially Christmas.
8. A feeling that the death occurred yesterday, even though the loss took place months or years ago.
9. Unwillingness to move the material possessions of the deceased.
10. Change in relationships following the death.
11. Diminished participation in religious and ritual activities.
12. The inability to discuss the deceased without crying or the voice cracking, particularly when the death occurred over 1 year before the interview.
13. Themes of loss.

person such as a sibling of the deceased.

11. Diminished participation in religious and ritual activities. These include attendance in church, visits to the grave, and participation in memorial services.

12. The inability to discuss the deceased without crying or the voice cracking, particularly when the death occurred over 1 year before the interview.

13. Themes of loss. The patient's associations may be marked by themes of loss: "I am losing my food . . . My wife is leaving me . . . I am sitting on a pyramid . . . I am living in a house that my grandmother owns . . . My grandmother died 10 years ago but the house was never probated . . . My wife will leave me if I don't move from the house . . . She thinks I have a peculiar attachment to the house."

In every interview, the clinician should actively consider the hypothesis of unresolved grief (see Chapter 7) since patients rarely present this directly as their problem. Such patients are more apt to complain of depression or interpersonal problems. I specifically inquire of each patient I evaluate what people important to him or her have died and whether there have been abortions or miscarriages. If the patient cries or is on the verge of tears during this discussion, I systematically pursue the 13 categories described above.

A more complex situation occurs when the issues of unresolved grief become accessible to the patient and clinician only after a significant time has passed in psychotherapy—months or years. I treated a patient for 2 years before she confronted me directly with her reluctance to grieve the death of her husband who had committed suicide 8 years previously. From that time until the present, she was hospitalized 4 times for major depression. Tricyclics, monoamine oxidase inhibitors, and lithium were attempted without success. She told me she would not grieve because she was like a 12-year-old in that she believed that her husband would walk in the door any minute. If she grieved, he would never return. This acknowledgment began the grieving process that lasted several months. In the 7 years that followed, there have been no major depressive episodes.

Two Conditions Which Are Not Unresolved Grief

There are two clinical conditions which may be mistaken for unresolved grief when they follow a loss through death. The first includes the major functional syndromes, such as primary affective disorders and schizophrenia. Although these conditions may be triggered by the stress of death, their diagnosis, treatment, and natural history differ from unresolved grief. The manner in which people who suffer from these disorders deal with the stress of bereavement, however, remains an important but overlooked clinical problem.

The second clinical condition which is often mistaken for unresolved grief is the depression which results from the social deprivation and isolation of the bereaved—the lonely widow/widower whose primary source of social support and interpersonal gratification was his or her spouse. For these people, the grieving might be quite satisfactory from the clinician's perspective, but the depression persists. Successful treatment must include a restructuring of the social network.

The Treatment of Unresolved Grief

General Principles

Little has been written about the treatment of unresolved grief, with the notable exceptions of Volkan and Showalter (35), Raphael (7), Paul and Grosser (41), and Klerman et al. (36). There has been no research on the effectiveness of treatment for unresolved grief although, in my opinion, this condition is usually more easily and successfully treated than any of the neuroses or personality disorders. What follows are recommendations from my own experience based on the classification outlined in Table 37.1.

The goal of treatment is to help patients accomplish what they were unable to do immediately following the death—the cognitive and affective work of bereavement. Since the failure to adequately mourn resulted from the complex interaction of supportive social milieu, the nature and meaning of the loss, and the characterology of the bereaved, the specific techniques for treatment are complex and will vary from one patient to another.

At some point in the therapeutic relationship, whether the first or the twentieth interview, the patient's voice cracks and the facial muscles quiver, the eyes water and quickly turn away from the therapist. This is a critical moment, for the patient is asking the clinician to tolerate and support the painful feelings and the entire process of bereavement. The patient hopes for a compassionate supportive response communicated via the clinician's facial and verbal expression. The therapeutic process stops if the clinician looks uncomfortable, leans away, changes the subject, smiles out of anxiety, tells the patient to be strong, or urges him or her not to cry.

With patients suffering from unresolved grief, I am more directive than I am with patients in traditional psychodynamic psychotherapy. When it seems appropriate, for instance, I describe the grief work they need to do, recommend they visit the cemetery, and encourage them to speak with friends and relatives about the deceased. Such an attitude not only catalyzes the mourning process directly but also communicates to patients that I know what I am doing and can be counted on should they feel out of control.

In spite of this directive approach, the clinician must not impose on the patient a predetermined timetable for "the cure" or a specific set of treatment strategies. The clinician must be psychologically available, ready to facilitate but not force the therapeutic work.

Inadequate Social Support System

The delayed grief reactions that are easiest to treat are those that result from an inadequate social support system in rela- tively healthy individuals. The treatment is the same as that for normal grief. For these patients an interest in them, an ability to bear their painful feelings, and some gentle urging often initiate the therapeutic process. When patients begin to appear sad or tearful, I often acknowledge their "heartache," the "tears inside," or the "crying and aching inside." Patients may mourn for the entire hour or for a part of that time. They often pursue their recollections of the bereaved throughout the week by reviewing photograph albums, rummaging through attics, and speaking with other people who knew the dead relative.

When patients seem "stuck," the clinician may inquire about the deceased and his or her relation to the bereaved. "What was he like?" "What did she look like?" "What kind of person was she?" "How long was he ill?" "When did she die?" "What were his last words?" "Where were you standing in the hospital room?" "What do you wish you could have said to him?" "With whom did you ride to the cemetery?" "Where were you standing in relation to the grave?" "Which of his belongings do you cherish the most?" "What do you most miss about her?" "Do you have any photographs of her?" The purpose of such questions is to encourage the patient to recall many specific affect-laden details of the deceased. This recollection is usually accompanied by surges of emotion. I use this approach with all patients and employ alternative techniques described below only when this fails.

Ambivalence and Repressed Hostility

For patients who have difficulty grieving because of their hostility and subsequent guilt over their unconscious wishes, there are some specific techniques, in addition to those described in the two previous sections, which facilitate the therapeutic process. Although it is often important for patients to verbalize and ultimately make peace with their hostility, it is ill advised and even dangerous to unthinkingly encourage patients to simply express all of their hateful and murderous wishes and feelings. If the patients were to do this, they might feel overwhelmed and out of control; they might conclude they are hateful, evil people; or they might become frightened over losing their psychologic attachment to the person who has meant so much.

The therapist can help patients comfortably acknowledge their ambivalence without feeling like a murderer or someone out of control in several ways: (*a*) The therapeutic alliance must be adequately established. This may occur during the initial interview or after 1 year, depending on the patient's capacity for trust and the therapist's skill. (*b*) The therapist can teach the patient the meaning of ambivalence. "I know your father must have meant a great deal to you, that you loved him very much. Otherwise you could not be so upset over losing him. But when someone loves someone else so much, it is normal for there to be other kinds of feelings, disappointment, resentment, anger, for instance. It always happens, it's normal." When the patient then verbalizes some negative feelings ("I suppose he did boss me around and get under my skin. Sure I resented him."), the therapist reaffirms the positive side of the ambivalence ("Yes, and your resentment was all the more difficult for you because of how much you cared for him."). Patients, assured of the clinician's belief in them as a good and loving person and assured that their hostility did not destroy the dead person, often begin a mourning process which is highlighted by frequent comments about their ambivalent feelings. (*c*) The therapist's choice of words can be useful in helping patients comfortably talk about their ambivalence. If at the beginning of treatment the therapist encourages patients to discuss their anger, hate, or murderous wishes toward the deceased, patients are apt to deny these feelings and resent the therapist. On the other hand, patients are more apt to willingly discuss "disappointment," "irritation," "annoyance," and "aggravation." (*d*) With patients who fear that dwelling on their "bad" feelings will leave them with nothing, I offer some assurance from my experience that they will likely rediscover a

positive side of the relationship when they have made peace with their negative feelings.

Inadequate Ego Development

For patients who fail to grieve because the psychic apparatus necessary for this process is not adequately developed, the goal of therapy is overall psychologic growth, not grief work over the specific loss. If therapy is successful, the first person the patient may mourn is the therapist—at the time of termination.

Other Clinical Situations

For patients whose loss awakens a previous unresolved grief, the earlier loss may need to be mourned. This may occur before, after, or at the same time the patient deals with the current loss. When the patient is overwhelmed by multiple loss or has suffered, in the loss, a severe narcissistic injury, therapy may be painstakingly slow, lasting for many months or years. For those who cannot mourn for fear of hurting others, being abandoned, losing control, or being attacked, the clinician, as in any other psychotherapy, helps the patient verbalize these concerns, trace their historical roots when possible, and, it is hoped, work through the resistance.

For many patients their unresolved grief does not become an apparent issue until other complex psychotherapeutic issues have been dealt with over a period of months to years.

Termination

Whether the grief work is accomplished in 10 sessions or 10 months, the work of termination is an essential part of the treatment process. To ensure the work gets done, therapists must always set a date for termination far enough in advance to leave time for the therapeutic work of termination. They must avoid deciding to terminate on the day the decision is reached. When the patient cannot understand this procedure ("I feel fine. So why don't we end today?"), the therapist may explain that the very decision to stop usually awakens in people painful feelings and memories of leavings from the past and that this is an important opportunity to deal with these issues. It is not uncommon, when termination is announced, for patients to reexperience the symptoms that initially brought them to therapy. ("I feel depressed and guilty all over again. You have not helped me at all.") The clinician may feel momentarily that he or she has failed and that all the hard work has been for naught. In the subsequent therapy hours, the patient often experiences new memories and intense feelings about past losses. During this period of termination, several patients have become so distraught that they requested (or I suggested) extra interviews. After these critical weeks, patients tell me they were appreciative of my explaining to them the termination process. "It somehow made it easier to go through."

Medication

To the best of my knowledge, there are no studies of the efficacy of psychotropic agents for the depression of bereavement. In my clinical experience the vast majority of patients suffering from the depression of unresolved grief respond to the psychotherapeutic techniques previously described. If depressive symptoms do not improve or worsen, I treat the symptoms with antidepressant agents.

Countertransference

Clinicians who are most effective in treating the bereaved are those who have grieved and have enjoyed the sense of well-being and peace that has come from the process. Therapists who have the greatest difficulty are those who themselves suffer from unresolved grief and must use a great deal of energy to avoid the pain of their own feelings. Therapy may also be difficult for the therapist when the person who died is of the same age as the therapist or the therapist's spouse or children.

Criteria for Successful Treatment

The results of treatment of unresolved grief can be extraordinarily gratifying, par-

ticularly when the symptoms and behavior which may have been present for many years subside in a relatively brief period of time (2–12 months).

In addition to the resolution of the depression of bereavement, I have observed other clinical phenomena which are indicative of successful treatment.

1. Patients may verbalize how the clock of life has resumed after feeling for years that time has stood still. One patient said, "On New Year's Eve, I said goodbye 1987, goodbye 1967 (the year her husband died). I feel like I've been Rip Van Winkle all these years." Another patient who had recently begun to mourn for her son who died 1 year before said, "I think I can begin to let time go on. But that is so hard because it means that I am going on without him."

2. Following the grief work, patients often experience and describe a different kind of sadness. "Before it was a bitter sadness; now it is a sweet sadness; the axe is out of my heart." Another patient said, "There are two ways of missing something. You can feel guilty and wish it were different. Now I feel good about the relationship and wish I could have it again."

3. The patient is able to discuss the deceased with relative equanimity and with the sweet sadness or nostalgia described above.

4. Holidays, particularly Christmas and Thanksgiving, become as enjoyable as they were prior to the loss.

5. Patients who expended considerable energy searching for the deceased discontinue the search.

6. Following the resolution of unresolved grief, the patient often relates in a more healthy way to the survivors. A patient who had difficulty relating to her 2-year-old following a miscarriage that she failed to grieve felt now that her 2-year-old seemed to be "an entirely different person." Other patients have described how those close to them seem to become more distinct from others, in

sharper focus. Previously, everyone seemed to blur into one.

7. One of the most gratifying changes that occurs as a result of treatment is a discovery of and an identification with positive aspects of the deceased. The patient previously described as insisting his mother have an autopsy and be buried without clothes described the following dream near the end of treatment: "I discovered a third floor in my house. It was lovely. It was mother's room. She was making gifts. I cried because I hadn't known this human being. I didn't know there was so much good stuff there. I found a great room. I woke up crying because I hadn't known my mother." Another patient, whose deceased mother was a gifted Italian cook, dreamt of throwing dirty socks in the minestrone soup while she experienced her hostility during therapy. As she improved, she began to take great pleasure in cooking as well as make periodic visits from Boston to a famous Italian restaurant in New York City. Just before completing treatment, she related the following: "I went up to the attic and found hundreds of pounds of rags that mother had left. I sorted through all of the piles and threw away all the bad ones—but I kept the good ones."

References

1. American Psychiatric Association: *Diagnostic and Statistical Manual of Mental Disorders (Third Edition-Revised.)* Washington, DC, American Psychiatric Association, 1987.
2. Van Eerdewegh M, Clayton PJ: Bereavement. In Michels R, Cafenar JO, Brodie HK, et al (eds): *Psychiatry.* Philadelphia, J.B. Lippincott, 1988, vol 1, Chapter 67, pp 1–11.
3. Osterweis M, Solomon F, Green M (eds): *Bereavement: Reactions, Consequences, and Care.* Washington, DC, National Academy Press, 1984, pp 15–44.
4. Frost NR, Clayton PJ: Bereavement and psychiatric hospitalization. *Arch Gen Psychiatry* 34:1172–1175, 1977.
5. Lindemann E: The symptomatology and management of acute grief. *Am J Psychiatry* 101:141–148, 1944.
6. Parkes CM: Bereavement: *Studies of Grief in Adult Life.* New York, International Universities Press, Inc., 1972.
7. Raphael B: *The Anatomy of Bereavement.* New York, Basic Books, 1983.
8. Marris P: *Widows and Their Families.* London, Routledge & Kegan Paul, 1958.
9. Kubler-Ross E: *On Death and Dying.* London, Tavistock, 1970.
10. Clayton PJ, Desmarais L, Winokur G: A study of normal bereavement. *Am J Psychiatry* 125:168–178, 1968.
11. Clayton PJ, Halikas JA, Maurice WL: The depression of widowhood. *Br J Psychiatry* 120:71–77, 1972.
12. Clayton PJ: The clinical morbidity of the first year of bereavement: a review. *Compr Psychiatry* 14:151–157, 1973.
13. Bornstein PE, Clayton PJ, Halikas JA, Maurice WL, Robins E: The depression of widowhood after thirteen months. *Br J Psychiatry* 122:561–566, 1973.
14. Feighner JP, Robins E, Guze SB, Woodruff RA Jr, Winokur G, Munoz R: Diagnostic criteria for use in psychiatric research. *Arch Gen Psychiatry* 26:57–63, 1972.
15. Das M, Berrios Ge: Dexamethasone suppression test in acute grief reaction. *Acta Psychiatr Scand* 70:278–281, 1984.
16. Kosten TR, Jacobs S, Mason JW: The dexamethasone suppression test during bereavement. *J Nerv Ment Dis* 172:359–360, 1984.
17. Shuchter SR, Zisook S, Kirkorowicz C, et al: The dexamethasone suppression test in acute grief. *Am J Psychiatry* 143:879–881, 1986.
18. Schleifer SJ, Keller SE, Camerino M, et al: Suppression of lymphocyte stimulation following bereavement. *JAMA* 250:374–377, 1983.
19. Schleifer SJ, Keller SE, Meyerson AT, et al: Lymphocyte function in major depressive disorder. *Arch Gen Psychiatry* 42:484–486, 1984.
20. Schleifer SJ, Keller SE, Siris SG, et al: Depression and immunity. *Arch Gen Psychiatry* 42:129–133, 1985.
21. Freud S: Mourning and melancholia (1917). In *Collected Papers.* New York, Basic Books, 1959, vol 4, pp 152–180.
22. Abraham K: A short study of the development of the libido, viewed in the light of mental disorders. In *Selected Papers on Psycho-Analysis.* London, Hogarth Press, 1927, pp 418–501.
23. Bowlby J: Processes of mourning. *Int J Psychoanal* 42:317–340, 1961.
24. Bowlby J: Pathological mourning and childhood mourning. *J Am Psychoanal Assoc* 11:500–541, 1963.
25. Fenichel O: *The Psychoanalytic Theory of Neurosis.* New York, W. W. Norton, 1945.
26. Loewald H: Internalization, separation, mourning, and the superego. *Psychoanal Q* 31:483–504, 1962.
27. Siggins LD: Mourning: a critical survey of the literature. *Int J Psychoanal* 47:14–25, 1966.
28. Osterweis M, Solomon F, Green M (eds): *Bereavement: Reactions, Consequences, and Care.* Washington, DC, National Academy Press, 1984, pp 199–214.

29. Kaplan BH, Cassell JC, Gore S: Social support and health. *Medical Care* 15:47–57, 1977.

30. Maddison D, Raphael B: Death of a spouse. In Grunebaum H, Christ J (eds): *Contemporary Marriage: Structure, Dynamics, and Therapy*. Boston, Little, Brown, 1976, pp 187–227.

31. Lopata H: The social involvement of American widows. *Am Behav Sci* 14:41–49, 1971.

32. Lopata H: *Widowhood in an American City*. Cambridge, MA, Schenkman Publishing, 1973.

33. Raphael B: Preventive intervention with the recently bereaved. *Arch Gen Psychiatry* 34:1450–1454, 1977.

34. Deutsch H: Absence of grief. *Psychoanal Q* 6:12 1937.

35. Volkan V, Showalter CR: Known object loss, disturbance in reality testing, and "re-grief work" as a method of brief psychotherapy. *Psychiatr Q* 42:358–374, 1968.

36. Klerman GL, Weissman MM, Rosaville BJ, et al: *Interpersonal Psychotherapy of Depression*. New York, Basic Books, 1984.

37. Grayson H: Grief reactions to the relinquishing of unfilled wishes. *Am J Psychother* 25:287–295, 1970.

38. Anable WR: Homicidal threat as grief work. *Psychiatr Opinion* 15:43–46, 1978.

39. Masterson JF: *Psychotherapy of the Borderline Adult. A Developmental Approach*. New York, Brunner Mazel, 1976.

40. Zetzel ER: Depression and the incapacity to bear it. In Schur M (ed): *Drives, Affects, Behavior*. New York, International Universities Press, vol 2, 1965.

41. Paul NL, Grosser GH: Operational mourning and its role in conjoint family therapy. *Community Ment Health J* 1:339–345, 1965.

33

Anorexia Nervosa and Bulimia Nervosa

David B. Herzog, M.D.
Andrew W. Brotman, M.D.
Aline L. Bisgaier, B.A.

Anorexia nervosa and bulimia nervosa are syndromes describing disturbances in appetite, eating behavior, and body image. The terms *anorexia nervosa*, meaning "a nervous loss of appetite" and *bulimia*, which translates as "ox hunger" reflect early attempts to describe these disorders. Criteria for anorexia nervosa and bulimia, Axis I syndromes, were delineated in the *Diagnostic and Statistical Manual of Mental Disorders (Third Edition)* (DSM-III) in 1980, and revised for the DSM-III-Revised (DSM-III-R) (see Tables 33.1 and 33.2). Revisions in DSM-III-R criteria for anorexia nervosa include the addition of amennorhea (in females) for 3 consecutive months, a reduction of the weight loss criteria from 25% to 15%, and the deletion of the criteria excluding physical causes for weight loss, since anorexia nervosa can coexist with disorders such as Crohn's disease and diabetes mellitus. Bulimia is now classified in the DSM-III-R as "bulimia nervosa," a distinct disorder from anorexia nervosa, and both disorders can coexist. The revised criteria continue to include episodic binge eating and feelings of lack of control, but eliminate weight fluctuations, inconspicu-

Table 33.1   Anorexia Nervosa[a]

DSM-III criteria
1. Refusal to maintain normal body weight.
2. Loss of more than 25% of original body weight.
3. Disturbance of body image.
4. Intense fear of becoming fat.
5. No known medical illness leading to weight loss.

DSM-III-R criteria
1. Refusal to maintain body weight over a minimal normal weight for age and height, e.g., weight loss leading to maintenance of body weight 15% below expected.
2. Intense fear of becoming obese, even when underweight.
3. Disturbance in the way in which body weight, size, or shape is experienced, e.g., the individual claims to "feel fat" even when emaciated, believes that one area of the body is "too fat" even when obviously underweight.
4. In females, absence of at least three consecutive menstrual cycles when otherwise expected to occur (primary or secondary amenorrhea). A woman is considered to have amenorrhea if her periods occur only following hormone, e.g., estrogen, administration.

[a] Reprinted with permission from American Psychiatric Association: *Diagnostic and Statistical Manual of Mental Disorders (Third Edition-Revised)*. Washington, DC, American Psychiatric Association, 1987. Copyright 1987 American Psychiatric Association.

Table 33.2   Bulimia Nervosa[a, b]

DSM-III criteria

1. Recurrent episodes of binge eating.
2. At least three of the following:
   a. consumption of high-calorie, easily ingested foods during a binge;
   b. termination of binge by abdominal pain, sleep, or vomiting;
   c. inconspicuous eating during a binge;
   d. repeated attempts to lose weight;
   e. frequent weight fluctuations of more than 4.5 kg.
3. Awareness of abnormal eating patterns and fear of not being able to stop voluntarily.
4. Depressed mood after binge.
5. Not due to anorexia nervosa or any physical disorder.

DSM-III-R criteria

1. Recurrent episodes of binge eating (rapid consumption of a large amount of food in a discrete period of time).
2. During the eating binges there is a feeling of lack of control over eating behavior.
3. The individual regularly engages in either self-induced vomiting, use of laxatives, strict dieting, fasting, or vigorous exercise in order to prevent weight gain.
4. A minimum average of two binge-eating episodes per week for at least 3 months.
5. Persistent overconcern with body shape and weight.

[a] Reprinted with permission from American Psychiatric Association: *Diagnostic and Statistical Manual of Mental Disorders* (*Third Edition-Revised*). Washington, DC, American Psychiatric Association, 1987. Copyright 1987 American Psychiatric Association.

[b] Referred to in DSM-III as bulimia.

ous eating, and depressed mood following a binge from the diagnostic criteria.

Eating disorders may affect as many as 5% to 10% of adolescent girls and young women (1). Morbidity and mortality rates associated with anorexia nervosa are among the highest recorded for psychiatric disorders. Despite substantial scientific and public interest in these disorders during the past two decades, they remain enigmas. This chapter describes the epidemiologic, pathophysiologic, and treatment aspects of anorexia nervosa and bulimia nervosa.

EPIDEMIOLOGY

Studies indicate that the incidence of anorexia nervosa has doubled over the past two decades. A retrospective study of treated cases in Monroe County, New York shows an increased incidence from 0.35 per 100,000 population in 1960–1969 to 0.64 per 100,000 population in 1970–1976 (2). In a defined region of Switzerland, the incidence of treated cases increased from 0.38 per 100,000 in the 1950s to 1.12 per 100,000 in the 1970s (3). There is considerable evidence that this increased incidence reflects an actual rise in the number of cases and cannot be explained by increased recognition or hospitalization for less serious illness. In 1976, Crisp et al. estimated the prevalence of anorexia nervosa (treated and untreated cases) in British private secondary school populations to be 1% (4).

Reports on the incidence of bulimia nervosa have varied. Studies of female high school and college students have found that between 4.5% and 18% of the students suffer from bulimia (5, 6). In a recent survey of medical students we found that almost 12% of the female students had a lifetime history of bulimia (7). Although a lesser frequency in nonuniversity settings has been noted, Pope et al. found that 10% of female shoppers surveyed at a suburban mall had a lifetime history of bulimia nervosa (1).

Between 90 and 95% of the anorectic and bulimic population is female. Although most anorectics are reported to be from White, upper class families, recent studies have indicated an increasingly varied population across social classes and races. Eating disorders occur over a wide age spectrum, from preadolescence to well into adulthood. The onset of anorexia nervosa tends to be at a younger age than bulimia nervosa. Anorexia nervosa has a bimodal age of onset at 13 to 14 years and 17 to 18 years (8), whereas the onset of bulimia nervosa usually occurs in late adolescence or young adulthood.

CLINICAL PICTURE

Anorexia Nervosa

Case Vignette

Fourteen-year-old Cathy had always been a shy, well-behaved child who worked hard to maintain a straight-A average in school. Other students teased her about being a book worm, but she claimed their ridicule didn't bother her. She was, however, very sensitive to her classmates' comments about her body, which was developing much faster than most of the other girls. Cathy decided that in order to avoid being teased, she would go on a strict diet and lose 10 pounds. At first her efforts were modest; she ate only half of her lunch and claimed she was too full to finish dinner. In a couple of months, Cathy had lost 8 pounds and her diet began to gain momentum. She resolved to lose even more weight, and began to skip lunch altogether and eat as little as possible at dinner.

Every morning, Cathy would weigh herself and examine her body in a full length mirror. Although she was pleased that her breasts were getting smaller, she wanted her hips, chest, and stomach to be completely flat. Cathy's parents began to worry about her weight loss and eating habits, but whenever they succeeded in getting her to eat, she would carefully calculate the number of calories she had ingested and attempt to burn them off with rigorous exercise. Before her parents insisted she see a pediatrician, Cathy's weight had dropped from 118 to 88 pounds, dangerously low for her 64" frame, and signs of severe malnutrition (her body temperature was 96°F, her pulse 43) were apparent.

Initially in individual psychotherapy, Cathy would not engage in any spontaneous talk. However, in family sessions, it became apparent that Cathy was seen as the perfect child in a family that valued accomplishments, not feelings, and she had never felt understood. Gradually, the family was able to acknowledge each other's strengths and weaknesses, and Cathy developed healthier strategies to help her separate from her parents.

Anorexia nervosa typically begins in a teenager who is slightly overweight or perceives herself to be overweight. The initial diet, which may be moderate, escalates into an obsessive preoccupation with thinness. Weight loss is achieved by severe restriction of caloric intake or through purging techniques (vomiting, laxatives, ipecac, or diuretics) to compensate for calories consumed. Excessive physical activity to achieve or maintain weight loss is also common in anorectics and may be an early sign of incipient anorexia nervosa.

Clinically these patients may appear either cheerful and alert or withdrawn and sad. They often are controlling and manipulative in their behavior, think only in terms of good/bad or black/white, and deny the severity of their illness. Like Cathy, anorectics are frequently achievement oriented and socially isolated. Studies have found between 25% and 74% of anorectic patients to be depressed (9, 10).

Peculiar behavior concerning food is also common in individuals with anorexia nervosa. They often prepare elaborate meals for others, but tend to restrict themselves to a narrow selection of low-calorie food. In addition, food may be hoarded, concealed, crumbled, or thrown away.

Anorexia nervosa may begin abruptly or may be an insidious process lasting months to many years. It may manifest as a single circumscribed episode; in a cyclical fashion, with several exacerbations and remissions; or in a chronic, unremitting course, leading to death. Suicide has been reported in 2% to 5% of patients with chronic anorexia (11, 12). Follow-up studies at 2 years indicate that despite weight gain and resumption of menses in most cases, social maladjustment in family relationships and pathologic eating habits persist in more than half the patients. Furthermore, vocational functioning is good, but more than one-third of the patients have recurrent affective illness and one-fourth do not regain menses or attain 75% of their ideal weight (13).

Bulimia Nervosa
Case Vignette

Andrea, a 28-year-old sculptress, presented for treatment with a 7-year history of almost daily bingeing and purging. Abnormal eating behaviors began at around age 10 when Andrea would sneak whole boxes of crackers, stuffing them into her mouth. She later remembered that "it felt calming—it was something just for me."

The patient is the second oldest of five children. Her mother was a successful writer, but was frequently depressed, occasionally suicidal, and generally overwhelmed with the responsibility of taking care of five children. She described her father, an alcoholic lawyer who had frequent extramarital affairs, as inconsistent and unavailable.

The initial phase of therapy was stormy, with Andrea oscillating between being sexually seductive and angry. The therapist's vacations were experienced as abandonment and responded to with missed sessions, threatened termination of therapy, and exacerbation of bulimic symptoms. With frequent interpretations and confrontations, Andrea began to describe a "push–pull" inside of her—alternately drawing close to people then feeling overwhelmed and fleeing—using bulimia as a way of regulating her closeness to the people in her life.

The topic of antidepressant medication was introduced about a year and a half into treatment because of continued depression and bulimic behaviors. Andrea was originally resistant and 8 months later continued to be quite ambivalent about the medication, although she reported a notable decrease in her anxiety, depression, and urge to binge while on it. She initially portrayed the drug as an agent of the therapist's invasion and control, but gradually revealed fantasies of nurturance and impregnation—being attracted to the sense of being "fed" yet frightened that she would "lose herself" in the feelings of caring for and being cared about by the therapist.

After 3 years of therapy, Andrea began to describe the people in her life in a much more genuine fashion. She continued to binge and purge, although with much less frequency and intensity than before, and it no longer held the place in her life that it once did. Although she still struggled with issues of closeness and identity, this struggle lacked the sense of stormy confusion for her that it once had.

Bulimia nervosa typically begins in a late adolescent who has attempted various methods of weight loss without much success. Either accidentally or through a friend, the bulimic becomes aware of self-induced vomiting or laxative abuse as a means of weight loss. Bulimics usually binge on "junk food" high in carbohydrates and may set aside time each day for solitary bingeing. This preoccupation is exacerbated by the embarrassment frequently experienced by the bulimic woman about her food-related symptoms. After eating, she feels out of control and ashamed (14). Unlike the anorectic, the bulimic is usually distressed by her symptoms and willing to accept help.

There is a remarkable disparity between how good the bulimic appears on the outside and how inadequate she feels inside. She is superficially sociable and frequently involved in heterosexual relationships. Her peers perceive her as strong and giving, but in reality, the bulimic is often plagued by conflicts with intimacy and dependency, manifests intense mood swings, and has difficulties managing aggression.

Bulimia nervosa is a chronic episodic disorder. Studies have found a wide variance in recovery rates from bulimia, ranging from 13% to 71% after 2 to 5 years of follow-up (15, 16). Relapse rates are also quite high. Mitchell and colleagues (17) contacted 75 patients 12 to 15 months after an outpatient evaluation in an eating disorders unit and found that 40% of those who had recovered had relapsed. In a prospective naturalistic study of 30 bulimic patients, we found that at 18 months 57% had recovered (defined as a minimum of 8 weeks with no or only residual symptoms) from the index episode of bulimia. However, 53% of those who had recovered had relapsed (defined as at least 2 weeks of meeting full DSM-III criteria for the disorder). Seventeen of the 30 patients had had a concomitant affective illness at intake. Of these 17, only 8 had recovered from both conditions at 18 months, of which 88% (7 out of 8) had relapsed into one or both disorders. Notably, depression at intake did not affect the probability of recovery from bulimia—59% of those with concomitant depression recovered from bulimia, compared with 54% of the nondepressed bulimics.

PHYSICAL MANIFESTATIONS

Both anorexia nervosa and bulimia nervosa can cause potentially life-threatening medical complications. The complications of anorexia nervosa are largely those of starvation, while those of bulimia nervosa result from bingeing and purging. Anorexia nervosa has been associated with cardiovascular, hematologic, renal, endocrine, and skeletal changes. Physical manifestations include amenorrhea, hypotension arrythmias, hypothermia, anemia, delayed gasttric motility, growth failure, lanugo (neonatallike hair), and osteoporosis (18). The gastrointestinal abnormalities may produce an exaggerated sense of stomach fullness, abdominal pain, or constipation. It is noteworthy that with rapid refeeding peripheral edema is common (18).

The bulimic often presents with a medical problem that developed as a result of her bingeing and purging behavior. The diagnosis of bulimia nervosa may be suspected if there is dental enamel erosion, electrolyte abnormalities, abrasion of the knuckles from induced vomiting (Russell's sign), or otherwise unexplained parotidomegaly (18). Over 40% of bulimic patients experience menstrual irregularities, particularly if a past history of anorexia nervosa is present. Repeated use of ipecac to induce vomiting can lead to chronic absorption of the drug and cause a potentially fatal myocardial dysfunction (18). Electrolyte abnormalities can also result from chronic vomiting.

PATHOPHYSIOLOGY

Sociocultural Perspective

The cultural value placed on slimness in Western society has played an important role in the development of eating disorders. The current physical ideal for women is a healthy thin body. A study of *Playboy* centerfolds and Miss America winners found that their bust and hip measurements as well as their weight have gradually decreased over the last 25 years (19). At the same time, the American population as a whole has become heavier (20).

Although there is little question that women are at greater risk for eating disorders than men, the source of this difference is not known. Several investigators have suggested that our culture teaches women to define themselves in terms of how they are perceived by others, leaving them dependent on an external audience. The resulting overemphasis on physical appearance and weight may predispose young women to abnormal eating behaviors.

Certain populations may be more likely to develop eating disorders by virtue of their occupations. The emphasis on physical appearance in modeling and ballet dancers may increase the risk of eating disorders (21). Long-distance runners, in their preoccupation with food, emphasis on a lean body mass, and denial of physical discomfort, often resemble female anorectics. Though "obligatory runners" show considerably less psychopathology than anorectics when on the Minnesota Multiphasic Personality Inventory (22), poor eating habits developed in athletic training may result in an eating disorder that continues long after the runner has ceased competition.

Biologic Perspective

Several neurochemical abnormalities have been noted in both anorexia nervosa and bulimia nervosa. The search for a specific abnormality in anorexia is complicated by the accompanying state of starvation which alone produces extensive changes in hypothalamic and metabolic functioning. Complications of starvation include abnormalities in the cerebrospinal fluid levels of central nervous system metabolites, including 3-methoxy 4-hydroxyphenylglycol, homovanillic acid, 5-hydroxyindoleacetic acid, and tyrosine (18). Furthermore, the rate of cortisol production, which is decreased in starvation, is increased in anorexia nervosa and returns to normal with weight gain (23). Some changes, however, cannot be attributed to starvation alone. Twenty percent of anorectic patients lose menses before any significant weight loss occurs. Anorectics also exhibit decreased levels of cerebrospinal fluid arginine vasopressin long after weight recovery (24). These neurotransmitter disturbances may be indicative of an underlying neurochemical disturbance in patients with anorexia nervosa.

Studies of bulimic patients suggest possible central neurochemical disturbances of the serotonergic and noradrenergic systems. Manipulations that increase serotonin are known to produce satiety and decrease carbohydrate ingestion in several animal models (25). Research has suggested that bulimics have a low level of serotonin, predisposing them to binge (26). The noradrenergic system has only been implicated indirectly through imipramine, a norepinephrine reuptake inhibitor, which has been effective in reducing bingeing in some patients (27).

Psychologic Perspective

While impaired psychologic development is often viewed as the core of anorexia nervosa and bulimia nervosa, there has been no agreement as to the specific developmental lesion. Failure to progress at every developmental stage, from infancy to adolescence, has been observed. Bruch described the anorectic's sense of ineffectiveness, faulty interoceptive awareness, and body image disturbance, relating these symptoms to early childhood experiences (28). She theorized that if appropriate responses from the mother are chronically lacking, such as when the mother feeds the child primarily to keep her quiet or put her to sleep, the child cannot learn how to differentiate her own needs from those imposed by others. As the child grows older she achieves feelings of competence, effectiveness, and control

by rejecting her own appetitive needs and becoming thin. Distorted attitudes such as the superiority of asceticism to self-indulgence, perfectionism as an attainable goal, and that weight gain means one is bad or out of control may affect almost every aspect of their lives (29).

Palazzoli evolved a similar theory of the origins of anorexia nervosa (30). Her view, like Bruch's, focuses on the helplessness of the ego: The anorectic does not perceive her body as belonging to her but as a threat, something that must be controlled. Palazzoli, using Fairbairn's model of object relationships, suggests that the anorectic experiences her body as the maternal object from which the ego must separate. She then incorporates the dreaded maternal object in an effort to control it. Central to this formulation is a mother who rewards compliance to her wishes, is overprotective, and is unable to tolerate efforts of the child to separate.

Geist, following a self-psychology perspective, proposes that the mother of the anorectic child, while allowing her daughter to identify with her, is unable to mirror any thoughts or feelings different from her own (31). This leads to the subordination of the child's self to a narcissistic extension of the mother, as well as a turning toward the father for mirroring and empathy that was lacking in the maternal relationship. Geist believes that this father–daughter bond is threatened by the sexual maturation of the daughter, which explains in part the onset of anorexia nervosa in adolescence.

Ego psychologists propose an ego defect as causative in bulimia nervosa, theorizing a lack of object constancy (32). When separated from the symbiotic mother, the bulimic is unable to evoke a mental image of the good, soothing mother. Bingeing is used as a means to evoke this representation, since the patient is deficient in the internal structures needed to regulate herself which were originally provided by the mother.

The psychodynamic and object relations theories discussed above describe anorexia nervosa and bulimia nervosa as a failure to separate and individuate and gain a sense of autonomy. The bias that defines autonomy as the goal of development in our culture has been questioned by researchers studying normal female development (33). They propose that in contrast to boys, for whom identity development is the outcome of increasing separation and gained autonomy, the female personality naturally develops through attachment to others. One of the adolescent female's major challenges is to confirm her worth through interpersonal relationships. It follows that the negative or positive value that any given culture might place on relationships would affect her sense of self-worth. In the past 20 years, a shift in societal values toward women have led to devaluing of relationships in favor of autonomy and independence. Similarly, female adolescents must struggle to accept their changing bodies in a culture that encourages them to try to alter their bodies to fit a narrowly defined ideal of beauty. Steiner-Adair proposed that eating disorders have erupted in this culture because of an unrealistic overemphasis on autonomy in women (34). In a study testing the relationship of eating disorders to girls' perceptions of cultural values, Steiner-Adair found that teenage girls who could identify and challenge new societal values of autonomy and independence for woman scored in the non-eating-disordered range on the Eating Attitude Test. All but one of the girls who blindly identified with society's image of the new independent women at the expense of relationships and dependence scored in the eating-disordered range on this questionnaire. Steiner-Adair postulates that the onset of anorexia nervosa in adolescence may result from the developmental crisis in which females must shift from a relational approach to life to an autonomous one, a shift that can represent much pain if independence is associated with isolation. The rounded female body is universally associated with mothering and the interdependency of people. The anorectic, in rejecting the symbolic parts of her body, is colluding with the current cultural norm.

In contrast to therapists who study the individual's conflicts in the etiology of eating disorders, family therapists view the eating-disordered patient as using her symptoms as a way of crying for help for her conflict-ridden family. The families of anorectics are often characterized by enmeshment, oscillating between overprotectiveness and abandonment (35). The daughter's rigidity and perfection can reflect similar values in her mother. The parental relationship may be deeply troubled by mutual difficulties in intimacy and trust, but masked by a facade of smooth functioning and family loyalty. Minuchin observed that the symptomatic child often serves to diffuse parental conflicts and that the maturation of the symptomatic child disrupts the balance of the family system (36).

TREATMENT

The treatment of anorexia nervosa and bulimia nervosa is extremely challenging. The onset of these disorders frequently precedes presentation for treatment by several years. It is not uncommon for a bulimic to present for evaluation after struggling alone with the disorder for 5 to 8 years. While the bulimic is usually initially accepting of treatment, she may often have a low frustration tolerance and quickly may terminate treatment that does not provide immediate symptom relief.

The anorectic is generally more elusive to treatment than the bulimic. In her obsession with thinness, she has found a solution to her deep-seated feelings of sadness and inadequacy. She often denies the severity of her illness, as does her family, who may cling to the idea that there is a medical rather than psychologic reason for their daughter's problems. Furthermore, the family communication system is often pathologic. The families tend to recreate their home environment among the clinicians who are involved in the treatment. Rather than face divisive issues within the family, families tend to focus on differences of opinion among the treating clinicians and use this to split the physicians. For example, instead of talking about whether the parents are contemplating separation, the family will tell Dr. X that Dr. Y does not understand them as well as he does. It is imperative that clinicians communicate frequently so that they avoid being split and can help the family refocus their energy.

Hospitalization

The initial task of the clinician is to assess the patient's health status and risk of death. Suggested indications for hospitalization include

1. Weight loss greater than 30% over 3 months;
2. Severe metabolic disturbances (pulse less than 40 per minute, temperature less than 36°C, systolic blood pressure less than 70 mm / Hg, serum potassium less than 2.5 mEq/l despite oral potassium replacement);
3. Severe depression or suicide risk;
4. Severe bingeing and purging;
5. Failure to maintain outpatient weight contract;
6. Complex differential diagnosis;
7. Psychosis;
8. Family crisis;
9. Needs for confrontation of individual and family denial and initiation of individual therapy, family therapy, and pharmocotherapy.

Hospitalization may occur on a pediatric or psychiatric ward, depending on several factors. Patients with significant suicide risk or family crises are usually better managed on a psychiatric ward, while those hospitalized with the goal of nutritional rehabilitation can be adequately treated on a medical ward, if the staff feels comfortable treating these disorders and a behavior protocol exists.

Outpatient Treatment

The outpatient treatment program should be designed to meet the needs of the individual patient. Ideally, the patient's initial evaluation should include a physical exam, psychiatric evaluation, nutritional history, and in many cases a family evaluation. While some patients can be managed by one clinician, multiple treatment programs are often indicated. The severely ill patient will require a team of clinicians, including a psychiatrist and internist or pediatrician. For all patients, an initial approach should include medical monitoring and behavioral treatment for weight recovery or control of bingeing and purging.

Psychodynamic Psychotherapy

Individual psychotherapy is the most commonly employed modality for outpatient treatment. The therapist first must establish trust through the acknowledgment of the patient's ongoing pain and recognition of the multiple determinants of the disorder (social, psychologic, biologic, behavioral, and familial). The goal of therapy is to help the patient uncover her own inner resources and potential for thinking and feeling other than through her eating symptoms.

Dynamic psychotherapy is a common treatment modality. However, a traditional analytic mode of relating may prove more harmful than helpful with these patients. The anorectic frequently views her early development as a series of concessions to other people's demands and expectations. In a rigid psychoanalytic setting, she may experience the analyst's silence as rejection or his or her interpretations as intrusions. As Bruch has pointed out, the therapist may have to do much of the talking in the beginning stages of therapy (28).

The eating disorder may be viewed as a compromise solution to unsolvable psychologic conflicts. These may include a simultaneous desire for autonomy and dependence and the need to be in complete control of a body that refuses to cease having appetites. In the course of psychotherapy, erroneous attitudes and assumptions are recognized, defined, and questioned so that they eventually can be modified. The therapist must have the patience to proceed slowly, using small, concrete events to challenge deeply held beliefs. The treatment of these patients requires a great degree of flexibility on the part of the therapist, who at times may need to speak frequently, educate, offer support and encouragements, and set behavioral limits.

Many patients benefit from a thorough description of anorexia nervosa or bulimia nervosa. Often, they are surprised to learn that their ideas and feelings have been experienced by others. Painful as their symptoms may be, patients are often relieved to find that the therapist can value them as partial solutions to unresolvable psychologic dilemmas and will not force the patient to give up these symptoms without helping to install other coping mechanisms. The therapist, too, must listen to the patient's impressions about the etiology and function of her eating disorder; often these patients have remarkable insight concerning the nature of their dilemma, despite its tenacity. They are often reassured by the therapist's knowledge and curiosity about eating disorders since it contradicts the expectation that others will be disgusted and bewildered by the disorder.

In a study of the process of recovering from anorexia nervosa, we interviewed 16 former anorectics, who previously had met full DSM-III criteria for the disorder and now consider themselves recovered. When asked what advice they would give to others suffering from anorexia nervosa, the most frequent answer was to find a good therapist or friend "whom you can relate to, talk with; who confronts your feelings and helps you accept yourself for what you are and not what you are trying to be." Fifteen of the sixteen had had experience with individual psychotherapy, which was rated both the most helpful and most potentially harmful of treatment modalities. An honest, nonjudgmental therapist who could be firm yet empathic, provide explanations and encouragement, and validate and deal with current feelings was rated as most helpful. Harmful features of psychotherapy include a therapist who is overly formal, emphasizes behavioral change, has little knowledge of eating disorders, strictly adheres to his or her own theory, and has inexplicit goals.

In the overall treatment of anorexia nervosa or bulimia nervosa, psychotherapy can provide a matrix through which other modes of treatment are available. If individual therapy can lead to a relationship of mutual trust, the patient who initially refuses medication may accept it; those who feel isolated may enter a group. In general, patients require a therapeutic relationship over an extended period of time in order to effectively use group, family, and drug treatment.

Cognitive–Behavioral Therapy

Much of the work with behavioral therapy for eating disorders has been done on inpatient units where weight restoration has been the main goal of treatment. Most inpatient eating disorder units use therapeutic contracts which specify the amount of weight gain required each week and tie weight gain to greater privileges, while providing negative reinforcement for lack of compliance. Obviously, in an outpatient setting the clinician cannot attempt to monitor day-to-day variables as closely, but the idea of an outpatient therapeutic contract, behavioral goals, limit setting, and examination of underlying cognitive distortions is an approach gaining wider acceptance.

The concept of establishing an outpatient treatment contract with an anorectic or bulimic has been somewhat controversial in the past but is widely used today. For the anorectic, the central part of such a contract is establishing a minimum weight below which the therapist feels it is no longer safe to continue outpatient treatment and inpatient hospitalization would be required. Since most therapists believe that an inpatient hospitalization is required in the face of unchecked weight-loss, establishing this minimum weight in advance makes sense so that all parties recognize what the limits of their behavior can be.

The weight that is chosen is somewhat arbitrary in light of the fact that no studies have documented exactly what weight is medically dangerous. Two weights are usually chosen, the first being a goal weight which can be approximately 90% of the patient's ideal body weight and which provides a therapeutic goal for treatment, and the second being the minimum acceptable weight for outpatient treatment to continue. This weight depends on how emaciated the patient is when she begins outpatient treatment and is usually designed to prevent the individual from losing more weight. For example, a 5' 4" woman who premorbidly was 125 pounds may come into treatment having lost 35 pounds over the prior 8 months. The therapist might establish 80 pounds as the minimum weight below which outpatient treatment is no longer feasible and inpatient treatment is required. At the same time, weekly contracts for modest weight gain of a pound or two once stabilization has taken place should be established, with a goal weight of 105 pounds. The patient is asked to agree to accept a referral for inpatient hospitalization if she goes below the minimum outpatient weight, and this agreement should be made before treatment commences. In this way all parties know what the behavioral parameters are and that the consequence of not complying with this agreement is inpatient hospitalization. If the patient reneges on her agreement, the therapist should provide an appropriate inpatient referral anyway, evaluate the patient for involuntary commitment (a very rare occurrence), and tell the patient that outpatient treatment cannot continue until the minimum weight is established. This treatment plan requires that the patient be weighed on a regular basis by the therapist, internist, or nutritionist involved.

In bulimia the outpatient contract is not as straightforward because weight, in most cases, is not the predominant issue, since the majority of bulimics are of normal weight. However, in serious cases of bulimia other parameters, specifically, serum potassium determination and vital signs, may be useful to examine on a regular basis. Should these variables be in the dangerous range, the therapist might make a contract specifying at what point inpatient hospitalization would be required. However, contracts such as these and the necessity for inpatient hospitalization are usually much less frequent for normal-weight bulimics than for anorectics.

The principles of the cognitive–behavioral approach can be illustrated using the bulimic disorder where the initial goal is clearly symptom reduction rather than an insight-oriented understanding of the pathogenesis of the problem. Three stages of treatment are outlined by Fairburn (37). In the first stage there is an attempt to stop habitual overeating and purging by having the patient initially see the therapist two to three times a week while keeping a journal to monitor what food she eats, when it is eaten, and where it is eaten. After self-monitoring is established, the patient is asked to eat three to four planned meals a day at specified times regardless of hunger. She is told that her hunger cues have been disturbed by the bulimic disorder and in order to reestablish normal eating preplanned patterns must be in place. Under Fairburn's schema bingeing is addressed first with the assumption that self-induced vomiting will cease when bingeing is controlled. Early therapy sessions focus exclusively on attempts to control eating. This first stage may last for several weeks. In the second stage, appointments are weekly and the emphasis remains on reviewing the patients' eating habits. Cognitive approaches are introduced in an attempt to challenge the patient's distorted thinking. For example, if a patient believes she is fat one day and thin the next, she might be able to test this by weighing herself or measuring her waistline.

In the final stage of treatment appointments are every 2 to 4 weeks, with the focus of treatment on the maintenance of change. Patients are told to expect periods of dyscontrol, are assured this is not necessarily a setback, and are asked to prepare written lists of activities which they can employ to combat these episodes. Under Fairburn's schema, the course of therapy lasts approximately 4 to 5 months and the emphasis is almost exclusively on symptom control.

Short-term goal contracts, constructing lists of alternate activities, time-delay tactics, relaxation techniques, and log keeping are all employed in this type of treatment. Cognitive approaches modified from Beck's technique are used to treat low self-esteem, body-image distortion, hopelessness, and other self-destructive cognitive styles associated with anorexia nervosa and bulimia nervosa (38).

In our experience, a multidimensional approach in which aspects of cognitive–behavioral therapy are used, particularly early in treatment, but followed by more insight-oriented approaches, is most effective. Cognitive–behavioral and dynamic approaches are not mutually exclusive, and many therapists use aspects of both.

Group Therapy

Group therapy may be prescribed in conjunction with other modalities or as the sole treatment for the moderately ill eating-disordered patient. Three major models of outpatient group treatment include psychodynamic groups, self-help groups, and cognitive–behavioral groups.

The psychodynamic group initially offers a safe setting for members to discuss the illness and find relief from their feelings of shame and isolation. Over time, the group focuses more on inner experiences and interpersonal relationships, and the members explore the particular meanings behind their own eating symptoms. Through interpreting correlations between past experiences, current relationships, and interactions within the group, psychodynamic group treatment can be a powerful therapeutic tool (39).

Self-help groups, such as Overeaters Anonymous or the Anorexia Nervosa Aid Society, offer support and encouragement to people with eating disorders. Members can develop a degree of self-worth from contact with others who have recovered or improved as well as become aware that change is possible (40). Usually, these groups involve little or no financial cost and can also serve as a source of information about both the disorder and other treatment modalities.

The cognitive–behavioral therapist plays the same role in group and individual treatment. As described above, techniques such as journal keeping, meal planning, and time-delaying behavior are used (41). Similar to cognitive–behavioral groups are time-limited psychoeducational groups, which are based on the assumption that the symptoms of bulimia nervosa are learned behaviors which can be unlearned.

Family Therapy

Family therapy is often used in conjunction with individual therapy in adolescents or young adults with an eating disorder. The four approaches of family therapy that have been applied to the treatment of eating disorders are structural family therapy, structural–strategic therapy, systemic family therapy, and symbolic–experimental therapy.

Structural family therapy is commonly used to treat the families of anorectics. The therapist focuses on changing patterns of family behavior centered on the issues of competency and power, while at the same time reinforcing clear boundaries between family members (42). Anorexia nervosa is seen not as a disease leaving the patient helpless and unable to eat, but as a fierce rebellion to which the parents can respond with firmness.

In structural–strategic therapy, indirect intervention is used by the therapist as a means of altering rigid family beliefs and behavioral patterns. Indirect or "paradoxical" techniques are used when the more open structural approach is likely to provoke denial of the problem. (42). For example, discouraging change in a patient is one method that has been successfully used. Instead of encouraging the patient to give up her purging, the therapist stresses all the problems that might result if she were to give up the symptom "too quickly."

Systemic therapy redefines the eating-disordered patient's behavior as one of the many difficulties in the family. Rigid family belief systems and cross-generational coalitions are examined. The therapist attempts to "positively reframe" the symptom as it relates to other behavioral patterns in the family system which preserve cohesiveness and protect against change (35).

The symbolic–experimental family therapy approach centers on unresolved emotional issues dating from the parents' childhood and how these issues have been passed on to the children. The therapist helps to resolve issues involving the lack of individuation and separation in the family in an effort to help them achieve greater self-understanding (43).

Pharmacotherapy

Anorexia Nervosa

A number of medications have been tried in the treatment of anorexia nervosa, most prominently the antipsychotics, antidepressants, and cyproheptadine, an antihistamine. Chlorpromazine was probably the most used medication in the 1950s and 1960s. Although no controlled studies have ever been done using this medication for anorexia, a number of reports suggest that it may reduce resistance to weight gain and may have a direct appetite stimulation and weight-gain effect (44). Side-effects include weight gain, hypotension, akathisia, and tardive dyskinesia. It is rarely used today, except transiently and in low doses or for anorectic patients who have concomitant psychotic illness.

A number of higher potency antipsychotics have been used in placebo-controlled crossover studies for anorexia nervosa, including pimozide, sulpiride, and thiothixine (45). The short duration of treatment makes it difficult to interpret the results of these studies, except to say that the use of antipsychotics may have a clinically insignificant weight-gain effect and that they are not usually indicated. They might be used in patients with concomitant psychotic illness or in patients with overwhelming anxiety when minor tranquilizers fail. However, the distortion of

body image which is central to anorexia nervosa does not seem to respond to antipsychotic medications.

The literature describing the treatment of anorexia nervosa with tricyclic and heterocyclic antidepressants is actually quite sparse. This is true for both open and controlled studies. In the late 1970s case reports on successful treatment of anorectic patients with amitriptyline and imipramine appeared. These anecdotal reports noted that patients seemed to have a response rate to modest doses by gaining weight and having a decrease in depressive symptoms and abnormal attitudes toward food.

Hudson et al. recently published data on a series of nine patients meeting the criteria for anorexia nervosa, several of whom also had concomitant bulimia (46). The patients were treated with a variety of antidepressant medication including tricyclics, trazadone, and monoamine oxidase inhibitors. The authors found that four of these patients significantly improved by achieving weight gain and having a decrease in depressive symptomatology. Of interest is that all four of these responders had concomitant affective disorder.

In open studies, most patients were engaged in other psychotherapeutic treatment modalities, and most had been inpatients during some portion of the medication trial. There is a suggestion that anorectics with concurrent affective illness may do better on antidepressants than anorectics without such disorders; however, the numbers are small and no generalizable conclusions can be reached from these reports.

Controlled studies have used amytriptiline (47), clomipramine (48), cyproheptadine (49) and lithium carbonate (50). In one study, amitriptyline was found to be somewhat better than placebo, but in a second study there was no difference between amytriptiline and placebo. There have been several studies of cyproheptadine with conflicting results. The latest report shows that it may be moderately helpful for inducing weight gain and decreasing depressive symptoms in anorectics. However, this was an inpatient study, and the authors recommend the medication only as an adjunctive treatment and do not believe it has a substantial impact outside of a more comprehensive treatment program.

Lithium carbonate was found superior to placebo in an 8-week study, but the results were not clinically meaningful and investigators do not generally advocate the use of lithium for anorectics except in the context of manic–depressive illness.

Lacey et al. treated 16 anorectic patients for 10 weeks using 50 mg of clomipramine, a serotonergic reuptake inhibitor not currently available in the United States, and found the medication had no substantial effect on weight gain when compared with placebo.

Taken together, the results of these studies suggest that thymoleptic medications used in controlled trials do not generally show superiority over placebo for the treatment of anorexia nervosa. Statistical significance has not generally translated into clinical significance, and most of these studies were short-term, inpatient-based trials where other forms of nonpharmacologic treatment were the primary modalities being used. Long-term effects of psychotropic medications with anorectics are not known, and at this point in time pharmacologic treatment of the disorder is rather discouraging.

Bulimia Nervosa

In the last 10 years there have been more than 30 reports on the pharmacologic treatment of bulimia nervosa, of which approximately one-third have been controlled, double-blind studies. Most of the medications studied have been antidepressants, and the results to date are much more encouraging than studies conducted for anorexia nervosa.

When pharmacologic research on bulimia nervosa and compulsive eating began in the 1970s, most of the literature concerned phenytoin. Although early results were encouraging, further research proved equivocal and this medication is rarely used in clinical practice.

Five placebo-controlled, double-blind studies with antidepressants have been completed, of which three were strongly positive—desipramine (51), imipramine (27), phenelzine (52)—one was marginally positive—amitriptyline (53)—and one was negative—mianserin (54). Less than 100 patients have completed controlled trials with any medication for bulimia, but preliminary results tend to show that in therapeutic doses antidepressants can decrease bingeing and purging over the short term, even without the presence of concomitant depression.

Other double-blind studies with very few subjects have used d-amphetamine, fenfluramine, and carbamazepine (55), but the methodologic weaknesses of these studies prevent any generalization into clinical utility.

The available evidence on small numbers of patients suggests that antidepressants may be effective in treating bulimia nervosa. However, the outcome measure is usually the frequency of bingeing and purging, and even patients who "respond" may still have bulimia nervosa. Furthermore, some long term studies which are now being reported suggest that the antibulimic effect of antidepressants may not persist over time and that patients may require multiple successive antidepressant trials in order to maintain or have an improved response. Further, follow-up reports suggest that bulimics may be particularly susceptible to the side effects of medications, and may choose to go off these medications even if they are effective.

It also seems clear that the presence of major depression is not necessary for antidepressants to be helpful in this disorder. It is not now possible to predict which subgroups, if any, will preferentially respond to antidepressants. Their use is guided by clinical judgment, and we offer some guidelines for their use below.

Clinical Considerations in the Drug Treatment of Eating-Disordered Patients

Anorexia Nervosa

Anorectic patients will often refuse pharmacotherapy either because of the syntonicity of the disorder, fear of loss of control, fear that taking medication means they are crazy, or misinformation concerning effects and side effects of medication. Their families may also wish to deny that their child has a psychiatric disorder that may respond to medication and thus may collude with the patient in her refusal to take it. In addition, these patients may be exquisitely sensitive to side effects and frequently report excessive sedation, insomnia, or dizziness even at very low doses. It is important to spend time telling the patient about the medication and its uses. Most anorectics want to be well informed, and the therapist should ally with their cognitive style and respect their wish for information. We want to make clear that psychotropics should not be employed as the sole treatment modality for anorexia nervosa but only as an adjunctive therapy in the context of a psychotherapeutic relationship.

We recommend the use of an antidepressant as a first choice for pharmacotherapy for the anorectic with concomitant major depressive disorder. In addition, the anorectic with neurovegetative signs or recurrent dystonic preoccupations or rituals may benefit from a tricyclic antidepressants or monoamine oxidase inhibitor. The choice of the specific agent involves several factors. Although amitriptyline is the best studied tricyclic in anorexia nervosa, it frequently produces uncomfortable side effects, particularly excessive sedation and anticholinergic effects. Imipramine and desipramine have not been well studied in anorexia nervosa but are clinically useful in our experience.

We generally initiate treatment with either imipramine or desipramine. We have found desipramine produces fewer side effects than other tricyclics; however, it is more expensive and this may be an important consideration.

As discussed previously, anorectic patients may present with medical complications (56). Routine laboratory tests before initiating pharmacotherapy should include a complete blood count, serum electrolytes, liver function tests, blood urea nitrogen, creatinine, thyroid functions, and an electrocardiogram. Metabolic and physiologic abnormalities should be at least partially corrected prior to the administration of antidepressants. In general, medication should begin at a low dose (not more than 25 mg) and slowly be titrated upward. Plasma blood levels should be drawn to determine whether the patient has taken medication and whether the dose is adequate.

An adequate response should be evaluated by parameters which include weight gain, increased interest in eating, fewer obsessional thoughts and compulsive rituals, reductions in depressive symptomatology, decrease in anxiety, and willingness to participate in a treatment program.

Other medications including cyproheptadine and lithium could be tried with the anorectic patient who is not responding to psychotherapy or traditional antidepressant treatment. Antianxiety agents have not been well studied but can be useful, especially around meal time, to reduce food-related anxiety.

Bulimia Nervosa

Bulimic patients are also often resistant to accepting medication. They express concerns that they may get hooked on the drug, that drugs are an artificial way of treating the problem, that they may get fat, or that taking medication means that they are extremely disturbed. We have found that excessive weight gain and carbohydrate craving are not common side effects among bulimics treated with antidepressants. We believe that use of antidepressants plus psychotherapy is more effective than either modality alone in most conditions. We emphasize again that we usually do not recommend psychotropic medication as the sole intervention in bulimia nervosa, except in selected patients not appropriate for therapy, and only with close supervision. Bulimic patients require a thorough psychiatric evaluation, particularly because of the common association with affective illness, anxiety disorders, suicidality, substance use disorders, and severe character pathology. Furthermore, the patient deserves a medical screening because of the potential for medical complications.

We recommend pharmacotherapy for the bulimic who has concomitant major depressive disorder, substantial depressive or anxiety symptomology, or significant obsessive–compulsive symptomatology, or who has been resistant to the usual psychotherapeutic interventions. Extreme caution is recommended in the outpatient setting with bulimics who are unreliable, are suicidal, abuse drugs, or have severe character pathology when there is a poor therapeutic alliance.

We usually begin drug treatment for bulimia nervosa with desipramine or imipramine taken entirely at bedtime. We start with a low dose of 25 mg and gradually increase to about 3.5 mg / kg per day of body weight by the 3rd week. Medication is taken at bedtime since at that time it is unlikely to be lost through purging. We recommend monitoring tricyclic plasma levels in order to ensure that the medication is being taken and to determine if the dose is adequate. Responses to medication are evaluated by noting a lessening of bingeing and purging behaviors and a decrease in depressive symptomatology or obsessive or anxiety symptoms.

In those patients who do not respond to an adequate trial of a tricyclic we usually try another class of antidepressant such as a monoamine oxidase inhibitor. In our experience some depressed bulimics will have an excellent response only with respect to their depression, while others will get a response only with respect to their bulimic symptoms. Most will have some improvement even though less than one-third will be "cured" and the long-term outcome is currently not known. We recommend that bulimics who have not responded to psychologic treatments should be given a trial of medication regardless of the presence of depression.

THE CLINICAL INTERVIEW

The Nature of the Problem

Eating disorders have been widely publicized in the media over the last few years, and many patients present for an evaluation because they believe they have a definable syndrome. It is critical that the evaluator "play dumb" by asking questions and not assuming that words like "anorexia" or "bulimia" mean the same thing to all people. Some consider a "binge" to be three cookies, while others can consume 10,000 calories. Since "normal" eating is difficult to categorize, the evaluator needs to assess whether a particular patient has an eating disorder or is just overly concerned about food.

Generally, DSM-III-R criteria are useful guidelines to indicate pathology. However, motivation for treatment also involves the degree to which the disorder "gets in the way" of the individual's leading a gratifying life. Some patients are not terribly distressed or inconvenienced by the disorder, and this is a poor prognostic sign. Others use the eating disorder as a "ticket" to get into psychotherapy—a "legitimate" reason to seek help with issues that go beyond eating. Still others seek consultation with eating-disorder "experts" because they are dissatisfied or have transference problems in their current treatment.

Eating disorders are symptom complexes which do not imply a specific type of psychopathology—high-functioning neurotics, personality-disordered individuals, and low-functioning schizophrenics can all have "bulimia nervosa." The evaluator needs to understand what the eating disorder means to the patient, identify comorbid syndromes, understand the patient's request (or clarify it when appropriate), and only then make treatment recommendations.

Developing and Maintaining a Therapeutic Relationship

With anorexia and bulimia, we find it useful to define acceptable parameters of behavior within which outpatient treatment is possible and beyond which hospitalization is necessary (see section on cognitive–behavioral therapy). Weight, potassium level, laxative abuse, medication compliance, and medical condition are among the parameters which could be selected depending on the clinical presentation. Discussion of this plan with the patient and family (if appropriate) before treatment is agreed to can lessen problems in the future and limit the "Should I or shouldn't I hospitalize" dilemma which frequently occurs with eating-disordered patients.

We use long-term psychotherapy primarily with patients whose personality disorders are coexistent with the eating disorder. Transference relationships can be intense, and the patient may express herself by losing weight, testing a weight contract, purging, or using other behaviors peculiar to eating disorders.

Communication Information and Implementing a Treatment Plan

Some treaters are thoroughly convinced that a particular treatment modality is indicated for an eating disorder and communicate that commitment to the patient. Some clinicians feel, for example, that time-limited cognitive–behavioral treatment is *the* treatment for bulimia, while others have the same belief in medication. Some believe that family therapy is the only way to treat anorexia. They project utmost confidence in their approach based on research findings and / or experience and are frequently charismatic in style.

This "one disorder–one treatment" approach has several advantages. The clinician becomes expert in one treatment modality, clearly states the limits of what it does, is convinced of its efficacy, and knows when to stop treatment and refer elsewhere if the patient doesn't respond. There is clearly therapeutic value in adhering to a specific theory which can inspire confidence in the patient.

On the other hand, we have seen many patients who have failed a treatment thought to be definitive, only to become hopeless and demoralized. Further, many patients with eating disorders are well informed about treatment approaches and

have strong ideas regarding the type of treatment they seek. To this extent, patients are sometimes selecting the treatment on the basis of what modalities are offered.

We favor an eclectic, pragmatic approach wherein it is not unusual for a patient to be treated with individual therapy, a cognitive–behavioral group, and medication at the same time, depending on the clinical presentation and the patient's request. We believe that if one approach doesn't work, try another, because there is no definitive treatment. This philosophy does have pitfalls, in that it implicitly suggests to the patient that an answer exists and we will try endlessly to find it. In psychotherapy, promising more than one can deliver invariably is a mistake. This is especially true with severely ill eating-disordered patients.

CONCLUSION

Anorexia nervosa and bulimia nervosa are poorly understood disorders that must be viewed as multidetermined. There is currently extensive research on these disorders, and in the next decade or so there should be substantial advances in the knowledge of their epidemiology and treatment. As the medical profession and lay public have become increasingly informed about these disorders, the mortality rates for anorexia nervosa have declined. Evaluation of the eating-disordered patient should be comprehensive and include a nutritional history, medical exam, and psychiatric interview. Treatment should be multimodal and may include a combination of individual psychotherapy, pharmacotherapy, group therapy, nutritional counseling, ongoing medical management, and family therapy. The treating clinician should be well informed about the disorder, flexible in his or her approach, and modest in setting treatment goals. Furthermore, idiosyncratic eating behaviors and attitudes are prevalent in young women and merit assessment in all patients in this category.

References

1. Pope HG, Hudson JI, Yurgelun-Todd D: Anorexia nervosa and bulimia among 300 women shoppers. *Am J Psychiatry* 141:292–294, 1984.
2. Jones DJ, Fox MM, Babigian HM, et al: Epidemiology of anorexia nervosa in Monroe County, New York: 1960–1979. *Psychosom Med* 42:551–558, 1980.
3. Willi J, Grossman S: Epidemiology of anorexia nervosa in a defined region of Switzerland. *Am J Psychiatry* 140: 564–567, 1983.
4. Crisp AH, Palmer RL, Kalucy RS, et al: How common is anorexia nervosa? A prevalence study. *Br J Psychiatry* 128:549–554, 1976.
5. Halmi KA, Falk JR, Schwartz E: Binge-eating and vomiting: a survey of a college population. *Psychol Med* 11:697–706, 1981.
6. Pyle RL, Mitchell JE, Eckert ED, et al: The incidence of bulimia in freshmen college students. *Int J Eat Disord* 2(3):75–85, 1983.
7. Herzog DB, Pepose M, Norman DK, et al: Eating disorders and social maladjustment in female medical students. *J Nerv Ment Dis* 173:734–737, 1985.
8. Halmi KA, Casper RC, Eckert ED, et al: Unique features associated with the age of onset of anorexia nervosa. *Psychiatr Res* 1:209–215, 1979.
9. Kirstein L: Diagnostic issues in primary anorexia nervosa. *International Journal of Psychiatry in Medicine* 11:235–244, 1982.
10. Rollins N, Piazza E: Diagnosis of anorexia nervosa: a critical reappraisal. *J Am Acad Child Psychiatry* 17:126–137, 1978.
11. Seidensticker JF, Tzagournis M: Anorexia nervosa—clinical features and long term follow-up. *J Chron Dis* 21:361–367, 1968.
12. Stonehill E, Crisp AH: Psychoneurotic characteristics of patients with anorexia nervosa before and after treatment and at follow-up 4–7 years later. *J Psychosom Res* 21:187–193, 1977.
13. Hsu LKG, Crisp AH, Harding B: Outcome of anorexia nervosa. *Lancet* 1:61–65, 1979.
14. Abraham SF, Beumont PJV: How patients describe bulimia and binge eating. *Psychol Med* 12:625–635, 1982.
15. Abraham SF, Mira M, Llewellyn-Jones D: Bulimia: a study of outcome. *Int J Eat Disord* 2:175–180, 1983.
16. Lacey H: Bulimia nervosa, binge eating and psychogenic vomiting: a controlled treatment study and long term outcome. *Br Med J* 286: 1609–1613, 1983.
17. Mitchell JE, Davis L, Goff G, et al: A follow-up study of patients with bulimia. *Int J Eat Disord* 5:441–450, 1986.
18. Herzog DB, Copeland PM: Eating disorders. *N Engl J Med* 313:481–487, 1985.
19. Garner DM, Garfinkel PE, Schwartz D, et al: Cultural expectations of thinness in women. *Psychol Rep* 47:483–491, 1980.
20. *Build Study 1979.* Chicago, Society of Actuaries and Association of Life Insurance Medical Directors of America, 1980.
21. Frisch RE, Wyshak G, Vincent L: Delayed menarche and amenorrhea in ballet dancers. *N Engl J Med* 303:17–19, 1980.
22. Blumenthal JA, O'Toole LC, Chang JL: Is running an analogue of anorexia nervosa? An empirical study of obligatory running and anorexia nervosa. *JAMA* 252:520–523, 1984.
23. Doerr P, Fichter M, Pirke KM, et al: Relationship between weight gain and hypothalamic pituitary adrenal function in patients with anorexia nervosa. *J Steroid Biochem* 13:529–537, 1980.
24. Kaye WH, Ebert MH, Raleigh M, et al: Abnormalities in CNS monoamine metabolism in anorexia nervosa. *N Engl J Med* 308:1117–1123, 1983.
25. Wurtman RJ: Behavioral effects of nutrients. *Lancet* 1:1145–1147, 1983.
26. Kaye WH, Ebert MH, Gwirtsman HE, et al: Differences in brain serotonergic metabolism between nonbulimic and bulimic patients with anorexia nervosa. *Am J Psychiatry* 141:1598–1601, 1984.
27. Pope HG, Hudson JI, Jonas JM, et al: Bulimia treated with imipramine: a placebo-controlled double-blind study. *Am J Psychiatry* 140:554–558, 1983.
28. Bruch H: *Eating Disorders: Obesity, Anorexia Nervosa, and the Person Within.* New York, Basic Books, 1973.
29. Garner DM, Bemis KM: A cognitive–behavioral approach to anorexia nervosa. *Cog Ther Res* 6:123–150, 1982.
30. Selvini Palazzoli, M: *Self-starvation.* London, Chaucer Publishing, 1974.
31. Geist RA: Therapeutic dilemmas in the treatment of anorexia nervosa: a self-psychological perspective. In Emmett SW (ed): *Theory and Treatment of Anorexia Nervosa and Bulimia.* New York, Brunner/Mazel, 1985, pp 268–288.
32. Weiss SR, Ebert MH: Psychological and behavioral characteristics of normal-weight bulimics and normal-weight controls. *Psychosom Med* 173:395–400, 1983.
33. Gilligan C: *In a Different Voice.* Cambridge, MA, Harvard University Press, 1982.
34. Steiner-Adair C: The body politic: normal female adolescent development and the development of eating disorders. *J Am Acad Psychoanal* 14:95–114, 1986.
35. Selvini-Palazzoli M: *Self-Starvation: From Individual to Family Therapy in the Treatment of Anorexia Nervosa.* New York, Jason Aronson, 1976.
36. Minuchin S, Rosman BL, Baker L: *Psychosomatic Families: Anorexia Nervosa in Context.* Cambridge, MA, Harvard University Press, 1978.
37. Fairburn CG: Cognitive–behavioral treatment for bulimia. In Garner DM, Garfinkel PE (eds): *Handbook for Psychotherapy in Anorexia Nervosa and Bulimia.* New York, Guilford Press, 1985.
38. Garner DM, Bemis KM: Cognitive therapy for anorexia nervosa. In Garner DM, Garfinkel PE (eds): *Handbook of Psychotherapy in Anorexia Nervosa and Bulimia.* New York, Guilford Press, 1985.
39. Brotman AW, Alonso A, Herzog DB: Group ther-

apy for bulimics: clinical experience and practical recommendations. *Group* 9:15–23, 1985.

40. Malenbaum R, Herzog DB, Eisenthal S, et al: Overeaters Anonymous: a self-help therapeutic group with impact on bulimia. *Int J Eat Disord* 7:139–143, 1988.

41. Fairburn CG: A cognitive–behavioral approach to the treatment of bulimia. *Psychol Med* 11:707–711, 1981.

42. Schwartz R, Barrett MJ, Saba G: Family therapy for bulimia. In Garner DM, Garfinkel PE (eds): *Handbook of Psychotherapy in Anorexia Nervosa and Bulimia*. New York, Guilford Press, 1985.

43. White M: Anorexia nervosa: a transgenerational system perspective. *Fam Proc* 22:255–273, 1983.

44. Dally PJ, Sargant W: A new treatment for anorexia nervosa. *Br J Med* 1:1770–1774, 1960.

45. Hsu LKG: The treatment of anorexia nervosa. *Am J Psychiatry* 143:573–581, 1986.

46. Hudson JI, Pope HG, Jonas JM, et al: Treatment of anorexia nervosa with antidepressants. *J Clin Psychopharmacol* 5:17–22, 1985.

47. Biederman J, Herzog DB, Rivinus T: Amitriptyline in anorexia nervosa: a double-blind study. *J Clin Psychopharmacol* 5:10–16, 1985.

48. Lacey JH, Crisp AH: Hunger, food intake and weight: the impact of clomipramine on a refeed-ing anorexia nervosa population. *Postgrad Med J* 56:79–85, 1981.

49. Halmi KA, Eckert E, Falk JR: Cyproheptadine for anorexia nervosa. *Lancet* 1:1357–1358, 1982.

50. Gross HA, Ebert MH, Faden VB, et al: A double-blind controlled trial of lithium carbonate in primary anorexia nervosa. *J Clin Psychopharmacol* 1:376–381, 1981.

51. Hughes PL, Wells LA, Cunningham LJ, et al: Treating bulimia with desipramine: a placebo-controlled double-blind study. *Arch Gen Psychiatry* 43:182–186, 1985.

52. Walsh BT, Stewart JW, Roose SP et al: Treatment of bulimia with phenelzine: a double blind placebo controlled study. *Arch Gen Psychiatry* 41:1105–1109, 1984.

53. Mitchell JE, Groat R: A placebo controlled double blind trial of amitriptyline in bulimia. *J Clin Psychopharmacol* 4:186–193, 1984.

54. Sabine ET, Yonae A, Forringten AT, et al: Bulimia nervosa: a placebo controlled double blind trial of mianserin. *Br J Clin Pharmacol* 16:1955–2025, 1983.

55. Pope HG, Hudson JI: Antidepressant drug therapy for bulimia: current status. *J Clin Psychiatry* 47:339–345, 1986.

56. Brotman AW, Rigotti NA, Herzog DB: Medical complications of eating disorders. *Compr Psychiatry* 26:258–272, 1985.

34

Anxiety Disorders

John H. Krystal, M.D.
Wayne K. Goodman, M.D.
Scott W. Woods, M.D.
Dennis S. Charney, M.D.

INTRODUCTION TO THE ANXIETY DISORDERS

The anxiety disorders are perhaps the most common clinical condition diagnosed and treated by outpatient psychiatrists. In Chapter 18, the authors describe four states in which anxiety symptoms are prominent: (*a*) normal anxiety, (*b*) anxiety states with a known "organic" etiology, (*c*) other psychiatric diagnoses which are associated with anxiety, and (*d*) the anxiety disorders.

The anxiety disorders are clinically distinguished by the nature of the anxiety experience, its precipitants, and course. The cardinal diagnostic features for the anxiety disorders are panic attacks, anticipatory anxiety, generalized anxiety, obsessions, and compulsions. Panic attacks are sudden episodes of intense anxiety which may be associated with a feeling of impending doom, loss of control, or humiliation. Somatic symptoms are also prominent and the *Diagnostic and Statistical Manual of Mental Disorders* (*Third Edition-Revised*) (DSM-III-R) panic criteria require at least four of the following symptoms: dyspnea, dizziness, faintness, palpitations, tachycardia,

trembling, sweating, choking, nausea, abdominal distress, depersonalization, derealization, paresthesia, hot and cold flashes, chest pains, as well as the cognitive symptoms noted above. Anticipatory anxiety is a fear state generated by a predicted confrontation with an unpleasant stimulus. Generalized anxiety is defined in DSM-III-R as an "unrealistic or excessive worry about two or more life circumstances" (1). Unlike panic attacks, generalized anxiety does not have a sudden onset and tends to be long-lasting, so that a person may wake up in the morning and experience a steady level of discomfort throughout the day until going to sleep. Obsessions are egodystonic intrusive thoughts which are generally resisted by the sufferer. Compulsions are repetitive purposeful behaviors which may be performed in response to an obsession or without clear precipitants.

This chapter is organized into descriptive, theoretical, and therapeutic components. The descriptive sections, "Diagnosis" and "Epidemiology and Course," introduce the reader to the major anxiety diagnoses, their course, and their epidemiology. This review should facilitate differential diagnosis and clarify current thinking about difficult diagnostic issues, such as comorbidity.

The theoretical components are contained in the sections "Etiology and Pathogenesis," "Genetic Models," and "Integrating Etiologic Models." These sections begin to integrate diverse areas of research fundamental to the anxiety disorders including clinical neuroscience, developmental neurobiology, molecular biology, genetics, learning theory, and developmental psychology. These sections provide a neurobiologic framework for considering interactive contributions of genetic and environmental factors on the development of the anxiety disorders.

The treatment of the anxiety disorders is reviewed in the sections "Treatment" and "The Clinical Interview." In order to avoid overlap with other chapters, some aspects of the anxiety disorders were abbreviated in this review. The authors refer the reader to Chapter 18 for the medical differential diagnoses for the anxiety disorders and Chapters 45 and 48 for psychotherapeutic strategies for these patients.

DIAGNOSIS

In this section we shall discuss the importance of the symptoms described above in the differential diagnosis of the anxiety disorders, including panic disorder, phobic disorders, generalized anxiety disorder (GAD), post-traumatic stress disorder (PTSD), and obsessive–compulsive disorder (OCD).

Panic Disorder

Panic attacks are the cardinal symptomatic marker for panic disorder. Historically psychiatry initially resisted differentiating clinical anxiety syndromes by the presence or absence of panic attacks. For example, in 1894, Freud combined two forms of anxiety, panic attacks and chronic anxiety, under the rubric of anxiety neurosis (2). This pattern was continued in DSM (3) and DSM-II (4). However, Klein et al. (5) found that the tricyclic antidepressant imi-

pramine produced remission of panic symptoms in anxiety patients without altering the severity of their generalized anxiety. This finding suggested that panic attacks might distinguish "panic disorder" from a generalized anxiety syndrome. The DSM-III adopted this distinction and introduced the diagnoses of panic disorder and GAD (6). According to DSM-III, the criteria for panic disorder included at least three panic attacks within a 3-week period. These attacks could not occur during marked physical activity, during a life-threatening situation, or only during exposure to a circumscribed phobic stimulus. The last of these criteria was introduced to distinguish phobic syndromes with severe anticipatory anxiety from panic disorder.

The DSM-III-R criteria for panic disorder (1) are only slightly modified from the DSM-III criteria. The DSM-III-R adds the additional restriction that panic attacks must not be triggered by social attention or scrutiny, which might confuse panic disorder with social phobia. Further, in order to meet DSM-III-R panic disorder criteria, patients must have four attacks within a 4-week period or one or more attacks followed by at least 1 month of persistent fear of panic. The DSM-III-R also places temporal requirements on a panic attack: At least four symptoms of panic must occur within 10 minutes of the beginning of at least some of the panic attacks. Episodic anxiety which fails to meet panic disorder criteria is labeled a "limited symptom attack" (1).

Agoraphobia and Other Phobic Disorders

Agoraphobia

Agoraphobia, perhaps a misnomer, is essentially a fear of situations in which one might feel trapped including such places as crowded theaters, traffic jams, bridges, and elevators. Most commonly, agoraphobia develops in individuals already experiencing panic attacks; hence the shift from "agoraphobia with panic" in DSM-III to "panic disorder with agoraphobia" in DSM-III-R (1).

Social Phobia

Another common phobia is social phobia, a persistent and exaggerated fear of social situations (7). Unlike agoraphobics, social phobics fear scrutiny rather than the crowd itself. This anxiety concerning social scrutiny must be unrelated to a physical illness or psychiatric illness that might sensitize the individual to criticism. In order to meet the criteria for social phobia, the individual must suffer from some impairment in occupational or interpersonal functioning or marked distress (1).

Simple Phobia

Simple phobia is a persistent fear of a specified stimulus other than panic, entrapment, or social criticism. Usually such patients only have a single well-defined phobia, such as a fear of snakes.

The phobic disorders share many common features. First, exposure to phobic stimuli precipitates anxiety. Second, phobic individuals generally avoid direct contact with phobic situations, as well as reminders of these situations. Avoidance may result in striking constriction in the phobic individual's life-style. Agoraphobics, for example, frequently may be housebound. Such restrictions in behavior may protect patients from experiencing anxiety but may impede in seeking help or complying with treatment.

Generalized Anxiety Disorder

Generalized anxiety disorder is primarily distinguished from other anxiety disorders by the presence of prominent generalized anxiety and the absence of panic attacks. Thus, GAD tends to be associated with chronic worry and fewer somatic symptoms than panic disorder (8, 9). Coexistent depressive symptoms commonly occur and do not negate the GAD diagnosis in DSM-III-R (1). Symptoms such as chronic anxiety and mild–moderate depression are relatively common in other diagnoses, and as shall be reviewed later, the independent validity of this diagnosis has been questioned (10).

Post-Traumatic Stress Disorder

The formal recognition of PTSD by psychiatry has been a controversial process. Medical descriptions of wartime PTSD emerged from the Crimean War and American Civil War, and physiologic investigations continued through World War I (reviewed in 11). However, this diagnosis was omitted from DSM-II for unclear reasons and replaced by "transient adjustment reactions of adult life" (4). The diagnosis of "post-traumatic stress disorder" was first introduced in DSM-III in response to research carried out in veterans of the Vietnam War, survivors of the Nazi concentration camps, as well as the survivors of other man-made and natural disasters (6). The DSM-III-R criteria for PTSD specify that a person has experienced a traumatic event which must be beyond the range of usual human experience, such as sexual assault, physical trauma, or war (1).

Subsequent to traumatization, individuals generally report a spectrum of symptoms which may be clustered into four categories: reexperiencing, traumatophobia (12), physiologic arousal, and numbing. The reexperiencing symptoms include intrusive memories of the traumatic situation, intense or repetitive nightmares which generally depict aspects of the trauma, and flashbacks which are vivid, polysensory, dissociative-like states during which patients often report "reliving" aspects of their trauma while experiencing panic symptoms (13). When exposed to reminders of the trauma, individuals with PTSD frequently exhibit markedly increased responses including anxiety, depression, anger, guilt, and symptoms associated with sympathetic nervous activation. In response, patients develop a phobic-like avoidance of thinking about the trauma or exposing themselves to stimuli that might evoke memories of it. In addition, individuals with PTSD exhibit chronic autonomic activation manifested by symptoms previously linked with panic, hypervigilence, and enhanced startle response (11, 14).

The numbing symptoms of PTSD include a spectrum of cognitive and affective responses which seem to reflect an emotional constriction or depression. Particularly after massive psychic trauma, individuals with PTSD report feeling emotionally numb or mechanical or difficulty in experiencing loving feelings. This inhibition may be associated with social isolation, loss of trust, loss of empathy, a sense of impending death or shortened life, survivor guilt, and depressive-like dysphoria (11, 14, 15). The onset of PTSD may be immediate. However, it is frequently delayed, and decades after a technologic or natural disaster patients will continue to appear at treatment settings with their first clinical presentation for PTSD.

The differential diagnosis of PTSD is made difficult by the variety of symptoms which may dominate the clinical picture. The intrusive thoughts may suggest OCD. However, the intrusive thoughts of PTSD generally concern specific traumatic content which is ego syntonic although actively resisted. The tonic arousal may suggest the diagnosis of generalized anxiety disorder, but PTSD may be distinguished by the history of trauma and other attendant symptoms. As noted earlier, PTSD mimics panic disorder in some respects. However, spontaneous panic attacks are generally infrequent for individuals with PTSD. Post-traumatic stress disorder symptoms overlap somewhat with other diagnoses and severe environmental stress may exacerbate other comorbid pathology such as panic disorder, depression or schizophrenia. This overlap slowed the formal recognition of PTSD by psychiatry and often prevents its recognition in individual patients. However, it is one of the few psychiatric diagnoses whose pathogenesis is included in its definition, and recognition of PTSD may have important clinical implications, which are discussed later.

Obsessive–Compulsive Disorder

Obsessive–compulsive disorder is distinguished by its two cardinal features, the obsession and the compulsion (16). Obsessions, defined earlier, may be distinguished from delusions by the retention of reality testing which permits the sufferer to recognize the intrusive thoughts as irrational, excessive, or uncharacteristic, e.g., "I know I just washed my hands, but this thought keeps coming that they're dirty." Obsessions may also be distinguished from depressive ruminations which are characteristically "owned" by the individual, e.g., "I'm a terrible person because I failed my sister." Compulsions are rarely confused with symptoms of other diagnoses.

Rasmussen and Tsuang reported on the frequency of classes of obsessions and compulsions in their sample of 44 patients (16). The most common obsession (55%) was a fear of contamination by dirt, toxins, or germs. In 83% of these patients, the obsession was associated with cleaning rituals. Aggressive (50%) and sexual (32%) obsessions were also frequent and involved fears of sexually molesting children, fears of sexual perversions, or thoughts of directly harming people. A third of their patients also had intrusive thoughts of symmetricality or exactness which led them to fear asymmetry and to be disturbed by untidiness or disorder, while a smaller proportion hoarded or saved useless items. In addition to cleaning rituals, counting and repeating rituals, such as having to perform a behavior a set number of times, and checking rituals, such as repeatedly examining the stove before leaving home, were quite common and frequently occurred together. In order to meet DSM-III-R criteria for OCD, the obsessions and compulsions must cause marked distress, consume a great deal of time, or significantly interfere with normal routine (1). However, the degree to which OCD symptoms interfere with a patient's lifestyle may frequently be underestimated due to avoidance which develops in response to stimuli that trigger obsessive thoughts or compulsive behaviors.

EPIDEMIOLOGY AND COURSE

The anxiety disorders, as a group, tend to follow a similar pattern. With the possible exception of social phobia, they develop most frequently in young women (17) and generally have a poor overall prognosis and chronic unremitting course without appropriate treatment (10, 18). They occur relatively frequently. Some reports place their prevalence between 2% and 5% (10) while the Epidemiologic Catchment Area (ECA) study reported higher lifetime prevalence rates, between 10% and 25% (19). In the section below, we review the course and prevalence of the anxiety disorders.

Panic Disorder

Onset

In roughly three quarters of patients, panic disorder began with a spontaneous panic attack, an anxiety attack with no obvious environmental precipitant. Most frequently, this panic attack occurred in the 3rd decade of life and within 6 months of a major stressful life event (20). Breier et al. (20) reported that in 55 patients, the most common stressful event was marital separation. This was consistent with a larger self-report survey that reported increased prevalence of panic symptoms among divorced individuals (21). Generally, when individuals experienced this first panic attack they misinterpreted its significance. Patients frequently felt that they were dying or going crazy (20).

Environmentally precipitated attacks develop on confrontation with a phobic stimulus, such as traffic jams, or during settings where other experiences, such as heat or bright lights, act as triggers for anxiety. In addition, patients frequently report that panic attacks occurred at a particular time of the day or woke them from sleep. The diagnostic significance of these patterns of panic disorder are not clear at this time. However, some phobic individuals with predominantly spontaneous panic attacks appear to have a narrower range of phobic avoidance than the typical agoraphobics (22). These authors suggested a new diagnosis, mixed phobia, to label this group.

Course

After the first panic attack, most patients with panic disorder progress within 2 months to panic attacks of sufficient frequency and severity to meet DSM-III criteria for this illness (20). Subsequently, most patients have chronic panic disorder, although a small subset of patients will have periods of a year or more of spontaneous remission before relapsing (20, 23). The subsequent panic attacks may be spontaneous or environmentally precipitated but environmentally precipitated attacks tend to dominate later in the course of the disorder (20). In the first year after the onset of panic, almost all patients develop agoraphobia (20, 24). Ninety-three percent of patients in one sample also developed anticipatory anxiety, and 5% of patients developed social phobia (20). Seventeen percent of the individuals with panic also had histories of alcoholism. However, in all but 2% of cases, the alcoholism preceded the first panic attack (20).

Prevalence

The lifetime prevalence of panic disorder appears to range between 0.4% and 2.5% (17, 19). The actual frequency of panic attacks is somewhat higher since, under DSM-III, agoraphobia with panic was a separate diagnosis and had a lifetime prevalence which varied between .8 and 2.3% at the three ECA sites (19). Panic symptoms are two to three times more frequent in women. Also, in both men and women, panic is most prevalent in the 2nd through 4th decades and decreases in frequency subsequently (17, 19, 25), consistent with occasional reports from patients in our clinic that their parents "used to have panic attacks, but grew out of them." Further, Von Korff and his associates reported that when they adjusted the rate of panic attacks for age, sex, education, and marital status, individuals over 65 had 6-month prevalence rates of 0.0% in New Haven and St. Louis (25).

Phobic Disorders

Agoraphobia

Onset. Agoraphobia generally develops in the context of a major life event such as marital separation or death of a parent, (26) but most frequently as a learned fear response to panic attacks (20, 27). Subsequent to the onset of agoraphobia, individuals generally begin avoiding the setting of anxiety attacks. This avoidance generalizes as the disorder becomes more severe causing some individuals to become housebound (28).

A substantial body of evidence supports the causative link between panic attacks and agoraphobia. First, several studies retrospectively trace agoraphobia to the time period surrounding the first panic attack (20, 24, 27). Second, agoraphobia and panic have similar ages of onset (29, 30). Third, the Yale ECA researchers noted that the overlap between panic attacks and agoraphobia is often underestimated. In their sample, 47% of subjects reporting agoraphobia without panic disorder had histories of panic symptoms and 40% had an additional psychiatric disorder (31). Thyer et al. also noted that their agoraphobia patients who did not describe an overt link between their agoraphobia and any history of panic attack "often suffered some somatic ailment of an unpredictable or spasmodic nature such as epilepsy or a colitis." The authors suggested that the episodes, perhaps unrecognized panic states, served as the "functional equivalents" of panic attacks in producing agoraphobia (32).

Course. Like panic disorder, untreated agoraphobia tends to have a chronic course with few remissions (19, 29).

Prevalence. In the New Haven ECA site, the lifetime prevalence of agoraphobia without panic disorder was 2.9%, panic disorder with agoraphobia was 0.3%, and panic disorder alone 0.9% (31). As noted earlier, Klein and associates found that these figures underestimated the coexistence of panic and agoraphobia (31).

Social Phobia

Onset. Social phobia tends to develop, without clear precipitant, equally in males and females during late childhood through early adulthood (7, 28, 30).

Course. This disorder has a chronic course when untreated (7). Individuals with social phobia may experience marked impairment of social and occupational functioning and may have increased risk for secondary alcoholism (7).

Prevalence. Although the lifetime prevalence of social phobia is not clear, its 6-month prevalence in the ECA study was 2.2% in Baltimore and 1.2% in St. Louis (30) and was most common in women between the ages of 18 and 24 (4.3% in Baltimore, 2.2% in St. Louis). In contrast to some earlier studies (7), the ECA data suggest the presence of a female preponderance for social phobia (30). The reason for this discrepancy in sex distribution is unclear.

Simple Phobia

Onset. As a group, the majority of simple phobias tend to arise in the first two decades of life (27). However, Marks (28). noted that simple animal phobias tend to cluster in early childhood, whereas other simple phobias tend to appear throughout life without a clear age preference.

Course. Simple phobias tend to have less chronicity than the other phobic disorders (25).

Prevalence. Across the three ECA sites, simple phobia showed a 2:1 female predominance. In the St. Louis and New Haven sites, males showed approximately a 4% lifetime prevalence compared to 9% for females. Age was not a consistent factor influencing simple phobia prevalence in this study (19).

Generalized Anxiety Disorder

Onset

Psychiatry has had difficulty demonstrating that GAD is a distinct disorder from panic disorder and depression, and this lack of clarity is also reflected in confusion over its onset and course. Some studies suggest that GAD, like the other anxiety disorders, occurs in the 3rd decade of life (10). However, some groups (9, 30) reported that GAD had an earlier onset than panic disorder. Consistent with these findings, before developing panic disorder, many individuals have a history of excessive nervousness (20, 34).

Course

Untreated GAD typically has a chronic course. For example, Barlow and his associates reported that GAD patients reported being "tense and anxious" for more than half of their lives (8).

Prevalence

The prevalence of GAD has also been difficult to establish because of the low interrater reliability of early diagnostic instruments for GAD (35, 36). Using more conservative and reliable measures, Bresleau and Davis (37) reported a lifetime prevalence of GAD of 9.1%, quite a bit higher than most other anxiety disorders.

In addition to the confusion around onset, there is a high level of overlap in the incidence of GAD and panic disorder. One study which reported data on 100 outpatients at a psychosomatic clinic reported that all 100 of their patients simultaneously met the criteria for panic disorder, GAD, and agoraphobia (38). Barlow and his associates noted that 60 to 80% of patients with agoraphobia with panic or panic disorder also met GAD criteria (36). Similarly, 100% of their obsessive–compulsive patients and two-thirds of their depressed patients also carried the diagnosis of GAD.

Some studies have attempted to distinguish GAD and panic disorders based on developmental factors. Raskin et al. noted an increased incidence of grossly disturbed childhood environment in individuals who developed panic disorder relative to GAD (39). Interestingly though, the study reported a similar age of onset for the panic disorder and GAD. However, the presence of one to three stressful life events in-

creased risk for GAD threefold, whereas four or more life events increased the risk for this disorder 8.5 times (40). Other studies (9, 41) distinguished panic disorder and GAD patients by the nature of their somatic symptoms noting more symptoms associated with autonomic arousal in patients with panic disorder relative to generalized anxiety patients.

Panic Disorder, Generalized Anxiety Disorder, and Depression: Comorbidity and Differential Diagnosis

In treating anxiety disorders, one often elicits in patients a previous history of major depression or developed depression which has emerged after the onset of their panic attacks. Similarly, in treating depressed patients one often elicits a history of anxiety disorder. Breier and his colleagues (42) suggested that a history of panic attacks or agoraphobia, high scores on the Hamilton Anxiety Scale, and low scores on the Hamilton Depression Scale reliably differentiate panic disorder and agoraphobia from major depressive illness. However, some studies have been unable to distinguish GAD from depression using standard measures for anxiety and depression (reviewed in 10). Studying the temporal aspects of occurrence of anxiety and depressive symptoms in these patients further supports the validity of panic disorder and agoraphobia and questions the validity of GAD as an independent diagnosis. In their review of the literature, Breier et al. (42) point out that there is strong evidence supporting the temporal separation of panic and depression, but there is only suggestive evidence supporting the temporal separation between generalized anxiety and depression or panic.

These findings question GAD's existence as an independent disorder as opposed to its reflecting an underlying anxious depression or a variant of panic. Both generalized anxiety and major depression occur frequently in individuals with agoraphobia with panic. Breier et al. (42) found that 80% of their patients with agoraphobia with panic had a history of GAD and that in 63% of these cases the GAD developed after the panic disorder. Major depression occurred in 70% of the patients with agoraphobia with panic. However, there was no clear tendency for the depressive episodes to be temporally related to the onset or course of the anxiety disorder. In contrast to the course of the anxiety disorders which had a continuous course following the onset, the depressive disorders appear to be episodic in course. Thus, by reviewing the course of illness and attendant symptoms one can distinguish clearly panic disorder with agoraphobia from major depression. The inability to make such clear distinctions for GAD questions its validity as an independent diagnosis. The critical unresolved epidemiologic questions regarding GAD are, How often does it exist without a history of panic attacks or depression? And is the disorder similar in these "pure" GAD patients to those with other comorbid disorders? Further questions of the validity of GAD are raised in the section on genetic issues.

Post-Traumatic Stress Disorder

Onset

A number of factors have been described which appear to increase the incidence of traumatic disorder. In the Vietnam veteran populations the following factors were thought to be important: (*a*) the exposure to "abusive violence" or atrocities, (*b*) the death or wounding of friends, (*c*) isolation from peers during combat, and (*d*) contacts with dead and dying soldiers outside of combat settings (43, 44). Studies in both technologic and natural disasters concur that in response to traumas of sufficient severity, the majority, if not all individuals, will develop symptoms of PTSD (11).

Course

Traditional formulations emphasized stages of post-traumatic response (45, 46). More recently, Horowitz (47) suggested that after a severe trauma individuals initially react with outrage or denial followed by psychic numbing which may last years or even decades. The numbing phase is frequently followed by periods of oscillation between reexperiencing material related to the trauma, associated with a great deal of both anxiety and depression, and periods of numbing, during which people generally feel mechanical, unmotivated, and perhaps depressed. It is thought that during periods of reexperiencing, symptoms such as panic attacks, flashbacks, and nightmares occur. However, cross-sectional studies have had difficulty documenting a strict serial course of traumatic disorders (14).

A "phase-oriented" course may account for the frequent delay in the onset of PTSD symptoms. Also, there may be a delayed onset of substance abuse after traumatization, as was seen in veterans who returned from Vietnam. Epidemiologic data suggest that there was an average delay of approximately 4 years between the return of veterans to the United States and the onset of a new wave of substance abuse (reviewed in 48). It is possible to understand this 2nd wave of substance abuse as a response to the delayed surge of intrusive PTSD symptoms. These intrusive symptoms most closely resemble the other anxiety disorders, such as GAD and panic disorder, both of which are also associated with an increase in alcohol abuse in men (9, 10).

Obsessive–Compulsive Disorder

Onset

Many OCD patients can recall subclinical ritualistic behaviors dating to early childhood (16). Such behaviors include minor rituals, such as avoiding stepping on cracks in the sidewalk or touching a lucky book or chair when walking into a room. Other children exhibit a repetitive, almost mechanical, movement such as rubbing objects or a particular part of their body (49). The significance of such preclinical phenomena are unclear at this time. Generally, the onset of a syndrome which is more clearly recognized as OCD occurs in the 2nd to 3rd decade of life (16). Rasmussen and Tsuang reported that only 11 of 44

(25%) of their OCD patients described an environmental precipitant for their illness (16).

Course

Rasmussen and Tsuang found that in 44 OCD patients, 84% reported a continuous course of symptoms since the onset, 14% had a chronic deteriorative course, and only 2% had an episodic course (16). Environmental events were also reported to significantly exacerbate symptoms in "almost all" of their patients. Also, schizotypal features appeared to be a poor prognostic sign in OCD (50).

Prevalence

Obsessive–compulsive disorder was once thought to be an uncommon disorder with an incidence of 0.05%, comparable to schizophrenia (51). More recently, the ECA study found the lifetime prevalence of OCD was 2 to 3% and its incidence over 1%, approximately a 20-fold increase over previous figures (19). The large number of patients who have been applying for treatment over the last few years suggests that the higher estimates may be more accurate. Most studies suggest that males and females are approximately equally affected with OCD (16). However, the St. Louis site revealed a two- to threefold increase in this disorder among women (19), and the childhood form of this disorder appears to develop more frequently in males (52).

Several studies report a high incidence of major depression in patients with OCD (16). In one study, 74% of the patients with depressed mood reported that depressive symptoms appeared after OCD had already produced functional impairment. Obsessive–compulsive disorder may co-occur with panic disorder, one study reported that 17% of panic patients also met criteria for OCD (20). Also, as noted earlier, Tourette's syndrome may be genetically linked to OCD. As many as 50% of Tourette's syndrome patients had OCD symptoms, while 5% of OCD patients meet criteria for Tourette's syndrome (16, 49, 50).

ETIOLOGY AND PATHOGENESIS

Etiologic theories for anxiety disorders may be simplistically grouped into those that are fundamentally biologic or behavioral in their focus. The neurobiologic theories highlight the roles which central noradrenergic and benzodiazepine systems might play in the genesis and treatment of anxiety states. Other neurotransmitter systems, including serotonin, dopamine, and neuropeptides may also be involved in anxiety disorders. In addition, carbon dioxide inhalation and lactate infusion have been used as physiologic probes for abnormal neuroregulation in anxiety disorders. Behavioral models such as classical and operant conditioning have also been applied to the genesis of phobic disorders. In addition, psychiatric researchers have also studied the particular relevance of naturally occurring anxiogenic situations, such as parental separation or inescapable stress exposure (learned helplessness). Genetic and neurodevelopmental factors also contribute to the development of anxiety disorders. The neurobiologic and behavioral models may be integrated in the process of considering the relative contributions of genetic and environmental factors to the development of anxiety disorders. These models are reviewed below.

Neurobiologic Contributions

Norepinephrine Systems

Animal studies, primarily from the monkey and cat, provided a strong link between the activities of the noradrenergic system based in the locus coeruleus and fear and anxiety states (53, 54, 54a). On the basis of these preclinical studies, a series of clinical investigations have been carried out in patients with anxiety disorders and major depression (55–58). Yohimbine, an α_2-adrenoceptor blocking drug which disinhibits central noradrenergic systems and blocks postsynaptic α_2-receptors, precipitates panic-like anxiety in the majority of the patients with panic disorder, unlike healthy subjects, who rarely respond with significant anxiety. After an oral dose of 20 mg of yohimbine, approximately half of panic disorder patients will experience a paniclike state. In addition to the increase in anxiety, patients with panic disorder exhibit an exaggerated increase in their blood pressure and heart rate and greater rises in plasma levels of the noradrenergic metabolite, 3-methoxy 4-hydroxyphenyl-ethyleneglycol (MHPG) in response to yohimbine (56, 57). These marked responses rarely occurred in patients with GAD, OCD, schizophrenia, or major depression, suggesting the presence of a specific noradrenergic abnormality in panic disorder (58). Patients with panic disorder also exhibited more pronounced responses to the α_2-adrenergic agonist, clonidine (57).

The norepinephrine-sensitive β-adrenergic receptor also appears to be abnormally regulated in panic disorder. Rainey and his colleagues found that the peripherally acting drug isoproterenol precipitated Research Diagnostic Criteria panic attacks in 8 of 15 males and 21 of 24 females (59). Other groups report decreased physiologic sensitivity to β-agonist infusion. Nesse and his associates (60) found that individuals with panic disorder had an elevated resting heart rate and elevated resting levels of plasma epinephrine, cortisol, growth hormone, and norepinephrine. This group had a decreased heart rate response to isoproterenol. The authors suggested that individuals with panic disorder become hyposensitive to β-receptor stimulation due to chronic activation by high levels of endogenous catecholamines. This is supported by another study (61) which suggested that the plasma lymphocyte β-adrenergic receptors are down regulated in individuals with panic disorder. The functional significance of β-receptor down regulation is unclear at this time. The physiologic studies suggest that it may play an adaptive role for patients by decreasing reactivity to some stimuli, such as stress-induced catecholamine release. Overall, these findings suggest that there is a specific dysfunction of central noradrenergic regulation in a subset of in-dividuals with panic disorder but not in patients with GAD, OCD, or major depression. At this time the molecular mechanisms responsible for the abnormal regulation of noradrenergic function in panic disorder have not been identified.

Patients with PTSD also show evidence of noradrenergic dysregulation. They exhibit elevated 24-hour urinary norepinephrine levels, down-regulated platelet α_2-adrenoceptors, and down-regulated lymphocyte β-adrenoceptors (reviewed in 11). Reexposure to reminders of the trauma also elicits exaggerated autonomic activity and anxiety (11).

The Benzodiazepine–GABA Chloride Channel Complex

Despite evidence that benzodiazepine systems are involved in the genetic transmission of fear dysregulation (61a), to our knowledge, there have been no published reports directly assessing the functional status of the benzodiazepine systems in anxiety patients. However, suggestive evidence implicates this system in the genesis of anxiety disorders and extensive evidence implicates this system in their treatment. This system has been studied using three groups of benzodiazepine drugs: agonists, such as diazepam, which possess sedative, anxiolytic, and anticonvulsant actions; inverse agonists, such as the β-carboline FG 7142, which exhibit anxiogenic and proconvulsant capacities; and antagonists, such as RO 15-1788 (flumazenil), which have mild effects in healthy subjects but block agonist and antagonist actions (reviewed in 62). Dorow et al (63) administered the benzodiazepine inverse agonist FG7142 to healthy subjects and precipitated severe anxiety states comparable to panic anxiety. This study has many parallels in the primate literature where intravenous infusion of β-carboline has been shown to precipitate fear states (64).

One clinical study has been carried out in panic disorder that used the benzodiazepine receptor antagonist RO 15-1788. This drug appeared to precipitate a moderate level of anxiety and panic attacks in a subset of patients with panic disorder (65).

Although an endogenous benzodiazepine-displacing peptide has been described, "diazepam binding inhibitor," this peptide has anxiogenic effects suggestive of inverse agonist properties (66, 67). However, the RO 15-1788 effects in panic are not consistent with an abnormal action from an endogenous benzodiazepine inverse agonist. The data do not exclude, though, increased sensitivity to the direct partial inverse agonist effects of RO 15-1788 in this disorder.

The most striking finding, however, has been the ability of benzodiazepine agonists, most notably alprazolam, to decrease the symptoms of both general anxiety and panic (reviewed in 62). This ability, combined with the presence of the benzodiazepine receptors in the brain, suggests that possible abnormalities in this system could contribute to the spectrum of anxiety disorders. However, no specific link between this system and any particular anxiety disorder has yet been demonstrated.

Serotonin Systems

A series of preclinical studies have suggested that serotonergic neuronal systems may be involved in anxiety as well as in the mechanisms of action of antianxiety drugs (68, 69). Interest in the functional role of serotonergic systems in anxiety has increased recently as buspirone, a drug used to treat anxiety disorders, has been shown to be an agonist at the 5-HT_{1A} receptor (70). Clinical studies to date have been unable to demonstrate an unequivocal abnormality in the serotonin functions of individuals with panic disorder. The prolactin response to tryptophan infusion, for example, did not differentiate healthy subjects from individuals with panic disorder (68). Buspirone appears to be relatively ineffective in treating panic disorder (D. Charney et al., unpublished observations). However, a role for serotonergic dysfunction in some forms of panic anxiety is suggested by the observation that intravenous administration of the serotonin receptor agonist m-chlorophenylpiperazine (MCPP) produced anxiety in 12 of 23 patients with panic disorder and in 6 of 19 healthy subjects (69). In another study, oral MCPP elicited significantly greater anxiety in panic disorder patients compared to healthy subjects (235).

It is more likely that serotonergic dysfunction may be etiologically important in GAD, where buspirone and a related drug, gepirone, appear efficacious (71, 72). The questionable independent validity of the GAD diagnosis raises questions whether serotonergic systems may play a role in the common diathesis for GAD and depression. Such a hypothesis is consistent with the rather large literature suggestive of an etiologic role for serotonergic systems in depression (73–76). Serotonergic systems have not been studied systematically in PTSD.

Brain serotonergic systems may also play a role in the treatment and pathophysiology of OCD. There are three lines of evidence suggesting serotonin may be involved in OCD: (*a*) drug response data, (*b*) neurobiologic findings, and (*c*) animal models. The bulk of the evidence for a serotonin hypothesis for OCD is based on drug response data. Early case reports and subsequent clinical trials suggested that the potent 5-HT reuptake blocker clomipramine showed superior efficacy in OCD compared to less potent or selective antidepressants (reviewed in 77, 78). These reports found that therapeutic efficacy correlated with levels of the serotonergically selective compound clomipramine rather than its noradrenergically active metabolite, desmethylclomipramine. In addition, responders to clomipramine have been found to have higher baseline cerebrospinal fluid levels of the serotonin metabolite 5-hydroxyindoleacetic acid (5-HIAA) and platelet serotonin concentrations. The degree of improvement during clomipramine treatment also significantly correlated with the drug-induced decreases in both of these measures (79, 80). Additional support for serotonin's role in OCD is provided by reports of efficacy with drugs such as fluoxetine (81) and fluvoxamine, (82, 83) which are more selective blockers of serotonin uptake than clomipramine.

Clinical investigations designed to more directly evaluate serotonin function in OCD have generally yielded less consistent data than the treatment studies. Whole blood serotonin levels were reported decreased in OCD patients (84). Platelet imipramine binding, which may be an index of serotonin uptake mechanisms, has been reported as normal in one study, (85) but a subsequent study has demonstrated decreased binding in OCD patients compared with healthy controls (86). One study reported that cerebrospinal fluid levels of 5-HIAA were elevated (85), but they were no different than controls in another study (79).

Recently, several research groups took advantage of the stimulatory effects of serotonin agonists on prolactin release to assess serotonergic regulation in OCD. Charney and his collegues demonstrated that prolactin increases were blunted in female, but not male, OCD patients following administration of the 5-HT$_1$ agonist, MCPP, but not the serotonin precursor, tryptophan (87). These findings are suggestive of selective 5-HT abnormalities in this disorder, particularly in light of sex differences reported in animal studies of 5-HT function (reviewed in 87). Other techniques may be necessary to demonstrate serotonergic changes in males. Although no changes in obsessive or compulsive behaviors were noted in this study when intravenous MCPP was administered, two studies found significant exacerbations of OCD symptoms after oral MCPP administration (88, 89). The reasons for these discrepant findings are unclear, but they may relate to differing MCPP preparations or differing route of administration. Lastly, animal models for repetitive behaviors, perhaps analogous to compulsions, suggest that serotonin systems may play an important modulatory role. For example, serotonergic depletion in rats exacerbated the display of perseverative behaviors elicited by amphetamine (90, 91).

Other Biologic Measures

Lactate provocation tests and the carbon dioxide inhalation tests deserve special mention in considering the biologic mechanisms involved in anxiety. The particular mechanisms of action for these two provocative tests are unknown. Individuals with panic disorder are clearly more sensitive to the anxiogenic effects of lactate infusion, as well as carbon dioxide inhalation (92–94). In addition, the anxiogenic response to both tests is decreased by pretreatments that are clinically useful in treating anxiety disorders. As reviewed by Carr and Sheehan, (95) monoamine oxidase inhibitors, imipramine, and alprazolam, all have the ability to decrease lactate-induced anxiety. Similarly, imipramine, alprazolam, and valium appear to be effective in inhibiting carbon-dioxide-inhalation-induced anxiety, whereas clonidine and haldol are ineffective or inconsistent anxiolytic agents in this paradigm (96, 97).

Lactate infusion and carbon dioxide inhalation also produce abnormal anxiogenic effects in individuals with PTSD. In seven PTSD patients, six of whom also met panic criteria, lactate infusions precipitated flashbacks in all patients and panic attacks in all but one (98). The vivid and depictive nature of their flashbacks distinctly pertained to their individual traumas. An early report from World War I also reported that veterans with irritable heart were more sensitive to the anxiogenic effects of carbon dioxide inhalation (reviewed in 11).

Behavioral and Psychologic Models

A number of behavioral and psychologic models for the etiology of anxiety disorders have been proposed. These models range from psychodynamic and information-processing models which focus on psychologic mechanisms to models of operant learning which focus on external influences on behavior. In the section below we briefly review four behavioral and psychologic approaches to the etiology of anxiety disorders.

Naturalistic Models

Naturalistic models for anxiety disorders posit that illness arises in response to situations which are instinctively dangerous or threatening. Freud drew mainstream psychiatry to the importance of instinctual life (99). He focused on infancy and childhood, where instinct is most clearly observed. The expression of instinctive behavior lends to at least two prototype experiences relevant to the genesis of anxiety states: (a) Critical needs are frustrated, for example, feeding or other forms of nurturing, and (b) instinctive behaviors place the infant into conflict situations which potentially threaten its safety. The first of these prototypal experiences was first studied by Spitz and his colleagues (100) in their studies of institutionalized children. Their description of anaclitic depression was further developed by Bowlby, (101) who described three phases of separation anxiety: protest, despair, and detachment. In response to maternal separation, children initially appear quite distressed and will visibly protest separation. During the second phase, despair, although the child is still preoccupied with the missing parent, physical protestation begins to diminish. The child may withdraw and become inactive and appear to mourn. The third phase, detachment, is evident as the child no longer mourns the mother but seems to become attached to the new caregivers, such as nurses or health workers. Bowlby suggested that the anxiety demonstrated by the maternally deprived infant is not merely a signal of some other danger, but rather a primary quality of the experience of maternal deprivation.

The instinctual nature of this kind of anxiety was most clearly demonstrated in the subsequent studies in nonhuman primates. In the rhesus monkey, sensitivity to social isolation begins in infancy and lasts through adolescence (discussed in 102, 103). Maternal deprivation within this critical period produced a syndrome very similar to the protest–despair–detachment process described by Spitz and Bowlby. It also produced disturbed social behavior, including social withdrawal, self-mouthing and clasping, stereotypal rocking, heightened aggressiveness, disturbed sexual behavior, impaired maternal behavior, as well as severe states of arousal or fear when confronted by novel environmental challenges normally tolerated by rhesus monkeys (102–104). Maternal deprivation could be viewed as a special form of learning, a disruption of a critical period in neurodevelopment, or as a frustration of an instinctual need, as suggested by Freud.

Both social therapy and pharmacotherapy reduce the behavioral abnormalities observed after maternal deprivation. When isolated monkeys are returned to groups of healthy peers, the abnormal behaviors are actively confronted by group monkeys, facilitating the "rehabilitation" of the deprived monkeys (104, 105). However, these rehabilitated monkeys continue to have "latent" behavior disturbances which may be elicited by socially stressful experiences or amphetamine administration (104). The behavior abnormalities are also reduced by antidepressant treatment (106). Consistent with the sensitivity to pharmacologic probes or treatments, maternal deprivation produces abnormalities in central catecholamine function and hypothalmic–pituitary–adrenal axis disturbance (104, 107).

Parental separation or disturbance in the parental relationship has been considered an important etiologic factor in a number of psychiatric disorders. Most directly, school phobia parallels the protest–despair of separation anxiety and responds to treatment with imipramine (108). However, maternal deprivation also produces long-standing hyperreactivity to novel situations. Its relevance to phobic and posttraumatic disorders must be considered as well. The long-standing consequences of maternal deprivation appear to be a mixture of anxiety and depressionlike symptoms. These findings make this model particularly interesting for disorders such as GAD and panic disorder which may share a common diathesis with depressivelike disorders.

The second naturalistic approach has been to study anxiety elicited in conflict situations. Freud (99) pointed out that anxiogenic conflicts may occur between external events, internal wishes, and impulses. Animal models have been designed which mimic such conflicts. The two most carefully studied conflict models are the Geller-Seifter test, (109) in which mice are deprived of food and trained to press a lever for a reward, and conflict is produced by combining the food reward with an electric shock; and the Vogel "Punished Drinking Test," which is similar to the Geller-Seifter procedure (110) but water is substituted for food.

These conflict models are very sensitive to the anxiolytic effects of benzodiazepines, as well as the anxiogenic effects of benzodiazepine inverse agonists (111). Buspirone is also effective in this model. However, trazodone, amoxepine, maprotiline, and doxepin were ineffective with acute administration (112). Likewise, opiates, amphetamine, and neuroleptics are ineffective in this paradigm (reviewed in 113). The selective efficacy of agents such as buspirone and benzodiazepines, which are thought to be effective in GAD, suggest that the behavioral state generated by the conflict paradigms may be more similar to generalized or anticipatory anxiety rather than panic disorder.

A third naturalistic model has been the social interaction tests. In these texts, anxiogenic substances, such as the benzodiazepine inverse agonists, decreased the time spent in social interaction. Like the conflict paradigms, the social interaction paradigm appears to assess a tonic state of anxiety akin to anticipatory anxiety associated with agoraphobia or social phobia, rather than phasic phenomena such as panic attacks. Consistent with this, the social interaction paradigm shows a pattern of pharmacologic sensitivity which parallels the conflict paradigms (described in 100, 114).

Learning Theories

Watson and Rayner described a possible behavioral mechanism through which operant learning could produce a phobic disorder in the case of "Little Albert." (115). In this study, a 2-year-old boy developed a rat phobia as a result of exposure to a loud noise while playing with a white rat. He subsequently displayed a fear of rats and objects which looked like rats. In this case, the loud noise served as an unconditioned stimulus which elicited a fear response, the unconditioned response. The white rat, the conditioned stimulus, is paired with the loud noise and evokes a similar alarm response, the conditioned response. This rather specific process produced a specified fear response, such as simple phobia.

Two-staged behavioral theories have been advanced which are more readily applied to disorders such as agoraphobia (116). In the two-stage theories, a second instrumental learning process interacts with the initial classically conditioned stimulus, foremost among these being stimulus generalization and higher order conditioning. As a result of stimulus generalization, in the example above, the individual comes to fear ratlike objects such as small moving objects, small animals, and furry clothes. Through higher order conditioning, the individual acquires a fear of predictors of a rat encounter, such as dark corners or unknown places. Avoiding novel places is rewarding because encounters are prevented, consistent with the clinical dictum "avoidance reinforces avoidance." Ultimately, one could theoretically account for a housebound agoraphobic through simple learning processes. It would be a mistake to say, though, that these behavioral processes are devoid of biologic substrates or pharmacologic modulation. Clearly the cellular mechanisms for learning, as well as the mechanisms involved in alarm states which were highlighted above, would be implicated in these behavioral models (discussed in 11, 117, 118).

Psychologic Trauma

Psychodynamic contributions to PTSD theory have changed radically during their development. Although they initially focused on the capacity of traumatic settings to revive latent infantile conflicts, current theory has attempted to be more integrative, capable of interfacing with cognitive, developmental and biologic theories (15).

Krystal has suggested that a critical process in traumatization is the capacity of severe stress to generate both extreme levels of arousal accompanied by helplessness. In response, people respond by "shutting down" cognitively, affectively, and physiologically producing a dissociated "catatonoid" state, and it is out of this state that individuals develop massive psychic trauma. Krystal points out that such extreme states are relatively rare in adults, but may be more common in children who have less well developed cognitive defense mechanisms. In adults, the response to trauma is actually quite varied so that some individuals may only exhibit aspects of the traumatic picture, a "partial traumatic response" manifested by a post-traumatic inhibitions in affective experience and "self-caring" functions, symptoms of anxiety or depression, or somatic symptoms (15, 19, 47).

Behavioral theories for PTSD are founded in two-stage learning theories described earlier (116) and are particularly useful in describing the acquisition and treatment of phobic aspects of this disorder (120). Such theories also complement neurobiologic theories for PTSD which incorporate models of learned alterations in nervous function (11).

Obsessive–Compulsive Disorder

Psychodynamic theorists suggested that obsessions and compulsions arise as defensive compromises (e.g., doing–undoing, reaction formation) in attempting to control anxiety and rage arising from unresolved conflicts from early childhood (121, 122). Behavioral approaches have also applied the two-stage classical instrumental conditioning models to OCD (116, 123, 124). First, obsessions are thought to arise through classical conditioning from the pairing of mental stimuli with anxiety-provoking thoughts. Following this, neutral behaviors are instrumentally associated with the reduction of anxiety and thus reinforced as compulsions. Avoidance of anxiogenic stimuli is also instrumentally reinforced. These behavioral theories support the use of desensitization techniques in this disorder (123, 124). Pitman (125) based a suggested cybernetic formulation for OCD on observations that OCD patients experience their cognitive information-processing mechanism as defective or incomplete. Viewing the human cognitive apparatus as a control system for resolving conflict between the environment and one's referential world (i.e., wishes, hopes, beliefs, etc.), Pitman suggested that OCD symptoms arise out of the persistence of "high error signals" or mismatch between one's beliefs about the world and sensory data which cannot be resolved through behavioral interventions. He also explains compulsive behavior as repeated attempts to reduce the mismatch between internal reference signals and the perceived environmental information.

GENETIC MODELS

Clinical Evidence for a Genetic Contribution

Currently, two major approaches have been taken to study genetic contributions to anxiety disorders. The first, twin studies, assessed the relative contribution of environmental and genetic factors by assessing the within-twin pair differences between monozygotic and dizygotic twins. In this model, traits with a high heritability are frequently shared by both members of an identical twin pair but infrequently shared by a fraternal twin pair. Traits shared by both monozygotic and dizygotic twins are thought to be environmentally transmitted. A second approach taken to evaluate the inheritance of anxiety disorders has been to study the first- and second-degree relatives of individuals with anxiety disorders. Two other new genetic approaches are being developed for application to anxiety disorders. The pharmacogenetic approach involves assessing the heritability of biologic traits or pharmacologic responses fundamental to the anxiety disorders. The molecular genetic approach attempts to isolate the DNA segments responsible for the transmission of anxiety disorders.

Molecular genetic techniques, such as studying restriction-fragment-length polymorphisms, have been recently applied to panic disorder. Crowe and his associates found evidence excluding the pro-opiomelanocortin gene in one large family with members affected with panic disorder (126). This group also reported a study that found that panic disorder was linked to chromosome 16q22 in a cohort of 29 families with members affected by panic disorder (127). Molecular genetic techniques hold much promise in increasing the specificity of our diagnostic and pharmacologic treatment approaches.

Twin Studies

Twin studies support the notion that genetic factors contribute significantly to the incidence of panic disorder and some phobic disorders but raise questions whether GADs are genetically transmitted. Two general approaches have been taken in the twin studies conducted to date: (a) small-scale studies studying twin pairs with affected members in detail and (b) large-scale epidemiologic studies which are not based on clinical samples. Torgerson (128) reported that the cotwins of monozygotic twins with panic disorder or agoraphobic with panic attacks exhibit these disorders five times more frequently than the dizygotic cotwins of individuals afflicted with these disorders. In contrast, he did not find evidence for a genetic contribution to GAD. In later studies, Torgerson (129, 130) found that individuals with pure anxiety disorders showed evidence of a genetic contribution which was not present in twins with mixed anxiety depressive disorders, or in depressive disorders which do not meet the criteria for bipolar disorder or major depressive disorder. Twin studies also support the genetic inheritance of some specific phobia such as blood injury phobia and OCD (reviewed in 131).

Two reports from a large-scale twin study conducted by Kendler and his associates (132, 133) also support the genetic contributions to the incidence of anxiety disorders. In the second of these two reports, Kendler and his associates found

that although anxiety and depression form separate symptom clusters, it appeared that genetic contributions to depression in their sample also strongly influenced symptoms of anxiety. In contrast, the environment had specific effects in precipitating symptoms of depression. It should be pointed out that their study did not specifically assess the inheritance of panic attacks. Thus, it is not clear whether their study supports a common genetic loading for all anxiety disorders and depression or instead supports the overlap between depression, GAD, and perhaps other anxiety disorders.

Family Studies

Family studies beginning in the late 1940s support the genetic transmission of panic disorder and agoraphobia, whereas the inheritance of GAD is more controversial (10, 134, 135). Noyes and his associates reported that first-degree relatives of patients with panic disorder had increased risk for panic disorders (17.3%) and panic attacks (19.2%) but not agoraphobia (1.9%) (124). The relatives of agoraphobics showed increased risk for panic disorder (8.3%), panic attacks (19.9%), and agoraphobia (11.6%). Male relatives of agoraphobics also had a 30.8% increased risk for alcoholism. The relatives of agoraphobics also reported earlier onset of illness and more severe symptoms than relatives of panic patients, suggesting to the authors that agoraphobia was a more severe subtype of panic disorder.

The inheritance of GAD is less clear. Several studies were unable to show familial inheritance of GAD (reviewed in 10). In contrast, Noyes and his associates (135) reported that GAD patients show a distinct familial inheritance. In their study, first-degree relatives of 20 GAD patients showed increased prevalence of GAD and adjustment disorders but not panic or agoraphobia. The overlap between GAD and PTSD was not reported in this study. Similarly relatives of patients with panic and agoraphobia did not show an increased risk for GAD.

A series of family studies suggest that

first-degree relatives of individuals with OCD, as well as individuals with obsessive–compulsive traits, show an increased incidence of the OCD symptoms (reviewed in 131, 137). Twin studies also support genetic contributions to this disorder, but the extent of this effect is unclear at this time (137).

Pharmacogenetic Studies

Pharmacogenetic strategies have also supported a genetic contribution to the development of anxiety disorders. Evidence for genetically determined regulation of catecholamine systems implicated in anxiety disorders comes from a number of sources. In humans, the levels of the catecholamine synthetic enzymes dopamine β-hydroxylase, catechol-o-methyltransferase, and monoamine oxidase are substantially genetically influenced (reviewed by 138, 139). The behavioral response to amphetamine, which acts on both norepinephrine and dopamine systems, has a heritable component reflected in twin studies (140). This finding is particularly relevant to panic disorder where anxiety attacks which may be precipitated by cocaine intoxication (141).

A number of studies show a genetic contribution to noradrenergic function and, more specifically, α_2-receptor regulation. For example, the number of platelet α_2-receptors appears to be genetically influenced (142). Baseline MHPG levels in plasma (143) and cerebrospinal fluid (144) also show a heritable influence. Preliminary data also suggest that the MHPG response to 0.4 mg/kg of yohimbine, given intravenously, has a heritable component in identical twins (J. Krystal et al., unpublished data). The genetic influences on central noradrenergic activity may account for the heritable components of such anxiety-related behaviors as galvanic skin response, (145) the blood pressure and pulse response to mental exercise and ischemic pain, (146) and responses to alcohol and other sedatives (reviewed in 147).

Animal models have been useful to demonstrate the diversity of pharmacogenetic contributions. Focusing on noradrenergic and adrenergic systems, phenylethanolamine N-methyltransferase (PNMT) levels, the final synthetic step in epinephrine synthesis, are genetically determined in rat strains where they inversely correlated with levels of brain α-2-receptors (148). Inherited differences in tyrosine hydroxylase, norepinephrine reuptake, and β-adrenergic receptor regulation have also been described (148–151). These genetic differences have been linked etiologically to behavioral differences in environmental reactivity.

The pharmacogenetic strategies are an important contribution to clinical neuroscience for their utility in clarifying etiologic questions concerning the development of physiologic abnormalities documented by traditional cross-sectional research methods and for potentially increasing diagnostic specificity by highlighting distinct neurobiologic traits which "breed true."

INTEGRATING ETIOLOGIC MODELS

The precise interaction of genetic, developmental and environmental factors that precipitate anxiety disorders is still unclear despite several attempts at integration. The French Neuropsychiatric School, as typified by Charcot, (152) developed genetic models for the etiology of hysteria. Freud, whose theories developed out of this school, attempted to integrate intrapsychic models with genetic models for the development of psychiatric disorders (153). More recently, psychologists (154–156) and primatologists (157) have emphasized the complex interaction between genetic endowment and rearing in the development of long-standing patterns of arousal regulation and reactivity to environmental stimuli. Neurodevelopmental contributions to psychiatric pathogenesis have also been highlighted (158). In the sections below, we shall describe the possible contributions from genetic, developmental, and environmental factors influencing the genesis of spontaneous panic attacks and abnormally increased environmental reactivity.

Neurodevelopmental Theories for the Etiology of Panic Disorder

Etiologic and pathogenic models for panic disorder must explain how one can have the genetic propensity for panic from birth, manifest this disorder at adolescence or young adulthood, and, perhaps, outgrow it in old age. The mechanisms underlying the female predominance in the incidence of panic disorder must also be explained. In the following sections, we discuss possible contributions of genetic and environmental factors to brain development as it may pertain to the genesis and course of panic disorders. Unfortunately, these factors have only recently come to the attention of psychiatric researchers. As a result, many approaches and theoretical models discussed in the following sections are borrowed from internal medicine and neurology as well as from preclinical studies of neurodevelopment.

Congenital Brain Lesions

Genetic and environmental processes which produce congenital disturbances in brain function could produce panic disorder that presented as this clinical entity at young adulthood. Many individuals with panic disorder note a prior history of nervousness (42) or school avoidance (159, 160). A family study also noted increased neophobia or "behavioral inhibition" in children of panic disorder patients (161).

The connection between congenital lesions, childhood nervousness, and later panic disorder could be found in neurodevelopment. Weinberger recently highlighted a number of clinical examples which illustrated a general neurodevelopmental concept: The developmental stage at which a brain lesion produces a particular behavioral abnormality depends on both the level of development of the organism at the time of the lesion and the time in the life cycle when that brain region matures and is critical to normal function (158). Thus, he pointed out that cerebral palsy arises from a single brain insult at birth which produces hemiparesis in a 2-year old, atheosis in the same individual when 4 years old, and later, seizures. Similarly temporal lobe epilepsy is associated with seizures in childhood and also with psychosis in adolescence. In some cases, temporal lobe EEG abnormalities also may be associated with panic attacks in adulthood (162). He also implicated congenital lesions of the dorso–lateral prefrontal cortex in the development of schizophrenia in adolescence.

Before discussing mechanisms that may contribute to the neurodevelopment of panic, it is useful to review general patterns of neurodevelopment (163–165). Prenatally, neuronal determination, neuronal migration to appropriate sites, neuronal maturation, and the outgrowth of axons and dendrites are significant processes. These steps are "progressive" in that they provide for connections in the brain and "competitive" in that the growth of active pathways is facilitated and inactive pathways regress (165). The progressive processes begin in fetal life and taper during early childhood and adolescence. Regressive events, including cell death, axonal regression, and synapse degeneration parallel progressive processes and provide for the specificity of central nervous function (163, 166, 167). Although regressive processes begin in infancy, they continue throughout life. During most of adult life, regressive loss of neurons, neuronal projections, synapses and other microstructures do not produce appreciable loss of function. However, in both animals and humans, old age is associated with noticeable decrements in both brain structure and function (168–173). Also, neurons are generally genetically "preprogrammed" to follow specific developmental patterns. Despite this genetic program, the brain regions which underlie fear acquisition retain significant plasticity and may respond to environmental factors or developmentally-regulated alterations in gene expression with functional alteration, and even subtle structural changes which shall be reviewed later in this chapter.

Returning to processes more specifically

relevant to panic disorder, congenital disturbances in noradrenergic neurodevelopment could account for the onset of panic symptoms at various stages in the life cycle. A model for an inherited noradrenergic lesion producing abnormal behavior during infancy is provided by the "tottering" mouse where a single locus mutation abnormally increases the number of locus coeruleus axonal projections, producing heightened behavioral reactivity, associated with seizures (174).

Genetic or environmental factors which disturb normal noradrenergic neurodevelopment could produce panic later in life when modulated function is required for normal social behavior. Noradrenergic systems undergo functional alterations during neurodevelopment. Unlike adult neurons, neonatal locus coeruleus neurons do not show spontaneous activity, fire equally strongly to noxious and innocuous stimuli, and increase firing in response to α_1-agonists (175, 176). Central α_2-adrenergic receptors also undergo a functional shift. The α_2-agonist, clonidine, produces hyperactivity in 7-day-old rats and hypoactivity in 20-day-old rats (177). Congenital lesions which alter the shift from infant to adult patterns of noradrenergic function could contribute to subsequent panic attacks.

Age-specific behavioral display of abnormalities in brain "fear centers" is also indicated by lesion studies. Bilateral amygdalectomy in infant monkeys has no effect on the "protest–despair" response to maternal deprivation. However, alarm responses are significantly attenuated by similar brain lesions in older monkeys (178). Similarly, prefrontal lobectomy failed to disturb social behaviors in infant rhesus monkeys but grossly disturbed these behaviors in juveniles and adults (179).

Developmentally Regulated Gene Expression

Panic attacks may also arise as a disturbance in the normal shifts in gene expression which occur during neurodevelopment. These shifts contribute to the development of adult patterns of function of a variety of brain nuclei (175, 180) and may include shifts from fetal to adult forms of regulatory proteins (181) and receptors (182).

In this model, panic disorder might be developmentally expressed analogously to the hemoglobinopathies (183). Hemoglobin is composed of four subunits. In most healthy adults there are two α subunits and two β subunits. In fetal life, however, the primary hemoglobin has two α units and two δ units (hemoglobic F). The gene coding for the δ subunit is next to the β subunit gene on chromosome 11. However, hemoglobin F functions poorly in the adult and adults who continue to produce Hemoglobin F are functionally anemic. Other diseases also arise in the transition from the fetal to the adult form of hemoglobin. For example, some anemic individuals retain the fetal homoglobin and do not switch to the adult form. Other anemic individuals, those with β thalessemia, produce an abnormal δ subunit from a gene also located on chromosome 11 rather than the normal adult β subunit. A third group of anemics express the right genes, but there is a structural abnormality in the gene. For example, sickle cell disease arises out of a gene error which changes a single amino acid in the β sub-unit of hemoglobin. Sickle cell disease nicely illustrates the complex interaction of developmentally regulated gene expression and environmental factors. Although sickle cell anemia arises from a genetic abnormality, a second process, hypoxia, is required to bring about sickle crises. The hypoxia interacts specifically with the abnormal hemoglobin structure but may be caused by toxins, such as carbon monoxide, or behaviors such as exercise.

Similarly, sex steroids, which act primarily through altering gene expression (184) might contribute to the postpubertal incidence of panic disorder and, perhaps, its differential incidence between sexes. Prenatally, the sex steroids have a major role in the neurodevelopment of brain regions which contribute to fear regulation including the hypothalamus, amygdala, and brainstem regions (reviewed in 185, 186). In addition, androgens and estrogens influence the migration of neural crest cells and may specifically control the development of cerebral lateralization (163, 164).

Developmental alterations in gene expression mediated by sex steroids could also be important to sexual differences in the onset and course of panic disorder at puberty and throughout adulthood. Clinically, premenstrual increases in the frequency of panic attacks (42) may be mediated by ovarian steroid effects on neuroendocrine regulation neuronal function (185, 187–189). Ovarian steroids decrease β-adrenoceptor sensitivity and increase α-receptor sensitivity in the hypothalamus (190). Other brain regions relevant to anxiety regulation, such as the amygdala and hippocampus, also show sex steroid modulation of noradrenergic receptor function (188, 191, 192). Physiologically, this modulation occurs cyclically in females, (193) although one group has questioned the significance of estrous changes for second messenger function (194).

Environmental Factors

Panic disorder could also arise during adolescence from disruptive influences of environmental factors on normal neurodevelopment. Neuronal development is particularly sensitive to disruption during periods of rapid growth, "critical periods in development." Most critical periods are early in life as most progressive events in neurodevelopment occur prenatally or in infancy. However, some progressive processes, such as myelinization of the reticular activating system and frontal cortex, continue through the 3rd decade of life in humans (195). Also, some brain regions, such as the hippocampus and amygdala, where processes such as long-term potentiation and kindling occur, retain microstructural plasticity through adulthood (11, 196, 197). Environmental processes which disrupt normal neurodevelopment include alterations in the level of environmental stimulation, malnutrition, and toxin or drug exposure.

Abnormally low or high levels of environmental stimulation can have deleterious effects on normal brain development which could predispose individuals to disorders of arousal regulation. While the migration and general pattern of synaptogenesis of the cortex is largely genetically determined, dark rearing, a form of sensory deprivation, impairs the development of visual cortical neurons while moderate levels of environmental stimulation enhance cortical development (198–200). Monocular closure competitively enhances the inputs from the intact eye through noradrenergic-dependent mechanisms (201–203). Such shifts, though, increase the locus coeruleus innervation of brain nuclei affected by sensory deprivation (204). These alterations in noradrenergic innervation may have general consequences for alarm regulation of significance-highlighting functions attributed to the locus coeruleus (205, 206).

Abnormally high levels of environmental stimulation may be traumatic and contribute to the later appearance of panic disorder through neurodevelopmental mechanisms, such as transsynaptic regulation of gene expression (206a). Overly stressful environments stunt cortical development (207). Also, severe uncontrollable environmental events appear to be particularly potent stimuli for engendering long-lasting "post-traumatic" fear and avoidance learning. These learned responses are mediated by noradrenergic systems, among others. The traumatic learning involves alterations in neuronal plasticity at many levels including receptor regulation, second messenger function, regulatory phosphoproteins, gene expression, and regional microstructural alterations (reviewed in 11). Severe aversive uncontrollable stimulus exposure has been proposed as a model for PTSD (11, 15, 207a). Environmental stress contributes both generally and specifically to models for the onset of panic.

Stress diathesis models for panic disorder attribute the increased incidence of life stress associated with the onset of panic disorder, reviewed earlier in this chapter, to general mechanisms. A more specific neurodevelopmental model is needed for panic disorder which links specific neurobiologic genetic abnormalities manifested in abnormal neuronal function to the specific neurobiologic consequences of "overstimulation" or "trauma" from environmental stimulus exposure.

Malnutrition and toxins may also influence noradrenergic neurodevelopment and contribute to subsequent behavioral abnormalities. Prenatal (maternal) or infant malnutrition impairs cortical development (208, 209) and alters the regulation of cortical activity in developing rats (210). Early malnutrition also reduces the numbness of α- and β-adrenoceptors in the adult brain and increases brainstem concentrations of serotonin and its metabolite 5-HIAA (211, 212). These biologic changes are associated with heightened environmental reactivity or fear including decreased exploratory activity and behavioral inhibition in two-way avoidance tasks (212). Exposure to neurotoxins, such as 6-hydroxydopamine, during development produces localized noradrenergic hyperenervation of the brainstem (213). Preliminary evidence also suggests that chronic prenatal exposure to caffeine may also alter dendritic branching during development (214). Chronic intermittent cocaine use also produces context-dependent sensitization of brain catecholamine function through "kindling" (215, 216). Related processes may pertain to cocaine-induced panic attacks.

Regressive Events in Development, Old Age, and Outgrowing Panic

In old age, the unbalanced loss of neurons, synapses, and decreases in brain metabolic activity could contribute to the "outgrowing" of panic symptoms in elderly individuals with the disorder. Noradrenergic systems which may be relevant to the genesis of panic attacks are generally decreased in function in old age. In humans, the number of locus coeruleus neurons decreases in old age (cited in 172). In rats, there is a senescent decline in the number of catecholamine receptors, (217)

norepinephrine-sensitive second messenger function (218, 219), decreased hippocampal sensitivity to norepinephrine (220), and decreased circulatory reactivity to stress-induced increases in plasma catecholamines (221). However, presynaptic autoinhibition is also lost with senescent cell loss. Aged rats show greater central and peripheral noradrenergic responses to stress (221, 221a). Although elderly men exhibit smaller stress-induced increases in urinary epinephrine, baseline plasma catecholamines are elevated and stress-induced increases in catecholamines return to baseline more slowly in elderly men than in younger men (222, 223). Consistent with the loss of baseline autoinhibition, excessive baseline catecholamine stimulation produces an age-dependent decline in platelet α_2-adrenoceptors (223).

Genetic Endowment, Rearing, and Environmental Reactivity

There is substantial evidence that the degree of emotional reactivity to environmental stimuli is a stable trait which is genetically inherited but also influenced by upbringing. Kagan and his associates (161, 224) showed that the degree of behavioral inhibition in response to a novel stimulus correlates with the autonomic response to a mildly stressful situation. In these studies, autonomic response was assessed by changes in heart rate and pupillary diameter. Behavioral inhibition may also predispose for later panic disorder (61). The incidence of behavioral inhibition was higher in children of parents with major depression (50%) than in healthy subjects and higher still in children of patients with panic disorder or agoraphobia (greater than 70%).

The specific interaction of genetic endowment and rearing in determining the level of environmental reactivity of an organism has been studied most carefully in the nonhuman primate by Suomi and his colleagues (157). By studying groups of siblings and half-siblings, they distinguished strains of genetically anxious rhesus monkeys that exhibited greater behavioral and neuroendocrine reactivity to environmental stimuli than genetically calm monkeys. After maternal separation, both the anxious and calm monkeys exhibited initial alarm phase responses as described in children by Bowlby (101). However, only the genetically anxious monkeys subsequently developed long-term traumatic sequelae, described earlier. These anxious monkeys generally competed poorly for social dominance and exhibited abnormally heightened reactivity when raised by anxious mothers. The anxious mothers also made poor parents; they handled their infants clumsily and often neglected or injured their offspring during rearing. However, when genotypically anxious monkey infants were raised by calm mothers, they often became socially dominant and resisted exhibiting behavioral abnormalities as long as the calm mother was present. In other words, the genetically anxious monkeys who possessed an anxious genotype exhibited a calm or even a competitively superior phenotype in the presence of the calm mother. However, when separated from their calm mothers or returned to anxious mothers, the genetically anxious monkeys reverted to their anxious genotype and again showed increased stress sensitivity and the full range of anxiety- and depressionlike symptoms.

The Social Darwinists of the 19th and early 20th centuries suggested a simple model to explain dominance hierarchies: Successful people had better genes and, as a result, better brains (225). However, the primate studies by Suomi and his colleagues do not indicate the presence of a simple "constitutional" weakness in the genetically reactive monkeys. Their heightened neurobiologic reactivity predisposed these monkeys to traumatization when maternally deprived or raised by anxious mothers. However, as noted above, this trait appeared advantageous when the animals were raised by calm mothers. As with other superficially disadvantageous genetic traits, such as the sickle cell gene which protects heterzygous individuals from malaria infections, (183, 225, 226)

the specific implications of possessing the "reactivity" or "traumatization" gene depends on the particular interactions between genetic and environmental factors.

TREATMENT

Traditionally two groups of drugs have been used to treat the anxiety disorders, the antidepressants and the benzodiazepines (5). Subsequent advances include the introduction of the potent triazalobenzodiazepine alprazolam, which shows antipanic and antianxiety effects. Also, buspirone, which appears to possess antianxiety actions (71) without antipanic efficacy (D. Charney et al., unpublished data). As discussed below, the differential efficacy of pharmacotherapies and behavioral therapies supports biologic distinctions between panic disorder and GAD. Psychotherapeutic approaches to anxiety-disorder patients are explored in Chapters 45 and 48. This section will focus on pharmacologic treatments. Additional integrative management issues for anxiety-disorder patients are reviewed in the section entitled "The Clinical Interview."

Panic Disorder and Agoraphobia

Klein initially suggested that imipramine was effective in the treatment of panic disorder without effecting the level of generalized anxiety (5). Subsequent studies by other groups confirmed the efficacy of pharmacotherapeutic interventions in panic disorder and agoraphobia (22, 227, 228). One initial question concerning the heterocyclic antidepressants was whether these drugs possessed direct antipanic properties or whether the antipanic effects were secondary to their ability to alleviate depression. A growing body of evidence suggests that the heterocyclics alleviate panic attacks independently of their antidepressant effects. Several studies have reported dissociation between the antipanic and antianxiety actions of antidepressants (229, 230). Another study questioned whether lower imipramine levels are required to treat panic disorder than commonly needed in major depression (231).

Charney and his associates suggested that there might be a biochemical rationale for the dissociation between the antidepressant and antipanic actions of the antidepressants (227). They found that the noradrenergically active substances imipramine and alprazolam were effective in treating panic and phobic avoidance, whereas the serotonergically active drug trazodone was ineffective in treating panic attacks. Sheehan and his associates also noted that bupropion, whose mechanism of action may involve central dopamine systems, also showed antidepressant but not antipanic effects (232). However, recent reports of the efficacy of serotonergically selective antidepressants, fluoxetine, (233) trazodone (234), and fluvoxamine, (235) in panic disorder question the necessity of primary effects on noradrenergic function for the efficacy of antipanic drugs.

The clinical utility of the antidepressants in panic disorder may be improved by educating the patient about the likelihood of delayed efficacy and about possible side effects. Although the anxiolytic properties of the heterocyclic agents may differ from their antidepressant actions, there is still approximately a 4-week delay in efficacy when heterocyclics are used in the treatment of panic disorder and agoraphobia. Although imipramine is a highly effective treatment in panic disorder and agoraphobia, some patients with these disorders will have difficulty starting these medications because of a paradoxical anxiety which may be precipitated in the early phase of treatment (22). The mechanism of this paradoxical anxiety is unclear at this time but may have to do with the reuptake blockade actions which may functionally increase postsynaptic noradrenergic tone.

In order to minimize the anxiogenesis often associated with the initiation of heterocyclic treatment, treatment may start with very low doses of imipramine, such as 10 mg at bedtime. This dose should be increased gradually to a dose which often approximates the antidepressant range, between 150 and 300 mg. Some patients may do quite well, however, at doses usually believed too low to be effective in depressed patients. Other patients may need supplementation of antidepressants with benzodiazepines during the initial phases of treatment prior to the onset of antipanic and antiphobic actions. These benzodiazepines may be useful for controlling the "paradoxical" anxiety induced initially by the heterocyclic agents (see also 236).

The monoamine oxidase inhibitors are also highly effective treatments for panic disorder and agoraphobia. Sheehan and his associates found that some patients with panic disorder do better on monoamine oxidase inhibitors than on imipramine (228). Although some patients may initially resist these drugs because of the associated dietary restrictions, clinicians should keep these drugs in mind, particularly for treatment resistant patients. Other groups with related disorders, such as social phobia or atypical depressions with concomitant panic attacks, may also benefit by the introduction of a monoamine oxidase inhibitor (7, 237).

Although the anxiolytic actions of benzodiazepines were recognized early on, their antipanic effects were initially questioned (5). Alprazolam was the first benzodiazepine with documented efficacy in treating panic disorder (230). Subsequent studies have confirmed the efficacy of alprazolam in panic disorder (62). Unlike the antidepressants, alprazolam begins to have antipanic and antiphobic effects within the first week of prescription, which makes it quite attractive to many panic disorder patients (237). In addition, alprazolam continues to have antipanic efficacy during chronic treatment, as demonstrated in a recent 2½-year follow-up study (239). The effective dose range for alprazolam in treating panic is usually 2 to 6 mg/day. Other benzodiazepines, such as lorazepam, clonazepam, and diazepam, have also shown antipanic efficacy (62). The long half-life of clonazepam may be advantageous for patients who experience brief periods of discomfort between alprazolam doses (240). The doses of these drugs must be adjusted for their potency at the benzodiazepine receptor (roughly, 1 mg alprazolam = 2 mg lorazepam = 0.5 mg clonazepam = 10 mg diazepam) (62).

Recently there has been increased concern that chronic benzodiazepine prescription results in benzodiazepine addiction characterized by both physical and psychologic dependence (241). However, a recent follow-up study (239) found that many patients, even those who have been on alprazolam for an average of 2½ years, could taper their dose or discontinue benzodiazepine completely without significant resurgence of anxiety symptoms or withdrawal symptoms as long as the taper was sufficiently gradual. Some patients with panic disorder did experience a resurgence of symptoms when the drug was stopped and therefore required long-term prescription of benzodiazepines for the treatment of their anxiety disorder. In many patients, it is difficult to distinguish withdrawal from a return of panic symptoms. However, such distinctions are important for clinical management. The rate of the taper is a critical factor influencing the success of benzodiazepine discontinuation (241). Abrupt discontinuation of benzodiazepines can produce serious medical side effects such as hallucinations, nightmares, and seizures (62, 242).

Although many patients will receive significant clinical benefit from alprazolam with doses within the 2 to 6 mg/day range, some patients will require greater doses (8 to 10 mg/day) in order to adequately control panic attacks. The decision to exceed the usual clinical doses of benzodiazepines must be done on an individual basis and with great care for potential side effects such as sedation, ataxia, and memory loss. Many clinicians believe that ongoing psychotherapy can help to minimize the dose of benzodiazepines required for control of symptoms. Heterocyclic antidepressants or monoamine oxidase inhibitors may provide an alternative to high dose benzodiazepine treatment. Shehi and Patterson also suggested that concomitant prescription of propranolol and alprazolam to treatment-resistant patients may also permit use of lower alprazolam doses in patients with panic attacks (242). Overall, the benzodiazepines are highly effective treatments for panic disorder and agoraphobia whose risks for both abuse and side effects are minimal when monitored closely by a physician. Ongoing research, though, is directed toward finding anxioselective benzodiazepines which do not cause sedation, tolerance, or withdrawal.

Generalized Anxiety Disorder

Benzodiazepines are the most commonly prescribed treatment for GAD (reviewed in 62). The benzodiazepines with documented efficacy in GAD include diazepam, (243) alprazolam (244), lorazepam (Woods et al., unpublished data) and clonazepam (245). As in panic disorder, benzodiazepines have a rapid onset of efficacy in decreasing GAD symptoms.

Heterocyclic antidepressants have also been reintroduced as a treatment for GAD. Although Klein suggested that imipramine lacks anxiolytic effects on generalized anxiety symptoms (5), recent studies suggest that imipramine may also be an effective treatment for GAD. Hoehn-Saric and McCleod found that both imipramine and benzodiazepines were effective in the treatment of GAD (246). Further, a more recent study (247) suggested that imipramine may be more effective in the treatment of generalized anxiety symptoms than benzodiazepines. In this study, therapeutic effects on generalized anxiety were still present after patients with panic attacks were excluded.

Recently, serotonergically active drugs have been introduced as treatments for GAD. Buspirone, the best studied of these drugs, appears to possess efficacy in GAD but not panic disorder (71; Charney et al., unpublished data). Buspirone has no anticonvulsant, sedative, or muscle relaxant effects, nor does it interact with alcohol or have a high risk for abuse (248). Like the antidepressants, buspirone has delayed anxiolytic effects which appear approximately 2 to 3 weeks after starting medication and reach a level comparable to benzodiazepines (see 72, 248). Both buspirone and gepirone, a drug which has not yet been released (249), appear to produce their anxiolytic efficacy by acting at the inhibitory presynaptic serotonin receptor, the 5-HT$_{1A}$ receptor (70). Ritanserin, a 5-HT$_2$ receptor antagonist, has also shown some efficacy in GAD patients (250). The efficacy of buspirone, gepirone, and ritanserin in GAD supports a role for serotonin in this disorder, in contrast to panic disorder, where trazodone shows inconsistent efficacy (227). Buspirone appears to exert its optimal clinical effects at doses ranging between 30 and 50 mg/day. Most patients tolerate an initial dose of 15 mg/day (5 mg three times a day) which is gradually increased over 4 weeks or so. Side effects, such as nausea and dizziness are usually mild and dose related (251).

Another group of drugs currently in development, drugs which may be useful in the treatment of GAD, are the mixed agonist–antagonist benzodiazepines, which produce anxiolytic effects in animal models with a minimal degree of physical dependency (62). Animal studies indicate that the antagonist component of these drugs are responsible for minimizing the degree of physical dependence which develops during chronic administration (252).

Post-Traumatic Stress Disorder

The first step in treating post-traumatic stress disorders is terminating the trauma. For soldiers, this might mean leaving an area of immediate combat or, during peace time, terminating a process of victimization which might be ongoing (45, 46). In World War II, one of the first pharmacologic supports, sodium amytal, was used as an acute anxiolytic and as an agent to facilitate abreaction, that is, reexperiencing traumatic material in a controlled fashion (45, 46). To date, Frank and her associates have reported the only double-blind, placebo-controlled, study of pharmacotherapy for PTSD (253). In this study, patients were randomly assigned to placebo, phenelzine, or imipramine. Both imipramine and phenelzine were effective treatments for the spectrum of symptoms of PTSD. However, there was a trend for phenelzine to show higher efficacy for symptoms of anxiety and intrusive reexperiencing. Out-

side of this study, a number of case reports, trials, and retrospective studies support the efficacy of tricyclics and monoamine oxidase inhibitors in the treatment of PTSD (reviewed in 11).

A broad spectrum of other medications, however, have been employed and found useful in the treatment of PTSD. Van der Kolk reported the results of an open trial using lithium which suggested that this medication was particularly useful for affective and reexperiencing symptoms (254). Lipper at al. reported that tegretol (carbamazepine) showed a similar spectrum of efficacy to lithium in treating PTSD in an open medication trial (255). Alprazolam also showed efficacy in creating PTSD symptoms, particularly anxiety-related phenomena (256). However, clinicians have been somewhat reluctant to prescribe benzodiazepines in populations in whom substance abuse is a common problem. Thus, benzodiazepines are rarely prescribed on a chronic basis to Vietnam veterans with PTSD. Kolb and his associates have recently reported a small open trial of clonidine which suggested that this drug was efficacious in treating anxiety, sleep disturbance, and intrusive reminders of the trauma (257). The efficacy of clonidine in treating PTSD has been most interesting in light of hypotheses that some symptoms of PTSD may be produced by central noradrenergic hyperactivity (11, 107a). A number of groups have also reported that propranolol may relieve some symptoms of PTSD (254, 257). However, as reported for other disorders, propranolol is a relatively weak anxiolytic. Neuroleptics are also commonly prescribed for PTSD, particularly for individuals with poor impulse control or who have psychotic features with their PTSD.

Obsessive–Compulsive Disorder

As a rule, OCD is relatively resistant to treatment. Psychotherapeutic interventions based on traditional psychoanalytic interpretations of obsessive–compulsive symptoms are largely ineffective and, in some cases, may cause more distress for the patient without removing symptoms

(258). The introduction of behavior modification approaches, particularly those using exposure and response prevention techniques, have met with greater success (259). Unfortunately, many patients may not be suitable candidates for behavior therapy. OCD patients with depression or very severe symptoms may not be able to tolerate the additional anxiety generated during exposure to stimuli which provoke their symptoms. However, the fortuitous discovery that the potent serotonin reuptake inhibitor clomipramine was effective in obsessive–compulsive patients has led to trials of other agents that may be promising in the treatment of OCD.

The success of clomipramine in open trials of OCD has been confirmed in a number of double-blind placebo-controlled studies (260). In the majority of studies, response of OCD symptoms to clomipramine treatment was not related to the severity of depressive symptoms present at the start of treatment (260). Several studies showed that even when patients with prominent depressive symptoms were excluded, OCD symptoms significantly improved with clomipramine treatment. Although there is still debate, such studies provide evidence that clomipramine, and possibly other serotonergic agents, may possess specific antiobsessional effects in addition to their antidepressant properties. This serotonergic selectivity in OCD contrasts with depression where antidepressant drugs with differing profiles for monoamine uptake blockade seem roughly equivalent in efficacy.

In several studies of OCD, clomipramine was superior to drugs with less potent effects on serotonin reuptake (260). In one double-blind study, obsessive–compulsive symptoms improved after clomipramine treatment but did not change significantly during treatment with the less potent serotonin reuptake inhibitors amitriptyline (261) and noritriptyline (79). In double-blind crossover studies, clomipramine was found to be more effective than either desipramine or the monoamine oxidase inhibitor clorgyline (260). Two studies failed to demonstrate a clear advantage for clomipramine over the somewhat weaker serotonin reuptake inhibitor, imipramine (262, 263). However, in a recent placebo-controlled study imipramine was found to be ineffective in treating obsessive–compulsive symptoms (264). More comparison trials between clomipramine and other antidepressant agents with different reuptake blocking properties are needed. However, it is apparent that antidepressant agents like imipramine are not as effective in OCD as they are in depression.

Several trials have now been conducted with serotonergically selective antidepressant agents. Prior to the discovery of serious adverse side effects, zimelidine, a selective serotonin reuptake inhibitor, was found helpful in reducing symptoms of OCD in three out of four trials (260). Although, double-blind studies are awaited, fluoxetine, a selective and potent inhibitor of serotonin reuptake, has been shown to be helpful in reducing symptoms of OCD in two studies (260). Also, a related drug, fluvoxamine, a unicyclic agent which is still under investigation in the United States, was first shown helpful in reducing symptoms of severe inpatient obsessive–compulsives (82). Subsequently, fluvoxamine was demonstrated to be superior to placebo in two double-blind trials in OCD outpatients (83, 265). In neither of these studies was the response of obsessive–compulsive symptoms related to the presence of depression.

The addition of lithium carbonate to ongoing antidepressant treatment has proved to be an effective approach to the treatment of refractory depression, consistent with preclinical evidence that lithium enhances serotonergic transmission. Similarly, there have been reports that combining lithium with clomipramine, trazodone, or fluvoxamine may augment the antiobsessional effects of these agents. Although preliminary data suggest that lithium augmentation is helpful, it is not as clearly efficacious in OCD as in depression (83; Goodman et al., unpublished data). The serotonin precursor tryptophan, alone or in combination with clomipramine, may also reduce obsessive–compulsive symptoms (83). Thus, the addition of lithium or tryptophan to antidepressant treatment may be considered in selected treatment refractory cases of OCD. Caution should be exercised in using tryptophan with monoamine oxidase inhibitors. Also, lithium, by itself, is probably not helpful in treating OCD (266). Among the available tricyclic antidepressant agents, there is some evidence favoring the use of imipramine in OCD at higher doses and for longer durations than typically used to treat depression (261–263). Monoamine oxidase inhibitors may also be helpful in some cases of OCD, particularly those with a history of panic disorder (267).

In contrast to some of the other anxiety disorders, benzodiazepine therapy seems of limited usefulness in OCD. Although, there have been several case reports of alprazolam reducing obsessive–compulsive symptoms, the general consensus is that in most cases benzodiazepines do little more than reduce the derivative anxiety symptoms (268). The use of buspirone in OCD has not been adequately tested.

There have been few systematic studies of neuroleptics in OCD (269). However, the weight of clinical experience suggests that neuroleptics are not useful in most cases. In our experience, patients frequently enter our program after many years on neuroleptics despite the absence of demonstrable benefits associated with their use. Until further studies demonstrate otherwise, the use of neuroleptics alone in the treatment of OCD is probably not justified. However, there is some preliminary evidence that neuroleptics may provide a useful adjunct to antidepressant treatment in putative subtypes of OCD. For example, the combination of an antidepressant drug with a neuroleptic, such as pimozide, may be helpful in cases of OCD presenting with schizotypal features or brief psychotic episodes. Also, it is possible that patients who show symptoms of both OCD and Tourette's syndrome may benefit from a combination of neuroleptics and antidepressants. For example, a recent case report described a patient suffering from both OCD and Tourette's syndrome who required a combination of fluvoxamine and pimozide for adequate control of

his OCD symptoms (Delgado et al., unpublished data). Despite several case reports that electroconvulsive therapy may ameliorate OCD symptoms, it is largely ineffective in OCD, especially when contrasted with its potent antidepressant effects (260). In the most severe cases, those who do not respond to any medication, stereotactic psychosurgery such as limbic leucotomy may be considered (270). Unfortunately, as has been the case with neuroleptics, benzodiazepines, and electroconvulsive therapy, these treatments have not been studied systematically.

THE CLINICAL INTERVIEW

Determining the Nature of the Problem

The clinical interview is a critical step in diagnosis and treatment of anxiety disorders. The first diagnostic issue faced by clinicians working with anxiety disorder patients is to rule out medical illness mimicking anxiety disorders. Ordinarily a careful history, supplemented in relevant patients by a physical and laboratory evaluation, is sufficient to dismiss diagnoses such as partial complex seizures, hyperthyroidism, caffeine abuse, or pheochromacytoma. Next, the clinician should determine whether the patient experiences panic attacks. It is critical to elicit a history of panic attacks because they respond to appropriate treatment. Many patients will be able to provide a clear history of panic attacks which are sudden in onset and meet the four symptoms criteria outlined in DSM-III-R. Such patients would generally be able to provide the clinician with the date of onset of the panic attack, their frequency and severity, and a description of the settings in which attacks take place.

Many patients, however, do not connect their symptoms to an anxiety disorder. As a result, they will first present to nonpsychiatric professionals for a variety of somatic complaints, particularly in the cardiovascular, gastrointestinal, and neurologic spheres. For many patients, the labeling of their clinical state as an anxiety disorder and their collection of symptoms as panic attacks will have major clinical benefits in their ongoing treatment.

Generally, once the presence or absence of panic attacks has been determined, the next clinical step is to explore the extent of anticipatory anxiety or agoraphobia which accompanies the panic attacks. In doing so, the clinician needs to consider the factors which trigger anxiety. These triggers include a broad spectrum of stimuli, including biologic precipitants, such as caffeine, which may precipitate anxiety by a direct action on the central nervous system; indirect biologic precipitants, such as hot temperature or exercise, which may produce many symptoms associated with anxiety; environmental precipitants, such as being in places where the individual feels trapped, e.g., elevators or traffic jams; and interpersonal precipitants, such as marital separation. These stimuli, which might be called "primary triggers" frequently precipitate anxiety attributed to secondary factors which are important to the patient. These "secondary triggers" or, as they are called by our staff, "fears behind the fears," include such concerns as fear of death, fear of humiliation, and fear of loss of control. For example, patients may present with a fear of driving because they notice that when driving, their heart pounds and they are afraid of having a heart attack. Often such patients are aware of their heart pounding and the anxiety, but they may not be aware of the connection between those symptoms and their fear of death. Cognitively oriented interventions directly addressing the primary and secondary triggers are frequently useful for patients.

It is also useful to inquire about the extent of the patient's phobic avoidance. Most panic patients avoid situations associated with previous panic attacks or where attacks might be particularly threatening. Obtaining a list of patients' phobias is the first step in helping them to overcome them in systematic desensitization procedures (270).

For many individuals, distinguishing so-cial phobia and agoraphobia will facilitate treatment. Social phobics will particularly highlight their fear of scrutiny and concerns about performance, whereas agoraphobic often accentuate their concerns about being trapped and the precipitation of panic attacks in nonsocial settings. Also, social phobics should not report a history of multiple spontaneous panic attacks.

In diagnosing GAD, one must pay particular attention to obtaining a history of anxiety which occurs in the absence of panic attacks and which is tonic rather than phasic in nature. As noted earlier, individuals with generalized anxiety often describe waking with anxiety which stays at a relatively stable level of severity throughout the day and which they experience until they go to sleep at night.

Post-traumatic stress disorders are frequently missed by clinicians, even those clinicians who elicit a history of trauma. One reason for this lack of clinical recognition is that the patient may fail to connect these patients' symptoms to their psychologic trauma. In fact, some patients will be hesitant to discuss the traumatic incident with the interviewer because it is shameful to them, (271) because they are concerned that their material may overwhelm the therapist, (272) or because the material may be too upsetting for the patient to discuss. In addition, PTSD may be complicated by dissociative episodes at the time of the trauma, so that individuals may have cognitive difficulties recalling the trauma. Obtaining a thorough history of the trauma is an important aspect of diagnosis and treatment but it must be conducted with sensitivity for the patient's capacity to tolerate reviewing the clinical material.

Another possible reason for the underdiagnosis of PTSD is that patients may present during stages of significant emotional numbing which may mask other symptoms. When patients are reexperiencing the trauma, they report symptoms such as nightmares, intrusive thoughts, or flashbacks which clearly link the current content to a previous traumatic experience. However, while affectively constricted, individuals may report their emotional numbness or machinelike feeling, or they may have trouble recognizing or labeling how they feel (119, 273).

Obsessions and compulsions are hallmarks of OCD. Yet they are often present in the context of other diagnoses, such as panic disorder (20). Patients are often reluctant to reveal their symptoms spontaneously. In order to elicit a history of obsessions and/or compulsions, patients must be directly asked about these. The most common reason for the reluctance of patients to discuss obsessions or compulsions is that their content may be disturbing to patients. Also, obsessions may contain content which the patient considers socially unacceptable and, therefore, embarrassing. Alternatively, patients with OCD may have long-standing symptoms which have become incorporated into their life-style and are not recognized as part of the disorder. This incorporation may be particularly striking in patients who present primarily with avoidance symptoms. In our anxiety clinic, obsessions and compulsions are so common, and so disturbing for patients, that we advocate directly asking each new patient about their presence.

A thorough history is central to determining the nature of the presenting problem in patients with anxiety disorders. Substance abuse is an important factor influencing the course of anxiety disorders. Substances such as cocaine, alcohol, amphetamine, and caffeine may initiate or exacerbate severe anxiety disorders. Alternatively, opiate, alcohol, or marijuana use may be an attempt to self-medicate anxiety (48). A thorough medical history, as reviewed in Chapter 18, is also a critical factor in the differential diagnosis of anxiety disorders. Family history is an increasingly important part of the diagnostic interview for anxiety disorders, not only to determine the nature of ongoing environmental stress, but also to help inform the clinician concerning genetic issues pertinent to anxiety disorders. The developmental history is also an important component of the interview. As reviewed earlier, a history of childhood separation anxiety may be a prognostic factor for later anxiety disorders. In regard to PTSD, it would be important to know whether the individual had experienced previous traumas which might influence subsequent response to potentially traumatic events. Developmental history is also important for OCD because of the recent link between OCD and Tourette's syndrome (16, 49, 50). Also, individuals with OCD frequently report a history of minor behavioral symptoms such as culturally acceptable rituals or complex motor tics prior to their clinical presentation for OCD.

Developing and Maintaining a Therapeutic Relationship

The most important aspect of treating individuals with anxiety disorders is to maintain a calm empathic relationship in the face of the fluctuating anxiety levels in the patient. Anxiety patients present two particular problems to the therapeutic relationship: avoidance and dependence. As a result of dealing with severe uncontrollable anxiety, individuals with anxiety disorders often develop a sense of hopelessness and helplessness toward their disorder. Clinicians working with anxiety-disorder patients must not collaborate in the sense of hopelessness and helplessness but must help patients to refrain from their negative perceptions of their illness and facilitate the development of an active stance toward symptom control. In initiating the therapeutic relationship, it is useful to let the patient know that you understand the illness and the symptoms that he or she might be experiencing. This approach is useful for anxiety patients who experience their symptoms as isolating and beyond their control and patients who may consider their symptoms shameful. Early in treatment, when symptoms of panic or generalized anxiety are particularly problematic, patients may require substantial support from their clinicians. However, most of these patients reduce their demands on the therapist once their symptoms begin to respond to appropriate treatment. Increased support during the early phases of illness does not appear to be destructive to the long-term goal of facilitating the autonomy of patients.

Developing and maintaining a therapeutic relationship may be slightly modified in dealing with patients with PTSD. Having been victims in a traumatic setting, such individuals frequently experience themselves as victims in their relationship outside of the trauma. As a result, individuals with PTSD often experience the therapeutic relationship as one which threatens to repeat the victimization experience. In contrast to the somewhat "expert" stance, which is often useful in other anxiety disorders, in treating PTSD, it is often useful to present oneself as less authoritarian.

When introducing medications into the treatment of anxiety disorders, it is important that patients recognize that their medications will ultimately produce clinical benefits. If patients can be motivated by a sense of collaboration to comply with medications such as the tricyclics, which may initially exacerbate some anxiety symptoms, they may ultimately achieve the benefits which accrue from clinically appropriate anxiolytic trials. For such patients, it is often useful to highlight the synergistic contributions of pharmacotherapy and psychotherapy.

Communication, Information, and Implementing a Treatment Plan

Patients with anxiety disorders, particularly those without significant additional psychopathology, are generally quite allied with treatment. However, conflicts in the clinical setting do occasionally arise in a number of areas, including the recognition of their diagnosis and their compliance with treatment. Some patients are resistant to the idea that they carry a psychiatric diagnosis and prefer to think of themselves as having a medical illness which produces symptoms commonly associated with panic attacks. This conflict potentially influences treatment since many of the psychotherapeutic strategies for treating panic disorder rely on the patient's recognition of irrational beliefs associated with anxiety symptoms. For some patients this resistance is easily dealt with in group therapy, where they readily see that other people with anxiety disorders have similar symptoms and syndromes. In individual therapy, however, it is sometimes useful to develop an alliance with patients around the belief system of a biomedical disturbance which produces panic, agoraphobia, or social phobia. Many patients who would not accept treatment when offered in a more psychologically minded fashion can ally with both psychotherapeutic and psychopharmacologic treatment when presented in a biomedical context. As noted earlier, the treatment alliance is essential for maintaining compliance particularly with the antidepressant medications. Implementing treatment plans may also be facilitated by early reduction of symptoms which may be achieved through use of benzodiazepines.

Other chapters have focused on insight-oriented and behavioral therapies for anxiety disorders, and these approaches are not reviewed here. Psychoeducational approaches can be particularly useful to patients with panic disorders. Many patients report a qualitative improvement in their life after accepting the idea that their symptoms may be attributed to panic disorder, agoraphobia, or other anxiety disorders. Often education about anxiety disorders may be facilitated through books about these disorders aimed at the lay public. In addition, psychoeducational approaches involving the family may be helpful in order to enable family members to make a useful contribution to the patient's treatment. Family members frequently find themselves overwhelmed by the limitations placed on family activity when a family member has agoraphobia or other anxiety disorders. In response, family members may ignore or ridicule the patient, exacerbating the patient's distress. Family members who themselves suffer from untreated panic disorder may find it particularly difficult to support affected family members. Family interventions have been particularly helpful in increasing family support both for treatment and for reinforcing "homework" assignments in treatment programs involving desensitization, progressive relaxation, or other techniques.

As noted earlier, patients with PTSD often are sensitive to feeling dehumanized or victimized. As a result, conflicts may arise concerning pharmacologic treatments if these are presented to patients in an impersonal manner. For such patients, the utility of medications must be carefully explained in the context of their treatment program. Family interactions are also useful for diminishing isolation and problems with empathy. Patients with OCD may require an extensive degree of support while undertaking behavioral desensitization or psychopharmacologic therapy.

As outpatients, patients with OCD may find it difficult to confront stimuli which they have been avoiding. Unless patients attempt to face phobic situations, the anticompulsive effects of the pharmacologic treatments may be missed. Family interventions may be quite effective in helping the OCD patients confront phobic situations. These patients also frequently avoid informing the clinician when they are having difficulty with their treatment, particularly side effects from medications, because of concerns that such complaints would jeopardize their therapy. In response, clinicians must be informed of possible side effects of treatment and actively inquire about them early in the course of tretment. Sensitive management of patients will increase their sense of security, improve compliance, and ultimately improve the success of treatment.

References

1. American Psychiatric Association: *Diagnostic and Statistical Manual of Mental Disorders (Third Edition-Revised)*. Washington, DC, American Psychiatric Association, 1987.
2. Freud S: On the grounds for detaching a particular syndrome from neurasthenia under the description "anxiety neurosis." In Strachey J, Freud A, Strachey A, et al. (eds): *The Standard Edition of the Complete Psychological Works of Sigmund Freud*. London, Hogarth Press and the Institute of Psycho-Analysis, 1895 pp 84–117.
3. American Psychiatric Association: *Diagnostic and Statistical Manual of Mental Disorders*. Washington, DC, American Psychiatric Association, 1952.
4. American Psychiatric Association: *Diagnostic and Statistical Manual of Mental Disorders (Second Edition)*. Washington, DC, American Psychiatric Association, 1968.
5. Klein DF: Delineation of two drug-responsive anxiety syndromes. *Psychopharmacology* 5:397–408, 1964.
6. American Psychiatric Association: *Diagnostic and Statistical Manual of Mental Disorders (Third Edition)*. Washington, DC, American Psychiatric Association, 1980.
7. Liebowitz MR, Gorman JM, Fyer AJ, et al: Social phobia: review of a neglected anxiety disorder. *Arch Gen Psychiatry* 42:729–736, 1985.
8. Barlow DH, Blanchard EB, Vermilyea JA, Vermilyea BB, DiNardo PA: Generalized anxiety and generalized anxiety disorder: Description and reconceptualization. *Am J Psychiatry* 143:40–44, 1986.
9. Anderson DJ, Noyes R Jr, Crowe RR: A comparison of panic disorder and generalized anxiety disorder. *Am J Psychiatry* 141:572–575, 1984.
10. Breier A, Charney DS, Heninger GR: The diagnostic validity of anxiety disorders and their relationship to depressive illness. *Am J Psychiatry* 142:787–797, 1985.
11. Krystal JH, Kosten TR, Perry BD, et al: Neurobiologic aspects of PTSD: Review of clinical and preclinical studies. *Behav Ther* (in press).
12. Rado S: Pathodynamics and treatment of traumatic war neurosis (traumatophobia). *Psychosom Med* 42:362–368, 1942.
13. Mellman TA, Davis GC: Combat-related flashbacks in post-traumatic stress disorder: phenomenology and similarity to panic attacks. *J Clin Psychiatry* 46:379–382, 1985.
14. Silver SM, Iacono CU: Factor-analytic support for DSM-III's post-traumatic stress disorder for Vietnam veterans. *J Clin Psychol* 40:5–14, 1984.
15. Krystal H: Trauma and affects. *Psychoanal Study Child* 33:81–116, 1978.
16. Rasmussen SA, Tsuang MT: Clinical characteristics and family history in DSM-III obsessive-compulsive disorder. *Am J Psychiatry* 143:317–322, 1986.
17. Wittchen H-U: Epidemiology of panic attacks and panic disorders. In Hand I, Wittchen H-U (eds): *Panic and Phobias: Empirical Evidence of Theoretical Models and Longterm Effects of Behavioral Treatments*. Springer-Verlag, New York, 1986, pp 18–28.
18. Coryell W, Noyes R, Clancy J: Panic disorder and primary unipolar depression: a comparison of background and outcome. *J Affect Dis* 5:311–317, 1983.
19. Robins LN, Helzer JE, Weissman MM, et al: Lifetime prevalence of specific psychiatric disorders in three sites. *Arch Gen Psychiatry* 41:949–958, 1984.
20. Breier A, Charney DS, Heninger GR: Agoraphobia with panic attacks. *Arch Gen Psychiatry* 43:1029–1036, 1986.
21. Uhlenhuth EH, Balter MB, Mellinger GD, et al: Symptom checklist syndromes in the general

population: development, diagnostic stability, and course of illness. *Arch Gen Psychiatry* 40:1167–1173, 1983.

22. Zitrin CM, Klein DF, Woerner MG, et al: Treatment of phobias: I. Comparison of imipramine and placebo. *Arch Gen Psychiatry* 40:125–138, 1983.

23. Thyer BA, Himle J, Curtis GC, et al: A comparison of panic disorder and agoraphobia with panic attacks. *Compr Psychiatry* 26:208–214, 1985.

24. Garvey MJ, Tuason VB: The relationship of panic disorder to agoraphobia. *Compr Psychiatry* 25:529–531, 1984.

25. Von Korff MR, Eaton WW, Keyl PM: The epidemiology of panic attacks and panic disorder: results of three community surveys. *Am J Epidemiol* 122:970–981, 1985.

26. Klein DF: Anxiety reconceptualized. Klein DF, Raskin J (eds): In *Anxiety: New Research and Changing Concepts*. New York, Raven Press, 1981, pp 235–263.

27. Tearnan BH, Telch MJ, Keefe P: Etiology and onset of agoraphobia: critical review. *Compr Psychiatry* 25:51–62, 1984.

28. Marks IM: The classification of phobic disorders. *Br J Psychiatry* 116:377–386, 1970.

29. Sheehan DV, Sheehan KE, Minichiello WE: Age of onset of phobic disorders: a reevaluation. *Compr Psychiatry* 22:544–553, 1981.

30. Thyer BA, Parrish RT, Curtis GC, et al: Ages of onset of DSM-III anxiety disorders. *Compr Psychiatry* 26:113–122, 1985.

31. Klein DF, Weissman MM, Leaf PJ, et al: Panic disorder and major depression: epidemiology, family studies, biologic, and treatment response similarities. *Psychopharmacol Bull* 21:538–541, 1985.

32. Thyer BA, Himle J, Curtis GC, et al: A comparison of panic disorder and agoraphobia with panic attacks. *Compr Psychiatry* 26:208–214, 1985.

33. Myers JK, Weissman MM, Tischler GL, et al: Six-month prevalence of psychiatric disorders in three communities. *Arch Gen Psychiatry* 41:959–967, 1984.

34. Cloninger CR, Martin RL, Clayton P, et al: A blind follow-up and family study of anxiety neurous: preliminary analysis of the St. Louis 500. In Klein DF, Rabkin J (eds): *Anxiety: New Research and Changing Concepts*. New York, Raven Press, 1981, pp 137–154.

35. DiNardo PA, O'Brien GT, Barlow DH, et al: Reliability of DSM-III anxiety disorder categories using a new structured interview. *Arch Gen Psychiatry* 40:1070–1074, 1983.

36. Riskind JH, Bech AT, Berchick RJ, et al: Reliability of DSM-III diagnoses for major depression and generalized anxiety disorder using the structured clinical interview for DSM-III. *Arch Gen Psychiatry* 44:817–820, 1987.

37. Breslau N, Davis GC: DSM-III generalized anxiety disorder: an empirical investigation of more stringent criteria. *Psychiatry Res* 14:231–238, 1985.

38. Sheehan DV, Sheehan KH: The classification of anxiety and hysterical states. Part I. Historical review and empirical delineation. *J Clin Psychopharmacol* 2:235–244, 1982.

39. Raskin M, Peeke HVS, Dickman W, et al: Panic and generalized anxiety disorders: Developmental antecedents and precipitants. *Arch Gen Psychiatry* 39:687–689, 1982.

40. Blazer D, Hughes D, George LK: Stressful life events and the onset of a generalized anxiety syndrome. *Am J Psychiatry* 144:1178–1183, 1987.

41. Hoehn-Saric R: Comparison of generalized anxiety disorder with panic disorder patients. *Psychopharmacology* 18:104–108, 1982.

42. Breier A, Charney DS, Heninger GR: Major depression in patients with agoraphobia and panic disorder. *Arch Gen Psychiatry* 41:1129–1135, 1984.

43. Laufer RS, Brett E, Gallops MS: Post-traumatic stress disorder (PTSD) reconsidered: PTSD among Vietnam veterans. In van der Kolk BA (ed): *Post-Traumatic Stress Disorder: Psychological and Biological Sequela*. Washington DC, American Psychiatric Press, 1984, pp 59–79.

44. Breslau N, Davis GC: Posttraumatic stress disorder: the etiologic specificity of wartime stressors. *Am J Psychiatry* 144:578–583, 1987.

45. Bartemeier LH, Kubie LS, Menninger KA, et al: Combat exhaustion. *J Nerv Ment Dis* 104:358–389, 1946.

46. Bartemeier LH, Kubie LS, Menninger KA, et al: Combat exhaustion. *J Nerv Ment Dis* 104:489–525, 1946.

47. Horowitz MJ: Stress-response syndromes: a review of posttraumatic and adjustment disorders. *Hosp Community Psychiatry* 37:241–249, 1986.

48. Kosten TR, Krystal JH: Biological mechanisms in post traumatic stress disorder: Relevance for substance abuse. In Galenter M (ed): *Recent Advances in Alcoholism*. New York, Plenum Press, 1985, pp 49–68.

49. Pitman RK, Green RC, Jenike MA, et al: Clinical comparison of Tourette's disorder and obsessive compulsive disorder. *Am J Psychiatry* 144:1166–1171, 1987.

50. Jenike MA, Baer L, Minichiello WE, et al: Concomitant obsessive-compulsive disorder and schizotypal personality disorder. *Am J Psychiatry* 143:530–532, 1986.

51. Rudin E: Ein beitrag zur frage der zwangskrankheit insbesondere ihere hereditaren bezeihungen. *Arch Psychiatr Nervenkr* 191:14–54, 1953.

52. Flament M, Rapoport JL: Childhood obsessive-compulsive disorder. In Insel TR (ed): *New Findings in Obsessive-Compulsive Disorder*. Washington DC, American Psychiatric Press, 1984, pp 23–43.

53. Redmond DE Jr: New and old evidence for the involvement of a brain norepinephrine system in anxiety. In Fan WE (ed): *The Phenomenology and Treatment of Anxiety*. New York, Spectrum Press, 1979, pp 153–203.

54. Rasmussen K, Jacobs BL: Single unit activity of locus coeruleus neurons in the freely moving cat. II. Conditioning and pharmacologic studies. *Brain Res* 371:335–344, 1986.

54a. Abercrombie ED, Jacobs BL: Single-unit response of noradrenergic neurons in the locus coeruleus of freely moving cats. I. Acutely presented stressful and nonstressful stimuli. *J Neurosci* 7:2837–2343, 1987.

55. Charney DS, Heninger GR, Breier A: Noradrenergic function in panic anxiety: effects of yohimbine in healthy subjects and patients with agoraphobia and panic disorder. *Arch Gen Psychiatry* 41:751–763, 1984.

56. Charney DS, Heninger GR: Abnormal regulation of noradrenergic function in panic disorders. *Arch Gen Psychiatry* 43:1042–1054, 1986.

57. Charney DS, Woods SW, Goodman WK, et al: Neurobiological mechanisms of panic anxiety: biochemical and behavioral correlates of yohimbine-induced panic attacks. *Am J Psychiatry* 144:1030–1036, 1987.

58. Charney DS, Woods SW, Price LH, et al: *The specificity of noradrenergic dysregulation in panic disorder*. Presented at the 6th International Catecholamine Symposium, Jerusalem, Israel, 1987.

59. Rainey M Jr, Ettedgui E, Pohl B, et al: The β-receptor: isoproterenol anxiety states. *Psychopathology* 17:40–51, 1984.

60. Nesse RM, Cameron OG, Curtis GC, et al: Adrenergic function in patients with panic anxiety. *Arch Gen Psychiatry* 41:771–776, 1984.

61. Brown S-L, Charney DS, Woods SW, et al: Lymphocyte β-adrenergic receptor binding in panic disorder. *Psychopharmacology* (94:24–28, 1988.)

61a. Robertson HA: Benzodiazepine receptors in "emotional" and "non-emotional" mice: comparison of four strains. *Eur J Pharmacol* 56:163–166, 1979.

62. Woods SW, Charney DS: Benzodiazepine treatment of anxiety disorder: Pharmacology and implications for pathophysiology. In Last C, Hersen M (eds): *Handbook of Anxiety Disorders*. New York, Pergamon Press, 1988, pp 413–444.

63. Dorow R, Horowski R, Paschelke G, et al: Severe anxiety induced by FG7142, a β-carboline legand for benzodiazepine receptors. *Lancet* 2:98–99, 1983.

64. Insel TR, Ninan PT, Alio J, et al: A benzodiazepine receptor-mediated model of anxiety. *Arch Gen Psychiatry* 41:741–750, 1984.

65. Woods SW, Charney DS, Silver JM, et al: Benzodiazepine receptor antagonist effects panic disorder. In *1988 New Research Program and Abstracts, 141st Annual Meeting*. Washington, DC, American Psychiatric Association, 1988.

66. Ferrero P, Guidotti A, Conti-Tronconi B, et al: A brain octadecaneuropeptide generated by tryptic digestion of DBI (diazepam binding inhibitor) duncitons as a proconflict ligand of benzodiazepine recognition sites. *Neuropharmacology* 23:1359 1362, 1984.

67. Ferrero P, Costa E, Conti-Tronconi B, et al: A diazepam binding inhibitor (DBI)-like neuropeptide is detected in human brain. *Brain Res* 399:136–142, 1986.

68. Charney DS, Heninger GR: Serotonin function in panic disorders: the effect of intravenous tryptophan in healthy subjects and patients with panic disorder before and during alprazolam treatment. *Arch Gen Psychiatry* 43:1059–1065, 1986.

69. Charney DS, Woods SW, Goodman WK, et al: Serotonin function in anxiety. II. Effects of the serotonin agonist MCPP in panic disorder patients and healthy subjects. *Psychopharmacology* 92:14–24, 1987.

70. Dourish CT, Hutson PH, Curzon G: Putative anxiolytics 8-OH-DPAT, buspirone and TVX Q 7821 are agonists at 5-HT$_{1A}$ autoreceptors in the raphe nuclei. *TIPS* 7:212–213, 1986.

71. Rickels K, Wiseman K, Norstad N, et al: Buspirone and diazepam in anxiety: a controlled study. *J Clin Psychiatry* 43:81–86, 1982.

72. Csanalosi I, Schweizer E, Case WG, et al: Gepirone in anxiety: a pilot study. *J Clin Psychopharmacol* 7:31–33, 1987.

73. Charney DS, Menkes DB, Heninger GR: Receptor sensitivity and the mechanism of action of antidepressant treatment: implications for the etiology and therapy of depression. *Arch Gen Psychiatry* 38:1160–1180, 1981.

74. Young SN, Smith SE, Pihl RO, et al: Tryptophan depletion causes a rapid lowering of mood in normal males. *Psychopharmacology* 87:173–177, 1985.

75. Shopsin B, Fradman E, Gershan S: Parachlorophenylalanine reversal of tranzlcypromine effects in depressed patients. *Arch Gen Psychiatry* 33:811–819, 1976.

76. Heninger GR, Charney DS, Sternberg DE: Serotonergic function in depression: prolactin response to intravenous tryptophan in depressed patients and healthy subjects. *Arch Gen Psychiatry* 41:398–402, 1984.

77. Insel TR, Murphy DL: The psychopharmacological treatment of obsessive-compulsive disorder: a review. *J Clin Psychopharmacol* 1:304–311, 1981.

78. Zohar J, Insel TR: Obsessive-compulsive disorder: psychobiological approaches to diagnosis, treatment, and pathophysiology. *Biol Psychiatry* 22:667–687, 1987.

79. Thoren P, Asberg M, Bertilsson L, et al: Clomipramine treatment of obsessive compulsive disorder. II. Biochemical aspects. *Arch Gen Psychiatry* 37:1289–1294, 1980.

80. Flament MF, Rapoport JL, Murphy DL, et al: Biochemical changes during chlomipramine treatment of childhood obsessive-compulsive disorder. *Arch Gen Psychiatry* 44:219–225, 1987.

81. Turner SM, Jacob RG, Beidel, et al: Fluoxetin treatment of obsessive-compulsive disorder. *J Clin Psychopharmacol* 5:207–212, 1985.

82. Price LH, Goodman WK, Charney DS, et al: Treatment of severe obsessive-compulsive disorder with fluvoxamine. *Am J Psychiatry* 144:1059–1061, 1987.

83. Goodman WK, Price LH, Rasmussen SA, et al: Efficacy of fluvoxamine in obsessive compulsive disorder: A double-blind comparison with placebo. *Arch Gen Psychiatry*, in press.

84. Yaryura-Tobies JA, Beberian RJ, Nezerogler FA, et al: Obsessive–compulsive disorders as a serotonergic defect. *Res Commun Psychol, Psych, and Behav* 2:279–286, 1977.

85. Insel TR, Mueller EA, Alterman I, et al: Obsessive-compulsive disorder and serotonin: is there a connection? *Biol Psychiatry* 20:1174–1188, 1985.

86. Weizman A, Carmi M, Hermish H, et al: High affinity imipramine binding and serotonin uptake in platelets of eight adolescent and ten adult obsessive-compulsive patients. *Am J Psychiatry* 143:335–339, 1986.

87. Charney DS, Goodman WK, Price LH, et al: Serotonin function in obsessive compulsive disorder: a comparison of the effects of tryptophan and MCPP in patients and healthy subjects. Submitted.

88. Hollander E, Fay M, Liebowitz MR: *5HT and NE behavioral response in obsessive-compulsives.* Presented at the American Psychiatric Association annual meeting, Chicago, 1987.

89. Zohar J, Mueller EA, Insel TR, et al: Serotonergic responsivity in obsessive-compulsive disorder. *Arch Gen Psychiatry* 44:946–951, 1987.

90. Gately PF, Poon SL, Segal DS, et al: Depletion of brain serotonin by 5,7-dihydroxytryptamine alters the response to amphetamine and the habituation of locomotor definity in rats. *Psychopharmacology* 87:400–405, 1985.

91. Geyer MA, Puerto DB, Menkes DB, et al: Behavioral studies following lessons of mesolimbic and mesostimuli serotonergic pathways. *Brain Res* 106:257–270, 1976.

92. Pitts FN Jr, McClure JN Jr: Lactate metabolism in anxiety neurosis. *N Engl J Med* 277:1329–1336, 1967.

93. Gorman JM, Askanazi J, Leibowitz MR, et al: Response to hyperventilation in a group of patients with panic disorder. *Am J Psychiatry* 141:857–861, 1984.

94. Woods SW, Charney DS, Loke J, et al: Carbon dioxide sensitivity in panic anxiety: ventilatory and anxiogenic response to carbon dioxide in healthy subjects and patients with panic anxiety before and after alprazolam treatment. *Arch Gen Psychiatry* 43:900–909, 1986.

95. Carr DB, Sheehan DV: Panic anxiety: a new biological model. *J Clin Psychiatry* 45:323–330, 1984.

96. Woods SW, Krystal JH, D'Amico CL, et al: A review of behavioral and pharmacologic studies relevant to the application of CO_2 as a human subject model of anxiety. *Psychopharmacol Bull* 24:149–155, 1988.

97. Krystal JH, Woods SW, Charney DS, et al: The effects of diazepam and haloperidol on CO_2-induced anxiety. Manuscript in preparation.

98. Rainey JM Jr, Aleem A, Ortiz A, et al: A laboratory procedure for the induction of flashbacks. *Am J Psychiatry* 144:1317–1319, 1987.

99. Freud S: New introductory lectures on psychoanalysis. In Strachey J, Freud A, Strachey A (eds): *The Standard Edition of the Complete Psychological Works of Sigmund Freud.* London, Hogarth Press and the Institute of Psycho-Analysis, 1932, pp 81–111.

100. Spitz RA, Wolfe KM: Anaclitic depression: an inquiry into the geneus of psychiatric conditions in early childhood. II. *Psychoanal Study Child* 2:313–342, 1946.

101. Bowlby J: Separation anxiety. *Int J Psycho-Anal* XLI:89–113, 1960.

102. Suomi SJ, Mineka S, DeLizio RD: Short- and long-term effects of repetitive mother-infant separations on social development in rhesus monkeys. *Dev Psychol* 19:770–786, 1983.

103. Suomi SJ: Anxiety-like disorders in young nonhuman primates. In Sittelman R (ed): *Anxiety Disorders of Childhood.* New York, Guilford Press, 1986, pp 1–23.

104. Kraemer GW, Ebert MH, Lake CR, et al: Amphetamine Challenge: Effects in previously isolated rhesus monkeys and implication for animal models of schizophrenia. In Miczek KA (ed): *Ethopharmacology Primate Models of Neuropsychiatric Disorders.* New York, Alan R. Liss, 1983, pp 199–218.

105. Suomi SJ, Harlow HF: Social rehabilitation of isolate-reared monkeys. *Dev Psychol* 6:487–496, 1972.

106. Suomi SJ, Seaman SF, Lewis JK, et al: Effects of imipramine treatment of separation-induced social disorders in rhesus monkeys. *Arch Gen Psychiatry* 35:321–325, 1978.

107. Kraemer GW, Ebert MH, Lake CR, et al: Cerebrospinal fluid measures of neurotransmitter changes associated with pharmacological alteration of the despair response to social separation in rhesus monkeys. *Psychiatry Res* 11:303–315, 1983.

108. Gittelman-Klein R, Klein DF: Social phobia: diagnostic considerations in the light of imipramine effects. *J Nerv Ment Dis* 156:199–215, 1973.

109. Geller I, Seifter J: The effect of meprobamate, barbiturates, d-amphetamine, and promazine on experimentally-induced conflict in the rat. *Psychopharmacologia* 1:482–492, 1960.

110. Vogel JR, Beer B, Clody DE: A simple and reliable conflict procedure for testing antianxiety agents. *Psychopharmacologia* 21:1–7, 1971.

111. Pellow S, File SE: Multiple sites for action for anxiogenic drugs: behavioural, electrophysiological and biochemical correlations. *Psychopharmacology* 83:304–315, 1984.

112. Mason P, Skinner J, Luttinger D: Two tests in rats for antianxiety effect of clinically anxiety attenuating antidepressants. *Psychopharmacology* 92:30–34, 1987.

113. Iversen SD: Animal models of anxiety and benzodiazepine actions. *Arzneim-Forsch Drug Res* 30:862–868, 1980.

114. File SE: The use of sound interaction as a method for defecting anxiolytic activity of chlordiazepoxide-like drugs. *J Neurosci Meth* 2:219–238, 1980.

115. Watson JB, Rayner P: Conditioned emotional reactions. *J Exp Psychol* 3:1, 1920.

116. Mowrer OH: *Learning Theory and Personality Dynamics*. New York, Ronald, 1950.

117. Thompson RF: Neuronal substrates of simple associative learning: classical conditioning. *TINS* 6:270–275, 1983.

118. Davis M, Hitchcock JM, Rosen JB: Anxiety and the amygdala: Pharmacological and anatomical analysis of the fear-potentiated startle paradigm. In Bower GH (ed): *The Psychologic of Learning and Motivation*. New York, Academic Press, 1987, vol 21, pp 263–305.

119. Krystal H: *Integration and Self-Healing: Affect, Trauma, Alexithymia*. Hillsdale, NJ, Analytic Press, 1988.

120. Keane TM, Zimmering RT, Coddell JM: A behavioral formulation of post-traumatic stress disorder in Vietnam Veterans. *The Behavior Therapist* 8:9–12, 1985.

121. Freud S: Obsessions and phobias: their psychical mechanism and their aetiology. In Strachey J, Freud A, Strachey A (eds): *The Standard Edition of the Complete Psychological Works of Sigmund Freud*. London, Hogarth Press and the Institute of Psycho-Analysis, 1895, pp 68–82.

122. Freud A: *The Ego and the Mechanisms of Defense*. New York, International Universities Press, 1966.

123. Marks IM: Review of behavioral psychotherapy I: Obsessive-compulsive disorders. *Am J Psychiatry* 138:584–592, 1981.

124. Foa EB: Failures in treating obsessive-compulsives. *Behav Res Ther* 17:169–176, 1979.

125. Pitman RK: A cybernetic model of obsessive-compulsive psychopathology. *Compr Psychiatry* 28:334–343, 1987.

126. Crowe RR, Noyes R Jr, Persico AM: Pro-opiomelanocortin (POMC) gene excluded as a cause of panic disorder in a large family. *J Affect Dis* 12:23–27, 1987.

127. Crowe RR, Noyes R Jr, Wilson AF, et al: A linkage study of panic disorder. *Arch Gen Psychiatry* 44:933–937, 1987.

128. Torgersen S: Genetic factors in anxiety disorders. *Arch Gen Psychiatry* 40:1085–1089, 1983.

129. Torgersen S: Hereditary differentiation of anxiety and affective neuroses. *Br J Psychiatry* 146:530–534, 1985.

130. Torgersen S: Genetics of somatoform disorders. *Arch Gen Psychiatry* 43:502–505, 1986.

131. Marks IM: Genetics of fear and anxiety disorders. *Br J Psychiatry* 149:406–418, 1986.

132. Kendler KS, Heath A, Martin NG, et al: Symptoms of anxiety and depression in a volunteer twin population. *Arch Gen Psychiatry* 43:213–221, 1986.

133. Kendler KS, Heath A, Martin NG, et al: Symptoms of anxiety and symptoms of depression. *Arch Surg* 122:451–457, 1987.

134. Cohen ME, Badal DW, Kilpatrick A, et al: The high familial prevalence of neurocirculatory asthenia (anxiety neurosis, effort syndrome). *Am J Human Genet* 3:126–158, 1951.

135. Noyes R Jr, Clarkson C, Crowe RR, et al: A

136. Noyes R Jr, Crowe RR, Harris EL, et al: Relationship between panic disorder and agoraphobia: a family study. *Arch Gen Psychiatry* 43:227–232, 1986.

137. Rasmussen SA, Tsuang MT: Epidemiology and clinical features of obsessive-compulsive disorder. In Jenike MA, Baer L, Minichiello WE (eds): *Obsessive Compulsive Disorders: Theory and Management*. Littleton, MA, PSG Publishing, 1986, pp 23–44.

138. Weinshilboum RM: Biochemical genetics of catecholamines in humans. *Mayo Clin Proc* 58:319–330, 1983.

139. Winter H, Herschel M, Propping P, et al: A twin study on three enzymes (DBH, COMT, MAO) of catecholamine metabolism: correlations with MMPI. *Psychopharmacology* 57:63–69, 1978.

140. Nurnberger JI Jr, Gershon ES, Simmons S, et al: Behavioral, biochemical and neuroendocrine responses to amphetamine in normal twins and "well-state" bipolar patients. *Psychoneuroendocrinology* 7:163–176, 1982.

141. Aronson TA, Craig TJ: Cocaine precipitation of panic disorder. *Am J Psychiatry* 143:643–645, 1986.

142. Propping P, Friedl W: Genetic control of adrenergic receptors on human platelets. A twin study. *Hum Genet* 64:105–109, 1983.

143. Jimerson DC, Nurnberger JI, Post RM, et al: Plasma MHPG in rapid cyclers and healthy twins. *Arch Gen Psychiatry* 38:1287–1290, 1981.

144. Oxenstierna G, Edman G, Iselius L, et al: Concentrations of monoamine metabolites in the cerebrospinal fluid of twins and unrelated individuals—a genetic study. *J Psychiatr Res* 20:19–29, 1986.

145. Rachman S: Galvanic skin response in identical twins. *Psychol Rep* 6:298, 1960.

146. Shapiro AP, Nicotero J, Sapira J, et al: Analysis of the variability of blood pressure, pulse rate, and catecholamine responsivity in identical and fraternal twins. *Psychosom Med* 30:506–520, 1968.

147. Propping P, Friedl W: Pharmacogenetics in psychiatry and psychobiology. In Sakai T, Tsuboi T (eds): *Genetic Aspect of Human Behavior* Tokyo-New York, Igaku-Shion, 1985, pp 219–233.

148. Vantini G, Perry BD, Guchhait RB, et al: Brain epinephrine systems: detailed comparison of adrenergic and noradrenergic metabolism, receptor number and in vitro regulation, in two inbred rat strains. *Brain Res* 296:49–65, 1984.

149. Vadasz C, Baker H, Joh TH, et al: The inheritance and genetic correlation of tyrosine hydroxylase activities in the substantia nigra and corpus striatum in the CxB recombinant inbred mouse strains. *Brain Res* 234:1–9, 1982.

150. Schoemaker H, Nickolson VJ, Kerbusch S, et al: Synaptosomal uptake studies on recombinant inbred mice: neurotransmitter interaction and behavioral correlates. *Brain Res* 235:253–264, 1982.

151. Severson JA, Pittman RN, Gal J, et al: Genetic

influence on the regulation of beta adrenergic receptors in mice. *J Pharmacol Exp Ther* 236:24–28, 1986.

152. Charcot JM: *Clinical lectures on diseases of the nervous system.* Delivered at The Infirmary of La Salpetriere, New Sydenham Society, London, 1889.

153. Freud S: Heredity and the aetiology of the neuroses. In Strachey J, Freud A, Strachey A (eds): *The Standard Edition of the Complete Psychological Works of Sigmund Freud.* London, Hogarth Press and Institute of Psycho-Analysis, 1896, pp 141–156.

154. Langinvainio H, Kaprio J, Koskenvuo M, et al: Finnish twins reared apart III: Personality factors. *Acta Genet Med Gemellol* 33:259–264, 1984.

155. Abe K, Oda N, Hatta H: Behavioural genetics of early childhood: fears, restlessness, motion sickness and enuresis. *Acta Genet Med Gemellol* 33:303–306, 1984.

156. Reznick JS, Kagan J, Snidman N, et al: Inhibited and uninhibited children: a follow-up study. *Child Dev* 57:660–680, 1986.

157. Suomi SJ: Genetic and maternal contributions to individual differences in rhesus monkey biobehavioral development. In Krasnagor N (ed): *Psychobiological Aspects of Behavioral Development.* New York, Academic Press, in press.

158. Weinberger DR: Implications of normal brain development for the pathogenesis of schizophrenia. *Arch Gen Psychiatry* 44:660–669, 1987.

159. Deltito JA, Perugi G, Maremmani I, et al: The importance of separation anxiety in the differentiation of panic disorder from agoraphobia. *Psychiatric Dev* 4:227–236, 1986.

160. Berg I, Marks I, McGuire R, et al: School phobia and agoraphobia. *Psychol Med* 4:428–434, 1974.

161. Rosenbaum JF, Biederman J, Gersten M, et al: *Behavioral inhibition in children of parents with panic disorder and agoraphobia: a controlled study.* Presented in part at the annual meeting of the American Psychiatric Association, Chicago, May, 1987.

162. Edlund MJ, Swann AC, Clothier J: Patients with panic attacks and abnormal EEG results. *Am J Psychiatry* 144:508–509, 1987.

163. Geschwind N, Galaburda AM: Cerebral lateralization: biological mechanisms, associations, and pathology: I. A hypothesis and a program for research. *Arch Neurol* 42:428–459, 1985.

164. Geschwind N, Galaburda AM: Cerebral lateralization: biological mechanisms, associations, and pathology: II. A hypothesis and a program for research. *Arch Neurol* 42:521–552, 1985.

165. Purves D, Lichtman JW (eds): *Principles of Neural Development.* Sunderland, MA, Sinauer Associates, 1985.

166. Oppenheim RW: Naturally occurring cell death during neural development. *TINS* 8:487–493, 1985.

167. Purves D, Lichtman JW: Elimination of synapses in the developing nervous system. *Science* 210:153–157, 1980.

168. Heumann D, Leuba G: Neuronal death in the development and aging of the cerebral cortex of the mouse. *Neuropathol Appl Neurobiol* 9:297–311, 1983.

169. Markus EJ, Petit TL, LeBoutillier JC: Synaptic structural changes during development and aging. *Dev Brain Res* 35:239–248, 1987.

170. Cragg BG: The density of synapses and neurons in normal mentally defective and aging human brains. *Brain* 98:81–90, 1975.

171. Huttenlocher PR: Synaptic density in human frontal cortex—developmental changes and effects of aging. *Brain Res* 163:195–205, 1979.

172. Tomlinson BE, Irving O, Blessed G: Cell loss in the locus coeruleus in senile dementia of Alzheimer type. *J Neurol Sci* 49:419–428, 1981.

173. Feldman ML, Dowd, C: Loss of dendritic spines in aging cerebral cortex. *Anat Embryol* 148:279–301, 1975.

174. Levitt P, Noebels JL: Mutant mouse tottering: selective increase of locus ceruleus axons in a defined single-locus mutation. *Proc Natl Acad Sci USA* 78:4630–4634, 1981.

175. Kimura F, Nakamura S: Locus coeruleus neurons in the neonatal rat: electrical activity and responses to sensory stimulation. *Dev Brain Res* 23:301–305, 1985.

176. Williams JT, Marshall KC: Membrane properties and adrenergic response in locus coeruleus neurons in young rats. *J Neurosci* 7:3687–3694, 1987.

177. Nomura Y, Oki K, Segawa: Pharmacological characterization of central α-adrenoceptors which mediate clonidine-induced locomotor hypoactivity in the developing rat. *Naunyn-Schmiedebergs Arch Pharmacol* 311:41–44, 1980.

178. Kling A, Green PC: Effects of neonatal amygdalectomy in the maternally reared and maternally deprived macaque. *Nature* 213:742–743, 1967.

179. Franzen EA, Myers RE: Age effects on social behavior deficits following prefrontal lesions in monkeys. *Brain Res* 54:277–286, 1973.

180. Bernstein SL, Gioio AE, Kaplan BB: Changes in gene expression during postnatal development of the rat cerebellum. *J Neurogenetics* 1:71–86, 1983.

181. Kelly PT, Shields S, Conway K, et al: Developmental changes in calmodulin-kinase II activity at brain synaptic junctions: alterations in holoenzyme composition. *J Neurochem* 49:1927–1940, 1987.

182. Michina M, Takai T, Imoto K, et al: Molecular distinction between fetal and adult forms of muscle acetylcholine receptor. *Nature* 321:406–411, 1986.

183. Bunn HF: Disorders of hemoglobin structure, function, and synthesis. In Petersdorf RG, Adams RD, Braunwald E, et al (eds): *Harrison's Principles of Internal Medicine,* ed 10. New York, McGraw-Hill, 1983, pp 1875–1885.

184. Yamamoto KR: Steroid receptor regulated transcription of specific genes and gene networks. *Ann Rev Genet* 19:209–252, 1985.

185. Beyer C, Feder HH: Sex steroids and afferent

input: Their roles in brain sexual differentiation. *Ann Rev Physiol* 49:349–364, 1987.

186. Toran-Allerand CD: Gonadal hormones and brain development: implications for the genesis of sexual differentiation. *Ann NY Acad Sci* 435:101–111, 1984.

187. De Villalobos DB, Lux VAR, De Mengido IL, et al: Sexual differences in the serotonergic control of prolactin and luteinizing hormone secretion in the rat. *Endocrinology* 115:84–89, 1984.

188. Harrel A, McEwen B: Gonadal steroid modulation of neurotransmitter-stimulated cAMP accumulation in the hippocampus of the rat. *Brain Res* 404:89–94, 1987.

189. Kaba H, Saito H, Otsuka K, et al: Effects of estrogen on the excitability of neurons projecting from the noradrenergic A1 region to the preoptic and anterior hypothalamic area. *Brain Res* 274:156–159, 1983.

190. Etgen AM, Petitti N: Mediation of norepinephrine-stimulated cyclic SMP accumulation by adrenergic receptors in hypothalamic and preoptic area slices: effects of estradiol. *J Neurochem* 49:1732–1739, 1987.

191. Wilkinson M, Herdon HJ: Diethylstilbestrol regulates the number of α- and β-adrenergic binding sites in incubated hypothalamus and amygdala. *Brain Res* 248:79–85, 1982.

192. Johnson AE, Nock B, McEwen B, et al: Estradiol modulation of α_2-noradrenergic receptors in guinea pig brain assessed by tritium-sensitive film autoradiography. *Brain Res* 336:153–157, 1985.

193. Etgen AM, Petitti N: Norepinephrine-stimulated cyclic AMP accumulation in rat hypothalamic slices: effects of estrous cycle and ovarian steroids. *Brain Res* 375:385–390, 1986.

194. Kant GJ, Sessions GR, Lenox RH, et al: The effects of hormonal and circadian cycles, stress, and activity on levels of cyclic AMP and cyclic GMP in pituitary, hypothalamus, pineal and cerebellum of female rats. *Life Sci* 29:2491–2499, 1981.

195. Yakovlev PI, Lecours A-R: The myelogenetic cycles of regional maturation of the brain. In Minkowski A (ed): *Regional Development of the Brain in Early Life*. Philadelphia, F. A. Davis Company, 1967, pp 3–70.

196. Fifkova E: A possible mechanism of morphometric changes in dendritic spones induced by stimulation. *Cell Mol Neurobiol* 5:47–63, 1985.

197. Buell SJ, Coleman PD: Quantitative evidence for selective dendritic growth in normal human aging but not in senile dementia. *Brain Res* 214:23–41, 1981.

198. Borges S, Berry M: The effects of dark rearing on the development of the visual cortex of the rat. *J Comp Neur* 180:277–300, 1978.

199. Muller L, Pattiselanno A, Vrensen G: The postnatal development of the presynaptic grid in the visual cortex of rabbits and the effect of dark-rearing. *Brain Res* 205:39–48, 1981.

200. Sirevaag AM, Greenough WT: Differential rear-

ing effects on rat visual cortex synapses: II. Synaptic morphometry. *Dev Brain Res* 19:215–226, 1985.

201. Kasamatsu T, Itakura T, Johnson C, et al: Neuronal plasticity in cat visual cortex: a proposed role for the central noradrenaline system. In Descarries L, Reader TR, Jasper HH (eds): *Monoamine Innervation of Cerebral Cortex*. New York, Alan R. Liss, 1984, pp 301–319.

202. Nelson SB, Schwartz MA, Daniels JD: Clonidine and cortical plasticity: possible evidence for noradrenergic involvement. *Dev Brain Res* 23:39–50, 1985.

203. Mirmiran M, Uylings HBM, Corner MA: Pharmacological suppression of REM sleep prior to weaning conteracts the effectiveness of subsequent environmental enrichment on cortical growth in rats. *Dev Brain Res* 7:102–105, 1983.

204. Nakamura S, Shirokawa T, Sakaguchi T: Increased adrenergic projection from the locus coeruleus to the lateral geniculate nucleus of rats following one-eye-removal at birth. *Dev Brain Res* 15:283–285, 1984.

205. Woodward DJ, Moises HC, Waterhouse BD, et al: Modulatory actions of norepinephrine in the central nervous system. *Fed Proc* 38:2109–2116, 1979.

206. Sara SJ: The locus coeruleus and cognitive function: attempts to relate noradrenergic enhancement of signal/noise in the brain to behavior. *Physiol Psychol* 13:151–162, 1985.

206a. Comb M, Hyman SE, Goodman HM: Mechanisms of trans-synaptic regulation of gene expression. *TINS* 10:473–478, 1987.

207. Lindroos OFC, Riittinen M-LA, Veilahti JV, et al: Overstimulation, occipital/somesthetic cerebral cortical depth, and the cortical asymmetry in mice. *Dev Psychobiol* 17:547–554, 1984.

207a. van der Kolk B, Greenberg M, Boyd H, et al: Inescapable shock, neurotransmitters, and addition to trauma: toward a psychobiology of post traumatic stress. *Biol Psychiatry* 20:315–325, 1985.

208. Clark GM, Zamenhof S, van Marthens E, et al: The effect of prenatal malnutrition on dimensions of cerebral cortex. *Brain Res* 54:397–402, 1973.

209. Zamenhof S, van Marthens E, Margolis FL: DNA (cell number) and protein in neonatal brain: alteration by maternal dietary protein restriction. *Science* 160:322–323, 1968.

210. Stern WC, Pugh WW, Johnson A, et al: Spontaneous forebrain neuronal activity in developmentally protein malnourished rats. *Dev Brain Res* 9:95–98, 1983.

211. Keller EA, Munaro NI, Orsingher OA: Perinatal undernutrition reduces alpha and beta adrenergic receptor binding in adult rat brain. *Science* 215:1269–1270, 1982.

212. Sobotka TJ, Cook MP, Brodie RE: Neonatal malnutrition: neurochemical, hormonal and behavioral manifestations. *Brain Res* 65:443–457, 1974.

213. Levitt P, Moore RY: Organization of brainstem

noradrenaline hyperinnervation following neonatal 6-hydroxydopamine treatment in rat. *Anat Embryol* 158:133–150, 1980.

214. Burgess JW, Monachello MP: Chronic exposure to caffeine during early development increases dendritic spine and branch formation in midbrain optic tectum. *Dev Brain Res* 6:123–129, 1983.

215. Post RM, Rubinow DR, Ballenger JC: Conditioning and sensitization in the longitudinal course of affective illness. *Br J Psychiatry* 149:191–201, 1986.

216. Post RM, Lockfeld A, Squillace KM, et al: Drug-environment interaction: context dependency of cocaine-induced behavioral sensitization. *Life Sci* 28:755–760, 1981.

217. Misra CH, Shelat HS, Smith RC: Effect of age on adrenergic and dopaminergic receptor binding in rat brain. *Life Sci* 27:521–526, 1980.

218. Walker JB, Walker JP: Properties of adenylate cyclase from senescent rat brain. *Brain Res* 54:391–396, 1973.

219. Schmidt MJ, Thornberry JF: Cyclic AMP and cyclic GMP accumulation in vitro in brain regions of young, old and aged rats. *Brain Res* 139:169–177, 1978.

220. Bickford-Wilmer PC, Miller JA, Freedman R, et al: Age-related reduction in responses of rat hippocampal neurons to locally applied monoamines. *Neurobiol Aging* 9:173–179, 1988.

221. Yamamoto J, Nakai M, Natsume T: Cardiovascular responses to acute stress in young-to-old spontaneously hypertensive rats. *Hypertension* 9:362–370, 1987.

221a. Algeri S, Calderini G, Lomuscio G, et al: Differential response to immobilization stress of striatal dopaminergic and hippocampal noradrenergic systems in aged rats. *Neurobiol: Aging* 9:213–216, 1988.

222. Faucheux BA, Bourliere F, Baulon A, et al: The effects of psychosocial stress on urinary excretion of adrenaline and noradrenaline in 51- to 55- and 71- to 74-year-old men. *Gerontology* 27:313–325, 1981.

223. Brodde O-E, Anlauf M, Graben N, et al: Age-dependent decrease of α_2-adrenergic receptor number in human platelets. *Eur J Pharmacol* 81:345–347, 1982.

224. Reznick JS, Kagan J, Snidman N, et al: Inhibited and uninhibited behavior: a follow-up study. *Child Dev* 51:660–680, 1986.

225. Gould SJ (ed): *The Mismeasure of Man.* New York, W. W. Norton, 1981.

226. Brain P: Sickle cell anemia in Africa. *Br Med J* 2:880–881, 1952.

227. Charney DS, Woods SW, Goodman WK, et al: Drug treatment of panic disorder: the comparative efficacy of imipramine, alprazolam, and trazodone. *J Clin Psychiatry* 47:580–585, 1986.

228. Sheehan DV, Ballenger J, Jacobsen G: Treatment of endogenous anxiety with phobic, hysterical, and hypochondriacal symptoms. *Arch Gen Psychiatry* 37:51–59, 1980.

229. Nurnberg HG, Coccaro EF: Response of panic disorder and resistance of depression to imipramine. *Am J Psychiatry* 139:1060–1062, 1982.

230. Mavissakalian M: Initial depression and response to imipramine in agoraphobia. *J Nerv Ment Dis* 175:358–361, 1987.

231. Sweeney DR, Gold MS, Pottash ALC, et al: Plasma levels of tricyclic antidepressants in panic disorder. *Int J Psychiatry Med* 13:93–97, 1983.

232. Sheehan DV, Davidson J, Manschrek T, et al: Lack of efficacy of a new antidepressant (bupropion) in the treatment of panic disorder with phobias. *J Clin Psychopharmacol* 3:28–31, 1983.

233. Gorman, JM, Liebowitz MR, Fyer AJ, et al: An open trial of fluoxetine in the treatment of panic attacks. *J Clin Psychopharmacol* 7:329–332, 1987.

234. Mavissakalian M, Perel J, Bowler K, et al: Trazodone in the treatment of panic disorder and agoraphobia with panic attacks. *Am J Psychiatry* 144:785–787, 1987.

235. Kahn RS, Van Praag HM, Asnis GM, et al: *5HT receptor hypersensitivity and anxiety.* Presented at the annual meeting of the American Psychiatric Association, Chicago, 1987.

236. Liebowitz MR: Imipramine in the treatment of panic disorder and its complications. *Psychiatr Clin North Am* 8:37–47, 1985.

237. Liebowitz MR, Quitkin FM, Stewart JW, et al: Phenelzine v imipramine in atypical depression: a preliminary report. *Arch Gen Psychiatry* 41:669–677, 1984.

238. Sheehan DV: Panic attacks and phobias. *N Engl J Med* 307:156–158, 1982.

239. Nagy LM, Krystal JH, Woods SW, et al: Efficacy of alprazolam and behavioral group therapy in panic disorder: 2.5 year follow-up study. Submitted for publication.

240. Herman JB, Brotman AW, Rosenbaum JF: Rebound anxiety in panic disorder patients treated with shorter-acting benzodiazepines. *J Clin Psychiatry* 48:22–26, 1987.

241. Fyer AJ, Liebowitz MR, Gorman JM, et al: Discontinuation of alprazolam treatment in panic patients. *Am J Psychiatry* 144:303–308, 1987.

242. Lader MH: The biological basis of benzodiazepine dependence. *Psychol Med* 17:539–547, 1987.

242a. Shehi M, Patterson WM: Treatment of panic attacks with alprazolam and propranolol. *Am J Psychiatry* 141:900–901, 1984.

243. Feighner JP, Meridith CH, Hendrickson MA: A double-blind comparison of buspirone and diazepam in outpatients with generalized anxiety disorder. *J Clin Psychiatry* 43:103–107, 1982.

244. Chouinard G, Annable L, Fontaine R, et al: Alprazolam in the treatment of generalized anxiety and panic disorders: a double-blind, placebo-controlled study. *Psychopharmacology* 77:229–233, 1982.

245. Buschsbaum MS, Hazlett E, Sicotte N, et al: Topographic EEG changes with benzodiazepine administration in generalized anxiety disorder. *Biol Psychiatry* 20:832–842, 1985.

246. Hoehn-Saric R, McLeod DR: *Alprazolam versus*

imipramine: effects on anxiety. Presented at the Panic Disorder Biological Research Workshop, Washington, DC, 1986.

247. Kahn RJ, McNair DM, Lipman RS, et al: Imipramine and chlordiazepoxide in depressive and anxiety disorders. *Arch Gen Psychiatry* 43:79–85, 1986.

248. Eison AS, Temple DL Jr: Buspirone: review of its pharmacology and current perspectives on its mechanism of action. *Am J Med* 80:1–9, 1986.

249. Cott JM, Kurtz NM, Robinson DS, et al: Clinical anxioselective activity of gepirone. Presented at the annual meeting of the American Psychiatric Association, Washington, DC, 1986.

250. Ceulemans DLS, Hoppenbrouwers M-LJA, Gelders YG, et al: The influence of ritanserin, a serotonin antagonist, in anxiety disorders: a double-blind placebo-controlled study versus lorazepam. *Pharmacopsychiatry* 18:303–305, 1985.

251. Goa KL, Ward A: Buspirone: a preliminary review of its pharmacological properties and therapeutic efficacy as an anxiolytic. *Drugs* 32:114–129, 1986.

252. Gonsalves SF, Gallager DW: Spontaneous and RO 15-1788 induced reversal of subsensitivity to GABA following chronic benzodiazepines. *Eur J Pharmacol* 110:163–170, 1985.

253. Frank JB, Kosten TR, Giller EL, et al: *Antidepressants for post traumatic stress disorders.* Presented at the annual meeting of the American Psychiatric Association, Chicago, 1987.

254. van der Kolk BA: Psychopharmacological issues in posttraumatic stress disorder. *Hosp Comm Psychiatry* 34:683–691, 1983.

255. Lipper S, Davidson JRT, Grady TA, et al: Preliminary study of carbamazepine in post-traumatic stress disorder. *Psychosomatics* 27:849–854, 1986.

256. Dunner FJ, Edwards WP, Copeland PC: Clinical efficacy of alprazolam in PTSD patients. Presented at the annual meeting of the American Psychiatric Association, 1985.

257. Kolb LC, Burris BC, Griffiths S: Propranolol and clonidine in treatment of the chronic post-traumatic stress disorders of war. In van der Kolk BA (ed): *Post-Traumatic Stress Disorder: Psychological and biological sequelae.* Washington, DC, American Psychiatric Press, 1984, pp 98–105.

258. Nemiah J: Foreword. In Insel TR (ed): *New Findings in Obsessive-Compulsive Disorder.* Washington, DC, American Psychiatric Press, 1984, pp xi–xii.

259. Steketee G, Foa EB: Obsessive-compulsive disorder. In Barlow D (ed): *Clinical Handbook of Psychological Disorders: A Step-By-Step Treatment Manual.* New York, Guilford Press, 1985, pp 69–144.

260. Insel TR, Zohar J: Psychopharmacologic approaches to obsessive-compulsive disorder. In Meltzer HY (ed): *Psychopharmacology: The Third Generation of Progress.* New York, Raven Press, 1987, pp 1205–1210.

261. Ananth J, Pecknold JC, Van Den Steen N, et al: Double-blind comparative study of clomipramine and amitriptyline in obsessive neurosis. *Pro Neuro Psychopharmacol Biol Psychiat* 5:257–262, 1981.

262. Mavissakalian M, Turner SM, Michelson L, et al: Tricyclic antidepressants in obsessive-compulsive disorder: antiobsessional or antidepressant agents? II. *Am J Psychiatry* 142:572–576, 1985.

263. Volavka J, Neziroglu F, Yaryura-Tobias JA: Clomipramine and imipramine in obsessive compulsive disorder. *Psychiatry Res* 14:83–91, 1985.

264. Foa EF, Steketee G, Kozak MK, et al: Imipramine and placebo in the treatment of obsessive-compulsives: their effect on depression and obsessional symptoms. *Psychopharmacol Bull* 23:8–11, 1987.

265. Perse TL, Greist JH, Jefferson JW, et al: Fluvoxamine treatment of obsessive-compulsive disorder. *Am J Psychiatry* 144:1543–1548, 1987.

266. Marks I (ed): *Fears, Phobias, and Rituals.* New York, Oxford University Press, 1987, pp 524–559.

267. Jenike MA, Surman OS, Cassem NH, et al: Monoamine oxidase inhibitors in obsessive-compulsive disorder. *J Clin Psychiatry* 144:131–132, 1983.

268. Tollefson G: Alprazolam in the treatment of obsessive symptoms. *J Clin Psychopharmacol* 5:39–42, 1985.

269. Rivers-Bulkeley N, Hollender MH: Successful treatment of obsessive compulsive disorder with lozapine. *Am J Psychiatry* 139:1345–1346, 1982.

270. Mitchell-Heggs N, Kelly D, Richardson A: Stereotactic limbic leucotomy—a follow-up at 16 months. *Br J Psychiatry* 128:226–240, 1976.

270a. Wolpe J (ed): *The Practice of Behavior Therapy,* ed 2. New York, Pergamon Press, 1973.

271. Rose DS: "Worse than death": psychodynamics of rape victims and the need for psychotherapy. *Am J Psychiatry* 143:817–824, 1986.

272. Haley SA: When the patient reports atrocities. *Arch Gen Psychiatry* 30:191–196, 1974.

273. Krystal JH, Giller EL, Cicchetti DV: Assessment of alexithymia in posttraumatic stress disorder and somatic illness: introduction of a reliable measure. *Psychosom Med* 48:84–94, 1986.

35

Personality

Aaron Lazare, M.D.

Personality (or specific personality traits) refers to "enduring patterns of perceiving, relating to, and thinking about the environment and oneself, and is exhibited in a wide range of important social and personal contexts" (1). When specific traits such as orderliness, perseverance, rigidity, strict conscience, parsimony, and emotional constriction cluster together into recognizable patterns, they are referred to as personality types, patterns or styles (2, 3). When these personality types become inflexible and maladaptive and cause either significant impairment in social or occupational functioning or subjective distress, they are referred to as personality disorders. The behaviors or traits that define the personality disorder must be characteristic of both recent and long-term functioning with onset in childhood or adolescence. Recent changes in behavior, by this definition, are not considered part of a person's personality (1).

Personality consists of a combination of temperament and character in which temperament represents inborn, genetically based determinants of personality, and character represents learned attributes originating primarily from early life experience (4).

Hirschfeld describes four commonly held beliefs about personality disorders, not made explicit in the *Diagnostic and Statistical Manual for Mental Disorders (Third Edition-Revised)* (DSM-III-R), that distinguish them from other psychiatric conditions such as mood disorders and anxiety disorders. He then questions the universality of each of these beliefs. First, personality disorders are conditions which are chronic and long-standing, as opposed to symptomatic or episodic. Second, personality disorders represent a more basic dysfunction than the superimposed symptom or syndrome. Third, the personality disorders are more resistant to change than the symptom or syndrome. Treatment, therefore, is apt to be longer and more difficult. Fourth, personality disorders are ego syntonic, which means that the patients are relatively comfortable with their behavior and often do not wish to change. With ego dystonic behavior, in contrast, patients are in greater distress and this often brings them to treatment (4).

Value of Personality Assessment

For the practicing clinician there are several reasons to assess the personality of the patient:

1. The human suffering of patients with personality disorders as well as of those who suffer at their hands makes attempts at understanding and treatment worthwhile.
2. Having a personality disorder is significantly correlated with the presence of

455

an Axis I disorder as well as with other personality disorders. Such comorbidity often influences the overall treatment plan.

3. Patients' personality traits may influence their vulnerability and response to environmental stress.

4. Patients personality traits influence how they will present the historical material for Axis I conditions, relate to the clinician, and accept the treatment plan. Clinicians' personality traits similarly influence how they will relate to patients. This issue has been the subject of considerable discussion regarding medical patients. In particular, much has been written about the influence of the patients personality styles on their reactions to medical illness (5).

Rationale for This Chapter

Clinicians generally find single chapter discussions of all 11 DSM-III-R personality disorders unsatisfying for several reasons. First, there is not enough space to adequately present the necessary material for some of the well-studied disorders. Second, for those personality disorders for which the amount of available knowledge is limited, the reader is often subjected to unsubstantiated generalizations and clinical advice. Third, even where there is a rich literature about a personality disorder, there is much confusion resulting from varying theoretical approaches addressing different patient populations under the same diagnostic rubric. In addition, the names of many of the personality traits and disorders have changed over the last several decades. Finally, even comprehensive reviews of the personality disorders as defined by DSM-III-R often seem to have limited relevance to general outpatient practice where many patients have personality problems that do not meet the criteria for personality disorder.

This chapter will attempt to address some of these problems by presenting an overview of the concepts and accomplishments of DSM-III and DSM-III-R; a discussion of some of the problems surrounding

the definitions of the 11 DSM-III-R disorders, a review of psychodynamic, biologic, interpersonal, and behavioral approaches to personality; and a discussion of some of the conceptual issues involving personality that affect clinical practice. For comprehensive discussions of the DSM-III and DSM-III-R personality disorders and other formulations of personality, the reader is referred to Millon (6), Shapiro (7, 8), Horowitz et al. (9), Frances and Hales (Section III) (10), and Michels et al. (Chapters 1–28) (11).

DSM-III-R CATEGORIES, AXIS II, OVERLAP, EPIDEMIOLOGY

DSM-III-R lists 11 distinct personality disorders which it groups into three clusters. The first cluster includes paranoid, schizoid, and schizotypal personality disorders and is characterized as "odd or eccentric." The second cluster includes antisocial, borderline, histrionic, and narcissistic personality disorders and is characterized as "dramatic, emotional, or erratic." The third cluster includes avoidant, dependent, obsessive–compulsive, and passive aggressive personality disorders and is characterized as "anxious or fearful." These three DSM-III-R groupings are intuitive, not empirical. Finally, there is a category for personality disorders which do not meet the criteria for any one of the 11 categories but still cause significant social or occupational impairment or personal distress. This is termed "personality disorder not otherwise specified."

These 11 diagnostic categories are placed on a separate axis of DSM-III-R to remind the clinician that a patient suffering from an acute, episodic, and sometimes more florid Axis I diagnosis may also have a personality disturbance that causes distress and complicates treatment (12). Docherty et al. suggest that the personality axis may be conceived of as a vulnerability diagnosis for the Axis I syndrome. They also make the point that there is the implication, by the separate designation, that the personality disorders represent a different and differentiable level or dimension of disease structure (13).

There is a considerable degree of overlap of the personality disorders in various populations. In one study, 54% of patients with one personality disorder received diagnoses of one or more additional personality diagnoses (14). In particular, significant overlap has been noted between borderline and histrionic disorders, between narcissistic and borderline personality disorders, and between schizotypal, borderline, and avoidant disorders (12).

Epidemiologic data on these categories of personality disorders are sparse because of the recent introduction of the diagnostic criteria and the lack of established instruments for measuring the presence of the defining personality traits. Four studies, nevertheless, show that the total lifetime prevalence of personality disorders in general populations ranges from 6.0 to 9.8 per 100. The variability of prevalence of specific personality disorders in several studies is so great that the results are meaningless. The only exception is antisocial personality disorder, whose average prevalence rate in the total population is approximately 3 per 100. In treated populations, approximately one-half of patients are apt to have diagnosable personality disorders (15).

COMORBIDITY

The phenomenon of patients sufffering from Axis I disorders who simultaneously suffer from what appears to be personality disturbance has been explained and investigated using the concept of comorbidity. This views the phenomenon as the coexistence of two separate diseases.

Using the comorbidity concept, significant relationships exist between personality disorder and various Axis I diagnoses. Understanding their nature and extent has clinical usefulness in that the diagnosis of one condition should alert the clinician to the presence of another, and the presence of more than one condition may influence the treatment and outcome of either condition. For situations of comorbidity of personality disorders of Axis I diagnoses, Docherty et al. suggest five possible relationships between the conditions. The first is *causal*, whereby the personality, perhaps triggered by a precipitating event, generates the Axis I disorder. In the second model, referred to as *forme fruste,* the personality disorder represents an attenuated form of the syndromal disorder, and both are expressions of the hypothesized disease process. The schizotypal personality disorder, for instance, may represent an attenuated form of schizophrenia. Third, the personality disorder may represent a *complication* of the syndromal disorder. For instance, a major depression or anxiety disorder may cause certain maladaptive personality traits such as diminished self-confidence and fears of recurrence. Fourth, the personality disorder may represent an independent condition which arises from the same etiology as the syndromal disorder. This is referred to as *coeffect.* For instance, a particular form of child rearing may cause both a dependent personality disorder and a depressive disorder. The two disorders are regarded as correlates. Finally, in the *interactional* relationship, both disorders interact in ways that make each more noticeable and more likely. For instance, the narcissistic personality disorder may lead to life situations which aggravate a depressive disorder, which in turn may lead to an exaggeration of narcissistic traits (13).

Patients with major depression are apt to have rates of personality disorders ranging from 23% to 53%. The most frequent personality disorders in decreasing frequency are borderline, histrionic, dependent, and avoidant. Depressed patients with coexisting personality disorders are less likely to respond to antidepressants and more likely to have a family history of alcoholism. The prevalence rate of mood disorders in patients with borderline personality disorders ranges from 25% to 60%. Borderline patients with comorbid major depression have better outcomes than pure borderlines (16, 17), and patients with mood disorders have worse outcomes if associated with borderline personality. Patients with anxiety disorders are more apt to have comorbidity with personality disorders than patients with depression. The presence of personality disorder in patients with anxiety disorder worsens the prognosis for the latter. Several studies report a higher than expected comorbidity of antisocial personality with depression and alcoholism. For schizophrenia, the comorbidity is highest for borderline and schizotypal personality disorders (11). For schizophrenia, the presence of a personality disorder improves the outcome. For the personality disorder, the presence of schizophrenia worsens the outcome. (See Docherty et al. (13) and Pfohl (12) for reviews of comorbidity.)

SOME CONCEPTUAL ISSUES REGARDING THE 11 DSM-III-R DISORDERS

This section will discuss some of the problematic conceptual issues for each of the 11 DSM-III-R personality disorders in hopes of facilitating for the practicing clinician a more in-depth approach to any single disorder. The diagnostic criteria are reproduced for the convenience of the reader in Tables 35.1 through 35.11. The reader is referred to Millon (6) and Siever and Klar (18) for reviews of these conceptual issues.

The Odd or Eccentric Cluster

All three personality disorders of the odd cluster have been linked historically and phenomenologically with schiophrenia, and all three have in common a distancing and aloofness in interpersonal relations and constriction of affect. (This affective manifestation is not listed as a criteria for the paranoid personality disorder but, in my opinion, is a common clinical observation.) Both schizotypal and paranoid disorders share the criterion of suspiciousness or paranoid ideation. It is understandable, therefore, that there is considerable overlap among these three disorders. There is also overlap between these "odd" disorders and other personality disorders. For instance, there is overlap between schizoid and avoidant and between schizotypal and borderline (18).

Paranoid Personality Disorder

Of the three "odd" personality disorders, the literature on the paranoid is the oldest, most comprehensive, and has the greatest consistency as to the phenomena under consideration. The standard textbooks over the past few decades nearly always describe the same disorder. Shapiro offers useful and creative insights as to the personality style of paranoid patients (6, 7), Colby presents an excellent review of four psychological theories of paranoia (19), and Salzman (20), Bullard (21), and Meissner (22) offer psychotherapeutic insights for the treatment of such patients. Meissner attempts to show the universality of the paranoid process.

Table 35.1   DSM-III-R Diagnostic Criteria for Paranoid Personality Disorder

---

A. A pervasive and unwarranted tendency, beginning by early adulthood and present in a variety of contexts, to interpret the actions of people as deliberately demeaning or threatening, as indicated by at least *four* of the following:
   (1) expects, without sufficient basis, to be exploited or harmed by others
   (2) questions, without justification, the loyalty or trustworthiness of friends or associates
   (3) reads hidden demeaning or threatening meanings into benign remarks or events, e.g., suspects that a neighbor put out trash early to annoy him
   (4) bears grudges or is unforgiving of insults or slights
   (5) is reluctant to confide in others because of unwarranted fear that the information will be used against him or her
   (6) is easily slighted and quick to react with anger or to counterattack
   (7) questions, without justification, fidelity of spouse or sexual partner
B. Occurrence not exclusively during the course of schizophrenia or a delusional disorder.

Reprinted with permission from American Psychiatric Association: *Diagnostic and Statistical Manual of Mental Disorders* (*Third Edition-Revised*). Washington, DC, American Psychiatric Association, 1987. Copyright 1987 American Psychiatric Association.

Table 35.2   DSM-III-R Diagnostic Criteria for Schizoid Personality Disorder

A. A pervasive pattern of indifference to social relationships and a restricted range of emotional experience and expression, beginning by early adulthood and present in a variety of contexts, as indicated by at least *four* of the following:
   (1) neither desires nor enjoys close relationships, including being part of a family
   (2) almost always chooses solitary activities
   (3) rarely, if ever, claims or appears to experience strong emotions, such as anger and joy
   (4) indicates little if any desire to have sexual experiences with another person (age being taken into account)
   (5) is indifferent to the praise and criticism of others
   (6) has no close friends or confidants (or only one) other than first-degree relatives
   (7) displays constricted affect, e.g., is aloof, cold, rarely reciprocates gestures or facial expressions, such as smiles or nods
B. Occurrence not exclusively during the course of schizophrenia or a delusional disorder.

Reprinted with permission from American Psychiatric Association: *Diagnostic and Statistical Manual of Mental Disorders* (*Third Edition-Revised*). Washington, DC, American Psychiatric Association, 1987. Copyright 1987 American Psychiatric Association.

Table 35.3   DSM-III-R Diagnostic Criteria for Schizotypal Personality Disorder

A. A pervasive pattern of deficits in interpersonal relatedness and peculiarities of ideation, appearance, and behavior, beginning by early adulthood and present in a variety of contexts, as indicated by at least *five* of the following:
   (1) ideas of reference (excluding delusions of reference)
   (2) excessive social anxiety, e.g., extreme discomfort in social situations involving unfamiliar people
   (3) odd beliefs or magical thinking, influencing behavior and inconsistent with subcultural norms, e.g., superstitiousness, belief in clairvoyance, telepathy, or "sixth sense," "others can feel my feelings" (in children and adolescents, bizarre fantasies or preoccupations)
   (4) unusual perceptual experiences, e.g., illusions, sensing the presence of a force or person not actually present (e.g., "I felt as if my dead mother were in the room with me")
   (5) odd or eccentric behavior or appearance, e.g., unkempt, unusual mannerisms, talks to self
   (6) no close friends or confidants (or only one) other than first-degree relatives
   (7) odd speech (without loosening of associations or incoherence), e.g., speech that is impoverished, digressive, vague, or inappropriately abstract
   (8) inappropriate or constricted affect, e.g., silly, aloof, rarely reciprocates gestures or facial expressions, such as smiles or nods
   (9) suspiciousness or paranoid ideation
B. Occurrence not exclusively during the course of schizophrenia or a pervasive developmental disorder.

Reprinted with permission from American Psychiatric Association: *Diagnostic and Statistical Manual of Mental Disorders* (*Third Edition-Revised*). Washington, DC, American Psychiatric Association, 1987. Copyright 1987 American Psychiatric Association.

Schizoid Personality Disorder

The schizoid personality presents serious conceptual problems because of its varied use since the term "schizoid" was used by Bleuler. In the past, the term was applied to patients who currently are diagnosed as schizoid, schizotypal, and avoidant (6). Many of the schizoid patients eloquently described by Guntrip, Fairbairn, and Winnicott have been loosely referred to as borderline by psychodynamic clinicians of other schools and as avoidant personality by DSM-III-R. The clinical value of the more limited DSM-III-R definition of schizoid personality disorder remains to be determined.

Schizotypal Personality Disorder

The schizotypal personality disorder was based on attempts of Rado (23) and Meehl (24) to describe individuals who had a genetic disposition for schizophrenia but were not overtly psychotic. This idea was used by the planners of DSM-III to distinguish those patients with "borderline schizophrenia" (those with genetic predispositions) from borderline personality disorder patients whose chronic instability presumably is of a different etiology and shows different behavioral manifestations (25). The schizotypal personality disorder first appeared in the official nomenclature with the DSM-III.

Table 35.4 DSM-III-R Diagnostic Criteria for Antisocial Personality Disorder

---

A. Current age at least 18.

B. Evidence of conduct disorder with onset before age 15, as indicated by a history of *three* or more of the following:
  (1) was often truant
  (2) ran away from home overnight at least twice while living in parental or parental surrogate home (or once without returning)
  (3) often initiated physical fights
  (4) used a weapon in more than one fight
  (5) forced someone into sexual activity with him or her
  (6) was physically cruel to animals
  (7) was physically cruel to other people
  (8) deliberately destroyed others' property (other than by fire-setting)
  (9) deliberately engaged in fire-setting
  (10) often lied (other than to avoid physical or sexual abuse)
  (11) has stolen without confrontation of a victim on more than one occasion (including forgery)
  (12) has stolen with confrontation of a victim (e.g., mugging, purse-snatching, extortion, armed robbery)

C. A pattern of irresponsible and antisocial behavior since the age of 15, as indicated by at least *four* of the following:
  (1) is unable to sustain consistent work behavior, as indicated by any of the following (including similar behavior in academic settings if the person is a student):
    (a) significant unemployment for six months or more within five years when expected to work and work was available
    (b) repeated absences from work unexplained by illness in self or family
    (c) abandonment of several jobs without realistic plans for others
  (2) fails to conform to social norms with respect to lawful behavior, as indicated by repeatedly performing antisocial acts that are grounds for arrest (whether arrested or not), e.g., destroying property, harassing others, stealing, pursuing an illegal occupation
  (3) is irritable and aggressive, as indicated by repeated physical fights or assaults (not required by one's job or to defend someone or oneself), including spouse- or child-beating
  (4) repeatedly fails to honor financial obligations, as indicated by defaulting on debts or failing to provide child support or support for other dependents on a regular basis
  (5) fails to plan ahead, or is impulsive, as indicated by one or both of the following:
    (a) traveling from place to place without a prearranged job or clear goal for the period of travel or clear idea about when the travel will terminate
    (b) lack of a fixed address for a month or more
  (6) has no regard for the truth, as indicated by repeatedly lying, use of aliases, or "conning" others for personal profit or pleasure
  (7) is reckless regarding his or her own or others' personal safety, as indicated by driving while intoxicated, or recurrent speeding
  (8) if a parent or guardian, lacks ability to function as a responsibile parent, as indicated by one or more of the following:
    (a) malnutrition of child
    (b) child's illness resulting from lack of minimal hygiene
    (c) failure to obtain medical care for a seriously ill child
    (d) child's dependence on neighbors or nonresident relatives for food or shelter
    (e) failure to arrange for a caretaker for young child when parent is away from home
    (f) repeated squandering, on personal items, of money required for household necessities
  (9) has never sustained a totally monogamous relationship for more than one year
  (10) lacks remorse (feels justified in having hurt, mistreated, or stolen from another)

D. Occurrence of antisocial behavior not exclusively during the course of schizophrenia or manic episodes.

The Dramatic, Emotional, or Erratic Cluster'

Antisocial Personality Disorder

The antisocial personality disorder, formerly referred to as psychopathy and sociopathy, has been associated with mental illness as early as the 18th century. This may be the most carefully studied diagnostic group and the most reliably diagnosable personality disorder. It may

Table 35.5   DSM-III-R Diagnostic Criteria for Borderline Personality Disorder

A pervasive pattern of instability of mood, interpersonal relationships, and self-image, beginning by early adulthood and present in a variety of contexts, as indicated by at least *five* of the following:
 (1) a pattern of unstable and intense interpersonal relationships characterized by alternating between extremes of overidealization and devaluation
 (2) impulsiveness in at least two areas that are potentially self-damaging, e.g., spending, sex, substance use, shoplifting, reckless driving, binge eating (Do not include suicidal or self-mutilating behavior covered in [5].)
 (3) affective instability: marked shifts from baseline mood to depression, irritability, or anxiety, usually lasting a few hours and only rarely more than a few days
 (4) inappropriate, intense anger or lack of control of anger, e.g., frequent displays of temper, constant anger, recurrent physical fights
 (5) recurrent suicidal threats, gestures, or behavior, or self-mutilating behavior
 (6) marked and persistent identity disturbance manifested by uncertainty about at least two of the following: self-image, sexual orientation, long-term goals or career choice, type of friends desired, preferred values
 (7) chronic feelings of emptiness or boredom
 (8) frantic efforts to avoid real or imagined abandonment (Do not include suicidal or self-mutilating behavior covered in [5].)

Reprinted with permission from American Psychiatric Association: *Diagnostic and Statistical Manual of Mental Disorders* (*Third Edition-Revised*). Washington, DC, American Psychiatric Association, 1987. Copyright 1987 American Psychiatric Association.

Table 35.6   DSM-III-R Diagnostic Criteria for Histrionic Personality Disorder

A pervasive pattern of excessive emotionality and attention-seeking, beginning by early adulthood and present in a variety of contexts, as indicated by at least *four* of the following:
 (1) constantly seeks or demands reassurance, approval, or praise
 (2) is inappropriately sexually seductive in appearance or behavior
 (3) is overly concerned with physical attractiveness
 (4) expresses emotion with inappropriate exaggeration, e.g., embraces casual acquaintances with excessive ardor, uncontrollable sobbing on minor sentimental occasions, has temper tantrums
 (5) is uncomfortable in situations in which he or she is not the center of attention
 (6) displays rapidly shifting and shallow expression of emotions
 (7) is self-centered, actions being directed toward obtaining immediate satisfaction; has no tolerance for the frustration of delayed gratification
 (8) has a style of speech that is excessively impressionistic and lacking in detail, e.g., when asked to describe mother, can be no more specific than "She was a beautiful person."

Reprinted with permission from American Psychiatric Association: *Diagnostic and Statistical Manual of Mental Disorders* (*Third Edition-Revised*). Washington, DC, American Psychiatric Association, 1987. Copyright 1987 American Psychiatric Association.

lend itself lend itself better to the categorical approach than any of the other 11 personality disorders (26). The evidence of genetic transmission for this disorder is clearly established. Cadoret points out the heterogeneity of this condition (27), and Millon takes exception to what he believes is a too narrow view which places an overemphasis on delinquent, criminal behavior rather than the broader personality from which this behavior sometimes emerges (6). Cleckley's book, written almost 50 years ago is still a classic in the field (28).

Borderline Personality Disorder

There is a rich literature on borderline personality disorders dating from the 1960s. These descriptions, however, were of a heterogeneous population that currently includes schizotypal, avoidant, histrionic, and other personality disorders. The psychodynamic literature used the term "borderline" to refer to a particular set of psychic mechanisms characteristic of patients of various phenomenology but presumably from a particular level of development and "psychic structure." The current more limited criteria for borderline

Table 35.7   DSM-III-R Diagnostic Criteria for Narcissistic Personality Disorder

---

A pervasive pattern of grandiosity (in fantasy or behavior), lack of empathy, and hypersensitivity to the evaluation of others, beginning by early adulthood and present in a variety of contexts, as indicated by at least *five* of the following:
(1) reacts to criticism with feelings of rage, shame, or humiliation (even if not expressed)
(2) is interpersonally exploitative: takes advantage of others to achieve his or her own ends
(3) has a grandiose sense of self-importance, e.g.., exaggerates achievements and talents, expects to be noticed as "special" without appropriate achievement
(4) believes that his or her problems are unique and can be understood only by other special people
(5) is preoccupied with fantasies of unlimited success, power, brilliance, beauty, or ideal love
(6) has a sense of entitlement: unreasonable expectation of especially favorable treatment, e.g., assumes that he or she does not have to wait in line when others must do so
(7) requires constant attention and admiration, e.g., keeps fishing for compliments
(8) lack of empathy: inability to recognize and experience how others feel, e.g., annoyance and surprise when a friend who is seriously ill cancels a date
(9) is preoccupied with feelings of envy

Reprinted with permission from American Psychiatric Association: *Diagnostic and Statistical Manual of Mental Disorders* (*Third Edition-Revised*). Washington, DC, American Psychiatric Association, 1987. Copyright 1987 American Psychiatric Association.

Table 35.8   DSM-III-R Diagnostic Criteria for Avoidant Personality Disorder

---

A pervasive pattern of social discomfort, fear of negative evaluation, and timidity, beginning by early adulthood and present in a variety of contexts, as indicated by at least *four* of the following:
(1) is easily hurt by criticism or disapproval
(2) has no close friends or confidants (or only one) other than first-degree relatives
(3) is unwilling to get involved with people unless certain of being liked
(4) avoids social or occupational activities that involve significant interpersonal contact, e.g., refuses a promotion that will increase social demands
(5) is reticent in social situations because of a fear of saying something inappropriate or foolish, or of being unable to answer a question
(6) fears being embarrassed by blushing, crying, or showing signs of anxiety in front of other people
(7) exaggerates the potential difficulties, physical dangers, or risks involved in doing something ordinary but outside his or her usual routine, e.g., may cancel social plans because she anticipates being exhausted by the effort of getting there

---

Reprinted with permission from American Psychiatric Association: *Diagnostic and Statistical Manual of Mental Disorders* (*Third Edition-Revised*). Washington, DC, American Psychiatric Association, 1987. Copyright 1987 American Psychiatric Association.

Table 35.9   DSM-III-R Diagnostic Criteria for Dependent Personality Disorder

---

A pervasive pattern of dependent and submissive behavior, beginning by early adulthood and present in a variety of contexts, as indicated by at least *five* of the following:
(1) is unable to make everyday decisions without an excessive amount of advice or reassurance from others
(2) allows others to make the most of his or her important decisions, e.g., where to live, what job to take
(3) agrees with people even when he or she believes they are wrong, because of fear of being rejected
(4) has difficulty initiating projects or doing things on his or her own
(5) volunteers to do things that are unpleasant or demeaning in order to get other people to like him or her
(6) feels uncomfortable or helpless when alone, or goes to great lengths to avoid being alone
(7) feels devastated or helpless when close relationships end
(8) is frequently preoccupied with fears of being abandoned
(9) is easily hurt by criticism or disapproval

Reprinted with permission from American Psychiatric Association: *Diagnostic and Statistical Manual of Mental Disorders* (*Third Edition-Revised*). Washington, DC, American Psychiatric Association, 1987. Copyright 1987 American Psychiatric Association.

personality have good reliability. Its clinical value remains to be determined by future research (6, 18, 29).

Histrionic Personality Disorder

The histrionic personality disorder was first used as an official diagnostic label in

Table 35.10   DSM-III-R Diagnostic Criteria for Obsessive–Compulsive Personality Disorder

A pervasive pattern of perfectionism and inflexibility, beginning by early adulthood and present in a variety of contexts, as indicated by at least *five* of the following:
  (1) perfectionism that interferes with task completion, e.g., inability to complete a project because own overly strict standards are not met
  (2) preoccupation with details, rules, lists, order, organization, or schedules to the extent that the major point of the activity is lost
  (3) unreasonable insistence that others submit to exactly his or her way of doing things, or unreasonable reluctance to allow others to do things because of the conviction that they will not do them correctly
  (4) excessive devotion to work and productivity to the exclusion of leisure activities and friendships (not accounted for by obvious economic necessity)
  (5) indecisiveness: decision making is either avoided, postponed, or protracted, e.g., the person cannot get assignments done on time because of ruminating about priorities (do not include if indecisiveness is due to excessive need for advice or reassurance from others)
  (6) overconscientiousness, scrupulousness, and inflexibility about matters of morality, ethics, or values (not accounted for by cultural or religious identification)
  (7) restricted expression of affection
  (8) lack of generosity in giving time, money, or gifts when no personal gain is likely to result
  (9) inability to discard worn-out or worthless objects even when they have no sentimental value

Reprinted with permission from American Psychiatric Association: *Diagnostic and Statistical Manual of Mental Disorders* (*Third Edition-Revised*). Washington, DC, American Psychiatric Association, 1987. Copyright 1987 American Psychiatric Association.

Table 35.11   DSM-III-R Diagnostic Criteria for Passive Aggressive Personality Disorder

A pervasive pattern of passive resistance to demands for adequate social and occupational performance, beginning by early adulthood and present in a variety of contexts, as indicated by at least *five* of the following:
  (1) procrastinates, i.e., puts off things that need to be done so that deadlines are not met
  (2) becomes sulky, irritable, or argumentative when asked to do something he or she does not want to do
  (3) seems to work deliberately slowly or to do a bad job on tasks that he or she really does not want to do
  (4) protests, without justification, that others make unreasonable demands on him or her
  (5) avoids obligations by claiming to have "forgotten"
  (6) believes that he or she is doing a much better job than others think he or she is doing
  (7) resents useful suggestions from others concerning how he or she could be more productive
  (8) obstructs the efforts of others by failing to do his or her share of the work
  (9) unreasonably criticizes or scorns people in positions of authority

Reprinted with permission from American Psychiatric Association: *Diagnostic and Statistical Manual of Mental Disorders* (*Third Edition-Revised*). Washington, DC, American Psychiatric Association, 1987. Copyright 1987 American Psychiatric Association.

DSM-III, although its antecedent, the hysterical personality, was used in DSM-II. There are two serious problems with the defining criteria for the histrionic personality disorder. The first is the significant overlap of criteria with the narcissistic and borderline personality disorders. The second is the distinction between the histrionic and the hysterical personality. The latter, which is not an official diagnosis, has similar behavioral manifestations to the histrionic personality, but they are of lesser severity. The psychologic issues of these two groups are radically different. The failure to distinguish these two conditions has been a source of considerable confusion in the literature on the hysterical and histrionic personality (6, 18, 30, 31).

Narcissistic Personality Disorder

The narcissistic personality disorder first appeared in the official nomenclature with the DSM-III. Earlier descriptions can be found in Freud, Reich, and Horney (6). More recent works of Kernberg (32) and Kohut (33) have popularized this disorder in psychoanalytic circles. Although the clinical picture makes intuitive sense to the clinician, there are no empirical studies, to my knowledge, as to the validity of the criteria. There are two major concerns with the current psychodynamic literature. First, it is not clear whether the patients described meet the criteria for the personality disorder or represent milder forms. Second, the clinical material described by

Kohut is based not on manifest behavioral characteristics but rather on the predominant transferences that the patient forms. Adler questions whether Kernberg and Kohut are in fact comparing similar populations in their differing approaches to these patients (34). Millon is highly critical of psychoanalytic contributions to the narcissistic personality and argues that the syndrome as described in DSM-III reflects a more solidly rooted biosocial and learning theory (6).

The Anxious and Fearful Cluster

Avoidant Personality Disorder

The avoidant personality disorder, a term coined by Millon, was first included in the official nomenclature with the DSM-III. This disorder is characterized by oversensitivity to social stimuli and hypersensitivity to situations of possible rejection and humiliation. This is in contrast to the schizoid disorder, in which the person is socially detached and lacks the affective capacity and desire for social relationships. Some of the interpersonal issues in avoidant patients are similar to those described by Fairbairn, Winnicott, Guntrip, and Kohut (under the diagnoses of schizoid character and false self). Similar personality constellations have been described by Bleuler (under the diagnosis of schizoid) and Schneider and Kretschmer (under the diagnosis of aesthenic) (6).

Dependent Personality Disorder

The dependent personality disorder was first included in the official nomenclature with the DSM-III. Its precursors were the oral receptive character of Abraham, the inadequate personality of Sullivan, the compliant type of Horney, and the passive–dependent personality type of DSM-II (6). Clinical evidence does exist for a cluster of traits which are recognized as part of the personality definition (2, 3, 35).

Obsessive–Compulsive Personality Disorder

The obsessive–compulsive personality has been one of the most consistently described personality type since Freud's description in 1908 (36). The traits of orderliness, perseverance, severe superego, emotional constriction, parsimony, and rigidity were found to cluster using factor analytic techniques (2, 3). An unsolved problem is the issue of the adaptive aspects of this personality style. Is the difference between adaptive and maladaptive obsessional traits a quantitative matter or a qualitative one? In other words, is an adaptive obsessional personality style a different clinical phenomena from the maladaptive disorder or is the difference a matter of degree?

Passive Aggressive Personality Disorder

Of all the personality disorders, passive aggressive disorder is perhaps the least clearly delineated and the most controversial (6, 37). This is because the disorder is based on a specific and a single interpersonal mechanism as opposed to a constellation of traits. Diagnostic agreement on this disorder is poor. It may be that the concept of passive aggressive behavior is a useful one and that some people rely to a considerable degree on this type of behavior, but that does not warrant the status of an official diagnosis. This diagnostic category has been in use since DSM-I.

Comment

From the above review of the 11 personality disorders in DSM-III-R, I suggest they can be organized into three categories according to the available knowledge base and clinical usefulness:

1. There are three disorders based on long historical tradition. These are the paranoid, the antisocial, and the obsessive–compulsive.
2. There are five disorders which appear to be clinically useful but present the clinician with a great deal of confusion because of the shifting names, concepts, and defining criteria throughout their history. These are the borderline, narcissistic, histrionic, avoidant, and dependent.

3. There are three personality disorders that may turn out to have questionable value. The passive aggressive may be little more than a trait; the schizotypal may eventually be better conceptualized as an Axis I condition; and the relevance of the schizoid disorders is questionable after other disorders are separated from them. The reader is referred to Siever and Klar for a review of the unsolved issues and future directions of the DSM-III-R personality disorders (18).

PSYCHODYNAMIC, BIOLOGIC, INTERPERSONAL, AND BEHAVIORAL APPROACHES TO PERSONALITY

Following the overall organization of this book, personality and the personality disorders can be usefully explored and understood from several conceptual frameworks. Such frameworks, in my opinion, are necessary for general clinical practice to complement existing knowledge about the 11 diagnostic categories.

Psychodynamic Models

Much of contemporary psychodyamic theory attempts to address issues of personality or character which it regards as more fundamental than symptom formation. On the other hand, there is considerable pessimism over the psychodynamic treatment of many of the conditions that are severe enough to meet the criteria of the DSM-III-R personality disorders. From my own observations, I believe that most psycho-dynamically oriented psychotherapists spend much of their clinical time treating long-term maladaptive patterns of behavior which by definition is personality. Most of these patients, however, do not meet the criteria for personality disorders.

To address this wide range of personality psychopathology, many psychodynamic clinicians currently classify personality according to developmental theory. (In earlier times, Freud developed a classi-

fication around libidinal theory [38].) Kernberg's classification, for instance, incorporates three major pathological developments: "(1) pathology in the ego and superego structures; (22) pathology in the internalized object relations; and (3) pathology in the development of libidinal and aggressive drive derivatives" (39). Using these concepts, he divides personality pathology into those disorders with "higher level of organization," which include obsessive–compulsive and most hysterical characters; "intermediate level of organization," which includes passive-aggressive and many narcissistic characters; and "lower level of organization," which includes antisocial, schizoid, paranoid, and some narcissistic personality disorders. Binstock, in an adaptation of Kernberg's classification, proposes 3 levels of personality disturbance which lie between health and chronic psychosis. These levels are discussed in terms of "internalized relationships with objects" and in terms of whether the patient primarily seeks sustenance, support, or gratification in a relationship (see table 35.12) (40). The three levels are the neurotic character, which includes the hysterical and obsessive–compulsive; the preoedipal character, which includes the mild borderline, mild narcissistic, passive aggressive, and hysteroid; and the borderline psychotic character, which includes the schizoid, severe paranoid, severe narcissistic, and primitive hysteric. Blanck and Blanck propose an individualistic diagnostic formulation based on what they refer to as developmental object relations theory. Each of their three books has useful chapters which discuss the meaning of diagnosis from contemporary psychodynamic perspectives (41–43).

By applying the psychodynamic classifications described above, different patients from a single DSM-III-R category may be placed in two or three different diagnostic groupings depending on level of organization of personality pathology or the nature of internalized object relationships. Histrionic and narcissistic personality disorders are but two examples. According to this developmental approach to diagnosis, suc-

Table 35.12   Assessing Levels of Character Pathology

Level of Character Pathology	Borderline Psychotic Character (Sickest)	Preoedipal Character (Sicker)	Neurotic Character (Sick)
Critical Ego Task	Basic Mistrust/Basic Trust	Shame and Doubt/Autonomy	Guilt/Initiative
Some extant labels	Sociopathic Multiple addictions and perversions Impulsive (chaotic) Schizoid Cyclothymic Severe paranoid Severe narcissistic Psychotic Severe borderline Primitive hysteric Borderline hysteric Infantile As if	Mild borderline Mild narcissistic Mild paranoid Passive aggressive Oral Hysteroid	Depressive (masochistic) Phobic (counterphobic) Hysterical Obsessive-compulsive
Symptom illness, same level	Acute psychosis	Acute psychosis or neurosis	Neurosis
Seeks in a relationship	Sustenance	Support	Gratification
Self–Object differentiation	– +	+	+
Object constancy	– +	+	+
Part or whole objects	Part	Part/whole	Whole
Management of ambivalence	Awkward	Strained	Smoothly patterned
Ability to mourn	–	+	+
Sadomasochism	+ + +	+ +	+
Tolerance for painful affect	–	– +	+
Defensive strategy	Reality distorting	Reality respecting	Reality respecting
Sublimations	–	– +	+
Organization of thought	Primary process, dominant	Secondary process, dominant	Secondary process, dominant
Object relationship concept	Dyadic (one to one)	Dyadic	Triangular
Superego	Chaotic, totally undependable morality	Alternatively punitive and lax	Rigid and severe
Ego ideal	Projection, introjection, denial	Grandiose but inconsistent	Reasonably clear
Approach to moral dilemmas		Reaction–formation	Inhibition
Sense of self: self-esteem	+	+ +	+ + +

Note: No one is simply one of these. This classifies psychopathology, not people: Anyone who exists in society has attained the neurotic level to some extent. From Binstock WA: The psychodynamic approach. In Lazare A (ed): *Outpatient Psychiatry: Diagnosis and Treatment.* Baltimore, Williams & Wilkins, 1979, pp 19–70.

cessful treatment of one psychodynami- cally defined personality disorder may lead to the development of a different, healthier personality diagnosis. Adler, for instance, postulates that the successful treatment of borderline conditions can lead to the de- velopment of a narcissistic disorder (44). A final feature of psychodynamic diagnosis which differs from categorical diagnosis is that the manifest behaviors of a given di- agnosis may be quite diverse. What de- fines the category are inferred mental mechanisms. Disorders of the self, accord- ing to Wolf and Kohut, for instance, vary in manifest behavior while sharing com- mon dynamic features such as the emerg- ing transferences (45). The various types of self-disorders, as described by these au- thors, would fall under several DSM-III-R diagnostic categories for personality disor- ders.

Biologic Models

Following the outline of Chapter 3, sev- eral dimensions of the biologic model can be applied to disorders of personality: the organic differential diagnosis, psychophar- macologic response, and biologic etiology and mechanisms. With regard to known organic or neuroanatomical determinants, Bear has described a variety of organic causes of acute personality change, epi- sodic personality change, and specific be- havioral profiles (46, 47). None of the 11 DSM-III-R disorders has known neuroana- tomical determinants. With regard to phar- macologic treatments for personality disorders, it is of interest that some condi- tions for which psychotropic agents have proved value are no longer included in the personality disorders. These are the de- pressive and cyclothymic personalities, which are now regarded as part of Axis I. As to pharmacologic treatment of person- ality disorders, Liebowitz et al. suggest that the goals are to "decrease vulnerabil- ity to affective or cognitive decompensa- tion; enhance pleasure capacity; normalize activation; and correct dysregulation. These changes enable patients to function more normally and, where indicated, to

benefit more from psychotherapy" (48). Translated into clinical terms, this means that one should consider pharmacologic treatment for comorbid Axis I anxiety, mood, and thought disorders or for subcli- nical states of the same when they do not meet the criteria for Axis I disorders. When pharmacologic agent are helpful, there is symptomatic improvement which may im- prove functioning, but there is no funda- mental change in personality. It may appear, however, that the personality has changed because the patient's decompen- sated presenting clinical state often is mistaken for personality. Genetic con- tributions have been found in antisocial personality disorders and to a lesser de- gree in schizoptypic personality disorders. Kendler et al. suggest that schizophrenia may be genetically related to a spectrum of personality disorders that would now in- clude schizotypic and paranoid personal- ity disorders (49). Many studies of twins and sibs find that genetic factors explain much of the variance of dimensions such as extroversion, neuroticism and anxiety, and approach–withdrawal. These dimen- sions are not related to DSM-III-R (12).

Interpersonal Models

During the past several years, interper- sonal approaches have been used to char- acterize personality disorders. Such approaches are based on the assumption that personality functioning is basically in- terpersonal in nature (50). Because there is no comprehensive interpersonal approach or interpersonal school, the clinician must make his or her own integration of inter- personal approaches. I recommend the overview article by Kiesler which describes the diagnostic and therapeutic aspects of a particular interpersonal approach (51). He describes, through "the interpersonal circle," a range of individual differences in both normal and abnormal behaviors. Lo- cation on this circle leads to a description of the patient's maladaptive patterns of liv- ing as well as suggestions for the optimal treatment plan. Kiesler offers translations of the DSM-III personality disorders into profiles on the interpersonal circle. This interpersonal system combines both dimensional and typologic assessment classifications.

Behavioral Models

Behavioral models have only recently been applied to the diagnosis and treatment of personality disorders. This is understandable because behavioral therapists have not found the constructs of personality to be of much use. Nevertheless, behavioral formulations can be applied to an individual case to determine the etiology of, mechanism for, and treatment of the behavior in question (48). DSM-III and DSM-III-R have in fact stimulated the interest of behavioral clinicians in the understanding and treatment of the personality disorders. Currently, there is insufficient evidence as to the efficacy of behavioral therapy for any given personality disorder. As described in Chapter 8, behavioral models, like psychodynamic models, are individualistic approaches to psychopathology. Diagnosis and treatment are not directed at the personality per se but at the "mechanism for, etiology of and future course of the phenomenon of interest" (48).

THEORETICAL AND CLINICAL ISSUES

This section will present five points which have relevance for clinical practice.

The first has to do with the problematic nature of the defining criteria for personality disorders. It is often difficult to make the judgment that the personality traits in question are inflexible and maladaptive and cause either significant functional impairment or subjective distress. Along these parameters, the traits of the personality disorders are quantitatively not qualitatively different from normality. Problems in judging pathology result from the tolerance of the observer, the situational role of the subject, and the concurrent Axis I diagnosis. In other words, a person in a particularly stressful situation

or suffering from a (state) Axis I disorder is apt to manifest maladaptive personality traits that are not characteristic of (trait) long-term functioning. Under these conditions, clinicians are apt to mistakenly make the diagnosis of personality disorder (50). A second point is whether, as the designation of a distinct axis suggests, there is something unique and distinctive about personality disorders as compared to other DSM-III-R diagnoses. This is a very difficult question, as Hirschfeld points out: "They are not the only chronic or longstanding conditions; we have no evidence that they are not reflective of more basic emotional dysfunctions; they are not less amenable to change than many other psychiatric disorders; and the ego-syntonicity issue is not unique"(52).

A third issue is whether the personality disorders are best conceptualized as categories, as dimensions, or by other forms such as prototypes. Of all psychiatric problems, personality disorders suffer the most from the absence of clear boundaries and the heterogeneity of members of the category. One alternative to this categorical model are dimensional systems which view the variables as continuous rather than dichotomous. Using this approach, each patient would have a personality profile which would describe the degree to which he or she manifests maladaptive personality traits (50). I believe that by using a dimensional approach to personality assessment for each patient, the clinician avoids the common error of making the most obvious diagnosis and then ignoring other less obvious diagnoses or personality traits that nevertheless contribute to the formulation. For example, for patients who are both obsessional and histrionic, it is common for clinicians to attend to the most obvious and ignore the less obvious despite its importance.

The fourth point concerns the relevance of the 11 personality disorders to the study and treatment of patients with personality dimensions or styles that are less serious. As described earlier, most long-term psychologic treatments attempt to deal with long-standing maladaptive attitudes and behaviors which do not meet the criteria for personality disorder. These conditions are more prevalent and more treatable than the 11 conditions of DSM-III-R. They certainly differ from DSM-III-R quantitatively—they are less severe. It is also possible that many of the personality features differ qualitatively; they include phenomena and processes that are described and addressed not by the Manual but by concepts and processes from psychodynamic, interpersonal, and behavioral formulations. It may be that in a general outpatient practice, the diagnosis, formulation, and management of these nondiagnosable personality dimensions are more significant than those that meet the DSM-III-R diagnostic criteria. In other words, I believe that in our attempts to study and understand the 11 categorical diagnoses, we must be careful not to ignore observations and understanding of those less severe personality phenomena that affect large numbers of patients and occupy much of ambulatory practice.

The final point has to do with a missing piece of knowledge which has considerable relevance to the outpatient clinician. This is the relationship between the personality profile, the nature of the psychosocial stressors, the psychologic meaning of the stressors, the social support system, the patient's reaction to the stress, and the manner in which the patient is apt to relate to the clinician. These are the kind of data, more or less, that constitute psychodynamic, interpersonal, and behavioral formulations that clinicians deal with in everyday practice. Their measurement and interrelationships should be subjects for future research.

References

1. American Psychiatric Association: *Diagnostic and Statistical Manual of Mental Disorders (Third Edition-Revised)*. Washington, DC, American Psychiatric Association, 1987.
2. Lazare A, Klerman GL, Armor D: Oral, obsessive and hysterical personality patterns: an investigation of psychoanalytic concepts by means of factor analysis. *Arch Gen Psychiatry* 14:624–630, 1965.
3. Lazare A, Klerman GL, Armor D: Oral, obsessive and hysterical personality patterns: replication of factor analysis in an independent sample. *J Psychiatr Res* 7:275–290, 1970.
4. Hirschfeld RMA: Personality disorders. In Frances AJ, Hales RE (eds): *Annual Review*. Washington, DC, American Psychiatric Press, 1986, vol 5, pp 233–239.
5. Kahana RJ, Bibing G: Personality types in medical management. In Zinberg N (ed): *Psychiatry and Medical Practices in a General Hospital*. New York, International Unviersity Press 1964, pp 108–123.
6. Millon T: *Disorders of Personality DSM-III: Axis II*. New York, John Wiley and Sons, 1981.
7. Shapiro D: *Neurotic Styles*. New York, Basic Books, 1965.
8. Shapiro D: *Autonomy and Rigid Character*. New York, Basic Books, 1981.
9. Horowitz M, Marmar C, Krupnick J, et al: *Personality styles and Brief Psychotherapy*. New York, Basic Books, 1984.
10. Frances AJ, Hales RE (eds): *Psychiatry Update*, vol 5. Washington, DC, American Psychiatric Press, 1986.
11. Michels R, Cavenar J, Brodie HKH, et al (eds): *Psychiatry*, vol 1. Philadelphia, J.B. Lippincott Company, 1986.
12. Pfohl B: Personality disorders. In Winokur G, Clayton P (eds): *The Medical Basis of Psychiatry*. Philadelphia, W.B. Saunders Company, 1986, pp 442–457.
13. Docherty JP, Fiester SJ, Shea T: Syndrome diagnosis and personality disorder. In Frances AJ, Hales RE (eds): *Annual Review*. Washington, DC, American Psychiatric Press, 1986, vol 5, pp 315–355.
14. Pfohl B, Coryell W, Zimmerman M, et al: DSM-III personality disorders: diagnostic overlap and interanl consistency of individual DSM-III criteria. *Compr Psychiatry* 27:21–34, 1986.
15. Merikangas KR, Weissman MM: Epidemiology of DSM-III Axis II personality disorders. In Frances AJ, Hales RE (eds): *Annual Review*. Washington, DC, American Psychiatric Press, 1986, vol 5, pp 258–278.
16. Pope HG, Jonas JM, Judson JI, et al: The validity of DSM-III borderline personality disorders. *Arch Gen Psychiatry* 40:23–30, 1983.
17. McGlashan TH: The borderline syndrome, II: Is it a variant of schizophrenia or affective disorder? *Arch Gen Psychiatry* 40:1319–1323, 1983.
18. Siever LJ, Klar H: A review of DSM-III criteria for the personality disorders. In Frances AJ, Hales RE (eds): *Annual Review*, Washington, DC, American Psychiatric Press, 1986, vol 5, pp 279–314.
19. Colby KM: Appraisal of four psychological theories of paranoid phenomena. *J Abnormal Psychol* 86:54, 1977.
20. Salzman L: Paranoid state—theory and therapy. *Arch Gen Psychiatry* 2:679–693, 1960.
21. Bullard DM: Psychotherapy of paranoid patients. *Arch Gen Psychiatry* 2:137, 1960.
22. Meissner WW: *Psychotherapy and the Paranoid Process*. New York, Jason Aronson, 1986.
23. Rado S: Theory and therapy: the theory of schizo-

typal organization and its application to the treatment of decompensated schizotypal behavior. In Rado S (ed): *Psychoanalysis of Behavior*. New York, Grune and Stratton, 1962, vol 2, pp 127–140.

24. Meehl PE: Schizotaxia, schizotypy, schizophrenia. *Am Psychol* 17:827–838, 1962.

25. Siever LJ, Kendler KS: Schizoid/schizotypal/paranoid personality disorders. In Michels R, Cavenar J, Brodie HKH, et al (eds): *Psychiatry*. Philadelphia, J.B. Lippincott Company, 1986, vol 1, Chapter 16.

26. Reid WH: Antisocial personality. In Michels R, Cavenar J, Brodie HKH, et al (eds): *Psychiatry*. Philadelphia, JU.B. Lippincott Company, 1986, vol 1, Chapter 23.

27. Cadoret R: Antisocial personality. In Winokur G, Clayton P (eds): *The Medical Basis of Psychiatry*. Philadelphia, W.B. Saunders Company, 1986, pp 231–245.

28. Cleckley HM: *The Mask of Sanity*. St. Louis, C.V. Mosby, 1941.

29. Stone MH: Borderline personality disorder. In Michels R, Cavenar J. Brodie HKH, et al (eds): *Psychiatry*. Philadelphia, J.B. Lippincott Company, 1986, vol 1, chapter 17.

30. Lazare A: The hysterical character in psychoanalytic theory: evolution and confusion. *Arch Gen Psychiatry* 25:131–137, 1971.

31. Kernberg OF: Hysterical and histrionic per-sonality disorders. In Michels R, Cavenar J, Brodie HKH, et al (eds): *Psychiatry*. Philadelphia, J.B. Lippincott Company, 1986, vol 1, chapter 19.

32. Kernberg OF: *Borderline Conditions and Pathological Narcissism*. New York, Jason Aronson, 1975.

33. Kohut H:P *The Analysis of the Self*. New York, International University Press, 1974.

34. Adler G: Psychotherapy of the narcissistic personality disorder patients: two contrasting approaches. *Am J Psychiatry* 143:430–436, 1980.

35. Tyrer P, Alexander J: Classification of personality disorder. *Br J Psychiatry* 135:163–176, 1979.

36. Freud S: Character and anal erotism. In Jones E (ed): *Collected Papers of Sigmund Freud*. New York, Basic Books, 1959, vol 2, pp 45–50.

37. Esman AH: Dependent and passive-aggressive personality disorders. In Michels R, Cavenar J, Brodie HKH, et al (eds) *Psychiatry*. Philadelphia, J.B. Lippincott Company, 1986, vol 1, Chapter 26.

38. Freud S: Libidinal types. In Jones E (ed): *Collected Papers*. New York, Basic Books, 1959, vol 5, pp. 247–251.

39. Keinberg O: A psychoanalytic classification of character pathology. In Keinberg O (ed): *Object Relations and Clinical Psychoanalysis*. New York, Jason Aronson, 1976, pp 139–160.

40. Binstock WA: The psychodynamic approach. In Lazare A (ed): *Outpatient Psychiatry: Diagnosis and Treatment*. Baltimore, Williams & Wilkins, 1979, pp 19–70.

41. Blanck G, Blanck R: *Ego Psychology II*. New York, Columbia University Press, 1974.

42. Blanck G, Blanck R: *Beyond Ego Psychology*. New York, Columbia University Press, 1979.

43. Blanck R, Blanck G: *Beyond Ego Psychology*. New York, Columbia University Press, 1986.

44. Adler G: The borderline-narcissistic personality disorder continuum. *Am J Psychiatry* 138:46–50, 1981.

45. Kohut H, Wolf ES: The disorders of the self and their treatment: an outline. *Int J Psychoanal* 59:413–425, 1978.

46. Bear D: Alterations in personality. In Lazare A: *Outpatient Psychiatry: Diagnosis and Treatment*. Baltimore, Williams & Wilkins, 1979, pp 337–352.

47. Bear D, Freeman R, Greenberg M: Changes in personality associated with neurologic disease. In Michels R, Cavenar J, Brodie HKH, et al (eds): *Psychiatry*. Philadelphia, J.B. Lippincott Company, 1986, vol 1, Chapter 28.

48. Liebowitz MR, Stone MH, Turkat ID: Treatment of personality disorders. In Frances AJ, Hales RE (eds): *Annual Review*. Washington, DC, American Psychiatric Press, 1986, vol 5, pp 356–393.

49. Kendler KS, Gurenberg AM, Strauss JS: An independent analysis of the Copenhagen sample of the Danish adoption study of schizophrenia, II: The relationship between schizotypal personality disorder and schizophrenia. *Arch Gen Psychiatry* 38:982–984, 1981.

50. Francis AJ, Widiger T: The classification of personality disorders: an overview of problems and solutions. In Frances AJ, Hales RE (eds): *Annual Review*. Washington, DC, American Psychiatric Press, 1986, vol 5, pp 240–257.

51. Kiesler DJ: Interpersonal methods of diagnosis and treatment. In Michels R, Cavenar J, Brodie HKH, et al (eds): *Psychiatry*. Philadelphia, J.B. Lippincott Company, 1986, vol 1, chapter 4.

52. Hirschfeld RMA: Afterword. In Frances AJ, Hales RE (eds): *Annual Review*. Washington, DC, American Psychiatric Association, 1986, vol 5, pp 394–395.

36

Psychoactive Substance Use Disorders: Alcoholism

Steven A. Adelman, M.D.
Roger D. Weiss, M.D.

Alcoholism is a complex problem with biologic, psychologic, and social dimensions. At various times alcoholism has been referred to as a disorder, a syndrome, a criminal offense, a social disease, an addiction, and an illness. The conceptual confusion suggested by this variety of terms reflects the complexity of alcoholism and illustrates the importance of approaching it from a number of different perspectives.

A logical starting point is to survey the extreme public health consequences of alcoholism. In the United States today, approximately 15% of health care dollars are spent on the treatment of alcohol-related illness (1). Alcohol contributes to 28,000 motor vehicle fatalities each year (2) and to one-third of all suicides (3). In addition, alcoholic women give birth to numerous babies with the fetal alcohol syndrome. These infants are born with a host of congenital abnormalities, including retarded growth and development, hyperactivity, and frank mental retardation. The aforementioned consequences of alcohol abuse may be significantly reduced by clinicians who are trained to recognize the initial stages of alcoholism and to intervene early, when treatment is most effective (4).

This brief survey of alcohol-induced morbidity serves to introduce the idea that alcoholism can be defined largely by the consequences of drinking. When an individual's repeated use of ethanol leads to medical, interpersonal, vocational, or legal problems, that person can be thought of as an alcoholic. This working definition of alcoholism as a "pattern of drinking which causes problems" simplifies the task of defining alcoholism in different cultures and at different times in history. It is a definition well suited to general psychiatric and medical practice.

HISTORICAL OVERVIEW

It is instructive to trace the concepts of alcoholism and alcoholism treatment historically (5). In colonial America drinking was common and drunkenness was frowned upon. The Puritans equated intoxication with sin and implicated Satan as its cause. The treatment of inebriation was religious and moralistic in tone, including social disapproval, whippings, imprisonment, and excommunications. In the late 1700s Dr. Benjamin Rush combined this moralistic approach with a medical one and deemed inebriety an odious disease process with moral underpinnings.

Rush set the tone for the temperance movement which was founded in 1826. Crusades for temperance and abstinence were a response to the increased use and abuse of alcohol which accompanied industrialization and the move westward in the 19th century. By the early 1900s the spiritual drive to end drinking, spearheaded by groups like the Women's Christian Temperance Union, had given rise to a political campaign to close saloons and ban alcohol. This culminated in the ratification of Prohibition in 1919. Thus, until the early part of this century, religious and political approaches to alcoholism prevailed, while the American medical community displayed relatively little interest in the problem.

The modern concept of alcoholism as an illness arose not in the United States but in Europe. As early as 1852 Magnus Huss in Sweden coined the term "chronic alcoholism," recognizing that it was distinct from other mental disorders. Although the early European notion that alcoholism was caused by a well-defined central nervous system lesion has never been substantiated, the concept of alcoholism as a disease with a understandable etiology, course, prognosis and treatment took root in the United States. The disease concept helped to organize American thinking about alcoholism. It was embraced first by Alcoholics Anonymous (AA), founded in 1935, and later by physicians, starting with Jellinek in the 1940s.

This lag in the medical community's acceptance of the disease concept is the source of what many have perceived as tension between physicians and AA. As the medical community and AA have grown to appreciate their common goals and mutual contributions, this tension has begun to recede. Over the past 40 years, health professionals and researchers in the United States have continued to refine the concept of alcoholism as a medical disorder by focusing attention on its diagnosis, etiology, concomitant disorders, clinical course, and treatment. Current understanding of these aspects of alcoholism is described in this chapter.

DIAGNOSIS

Although groups such as the American Psychiatric Association, the World Health Organization, and others have established diagnostic criteria for alcoholism based on methodologically rigorous studies, several factors combine to make the diagnostic process quite difficult at times. First, drinking patterns and problems occur along a continuum ranging from abstinence, to moderate social drinking, to episodic alcohol-induced difficulties, to chronic alcohol dependence. In addition, patterns of drinking which qualify as alcoholism according to some diagnostic instruments are seen as normal in some cultural contexts. Because of the wide variation in drinking patterns and cultural norms, one must rely on a largely functional approach to drinking. In general, then, when a person, his family or his employer suspect that alcohol has caused some dysfunction, then an alcohol problem usually exists. Because the progression of alcoholism may be most effectively halted in the early stages with rather modest therapeutic interventions, it is generally useful to have a very high index of suspicion and low threshold in making the diagnosis of an alcohol problem. Formal diagnostic instruments, such as the *Diagnostic and Statistical Manual of Mental Disorders (Third Edition-Revised)* (DSM-III-R) and the Michigan Alcoholism Screening Test, familiarize clinicians with important diagnostic features, and are often useful for convincing doubting patients that their problem is alcohol related.

Current work in the field has shifted clinicians' traditional reliance on the presence of physical dependence as the major feature of alcoholism. It is now clear that pathologic drinking, defined loosely as alcohol-induced impairment of social or occupational functioning, may precede physical dependence by a number of years. Similarly, alcohol-induced blackouts, which are amnestic periods occurring during intoxication, often do not occur until a long-standing pattern of pathologic drinking has been established. Rounsaville et al. (6) have described the rationale behind the DSM-III-R criteria for the diagnosis of alcohol dependence. These revised criteria broaden the concept of dependence to include pathologic behavior related to drinking and the use of other psychoactive drugs. Of the nine diagnostic criteria listed (see Table 36.1), the presence of three qualifies an individual as being dependent. Tolerance and withdrawal are neither necessary nor sufficient for the diagnosis of alcohol dependence. The DSM-III-R also includes a rating system for the severity of psychoactive substance abuse.

The Michigan Alcoholism Screening Test or MAST (7, 8) is a sensitive diagnostic tool, commonly used both by clinicians and researchers (see Table 36.2). The primary advantage of the MAST is its simplicity. It consists of a series of weighted yes/no written questions about the pattern and consequences of a person's drinking. Patients may score the questionnaire and see for themselves whether or not they meet the MAST criteria for the diagnosis of alcoholism. Many patients who initially reject the suggestion that they have a drinking problem score significantly more

points than the MAST requires to qualify them as alcoholic. The results of this objective test may represent the beginning of an indivdual's acceptance that he or she does indeed have a drinking problem.

A second screening test, which can be incorporated into a medical or psychiatric interview, is known by the useful mnemonic CAGE (9), which consists of the following four questions:

1. Have you ever felt the need to — *C*ut down on drinking?
2. Have you ever felt — *A*nnoyed by criticism of your drinking?
3. Have you ever had — *G*uilty feelings about drinking?
4. Have you ever taken a morning — *E*ye-opener?

The authors who designed the instrument contend that affirmative answers to three of these four questions confirm the diagnosis of alcoholism, while two affirmative answers are suggestive. Although the diagnostic validity of CAGE has not been

Table 36.1   Diagnostic Criteria for Psychoactive Substance Dependence[a]

A. At least three of the following:
   (1) substance often taken in larger amounts or over a longer period than the person intended
   (2) persistent desire or one or more unsuccessful efforts to cut down or control substance use
   (3) a great deal of time spent in activities necessary to get the substance (e.g., theft), taking the substance (e.g., chain smoking), or recovering from its effects
   (4) frequent intoxication or withdrawal symptoms when expected to fulfill major role obligations at work, school, or home (e.g., does not go to work because hung over, goes to school or work "high," intoxicated while taking care of his or her children), or when substance use is physically hazardous (e.g., drives when intoxicated)
   (5) important social, occupational, or recreational activities given up or reduced because of substance use
   (6) continued substance use despite knowledge of having a persistent or recurrent social, psychological, or physical problem that is caused or exacerbated by the use of the substance (e.g., keeps using heroin despite family arguments about it, cocaine-induced depression, or having an ulcer made worse by drinking)
   (7) marked tolerance: need for markedly increased amounts of the substance (i.e., at least a 50% increase) in order to achieve intoxication or desired effect, or markedly diminished effect with continued use of the same amount
   Note: The following items may not apply to cannabis, hallucinogens, or phencyclidine (PCP):
   (8) characteristic withdrawal symptoms (see specific withdrawal syndromes under psychoactive substance-induced organic mental disorders)
   (9) substance often taken to relieve or avoid withdrawal symptoms
B. Some symptoms of the disturbance have persisted for at least one month, or have occurred repeatedly over a longer period of time.

[a] Reprinted with permission from the *Diagnostic and Statistical Manual of Mental Disorders* (*Third Edition-Revised*). Washington, DC, American Psychiatric Association, 1987.

Table 36.2   Michigan Alcoholism Screen Test[a]

Points for "Yes" Answer			Yes	No
	0.	Do you enjoy a drink now and then?	—	—
(2)[b]	1.	Do you feel you are a normal drinker? (By normal we mean you drink less than or as much as most other people).	—	—
(2)	2.	Have you ever awakened the morning after some drinking the night before and found that you could not remember a part of the evening?	—	—
(1)	3.	Does your wife, husband, a parent, or other near relative ever worry or complain about your drinking?	—	—
(2)[b]	4.	Can you stop drinking without a struggle after one or two drinks?	—	—
(1)	5.	Do you ever feel guilty about your drinking?	—	—
(2)[b]	6.	Do friends or relatives think you are a normal drinker?	—	—
(2)[b]	7.	Are you able to stop drinking when you want to?	—	—
(5)	8.	Have you ever attended a meeting of Alcoholics Anonymous (AA)?	—	—
(1)	9.	Have you gotten into physical fights when drinking?	—	—
(2)	10.	Has your drinking ever created problems between you and your wife, husband, a parent, or other relative?	—	—
(2)	11.	Has your wife, husband (or other family member) ever gone to anyone for help about your drinking?	—	—
(2)	12.	Have you ever lost friends because of your drinking?	—	—
(2)	13.	Have you ever gotten into trouble at work or school because of drinking?	—	—
(2)	14.	Have you ever lost a job because of drinking?	—	—
(2)	15.	Have you ever neglected your obligations, your family, or your work for two or more days in a row because you were drinking?	—	—
(1)	16.	Do you drink before noon fairly often?	—	—
(2)	17.	Have you ever been told you have liver trouble? Cirrhosis?	—	—
(2)[c]	18.	After heavy drinking have you ever had delirium tremens (DTs) or severe shaking, or head voices or seen things that really weren't there?	—	—
(5)	19.	Have you ever gone to anyone for help about your drinking?	—	—
(5)	20.	Have you ever been in a hospital because of drinking?	—	—
(2)	21.	Have you ever been a patient in a psychiatric hospital or on a psychiatric ward of a general hospital where drinking was part of the problem that resulted in hospitalization?	—	—
(2)	22.	Have you ever been seen at a psychiatric or mental health clinic or gone to any doctor, social worker, or clergyman for help with any emotional problem, where drinking was part of the problem?	—	—
(2)[d]	23.	Have you ever been arrested for drunk driving, driving while intoxicated, or driving under the influence of alcoholic beverages? (IF YES, how many times? ___)	—	—
(2)[d]	24.	Have you ever been arrested, or taken into custody, even for a few hours, because of other drunk behavior? (IF YES, how many times? ___)	—	—

[a] Reprinted with permission from Selzer ML, Vinokur A, van Rooijen L: A self-administered short version of the Michigan Alcoholism Screening Test (SMAST). *Journal of Studies on Alcohol* 36:117–126, 1976.
[b] Points are for "no" answer.
[c] 5 points for delirium tremens.
[d] 2 points for each arrest.
SCORING SYSTEM: In general, five points or more would place the subject in an "alcoholic" category. Four points would be suggestive of alcoholism, and three points or less would indicate the person was not alcoholic.

rigorously demonstrated, it remains a useful clinical device.

The prevalence of alcoholism within a given population will vary with the diagnostic tool employed. In one study seven different diagnostic schemes were utilized to evaluate a population of more than 500 patients (10). Depending on the diagnostic tool employed, the current prevalence of alcoholism varied from 1.6 to 2.4%, and lifetime prevalence varied in the same population from 3.1 to 6.3%. In two more recent studies, DSM-III criteria were employed in determining 6 month and lifetime prevalence rates of alcohol abuse and alcohol dependence in three United

States inner-city populations. The 6-month prevalence was approximately 5% for women and about 9% for men (11). Lifetime prevalence rates varied between 11 and 15% (12). The contrasting results in these studies illustrate how powerfully research methodology can affect prevalence rates.

ETIOLOGY

Clinicians and researchers from a wide variety of disciplines have attempted to investigate the causes of alcoholism from a number of different perspectives. Research in the field is necessarily complex, because of the probable multifactorial etiology of alcoholism and the clinical heterogeneity of most patient populations studied. An additional methodologic problem, often unavoidable, is the difficulty in distinguishing the causes of alcoholism from the effects of alcohol in individuals with a history of a long-standing alcohol problem. For all these reasons, current knowledge of what actually causes people to drink remains rudimentary. The following discussion focuses on three types of etiologic hypotheses: psychologic, biogenetic, and sociocultural

Psychologic Hypotheses

Psychodynamic

One oft-quoted theory of alcoholism is the psychoanalytically based description of the "alcoholic" or "oral" personality. This theory posits that unresolved psychologic conflicts traceable to the oral stage of psychosexual development cause people to become dependent on alcohol. Careful research, however, has never substantiated this hypothesis. Indeed there is no evidence that a single constellation of personality traits causes or leads to the development of alcoholism (14). Although an association between alcohol dependence and antisocial personality exists in a minority of cases, it remains uncertain whether or not sociopathy actually causes alcoholism (15).

Tension Reduction Hypothesis

Another psychologic hypothesis which has failed the test of research scrutiny is the so-called tension reduction hypothesis, which posits that alcoholics drink in order to suppress unwanted symptoms such as anxiety or depression. Although individuals who drink in moderation may experience some reduction in tension, studies examining this hypothesis in alcoholics indicate that alcohol augments, rather than reduces, their experience of unpleasant affects. Similarly, the idea that alcoholics drink simply to avoid the unpleasant effects of alcohol withdrawal has also been refuted (14).

Biogenetic Hypotheses

Family studies have shown that having alcoholic first-degree relatives increases an individual's chance of developing alcohol dependence by a factor of four (17). Adoption studies and high-risk studies strongly suggest a genetic component to this risk. The adoption studies of Bohman (18) and Cloninger (19) indicate that the genetic susceptibility to alcoholism takes different forms. One inherited form of alcoholism is mild, tends to affect members of both sexes, and is associated with little criminality. The other type of inherited alcoholism tends to be more severe and recurrent and is found mostly in males. The effects of environment suggested by these studies are discussed below.

The observation that in some cases alcoholism appears to be genetically transmitted has led researchers to look for what is actually inherited. Recent research has focused on examining the effects of ethanol on nonalcoholic individuals who are at high risk by virtue of strongly positive family histories. Such research thus averts the confounding problem of having to account for the effects of chronic alcohol intake on the variable being investigated. In such a study, Pollock et al. (20) showed that the sons of male alcoholics experienced greater augmentation of slow alpha activity on their electroencephalograms following an oral dose of alcohol than did controls. This study may suggest at why individuals with a positive family history of alcoholism might find ethanol particularly reinforcing.

In a related study, Schuckit (21) found that a given dose of alcohol produced less subjective intoxication in family-history-positive individuals that it did in family-history-negative controls. Schuckit (22) also determined that the amount of body sway induced by alcohol was less in the experimental group than in the control group. These studies all point to the possibility that the hallmark of familial alcoholism is the inheritance of the propensity to experience more pleasant effects and fewer adverse effects from a given amount of alcohol.

Although studies of the biology of alcoholism have yielded a great deal of information, even a complete understanding of familial alcoholism will not explain why some individuals with strong genetic loading do not develop alcoholism. It also does not shed light on why half of the population of alcoholics may have no family history of the illness. Experts have looked at sociocultural factors to explain those aspects of alcoholism which cannot be accounted for by biogenetic and psychologic mechanicms.

Sociocultural Hypotheses

It has long been known that certain religious, ethnic, national, and class groups have more alcoholism than others. Although most explanations of this phenomenon have been impressionistic and unscientific, some studies have been illuminating.

Bohman (18) and Cloninger (19), for example, have conducted careful adoption studies which clearly indicate that low occupational status in adoptive parents is associated with alcoholism in their adopted children, independent of genetic factors. However, observations linking low socioeconomic status and early family and school problems with alcoholism do not explain why this disorder afflicts individuals without such backgrounds.

Zinberg (23) has stressed the important effect of social controls on drinking behav-

ior. His work indicates that cultural groups with low rates of alcoholism share a number of common features. For example, alcoholism is rarely seen in groups that use alcohol for religious celebrations, in groups that include members of both sexes and different generations in the drinking situation, and in groups that view drunkenness (as opposed to drinking) with opprobrium. A sociocultural group may thus evolve certain norms that in large part protect its members from developing alcoholism.

Zinberg's ideas shed light on concurrent changes which Americans are experiencing in the social context of drinking alcohol. Groups such as Mothers Against Drunk Driving and Students Against Drunk Driving, reacting to the unacceptably high toll of alcohol-related traffic fatalities, are actively working to alter the public's perceptions about drinking and driving in order to reduce alcohol abuse. It may take years to measure the effects obtained by these concerted efforts to change people's attitudes and habits. Psychiatrists and other health care providers may contribute to this change by focusing on both early identification and aggressive treatment of drinking problems.

CONCOMITANT DISORDERS

Alcoholism frequently occurs in conjunction with other physical and psychiatric problems. Clinical experience indicates that although a number of psychiatric disorders may precipitate, exacerbate, or coexist with alcohol dependence, it is usually safest to assume that the patient's alcohol problem has taken on a life of its own. In other words, alcoholism should be regarded as a primary problem requiring specific therapeutic intervention. Attempts to treat a drinking problem by focusing on the "underlying" depression or other psychiatric problem are almost always unsuccessful unless there is a concerted treatment effort directed towards the alcoholism itself.

The above qualifying statements notwithstanding, it is of both clinical and theoretical interest to review the evidence linking alcoholism to other psychiatric disorders. Because alcoholism is not a unitary illness with a single, clearly identifiable lesion, the role of concomitant disorders is more contributory than causal. No one underlying disorder has been found to explain the existence of alcoholism in a sizable percentage of the alcoholic population. However, the ability to recognize and treat the spectrum of associated disorders may augment a clinician's effectiveness in many cases of alcohol dependence.

Essential Tremor

The link between alcoholism and this nonpsychiatric disorder is of theoretical interest. Schroeder and Nasrallah (24) demonstrated a high rate of alcoholism in patients with essential tremor. Some such individuals find alcohol's suppression of their endogenous tremor reinforcing, and this may lead to excessive drinking. When treated with β-blockers to eliminate the tremor, a significant proportion of these patients are able to successfully give up alcohol. This association between alcoholism and essential tremor serves as an attractive model of how alcohol dependence may evolve as a consequence of an underlying physiologic defect. This type of link is not nearly as clear in most of the other concomitant disorders.

Panic Disorder

People who suffer from spontaneous panic attacks are prone to paroxysms of anxiety and autonomic arousal. They commonly develop anticipatory anxiety and phobic avoidance, sometimes progressing to frank agoraphobia. Studies indicate that panic disorder is complicated by alcoholism more than would be expected by chance (25). This may be the case because alcohol may block panic attacks and lessen anticipatory anxiety in some cases. Quitkin et al. (26) have examined the effect of imipramine on individuals with panic disorder complicated by alcoholism. This study indicated that such patients treated with imipramine did well and did not have

recurrent alcohol abuse, whereas those not treated with imipramine tended to relapse. Although tricyclic compounds like imipramine and monoamine oxidase inhibitors like phenelzine may be valuable in the treatment of panic disorder complicated by alcoholism, clinicians should avoid using potentially addictive benzodiazepines like clonazepam and alprazolam in patients with these two disorders.

Mood Disorders

Fueled by the hope that treatment of affective illness in an alcoholic might alleviate the individual's alcoholism, much research has focused on determining the relationship between these two disorders. Currently, this link appears to be much more tenuous than it was believed to be in the past. Merikangas et al. (27) have refuted the common assumption that major depression and alcoholism are manifestations of a common underlying disorder. If these two disorders are at all connected, the data suggest that this is so in women but not in men (28). Although many alcoholics manifest symptoms identical to those of a major depression upon admission to treatment programs, the overwhelming majority of these symptoms are alcohol induced and resolve spontaneously within 4 weeks of cessation of drinking. When alcoholism and major depression do coexist, it is clinically most appropriate to render specific treatment for each disorder. In contrast to unipolar depression, patients with bipolar disorder manifest increased alcohol consumption during the manic phase of illness.

Attention Deficit–Hyperactivity Disorder

This disorder, alternatively referred to as minimal brain dysfunction and the hyperactive child syndrome, frequently persists into adulthood. Several studies suggest that adolescents and young adults with residual symptoms of attention deficit–hyperactivity disorder (ADHD) are at increased risk for developing alcohol dependence (29). Theoretically, the pharmacologic treatment of residual type ADHD with psychostimulant medications like pemoline may facilitate the treatment of concomitant alcoholism.

Personality Disorders

There is a well-known association between antisocial personality disorder and alcohol dependence. Although some studies indicate a familial relationship between these two disorders, recent evidence suggests that they are genetically independent (30). Vaillant (15) posits that antisocial personality features are more often a consequence of alcoholism rather than a cause. Recent work on borderline personality disorder and alcoholism delineates a possible association between these two disorders as well (31). Overall, however, there is no clear evidence to suggest that particular personality traits predispose an individual to developing alcoholism.

This brief review of concomitant disorders underscores the heterogeneity of alcoholism and emphasizes certain potential etiologic links to other forms of psychopathology. Future research will elaborate more fully the relationship between alcoholism and other psychiatric disorders.

CLINICAL COURSE

The course of alcohol dependence is best typified by its variability. Individuals may progress from social drinking to problem drinking, alcohol abuse, and alcohol dependence in different ways and at different rates, because of the variety of cultural, biologic, familial, and psychologic factors which interact in each case.

Binge drinking, for example, is a common form of alcoholism. Binge drinkers commonly abstain for weeks at a time, only to periodically imbibe huge quantities of alcohol in a very brief period, often to the point of intoxication. Although binge drinkers may escape some of the deleterious medical effects of chronic, daily alcohol abuse, they often behave impulsively and erratically while drunk. This places

them at particularly high risk for alcohol-induced accidents, suicide, and other forms of violence. In these individuals, it is the consequences of their drinking rather than any particular pattern or quantity of usage that make them alcoholics.

The variability of the course of alcoholism is further illustrated by comparing different alcoholic subpopulations. For example, individuals with a positive family history of alcoholism generally start drinking earlier, progress faster, and develop more severe drinking problems than people with a negative family history. Men and women drink differently as well, as pointed out in a review by Lex (16):

1. Women usually consume less alcohol than men. They are less likely to drink everyday, to drink continuously, or to binge drink. They usually prefer spirits or wine to drinking beer.
2. Women typically begin drinking and develop drinking problems at a later age than men.
3. Compared with men, women tend to progress more quickly to alcoholism, a phenomenon known as "telescoping."
4. Women are more likely than men to attribute the onset of problematic drinking to stressful life situations. These events are often associated with uniquely female experiences such as menses and menopause.

Age of onset of drinking appears to influence subsequent drinking patterns. At least one study indicates that the younger individuals are when they take their first drink, the greater the likelihood that they will subsequently develop alcoholism (32). Many alcoholics vividly recall the circumstances and effects of their first drink. Early onset of heavy drinking frequently predicts the evolution of frank alcohol dependence (33).

So-called normal drinking is usually sporadic and consists of moderate amounts of ethanol. As an alcohol problem typically progresses, sporadic moderate drinking becomes regular, heavy drinking. For instance, a young man who began drinking beer at monthly parties may escalate, in the course of a year, to drinking a six-pack of beer on both Friday and Saturday nights. After some months he may drink a six-pack each weeknight and a case of beer each weekend day. Eventually, his drinking may affect his relationships, family life, and work. Eventually, he may become increasingly tolerant to the effects of alcohol and begin experiencing morning shakes. This may precipitate morning drinking in order to ameliorate the symptoms of alcohol withdrawal. This pattern of drinking may be accompanied by amnestic periods called "blackouts." For example, he may drive while drinking and awaken the next morning, not knowing where he had parked his car.

Physical Dependence

Tolerance and withdrawal are the hallmarks of physiologic dependence on alcohol; they signify an advanced and chronic alcohol problem. Tolerance refers to the need for progressively larger quantities of alcohol to produce its desired effect. Tolerance to alcohol may have a metabolic and pharmacodynamic basis (34). Metabolic tolerance refers to the enhancement of enzymatic degradation of alcohol which occurs with regular consumption. The upper limit of metabolic tolerance occurs quickly, peaking at about 3 weeks. Pharmacodynamic tolerance refers to end-organ adaptation to the effects of alcohol, such that progressively higher alcohol levels are necessary in the brain to produce a given degree of intoxication. This habituation of neurons and other cells to the effects of alcohol proceeds much more slowly than metabolic adaptation of degradatory liver enzymes.

Alcohol Withdrawal Syndrome

The alcohol withdrawal syndrome consists of symptoms of autonomic hyperactivity occurring shortly after a person cuts down or stops drinking (35). The most prominent features of the syndrome are tremulousness, diaphoresis, anxiety, fever, nausea and vomiting, weakness, tachycardia, and unstable blood pressure. Many advanced alcoholics experience symptoms of withdrawal upon awakening, until they imbibe their first drink. Some alcoholics suffer seizures, commonly referred to as "rum fits," during the withdrawal syndrome. A small percentage experience severe autonomic instability and disorientation, a syndrome known as delirium tremens or alcohol withdrawal delirium. The mortality rate of this severe form of alcohol withdrawal approaches 15% (36).

Alcohol-dependent individuals suffer from a host of concomitant vocational, family, legal, psychologic, and medical problems. The medical complications associated with alcoholism are listed in Table 36.3. The idea that persons dependent on alcohol suffer uniform decline in all arenas has not been substantiated. One recent study (37) suggests that a number of dif-

Table 36.3   Medical Complications of Alcoholism

Nervous system
   Amblyopia
   Cerebellar degeneration
   Cerebral atrophy
   Polyneuropathy
   Seizures
   Wernicke-Korsakoff syndrome
Gastrointestinal tract
   Alcoholic hepatitis
   Cirrhosis
   Esophageal carcinoma
   Gastritis
   Hepatocellular carcinoma
   Malabsorption
   Mallory-Weiss syndrome
   Pancreatitis
   Peptic ulcer disease
Endocrine system
   Hypocalcemia
   Hypoglycemia
   Hypogonadism and feminization
Heart
   Arrhythmias
   Cardiomyopathy
Blood
   Anemia
Muscle
   Myopathy
Fetal alcohol syndrome
Malnutrition
Sexual dysfunction

ferent patterns of alcohol-induced problems exist, negating the concept of a general, progressive disease which cannot be treated until those who suffer from it are most symptomatic. Despite the lack of uniformity in alcohol-induced morbidity, a brief survey of the spectrum of problems encountered is instructive.

The effects of an alcohol problem often occur initially at home. The families of alcoholics function poorly (38). Alcoholics experience anxiety, depression, and loss of impulse control due to drinking; these negative affects are transmitted to other family members, upsetting the balance in even the best functioning families. In many cases alcoholism has been associated with frank spouse and child abuse. Children of an alcoholic parent may switch roles with their impaired mother or father and commonly experience feelings of shame, mistrust, anger, embarrassment, and fear which they may adopt in their dealings with people outside the family. It appears that when a parent abuses alcohol during a significant period of a child's formative years, that child may grow up with significant psychological and interpersonal difficulties. Children of alcoholic parents may blame themselves for their parents' drinking. They experience frequent disappointments, even in the absence of physical abuse. For all of these reasons, there is a burgeoning interest in the children of alcoholics at this time.

In its latter stages, alcohol dependence may adversely affect job performance, leading to lowered productivity, absenteeism, and industrial accidents. However, the absence of these complications does not rule out the existence of a serious alcohol problem. In addition to the role alcohol plays in harming people on the roads, at home, and in the workplace, a majority of violent crimes are committed by men under alcohol's influence. Thus, alcohol's adverse consequences range from individual medical problems to major societal hazards.

Detailed delineation of the entire spectrum of alcohol-induced medical problems is beyond the scope of this chapter. Table 36.3 indicates that alcohol's toxic effects damage many of the body's organ systems. Alcohol can cause many types of cognitive impairment, adversely affecting learning, psychomotor skills, and memory. Long term memory impairment appears to be relatively permanent, whereas short-term memory deficits tend to improve over several years of prolonged abstinence (39). As noted above (4), treatment is least effective when an individual has already suffered cognitive impairment. This underscores the importance of early detection and early intervention.

TREATMENT

It is striking how responsive some individuals are to rather modest therapeutic interventions early in the course of alcoholism. In a well-controlled Swedish study (40), a large group of alcoholics were detected by screening with the γ-glutamyl transferase liver function test. The members of the experimental group were encouraged to stop drinking by means of monthly appointments, during which their abnormal blood test was repeated. The control group received a letter mentioning the abnormal blood test and its probable connection to alcohol, with no further intervention. When compared with controls, the experimental group had an 80% reduction in absenteeism at work at 4 years, a 60% lower rate of hospitalization at 5 years, and a 50% lower mortality rate at 6 years.

For individuals with alcohol problems of longer duration and greater severity, simple interventions frequently do not suffice. In assessing such a patient, it is essential to determine if the individual experiences symptoms of alcohol withdrawal when he or she attempts to reduce alcohol consumption. If the person does not have a history of severe withdrawal symptoms, withdrawal seizures, or alcohol withdrawal delirium, then outpatient detoxification may be attempted. Feldman (41) demonstrated the safety and efficacy of outpatient detoxification in a sample of 564 alcoholic patients. Unfortunately, few clinicians or clinics are properly set up to perform this outpatient procedure, and consequently most physiologically dependent alcoholics seeking treatment are hospitalized for detoxification. Sedative–hypnotic compounds with relatively long serum half-lives are the treatment of choice for the alcohol withdrawal syndrome (36); the drug most often prescribed is chlordiazepoxide (see Table 36.4). Oxazepam is frequently used to detoxify alcoholics with hepatic dysfunction.

Physical detoxification can ordinarily be completed in 2 to 5 days. However, unless

Table 36.4   Sample Alcohol Detoxification Protocol[a]

Thiamine 100 mg intramuscularly or orally on admission, then 50 mg orally every day after that.
Folic acid 1 mg orally every day
Multivitamins—1 tablet orally every day

Day 1
Chlordiazepoxide (Librium) 25–100 mg orally every 4 hours as needed for signs and symptoms of withdrawal, to a maximum of 600 mg in 24 hours.
Signs of withdrawal: Elevated pulse
                       Blood pressure elevated when adjusted for age
                       Tremulousness
                       Sweating
                       Restlessness, anxiety, insomnia
                       Nausea and/or vomiting
                       Hyperreflexia
ALL doses of chlordiazepoxide in the first 24 hours are given as needed, rather than regularly scheduled.

Day 2
(After chlordiazepoxide has been given for 24 hours) Give approximately 75% of the total Day 1 dose, in three or four divided doses.

Day 3
Give approximately 50% of the total Day 1 dose, in divided doses.

Day 4
Give approximately 25% of the total Day 1 dose, in divided doses (if possible).

Day 5
Discontinue chlordiazepoxide.

Example
A patient is admitted and receives four 50 mg doses of chlordiazepoxide in a 24-hour period. On Day 2, the patient receives 50 mg orally three times. On Day 3, the patient receives 25 mg orally four times. On Day 4, the patient receives 25 mg orally twice.

---

[a] This sample protocol is for illustration only. In clinical practice, the determination of a specific protocol rests on the assessment of each individual patient.

detoxification is coupled with a rehabilitative treatment program, most recently detoxified alcoholics will resume drinking. The "revolving door alcoholic," an individual who frequents detoxification facilities with alarming regularity, is testimony to the lack of efficacy of detoxification as the sole form of treatment.

Both types of alcoholics, those who experience withdrawal symptoms and those who do not, benefit from alcohol rehabilitation programs which employ a variety of different therapeutic modalities. An ideal program has both outpatient and inpatient treatment options, with the latter being reserved for individuals who have failed the former or who cannot be safely or effectively treated as outpatients.

The many studies which examine the efficacy of alcohol treatment programs concur that patient variables have more bearing on outcome than program variables. In other words, individuals with mild to moderate drinking problems and viable support systems do well in most forms of treatment, whereas those with severe alcohol dependence and poor social supports have generally poor outcomes. One study (42) suggests that programs with medical forms of intervention have better treatment outcome records than those which shun medication and medical assessment.

One methodologic difficulty in assessing the efficacy of alcohol treatment programs is that most studies examine patient and program variables separately. A recent well-designed study (43) look at both sets of variables simultaneously and concluded that patients can be matched to different types of treatment programs on the basis of their degree of psychiatric severity. Such matching steers patients to the type of program best suited to their specific set of alcohol-related problems.

In most current multimodality alcohol rehabilitation programs a type of internal matching exists. This refers to the differential use of multiple treatment modalities in a heterogeneous patient population. In other words, each patient may benefit more from some treatment components than from others. Abstinence is the goal of virtually all rehabilitation programs. Those programs which appear to be most successful are those which offer patients a vast array of efficacious therapies. These include group therapy, participation in Alcoholics Anonymous, family therapy, vocational liaison and medications. In the following paragraphs each of these standard alcohol rehabilitation treatment modalities is described.

Group Therapy

Group meetings form the cornerstone of most alcohol rehabilitation programs. In the early phases of treatment, groups are predominantly educative, focusing on the dissemination of facts about the nature of alcoholism and recovery. Many programs also utilize interactional groups which facilitate the sharing of common experiences, feelings, and coping strategies (44). Many alcoholics are enormously relieved to discover that others have had similar experiences. Groups comprised of individuals at different stages of recovery serve to acquaint new members with the difficulties and benefits associated with abstinence.

Alcoholics Anonymous

Most successful alcohol treatment programs stress involvement with AA—some even require program participants to attend daily meetings. There is no question that hundreds of thousands of recovered alcoholics around the world attribute their recovery to AA. However, it is still uncertain whether affiliation with AA actually promotes recovery or whether the converse is true, and the recovery process itself promotes affiliation with AA. Because of a historical rift between AA and the medical/psychiatry community (which is currently healing), and due to the anonymous nature of the organization, it has been difficult for researchers to study AA. For this reason, a relatively recent review (45) of the research literature suggests that AA's efficacy remains to be proved by the usual scientific research methods. AA appears to appeal particularly to those who possess the capacity to work well in group situations (46).

Despite these qualifying comments, it is clear that AA's firm, pragmatic, hopeful, self-help approach is a useful component in most alcohol treatment programs. Vaillant (47), who prospectively studied a cohort of 110 inner-city men, found abstinence to be associated with involvement in AA, religious groups, and new relationships. In this population, conventional clinic treatment did not predict abstinence.

Family Therapy

Interactional patterns in the families of alcoholics are often pathologic. When treatment is finally initiated, these family difficulties may be quite prominent, with a low likelihood of spontaneous resolution accompanying the cessation of drinking of the alcoholic family member. In such cases, family meetings that attempt to change these disturbed interactional patterns may significantly increase the prospects for recovery (48).

Vocational Liaison

Employee Assistance Programs are sponsored by industry to help workers with alcoholism and other problems, and to make appropriate treatment referrals. When employees are in need of rehabilitation programs, collaboration between the Employee Assistance Program and the rehabilitation facility increases the chances of success. Alcoholics who have a job to return to fare better than those who do not. Programs which provide occupational therapy and rehabilitation are especially effective for individuals who have left the work force because of alcohol-related problems.

Medication

Although the idea of prescribing medications to alcoholics as part of the treatment process is disturbing to those who believe that abstinence from all drugs is necessary, this position is as extreme as the opposite one, whereby a misguided physician substitutes an addictive sedative–hypnotic drug like diazepam (Valium) for alcohol. Medication should not be used to substitute for alcohol, nor should it be categorically excluded from alcohol treatment programs. The medications described below offer clinical benefits when prescribed judiciously for selected groups of patients.

Sedative–Hypnotics

The use of sedative–hypnotics is limited to the management of the alcohol withdrawal syndrome. Because they possess the propensity to lead to physiological dependence, the sedative–hypnotics should not be used in the treatment of anxiety or insomnia in the alcoholic population.

Disulfiram (Antabuse)

Disulfiram blocks the metabolism of acetaldehyde, an intermediate compound in the breakdown of ethanol. Relatively high concentrations of acetaldehyde cause extremely distressing physical symptoms; the avoidance of these symptoms supplies an immediate motivation for abstinence. Although the use of disulfiram alone is not a complete treatment for alcoholism, its efficacy has been demonstrated as one component of a multimodal treatment program (49). Rehabilitation programs which include the prescription of disulfiram as one of many therapeutic tools have better success rates than those which do not.

Heterocyclic Antidepressants

None of the seven controlled studies that have investigated the efficacy of heterocyclics in the treatment of alcoholism have demonstrated any benefit (50). Therefore, their use should be restricted to individuals who meet DSM-III-R criteria for either major depression or panic disorder once they have been free of alcohol and drugs for several weeks or more.

Lithium

In addition to its utility in the management of individuals who suffer from both bipolar disorder and alcohol dependence, lithium may someday also play a more universal role in alcoholism treatment. Judd and Huey (51) demonstrated in a double-blind study that detoxified alcoholics on lithium who were challenged with alcohol experienced less intoxication, a diminished desire to continue drinking, and reduced cognitive dysfunction when compared with a placebo group. Other more recent studies have also documented lithium's therapeutic effects in alcohol treatment (52).

Controlled Drinking

No discussion of alcohol treatment would be complete without addressing the issue of "controlled drinking"—that is, the attempt to train alcoholics to substitute moderate, nonpathological drinking for their previous pattern of excess. Although the notion of controlled drinking gained favor with the original publication of the RAND report in 1976 (53), subsequent studies have refuted the initial conclusion that alcoholics could learn to safely drink in a controlled fashion. Recently, Helzer et al. (54) published impressive evidence that alcoholics are not able to modify their drinking patterns and learn to drink in moderation. Thus, abstinence continues to be the goal of alcoholism treatment.

Outcome Assessment

Because of extensive differences in diagnostic criteria, dropout rates, treatment methods, follow-up periods, and definitions of successful outcome, treatment outcome studies have reported success rates ranging from 10 to 90%. In his survey on the evaluation of treatment methods in chronic alcoholism, Baekland (55) reviewed 30 outcome studies with an average follow-up of 2.2 years. In correcting for both dropout rates and spontaneous remissions, he established that the overall improvement rate across these many studies was approximately 30%. Saxe et al. (56) have demonstrated that the overall benefits of alcoholism treatment far outweigh the costs (56). And McLellan et al. (43) have demonstrated that individuals with moderately severe problems have better outcomes when treated on an intensive inpatient basis than when they are treated in outpatient treatment programs. However, if clinicians follow the strategy of early identification and aggressive treatment of alcoholism as described throughout this chapter, the heavy toll imposed by alcoholism can be reduced significantly, often with outpatient intervention and management alone. In the concluding section of this chapter, we describe our clinical approach to alcoholic outpatients.

THE CLINICAL INTERVIEW

Determining the Nature of the Problem

Alcoholism is psychiatry's great masquerader. Individuals with primary alcoholism may present to the psychiatrist appearing depressed, anxious, psychotic, or confused; their chief complaints may suggest marital problems, vocational difficulties, or characterologic issues. Since so many alcoholics either fail to appreciate or do not wish to discuss the relationship between their emotional difficulties and drinking, it is incumbent upon the psychiatrist to inquire directly about a person's pattern of drinking and its consequences in every initial psychiatric interview. Multiple psychiatric diagnoses, always including the possibility of substance abuse, should be considered in every comprehensive psychiatric assessment.

In determining the scope of a patient's alcohol problem, it is useful to focus on the adverse consequences of his or her drinking. Has alcohol contributed to any medical problems? To any legal, marital, financial, or occupational difficulties? Has drinking resulted in changes in the person's sleep pattern, sexual performance, social life, or sense of well-being? While

focusing on how alcohol has hurt the patient, the clinician should be careful to proceed in a matter-of-fact, nonjudgmental fashion. This initial approach facilitates the establishment of a therapeutic alliance in which patient and clinician work together to help the patient eliminate the problems caused by alcohol.

Developing and Maintaining a Therapeutic Relationship

Developing a therapeutic relationship with an alcoholic is easiest when the patient acknowledges the existence of an alcohol problem and accepts abstinence as the goal of treatment. However, in the outpatient setting a large number of alcoholic patients initially deny the seriousness of their drinking problem and do not readily accept abstinence as a treatment goal. In the majority of cases, this denial is partial rather than complete. In order to develop a therapeutic relationship with the alcoholic patient, then, the clinician's primary task is to ally him- or herself with that part of the patient which realizes that alcohol is adversely affecting him or her.

It is important to avoid creating an adversarial relationship in which the clinician authoritatively tells the patient, "You're an alcoholic," and the patient defensively counters, "No I'm not." Terms such as "drunk" and "alcoholic" with pejorative connotations should be avoided in the initial stages. Clinicians should freely acknowledge that they and the patient need not agree on everything in order to work together. At the same time, the clinician's focus in the initial sessions should be educative, focusing on the adverse effects that drinking has had on the patient. "Let's look at what drinking alcohol is doing to you," is a useful approach. While focusing on drinking, its consequences, and abstinence as the most effective solution, the clinician can take time to get to know the patient's life story. Rapport developed around neutral topics may help in addressing the more difficult ones.

In this initial negotiating period, which is typically characterized by an attempt by the clinician and patient to reach a mutually acceptable definition of the problem and a reasonable plan for attacking it together, stalemates are frequently reached. In such cases the clinician may recommend bringing a close relative or friend in order to lend a different perspective on the problem. Another alternative is to enlist the services of a consultant. In these cases, the developing therapeutic alliance is frequently strengthened by the clinician's timely suggestion to involve others in the evaluation process.

Communicating Information and Implementing a Treatment Plan

Individuals with drinking problems usually respond well to clinicians who communicate in an open, clear, and straightforward manner. Although "telling patients what to do" is a technique which may run counter to some of the goals and methods of traditional psychodynamic psychotherapy, many alcoholic patients whose lives are fragmented and disorganized require the structure and direction provided by a clinician who is able to play an active role in guiding the way toward recovery.

With the clinician providing as much guidance as necessary to set the recovery process in motion, it is essential that the patient and doctor collaborate in fashioning a treatment plan aimed at curtailing the patient's drinking. Ideally, patients actively contribute to the plan themselves; their ideas may be elicited by asking questions such as "What do you think you need to do in order to stop drinking?" If patients are initially unwilling to commit themselves to a very extensive treatment program, the clinician may counter by saying, "We can go ahead and try it your way. But if we find that you start drinking again, then I'd like you to add the following [e.g., disulfiram, more AA meetings]." By adding further treatment supports as needed, the treatment needs of each individual patient may be met. When outpatient treatment strategies have been nearly exhausted, it is wise to lay the groundwork

for hospitalization as a step to take when other measures have failed.

It is important to help alcoholic patients realize that the treatment process works best if they are open and honest with their physician about their drinking. Rather than responding to "slips" punitively or judgmentally, one should take them as an indication that the current treatment strategy needs to be reexamined and possibly amended. For patients who are engaged with multiple treatment providers (e.g., a psychiatrist, alcohol counselor, and group leader), it is important that the different treatment providers communicate freely with one another and, as much as possible, present a united front to the patient. Splitting benefits no one.

Once an alcoholic patient has been abstinent for several weeks and the treatment program appears to be working, patient and physician may together discuss the possibility of widening the focus of treatment. In this way a treatment which begins as an effort to curtail dysfunctional drinking may lead into psychotherapy to examine a disturbed pattern of relationships, or into a medication trial for cyclothymic mood swings. Even after the focus of treatment shifts away from drinking, the clinician should make it clear that the patient's ongoing sobriety is essential to the success of his or her psychiatric treatment.

The approach to treating alcoholism presented in this chapter can be mutually gratifying to patients and psychiatrists alike. When identified early, and addressed directly and sympathetically by a caring clinician, alcoholism is a very treatable disorder. The remarkable gains made by successfully treated alcoholic patients are among the most dramatic in all of medicine.

References

1. Secretary, Department of Health, Education and Welfare: *Third Special Report to the U.S. Congress,* Washington, DC, U.S. Government Printing Office, 1978.
2. Barchas JD, Elliott GR, Berger PA, et al: Research on mental illness and addictive disorders:

progress and prospects. *Am J Psychiatry* 142:8–41, 1985.

3. Eckardt MJ, Hartford TC, Kaelber CT, et al: Health hazards associated with alcohol consumption. *JAMA* 246:648–666, 1981.

4. Gregson RAM, Taylor GM: Prediction of relapse in male alcoholics. *J Stud Alcohol* 38:1749–1760, 1977.

5. Paredes, A: The history of the concept of alcoholism. In Tarter RE, Sugerman AA (eds): *Alcoholism: Interdisciplinary Approaches to An Enduring Problem*. Reading, MA, Addison-Wesley, 1978, pp. 9–52.

6. Rounsaville BJ, Spitzer RL, Williams JBW. Proposed changes in DSM-III substance use disorders: description and rationale. *Am J Psychiatry* 143:463–468, 1985.

7. Selzer ML: The Michigan Alcoholism Screening Test (MAST): the quest for a new diagnostic instrument. *Am J Psychiatry* 3:176–181, 1971.

8. Gibbs LE: The validity and reliability of the Michigan alcoholism screening test: a review. *Drug Alcohol Depend* 12:279–285, 1983.

9. Ewing J, Mayfield D: CAGE. *Am J Psychiatry* 131:1121–1122, 1974.

10. Boyd JH, Weissman MM, Thompson WD, et al: Different definitions of alcoholism. I: Impact of seven definitions on prevalence rates in community survey. *Am J Psychiatry* 140:1309–1313, 1983.

11. Myers JK, Weissman MM, Tischler GL, et al: Six-month prevalence of psychiatric disorders in three communities. *Arch Gen Psychiatry* 41:959–967, 1984.

12. Robins LN, Helzer JE, Weissman MM, et al: Lifetime prevalence of specific psychiatric disorders in three sites. *Arch Gen Psychiatry* 41:949–958, 1984.

13. Frances RJ, Timm S, Bucky S: Studies of familial and non-familial alcoholism. *Arch Gen Psychiatry* 37:564–566, 1980.

14. Mello NK: The role of aversive consequences in the control of alcohol and drug self-administration. In Meyer RE (ed): *Evaluation of the Alcoholic: Implications for Research Theory, and Treatment*. Washington, DC, National Institute of Alcohol Abuse and Alcoholism, 1981.

15. Vaillant GE: Natural history of alcoholism V: Is alcoholism the cart or the horse to sociopathy? *Br J Addict* 78:317–326, 1983.

16. Lex BW: Alcohol problems in special populations. In Mendelson JH, Mello NK (eds): *The Diagnosis and Treatment of Alcoholism*. New York, McGraw Hill, 1985, pp 89–187.

17. Goodwin DW: Alcoholism and genetics. *Arch Gen Psychiatry* 42:171–174, 1985.

18. Bohman M, Sigvardsson S, Cloninger CR: Maternal inheritance of alcohol abuse. *Arch Gen Psychiatry* 38:965–969, 1981.

19. Cloninger CR, Bohman M, Sigvardssons: Inheritance of alcohol abuse. *Arch Gen Psychiatry* 38:861–868, 1981.

20. Pollock VE, Volarka J, Goodwin DW: The EEG after alcohol administration in men at risk for alcoholism. *Arch Gen Psychiatry* 40:857–861, 1983.

21. Schuckit MA: Subjective responses to ethanol in sons of alcoholics and control subjects. *Arch Gen Psychiatry* 41:879–884, 1984.

22. Schuckit MA: Ethanol induced changes in body sway in men at high risk for alcoholism. *Arch Gen Psychiatry* 42:375–379, 1985.

23. Zinberg NE: Social interactions, drug use, and drug research. In Lowinson JH, Ruiz PR (eds): *Substance Abuse: Clinical Problems and Perspectives*. Williams & Wilkins, Baltimore, 1981, pp 91–108.

24. Schroeder D, Nasrallah HA: High alcoholism rate in patients with essential tremor. *Am J Psychiatry* 139:1471–1743, 1982.

25. Quitkin FM, Rubkin JG: Hidden psychiatric diagnoses in the alcoholic. In Solomon J (ed): *Alcoholism and Clinical Psychiatry*. New York, Plenum, 1982, pp 129–140.

26. Quitkin FM, Rifkin A, Kaplan J, et al: Phobic anxiety syndrome complicated by drug dependence and addiction. *Am Geo Psychiatry* 27:159–162, 1972.

27. Merikangas KR, Leckman JF, Prusoff BA, et al: Familial transmission of depression and alcoholism. *Arch Gen Psychiatry* 42:367–372, 1985.

28. Schuckit MA, Winokur G: A short-term follow-up of female alcoholics. *Dis Nerv Syst* 33:672–678, 1972.

29. Goodwin DW, Schulsin F, Hermansen L, et al: Alcoholism and the hyperactive child syndrome. *J Nerv Ment Dis* 160;349–353, 1975.

30. Cloninger CR, Vonknerring AL, Sigvardsson S, et al: Gene–environment interaction in the familial relationship of alcoholism, depression, and antisocial personality. In Edwards G, Littleton J (eds): *Pharmacological Treatments for Alcoholism*. London, Croom Helm, 1983, pp 417–444.

31. Loranzer AW, Tulis EH: Family history of alcoholism in borderline personality disorder. *Arch Gen Psychiatry* 42:153–157, 1985.

32. Schuckit MA, Russell JW: Clinical importance of age at first drink in a group of young men. *Am J Psychiatry* 140:1221–1223, 1984.

33. Goodwin DW: Genetic factors in alcoholism: In Mello NK (ed): *Advances in Substance Abuse*. Greenwich, CT, JAI Press, 1980, Vol 1, pp 305–326.

34. Mirin SM, Weiss RD: Substance abuse. In Bassuk EC, Schoonover SC, Gelenberg AS (eds): *The Practitioner's Guide to Psychoactive Drugs*. New York, Plenum, 1983, pp 221–292.

35. Sellers EM, Kalant H: Alcohol intoxication and withdrawal. *N Engl J Med* 794:757–762, 1976.

36. Thompson WL: Management of alcohol withdrawal syndromes. *Arch Intern Med* 138:278–283, 1978.

37. McLellan AT, Luborsky L, Woody GE, et al: Are the "addiction-related" problems of substance abusers really related? *J Nerv Ment Dis* 169:232–239, 1981.

38. Moos RH, Moos BS: The process of recovery from alcoholism: III. Comparing functioning in fami-

lies of alcoholics and matched control families. *J Stud Alcohol* 45:111–118, 1984.

39. Brandt J, Butlers N, Ryan C, et al: Cognitive loss and recovery in long-term alcohol abusers. *Arch Gen Psychiatry* 40:435–442, 1983.

40. Kristenson H, Ohlin H, Hulten-Nosslin MJ, et al: Identification and intervention of heavy drinking in middle-aged men: results and follow-up of 24–60 months of long-term study with randomized controls. *Alcoholism: Clin Exp Res* 7:203–209, 1983.

41. Feldman DJ, Pattison EM, Sebell LC, et al: Outpatient alcohol detoxification: initial findings on 564 patients. *Am J Psychiatry* 132:407–412, 1973.

42. Smart RG: Multiple predictors of dropout from alcoholism treatment. *Arch Gen Psychiatry* 35:363–367, 1978.

43. McLellan TA, Luborsky L, Woody GE, et al: Predicting response to alcohol and drug abuse treatments: role of psychiatric severity. *Arch Gen Psychiatry* 40:620–625, 1983.

44. Yalom ID, Bloch S, Bond G, et al: Alcoholics in interactional group therapy: an outcome study. *Arch Gen Psychiatry* 35:419–425, 1978.

45. Glaser FB, Osborne AC: Does AA really work? *Br J Addict* 77:123–129, 1982.

46. Patterson EM (ed): *Selection of Treatment for Alcoholics*. New Brunswick, NJ, Rutgers Center of Alcohol Studies, 1982.

47. Valliant GE, Milofsky ES: Natural history of male alcoholism IV. Paths to recovery. *Arch Gen Psychiatry* 39:127–133, 1982.

48. Kauffman E, Kaufmann P: Multiple family therapy: a new direction in the treatment of drug abusers. *Am J Drug Alcohol Abusers* 4:467–478, 1977.

49. Fuller RK, Roth HP: Disulfiram for the treatment of alcoholism. *Ann Intern Med* 90:901–904, 1974.

50. Goodwin DW: Alcoholism and affective disorders—the basic questions. In Solomon J (ed): *Alcoholism and Clinical Psychiatry*. New York, Plenum, 1982, pp 87–95.

51. Judd LL, Huey LY: Lithium antagonizes ethanol intoxication in alcoholics. *Am J Psychiatry* 141:1517–1521, 1984.

52. Fawcett J, Clark DC, Aagesen CA, et al: A double-blind, placebo-controlled trial of lithium carbonate therapy for alcoholism. *Arch Gen Psychiatry* 44:248–256, 1987.

53. Polich JM, Armor DJ, Braiker HB: *The Course of Alcoholism: Four Years After Treatment* (R-2433-NIAAA). Santa Monica, CA, Rand Corporation, 1980.

54. Helzer JE, Robbins LN, Taylor JR, et al: The extent of long-term moderate drinking among alcoholics discharged from medical and psychiatric treatment facilities. *N Engl J Med* 312:1678–1682, 1985.

55. Baekeland F: Evaluation of treatment methods in chronic alcoholism. In Kissin B, Begleiter H (eds): *The Biology of Alcoholism*. New York, Plenum, 1977, pp 385–440.

56. Saxe L, Dougherty D, Esty K: The effectiveness and cost of alcoholism treatment: a public policy perspective. In Mendelson JH, Mello NK (eds): *The Diagnosis and Treatment of Alcoholism*. New York, McGraw Hill, 1985, pp 485–540.

37

Psychoactive Substance Use Disorders: Drug Abuse

Thomas R. Kosten, M.D.
Herbert D. Kleber, M.D.

After psychiatry residents complete a rotation in our substance abuse treatment unit, they consistently report uncovering substance abuse among a large percentage of their "regular" psychiatric patients. Covert substance abuse is a major issue among general psychiatric patients and much is being made of the "dually diagnosed" psychiatric patient. These dually diagnosed patients have substance abuse along with another major psychiatric disorder such as schizophrenia or major affective disorder. This concurrence of disorders has been repeatedly demonstrated by inpatient studies of general psychiatric patients, by systematic evaluations of outpatients, and by surveys of general populations such as the Epidemiological Catchment Area (ECA) study (1–3). In one of the earlier inpatient studies, 28% of 50 consecutive admissions were found to have illicit drug use on laboratory urine testing, although drug abuse was not an admitting diagnosis (1). In an outpatient setting, a similar survey of 195 general psychiatric outpatients based on urine toxicology found that 13% were covert drug abusers (2). More importantly in that outpatient study, drug abuse was a major factor distorting the accuracy of diagnosis,

and treatment was significantly less likely to help these covert drug abusers than non-abusers. The major misdiagnoses were that covert drug abusers were labeled either schizophrenic or depressed, when on careful structured interview they did not meet the criteria for these disorders. Poor treatment outcomes among the covert drug abusers were due to a six-times higher premature termination rate and a substantially higher rate of prescribed (as well as illicit) medications (an average of 3.8 different prescribed medications per patient for the covert drug abusers). Finally, in the recently completed ECA population survey, substance abuse was the most commonly diagnosed disorder (13 to 18% at various sites) (3). Thus, substance abuse is common and needs specific attention during psychiatric evaluation in order to provide proper diagnosis and effective treatment.

The first step in understanding drug abuse and its treatment is clear definition of the problem. Because "drug abuse" is one of the most value-laden terms in medicine, many writers have urged that it not be used. However, the World Health Organization (WHO) has developed several definitions, as follows (4). *Drug abuse* has been defined by the WHO as the taking of any psychoactive substance in any quantity not under medical auspices and/or not for a medical purpose. The concept of abuse lies in the *intention* of the user. Thus, a person who takes an amphetamine under a physician's direction to help lose weight is a drug user, but if the person takes the drug to promote a "speeding" feeling rather than weight loss, he or she is a drug abuser. By this definition, any use of an illegal drug such as heroin equals abuse. In this chapter, we shall use a somewhat more restrictive or medical definition of drug abuse. According to this definition, the nonprescriptive use of psychoactive chemicals to alter psychologic state, must also lead to some *harm* to the person, others, or society. Occasional use with no harm incurred would not be considered drug abuse, although it might meet a legal definition of drug abuse.

Another important term is *drug dependence*, since the "dependence syndrome" is now the basis for the *Diagnostic and Statistical Manual of Mental Disorders (Third Edition-Revised)* (DSM-III-R) criteria in this area. Drug dependence is defined by the WHO as

a state, psychic and sometimes also physical, resulting from the interaction between a living organism and a drug, characterized by behavioral and other responses that always include a compulsion to take the drug on a continuous or periodic basis in order to experience its psychic effects and sometimes to avoid the discomfort of its absence. Tolerance may or may not be present. A person may be dependent on more than one drug.

The characteristics of the dependent state vary with each class of drugs. The term "drug dependence" has now replaced the earlier terms, *addiction* and *habituation*, because these older terms had acquired too many negative connotations.

Two types of dependence are included in the definition: psychic and physical. *Psychic* or *psychologic dependence* is a state in which a drug produces "a feeling of satisfaction and a psychic drive that requires periodic or continuous administration of the drug to produce pleasure or to avoid discomfort." *Physical dependence* is a condition that "manifests itself by intense physical disturbances when the administration of the drug is suspended. . . . these disturbances, i.e., the withdrawal or abstinence syndromes, are made up of specific arrays of symptoms and signs of a psychic and physical nature characteristic of each drug type."

THEORIES OF ETIOLOGY

Theories about the etiology of drug abuse abound. While at times the theories are complementary to each other, they are often contradictory and leave unclear the best course of action to follow for treatment or prevention. Several etiologic theories shall be discussed. Kleber offers a more extensive review (5).

Availability

In one sense availability can be viewed as the primary cause of drug abuse since without access to suitable drugs, there can be no drug abuse. (Of course, it has been noted that where drugs are not available, individuals may resort to other means of altering consciousness, such as sensory deprivation, self-flagellation, or fasting.) The high incidence of drug abuse in certain populations (e.g., inner-city areas or among medical personnel) emphasizes the importance of availability to explain individual drug abuse, while sudden easy access to drugs (as with amphetamines in Japan after World War II) is an explanatory concept for epidemics of drug abuse.

Psychologic Deficit

After availability, the most common theory of the cause of drug abuse relates to psychologic problems in the user. Personality disturbances, especially in the handling of aggressive or sexual impulses or conflicts around dependency strivings, are frequently seen in individuals with drug problems. Depression is quite common, and much illicit drug use may represent an attempt at self-medication. Some personality types described among drug abusers include alienated, aggressive, psychopathic, emotionally unstable, immature, hedonistic, cyclothymic, narcissistic, and passive–aggressive. Epidemics are explained, according to this view, by postulating the existence in the population of many disturbed individuals who have access to an increased availability of a particular drug. It is, of course, often unclear whether a certain psychological picture preceded or followed the drug use.

Pharmacologic Disturbance

Early in this century narcotic addiction was seen by some medical personnel as due to autotoxins. About 50 years later the concept of metabolic deficiency was popularized by the founders of the methadone maintenance approach to treatment and, most recently, by the discovery of opiate receptor sites and the endogenous opiate-like substances (endorphins and enkephalins) in the brain. Receptor sites have also been found for nicotine and diazepam, two other substances that are widely used in our society. Like the psychologic theories, however, it is unclear whether drug abuse is a cause or result of the metabolic disturbance.

Socioeconomic Factors

Certain kinds of drug use are much more common in ghetto areas—regardless of which minority group predominates in the ghetto at the time. This ideas has focused attention on the role of poverty and its frequent concomitant, hopelessness, in the etiology of drug problems. Epidemics may be explained by noting that the drug use in these areas is usually very high, but ignored by society in general until something happens to bring it to their attention, at which point it is labeled an epidemic. The "something" may be crime spilling out of the ghetto into the affluent suburbs or drug use occurring in middle-class youngsters.

Social Factors

To find a single explanation for drug use by a group of individuals so diverse as to include the housewife using tranquilizers, ghetto residents using heroin, and middle-class adolescents using psychedelics, some theorists have invoked the evils of American society. Issues such as economic inequality (or capitalism per se), materialism, sexism, racism, the Vietnam War and its aftermath, and governmental hypocrisy and mendacity have all been put forward as causing drug abuse. These social evils are seen as providing a breeding ground for disturbed individuals who then use drugs to cope with or escape from the disturbing environment. Difficulty with this theory arises from the existence of drug abuse of various kinds in every society where abusable substances exist, regardless of the social or economic structure of the country. Socialist Sweden has major problems with amphetamine abuse, while communist Russia has an alcohol problem.

Biopsychosocial Model

An integration of these various etiologic theories is an important conceptual task for the clinician, and even then the exact combination of factors will vary among patients seeking treatment. The clinician needs a broad view of etiology for each patient and should consider all these areas when developing a formulation. No single theory is likely to fit the individual patient, but attempting to develop a comprehensive picture of the biologic, psychologic, and social aspects of etiology in a patient will ensure that major gaps in treatment planning do not occur. We shall return to this at the end of the chapter in the section on the clinical interview.

THE DIAGNOSIS OF SUBSTANCE USE DISORDERS

In the DSM-III-R, the diagnosis of substance use disorders has been substantially modified and now is based on a more coherent model of addiction. This model, which has been called the dependence syndrome, was originally developed for alcoholism by Edwards and Gross (6). It includes six major elements that together form a measure of severity of drug dependence: (*a*) salience of substance-taking behavior such that despite negative consequences substance abuse is given higher priority than other activities which had previously been important, (*b*) increased tolerance with repeated drug use, (*c*) withdrawal symptoms after discontinuing use, (*d*) substance use to avoid withdrawal, (*e*) subjectively experienced compulsion to use the drug, and (*f*) readdiction liability. These six elements have been operationalized into nine criteria for DSM-III-R, as shown in Table 37.1. In order to meet the diagnosis for drug dependence, a patient must have at least three of these criteria for at least a month. Furthermore, a patient having a greater number of these criteria (e.g., four to nine) is considered to have more severe drug dependence.

These new criteria include four changes from DSM-III. First, the format of the criteria has been changed to a diagnostic index in which no single symptom is required for a diagnosis of psychoactive substance dependence. Second, the same set of criteria applies to all substances. Third, the criteria for dependence has been broadened to include cognitive and behavioral symptoms. Fourth, a system has been provided for denoting severity of dependence as "in remission," "mild," "moderate," and "severe." These changes address some key criticisms of the DSM-III, including too great an emphasis on tolerance as a criterion and basing diagnoses on social consequences of a disorder. In the DSM-III-R, social consequences are not a part of the criteria, and in fact the dependence syndrome postulates that social consequences are independent of severity of drug dependence. While complete independence is unlikely to occur in the real world, some patients may be protected from social consequences, and other psychiatrically impaired patients such as schizophrenics may have severe social disruption with minimal substance abuse. Severe drug abusers in need of intensive drug abuse treatment may not experience severe social consequences, because of protection by family or social position. This recognition of independence will improve our ability to classify and plan treatment for all substance abusers.

As a first step in treatment planning, the clinician needs to recognize a variety of specific drug abuse syndromes; we shall now review them.

SPECIFIC DRUG SYNDROMES

Narcotics

For more detailed description of the signs and symptoms related to drug intoxication, withdrawal, and overdose, the reader is referred to Inaba et cl. (7).

Intoxication

Narcotics such as heroin, morphine, meperidene, codeine, and methadone are usually taken by injection—either subcutaneous, intramuscular, or intravenously. Nicknames for narcotics include "horse," "scag," "junk," and "Blue Thunder." The signs and symptoms of intoxication from narcotics are as follows.

Symptoms of Intoxication

The symptoms of intoxication are euphoria, drowsiness (an addict may be "on the nod," i.e., the head falls to the chest and then snaps back up as the user tries to stay awake and enjoy the high rather than sleep), and scratching (usually a slow sensual scratching).

Signs of Intoxication

The signs of intoxication are decreased respiratory rate and depth, decreased blood pressure and pulse, and miosis (contracted or pinpoint pupils). Although the effects of the drug may last a number of hours, often the only sign visible after the first 30 to 60 minutes is pinpoint pupils. Except for contracted pupils, the narcotic addict may talk and act in a seemingly normal fashion.

Table 37.1   Relationship of DSM-III-R Substance Dependence Criteria to World Health Organization (WHO) Drug Dependence Syndrome Elements

DSM-III-R Criteria	WHO Dependence Syndrome Elements
1a. Often intoxicated or impaired by substance use when expected to fulfill social or occupational obligations or when substance use is a hazard. (e.g., goes to work high, drives while drunk).	Salience
1b. Has given up some important social, occupational, or recreational activity in order to seek or take the substance.	Salience
1c. Continuation of substance use despite a physical or mental disorder or a significant social or legal problem that the individual knows is exacerbated by the use of the substance.	Salience
2. Tolerance: Need for increased amounts of substance in order to achieve intoxication or desired effect, or diminished effect with continued use of same amount.	Tolerance
3. Withdrawal: Substance specific syndrome following cessation or reduction of intake of substance.	Withdrawal
4. Often uses a psychoactive substance to relieve or symptoms (e.g., takes a drink or diazepam to relieve morning shakes).	Withdrawal avoidance
5a. Frequent preoccupation with seeking or taking the substance.	Compulsion
5b. Often takes the substance in larger doses or over a period than he or she intended.	Compulsion
6a. Repeated effort or persistent desire to cut down or control substance use.	Readdiction liability
6b. Reinstatement of excessive substance use after a period of abstinence is much more rapid than initial development (Dropped from final DSM-III-R.)	Readdiction liability

Overdose

While there is some controversy over whether the usual picture of heroin overdose is actually due to an excessive amount of heroin or to an acute hypersensitivity or allergic reaction, there is no question that the condition is an extremely serious one with a possibly fatal outcome. Overdose can occur so swiftly that the addict may be found with the needle still in the vein. More often, the patient is brought to the emergency room in a comatose state with pinpoint pupils; pale, cool damp skin with a cyanotic hue; severe respiratory depression ranging from apnea to a few shallow gasping breaths per minute; and arreflexia. Frothy pink-tinged sputum indicative of pulmonary edema may be noted. Pinpoint pupils may not be present because of either anoxia or the concurrent use of other drugs such as atropine or glutethimide. Pinpoint pupils, on the other hand, may be the result of nonnarcotic drugs such as pilocarpine or of farsightedness.

Withdrawal

The appearance of the first signs and symptoms of narcotic withdrawal, their peak, and their remission depend on the duration of action of the drug. Thus, signs and symptoms of heroin or morphine withdrawal begin approximately 12 hours after the last dose, peak at 36 to 72 hours, and disappear for the most part by the fifth day. With methadone, withdrawal begins at 24 to 48 hours and peaks at 96 to 120 hours; symptoms may still be evident as long as 3 weeks. In general, with addiction to equivalent doses, the withdrawal of longer acting narcotics are less intense but last longer.

A common classification of narcotic withdrawal signs and symptoms is described using a grade system to express increasing severity:

Grade 0—Craving for drugs; anxiety; drug-seeking behavior.

Grade 1—Yawning; perspiration; lacrimation; rhinorrhea; "yen" (light, restless, broken sleep); irritability.

Grade 2—Mydriasis with progressive decreased reaction to light; at peak of withdrawal, pupils are dilated and unreactive to light. Muscular twitches (hence the term "kicking" the habit); piloerection or "gooseflesh" (hence the term "cold turkey"); hot and cold flashes; abdominal cramps; aching joints and muscles; anorexia; chills; and lack of energy.

Grade 3—Insomnia, low-grade fever, increased respiratory rate and depth, increased pulse rate and increased blood pressure, nausea, vomiting, diarrhea, and weight loss.

The grades outlined are arbitrarily selected, and not all signs are necessary to diagnose each grade. The signs will sometimes overlap between the grades, and individuals differ as to which signs and symptoms they display. There is a tendency for individuals to manifest similar signs and symptoms each time they withdraw. Thus, one individual will have predominant gastrointestinal symptoms, while another will be bothered by musculoskeletal problems.

Convulsions are not characteristic of opiate withdrawal or intoxication with the exception of meperidene intoxication. If a patient has a seizure, therefore, it usually signifies undiagnosed barbiturate–sedative withdrawal, another medical condition such as epilepsy, hysteria, or a faked convulsion in an attempt to obtain drugs. Since mixed addiction is quite common, the possibility of abuse of barbiturate-type drugs should always be kept in mind when dealing with any narcotic addict.

Even after most withdrawal signs and symptoms have passed, aching muscles, irritability, insomnia, and lack of energy may persist for weeks. A "protracted abstinence syndrome" has been described in which as late as months after the last dose, some subclinical signs of withdrawal can still be found.

Sedatives

Sedatives, such as barbiturates, glutethimide, and methaqualone, and minor tranquilizers such as diazepam are usually taken orally or by injection. Since there is a tendency for these drugs to scar the veins, intravenous injection is usually replaced by intramuscular use in regular users. Some nicknames for sedatives are "ludes," "downers," and "reds."

Intoxication

Signs of progressive barbiturate intoxication include depression of superficial skin reflexes, horizontal nystagmus (first present only on extreme lateral gaze but as intoxication deepens, it will eventually be found on forward gaze), decreased alertness, ataxia, slurred speech, positive Romberg sign, and excitement followed by depression and drowsiness.

Overdose

The signs of sedative–hypnotic overdose include the signs of intoxication described above accompanied by thick speech, marked ataxia with falling, confusion, sleep with difficulty in arousing, semicoma with constricted pupils, marked respiratory depression, and shock with dilated pupils. Overdose of sedatives can lead to death, if untreated.

Withdrawal

Unlike narcotic withdrawal, which can be painful but is not medically serious, except in the presence of complicating physical illness, sedative withdrawal has a significant fatality rate if untreated. Because of this, it is important to have a high index of suspicion, especially if any of the following features are present.

1. Present or past history of excessive use of any of the drugs in the sedative–barbiturate hypnotic class.
2. Present or past history of excessive use of alcohol.
3. Signs of barbiturate withdrawal.
4. History of recent seizure.
5. Patient is a physician.
6. Multiple drug use.
7. Complaint of chronic insomnia.

Minor signs and symptoms of sedative withdrawal appear within 24 hours and last 3 to 14 days. They are anorexia, anxiety, insomnia, muscular weakness, nausea, orthostatic hypotension, tremors of upper extremities, and twitching movements. The major signs and symptoms appear within 48 to 72 hours and may last 3 to 14 days. They are confusion, convulsions (usually grand mal type seizures, which may be single or status epilepticus), delirium (includes disorientation, delusions, visual hallucinations), formication, hyperthermia (fever as high as 105 to 106° F is possible), and paranoid ideation. Convulsions usually do not occur before 16 hours of withdrawal and psychotic behavior usually not before 36 hours. If these symptoms become severe, they may not be reversed simply by giving barbiturates, but may follow the pattern of many toxic psychoses in which death may occur.

It is important to keep in mind that diazepam withdrawal may not occur until 3 to 5 days after abrupt discontinuation. The symptoms of mild withdrawal—irritability, anxiety, trouble with sleeping—may be confused with the initial reasons for which the patient took the drug. This may lead both patient and doctor to believe that the drug needs to be restarted. These mild withdrawal symptoms may occur at relatively low-dosage levels, for example, 40 to 60 mg per day, while the more serious conditions of seizure and delirium usually do not occur below doses of 80 to 100 mg per day.

Stimulants and Cocaine

Stimulants, such as dextroamphetamine, methamphetamine, methylphenidate and cocaine, are usually taken by inhaling, intramuscular or intravenous injection, or ingestion. Cocaine or "crack" is increasingly used by freebase smoking. Some nicknames are "uppers, "speed," and "black beauties."

Intoxication

Low doses of stimulants produce elevated mood with mild euphoria, increased alertness and self-confidence, increased concentration, decreased appetite, talkativeness, decreased awareness of fatigue (sometimes with enhanced performance) increased pulse and blood pressure, and increased respiration.

High doses can produce irritability, restlessness, insomnia, tremors, hyperreflexia, palpitations, paranoid ideation with or without confusion, dry mouth with frequent licking of lips and cheilosis, cardiac arrhythmias, and dilated but reactive pupils. Chronic high doses may lead to the symptoms just listed, along with a paranoid or toxic psychosis that may be very difficult to distinguish from paranoid schizophrenia. Visual and tactile hallucinations may occur as well as auditory ones. The combination of paranoia with physical hyperactivity may lead to the occurrence of violent behavior. Chronic stimulant use may also be associated with compulsive behavior in which the individual engages in an activity for hours at a time. These range from simple acts like tying and untying shoelaces to complex ones like taking apart and putting together alarm clocks. Chronic inhalation of cocaine may lead to necrosis of the nasal septum and eventually perforation. Other physical side effects of chronic stimulant abuse may include necrotizing angiitis and cerebral vascular damage.

Overdose

Overdose of stimulants includes the signs of high-dose intoxication along with hyperthermic convulsions, circulatory collapse, and cerebral hemorrhage. Coma may occur, and death can quickly follow.

Withdrawal

Until recently it was believed that stimulants were not physically addicting and that there was no true withdrawal syndrome. It is now felt that there is some degree of physical dependence. Typically when the chronic abuser abruptly stops, there is a period of profound fatigue that may manifest itself in sleeping for 24 hours or more. Upon awakening, the individual is still fatigued and, in addition, may be quite depressed. The severity of depression may be such that suicide is a possibility and withdrawing patients must be watched for this. The worst fatigue and depression is over within a week, but may persist for months at a lower level.

With severe cocaine abusers, use tends to occur in episodic prolonged binges that last up to several days. Immediately following discontinuation, irritability and anxiety called a "crash" begin and last for several hours to days followed by prolonged sleep. More protracted postuse symptoms have also been noted including an anhedonic "withdrawal" with high cocaine craving. This withdrawal lasts from 1 to 10 weeks, and relapse to cocaine use is high. To manage this syndrome a number of medications have been used. The use of tricyclic antidepressants such as desipramine appears to be generally efficacious in reducing cocaine craving and relapse. Other medications with possible efficacy are dopamine agonists such as amantadine and bromocriptine and lithium for cocaine abusers with cyclothymia. Further work is needed with these pharmacologic approaches, but they do hold promise for prevention of relapse (8).

Hallucinogens

Hallucinogens—lysergic acid diethylamide (LSD), mescaline, psilocybin, 2, 5-dimethoxy-4-methylamphetamine (DOM or STP), dimethyltryptamine (DMT), 3, 4-methylene dixoyamphetamine (MDA, or "love drug")—are usually taken orally. "Acid" and "magic mushrooms" are two nicknames for psychedelic substances.

Intoxication

The psychedelic experience brought on by hallucinogenic drugs includes changes in perception, mood, consciousness, and judgment. An initial period of giddiness and euphoria is followed by profound alterations in consciousness. Synesthesia—a phenomenon in which stimulation of one sensory modality leads to changes in another, for example, seeing music, hearing colors—is a common experience. Physical signs include hyperreflexia, dilated pupils, increased pulse and blood pressure, and increased temperature. Anxiety, anorexia, rambling speech, increased suggestibility, and changes in body image may be noted. Illusions and hallucinations are common. Fear of death is often markedly diminished and the whole attitude towards dying sig-

nificantly altered so that "inadvertent" suicide attempts may occur. Paranoia is not uncommon.

The most common serious untoward event associated with hallucinogenics is a panic reaction or "bad trip." This is usually temporary, lasting less than 24 hours, but it can persist, worsen, and become a full-blown psychotic episode. It is controversial whether a prolonged psychotic state is due to the drug's toxicity or to the unmasking of already existing traits. The relation to dose is also unclear. Flashbacks, the recurrence of part of the psychedelic experience days, weeks, or even months after the last use of the drug, usually occur in an individual who has had multiple experiences with hallucinogens, but occasionally happen after only one experience. They usually fade over time if the drugs are no longer used, but can apparently be restimulated by marijuana. At times, the flashbacks are viewed as pleasant but more often they are frightening and raise fears in the individual that he or she is "going crazy."

Overdose

In hallucinogenic overdose, all of the signs mentioned, plus grand mal seizures, delirium, nausea, and vomiting, can take place. Whether the psychotic state is an overdose phenomenon or an uncovering of a preexisting personality trait is uncertain. Unlike narcotics or sedatives, overdose is usually not associated with a fatal outcome unless delusions of grandeur (for instance, belief in ones ability to fly) lead to a fatal accident.

Withdrawal

Tolerance develops rapidly to psychedelic drugs so that daily usage for only 3 to 4 days will markedly diminish the effect of the same dose. Tolerance is lost just as rapidly. Since use is usually episodic rather than continuous, physical withdrawal is uncommon.

Phencyclidine

Phencyclidine, or PCP, is nicknamed "angel dust," "*PeaCe Pill*," "hog," "rocket fuel," and "monkey dust." Sometimes classed as a central nervous system depressant and sometimes as a hallucinogen, PCP has enough special features to warrant discussion of its own. Developed as a general anesthetic for humans, the frequency and seriousness of side effects led to its being used only in veterinary medicine under the brand name Serynlan. Apparently PCP first emerged as a drug of abuse in 1967 under the name "*PeaCe Pill*," but the frequency of adverse affects soon diminished its popularity. In the early to mid-1970s, it began to be used again, often sold under false pretenses. It is sold as tetrahydrocannabinol (THC) or substituted for LSD or mescaline or sprinkled on marijuana. Phencyclidine is easily and cheaply manufactured from easily obtained chemicals, and today it is often taken knowingly in spite of or even because of its bad reputation. It is related chemically to the anesthetic ketamine.

Phencyclidine may be ingested, injected, snorted, or smoked. A common method is to sprinkle it on parsley and smoke it. Other forms of PCP beside powder include tablets, capsules, rock crystal, and liquid.

Intoxication

Signs and symptoms of PCP intoxication include horizontal and vertical nystagmus, analgesia, tachycardia, increased deep tendon reflexes, muscle rigidity, ataxia, flushed skin, sweating, blank stare, calmness and apathy or agitation and excitement, body image distortion, floating feeling, hostility and possible violence, and fever.

Overdose

Besides the signs of intoxication, the indications of PCP overdose are coma or stupor with fluctuating levels of consciousness, eyes may be open in coma or closed, pupils miotic but reactive, hypertension, convulsions, decreased or absent reflexes, hypersalivation and drooling, sweating, opisthotonic posture, inability to speak, labile affect, disorientation, hallucinations, amnesia, and fever.

The PCP-intoxicated individual may mimic a person having a schizophrenic reaction. Symptoms typically include several days of confusion, paranoid ideation, insomnia, restlessness with intermittent aggressive or violent behavior and delusions of grandeur, but no systematized delusional system. Although recovery is usually complete after days or weeks, patients may have recurring episodes of schizoid behavior, not drug-related. Chronic PCP users may show memory gaps with some disorientation, visual, and speech difficulties even when not using the drug.

In addition to the psychologic and physical dangers associated with PCP, there is a significant risk of what has been called *behavioral toxicity*. Because of impaired perception or delusional beliefs, PCP users have died by fire, falls from heights, burns, and drowning even in quite shallow water. Phencyclidine-intoxicated persons have been known to show extraordinary strength which, when combined with the loss of pain sensation, may mean that three or four persons may be needed to control a person under the influence of PCP.

Treatment of Phencyclidine

In acute intoxication and early stages of PCP-induced acute psychosis, patients need to be isolated from environmental stimulation, with care taken that they do not harm themselves or others. Because of the analgesia and distorted body image, patients have been known to severely mutilate themselves. The propensity to violence against others is also well known. Sedative drugs may be helpful in controlling seizures, violent behavior, agitation, muscle rigidity, and insomnia. Diazepam, 10 to 30 mg intravenously, is often preferred for these states. "Talking down," which can be useful in treating "bad trips" that result from LSD and other hallucinogens, is likely to make matters worse in cases of PCP overdose and should not be used. Phenothiazines should be avoided while the patient is still acutely intoxicated.

If ingestion of PCP was recent, gastric lavage is a worthwhile procedure. Acidification of the urine with ammonium chloride, 2 to 3 mEq/kg every 6 hours, or ascorbic acid, 2 g every 6 hours, is said to greatly increase urinary PCP excretion. As the urine pH is decreased from 7 to 5, PCP clearance is increased by as much as 100 to 300 times. Acidification is contraindicated in the presence of severe liver disease, renal insufficiency, or when the patient has ingested large amounts of drugs, such as barbiturates or salicylates, and excretion of them would be adversely affected by acidification.

Depression can occur several weeks after the acute PCP episode and has been associated with suicide attempts. It is important to be aware of this possibility. Any hospital discharge should include a follow-up treatment plan that provides for ongoing contact and support.

Marijuana

The main mode of ingestion of marijuana is smoking. At times it is taken orally, and very uncommonly it is injected intravenously. "Pot," "grass," "weed," and "reefer" are some nicknames for marijuana. For more details, see Petersen (9).

Marijuana comes from a hemp plant called *Cannabis sativa* cultivated in many parts of the world. Although the principle active ingredient is tetrahydrocannabinol (THC), there are over 400 chemicals in the plant. The THC content is determined by the plant strain, climate, soil conditions, and harvesting. Typically the marijuana used in cigarettes or "joints," is made from particles of the whole plant, especially the leaves and flowers at the top. Potency may vary considerably. For example, in 1975, the average THC content of the confiscated marijuana was 0.5%. In 1978 this had increased to 3% as the source shifted from Mexico to Columbia. California *Sinsimmela* may contain as much as 7% THC. Hashish (hash) is a dark brown or black resin extracted from the plants and smoked to produce a high. Its average THC content is about 2%. Hash oil, an even stronger extract of the plant, may contain up to 35% THC. Hash looks like a tarlike substance and usually is smoked in small amounts on tobacco or marijuana cigarettes to enhance the effect, or it may be smoked in pipes, sometimes called "bongs."

Intoxication

The most common effects of smoking marijuana are feelings of euphoria and relaxation. Users may also experience an increase in pulse rate, reddening of the eyes, dryness of the mouth and throat, and a mild decrease in body temperature. There is also often an associated increase in appetite called "the munchies." High doses may result in image distortions as well as hallucinations. Marijuana has been claimed by users to enhance tactile, auditory, and visual sensations. Research studies have indicated that marijuana may temporarily interfere with memory and may alter the sense of time, making it seem to pass more slowly. It also may decrease the ability to perform tasks requiring concentration, swift actions, and coordination such as driving.

The most common adverse reaction to marijuana is a panic anxiety state sometimes accompanied by paranoia. The symptoms which are more common in novice users generally wear off in a few hours and respond well to reassurance. Marijuana has been reported to exacerbate psychotic symptoms in schizophrenic patients in remission, and has been noted in case reports from India to produce a psychotic state. Such states are apparently very rare in the United States. Because of the sedative and euphoric effects of marijuana, frequent use may be associated in some individuals with decreased interest in academic and occupational achievement, a situation that has been labeled the "amotivational syndrome." It is likely that heavy daily use of sedative drugs other than marijuana would produce a similar situation. The "burn-out-syndrome" is used to describe a situation in which an individual who has been smoking marijuana, usually for 5 years or more, appears to have symptoms suggestive of a chronic brain syndrome. Individuals with this syndrome appear dull, slow moving, and inattentive. There are memory and attention deficits and the effects may last for weeks or months after marijuana is discontinued. It should be noted in this regard that the active ingredient of marijuana, THC, is fat soluble and can be stored in the body for up to 30 days.

The major physical effect demonstrated to date has to do with the pulmonary system, since many users inhale the smoke deeply and hold it in their lungs as long as possible. Signs of airway obstruction in chronic users have been noted. Certain animal tests raise the possibility of lung cancer, but as yet the results have been inconclusive. As for the effects of marijuana on the immune system and on chromosomes, tests results are inconclusive. Although marijuana has been shown to decrease the testosterone level in males to low-normal levels and to increase the number of defective cycles in women, the implications of these findings are unclear.

Withdrawal

The increased potency of marijuana currently in use together with increased frequency of use has been associated with more individuals reporting problems in stopping use of marijuana. There is, however, little evidence in humans that there is physical dependence or physical withdrawal from marijuana in the usual doses.

Overdose

Although injected marijuana extract has been associated with cardiovascular collapse, it is more difficult to overdose by the inhalation route and more possible but still uncommon via the ingestion route. High doses of THC given orally in laboratories have been shown to produce an acute psychotic syndrome. A potentially serious interaction with alcohol is the suppression by marijuana of nausea and vomiting which are body defenses against ingesting too much alcohol. This suppression results in higher blood alcohol levels and the possibility of alcohol poisoning, sometimes leading to death.

LABORATORY TESTS

Many laboratories are able to do a "toxicologic screen" of urine or blood for the presence of many of the drugs of abuse. Such tests can be useful both because of what they may show and because patients may become more truthful when they know that such tests are being done. It is important to keep in mind the following points: Positive test results for the presence of drugs indicate use, but cannot indicate how long or how often the individual may be using that drug—that is, they can define use but not abuse. Negative test results may mean the individual is not using the drug or that the drug is no longer detectable in the urine. For example, traces of cocaine last a relatively short period of time, heroin (in the form of morphine) can be detected in the urine often up to 48 hours after use, and quinine, a diluent often used with both these drugs, can last 5 to 8 days. Since quinine is also found in soft drinks and cold remedies, its presence is at best suggestive. While the presence of a drug in the urine may be helpful in deciding on an overall treatment approach (for example, PCP in the urine of an acutely psychotic patient), such findings usually are not available soon enough to aid in the management of acute situations such as coma. In these cases, diagnosis on the basis of signs and symptoms and symptomatic management are usually necessary.

To uncover possible medical complications of the drug use, studies of blood constituents, including a complete blood cell count, SMA 12/60 (Sequential Multiple Analyzer [by Technicon], 12 constituents per specimen per minute), serology, and Australia antigen should be done. A positive serologic finding (Venereal Disease Research Laboratory Test) should be further evaluated with a fluorescent treponema antibody test because of the frequency of false-positive results. Testing for human immunodeficiency virus antibody is particularly indicated in intravenous drug users considering pregnancy and in users having symptoms of aquired immunodeficiency syndrome. Chest roentgenograms and electrocardiograms are done when medically indicated, the former especially if one has not been done in the past 6 to 12 months and the latter especially in patients over age 35. Because of the deleterious effect of many drugs on the fetus and because drug use may lead to irregular menstrual cycles, a pregnancy test should be performed on any female patient with missed or irregular periods where drug use is suspected. A history of seizures that has not been previously investigated calls for an electroencephalogram. Additional laboratory tests may be suggested by the history or physical examination.

SPECIALIZED TREATMENT APPROACHES

Detoxification

Although in the past, detoxification was often considered treatment in and of itself, most experienced clinicians now regard withdrawal from drugs as pretreatment or as the first step in treatment. Withdrawal from narcotics without medical help is painful but rarely life threatening. With medical support it becomes relatively easy to do. It can take place on an inpatient, residential, or outpatient basis. Outpatient withdrawal is usually difficult without strong family support, because the individual remains in more or less the same environment and is able to obtain drugs. The first signs of discomfort under such circumstances are often enough to send him or her searching for more chemicals. On an inpatient or residential basis, through methadone substitution of 20 to 25 mg daily for the heroin, and then withdrawal, detoxification becomes a relatively simple procedure lasting 5 to 10 days. Methadone can also be given on an outpatient basis.

More recently, clonidine, an α-adrenergic agonist, has been shown to be effective in the rapid detoxification from opiates (10). Because clonidine is an antihypertensive agent, blood pressure should be monitored carefully during withdrawal, especially in medically ill patients.

Withdrawing an individual from barbiturates, or similar sedative drugs, on the other hand, carries with it the possibility of a fatal outcome. Because of this, withdrawal should be carried out on an inpatient basis. Detoxification from barbiturates is usually carried out by initially giving individuals an intermediate-acting barbiturate such as pentobarbital, stabilizing them for a few days, and then withdrawing usually no faster than 10% of the dose a day. Some clinicians prefer the longer acting drug, phenobarbital to provide a smoother withdrawal pattern. However, when adjusting the dosage needed to cover withdrawal, the longer acting properties of phenobarbital may complicate patient management and dosage adjustment. Patients who are addicted to the benzodiazepines should be withdrawn using those drugs rather than barbiturates. The mechanics of gradual withdrawal remain the same.

Abrupt cessation of amphetamines and some stimulants can lead to severe depression and suicide requiring inpatient treatment, although cocaine withdrawal usually does not require an inpatient program. There has been fairly good success in detoxifying cocaine-dependent individuals on an outpatient basis, and there appears to be an important role for pharmacologic agents such as desipramine or dopamine agonists to reduce cocaine relapse. There is some controversy over whether stimulant dependency should be handled by abrupt or gradual withdrawal. The former has been the preferred approach for years and is preferable with cocaine abusers, but gradual withdrawal may have a role with abuse of other stimulants.

Individuals dependent on multiple drugs usually need to be detoxified on an inpatient basis, as outpatient withdrawal usually means the individual switches over to another drug or intensifies the use of one drug, while he is being medically withdrawn from another. Individuals with serious medical problems should almost always be detoxified in an inpatient setting.

The Therapeutic Community

Residential therapeutic communities have been used during the past few decades for the treatment of drug abuse. Key elements of their program usually include emphasis on confrontation, group therapy, a relatively rigid hierarchial structure, a reward and a punishment system based on a fairly strict value code which emphasizes honesty, openness, family feeling, accepting responsibility, and prohibitions against violence or drug use. Although originally they were operated exclusively by ex-addict staffs who had themselves gone through the program, more recently there has been an increase in the active participation of mental health care professionals. There has also been an increase in educational and vocational training during the residential stay. The programs seem to be especially useful for substance abusers without serious psychiatric problems. Since many adolescent and young adult abusers have serious psychiatric difficulties, however, and probably would not do well in an environment that is confrontation oriented and where mental health care professionals are not available, the practitioner making a referral must be aware of the program and staff in each facility to be considered. Such patients may do better in programs where the approach is more supportive than confrontational.

Outpatient and Day Programs

Outpatient and drug-free day programs often have little in common with each other besides not using methadone or narcotic antagonists and not being residential. They represent the largest number of drug treatment programs in the country today and differ enormously in the kinds and quality of services offered. Their approach may be most appropriate for four groups of clients: people seeking their first treatment experience; those who have successfully completed other treatment modalities; clients who have relapsed following other treatments; and, finally, drug abusers requiring treatment after prison or

hospital stays. Approaches include group therapy, individual counseling, vocational training, family therapy, job counseling, and in some cases specialized programs such as transcendental meditation, art therapy, music therapy, and yoga. If there are medical consultants available to the program, psychotropic drugs such as antidepressants may also be used. At times group therapy is more effective than traditional one-to-one counseling because of the peer-pressure that can be exerted on the individual and because the group may more effectively cut through many of the denials, rationalizations, and manipulations employed by the drug abuser.

Methadone Maintenance

Methadone maintenance involves the use on a daily basis of the synthetic narcotic, methadone, as a replacement for heroin. At the usual dosage range, 50 to 100 mg once daily, it reduces or eliminates drug-seeking behavior, blocks the effect of the average street amounts of heroin, and permits the individual to function without undue drowsiness or euphoria and with a minimum of other side effects. Since its introduction in the mid 1960s, it has become one of the more widely used treatments for narcotic addicts and one of the most controversial.

In general, programs that employ ancillary supports such as counseling or vocational and educational help seem to do better than those that provide methadone alone. These multimodality programs often have a complex therapeutic structure with a variety of limit-setting mechanisms to help patients internalize controls for their aggression and anxieties (12). Individuals who start on methadone maintenance should have been using heroin on a more or less regular basis for at least 2 years and have tried other methods of treatment before being placed on this maintenance drug. Minimum age under federal regulations is 18 years, and in some programs age 21 is required. Once started on methadone, clients should continue for at least 12 months before detoxification is attempted. Detoxification appears to be most successful when done on a slow, gradual basis over a 3 to 6 month period. Because even this gradual withdrawal is at times associated with low level symptoms that addicts do not tolerate well, many patients who otherwise seem ready to be drug free have been unable to stop taking methadone. Clonidine detoxification may be helpful for the final phases of detoxification by stopping methadone at 15 to 20 mg daily and substituting clonidine for the last 2 weeks of detoxification.

Narcotic Antagonists

Naltrexone is an agent which blocks the effects of narcotics without producing any addiction itself. It is long acting, has a minimum of side effects, and can be given on a Monday, Wednesday, and Friday basis to block the euphoric effects of street doses of heroin. Compliance with taking naltrexone is the major clinical problem in its use, and a variety of approaches have been used to improve compliance, including behavior therapy and family treatment (13). Patients are encouraged to continue on it for 6 to 9 months before stopping treatment. The groups of patients who may do best on naltrexone are those who are coming out of a drug-free environment such as prison or a hospital and need some help in remaining drug free; those who are leaving other treatment programs such as methadone or therapeutic communities; individuals who may be "chipping" but not addicted to narcotics or who have not been taking them for a long time; and business executives or professionals in health care. To start on naltrexone, individuals must be free of short-acting narcotics (e.g., free of heroin for at least 5 to 7 days and free of methadone for at least 10 days).

The last two methods, methadone maintenance and narcotic antagonists, are clearly indicated for the individual with an opiate-abuse problem. Stimulant, depressant, and polydrug abusers need to be treated within the therapeutic community or any of the outpatient approaches. Alcoholics Anonymous (AA), while useful for alcoholics, has not been shown to be particularly helpful with adolescent polydrug users or with adult heroin users. Recently some AA groups have been formed that specialize in working with opioid and cocaine abusers, and Cocaine Anonymous and Narcotic Anonymous groups have begun to appear around the country.

THE CLINICAL INTERVIEW

Determining the Nature of the Problem

Among general psychiatric patients the first problem in making a correct diagnosis of drug abuse or dependence is eliciting the use of the particular drug. The clinician must ask about the various drugs of abuse in a nonjudgmental way, assuring the patient that what is told will be held in confidence and that the primary goal is to help the patient, not the police. This is a particular issue outside of specialized treatment programs for drug abuse, since the drug abuser has often encountered rejection and hostility when he has revealed his drug abuse. In many cases, there is a real conflict between a desire for help and a fear of arrest.

Drug History

In those cases in which the use or abuse of drugs is the overt reason the client is seeing the clinician, the interview should begin with a discussion of why the patient is coming now rather than earlier. Some reasons may be legal pressure, family, peer, or job pressure, medical problems, or self-decision. For the patient's history of drug use, the following information for each drug provides necessary data for evaluation. Whether the clinician needs to obtain a drug history as detailed as outlined here depends on the nature and circumstance of the evaluation.

In asking about current use, for each drug the clinician should ask for the name of the drug, length of time used, frequency of use, route of administration, amount, cost, and purpose (to get high, to relieve boredom, to sleep, for energy, socialization, to relieve depression or nervousness, and so on). To determine previous use, the clinician asks for the name, the age the drug was started, length of time used, any adverse effects, and previous treatment experiences (where, what kind, and outcome) about each drug used in the past.

A clinician's suspicion of a drug abuse problem should be high among adolescents and young adults with nonspecific medical or psychological problems. Furthermore, if any major medical indications of drug abuse are evident, such as hepatitis, needle track marks, or withdrawal symptoms, then careful and detailed questioning is indicated. Denial of drug abuse along with minimization of the amount of drug use and its social complications is common. Polydrug abuse has also become the norm rather than the exception, so that multiple drugs must be considered in any evaluation. Polydrug abuse involving cocaine has become a recently increasing problem. The most common drug combinations with cocaine are alcohol, marijuana, and opioids (heroin). The intravenous cocaine abusers frequently "speedball" by combining cocaine with heroin, while freebase cocaine smokers often use substantial amounts of alcohol to ameliorate the cocaine crash.

In some cases a urine toxicology can be helpful to identify the range and recentness of abused drugs. When using toxicology results, it is important to be aware of the duration of positive tests and that single usage can produce a positive test. The length of time that these tests remain positive after drug use is quite variable. Among various drugs, marijuana or THC is at the long end, with positive tests lasting for sometimes weeks since last use, while cocaine is at the short end with positive tests lasting for only 24 to 48 hours since last use, even for heavy users. No urine test substitutes for a careful interview covering drug dependence, since positive urine tests can occur after a single use of a drug, and a positive urine test does not necessarily indicate drug dependence. For opioids and sedatives, laboratory tests of dependence are available (e.g., naloxone challenge and the barbiturate tolerance test), but these tests have a limited utility in clinical practice. Family members are more reliable sources of diagnostic information than these laboratory tests, particularly for indications of social disruption.

Social Situation

After obtaining a picture of the current and past drug use, the interview should move into the area of social functioning. Information about the following material should be elicited: living arrangements (alone, with family, or with other), marital status, sexual orientation and functioning, employment and/or educational status, family members (parents, siblings, spouse, other key members), occupation, education, psychologic state, friends, and recreational activities. The clinician should try to understand not only the factual aspects of these areas, but also the emotional ones, i.e., the quality of the patient's relation with his or her parents or spouse should be probed as well as the attitude toward a job or schooling. Does the patient have close friends, hobbies, or sports interests? The nature and degree of the patient's social supports should become clear—is the drug use jeopardizing them or is it taking their place because of their meagerness? The presence of adverse family conditions, currently or in the past, such as alcoholism, mental illness, brutality, compulsive gambling, or the like, should be looked for and noted. Recent changes in the patient's behavior should be taken as clues to either antecedents or sequelae to the drug abuse. Did a divorce precede or follow the increased use of barbiturates? Did the heavy marijuana use precede or follow a fall in grades and decision to drop out of school? Did the cocaine use occur after or before taking up with a new group of friends? Although it is tempting to associate calamitous occurrences as a result of drug abuse, careful questioning may reveal they were prior events.

Psychologic Status

Elsewhere in this book there is a detailed description of comprehensive psychologic evaluation of patients. In dealing with drug abusers, such evaluation has several purposes. It aids in deciding who may need to be referred for specialized help as opposed to more nonspecific counseling. It may also highlight the existence of conditions for which there is appropriate psychoactive medication. Of course, in dealing with a drug-abusing population, the physician must be very cautious in prescribing such drugs, but they need not be withheld where appropriate. Certain drugs, such as lithium and monoamine oxidase inhibitors, may be risky to use, because a careless life-style or haphazard approach to dosage can create serious hazards when these substances are being taken. Other drugs, such as the minor tranquilizers, are often abused for their psychoactive effects. Certain categories, such as the phenothiazenes, on the other hand, are rarely abused by these patients and the problem more often is how to get the patient to keep taking such agents when they are prescribed.

As with social supports, it is important to ascertain whether detectable psychiatric conditions predate or postdate the drug abuse. Certain people take drugs on a self-medicating basis to deal with unbearable states of loneliness, depression, or anxiety, or to control unacceptable aggressive or sexual drives. Conversely, continued use of certain drugs may lead to or exaggerate psychiatric states not evident before. For example, chronic cocaine use may lead to depression, paranoid feelings, and even frank psychosis. Personality factors play a role in determining which drug will be used, the pattern of use, and to some extent psychoactive effects. While, in general, experimental or occasional use of drugs may not indicate any psychopathology, heavy or compulsive use is usually associated with serious problems. However, at present there is no good way to predict whether or not a person with certain characteristics will become a compulsive user or which people will use a particular category of drugs. As one example, although a number of heroin addicts may have passive–aggressive personality features, most passive–aggressive people are not heroin addicts (or even drug abusers) and most heroin addicts are not passive–aggressive.

In formulating a clinical hypothesis about the nature of the drug abuser's problems, it is most important to recognize that almost 90% of drug abusers have concomitant psychiatric problems (14). Most commonly these are depression and antisocial personality disorder. Depression is particularly important, because it is associated with suicidality (a major cause of death in young adults) and quite treatable with either psychotherapy or pharmacotherapy. With any drug abuser it is useful to wait until detoxification is complete, and he or she has been drug free for several days to a week, before making a firm diagnosis or instituting pharmacotherapy for an affective disorder. Many times patients will initially appear to have a depressive or even psychotic disorder that will clear after a few drug-free days.

Antisocial personality can be a difficult disorder for psychotherapists to manage. We shall return to its management below in the section on the therapeutic relationship, but it may help to recognize that many antisocial activities are directed toward obtaining money to buy drugs, and with drug abstinence these antisocial activities will often disappear. An important distinction should be made between those antisocial patients where antisocial activity is confined to obtaining drugs and those whose antisocial activity extends far beyond the need to obtain drugs. Furthermore, drug abusers having both depression and antisocial personality appear to have the relatively good prognosis of depressives rather than the poorer prognosis of "pure" antisocial personality disorder (15).

Medical Evaluation

Medical problems also need careful attention. Drug abusers generally obtain very little medical care, in spite of these drugs' having major medical complications. The recent emphasis on AIDS (acquired immunodeficiency syndrome) among intravenous drug abusers has raised the awareness of health care providers to the medical needs of these patients, but many other infectious diseases are common. Among drug abusers there have been high rates of veneral diseases and tuberculosis. Axis III of the DSM-III-R will almost always include significant illnesses among drug abusers, and denial of medical illnesses among these patients should not be accepted uncritically.

Although there is no special physical examination for drug abusers, it is useful to keep in mind certain conditions which can be either direct or indirect sequelae of drug abuse. While many of them can be found in nonabusers and many abusers may have few or none of them, the presence of certain signs should raise one's index of suspicion.

Some *cutaneous signs* directly or indirectly associated with drug abuse are needle *puncture* marks—usually found over veins especially in the antecubital area, dorsum of the hands, and forearms, but they can be found anywhere on the body where a vein is reachable, including the neck, tongue, and dorsal vein of the penis.

Tracks are one of the most common and readily recognizable signs of chronic injectable drug abuse. They are scars located along veins and are usually hyperpigmented and linear. They result both from frequent unsterile injections and from the deposit of carbon black from attempts to sterilize the needle with a match. Tracks tend to lighten over time but may never totally disappear. Because tracks are such a well-known indication of drug abuse, addicts may hide them by having a *tattoo* over the area. Tattoos in general are not uncommon among certain groups of drug abusers.

When addicts run out of antecubital and forearm veins they often turn to veins on the finger and dorsum of the hand, which can lead to *hand edema*. Such edema can persist for months.

Thrombophlebitis is commonly found in addicts on arms and legs because of the unsterile nature of the injections and the irritating quality of some of the adulterants mixed with the active drug. *Abscesses* and *ulcers* are particularly common among individuals who inject barbiturates because of the irritating quality of these chemicals. Those abscesses that are secondary to opioid or cocaine injection are more likely to be septic and occur around the veins.

Ulceration or perforation of the nasal septum is a frequent effect of inhalation or "snorting." Heroin can lead to ulceration of the septum, while similar chronic use of cocaine can cause perforation secondary to vasoconstriction and loss of blood supply.

Cigarette *burns* or scars from old burns are another sign of possible drug abuse. They can occur as a result of drug-induced drowsiness. Fresh burns are usually seen between the fingers while old scars are often seen on the chest as a result of the cigarette falling out of the user's mouth. It has been estimated that over 90% of addicts and alcoholics smoke.

Piloerection ("gooseflesh") is an opiate withdrawal sign, usually found on the arms and trunk. *Chelitis* (cracking of skin at corners of mouth) is especially seen in chronic amphetamine users and in opiate addicts prior to or during detoxification. Contact *dermatitis* is observed around the nose, mouth, and hands, in solvent abusers. Sometimes it is called "glue-sniffer's rash." In other drug abusers it may occur around areas of injection secondary to use of chemicals to cleanse the skin. *Jaundice*, due to hepatitis, in drug abusers is usually attributable to use of unsterilized shared needles and syringes. A common manifestation of AIDS is lymphadenopathy with emaciation.

Developing and Maintaining a Therapeutic Relationship

While assessing the types and patterns of drug abuse and the need for immediate medical treatment of withdrawal and drug abuse complications, the therapist must also be aware of potential conflicts in the expectations of the patient and the therapist. When patients feel that their only need is for drugs to relieve withdrawal, and the therapist focuses on long-term rehabilitation, the initial interview can break down into an angry confrontation. A first step in establishing a working relationship may be to provide some pharmacologic relief of withdrawal symptoms. With opioid (heroin) abusers, for example, this may take the form of clonidine rather than an opioid such as methadone. With abusers of other types of drugs, no immediate relief of withdrawal may be needed, but a promise of some medication for sleep may help the relationship. Clearly, the use of barbiturates for sleep would be a poor choice in a sedative abuser, but an antihistamine may be considered. The medication is part of a negotiation in which the therapist offers some recognition of the patient's genuine discomfort, using a symbol (the pill) that the patient readily understands. The patient may then be more receptive to discussing long-term rehabilitation.

Overall, the issue of trust is important, and the therapist may need to explicitly state that he or she will not report the patient's drug abuse to the police. For adolescents, the involvement of their parents is a somewhat different issue, and therapists should not lock themselves into a promise not to inform them. Early parental involvement in treatment has been repeatedly shown to improve treatment outcome, and this opportunity should not be given up without careful and extended discussion with the patient (16, 17). A similar statement can be made about spousal involvement in treatment, although married drug abusers frequently come in under the urging of their spouse so that involvement already exists.

The drug abuse itself often has a defensive function of helping maintain intrapsychic equilibrium. Thus, giving up the drug may expose patients to internal conflicts and affects with which they are ill prepared to cope. The therapist should try to work with the patient to uncover some of the defensive or coping strategies that the drug serves and not simply approach the drug use as a hedonistic attempt to "get high," even when patients say that is the reason for their drug use. The young adolescent who defiantly states that he only uses drugs to get high is usually the most seriously disturbed and threatened by life without drugs.

The stereotype of a street junkie who "pushes" drugs onto school children is a political overstatement, but drug dealers are common and do seek treatment. In the real world of drug abuse, there is often little distinction between the drug dealer and the addict. To obtain drugs regularly, the addict must have large amounts of money and often sells drugs and uses a portion of them himself. Among addicts, selling drugs, as a way of supporting a drug habit, is seen as less disreputable than stealing, and many of the heavier drug abusers will be drug dealers. Do not be caught in the fantasy that drug dealers are making great profits and need imprisonment, not treatment. There is a subpopulation of major drug dealers who generally do not use drugs and are very unlikely to come for treatment.

Sociopathic drug addicts most frequently seek help with their drug abuse after being arrested and given the option of treatment or imprisonment. Developing a therapeutic relationship with this type of patient requires that the therapist be comfortable with limit setting. Limit setting must be fair and presented in a nonangry way. When the therapist fails to set limits at the appropriate time, he or she will inevitably feel angry and misused by these patients. In managing the initial interview with these patients, the therapist should keep in mind that although such patients may appear composed, pleasant, and engaging at first, early confrontation with them about misrepresenting "facts" will usually lead to angry denial and a more difficult interview. Confrontation and limit setting may become important, but allowing the patient to "save face" is of equal use in conducting these interviews. The therapist also needs to avoid keeping any secrets given to him or her by family members, who may place the therapist in a double bind. The family may ask the therapist to take sides on many behaviors of the patient including the drug abuse. The therapist should try to stay neutral, but not support, by default, a position advocating abuse of drugs. Drug abusing antisocial parents will often ask some favor or permission just before the interview ends, thereby preventing full discussion of the issue. In general, try to delay your response until the next meeting, but if clinical judgment demands a more prompt response, then propose a compromise that imposes some frustration of the demand while providing for discussion at the next meeting. Be sure that you then bring up the issue at the next meeting, since the patient may not.

Communicating Information and Implementing a Treatment Plan

After the extent and complications of the drug abuse problem have been determined and while developing an emphatic yet firm therapeutic relationship, the therapist can begin implementing a treatment plan with the patient. As described in the earlier section on the therapeutic relationship, a real difference may exist between the perspectives of the clinician and the patient, and several educational and negotiating strategies may be useful in bridging this gap. In treating substance abusers, limits must be set on the self-destructive behavior associated with abusing drugs. Thus, the therapist must actively intervene and be prepared to use confrontation rather than interpretation to communicate the basics of an effective treatment plan. Active intervention may even extend to hospitalization including legal commitment, for example, if a "crashing" cocaine abuser is actively suicidal and refusing hospitalization because of acute paranoia. In general, the first part of an effective treatment plan is to establish control of the drug abuse itself, since any further treatment will be impossible without abstinence.

Roles of the Family

Family collaboration may also be helpful. Not infrequently the first complication in the treatment of the substance abuser is convincing the individual to seek help. A spouse, parent, or offspring often appears in the office and asks for help in getting the person to seek assistance. The individual who is abusing drugs may deny or minimize the existence of any substance abuse problem and may refuse to see a therapist. While this is a difficult situation, there are definite steps family members can take to increase the chances of the individual's seeking help.

First, the clinician should have the family members describe in detail the behavior that leads them to suspect substance abuse and the duration of time over which this has taken place. Despite the prevalence of chemical use in our society, one cannot assume that the family has always made the correct diagnosis. A sharp drop in an adolescent's grades may have more to do with depression or unrequited love than with drugs.

Second, family members should be encouraged to do some reading about the problem. Drug and alcohol treatment centers usually have literature about the nature of substance abuse (18, 19).

Third, the nature of the confrontation that may have to occur should be fully discussed. Role-playing may offer a rehearsal for what is usually a very difficult and painful situation. The meaning of the ultimatum should be very clear and related to the situation. With a spouse it may be, "See the doctor or leave the house" or "I'll leave if you don't see the doctor." With an adolescent the threat may have to do with loss of privileges or even the ultimate threat, "See the doctor or get out of the house." It is important not to have the confrontation until the family member is ready for it and has rehearsed ways of handling the usual replies. It is also important that they only make threats that have been fully thought through and that they are prepared to carry out. Idle threats worsen communication and may markedly prolong the period of time before the individual seeks treatment. Finally, when the family member is ready, a date is set for the appointment. This should be a realistic date that takes into account any other circumstances in the individual's life.

Role of Drugs in the Family

When the clinician meets with the family member or the drug-abusing client, it may be useful to think first about the role drugs may play in that particular family. Although almost always the family overtly condemns the drug or alcohol abuse, the covert processes may tell a different story. The drug use may serve as a problem that unifies the family and keeps it together. The drug user may be viewed as helpless and dependent, unable to live on his or her own. This attitude may keep adolescents home long beyond the time when they should leave. The parents may intuitively know that if their drug-abusing child left, their marriage would break up. In the marital situation, a husband or wife may covertly encourage the drug or alcohol use in a spouse, because it gives them the dominant role while at the same time they are able to portray themselves and think of themselves as the helpless victim. Physicians have been known to encourage their spouses' heavy use of sedative drugs or even narcotics as a way of forestalling complaints about the amount of time the physicians are out of the home and the lack of attention they give to the family. The sedated elderly parent may be easier to have around than the whining, querulous, unsedated one. These factors may lead the family to sabotage treatment, if the clinician is not alert to what may be going on in the family constellation. Before expending much effort on treatment, therefore, it behooves the clinician to try to understand the particular dynamics for each family in question. For a full discussion of the role of the family in drug abuse situations, see Stanton (17).

No matter what the role of the family may be, without their help referral or treatment may fail. Thus, it is important for the clinician to involve the family in the treatment process to whatever extent possible. The clinician may provide short-term crisis-oriented service to families and focus on improved communication skills, family negotiations, setting and achieving of realistic goals, and reasonable limit setting.

Parents are usually confused about how to react to and handle adolescent drug use. This confusion has led them to avoid taking stands or to pretend not to notice obvious drug-related behavior so as not to have to take a position or have a confrontation. This has been true about tobacco and alcohol as well as marijuana and other drugs. The younger adolescent is especially vulnerable to the effects of drug abuse and in this case parents may have to be especially forceful in their negative statements and limits.

Individual Treatment

The subsequent phases of therapy can then be targeted toward helping patients develop adequate defenses, since they frequently have only a few primitive defenses to protect them from relapse to drug abuse. The therapist can elicit feelings from the patient and help the patient label them by putting them into words. By sharing these feelings with the therapist, the patient will learn that painful affects can be tolerated. These painful affects may range from depression to anger and poorly controlled rage, and the patient needs help in sharing these feelings within the human relationship of the therapy.

In the outpatient setting medications can have a significant role. Although treating drugs with drugs can be a precarious position to maintain and is opposed by many self-help groups, judicious use of medications with virtually no abuse potential can help the patient tolerate the therapeutic process. The appropriate use of psychoactive medications might include tricyclic antidepressants for clinically depressed patients, or the short-term use of antipsychotic agents such as thioridizine in low doses for recent drug-induced psychoses. Specialized medication for managing the drug abuse itself, such as methadone maintenance and naltrexone for opioid addicts or desipramine for cocaine abusers, are also quite important in many cases of severe drug dependence.

Since depression is one of the most common secondary disorders among drug abusers, its management should be carefully considered. From a psychotherapeutic approach, many of these patients have low self-esteem and intense dependency needs. These needs may be masked by a hostile, independent demeanor, but this is a type of testing behavior used to establish the limits of the therapist's concern about them. The therapist should recognize this behavior, and by acknowledging anger at the patient for this, the therapist may lessen the tension. Therapists cannot be effective if they lose control of their anger. In general, the therapist needs to act as a model for the patient's identification, rather than a "blank screen" for the patient's projections. The patient needs active help in developing substitutes for rather primitive defenses, for example, in replacing acting-out with reaction formation and in replacing projection with altruism. From a pharmacologic approach, the use of antidepressants is indicated in those patients who remain depressed for more than 10 to 14 days after detoxification. However, monoamine oxidase inhibitors may be a high-risk choice and tricyclics are usually effective with depressed methadone or naltrexone maintained patients.

Individual or group treatment can have for its major focus the prevention of relapse. This type of therapy was initially developed for alcoholism by Marlatt, but has more general applicability in substance abuse (20). It includes a mixture of behavioral, cognitive, educational, and self-control techniques which addresses the following relapse issues: high-risk situations, conditioning factors, early warning signals, and the abstinence violation effect. Such therapy also focuses on stress reduction and life-style changes. While we cannot describe this approach in detail here, several points deserve emphasis. For each individual there are particular situations that present a high risk for relapse to drug use (e.g., parties where cocaine is available, cocaine paraphernalia at home or work). To deal with this problem, the patient needs to imagine potential risk situations and devise strategies for coping with or avoiding them (e.g., leave high-risk parties, discarding old paraphernalia). In gen-

eral, the former drug user must devise ways to say "no" when offered drugs. Ways to say "no" might include "I can't afford it anymore," or "I don't like the irritable feeling the next morning." The other parts of this comprehensive treatment are somewhat more complex, but are easily learned by therapists and patients and can be an important part of any therapy.

With any therapy for drug abusers, premature termination may occur, when the drug user is under good control and the abuser feels cured. The therapist needs to remind the patient that abstinence alone does not mean completion of the psychologic work needed to prevent relapse. If the patient insists on leaving treatment, the invitation to return to treatment should be stated such that the patient does not have to relapse into drug dependency before seeking treatment again. The concept of a chronic relapsing disorder can be tied to the idea of "slips" with drugs. The patient can be educated that these slips into single episodes of drug use can be considered indications that the psychologic work is not complete and that reentry into treatment is essential to prevent complete relapse. This has been called the abstinence violation effect by Marlatt (20). Self-help groups might also be considered for more long-term support after leaving treatment. These self-help groups such as AA can satisfy many dependency needs directly without the patient's exposing his or her desire for dependency. In general, the patients should leave treatment with a clear sense from the therapist that drug abusers can be treated successfully and that there is hope for them to lead productive and abstinent lives.

References

1. Crowley TJ, Ghesluck D, Hart R: Drug and alcohol abuse psychiatric admissions. *Arch Gen Psychiatry* 30:13–20, 1974.
2. Hall RCW, Popkin MK, Devaul R, Stickney SK: The effect of unrecognized drug abuse on diagnosis and therapeutic outcome. *Am J Drug Alcohol Abuse* 4:455–465, 1977.
3. Regier DA, Myers JK, Kramer M, et al: NIMH

Epidemiological Catchment Area Program. *Arch Gen Psychiatry* 41:934–941, 1984.

4. Eddy NB, Halbach H, Isbell H, et al: Drug dependence: its significance and characteristics. *Bulletin of the World Health Organization* 37:721–733, 1965.

5. Kleber HD: Drug abuse. In Bellack L (ed): *A Concise Handbook of Community Psychiatry and Community Mental Health*. New York: Grune & Stratton, 1974, pp 129–162.

6. Edwards G, Gross MM: Alcohol dependence: provisional description of the clinical syndrome. *Br Med J* 1:1058–1061, 1976.

7. Inaba DI, Way EL, Blum K, et al: Pharmacological and toxicological perspectives of commonly abused drugs. *National Institute of Drug Abuse Medical Monograph Series* 1: 1978, pp 1–40.

8. Gawin, FH, Kleber HD: Cocaine abuse treatment: an open pilot trial with lithium carbonate and desipramine. *Arch Gen Psychiatry* 41:903–910, 1984.

9. Petersen RC (ed): *Marijuana and Health 1977* (7th annual report to the U.S. Congress from the Secretary of Health, Education and Welfare). Rockville, MD, National Institute on Drug Abuse, 1979.

10. Gold MS, Redmond DE Jr, Kleber HD: Clonidine in opiate withdrawal. *Lancet* 1:929–930, 1978.

11. Kleber HD, Riordan CE, Rousaville BJ, et al: Clonidine in outpatient detoxification from methadone maintenance. *Arch Gen Psychiatry* 42:391–395, 1985.

12. Kosten TR, Astrachan BM, Riordan C, et al: The organization of a methadone maintenance program. *Journal of Drug Issues* 12:333–342, 1982.

13. Kosten TR, Kleber HD: Strategies to improve compliance with narcotic antagonists. *Am J Drug Alcohol Abuse* 10:249–266, 1984.

14. Rounsaville BJ, Weissman MM, Kleber HD, et al: Heterogeneity of psychiatric diagnosis in treated opiate addicts. *Arch Gen Psychiatry* 42:161–166, 1982.

15. Woody GE, MCLellan AT, Luborsky L, et al: Sociopathy and psychotherapy outcome. *Arch Gen Psychiatry* 42:1081–1086, 1985.

16. Kosten TR, Jalali B, Hogan I, et al: Family denial as a prognostic factor in opiate addict treatment outcome. *J Nerv Ment Dis* 171:611–616, 1983.

17. Stanton MD, Todd TC, Heard DB, et al: Heroin addiction as a family phenomenon: a new conceptual model. *Am J Drug Alcohol Abuse* 5:125–150, 1978.

18. Bair GO, Elder C, Wallsmith P: *When It's Your Kid: The Crisis of Drugs*. Kansas City, Lowell Press, 1978.

19. Manatt M: *Parents, Peers, and Pot*. Rockville, MD, National Institute on Drug Abuse, 1979.

20. Marlatt GA, Gordon, JR: Determinants of relapse: implications for the maintenance of behavior change. In Davidson PO, Davidson SM (eds): *Behavioral Medicine: Changing Health Lifestyles*. New York, Brunner Mazel, 1980, pp 410–452.

38

Schizophrenic Disorders

Theo C. Manschreck, M.D.

Schizophrenic disorders represent a major public health problem. They affect approximately 1% of the adult population and impair social, occupational, and intellectual functioning, often for years. While the dramatic nature of florid psychosis in such individuals has received the most attention, the lifelong disabilities in cognitive and perceptual function, coordination, emotional expression and experience, thinking, speech, and reduced ambition represent the main burden of suffering. The resulting social losses in productivity and creativity are staggering.

Patients with these disorders are among the most challenging to evaluate and to treat. There are few recipes for successful intervention, and our ignorance is a serious limitation in selecting treatments. In short, much needs to be learned about the nature of these disorders and how to manage their impact. The situation is more serious: many of these patients are poor, frequently indigent, if not homeless or institutionalized. All too often, despite the complexity of their illnesses they receive minimal care, or care in its least sophisticated forms. As a rule, patients with these disorders have been underserved.

This chapter attempts to provide a framework relevant to the activities of diagnosis, differential diagnosis, treatment, and long-term planning in schizophrenic disorders. Increasingly in the last several

decades, these tasks have centered in outpatient settings.

DEFINITION

The adoption of the third edition of the *Diagnostic and Statistical Manual* of the American Psychiatric Association (DSM-III) (1) in 1980 revitalized the diagnosis of schizophrenia. While these disorders remain poorly understood, they are more carefully defined and clinical discourse about them is clearer.

The essential features of this group of disorders are: the presence of certain psychotic features during the active phase of the illness, characteristic symptoms involving multiple psychological processes, deterioration from a previous level of functioning, onset before age 45, and a duration of at least six months. The disturbance is not due to an affective disorder or organic mental disorder. At least some phase of the illness schizophrenia always involves delusions, hallucinations, or certain disturbances in the form of thought.

This definition, elaborated in Table 38.1, reflects several developments in views about these conditions. First, the criteria made it explicit that schizophrenia is an *idiopathic syndrome* with heterogeneous causes: It is schizophrenic disorders. Second, there was a more balanced emphasis

Table 38.1   DSM-III Criteria for Schizophrenic Disorders (1980)

A. At least one of the following during a phase of the illness:
1. Bizarre delusions (content is patently absurd and has no possible basis in fact), such as delusions of being controlled, thought broadcasting, thought insertion, or thought withdrawal.
2. Somatic, grandiose, religious, nihilistic, or other delusions without persecutory or jealous content.
3. Delusions with persecutory or jealous content if accompanied by hallucinations of any type.
4. Auditory hallucinations in which a voice keeps up a running commentary on the individual's behavior or thoughts or two or more voices converse with each other.
5. Auditory hallucinations on several occasions with content of more than one or two words, having no apparent relation to depression or elation.
6. Incoherence, marked loosening of associations, markedly illogical thinking, or marked poverty of content of speech if associated with at least one of the following:
   a. blunted, flat, or inappropriate affect
   b. delusions or hallucinations
   c. catatonic or other grossly disorganized behavior
B. Deterioration from a previous level of functioning in such areas as work, social relations, and self-care.
C. Duration: Continuous signs of the illness for at least 6 months at some time during the person's life, with some signs of the illness at present. The 6-month period must include an active phase during which there are symptoms from A, with or without a prodromal or residual phase.
D. The full depressive or manic syndrome, if present, developed after any psychotic symptoms, or was brief in duration relative to the duration of the psychotic symptoms in A.
E. Onset of prodromal or active phase of the illness before age 45.
F. Not due to any organic mental disorder or mental retardation.

Reprinted with permission from American Psychiatric Association: *Diagnostic and Statistical Manual of Mental Disorders (Third Edition)*. Washington, DC, American Psychiatric Association, 1980. Copyright 1980 American Psychiatric Association.

on symptoms and course factors because neither alone sufficiently distinguishes the schizophrenic group (2, 3). Third, the criteria narrowed the boundaries of schizophrenia as defined by Bleuler (4) in 1911 and DSM-II (5) in 1968. Fourth, the requirement that affective and organic mental disorder be ruled out made schizophrenic disorder a diagnosis of exclusion. Fifth, the traditional phenomenologic subtypes (e.g., paranoid, catatonic, and hebephrenic) were deemphasized, owing largely to lack of validation (6). Sixth, in extensive field trials (1) this 1980 definition was applied with a high degree of reliability, comparable to that achieved in diagnoses of many medical diseases. In short, it made the identification of cases more effective. The achievements associated with these criteria represent one of the most significant research advances in this area of psychopathology.

Revisions of the DSM-III criteria (7) (see Table 38.2) have recently been adopted and shall be the guiding definition for this chapter. For schizophrenic disorders, the changes are generally minimal: the one major alteration is that the age of onset criterion is no longer part of the definition.

A summary of differences from DSM-III is presented in Table 38.3. For professionals new to the field, careful study of the revised definition makes sense.

These definitions have had an important impact already. The percentage of psychiatric inpatients who meet the criteria for schizophrenic disorders is substantially lower than the 30 to 40% previously reported (8). Many patients may fit into other categories, particularly that of mood disorder, for which treatments are generally more effective and the prognosis is less pessimistic.

The focus on the course of schizophrenic disorder may be associated with a major reorientation away from viewing schizophrenic disorders almost exclusively in terms of their acute or florid psychotic symptoms toward greater awareness of the more chronic features and their associated impairments. And, because of its relatively recent adoption, many current concepts may be modified as research using DSM-III-R criteria expands.

One of the most important advances in the definition of schizophrenic disorders is the delineation of phases of the illness: *prodromal*, *active*, and *residual*. A prodromal

Table 38.2 DSM-III-R Criteria for Schizophrenia (1987)

A. Presence of characteristic psychotic symptoms in the active phase: Either (1), (2), or (3) for at least 1 week (unless the symptoms are successfully treated):
   (1) Two of the following:
      (a) delusions
      (b) prominent hallucinations (throughout the day for several days or several times a week for several weeks, each hallucinatory experience not being limited to a few brief moments)
      (c) incoherence or marked loosening of associations
      (d) catatonic behavior
      (e) flat or grossly inappropriate affect
   (2) Bizarre delusions (i.e., involving a phenomenon that the person's culture would regard as totally implausible, e.g., thought broadcasting, being controlled by a dead person)
   (3) Prominent hallucinations (as defined in [1b] above) of a voice with content having no apparent relation to depression or elation, or a voice keeping up a running commentary on the person's behavior or thoughts, or two or more voices conversing with each other
B. During the course of the disturbance, functioning in such areas as work, social relations, and self-care is markedly below the highest level achieved before onset of the disturbance (or, when the onset is in childhood or adolescence, failure to achieve expected level of social development).
C. Schizoaffective disorder and mood disorder with psychotic features have been ruled out, i.e., if a major depressive or manic syndrome has ever been present during an active phase of the disturbance, the total duration of all episodes of a mood syndrome has been brief relative to the total duration of the active and residual phases of the disturbance.
D. Continuous signs of the disturbance for at least 6 months. The 6-month period must include an active phase (of at least 1 week, or less if symptoms have been successfully treated) during which there were psychotic symptoms characteristic of schizophrenia (symptoms in A), with or without a prodromal or residual phase.
E. It cannot be established that an organic factor initiated and maintained the disturbance.
F. If there is a history of autistic disorder, the additional diagnosis of schizophrenia is made only if prominent delusions or hallucinations are also present.

Reprinted with permission from American Psychiatric Association: *Diagnostic and Statistical Manual of Mental Disorders (Third Edition-Revised)*. Washington, DC, American Psychiatric Association, 1987. Copyright 1987 American Psychiatric Association.

Table 38.3 Summary of Differences Between DSM-III and DSM-III-R Definitions

DSM-III	DSM-III-R
A. Only one active phase symptom required for 2 weeks	Several choices for the characteristic psychotic symptom for 1 week
B. Deterioration required	Less serious change in functional ability: that is, markedly below best premorbid achievement
C. Duration 6 months	Unchanged
D. Rule out affective disorders	Unchanged
E. Age criterion less than 45	Age criterion eliminated
F. Rule out organic disorder	Unchanged. Autistic disorder should be considered
Phases	
Prodromal, residual	An additional prodromal and residual feature: marked lack of initiative, interests, or energy
Active	Unchanged
Phenomenologic subtypes	The paranoid subtype is changed: specification of stable type when all exacerbations meet the criteria. Otherwise, unchanged

phase not due to a psychoactive substance abuse disorder may precede the active phase and is characterized by impaired social functioning, withdrawal, eccentric behavior, perceptual disturbances: but it does not usually include psychotic symptoms. The active phase is the phase of *psychotic features:* delusions, hallucinations, marked disturbances of affect, thinking, motor and volition. It is essential for this phase to have been present for the diagnosis to be applied. The residual phase follows the active phase and has the same features as the prodromal phase. The

Table 38.4   Phases of Schizophrenia (DSM-III-R)

Prodromal phase:	A clear deterioration in functioning before the active phase of the disturbance that is not due to a disturbance in mood or to a psychoactive substance use disorder and that involves at least two of the symptoms listed below.
Active phase:	See A(1), (2), (3) in Table 38.2.
Residual phase:	Following the active phase of the disturbance, persistence of at least two of the symptoms noted below, these not being due to a disturbance in mood or to a psychoactive substance use disorder.

Prodromal or residual symptoms:
   (1) marked social isolation or withdrawal
   (2) marked impairment in role functioning as wage-earner, student, or homemaker
   (3) markedly peculiar behavior (e.g., collecting garbage, talking to self in public, hoarding food)
   (4) marked impairment in personal hygiene and grooming
   (5) blunted or inappropriate affect
   (6) digressive, vague, overelaborate, or circumstantial speech, or poverty of content of speech
   (7) odd beliefs or magical thinking, influencing behavior and inconsistent with cultural norms, e.g., superstitiousness, belief in clairvoyance, telepathy, "sixth sense", "others can change my feelings", overvalued ideas, ideas of reference
   (8) unusual perceptual experiences, e.g., recurrent illusions, sensing the presence of a force or person not actually present
   (9) marked lack of initiative, interests, or energy

Reprinted with permission from American Psychiatric Association: *Diagnostic and Statistical Manual of Mental Disorders (Third Edition-Revised)*. Washington, DC, American Psychiatric Association, 1987. Copyright 1987 American Psychiatric Association.

phases are defined in more detail in Table 38.4. The strong tendency to consider schizophrenia as a condition characterized primarily by psychosis (i.e., active phase disorders) has blurred the reality that the prodromal and especially residual phases may be the most lengthy in the course of the illness.

EPIDEMIOLOGY

Schizophrenia occurs in all cultures and international rates of incidence and prevalence, though approximate, are generally consistent (see Table 38.5). The disorder is characterized by intermittent exacerbations of psychosis (active phase), but it is likely that most morbidity is concentrated in the residual phase. This characteristic is critical to understanding the value and benefits of treatment.

Table 38.5   Epidemiologic Features of Schizophrenic Disorders

Incidence:	20 cases/100,000 per year
Prevalence:	2–4 cases/1,000
Lifetime risk:	approximately 1%
Male/female ratio:	1:1
Onset before age 40:	approximately 80%

Although males may experience earlier onset and a possibly more severe course, women are affected in roughly equal numbers, with some tendency for increased incidence in the 5th and 6th decades.

DIAGNOSIS

There is no diagnostic laboratory test for schizophrenic disorder. To make the diagnosis, the clinician must match the features of the patient's history and examination to the DSM-III-R criteria. A period of at least 6 months of continuous signs of the illness, which must include an active phase with prominent psychotic symptoms and may or may not include a prodromal or residual phase, is essential for diagnosis.

The prodromal phase of the disorder varies greatly in duration and is characterized by social withdrawal, impaired work functioning or self-care, markedly peculiar behavior (e.g., collecting garbage or hoarding food), a blunted or inappropriate affect, digressive, vague, overelaborate, circumstantial, or metaphorical speech, odd or magical thinking (e.g., clairvoyance, telepathy, or "sixth sense"), unusual perceptual experience, and a lack of initiative, interest, or energy. We know little about this phase.

The active phase may involve a number of characteristic symptoms. For instance, a variety of delusions (false, irrefutable beliefs) may be present. Delusions of persecution such as being spied on or conspired against are common. Certain delusions, such as the belief that one's thoughts are broadcast from one's head so that others can hear them ("thought broadcasting"), that thoughts are inserted into one's mind ("thought insertion"), that thoughts are being removed from one's mind ("thought withdrawal"), or that feelings, impulses, actions, or thoughts are not one's own but are imposed from external sources ("delusion of influence or being controlled"), are more common in schizophrenia than in other psychotic disorders. Less commonly, delusions of a somatic, grandiose, nihilistic, or religious nature are observed. A range of disturbances in the form of thinking, from mild vagueness and perseveration to neologisms and incoherence, may be encountered. These disturbances are different from disorders in the content of thought (e.g., delusions). The most common type is loosening of associations, sometimes referred to as derailment, in which ideas shift from one topic to another in an unrelated or obliquely related manner at best. Patients may show no awareness that their speech is so disconnected. If severe, this type of disturbance may make the speech incomprehensible (incoherent). Another type is poverty of content of speech, in which speech is adequate in amount, but conveys little information because of its vagueness, repetitiousness, or concreteness. This disorder is recognized by noting that little information has been conveyed despite the fact that the patient has been speaking at some length. The major perceptual disturbance is hallucinations; the most common are auditory, but visual, tactile, olfactory, and gustatory hallucinations can occur, although less often. The voice may be single or multiple, familiar, or insulting and critical. Frequently the voice(s) may provide a running commentary on the patient's behavior. Other abnormalities include increased sensitivity to sound, sight, and smell, sensations of bodily changes, illusions, and synesthesias. A reduced intensity (bluntness or flatness) of affective expression and an expression not consistent with the content of speech ("inappropriate affect") are frequently present. Also common are reduced interest and motivation ("volitional disorder") for carrying out various courses of action to their conclusion. This feature is especially characteristic of the residual phase (cf. below). Motor disturbances such as marked clumsiness, stereotypic, manneristic, or disorganized movements, occasionally reaching extremes such as catatonic stupor and excitement, may also be observed. The sense of self, that which provides the normal person with a feeling of uniqueness, individuality, and self-direction, may be impaired.

The residual phase usually follows the active phase. Its clinical picture may be similar to that of the prodromal phase, with the possible addition of lingering delusions and hallucinations or more pronounced difficulties in role functioning, affect, and volition.

Accurate diagnosis is vital. The purpose of the diagnostic process is twofold: first, to determine whether often treatable organic factors or medical or psychiatric conditions might account for the presentation, and second, to provide a more complete picture of the physical, cognitive, emotional, and social status of the patient. Evaluation requires consideration of the onset, duration, variety, and severity of the symptoms, the course and impact of the illness on daily activities; premorbid functioning; family history; and past medical and psychiatric history (including licit and illicit drug and alcohol intake). Information from family and others who know the patient is often more reliable than that provided by the patient. Physical, neurologic, and mental status examinations and laboratory studies are always required. For the latter, drug toxicology screens, electrolytes, liver function, blood count, serology, and endocrine examinations as well as routine electroencephalography are generally required. Computerized tomography and brain electrical activity mapping make sense to rule out space-occupying lesions and physiologic abnormality and to establish a baseline record of anatomic and electrophysiologic activity. Psychometric examination of intelligence (e.g., Wechsler Adult Intelligence Scale) and personality (e.g., Minnesota Multiphasic Personality Inventory) may also be valuable. Neuropsychologic testing focusing on cognitive functions can provide useful information for understanding deficiencies and strengths in mental abilities. This data can assist in diagnosis and in rehabilitation.

The diagnostic process must go beyond mere labeling to include assessment of educational and related competencies (e.g., reading and writing, high school or college diploma), vocational skills and interests, socialization, financial support, family's understanding and tolerance, and the patient's view of the illness (9). Following diagnosis, recommendations should be made for drug treatment and for measures to reestablish ability to function on the job, at school, and at home.

DIFFERENTIAL DIAGNOSIS

Careful differential diagnosis is essential; it is well known that many diseases mimic features of the active phase and even residual schizophrenic disorder. Moreover, no single feature of schizophrenia is unique to this illness (10). Overemphasis on dramatic symptoms can result in an inappropriate diagnosis. On the other hand, certain symptoms appear to be highly discriminating, particularly thought insertion, thought broadcasting, thought withdrawal, delusions of control, and certain types of auditory hallucinations (11).

Because there are so many conditions to consider, and because schizophrenic disorders should only be diagnosed when other conditions are excluded, the diagnostic process can appear overwhelming. Certain principles can simplify the diagnostician's task. The first is that there are only a few life-threatening disorders to consider (Table 38.6). Second, there are a host of disorders that have been reported

Table 38.6   Acute Potentially Life-Threatening Conditions to Differentiate from Schizophrenic Disorders

Delirium
Anticholinergic poisoning
Steroid poisoning
Hypoglycemia
Meningitis
Organic delusional syndrome
Others, including Wernicke-Korsakoff syndrome, hypertensive encephalopathy, carbon monoxide poisoning, intracranial hemorrhage, and subdural hematoma

to produce illnesses similar to schizophrenia; yet many are rare or uncommon. Most are relatively easy to rule out. Third, the diagnosis of schizophrenia is ultimately never secure. It should be made humbly and remain open to revision.

Organic mental disorders often present with features that suggest a schizophrenic disorder. For example, phencyclidine, cocaine, or amphetamine intoxication may induce a similar clinical condition (organic delusional syndrome). The presence of disorientation; memory impairment; visual and other types of hallucinations in the absence of auditory hallucinations; abrupt changes in mental state, mood, or personality; and failure to respond to treatment should spur the search for organic causes. Certain less acute conditions may produce features similar to active and residual phases of schizophrenia (see Table 38.7). These conditions can generally be ruled out with the strategy of assessments outlined above. The biggest obstacle to their diagnosis is considering them in the first place.

Table 38.7   Subacute/Chronic Conditions to Differentiate from Schizophrenic Disorders

TLE (complex partial seizure disorder)
Dementia
Hepatic encephalopathy
Brain tumors (particularly frontal and temporal lobes
Others, including porphyria, posterior aphasia, thyroid disease, narcolepsy, systemic lupus erythematosus, Huntington's chorea, Gilles de la Tourette disorder, renal failure, acquired immune deficiency syndrome

Other psychiatric disorders (Table 38.8) must also be excluded, especially mood disorders (manic and psychotic depressive disorders) and schizoaffective disorders; delusional disorders in which prominent hallucinations, incoherence, or bizarre delusions are absent; and schizophreniform disorders, which, by definition, have a duration of less than 6 months and in which prognosis is generally more favorable. Mental retardation, certain personality disorders (especially schizotypal and paranoid), and factitious conditions must also be considered. In autistic disorder there are disturbances in communication and in affect that suggest schizophrenic illness; however, the latter diagnosis is warranted only if prominent hallucinations or delusions are also present.

ETIOLOGY

The etiology of schizophrenic disorders remains obscure. Nevertheless, evidence from clinical, genetic, epidemiologic, and biochemical sciences is consistent with the concept that schizophrenia is a disease. A variety of diseases may mimic schizophrenia, particularly the psychoses associated with brain disease, especially temporal lobe epilepsy (12), intoxication disorders (e.g., amphetamine, cocaine, and phencyclidine) (13–15), and metabolic illnesses

Table 38.8 Psychiatric Conditions to Differentiate from Schizophrenic Disorders

Mania
Depression
Personality disorder—borderline personality
 schizotypal, schizoid, paranoid personality
Alcohol intoxication
Drug intoxication (phencyclidine, amphetamines,
 mescaline, lysergic acid diethylamide, bromides,
 cocaine, marijuana)
Drug withdrawal
Chronic auditory hallucinosis
Delusional (paranoid) disorders
Schizoaffective disorders
Schizophreniform disorder
Atypical psychosis
Brief reactive psychosis, factitious disorder,
 malingering, pervasive developmental disorder,
 obsessive–compulsive disorder

(e.g., porphyria) (16). Reports of electrodermal dysfunction, electroencephalographic evoked response changes, regional cerebral blood flow activity differences, position emission tomography differences, neurologic signs, motor abnormalities, smooth-pursuit eye tracking and optokinetic nystagmus disturbances, and radiographic evidence of anatomic abnormalities have strengthened the view that schizophrenic disorder is a disease (17).

Consistent with that concept is the observation that whereas the lifetime risk of schizophrenic disorders in the general population is about 1%, genetic studies indicate that the risk increases with the degree of biological relatedness to an affected family member (18, 19). Risk is adjusted up or down in order to reflect the number of relatives affected, the severity, and the age at onset of the illness. The mode of transmission is unclear. Monogenic (autosomal dominance with reduced penetrance) and polygenic theories appear to be partly supported by available evidence. Yet, large numbers of schizophrenic patients have no identifiable family members with the disorder. Moreover, although data from twin studies indicate genetic influence, environmental factors also contribute; about half the monozygotic twin pairs are concordant for schizophrenia. Studies of adopted persons provide the strongest evidence for genetic involvement, as they were designed to separate genetic and environmental influences. These studies showed that adopted children of schizophrenic parents have higher incidence of schizophrenia than adopted controls of normal parents. The biologic relatives of schizophrenic adopted children are more likely to be schizophrenic than those of normal adopted children. Normal children adopted by schizophrenic parents do not have increased rates of schizophrenia.

While the disease concept appears robust, it is generally believed that some of the variability in course is a function of circumstances and life events. Specification of environmental factors relevant to the development of schizophrenia remains limited, however. Studies of social class demonstrate a disproportionate rate of schizophrenia in lower class families that cannot be accounted for solely in terms of a downward social drift among schizophrenics (20). This work has stimulated investigations of stressful life events which occur at increased rates prior to episodes of acute psychosis. The study of family relationships (e.g., the "doublebind," "marital skew," and "schizophrenogenic" mother) has also been voluminous, but though it appears that families of schizophrenics have a wide range of deviances, the direction of causal influence is unclear. Some studies suggest that parental difficulties may be the result of living with disturbed children rather than the more popular view that parents' problems promote maladjustment in their offspring (21).

Recent interest has focused on several independent observations that the dates of birth of schizophrenics are more concentrated in the late winter and early spring months. The significance of these findings is unclear, but it may be that certain relevant obstetrical complications (e.g., infections) have a seasonal incidence.

Meanwhile, the study of biochemical aspects of schizophrenia has been influenced by new advances in neurosciences and by increased attempts to relate clinical to neurobiologic features. The hypothesis that certain central dopaminergic systems may be overactive in schizophrenia remains the main beacon for current investigation (22, 23). The consistent antidopamine effects of available antipsychotic drugs (phenothiazines, butyrophenones, thioxanthenes, dibenzoxazepines, and dihydroindolones) and the psychotic effects of dopamine-stimulating drugs such as amphetamine have supported this view. Antipsychotic drugs may work on the basis of dopamine receptor antagonism, or time-delayed dopamine neuronal changes, particularly in the mesolimbic dopamine system. Yet, the biology is far from simple to investigate; other neurochemical systems (e.g., acetylcholine, γ-aminobutyric acid) appear to influence dopamine transmission. There are several dopamine systems (e.g., mesocor-

tical, mesolimbic), and they do not respond to neuroleptics in precisely the same manner. Moreover, it is unclear whether overactivity results from changes in dopamine receptors or presynaptic activity. Estimates of dopamine turnover, gained from study of the dopamine metabolite homovanillic acid in cerebrospinal fluid, show no increase in schizophrenics. Because in vivo studies pose major methodologic barriers, researchers have carried out postmortem neurochemical studies in psychotic patients. Nor have these studies established that dopamine neurons are overactive in schizophrenia; but they indicate that dopamine receptors are increased, possibly as a result of chronic drug administration. Subtypes of dopamine receptor have been distinguished through radioimmunoassay techniques (24, 25), and some research has pointed to increased dopamine (D2) receptors in drug-naive schizophrenics (26). Because growth hormone and prolactin re partially regulated by central dopamine neurons and can be measured in the blood, neuroendocrine studies may help unravel these complex relationships.

Nevertheless, the connection between dopamine and the clinical phenomena of schizophrenia is not clear. The fact that antipsychotic drugs are useful in the treatment of affective, drug-induced, and organic psychoses suggests that dopamine disturbances are not unique to schizophrenia. Certainly the "positive" symptoms of active phase schizophrenia (delusions, hallucinations, derailed thinking) are responsive to these agents. Yet, interestingly, the "negative" symptoms (flat affect, loss of drive, impoverished thought) are probably little affected by drugs; because of their association with intellectual changes and increased ventricular size, these symptoms may represent a subtype of schizophrenic disorder (27).

Despite reports of low platelet monoamine oxidase (MAO) activity in schizophrenic disorder, current evidence suggests that MAO biochemistry is more complex than previously believed and that MAO changes may be associated with vulnerability to a number of chronic disorders, including alcoholism. The discovery of endorphins and endorphinlike compounds has not led as yet to major insights regarding schizophrenic pathophysiology. Other interesting leads include the possibility of a slow virus or viral-like infection etiology, the association of increased creatine kinase with psychosis, and the possible roles of human leukocyte A (HLA) antigens and endogenously formed hallucinogens.

Investigations of cognitive deficiency in schizophrenics suggest several loci of information processing disturbance occur in this disorder, including operations associated with short-term memory and selective attention. A major focus of this work is disturbed linguistic performance (thought disorder) which schizophrenics frequently exhibit, despite their appropriate use of syntax and general competence as speakers. The fact that irrelevant associations tend to occur at terminal points of utterances (periods and clausal boundaries) may represent a failure of selective attention in inhibiting the intrusions of distractions. The density of repetitiousness in schizophrenic speech and movement also suggests a common pathogenic factor that operates to maintain the patient in "the same circle of ideas," as Bleuler put it (4, 28, 29).

Studies of neuropathology, long dormant, now enjoy new enthusiasm. Published reports indicate a variety of postmortem changes in the brain of schizophrenic patients. Periventricular pathology of a nonspecific type had been described by several investigators, and a number of studies have implicated specific limbic and diencephalic structures. Whether these changes are the cause of, the result of, or a coincidence with the illness is not determined.

Computed tomographic (CT) studies of the brains of schizophrenic patients point to a consistent pattern of findings, many made earlier in this century with pneumoencephalography. These include enlargement of the lateral and third ventricles and signs of cortical atrophy. The findings

are present in a proportion of schizophrenic patients, perhaps as much as 40%. Other features, such as cerebellar vermis atrophy and reversed neuroanatomic asymmetries, have also been reported, but less firmly. These findings are nonspecific; they indicate that a neuropathologic process involving reduced brain mass is associated with the diagnosis of schizophrenia. The cause of these changes is also unknown, but they are not thought to be the result of neuroleptic therapy. They appear to be present early in the illness, and to neither progress nor reverse. They also appear to be associated with increased deficit or negative symptom patterns (loss of volition, impoverished thought), poor premorbid adjustment, poorer prognosis, and poor response to neuroleptics. These observations, though intriguing, are in the realm of research and do not provide assistance in the diagnosis of schizophrenia or in attempts to predict outcome or response to treatment in individual cases.

Although research is promising, the hope of discovering a biochemical origin or marker, a unique cognitive deficit, a common neuropathologic lesion, a distinctive psychophysiologic test, or any assessment technique more objective than the DSM-III-R criteria remains unfulfilled. Evidence for brain dysfunction (especially in frontal areas) and structural changes are changing the prospects for clarification of the nature of these disorders.

COURSE AND PROGNOSIS

The age at onset varies, usually occurring during adolescence or early adulthood. Nevertheless, the disorder may begin in middle or late adult life. Many studies suggest an earlier onset and a possibly more severe course in males than in females.

The course of schizophrenic disorders varies greatly, but recurrent episodes of active psychosis and persistent impairment are common (Table 38.9). The vulnerability to relapse is also reflected in difficulty in handling anxiety, a relative lack of emotional maturity and experience

Table 38.9   Course of Schizophrenic
Disorders

Variable
25% will experience improvement in social functioning.
25% will remain ill, often severely so, with mental as well as social impairment.
50% will be subjected to intermittent, recurrent disturbances and a range of residual features.

compared to peers, social isolation, cognitive inefficiency, and increased suicide risk. Ten percent of schizophrenics die by their own hands. As many as 40% of schizophrenic patients will attempt suicide. Because these risks are not well known, education about them is important. The clinician must be vigilant to recognize potential suicidal behavior. The reasons for such behavior include the desperation of awareness of the illness, depressed mood, and a variety of psychosis related behaviors such as responses to auditory hallucinations that berate, criticize, or even encourage self-destruction. Other factors still not well understood may operate as well, such as isolation, life events, and delusional thinking.

Schizophrenic patients may have much to be depressed about, yet are no less at risk than the rest of the population for depressive illness and generally have less capacity to adapt to intense changes in affective response. Clinically diagnosable depression therefore can complicate the course of the illness but subclinical depressive changes can disturb the patient's functioning dramatically.

Closely associated with depressed mood are other characteristics that complicate the course of schizophrenic patients. Drug and alcohol abuse, another form of serious self-destructive behavior, are common and can lead to diagnosable disorders as well as to major exacerbations of active psychosis. Poor hygiene, reduced nutritional intake, and a tendency to ignore infectious disease add to the list of serious complications.

Residual impairments fall into two main groups which often overlap, have varying degrees of severity, and may fluctuate widely. One group consists of symptoms associated with active psychosis, including the disabling effects of incoherence and unpredictable associations in speech, chronic delusions, and hallucinations. The other group consists of apathy, lack of ambition (volitional disorder), slowed, impoverished thought, underactivity, and withdrawal. While both groups are disabling, the second group, not surprisingly, is especially associated with poor social performance. Schizophrenic patients are frequently unemployable, less likely to be skilled or highly trained, and more likely than peers to lose jobs if they have them. They are most often single, frequently live with aging parents, and have few friends or intimate relationships. Indeed, a lack of trusting relationships is common and in the extreme leads to more pronounced withdrawal and isolation from other people. These individuals constitute a major proportion of the homeless population.

Prognosis has improved, largely as a result of the benefits of antipsychotic medication in alleviating and preventing episodes of active psychosis. Full recovery is uncommon and usually occurs within the first two years; after 5 years of illness, few recover. Some long-term studies suggest that residual symptoms attenuate with time and that a positive outcome is more common than previously thought. Definitions of recovery vary, and this makes generalizations difficult. Factors assisting in predicting outcome are not clearly understood and provide estimates at best (Table 38.10). Social recovery, de-

Table 38.10   Factors Affecting Outcome

Somewhat More Favorable	Somewhat Less Favorable
Acute onset	Insidious onset
Normal premorbid status	Premorbid abnormalities ? personality disorder
Social atmosphere of relatively lower expressed emotion	Higher expressed emotion
Later age of onset	Earlier age of onset
Female	Male
Marriage	Drug, alcohol abuse
Illness experienced in developing countries	Illness experienced in industrialized countries

fined usually as ability to function outside the hospital, takes many forms. Some patients may need supervised housing; others may live independently and require only infrequent psychiatric attention. Cultural factors, perhaps greater tolerance and less social pressure, may influence outcome; a more benign course has been associated with cases occurring in nonindustrialized countries (11, 30). Certainly, personal and social reactions to the illness have impact on the self-esteem and status of the patient in a way that may enhance or worsen chances of recovery. The social effects of schizophrenic disorder are devastating. Its consequences, in terms of individual productivity, family stability, and the use of social and health services, not to mention personal tragedy and suffering, are monumental.

TREATMENT

During the 1950s, nearly half of U.S. hospital beds were filled with patients suffering from a disorder labeled schizophrenia. Lengths of stay in excess of 6 months were common. This picture began to change dramatically with the advent of antipsychotic drug treatment which rapidly became the foundation of therapy of schizophrenic disorder and hospital stays came down to several weeks. Other treatments such as insulin coma, psychosurgery of the frontal lobe, and related procedures are no longer considered useful. Although electroconvulsive therapy is effective in some cases, it has fallen out of fashion in part because of poor acceptance and to a limited literature on its efficacy compared to drugs.

It is no longer practical to speak of the treatment of schizophrenia without specifying whether the focus is the active (i.e., psychotic) or residual phase or the liability to relapse, associated with the chronic illness (see Table 38.11). Antipsychotic medications are particularly successful in improving symptoms associated with the active phase, including hallucinations, verbal incomprehensibility, delusions, agitation, perplexity, insomnia, and anxiety

(31). Patients receiving maintenance antipsychotic medication relapse less often than those treated with placebo. Moreover, the prophylactic value of antipsychotic drugs may be enhanced with counseling and rehabilitative interventions (32).

Yet, the limitations of antipsychotic drugs are also apparent. For example, many patients recover from the active phase of illness but do not satisfactorily readjust to the demands of their previous routine. Residual symptoms, subtle deficiencies in cognitive and motor performance, and affective response, may simply be refractory to these agents. The reasons why many patients (up to 30% or more) fail to relapse while taking placebo also remain unclear. Attempts to distinguish particular subgroups of schizophrenic patients on the basis of drug responsiveness have been unsuccessful. Yet one series of investigations indicates that the effectiveness of maintenance medication may be influenced by social environment. In living situations (at home or in an institution) characterized by low levels of expressed emotion, relapse rates appear to be low, at least in the short run, regardless of medication treatment. In environments with high levels of expressed emotion, drugs exert a preventive effect only to an extent and relapse can occur even during treatment (33). These observations have formed the basis for family-based behavioral treatment intervention, now shown to be useful in preventing relapse in several independent studies. (32, 34).

Another limitation in the use of antipsychotic medications are their multiple and frequent side effects, notably the extrapyramidal disturbances and tardive dyskinesia. The latter remains only partially understood: Some evidence indicates that

Table 38.11   Phase-Related Treatment Issues

Prodromal—careful evaluation, follow-up
Active—management and alleviation of psychotic
  features, thorough diagnostic workup
Residual—prevention of relapse, rehabilitation,
  maintenance of sound medical care

it is related to aging and the disease process as well as exposure to medication. In any case, it is difficult to treat. For younger patients who possibly face years of treatment, these risks pose particular concern. Compliance problems often prompt the use of newer high potency intramuscular depot medications (e.g., haloperidol decanoate and fluphenazine enanthate and decanoate). These drugs are convenient and useful, but like oral preparations should be administered with clear guidelines for monitoring efficacy and for discontinuation.

Although research on psychotherapy of schizophrenia is blossoming, especially in family-based approaches, to offer traditional psychotherapy as the only treatment in schizophrenic disorder is generally regarded as inadequate and possibly negligent. On the other hand, the value of the doctor–patient relationship is as critical to treatment success as anywhere in medicine. Its aims are monitoring the course of illness, encouraging social relations, developing interests, maintaining employment, and helping the patient and family to understand the illness (35). Frequently this dimension of treatment takes the form of counseling and directive therapy.

Various social rehabilitation therapies (e.g., anxiety management, day treatment, skills development, sheltered workshops for vocational training) have demonstrated some value in assisting readjustment outside hospital. These aim to provide satisfaction from social and occupational activity as well as to prevent or curb apathy, anxiety, and frustration with which are associated isolation, withdrawal, and potential relapse. Behavioral treatments, based on learning theory, have enjoyed some success in schizophrenia and often are the main applied science in rehabilitative efforts (36). The theory suggests that whatever the origin of the appearance of abnormal behavior, its maintenance is affected by the external environment. Because external environmental factors can be changed, abnormal behavior can also be modified. Numerous techniques (e.g., shaping, generalization, extinction) have been applied following careful analysis of the antecedents and consequences of the relevant maladapted behavior.

There has been a decreased amount of hospitalization in the treatment of schizophrenic disorders. Hospitalization may still be useful for the short-term evaluation and treatment of active psychosis. However, relatively few patients are now institutionalized chronically. Controversy about deinstitutionalization of patients is partially the consequence of inadequate treatment programs outside the hospital and the naive theory that less restrictive environments reduce chronicity in mental illness. Institutional life, provided without care or thought for its consequences, may create problems for patients, since it can be associated with boredom, neglect, withdrawal, isolation, lack of spontaneity, and generally socially maladaptive behavior; the effect may be perpetuation or worsening of the illness (30). However, inappropriate discharge to the community for those lacking minimal social competence may be equally disastrous.

The focus of treatment outside hospital is to prevent relapse and enhance or maintain adjustment. The most difficult management problem is the tendency to stop taking medication, leading to relapse and often readmission to hospital. Improving personal hygiene and self-awareness, reducing the impact of diagnosis on employability, and assuaging the family's guilt are critical treatment issues. But there are other problems. For example, schizophrenic patients receive less than optimal medical care generally, in part because of reluctance to use services, inability to express specific complaints clearly, and the tendency of health professionals to attribute vague somatic complaints to psychopathology. The practitioner may be able to play a key role by anticipating these difficulties. The problems are vital: Schizophrenic patients on the average are more likely to die at an early age and may be more likely to die of the complications of routine medical illness (37).

Professional intervention early in the course of the disorder can reduce the uncertainty, guilt, and embarrassment experienced by patient and family. With skill and with the support of family or those who live with the patient, recurrent active phase episodes can be minimized and better adjustment achieved. In milder cases especially, specialist backup is enough to permit the general physician or nonpsychiatrist to manage the case. It is essential, however, to be aware that the patient has a complex disorder with multiple psychologic and social problems, that medications alone are generally not sufficient therapy, and that it is common for families to become discouraged and frustrated, no matter how sophisticated the care. It should be noted that much of the therapeutic work in schizophrenia is painstaking and laborious (35). Psychiatrists often coordinate the services of other professionals (social workers, clinical nurse specialists, vocational counselors, behavioral therapists, family counselors, etc.) to provide programs that meet the multiple needs of their patients and share the responsibilities (and burdens) of care.

PREVENTION

Genetic counseling is a potential preventive tool. However, our understanding of genetic risk and psychopathology remain imprecise because the mode of transmission of schizophrenia is not known. This fact in itself is enough to warrant caution in counseling would-be parents affected by these disorders (18). At present prevention must be directed largely to known cases; hence the most important preventive measures are early diagnosis and attempts to reduce risk factors (sources of severe anxiety, intercurrent medical illness, drug and alcohol abuse, poor social adjustment, etc.) that are likely to increase morbidity and mortality.

THE CLINICAL INTERVIEW

Determining the Nature of the Problem

The fundamental task in the initial assessment of the patient is to ensure an accurate diagnosis. The best guide to this diagnosis is the DSM-III-R criteria. In particular, these criteria place major emphasis on excluding alternative diagnoses. The requirement for this task is to be organized and aware of the differential diagnostic process and to put the patient at ease. If the clinician has a clear strategy, he or she can comfortably examine the patient and remain able to hear the patient's story as well as collect data relevant to the diagnostic process. Ideally, the patient may become a collaborator, collecting information relevant to diagnosis as well as establishing a relationship with the clinician. The keys to differential diagnosis have been presented in an earlier section of this chapter.

To establish a working base of information from the patient requires attending first to the patient's concerns. What is the complaint? The worry? The hope? Patients who have psychotic disorders in general are unlikely to understand the depth of their psychopathology and may even deny its presence. If they present with paranoid features, they may be remarkably humorless and unspontaneous. On the other hand, such patients may be intensely emotional and provocative. In short, they can test the skills of the most seasoned among us.

To get a sense of the nature of the psychopathology, it is often useful for clinicians to listen to the patient as they would the "man on the street," rather than trying to interpret associations and other features of the patient's behavior—in other words, to simply listen carefully. Clinicians should follow the logic of what is said and explore the phenomenology of the psychopathology in some detail, including, for example, detailed descriptions of hallucinations and affective responses.

One of the key problems in assessing psychopathology and in making a diagnosis of schizophrenic disorders is the clinical information gap. Because patients are frightened, cognitively disabled, paranoid, or simply unknowing, the information required for a careful and accurate assessment may simply be unattainable.

Certainly objective examination and mental status testing can provide useful data, but as in most areas of medicine, the diagnosis rests fundamentally on the history. Hence, the need to draw on other sources of information, especially from those people who live or are with the patient.

Developing and Maintaining a Therapeutic Relationship

Perhaps the most important principle in developing and maintaining a therapeutic relationship with a patient is to convey a sense of caring and concern. At the same time, appropriate distance is necessary in accomplishing this goal. Confrontational tactics with psychotic patients rarely work. To have the patient feel comfortable and able to express concerns is no easy task. It requires judicious use of many therapeutic skills. It may also require the effective use of humor. Fundamentally, caring is expressed or is most successful when it is focused around the specific concerns that a patient brings to the clinic. The patient's lack of insight is a potential problem in maintaining the therapeutic relationship. It is probably wiser to develop a collaborative relationship with the patient until a true alliance results. A collaborative relationship means that the patient comes to believe in the shared goals of the professional consultation, namely, to alleviate suffering, pain, and the other forces that create the complaints that the patient has in the first place.

Communication of Information and Implementation of a Treatment Plan

It is essential to maintain good communication throughout the diagnostic process. Concretely, the diagnostic process should be explained in its entirety to the patient and others who are involved in the diagnostic process. An explanation of the particular procedures for further testing, the reasons that a detailed history are required, the process of integrating the information and educating the patient as well the nature of the questions being asked, all constitute the basis for effective communication and the foundation for implementing a treatment plan. In effect, treatment begins with the diagnostic process and the channels of communication which are opened in that process become the channels of communication for the initiation, continuation, and the long-term planning of treatment.

It is useful to keep the patient informed about the progress of the diagnostic process as the evaluation proceeds. As hypotheses are entertained and discarded on the basis of accumulated evidence, the patient should be informed. If the diagnosis does go in the direction of schizophrenic disorders, the clinician should carefully inform the patient. As noted above, a professional approach to diagnosis in this disorder is to be open about diagnostic conclusions; therefore, the patient should be told that this diagnosis is not written in stone and that it may be modified in light of additional information that can be gathered. This serves the purpose of keeping the patient involved in the diagnostic process while providing some closure so that treatment can proceed. Should the diagnosis be given to the patient? In most cases, the patient should be informed about the diagnosis. Occasionally, a variety of reasons may make that decision problematic. The diagnosis is an important step in giving the patient and family the information required to plan and support further action. Leaving matters vague (i.e., not supplying a diagnosis or giving an uninformative one) is as bad as making an incorrect diagnosis.

There is perhaps no other condition in psychiatry in which it is more important to involve family members and other close relations in treatment planning. Sometimes, of course, this is not possible because of feuds, distance, or lack of family that may influence the situation. But where at all possible, the family can be both a great resource and strength to the patient and can help make possible optimal and effective implementation of treatment. Patients with schizophrenic disorders are among the disenfranchised politically and economically. In recent years, various groups, such as the Alliance for the Mentally Ill, have focused efforts on improving institutional care and support for patients with severe and chronic mental illnesses. The efforts of this organization and others like it are to be applauded. Family members with individuals who suffer from schizophrenic disorders may find involvement with such groups to be a productive and satisfying activity to counter some of the helplessness and frustration associated with the illness. The use of various books and pamphlets that are available for the lay public can also be of some help in providing additional information and knowledge about these conditions. In general, an attitude of active encouragement, and clear provision of information on the part of the clinician are sound approaches. Reducing the alienation and isolation of family members promotes the cause of the patient.

SUMMARY

Schizophrenic disorders is a serious illness that continues to elude simple solutions. Contemporary criteria have enhanced our ability to identify cases and have also established a basis for much-needed research. Nevertheless, understanding of the nature of schizophrenic disorders remains crude, and ability to treat them successfully remains limited. A rational approach encompassing accurate diagnosis, control of symptoms, and careful planning for what may be long-term treatment, is fundamental to effective intervention.

References

1. American Psychiatric Association: *Diagnostic and Statistical Manual of Mental Disorders (Third Edition)*. Washington, DC, American Psychiatric Association, 1980.
2. Pope HG, Lipinski JF: Diagnosis in schizophrenic and manic–depressive illness. *Arch Gen Psychiatry* 35:811–828, 1978.
3. World Health Organization: *The International Pilot Study of Schizophrenia*. Geneva, World Health Organization, 1973.
4. Bleuler E: *Dementia Praecox or the Group of Schizophrenias*. New York, International Universities Press, 1950.
5. American Psychiatric Association: *Diagnostic and Statistical Manual of Mental Disorders (Second Edition)*. Washington, DC, American Psychiatric Association, 1968.
6. Carpenter WT Jr, Strauss JJ, Carpenter CC, et al: Another view of schizophrenic subtypes. *Arch Gen Psychiatry* 33:508–516, 1976.
7. American Psychiatric Association: *Diagnostic and Statistical Manual of Mental Disorders (Third Edition-Revised)*. Washington, DC, American Psychiatric Association, 1987.
8. Taylor MA, Abrams R: The prevalence of schizophrenia: a reassessment using modern diagnostic criteria. *Am J Psychiatry* 135:945–948, 1978.
9. Kleinman AM: Recognition and management of illness problems: therapeutic recommendations from clinical social science. In Manschreck T, et al (eds): *Psychiatric Medicine Update: Massachusetts General Hospital Reviews for Physicians*. New York, Elsevier North-Holland, 1979, pp 23–32.
10. Fish F: *Schizophrenia*. Bristol, John Wright, 1976.
11. World Health Organization: *The International Pilot Study of Schizophrenia*. Geneva, World Health Organization, 1973.
12. Davison K, Bagley CR: Schizophrenia-like psychoses associated with organic disorders of the central nervous system: a review of the literature. In Herrington RN (ed): *Current Problems in Neuropsychiatry*. Ashford, England, Healey Press, 1969.
13. Ellinwood EH: Amphetamine psychosis I: Description of the individuals and process. *J Nerv Ment Dis* 144:273–283, 1967.
14. Manschreck TC, Laughery J, Weisstein C, et al: Characteristics of freebase cocaine psychosis. *Yale Journal of Biology and Medicine*, 61:115–122, 1988.
15. Allen RM, Young SJ: Phencyclidine-induced psychosis. *Am J Psychiatry* 135:1081–1084, 1978.
16. Reid AA: Schizophrenia—disease or syndrome? *Arch Gen Psychiatry* 28:863–869, 1973.
17. Nasrallah HA, Weinberger DR (eds): *The Neurology of Schizophrenia*. Amsterdam, Elsevier, 1986.
18. Tsuang MT, Vandermay R: *Genes and the Mind: Inheritance of Mental Illness*. New York, Oxford University Press, 1980.
19. Kendler KS: Genetics of schizophrenia. In Frances AJ, Hales RE (eds): *Psychiatry Update: American Psychiatric Association Annual Review*. Washington, DC, American Psychiatric Press, 1986, vol 5, pp 25–41.
20. Neale JM, Oltmanns TF: *Schizophrenia*. New York, John Wiley and Sons, 1980.
21. Hirsch SR, Leff JP: *Abnormalities in Parents of Schizophrenics*. London, Oxford University Press, 1975.
22. Meltzer HY, Stahl SM: The dopamine hypothesis of schizophrenia. *Schizophr Bull* 2:19–76, 1976.
23. Pickar D: Neuroleptics, dopamine and schizophrenia. *Psychiatr Clin North Am* 9:35–48, 1986.
24. Snyder SH: Dopamine receptor, neuroleptics,

and schizophrenia. *Am J Psychiatry* 138:460–464, 1981.

25. Weinberger DR, Kleinman JE: Observations on the brain in schizophrenia. In Frances AJ, Hales RE (eds): *Psychiatry Update: American Psychiatric Association Annual Review.* Washington, DC, American Psychiatric Press, 1986, vol 5, pp 42–67.

26. Wong DF, Wagner HN, Tune LE, et al: Positron emission tomography reveals elevated D_2 dopamine receptors in drug-naive schizophrenics. *Science* 234:1558–1563, 1987.

27. Crow TJ: Molecular pathology of schizophrenia: more than one disease process? *Br Med J* 280:6668, 1980.

28. Maher BA: The language of schizophrenia: a review and interpretation. *Br J Psychiatry* 120:3–17, 1972.

29. Manschreck TC: Motor and cognitive disturbances in schizophrenic disorders. In Schulz SC, Tamminga C (eds): *Schizophrenia: A Scientific Focus.* New York, Oxford University Press, in press.

30. Wing JK: *Reasoning About Madness.* New York, Oxford University Press, 1978.

31. National Institute of Mental Health, 1964 Collaborative Study Group: Phenothiazine treatment in acute schizophrenia: effectiveness. *Arch Gen Psychiatry* 10:246–261, 1964.

32. Falloon IRH, Boyd JL, McGill CW, et al: Family management in the prevention of exacerbation of schizophrenia: a controlled study. *N Engl J Med* 306:1437–1440, 1982.

33. Vaughn CC, Leff JP: The influence of family and social factors on the course of psychiatric illness: a comparison of schizophrenic and depressed neurotic patients. *Br J Psychiatry* 129:125–137, 1976.

34. Leff S, Kuipers L, Berkowitz R, et al: A controlled trial of social intervention in the families of schizophrenic patients. *Br J Psychiatry* 141:121–134, 1982.

35. Mendel WM: *Schizophrenia: The Experience and its Treatment.* San Francisco, Jossey-Bass, 1976.

36. Liberman RP: Behavioral modification of schizophrenia: a review. *Schizophr Bull* 6:37–48, 1972.

37. Tsuang MT, Woolson RF, Fleming JA: Premature deaths in schizophrenia and affective disorders. *Arch Gen Psychiatry* 37:979–983, 1980.

39

The Paranoid Syndrome and Delusional (Paranoid) Disorders

Theo C. Manschreck, M.D.

Paranoid features, including delusions, are common and cardinal manifestations of severe psychopathology. It is now well known that paranoid characteristics are nonspecific. That is, they arise in multiple medical and psychiatric diseases and certainly are not limited to schizophrenic or delusional disorders. Indeed, the list of reported clinical conditions associated with paranoid behavior is growing. The psychiatric diagnostician must launch a thorough assessment.

"Delusional disorders" is the new designation for a group of clinical conditions of unknown etiology whose cardinal feature is the delusion. In these conditions, the source of the delusion cannot be attributed to other organic or psychiatric disorders. The critical task in diagnosing these disorders is to rule out alternative disorders. In short, the task is to know and carry out the differential diagnosis of paranoid features.

The first portion of this chapter shall be devoted to a discussion of paranoid features, including their recognition, appropriate assessment, and differential diagnosis. The second portion is devoted to a discussion of delusional disorders.

THE PARANOID SYNDROME AND CLARIFICATION OF THE PARANOID CONCEPT

Paranoid features (signs and symptoms) are among the most serious disturbances in psychiatry. Nevertheless, the term "paranoid" refers to a *variety of behaviors* that are often not psychopathologic and are not necessarily related to schizophrenia. Unfortunately, the use of the word has become so varied that its meaning has become obscure. Some label ordinary suspiciousness paranoid. Others restrict its use to persecutory delusions, and yet others apply it to grandiose, hostile, litigious, and jealous behavior, despite the fact that all of these may be within the normal spectrum. Clearly, "paranoid" describes or refers to a plethora of behaviors.

To make the paranoid concept more clinically useful and less confusing requires consideration of several points. First, the paranoid concept is a clinical construct and is therefore used to interpret observations. To apply it effectively, the clinician must know the meaning of this concept and be able to make accurate observations of potentially paranoid features. Second, the

Table 39.1 Paranoid Features

Objective features	
Anger	Hypersensitivity
Sullenness	Defensiveness
Hate	Resentment
Suspiciousness	Irritability, quick annoyance
Critical, accusatory behavior	Inordinate attention to small
Self-righteousness	details
Guardedness, evasiveness	Humorlessness
Grandiosity or excessive	Litigiousness (letter writing,
self-importance	complaints, legal action)
Hostility	Violence, aggressiveness
Obstinance	Seclusiveness

Subjective features[a]

Overvalued ideas; delusions of self-reference, persecution, grandeur, infidelity, love, jealousy, imposture, infestation, disfigurement

[a] Part of private mental experience. The patient often discloses these features during the clinical interview, but may not do so, even with specific questioning.

term means that the behavior is psycho-pathologic. This is a judgment, usually based on the discovery that the patient is either disturbed or is disturbing to others. Third, although many references to the paranoid concept focus on its centrality to conditions such as schizophrenia, the features which we label paranoid are not necessarily associated with schizophrenia and can appear in a number of other psychiatric and medical disorders. Therefore, paranoid features indicate psychopathology, but *no specific etiology, chronicity, or reversibility*. Fourth, two kinds of observations form the basis for judging behavior to be paranoid: subjective, meaning that the observations are part of the private mental experience of the patient, for example, a delusion; and objective, referring to observations of features in manifest behavior, for instance, guardedness, grandiosity, litigiousness. Table 39.1 lists the subjective and objective features that have traditionally been labeled paranoid. Frequently, they are found in association, and form a constellation referred to as the *paranoid syndrome*. Some of them can be entirely normal features of behavior. Therefore, the judgment that they are paranoid rests on (*a*) their extremeness or inappropriateness, (*b*) their presence in association with other behaviors considered to be paranoid; or (*c*) the presence of delusions. Finally, paranoid de-lusions have traditionally referred to a wide variety of delusions, not simply those of persecution, grandeur, or jealousy. Unfortunately, there has been recent confusion regarding this point and the term "paranoid delusion" probably should not be used; the particular delusion should be more specifically characterized. A glossary of the paranoid terminology is found in Table 39.2 (1).

PARANOID SYNDROME

Published reports indicate that medical and other conditions have been associated with paranoid features (2). These include such features as persecutory and grandiose delusions, suspiciousness, sensitivity, resentment, sullenness, hate, jealousy, guardedness, evasiveness, humorlessness, and litigiousness. Since these characteristics are often found together, they should be treated as a syndrome, which may be due to a number of causes, as was recognized very early by Kahlbaum, Kraepelin, and Bleuler. There has been a tendency to forget that paranoid features are seen in many conditions. The conditions in which paranoid features may be found include psychiatric, neurologic, sex chromosome, metabolic and endocrine disorders as well as drug abuse, pharmacologic toxicity, and other kinds of abnormalities. A listing of

Table 39.2   Paranoid Terminology

Delusional (paranoid) disorders	—DSM-III-R category emphasizing that the cardinal feature of these conditions is delusions.
Paranoia	—Old term for an insidiously developed disorder in which individuals suffer from an unshakable delusions system but have no disturbance in the clarity or form of their thinking. Also known as *paranoia vera*, simple delusional disorder, or delusional monomania.
Paranoiac	—Old adjective used to describe individuals with paranoia.
Paranoid	—Broad term meaning suspicious to most people. In psychiatry, however, it is a clinical construct used to describe various objective and subjective features of behavior deemed to be psychopathologic. (See Table 39.1 for a list of such behaviors.) It refers to no specific condition (e.g., to be paranoid does not mean that schizophrenic disorder is present).
Paranoid delusion	—Older term used to refer to persecutory and grandiose delusions because of their occurrence in the paranoid subtype of schizophrenia. This term has suffered from the confusion associated with the paranoid concept. DSM-III recommends it not be used.
Paranoid disorders	—DSM-III term for an idiopathic group of conditions including paranoia, acute paranoid disorder, shared paranoid disorder, and atypical paranoid disorder.
Paranoid personality	—Enduring traits of paranoid behavior not due to schizophrenia or other mental disorder. Generally, there is no evidence of delusions or other features of psychosis.
Paranoid syndrome	—Term applied to constellations of paranoid features that occur together and can arise from multiple sources, including depression, organic disorder, and schizophrenic disorders.
Paraphrenia	—Old term for conditions lying theoretically between schizophrenia and paranoia and sharing features of both (e.g., hallucinations but no deterioration). It, too, remains controversial and probably should not be used until research validates its meaning.

reported sources of paranoid features is presented in Table 39.3.

It is essential to investigate all cases with paranoid features carefully. Certain principles can guide an accurate and effective assessment. First, it is important to know the range of paranoid features and the variety of clinical conditions in which they occur. Second, the premorbid status of the patient should be determined. Generally, a normal premorbid status suggests that acute paranoid features are the consequence of medical disease. Third, abrupt changes in personality, mood, and the ability to function also strongly hint at complications resulting from medical disease. Fourth, fluctuation in the mental state that occurs acutely should make the clinician suspect not psychiatric disorder, but medical illness. Fifth, in those cases in which there is evidence that the patient has been refractory to psychotropic medication or psychotherapy, the continuing presence of paranoid features should alert the clinician

to consider alternative diagnoses such as thyroid disorder or dementia.

The final diagnosis in cases where paranoid features occur should be made following (*a*) a complete medical and psychiatric history, with special attention paid to alcohol and drug history, including both drugs of abuse and current medication history (this should also include over-the-counter preparations); (*b*) a thorough physical examination including neurologic and mental status assessments; and (*c*) appropriate laboratory studies, particularly serologic, toxicologic, endocrine, microbiologic, and encephalographic and other imaging investigations.

These principles and a high index of suspicion that paranoid features do not represent schizophrenia or, for that matter, any of the major psychiatric disorders that have paranoid features, until specific evidence is gathered to refute or support that claim, remain the best guides to differential diagnosis of paranoid features.

DELUSIONAL DISORDERS

Delusional (paranoid) disorders represent a heterogeneous group of clinical conditions of unknown etiology, whose chief feature is the delusion. The *Diagnostic and Statistical Manual of Mental Disorders (Third Edition-Revised)* (DSM-III-R) criteria (3) (Table 39.4) provide a reliable basis for identifying cases with such disorders and for developing systematic research information about these conditions. Delusional disorders has replaced the DSM-III category "paranoid disorders" (4). The term "delusional" was selected to avoid confusion about the term "paranoid" as discussed above and to emphasize that the category includes disorders in which delusions other than the persecutory or jealous type are present. The validity of these criteria is at this point only partially established. Our knowledge must grow substantially if we are to master this area of psychopathology. Nevertheless, these criteria represent distinct progress.

Because delusional disorders are uncommon, and because paranoid features are ubiquitous in medical and psychiatric disorders, it is critical to be aware of the importance of careful diagnosis, especially differential diagnosis in these conditions.

Definition

Delusional disorder is diagnosed, according to DSM-III-R, when an individual exhibits nonbizarre delusions of at least 1 month's duration that cannot be attributed to other psychiatric disorders. The features of delusional disorder are presented in Table 39.5. Nonbizarre means that the delusions must be about situations that can occur in real life, such as being infected, loved, followed, and so on. There are sev-

Table 39.3   Conditions Associated with Delusions and Other Paranoid Features

Neurologic

Temporal lobe epilepsy	Multiple sclerosis
Huntington's chorea	Senile psychoses
Presenile psychoses (Alzheimer's and Pick's diseases)	Arteriosclerotic psychoses
	Hypertensive encephalopathy
Brain tumors	Postencephalitic parkinsonism
Subdural hematoma	Subarachnoid hemorrhage
Fat embolism	Menzel-type ataxia
Roussy-Lévy syndrome	Motor neuron disease
Muscular dystrophy	Narcolepsy
Delirium	Dementia
Hearing loss	Blunt head trauma
Migraine	Intracranial hemorrhage
Idiopathic Parkinson's disease	Spinocerebellar degeneration
Idiopathic basal ganglia calcification	Metachromatic leukodystrophy
Hydrocephalus	Marchiafava-Bignami disease
	Cerebrovascular disease

Metabolic and endocrine disorders

Uremia	Pellagra
Wilson's disease	Systemic lupus erythematosus
Acute intermittent porphyria	Pernicious anemia
Hypopituitarism	Cushing's syndrome
Thyroid disorders	Liver failure
Hemodialysis	Hypoglycemia
Complication of surgical portacaval anastomosis for cirrhosis	Vitamin B_{12} deficiency
	Addison's disease
Malnutrition	Pancreatic encephalopathy
Hypercalcemia	Hyponatremia
Parathyroid disorders	Niacin deficiency
Folate deficiency	Thiamine deficiency
Phenylketonuria	

Table 39.3   *(Cont.)*

Infections	*Psychiatric*
Syphilis	Schizophrenic disorders, all subtypes
Malaria	Delusional disorders
Encephalitis lethargica	(including classical paranoia)
Typhus	Induced psychotic disorder
Trypanosomiasis	Affective disorders (including mania)
Acquired immune deficiency disorder	Schizophreniform disorder
Jakob-Creutzfeldt's disease	Schizoaffective disorder
Viral encephalitides	Brief reactive psychosis
Toxic shock syndrome	
Meningitis	

Sex chromosome	*Toxic*
Klinefelter's syndrome	Mercury
Turner's syndrome	Arsenic
47 XXY	Thallium
	Manganese
	Carbon monoxide

Alcohol and drug abuse	*Pharmacologic agents*
Alcohol withdrawal	Amphetamine and related compounds
Chronic alcohol hallucinosis	Phenylpropanolamine
Marijuana	Mephentermine
Chronic bromide intoxication	Prophylhexedrine
Amphetamine	Methyldopa and imipramine (combination)
Barbiturate abuse	Pentazocine
Cocaine abuse	Adrenocorticotropic hormone
Mescaline and other hallucinogens	Cortisone
Perbitine	L-dopa
Ephedrine	Methyltestosterone
Withdrawal from minor tranquilizers and	Imipramine
hypnotic medications	Diphenylhydantoin
Anesthetic nitrous oxide	Cimetidine
Atropine toxicity	Buproprion
	Disulfiram
	Bromocriptine
	Anticholinergic drugs
	Antitubercular drugs
	Antimalarial drugs

eral types of such delusions, and the predominant type is specified in making the diagnosis. Generally, the nonbizarre delusions in delusional disorders are well systematized and logically developed. A patient with these disorders may experience auditory or visual hallucinations, but they are usually not prominent features. In fact, the behavioral and emotional responses of the individual to the delusion appear to be appropriate. Impairment of functioning and personality deterioration is in general minimal, if it occurs at all.

Induced psychotic disorder (shared paranoid disorder) is an unusual condi-tion, which has also been termed *folie á deux*. It requires the absence of a psychotic disorder prior to the onset of the induced delusion. It has generally been classified with paranoid disorder, and was so in the DSM-III criteria. However, in DSM-III-R, it is separately classified in the category "psychotic disorders not elsewhere classified," along with schizophreniform and schizoaffective disorders and brief reactive psychosis.

Epidemiology

Delusional disorders have been considered uncommon if not rare conditions. We know little about their epidemiology. Demographic information covering the period from 1912 to 1970 has provided an estimate of their incidence and prevalence and related statistics (5). However, this evidence was assembled using definitions that are not the same as those of DSM-III or DSM-III-R, and the figures will, in all likelihood, be different using these newer criteria. Clearly, they are merely indications in anticipation of future knowledge about these conditions (see Table 39.6). Certain features are remarkable nonetheless. For instance, incidence has remained stable over extended periods of time in this century. Prevalence also substantiates the widely held impression that these disorders are uncommon compared to affective and schizophrenic disorders, but it also indicates that they are not rare. Patients with delusional disorders are somewhat more likely to be female, but this is a feature with some degree of controversy associated with it, and patients are considered to be relatively more disadvantaged socially and educationally compared to patients with affective illnesses. There is some suggestive evidence that immigrant status is associated with delusional disorder.

Etiology

The etiology of delusional disorders is unknown. Controversy in classifying disorders with paranoid features has added problems to understanding the etiology of delusional disorders. Theories and explanations of delusions abound in the literature, and yet evidence to support them is limited (6, 7). Because of these uncertainties, statements concerning etiology represent no more than speculation.

Clinical Description

The core feature of delusional disorders is the persistent, nonbizarre delusion, not explained by other psychotic disorders. In some cases, there is evidence of precipitating events which may be associated with the acute formation of the delusional thinking, but the disorder may emerge gradually and become a chronic disorder, without any acute precipitants. Emotional and behavioral responses are generally appropriate with depressed mood a common feature. Neither an affective syndrome nor the features of a schizophrenic illness are present, however.

The delusions in delusional disorder are unusual, yet they refer to aspects of life that could be real, such as being cheated on by someone, conspired against, physically ill, in love with someone, jealous of someone, and the like. Winokur (8) has suggested that such delusions are possible, rather than totally incredible and bizarre, like many of the delusions of schizophrenia, for example. The types of delusions are specified according to their content. There are several types, and they have also been the sources of somewhat separate eponyms in the past, such as erotomania or de Clerambault's syndrome. The most common delusions concern persecution and jealousy. They are fixed, that is, persistent and unarguable. The patient interprets facts to fit the delusion rather than modifying the delusion to fit the facts. There is systemization in the delusional thinking, meaning that a single theme, or a series of connected themes is present and links to the predominant delusion. The delusions are not shared with members of the patient's social group. While many have pointed to a descriptive continuum between paranoid personality disorder, delusional disorders, and the paranoid subtype of schizophrenia in terms of degree of disorganization and impairment, there is little evidence to support the concept that these disorders share more than overlapping psychopathology.

Patients with delusional disorder show little disorganization or impairment of their behavior or thinking. Infrequent, often transitory hallucinations appear in at least some cases of delusional disorder. Usually, these hallucinations are auditory, but they may be visual, and they tend to be more common in acute cases. Other types of hallucinations are rare. Emotional responses are frequently consistent with the delusional concerns. Restlessness and agi-

Table 39.4   Diagnostic Criteria for Delusional Disorder

A. Nonbizarre delusion(s) (i.e., involving situations that occur in real life, such as being followed, poisoned, infected, loved at a distance, having a disease, being deceived by one's spouse or lover) of at least one month's duration.
B. Auditory or visual hallucinations, if present, are not prominent [as defined in schizophrenia, A(1)(*b*)].
C. Apart from the delusion(s) or its ramifications, behavior is not obviously odd or bizarre.
D. If a major depressive or manic syndrome has been present during the delusional disturbance, the total duration of all episodes of the mood syndrome has been brief relative to the total duration of the delusional disturbance.
E. Has never met criterion A for schizophrenia, and it cannot be established that an organic factor initiated and maintained the disturbance.
Specify type: The following types are based on the predominant delusional theme. If no single delusional theme predominates, specify as *unspecified type.*
Erotomanic type
Delusional Disorder in which the predominant theme of the delusion(s) is that a person, usually of higher status, is in love with the subject.
Grandiose type
Delusional disorder in which the predominant theme of the delusion(s) is one of inflated worth, power, knowledge, identity, or special relationship to a deity or famous person.
Jealous type
Delusional disorder in which the predominant theme of the delusion(s) is that one's sexual partner is unfaithful.
Persecutory type
Delusional disorder in which the predominant theme of the delusion(s) is that one (or someone to whom one is close) is being malevolently treated in some way. People with this type of delusional disorder may repeatedly take their complaints of being mistreated to legal authorities.
Somatic type
Delusional disorder in which the predominant theme of the delusion(s) is that the person has some physical defect, disorder, or disease.
Unspecified type
Delusional disorder that does not fit any of the previous categories, e.g., persecutory and grandiose themes without a predominance of either; delusions of reference without malevolent content.

Reprinted with permission from American Psychiatric Association: *Diagnostic and Statistical Manual of Mental Disorders* (*Third Edition-Revised*). Washington, DC, American Psychiatric Association, 1987. Copyright 1987 American Psychiatric Association.

Table 39.5   Features of Delusional Disorders

Essential Features	Associated Features
Nonbizarre delusions (especially persecutory, jealousy)	Anger, litigiousness, hostility, humorlessness, suspiciousness
Absence of schizophrenic disorder	Social isolation, eccentric behavior
Absence of affective disorder	Ability to organize action in response to delusion (e.g., litigious behavior)

tation may be present. Loquaciousness and circumstantiality (usually accompanying descriptions of the delusions) are found in some patients, but formal thought disorder is absent. Associated features in delusional disorders include those of paranoid syndrome, as discussed earlier in this chapter. The degree of hostility and suspiciousness may be such that violent or aggressive behavior can result. Litigious behavior (e.g., letter writing, threats of legal action) is common.

Diagnosis

The diagnosis of delusional disorders requires a match between the features of the case and the DSM-III-R criteria. When alternative sources for the delusional illness can be successfully ruled out, certain fea-

Table 39.6 Epidemiologic Features of
Delusional Disorders

Incidence	0.7–3.0
Prevalence	24–30
Age at onset (range)	35–45 (18–80)
Sex ratio M:F	.85

Incidence and prevalence figures represent cases per 100,000 population. Data are from Kendler (5).

tures of the case can help substantiate the diagnosis of delusional disorder.

Often the patient's complaints are brought to clinical attention by the patient or a third party, such as family, neighbors, or the police. The patient may have acted to draw attention by asking the police for protection or quarreling with neighbors. The complaint often focuses on the patient's distressing behavior and possibly on incidental symptoms. As a rule, the patient will not complain about psychiatric symptoms. The patient's examination often reveals that thinking, affect, orientation, attention, memory, perception, and personality are intact. In fact, the patient's thinking may be so clear, and the delusional features so central to the patient's concerns, that the clinician can begin to anticipate precisely the responses of the patient, to the point that accurate predictions of specific actions and reactions are possible. This predictability may distinguish the behavior of a delusional disorder patient from that of patients with other psychotic conditions in which disorganization and confusion are more characteristic.

There may be a lack of cooperation, presence of hostility or anger, and a sarcastic or challenging quality to most of what is said. The capacity to act in response to delusions is an important dimension of the evaluation. Impulsiveness should be assessed and related to the potential for violence or suicidal behavior. The patient's self-righteousness and the intensity of the delusional experience may be clues to the possibility of violent behavior, and any plans for harming others, including homicide, should be inquired about. If such plans exist, the patient should be asked how they were handled in the past.

A range of laboratory assessments is of-ten necessary, but several have a higher likelihood of detecting key factors in the case. The use of drug screening measures is particularly valuable given the marked delusional responses induced by drugs, particularly central nervous system stimulants. Neuropsychologic assessment may help disclose evidence of impaired intellectual functioning that suggests brain abnormality. The assessment of intelligence may show discrepancies between performance and verbal scores as well as scatter in overall performance. We do not have extensive data on this matter, but that which exists suggests that average or marginally low intelligence is characteristic in delusional disorders. Projective testing may have value in making the diagnosis, in that it may confirm features consistent with the clinical diagnosis. The Minnesota Multiphasic Personality Inventory has a number of clinical scales, including the Pa, or paranoia scale, developed to identify paranoid symptoms. Deviation on this scale is correlated with the presence of paranoid features. Again, this may help to substantiate the diagnosis or raise it as a possibility.

Differential Diagnosis

Because delusional disorders are uncommon if not rare, because they are idiopathic, and because they possess features characteristic of the full range of paranoid illnesses, differential diagnosis has a clear strategy. Namely, delusional disorders is a diagnosis of exclusion. There are many conditions to consider. In order to avoid premature diagnosis, careful evaluation is required.

The clinical assessment of paranoid features requires three steps. (a) The clinician must recognize, characterize, and judge as pathologic the presence of the paranoid features. (b) The clinician should determine whether they form part of a syndrome or are isolated. And (c) the clinician should develop the differential diagnosis.

The first of these three steps can be pursued systematically. The clinician needs to be aware that a range of objective traits or behaviors (see Table 39.1) are often found in paranoid illness. It may be difficult at times to determine that paranoid illness is present because patients may be unwilling to reveal their subjective concerns. Nevertheless, the interview and information gathered from other informants may disclose critical evidence that the behavior is clearly psychopathologic. In some cases, however, this conclusion must await further observations. Delusional thinking should be examined for its logic, fixedness, encapsulation, degree of systemization and elaboration, and effect on action and planning. Once it has been determined that a paranoid condition is present, the clinician should attend to the premorbid characteristics, the course, and the associated symptomatology of the disorder in order to detect patterns of psychopathology. For example, discovering disorientation, disturbances in perception, other psychopathology, physical signs, or confusing symptoms may suggest different possibilities for paranoid features. Isolated or acute paranoid symptoms may appear in early medical illness. Finally, the clinician should avoid an early temptation to diagnose schizophrenia and delusional disorders in cases where paranoid features are present. These features occur in such a variety of conditions that awareness of the multiple causes of paranoid features is essential to completing this differential process.

Treatment

The goals of treatment in delusional disorders are to establish the diagnosis, decide on appropriate intervention, and manage the complications. The doctor–patient relationship is absolutely fundamental to the successful achievement of these goals. Establishing an effective doctor–patient relationship is, however, far from simple. These patients do not complain about psychiatric symptoms and generally enter treatment against their will. Even the psychiatrist may be brought into the delusional net.

Considerable skill is required in dealing with the profound and intense feelings of these patients. There is not enough evidence to substantiate the claim for any particular approach to talking with the patient. Insight-oriented treatment is generally contraindicated, but a combination of supportive approaches is sensible. Awareness of the fragile self-esteem and sensitivity of these patients is essential for their management and somatic treatment. It is seldom helpful to directly question the patient about the veracity of the delusion, apart from establishing the diagnosis during the initial clinical evaluation. Achieving an alliance may be especially difficult, but responding to the patient's concerns rather than the delusional thinking may be effective. Understanding that fear and anxiety serve to stimulate hostility may promote empathy while maintaining appropriate distance. Patients with these disorders are demoralized, isolated, and miserable, and feel abandoned. They often face rejection. They can be approached and their treatment focused on these types of experiences. The goals of therapy are to allay anxiety, initiate discussion of troubling experiences, and thereby gradually develop rapport and alliance. The aim of such interventions is to assist in a more satisfying general adjustment.

Delusional disorders are psychotic disorders by definition, and it is reasonable to presume that they might respond to antipsychotic medication. However, there is no clear evidence that this is the case. Nonetheless it seems reasonable to suggest trials of antipsychotic medication when the agitation, apprehension, and anxiety that accompany delusions are prominent. There is evidence that delusional disorders respond less well generally to electroconvulsive treatment than do major affective disorders with psychotic features. A trial of antipsychotic and antidepressant therapy may be worthwhile if the differential diagnosis is unclear between delusional disorders and psychotic depression. It has been suggested that where standard strategies are unsuccessful, trials of lithium and/or anticonvulsive medication might be considered.

The use of somatic therapies is difficult

on two levels in such patients. Their insistence on the lack of psychiatric difficulties may be a barrier to the initiation of treatment, and their sensitivity to side effects may constitute an additional frustrating factor in their care. An open attitude and clear explanations about such possibilities, as well as a willingness to assist them through unpleasant experiences, is essential.

Hospitalization is usually unnecessary, since most patients with delusional disorder can be treated as outpatients. However, inpatient care may be necessary to manage aggressiveness or potentially dangerous behavior as well as suicidal ideation and planning. It is preferable to inform the patient through a process of tactful persuasion that voluntary hospitalization is necessary should that be the case. If this fails, legal means to commit the patient must be undertaken.

Course and Prognosis

Factors associated with a more favorable course are listed in the Table 39.7. Most studies generally indicate that delusional disorders do not lead to severe impairment, and the base rate of spontaneous recovery, though not known, may not be as low as previously believed. Most patients live a normal life span, although there have been reports of suicide. The more chronic forms of the illness (i.e., patients ill for more than 6 months) appear to have their onset early in the 5th decade, based on Retterstol's (9) personal follow-up investigation of a large series of cases. Here, the onset was acute in nearly two-thirds of the cases, gradual in the remainder. At follow-up, in 53% of the cases the delusion had disappeared, in 10% it was improved, and in 31% it was unchanged. In more acute cases, with the age of onset in the 4th decade, a lasting remission occurred in over half the patients and a pattern of chronicity occurred in only 10% of the cases. Some 37% did have a relapse in course. The earlier and more acute the onset, the more generally favorable the prognosis. The presence of precipitating and other factors may signify a more positive outcome. These observations provide a basis for some optimism: Perhaps half of cases with delusional disorders may eventually remit. However, relapse and chronicity are common.

Prevention

Because so little is known about these disorders, it would be premature to suggest the means of primary prevention. Although concentrations of paranoid personality patterns in the relatives of individuals with delusional disorders have been observed, the evidence for genetic factors is far from robust. A host of factors, including sensory impairment, immigrant status, physical illness, and aging itself, have been associated with these disorders, but we do not yet know how to unravel the causal tangle. Nevertheless, secondary prevention, that is identifying and reducing sources that may increase clinical morbidity, is feasible. Reducing the effects of various forms of stress might improve the patient's course. Again, this is an optimistic claim and remains to be evaluated.

The Clinical Interview

Determining the Nature of the Problem

This chapter has focused on the process of establishing the diagnosis of delusional disorders. Fundamentally, that process involves the task of careful differential diagnosis. Because delusional disorders is a diagnosis of exclusion, and because the disorder is idiopathic, the clinician needs

Table 39.7   Factors Affecting Outcome

More favorable	Less favorable
Acute onset	Insidious onset
Short duration	Longer duration
Younger age	Older age
Married	Single status
Recent immigration	Sensory
Affective features	impairment
(depressed mood,	Seclusiveness
irritability)	

to keep open the possibility that delusional disorders is not the correct diagnosis.

Knowledge of the DSM-III-R criteria is essential in understanding how to make this diagnosis. There are a number of features in the mental status examination and interview which suggest delusional disorders. For example, such patients exhibit remarkably intact cognitive functions despite the nonbizarre delusion which is their focus and the central feature of the illness. This fundamental observation is the one that usually provides the stimulus for an even more thorough description and assessment since it seems strange not to see more psychopathology. *Most clinicians find it difficult to believe that delusional disorder is not another psychotic disorder.* However, if the patient's delusions cannot be attributed to schizophrenic disorders, other psychopathologic conditions, or organic factors, this diagnosis becomes more plausible.

In patients with delusional disorders, the exploration of various hypotheses which may account for the illness proceeds as indicated above. However, the patient's own complaint is not likely to be a psychiatric symptom. To establish an appropriate level of involvement and to increase the likelihood that the full nature of concerns and diagnosis is fully understood, it is useful for the clinician to be aware that confrontation about the delusion is rarely a successful strategy for improving the database. Careful questioning, with heightened awareness of the patient's sensitivity, is required. The patient's life story and concerns may be the features which permit a connection to develop with the clinician and an opportunity to gain other relevant diagnostic interview data. This connection or collaboration becomes the basis for therapeutic intervention and the development of an alliance.

Developing and Maintaining a Therapeutic Relationship

Many of the features of the clinical interview that relate to these goals have been discussed. It is useful here to repeat that the patient has come to the situation not to be treated for a psychiatric disorder, but because of some other specific complaint. Recognition of this fact; recognition that the patient is likely to have a number of associated paranoid features, such as hostility, obstinance, lack of humor, and the like; and recognition that most patients will be unwilling to accept a psychiatric diagnosis are the fundamental bases from which to proceed. In short, the patient should not be told that he or she is psychiatrically ill in a confrontative manner. Rather, there should be an attempt to empathize with and alleviate the presenting concerns and symptomatic experiences. It is on this basis, rather than on any intellectual diagnostic basis, that the patient is likely to be responsive in a therapeutic relationship.

A collaborative relationship in which the issues that lead to and perpetuate the delusional thinking are sensitively explored is most helpful. Despite the best efforts, a patient with delusional disorders is unlikely to feel satisfied in a treatment situation. It is probably the degree to which dissatisfaction is limited that will determine the interest and connectedness to the therapist in both the diagnostic and treatment process. Nevertheless, every attempt should be made to listen to the patient's story, to hear and tolerate the patient's expression of painful feelings, and to express genuine interest and empathy toward the patient's concerns.

Communicating Information and Implementing a Treatment Plan

The nature of delusional disorders is such that the patient's understanding and acceptance of the diagnosis and the treatment plan will be difficult to achieve. In most situations, telling patients that they have the specific disorder will lead to a negative reaction. It is, however, necessary to convey directly the diagnostic impression that the clinician entertains. However, once done, it is counterproductive to refer to that particular fact repeatedly. Rather, address the issues that most complicate and disrupt the patient's life. The patient's involvement in the diagnostic process and ultimately the treatment process can be enhanced if the patient is made a full partner in an exploration of reasons for various tests, questions, and ultimately, the differential diagnostic process itself. As conditions are ruled out one by one, it would be helpful to explain to the patient that whatever is ailing him or her is not the result of a particular disorder. This kind of information exchange in an atmosphere of caring and reasonable warmth constitutes the basis for a successful intervention with such patients. As a treatment plan is devised and clinical interventions are suggested, it is useful to keep the patient informed of the specifics of any proposed treatment. Suggestions about the use of medication have already been indicated above, but the same principles apply to any form of intervention in the treatment of this disorder.

Clearly, communicating with a patient with delusional disorders is a task requiring considerable skill. There are many pitfalls. In summary, a sensitive yet always clear and consistent approach is the best medicine.

CONCLUSION

Delusional disorders are uncommon, although probably not rare. On the other hand, the features of paranoid behavior are ubiquitous, found in a large variety of medical and psychiatric conditions, and certainly not confined to delusional, schizophrenic, or affective disorders. Because of the cardinal nature of paranoid symptoms and signs in psychopathology, clinicians are urged to be particularly careful in assessing and assigning diagnoses in conditions in which such features occur. Through the elaboration of our understanding and knowledge, we will be more effective in diagnosis and treatment.

References

1. Manschreck TC: The assessment of paranoid features. *Compr Psychiatry* 20:370–377, 1979.
2. Manschreck TC, Petri M: The paranoid syndrome. *Lancet* 2:251–253, 1978.
3. American Psychiatric Association: *Diagnostic and Statistical Manual of Mental Disorders (Third Edition-Revised)*. Washington, DC, American Psychiatric Association, 1987.
4. American Psychiatric Association: *Diagnostic and Statistical Manual of Mental Disorders (Third Edition)*. Washington, DC, American Psychiatric Association, 1980.
5. Kendler K: Demography of paranoid psychosis (delusional disorder): a review and comparison with schizophrenic and affective illness. *Arch Gen Psychiatry* 39:890–902, 1982.
6. Manschreck TC: Delusional disorders. In Sadock B, Kaplan K (eds): *Comprehensive Textbook of Psychiatry V*. Baltimore, Williams & Wilkins, in press.
7. Arthur AZ: Theories of delusions: a review. *Am J Psychiatry* 121:105–115, 1964.
8. Winokur G: Delusional disorders (paranoia). *Compr Psychiatry* 18:511–521, 1977.
9. Retterstol N: *Paranoid and Paranoiac Psychoses*. Springfield, IL, Charles C. Thomas, 1966.

40

Psychiatric Illness in the Elderly

Merle Ingraham, M.D.

Senescence: "It is the best of times; it is the worst of times."

The mental health status of the individuals who make up the heterogeneous group called the elderly will be determined by their ability or inability to surmount the vicissitudes of their lives. For the majority of persons in their later years life will be "all right" if not reasonably happy. Many of them, enjoying the freedom from the work role and parenting responsibilities, will describe community and family participation and pursuit of avocations and will consider themselves productive and satisfied with their lives.

As many as 20% to 25% of our elderly, however, will exhibit maladaptive behavior patterns which will fall into variously described mental illness categories. In general, this group of persons will be dissatisfied with their lives. Not a few of them will end their lives by their own hands overtly or will succumb to diverse organic illnesses toward which unhealthy living habits and attitudes or loss of the will to survive have contributed.

Of the group with definable mental illnesses an unmeasured number will have experienced these illnesses before they became old and will carry them into senescence shaped and altered by the aging

process. At times the presentation of illness will be quite different from what it had been earlier in life. Other patients may have carried the underlying intrapsychic dynamics and other etiologic factors of their mental illnesses throughout early life without manifestations until failing defenses lead to the appearance of symptoms. There are relatively few new major emotional disorders in later years. A few elderly, nevertheless, will develop mental illness which appears to be unique to the old-age period itself. Examples are paraphrenia, dementia, delirium, first episode of depression, and those many other medical illnesses seen more often in later life with their accompanying psychosyndromes of anxiety, depression, and diminished coping.

Numerous elderly who are lonely and unhappy but do not have a definitive *Diagnostic and Statistical Manual of Mental Disorders (Third Edition-Revised)* (DSM-III-R) (1) diagnosis often find their way to the professional caretaker. These more modestly "disturbed" elderly may be helped both therapeutically and preventatively, depending on the caretaker's judgment, temperament, perceived role and interest, and

538

the health system's policies and reimbursement patterns.

Another subpopulation of the elderly are those men and women who are sufficiently dysfunctional as to require nursing home residency. Perhaps they have exhausted the caring energies and skills of their families. In the best circumstance they remain supported by their families, who find an excellent nursing home and continue to take them out for rides and for Sunday dinners and make frequent visits. The managers of the nursing home, if enlightened, allow their residents to bring with them treasured personal posessions in order to preserve, at least symbolically, a piece of their former lives. The staff of such homes facilitate their patient's transition to a communal life while allowing as much autonomy as possible, addressing the person's strengths, and offering a variety of menus, "people spaces," and imaginative stimulating programs designed more around the patient's needs than the staff's needs. The attending physicians of such fortunate patients make meaningful rounds as often as is medically necessary rather than as often as Medicare provisions require. These physicians are by nature generalists regardless of their avowed specialties and are ever mindful of the challenging diagnostic presentations of the elderly, such as the pneumonia appearing only as fatigue, the dehydration as apathy, and the abnormal electrolytes as behavioral agitation. Such physicians will take time to consider their patients from a psychobiologic and social reference.

Regrettably, the above-described environment is not the prevailing one among nursing homes. Impersonal and third-rate attention to the needs of our chronically institutionalized elderly, whether in chronic state hospitals or nursing levels 2, 3, or 4 placement, is more often the case in the United States.

Laws behoove an elderly person to spend down his or her life savings prior to eligibility for Medicaid. Unless the person is rich this process often jeopardizes the noninstitutionalized spouse's financial abilities. Once granted, Medicaid status often relegates patients needing long-term care to less favored status regarding housing, admission to nursing homes, general medical care, and mental health care. The damages to the self-image of the elderly person by pauperization and resultant disenfranchisement, embarrassment, and feelings of worthlessness can scarcely be imagined. Many elderly have already come to feel severely diminished by waning vigor, reduced hearing and vision, and loss of useful function in society. Such bureaucratic financial requirements and lack of support for the families of the elderly (who render without acknowledgment most of the long-term care) become stultifying.

Only belatedly is protest beginning to swell to rectify our society's inadequate provisions for its elderly. Long-term-care insurance and social Medicare recommendations are being proposed. The outcry of the elderly themselves is beginning to be recognized. Winston Churchill said that you can judge the maturity of a country by the way it takes care of its elderly. The United States is falling woefully short on this measure at this point in time.

WORKING WITH MENTALLY ILL ELDERLY

Working with the mentally ill elderly, as with the physically ill elderly, warrants a broader intervention by the clinician than is usually used with a younger population. Interviews with caretakers, family, neighbors, home health personnel, other physicians, nurses, and social service personnel are often necessary to make an assessment not only of the patient's ego strengths, defenses, interpersonal skills, and symptomatology, but also of the current support system, premorbid behavior, and functioning as viewed by others as well as by the patient. The life review as emphasized by Robert Butler (2) of the numerous biologic, psychologic, and environmental data to establish the fabric of the patient's life is very valuable in furthering understanding of the maladaptive behavior (the mental illness) pattern by the patient, the patient's kith and kin, and other caretakers. Such an understanding is especially valuable for the elderly as opposed to patients in other age groups because they frequently feel their symptoms to be stigmatizing and reflective of moral weakness. Harry Stack Sullivan's view that we are all more nearly human than otherwise may be a helpful attitude to share in working with elderly patients.

Working with the elderly takes time. In an economy where professional caretakers grow ever more conscious of the meter ticking during the complex processes of assessment and intervention, the ideal amount of time necessary in working with elderly patients is seldom available. Yet shortening these processes may be in the long run more time consuming as diagnoses are missed and the psychosocial supports of medical care are experienced as inadequate.

There are a number of features about our elderly which may require a lengthening of the evaluative process. Many elderly are slower to accept psychiatric diagnoses and treatment because of the perceived negative stigma. Many have communication difficulties caused by vision and hearing impairment. Many move into and out of the consulting rooms more slowly and adapt to strange environments less easily, delaying an orderly scheduling. Their thinking is slower and they are less able to organize a good history. Pressure of time constraints or expectations for rapid change can cause great frustration for patient and caregiver. Many, especially those referred from general medical settings, are physically handicapped, more somatically concerned, and less psychologically reflective than would be ideal for psychotherapeutic intervention.

It is important to recognize that not all of the elderly have difficulty accepting psychotherapy and change. Psychiatrists should not permit an ageist bias by accepting the myth that psychotherapy is ineffective in older people (3). In this regard, Sobel has described two types of countertransference difficulties that therapists experience with later life patients (4). First, the therapist may be biased toward the use of drugs and consider regressive behavior to be invariably due to organic brain changes. Second, the therapist may resist intensive psychodynamic psychotherapy ("transference-indulgent psychotherapies"), when in a younger person the same therapist would regard it as the treatment of choice.

Implicit in working with the elderly is the need to establish an enduring relationship. The value of such a relationship is in establishing trust, replacing lost objects, and providing continuing support. Such support may serve a wide variety of purposes, ranging from organizing the patient's use of money, clarifying the nature of illnesses, and informing patients of the network of health and recreational services to telling patients that the explanation of the benefit form is not a bill. The effective therapist for the elderly, in contrast to traditional therapists, is usually less distant, less hidden, more self-disclosing, and less enamored of his or her familiarity with the unconscious mental life and the need for interpreting the transference in a dogmatic manner. The psychotherapist for the elderly is more of a "real person," coming together with his or her patient to share feelings in the alliance; to comfort, explain, and help prepare for the ultimate end of life; and to help enhance the life remaining until that time.

CONDITIONS COMMONLY ENCOUNTERED IN THE ELDERLY

Dementia and Deliria

The organic psychosyndromes of dementia and delirium are very common. They often are accompanied by anxiety and depression, depending on the particular disorder and on the degree of the patient's awareness of what is happening. Mixtures of organic and functional disorders are the common pattern. In this day of "Alzheimerism," as Alex Comfort writes, senile dementia, Alzheimer's type lies within everyone's mind as a diagnosis of exclusion. Fortunately, those organizations popularizing the disorder as a disease state have helped to dispell the myth that all old persons are destined to become demented. The insidious onset in late middle and older ages of Alzheimer's disease with its gradual disturbance of memory, orientation, and judgment leading to a variety of aphasias, agnosias, and apraxias is a familiar pattern. The increasing loss of self-care skills poses an enormous blow to the victim's perception of themselves and an equally enormous task for caretakers within the private home or in the long-term-care facilities. As more people live to those ages which seem most vulnerable to Alzheimer's disorders, caretaking sons and daughters, themselves often elderly, are faced with the possibility of a growing burden, which can provoke emotional illness in them as well.

While Alzheimer's disease is definitively diagnosed only on postmortem examination of the central nervous system tissue, characterized by a neuropathologic picture of neurofibrillary tangles, senile plaques, and granulovacular changes of great profusion in the brain, its usual antemortem diagnosis is one of clinical judgment. Review of the family history where the presence of Alzheimer's disease is more common (or is at least more common in one of the types of Alzheimer's disease where a biogenetic history is strong), observation of the clinical features of a growing loss of memory, increased apathy, language difficulties, loss of urinary control, reduced energy, and disinhibition behavior should point to the diagnosis.

The good clinician will want to rule out a variety of other degenerative disorders such as multiinfarct dementia, Jakob-Creutzfeld's disease, dementia associated with head trauma, normal-pressure hydrocephalus, alcohol use, parkinsonism, Huntington's disease, or viral disease. Each condition must be looked at from a genetic, developmental, clinical-onset, and natural-history points of view. Patients and their families have a right to know what kind of degenerative disorder exists, what the probable prognosis is even where definitive intervention is unavailable.

Management, estate planning, mobilization of support services, preparation for role reversal, and family decision making are but a few processes initiated by the development of dementia.

However important it may be for the physician to diagnose a specific dementia, it is imperative to rule out reversible dementiform disorders lest the victim be consigned to a progressive degenerative course irrespective of the possibility of helpful interventions.

Statistics vary regarding the percentage of patients with a dementiform picture who suffer from a reversible illness. Ten to fifteen percent of such patients is often quoted as having a reversible condition. The enormous variety of medical and psychiatric disorders which may provoke a dementia-like picture can only be briefly listed within the scope of this chapter. These include thyroid, B_{12}, folate deficiencies, malnutrition, congestive heart failure, electrolytic disturbances, sepsis, and neoplasms, to mention a few. The routine dementia workup protocol will usually screen out these medical conditions (see Chapter 23).

Such protocols usually include a chemistry profile; electrolytes, including magnesium studies; thyroid panel; complete blood count; B_{12} and folate analysis; and computerized axial tomographic (CAT) scans of the brain. A study conducted at the Psychogeriatric Unit of the Royal Edinburgh Hospital and reported by Kolman (5) suggests that the most "useful" tests are the midstream urine catch, chest x-ray, serum B_{12}, electrocardiogram (ECG), and blood urea, for the detection of a previously unknown disease. Kolman states along with other clinicians that the value of a history and physical in the assessment of the elderly psychiatric patient is absolutely fundamental.

In the view of Dubin et al., reporting from Jefferson Hospital Psychiatric Emergency Service in Philadelphia, the value of laboratory tests in the initial emergency department assessment is unresolved (6). These authors found that of 1140 patients the cause of organic brain syndrome in only 6 patients (3 with hypoglycemia and 3 with azotemia) was established by laboratory tests. Rather than relying on laboratory tests, these authors recommend use of four screening criteria: presence of disorientation, vital signs, clouded consciousness, and the fact of the patient's being older than age 40 without previous psychiatric history. In Dubin et al.'s study, both delirious and demented organic brain syndromes were included for discussion.

At least as common a condition as dementia in the elderly is that of delirium. Neurologists are fond of referring to this disorder as acute confusional episodes. Lipowski argues that all deliria should by definition be considered to be organically caused, whereas those deliria induced by sensory deprivation, emotional stress, and environmental disruption and sleep loss should be called pseudodeliria (7).

"There is reason to argue," however, "that the dichotomy between functional and organic dysfunctions is both unwarranted and unhelpful, particularly in the elderly," writes Wells (8). Wells questions the merit of a specific disease diagnosis, favoring a functional assessment of the patient which can provide a more adequate basis for care.

The reader is referred to the DSM-III-R for criteria lists for delirium and for dementia (see Chapter 23). While disorientation and memory impairment occur in both conditions, the consciousness of the dementia patient is not impaired, whereas the delirious patient is often referred to as having clouding of consciousness with a reduced attentional capacity. Delirium, furthermore, has an acute or subacute progression with variability in clinical features from time to time that is not usually shared by the dementia patient. Dementia and delirium can coexist, and the delineation of the syndromes may be difficult to tease out despite a thorough review of onset and duration; assessment of consciousness, attention, perception, thinking, judgment, insight, sleep; and electroencephalographic (EEG) patterns.

Perhaps the most common cause for delirium in an elderly population is the use of prescribed and over-the-counter drugs. While problematic in the drug regimens in one's own home, a greater risk applies in many a long-term care setting where monitoring of medication intake of a more disabled elderly population may be lax. All would agree that elderly persons are very sensitive to nearly all medications. Because physiologic changes exist such as reduced lean body mass and reduced ability for detoxification, metabolism and excretion, and because there is a wider volume of distribution of drugs, drugs should be sparingly and cautiously used. The slogan "Start slow, go slow," while hackneyed, is well worth repeating. Psychoactive drugs, hypotensive drugs, anticholinergic and sedative drugs have an especially great potential for provoking delirium.

A wide variety of general medical abnormalities of electrolytes, water balance; acid–base balance; hormonal, infectious, and nutritional disorders; metabolic disorders; neoplasms; and withdrawal syndromes may contribute to delirium. Estimates of 5 to 15% incidence of delirium for all patients on general medical surgical wards is noted. For patients 60 years of age or older an incidence of 40 to 75% of delirium exists.

Depression

There is value in clarifying the matrices in which depression exists. Is it an adjustment disorder with depressed mood? A dysthymic disorder? A major affective disorder? Are there elements of autonomous, biologic changes? Is it reactive to influenza or other viral disorder? Is it due to the recent myocardial infarction, stroke, or cancer? Is it part of an alcoholism condition (see Chapter 36)? How much of the depression may be unresolved grief (see Chapter 32)? Only by careful inquiry can the nature of the depression be determined, and as with every other emotional disorder in the elderly, a holistic and longitudinal perspective is warranted.

Aspects of the depressive matrix that are unique to the elderly are particular psychologic issues that have to do with decreasing social and biologic functioning, frailty, and anticipation of death. Gotjahn puts it well: "I used to think old age was an achievement in itself. I now know better: to get sick and to live on, that is an achievement"(9). Senescence at its worst is a season of loss and not everyone has the fortitude to surmount the loss of work role identity, let alone transcend preoccupation with one's body or overcome one's preoccupation with oneself (10).

The DSM-III-R criteria for a major depressive episode include, in addition to a dysphoric mood or loss of interest or pleasure, at least four symptoms, existing for at least 2 weeks, from the following list: poor appetite, insomnia or hypersomnia, psychomotor agitation or retardation; loss of energy; loss of interest or pleasure; feelings of worthlessness, self-reproach, or excessive guilt; complaints of diminished ability to think or concentrate; recurrent thoughts of death or suicidal ideation; or wishes to be dead or suicide attempt. Although clinicians are additionally reminded that the diagnosis for major depressive disorder should not be made when an organic mental disorder or normal bereavement exists, the mixture of organic and functional disorders is commonly seen. Within the subclassification of major depression the presence of psychotic or melancholic phenomena (that is, delusions and hallucinations) and/or early morning awakening, diurnal mood shift, marked agitation or retardation, and weight loss and excessive guilt have value in the determination of treatment interventions.

Elderly depressed patients are more often agitated and more often suffer from cognitive impairment, making differentiation from organic dementia a difficult task. Feinberg and Goodman propose four "ideal types" of patients spanning the spectrum of these illnesses (11). These authors identify four types of mixtures of depression and dementia. The first is depression initially diagnosed as dementia but on extensive clinical examination and evaluation no intellectual deficit is found, affective illness is found, and the entire syndrome is reversible with successful treatment. The second type is depression with secondary dementia, in which the patient presents as primarily depressed, and on examination and evaluation intellectual deficit is found, affective illness is confirmed, and the entire syndrome is reversible with successful treatment. The third type is dementia presenting as depression "pseudodepression," in which the patient presents as depressed and clinical examination and evaluation reveal intellectual deficit, but no affective illness is found and the syndrome may or may not be reversible. The last type is dementia with secondary depression, in which the patient presents as primarily demented and examination and evaluation reveal both affective illness and dementia.

In the United States, in contrast to London and Toronto, clinicians are more apt to diagnose dementia than depression where the two presentations coexist. This risks inadequate treatment for some patients with depression. Psychiatrists who trust their own emphatic responses to these patients are often able to effectively differentiate between the two presentations (12).

When depression exists in the elderly patient, it may present itself differently from its presentation in other age groups. Charatan alleges that "older depressives report more physical symptoms and complaints, express less guilt, [and] rarely report feeling depressed" as such. Apathy and paranoid symptoms are commoner in the elderly depressions (13).

When endogenous depressive illness exists, somatic treatment has much to offer. Electroconvulsive treatment may be even a safer treatment than antidepressant drugs, but both have a definite place in the treatment of depression. There is controversy among psychiatrists as to the priority of choice of these measures. Certainly an acutely agitated, suicidal and delusionally depressed elderly man warrants immediate protection and hence probably electroconvulsive treatment. The high suicidality of our depressed elderly requires prompt assessment and intervention. Data from the 1975 National Center for Health Statistics reveal that those over age 60 represented 18.5% of the United States population but this population committed 23% of all suicides (14).

The recommendation for antidepressant medications, whether tricyclics, monoamine oxidase inhibitors (MAOIs), or central nervous system stimulants, with or without adjunctive medications, varies from author to author. The concept of atypical depression as described by Friedel (15) and Sovner (16) has heuristic and treatment value, but remains controversial. These authors describe a clinical picture of hypersomnia, hyperphagia, phobic anxiety, fatigue, and anhedonia in the atypical depression. They further allege that a significant number of patients given the diagnosis of dysthymic disorder or depressive character may be suffering from atypical depression. Comfort (17) and Georgotas et al. (18) would select MAOIs for treating these resistant geriatric depressions.

Whenever drug therapy and electroconvulsive and supportive therapy may have been administered to elderly depressed patients, prognosis may be poor to fair according to Millard's study of 124 patients between the ages of 65 and 89 years (19).

The diagnostic use of the dexamethasone suppression test in the elderly has become less popular recently because of the difficulties in interpreting the findings. The use of a Ritalin probe for assessment of the probable value of tricyclic antidepressants also remains controversial, but there is clearly a subgroup of depressed elderly who respond positively to this psychostimulant.

Another type of depression occurring in the elderly is bipolar depressive disorder. It seldom takes its onset in this era, but may be persistent from early middle life. In this situation the patient will have had one or more manic episodes by history and will be currently undergoing a major depressive episode.

The use of lithium in bipolar illness calls for caution in elderly patients because of their greater neurologic sensitivity to the cognitive dulling features of the drug and their frequently diminished renal clearance ability. Carbamazepine is being used in-creasingly in the management of manic–depressive illness, particularly in those patients who fail to respond to lithium. Careful blood monitoring is necessary when either drug is used.

When a manic presentation occurs in the elderly patient, the possibility of organic brain syndrome must be ruled out. In contrast to 19th-century neuropsychiatrists' belief that aged bipolar patients usually developed chronic mania which eventually turned into dementia, Himmelhock et al. (20) have found that advanced age has no effect on the course or the outcome. Some manic elderly patients present as manic pseudodementia, a condition comparable to depressive pseudodementia (21).

Medications, electronconvulsive treatment, and support treatment may not be the only interventive measures to be considered in working with the depressed elderly. Families and long-term-care personnel need to be taught attitudes which do not lead to learned helplessness and do not scold or whip the patient. Therapists would do well to encourage patients' retention of as much control and responsibility for themselves as possible since these are key factors in their prognosis. Therapists should encourage patients to label the subjective components of depression and identify the associated thoughts. The therapist can then assist the elderly patient to break up negative views about him- or herself, the world, and the future, by persuasion and education (22). In the successful management of the elderly patient, a high degree of negotiation surrounding medications and non-medication interventions will achieve greater compliance, more positive therapeutic relationships, and a greater likelihood of good results (see Chapters 9 and 10). This skill in the treatment setting often must be exercised with numerous collateral interviews with the patient's family as well as with other caretakers.

Anxiety

Impaired defenses associated with frailty, losses, and other stresses commonly impair the older adult's security, with the resultant emergence of anxiety. Sudden anxiety may also herald the development of an organic illness. It is nearly always an accompaniment of depressive illness as well. Post-traumatic stress disorders associated with specific emotional vulnerabilities and at times seemingly insignificant traumata are seen. Panic disorders and agoraphobic symptoms may blur with disengagement behavior so common in older persons. A frequent denominator to many of these variable presentations of anxiety is the loss or perceived loss of control over one's life. When a measure of control can be restored, anxiety symptoms have a greater chance of subsiding.

The use of anxiolytic drugs can often be counterproductive because of the risk of excessive sedation and falling or paradoxical aggravation of existing symptoms and creation of confusion or hostility. The therapists themselves, by virtue of a supportive relationship of an enduring nature, may do a great deal more to quell the anxiety. Many patients can benefit from relaxation training and desensitization if a phobic object or situation exists. If drugs are used, they should not be the first consideration. They should be used in low dosages, for short periods of time, with an intelligent choice of product based on knowledge of the half-life, side effects, and compliance pattern. It is often the symbolic features of the medication rather than the pharmacologic properties which justify drug use in the control of anxiety.

Paranoia

While the persistence of paranoid schizophrenia into the elderly period is common in some settings, e.g., long-term-care facilities, the more common paranoid presentment is that which accompanies brain failure or delirium. Comfort (23) lists a variety of diagnoses of "nonpsychiatric" causes of paranoid symptoms (see also Chapter 39). Accusations of stealing money or hiding personal possessions made against the caretaker lead to strain, and rational denials fail to alter the suspicious posture. One can understand this phenomenon arising in the older adult who has forgotten where he or she put something and needs to explain the loss in order to deny his or her cognitive failure. The therapist may be most useful in working with caretakers around this issue.

Paraphrenia (atypical paranoid disorder) is considered by many to be a functional paranoid disorder unique to elderly persons who do not exhibit schizophrenic affective and cognitive symptoms. Social isolation and hearing loss are common accompaniments. Unresolved is the possibility that paraphrenia (Kraeplin's term) may be a late-onset schizophrenia although the DSM-III-R recognizes the possibility that the onset of schizophrenia may occur after age 45.

Paranoia is also a frequent accompaniment of major affective disorder and may be a harbinger presentation. Alcohol abuse may favor paranoid thinking.

The rise in criminal attacks on elderly victims may provide a "normal paranoia" or at least suspicions and highly wary postures.

Hypochondriasis

Hypochondriasis is described in DSM-III-R as "an unrealistic interpretation of physical signs or sensations as abnormal, leading to preoccupation with the fear or belief of having serious disease"(1). The tendency toward preoccupation with one's body increases with advanced age, particularly when one system or another exhibits dysfunction, but it is unfair to label this tendency per se hypochondriasis. It is only after the preoccupation has robbed the patient's mind of interest in other matters, has sapped the individual's energy for life-affirming pursuits, and has caught him or her up in a constant search for organic illness that the label "hypochondriasis" is appropriate.

In the elderly person, because of the greater likelihood of occurrence of organic failure, the astute clinician can be faced with a dilemma. Should a casual, minimizing response to the patient's complaints be made, the clinician may miss an important, treatable condition. Yet, an aggressive pursuit of the disease in the patient may compound the plight of the hypochondriacal patient by intimating that there really must be something terribly wrong to warrant all these tests . . . and there are always other doctors and clinics, and repeated tests. . . . The patient meanwhile is taught an entire idiom of part-knowledge about medicine, and his or her anxiety titer mounts. Treatment is more often successfully managed by a primary care physician whose concern is for the whole person, who is less concerned about the disease in the patient, and who listens patiently for the frequent hidden agenda of need for confirmation and worth. The caretaker strain of many of these patients because of their demandingness, hostility, and modest to poor responsiveness to reassurance can easily lead to their rejection. Such patients become the "rotating" patients about whom Lipsitt has written (24).

THE CLINICAL INTERVIEW

Determining the Nature of the Problem

Determining the nature of the problem to be addressed is often more complex than at first thought. The elderly patient in particular often has a different presentation from that of younger adults. There may be a silent coronary, a painless acute abdomen, an afebrile infectious disorder. What the geropsychiatrist must realize again and again is that a psychiatric presentation may indicate a medical/surgical problem. That such a hidden problem may exist is made the more difficult by a patient who may belittle his condition and would have the clinician believe that it is nothing serious at all.

The dynamics of the diminished complaint can indicate reduced systemic response, reduced pain perception, or even the denial of a tired old person who secretly hopes that whatever the condition is, it will bring on his or her own demise simply out of a sense of having lived about as long as he or she feels is necessary. This sense of diminished self-worth may lead the patient to not want to bother the doctor about his or her plight.

Conversely, many older men and woman somatize, whether this be a conscious or unconscious process. A hypochondriacal older patient is often depressed. Increased fixation on the body may be a maladaptive aging process. In general, the clinician treads a narrow path with such patients, wanting on the one hand to treat the medical/psychiatric problem, whether specifically articulated or not, but on the other hand, not wanting to reinforce unhealthy obsessional body preoccupation.

The clinician should be aware of surrogate symptoms put forth by the patient who may be embarrassed to talk about a sexual problem, an untenable home situation, or a more ominous symptom which is perceived as being life threatening. Indeed, the clinician needs to listen with a third ear to determine the nature of the problem.

Developing and Maintaining a Therapeutic Relationship

A therapeutic relationship develops not only between the physician and the patient but between the physician and the patient's spouse, children, or caretaker. Each of the persons presenting at the interview is likely to have a different agenda, and much can be learned about familial interactions, needs and power systems, as well as about the identified patient by simply allowing all parties to talk. The identified patient may be the one whose name appears on the clinician's appointment schedule but may not be the real patient in this scenario.

Many older men and women today are very uncomfortable attending a psychiatrist because of the expectation of being considered "crazy" and automatically being sent off to a mental hospital. Most of them find it difficult to talk about intimate personal, emotional, conflictual material;

many want a quick fix for the presenting symptoms of anxiety or irritability without understanding the necessity for any orderly assessment of the matrices in which these symptoms take place. Our current elderly are far more likely to take their problems to a primary care physician, to their pastor, or to a friend than to a psychiatrist. It will be necessary for primary physicians to recognize the limitations of their abilities and interests and to facilitate referrals to psychiatric consultants with an open explanation of what special skills today's psychiatrists have. Not to prepare the patient for a psychiatric evaluation is quite likely to lead to a poor relationship even if the patient appears for the appointment.

Not only the general medical population but the elderly patients, themselves, frequently do not realize the possible value of psychotherapy in its various settings of individual, couple, and group therapy; the judicious use of neuroleptics, antidepressants, newer tranquilizers, and antimanics; and a session or two with a psychotherapist familiar with developmental issues and the common problems of aging.

Not all elderly are energetic gray panthers insisting on being considered equally with their younger friends in an ageist society; many are quite ashamed of simply being old. A clinician wishing to establish a therapeutic relationship needs to be gentle, supportive, patient, and appreciative of the psychologic issues of aging.

Because the elderly comprise such a heterogeneous group, however, it must be stated that some enlightened older adults are ready and willing to enter into dynamic psychotherapy. Such persons are often less defensive and work harder than many a younger patient.

For the maintenance of a therapeutic relationship with older persons it is recommended that the relationship be an abiding one. Most older patients have suffered the loss of siblings, friends, and spouses. The total loss ought not to be compounded by therapists who are here today and gone tomorrow.

This recommendation for constancy and abidance flies in the face of health care delivery systems which dictate how many days a patient may remain in a hospital and similarly ration psychiatric outpatient care. Whatever merit such nonclinical regulation may have in general, it is decidedly countertherapeutic for most elderly patients. Such patients need the security of a relationship which can reasonably be expected to persist for a long time. Where the number of visits are arbitrarily limited, however, it may be appropriate for the clinician to space them further apart than one might normally do with a younger clientele.

Attitudes in the clinician which encourage the older person to assume responsibility, make decisions, expect full explanation of his or her problems serve to empower the patient. The patient-centered, negotiated approach to interviewing fosters an enhanced executive ego function in the patient (see Chapters 9 and 10). The doctor-centered authoritative approach, if used exclusively, may impair rapport and lead to feelings of infantilization and anger.

Relationships with elderly patients can be enhanced by touching the patients, greeting them, bidding them farewell, and taking an occasional pulse and blood pressure to provide socially acceptable opportunities for such touching. The elderly are usually very hungry for touch since there often are few people in their lives who might provide that touch, and since so many people have come to find touching a wrinkled elderly person as something to be avoided.

Elders, like other adult patients, should be addressed initially at least, by their proper name as a respectful gesture (25).

Clinicians should give more of themselves as they collaborate with their older patient to find, beyond the particular symptomatology, the meaning, the ultimate concerns, and the drama of the patient's life.

The placement of the clinician in a position where the older person can see and hear him or her is vital to the relationship because clearer communication is facilitated.

Reminiscing gives value to the patient's life, and the clinician will do well to attend. Let the patient begin where he or she wants to, but look for innner desires, drives, and dreams behind the manifest content.

Communicating Information and Implementing a Treatment Plan

Negotiating with the elderly patient around treatment issues may mean relinquishing an authoritarian attitude and a desire to be overzealous in treatment, replacing these with a more modest and humble intervention, if that is what the patient wants. Short, frequent chats may be more beneficial to some severely incapacitated elders than the most carefully chosen treatment plan. The clinician would do well to recognize how frightening medical jargon can be to many a patient and should use the language of the home or more simple conceptualizations in describing diagnosis.

Our health care system relies on patients to initiate care, but our elderly are not as proactive regarding their care as are younger people, and clinicians may need to reach out to them more aggressively than is customary. This may warrant house calls, consultation at neighborhood health centers, talks at senior citizen centers, and other similar endeavors. In general, our elderly underreport their illnesses and their needs, but we need to remember always that sick old people are sick because they are sick and not just because they are old.

It will often be helpful to tell the caretaker of your elderly patient as well as the patient him- or herself what your treatment plan is. Writing your instructions legibly, unambiguously, and simply for the patient will be helpful, especially where some cognitive or hearing impairment exists. All diagnostic procedures should be carefully explained to both the patient and caretaker. It is to be expected that most elderly will not retain what you have stated after the assessment. Repetition of your diagnosis and treatment plan during the initial visit and at later visits and possibly over the telephone is to be recommended. Pillbox dispensing systems for times of administration and the assistance of home health personnel in medication supervision are often necessary. The use of as few pills as possible to be taken as few times a day as possible will enhance patient compliance with medications.

The sick elderly are one of the most difficult patient populations to work with. Formal diagnosis and often multiple diagnoses featuring contributions and shaping from normal aging processes, organic illnesses, and many other stressful psychosocial current and past life events present a demanding challenge. But the sick and elderly are a most gratifying population to work with in this author's opinion. Whatever the difficulties which may arise in attending the elderly, their appreciation for our interest is clear and rewarding.

References

1. American Psychiatric Association: *Diagnostic and Statistical Manual of Mental Disorders (Third Edition-Revised)*. Washington, DC, American Psychiatric Association, 1987.
2. Butler R: The life review, an interpretation of reminiscence in the aged. *Psychiatry* 26:65–76, 1963.
3. Ford CV, Sbordone RJ: Attitudes of psychiatrists toward elderly patients. *Am J Psychiatry* 137:571–575, 1980.
4. Sobel E: Countertransference issues with the later life patient. *Contemp Psychoanal* 16:211–222, 1980.
5. Kolman PB: The value of laboratory investigations of elderly psychiatric patients. *J Clin Psychiatry* 45:112–116, 1984.
6. Dubin WR, Weiss KJ, Zeccardi A: Organic brain syndrome, the psychiatric imposter. *JAMA* 249:60–62, 1983.
7. Lipowski ZJ: Transient cognitive disorders in the elderly. *Am J Psychiatry* 140:1426–1436, 1983.
8. Wells C: Diagnosis of dementia: a reassessment. *Psychosomatics* 3:183–190, 1984.
9. Grotjohn M: An editorial. *Lancet* 1:441–442, 1982.
10. Peck RC: *Psychological Developments in the Second Half of Life: Middle Age and Aging*. Chicago, University of Chicago Press, 1968.
11. Feinberg T, Goodman B: Affective illness, dementia and pseudodementia. *J Clin Psychiatry* 45:99–103, 1984.
12. Cavenar JO, Maltbie AA, Austin L: Depression simulating organic brain disease. *Am J Psychiatry* 136:521–523, 1979.
13. Charatan F: Depression in the elderly: diagnosis

and treatment. *Psychiatr Ann* 15:313–316, 1985.

14. Osgood N: *Suicide in the Elderly.* Rockville, MD, Aspen Publications, 1985.

15. Friedel R: Subtypes and lab measures of autonomous depression. *J Clin Psychiatry* 43:28, 1982.

16. Sovner R: The clinical characteristics and treatment of atypical depressions. *J Clin Psychiatry* 42:285, 1981.

17. Comfort A: Phenelzine therapy, the doctor, the patient and the wine and cheese party. *J Operational Psychiatry* 13:37–40, 1982.

18. Georgotas A, Freedman E, McCarthy M, et al: Resistant geriatric depressions and therapeutic response to MAOI. *Biol Psychiatry* 18:195–205, 1983.

19. Millard PH: Depression in old age. *Br Med J* 287:375, 1983.

20. Himmelhoch JM, Neil JF, May SJ, et al: Age, dementia, dyskinesia and lithium response. *Am J Psychiatry* 173:941–945, 1980.

21. Tease M, Reynolds C: Manic pseudodementia. *Psychosomatics* 25:256–260, l984.

22. Beck AT: *Cognitive Therapy and the Emotional Disorders.* New York, International Universities Press, 1976.

23. Comfort A: *Practice of Geriatric Psychiatry.* New York, Elsevier, 1980.

24. Lipsitt DR: The rotating patients: a challenge to psychiatrists. *J Geriatr Psychiatry* 69:51–61, 1968.

25. Lazare A: Shame and humiliation in the medical encounter. *Arch Intern Med* 147:1653–1658, 1987.

41

The Mentally Retarded/Mentally Ill

Mai-Lan Rogoff, M.D.

Between one and three percent of the U.S. population is estimated to be mentally retarded (up to six million people). Between 30% and 60% of this group are believed to be suffering from emotional disturbance and therefore potentially in need of psychiatric services. The number of these patients in need, particularly in outpatient settings can be expected to increase over the next decade for several reasons: (a) Deinstitutionalization and "normalization" have raised the number of mentally retarded adults living outside of institutions. (b) Improved standards of medical care for retarded individuals have lengthened their lifespans. (c) Improved survival of very ill infants through neonatal intensive care has increased the number of individuals who are mentally retarded due to pre- and perinatal insult. And (d) mentally retarded individuals as well as those who staff the residences which care for many of them are increasingly aware both of mentally retarded persons' "normal" ability to develop emotional disorders and of their right to seek appropriate care for psychiatric complaints.

MENTAL RETARDATION IN ADULTS

Mental retardation is generally classified according to four levels of intellectual func-
tion: mild, moderate, severe, and profound. Mildly retarded individuals have an IQ measured from approximately 70 to 55–50 (greater than 2 standard deviations below the mean). They may be capable of a 4th- to 5th-grade education, account for about 80% of the mentally retarded population, and often live independently in the community. Moderately retarded individuals have an IQ of 55–50 to 40–35, may achieve up to 2nd grade academically, and require some community support as adults. Severely retarded individuals have an IQ of 40–35 to 25–20, or about a 3-year cognitive level. Profoundly retarded individuals (about 1% of the mentally retarded population) have an IQ below 25–20 or approximately an 18-month cognitive level. Most of the mentally retarded people still living in institutions have severe or profound levels of retardation. Increasing availability of supported community living, however, has allowed many of these individuals to be "deinstitutionalized."

The *Diagnostic and Statistical Manual of Mental Disorders* (*Third Edition-Revised*) (DSM-III-R) (1) defines the essential features of mental retardation as

1. Significantly subaverage intellectual functioning resulting in, or associated with,

550

2. Deficits or impairments in adaptive behavior,
3. With onset before the age of 18.

This definition contains the major elements contributing to the vulnerability of mentally retarded children and adults to emotional and behavioral disturbance. Subaverage intelligence function, generally measured by IQ test scores as 2 standard deviations or more below the mean, compromises the individual's ability to comprehend events and their consequences. Deficits in adaptive ability include difficulties in developmental skills necessary for independent functioning, such as meeting basic physical needs, and ability to function as a member of a community. The latter skills include ability to cooperate, persist at a functional task, or to chain several tasks in sequence. Adaptive behavior may be measured relatively objectively through the American Association on Mental Deficiency (AAMD) (2) or Vineland (3) scales of adaptive behavior. Neuropsychologic tests may also provide an indication of adaptive abilities. Deficiencies in adaptive behavior tend to alter judgment, insight, the ability to learn from mistakes, and flexibility. The ways in which peers and teachers will interact with the mentally retarded individual, whether or not the individual has been labeled as mentally retarded, are also influenced both by adaptive and by intellectual deficits. Perhaps most importantly, mental retardation is a disorder of the developmental stage of life. The other conditions and social consequences of the disorder, sub-average intellectual functioning and deficits in adaptive behavior, thus affect the child as he or she grows up, forms a sense of self, and develops ways of coping and interacting with the world.

Emotional disturbance may be more problematic for the mentally retarded individual than any intellectual deficit. Socially unacceptable behavior is more detrimental to community and vocational acceptance than are low skill levels (4, 5). Behavioral problems are a major cause of continued need for institutional or highly supervised care.

DEINSTITUTIONALIZATION AND "NORMALIZATION"

Public policy since the 1970s has emphasized care of the mentally retarded individual outside of institutions, with "mainstreaming" and "normalization" as the guiding principles (6). The mandate of Public Law 94-142 (1975) is to educate all children, including retarded children, within the "mainstream" of the public school system, providing alternatives only if necessary. This mandate has also meant a change in residential placement keeping developmentally delayed children out of large institutions and raising them with biologic parents if possible, or in the "least restrictive environment." Early studies suggest that mentally retarded children raised in foster homes do better as adults than those raised in institutions with custodial care and that "normalizing" the environment even of institutionalized children improves functioning in various areas (7–10). On the other hand, the current data on effects of educational mainstreaming as opposed to specialized education are equivocal, with most studies showing no diference in academic ability, mixed effects on self-esteem, and no decrease in stigmatization compared with children in self-contained classrooms (11, 12). Some caution must also be exercised in using earlier studies regarding residential setting which essentially compared foster families with large institutional care, to argue for policy which labels any rearing away from biologic parents as "institutional care." Even in large institutions, the effect of such placements vary; some work suggests that residents who came from socially deprived homes prior to institutionalization showed significant improvement in IQ scores after being placed in the institution (13). Generally, research seems to support the benefits of raising mentally retarded children, as all children, in small loving environments, groups or families. There are incomplete answers as to the relative merits of education in regular versus specialized environments. Current policy increasingly keeps mentally retarded children, adolescents, and ultimately adults in the mainstream of society as much as possible.

Normalization of retarded adults has meant maintaining the usual, "normal" phases of adult life, including movement away from home toward independent living in the community and going to work during the day. For those unable to maintain a job in "competitive" (regular) employment, work is achieved through a sheltered workshop system including a system of "supervised employment." In supervised employment, jobs in a regular competitive environment are supervised by vocational rehabilitation staff, assuring the employer of job completion without concerns about performance level, absenteeism, or hiring/firing for that position. The benefit to the retarded employee is that he or she is performing a regular job in a regular job environment but is provided with additional structure and support. The effort to normalize living situations involves progressively increasing independence and movement from sheltered group living through staffed apartments to independent living. This progression is intended to provide the mentally retarded individual with steadily increasing responsibility together with the accompanying feelings of accomplishment.

Normalization and mainstreaming are not without problems. Since mainstreaming keeps developmentally delayed youngsters in their own schools as much as possible, and since only 2 to 3% of the children in any given school system will be developmentally delayed, one effect of mainstreaming is to limit the number of developmentally disabled children and adolescents at any one school. Insufficient numbers together with the desire to "mainstream" lowers the availability of specialized after-school activities. When the mentally retarded youngster is unable to make the varsity or the cheerleader squad, fails the auditions for the orchestra or drama group, and is unable to keep up in French club, he or she may end up with few after-school activities. One consequence of this situation is a further increase in the social isolation which mentally retarded people commonly experience. Mainstreaming of adolescents generally means fewer opportunities for romantic involvements, with less time to learn how to accomplish common social maneuvers such as indicating to a likely prospect that one is interested. This may later result in inappropriate social behavior through ignorance and lack of opportunities to practice.

Mentally retarded adults are apt to experience relatively frequent transitions both in living environment and in employment as they move through the system and become increasingly "normalized." If the movement is to a level of structure which is less than optimal for that person, it is often difficult to move "backwards" to a more structured situation. Normalization, then, may become a stress which leads to regression. Under this stress an individual who had functioned well in a structured environment may become disorganized and show inappropriate behavior while being "normalized." In such an instance, the process may paradoxically threaten his or her job or even ability to remain in the community at all. A request for psychiatric intervention often follows.

OCCURRENCE OF MENTAL ILLNESS IN MENTALLY RETARDED PERSONS

Individuals with mental retardation have a higher incidence of mental illness than do nonretarded individuals. Using standardized criteria, Rutter et al. (14) found that as many as 50% of the severely retarded children on the Isle of Wight showed psychiatric disorder compared with 7% of those without central nervous system dysfunction. Corbett (15) found a similar figure of 43%. Most research shows a greater prevalence of emotional disturbance in mentally retarded populations, with reported incidence varying from 30 to 60% (16–18).

The higher reported percentages of mentally retarded individuals with emotional disorders tend to occur in studies looking at "behavioral disorders" as opposed to major psychiatric diagnoses, and in institutionally based rather than community-based studies. Parsons (19) estimated that of institutionalized adults, 10% were psychotic and up to 60% had behavioral problems sufficient to interfere with functioning. Tu and Smith (20) studied 2158 institutionalized residents, of whom 43% were identified as problem cases. Aggressive behavior, hyperactivity, and self-injury were the most prevalent problems cited. Mentally retarded individuals can be diagnosed as having major psychotic disorders which respond favorably to appropriate psychotropic medications (21–25). Institutionalized adults have historically had more severe disturbances than mentally retarded individuals living in the community. While this will probably always be so, one effect of deinstitutionalization has been to move many of these individuals to the status of outpatients. Many problems formerly seen primarily in institutionalized patients are now being seen by outpatient psychiatrists.

Significant levels of psychopathology have been found in outpatient as well as in institutionally based samples. Matson (26) cited an overall figure for all psychiatric disorders as four to five times more frequent in the retarded than in the non-retarded group. Aman et al. (27) found that in a community-based mentally retarded population, 2% of preschoolers, 3% of special school students, and 14% of the adults were receiving psychotropic drugs. Personality disorders are also a significant problem in outpatient mentally retarded groups: Eaten and Menaloscino (28) found in a community-based population that 27% of the psychiatric diagnoses were personality disorders. On the other hand, completed suicide has been relatively rare. This may be a product of the supervision with which many mentally retarded individuals live, as well as lack of access to means (e.g., firearms) to commit suicide.

VULNERABILITY TO MENTAL ILLNESS IN MENTAL RETARDATION

Intrapsychic and Social Factors

Mentally retarded individuals have a high probability of having experienced failure in social as well as academic conditions. Academically, many will have been diagnosed through the experience of school failure and suffer both the stigmatizing effects of being labeled "retarded" and perhaps the more stigmatizing effects of self-labeling as "lazy" or "stupid." In one study, retarded children tended to blame themselves if unable to complete a task and settled for strategies which did not yield as high a degree of success as normal children. The nonretarded children, in contrast, tended to blame the tester or the test rather than themselves for failure to complete tasks (29) The expectation of failure often discourages retarded individuals from seeking out new problems to solve, even those within their capabilities. This further deprives those individuals of learning experiences. Socially they are often exposed to and aware of negative social conditions such as rejection and ridicule, isolation, infantilization, and restricted social and job opportunities (30). The diagnosis of mental retardation in a child is a very difficult one for most parents and frequently brings on a period of grief. The child will then have to cope with the effects of this grief, which may be expressed in pathologic ways, such as rejection or oversolicitousness, as well as in appropriate concern and advocacy. School-aged and adolescent mentally retarded children also frequently experience exclusion and teasing by peers. Mentally retarded people are as vulnerable as non-retarded individuals to depression, anxiety, and other dysphorias. They are more likely than the general population to encounter situations which tend to elicit loss of self-esteem with the associated affects of shame and humiliation. Those who have been placed in institutions may additionally show "institutionalization," behaviors characterized by dependence and sometimes by attention-seeking rituals or imitation of behaviors (such as seizures) observed in other residents.

As mentally retarded children become adults, they are likely to experience social disruption and object loss as they progress through work and residential programs. Residential staffs are particularly susceptible to burnout and rapid turnover of personnel due to large amounts of responsibility, poor pay, poor support and inadequate training. Staff turnover combined with the movement of clients through various placements often contributes to an experience of repeated loss and transitory relationships for mentally retarded adults. Restricted job, social, and, particularly, romantic opportunities also contribute to social isolation. Mentally retarded people often live in less prosperous neighborhoods and become subject to the problems and stresses associated with lower socioeconomic status. They may be victimized both by being interpersonally "used" through their normal desire to be accepted, and as victims of crimes. Mentally retarded individuals are subject to a great deal of social stress, much of which involves experiences of failure and loss of self-esteem which contribute to a sense of the self as unable to modify and influence the environment to satisfy wants and needs.

Developmental as well as social stresses impinge on the mentally retarded individual. Emotional development tends to proceed at chronological age-appropriate times, particularly in mild–moderate mental retardation, while cognitive development is delayed. This results in mentally retarded persons' having to cope with normal developmental issues with a decreased capacity to understand and assess them. Normal desires to form an identity, be accepted by the group, have friends, explore career choices, and cope with budding sexual urges may occur in a moderately retarded adolescent with a cognitive age of 6 years. Deficits in judgment may combine with the intense age-appropriate desire for peer acceptance to result in inappropriate

and ultimately maladaptive behavior. Deficits in cognitive capacity impair the ability to develop alternative solutions to problems and crises. Deficits in verbal abilities compromise the ability to label and talk about feelings or to develop friends who are also confidants. Mental retardation itself involves deficits in flexibility and problem solving (essential features of "intelligence"), leading to limited and relatively rigid repertoires of responses. Mentally retarded people thus often have to cope with increased sources of social and developmental stress in the face of reduced capacity to cope with those stresses.

Biologic Factors

Many mentally retarded individuals, particularly those with moderate to profound levels of retardation have a biologic burden in addition to psychologic and social vulnerabilities. Animal studies and neuropsychologic investigations of stroke and head injury patients have shown that damage to certain parts of the brain may predispose to maladaptive behaviors. Frontal lobe damage, for example, may lead to apathy or loss of judgment and impulsivity (31). Temporal lobe damage may be related to rage reactions (32). Neurologic disorders may also directly predispose the individual to major psychiatric disorders (33).

In addition to specific central nervous system damage, many mentally retarded individuals have associated deficits which compromise adaptive functioning. Sensory deficits such as hearing or visual problems impair the ability to understand events. Communication problems often found in association with mental retardation such as language delay or even simple dysarthria have been found to be associated with the development of behavior problems even in the absence of mental retardation (34, 35). Specific learning disabilities and auditory-processing problems hamper learning and problem solving. Seizure disorders, more common in individuals with mental retardation than in the general population, make it more difficult to learn and generalize responses in childhood because of the interruptions in attention and amnesia associated with each seizure. The proportion of persons with seizures increases as intellectual level decreases (14, 15, 36). This is probably due to the increasing incidence of central nervous system anomalies as a major causative factor in mental retardation at increasing levels of developmental delay.

Emotional disorders are thus a significant problem in mentally retarded individuals, for biopsychosocial reasons. Mentally retarded individuals are more likely than nonretarded individuals to carry a high burden of social stress and experience of failure and stigmatization. They may also be biologically vulnerable, have associated problems which complicate problem solving, and have fewer coping strategies available to deal with these stresses.

CHALLENGES IN OUTPATIENT PSYCHIATRIC CARE

Patient Characteristics

Dually diagnosed individuals (mentally retarded individuals with mental illness) may have characteristics which are also problematic in the general population, such as chaotic behavior, assaultiveness, sexually inappropriate behavior, or fire setting. While these present obvious difficulties in management, nondangerous but difficult to contain behaviors and feelings are probably more common. These include depression and social withdrawal, aggressive behavior such as verbal threats of assault or damage to property, and oppositional behavior (e.g., refusal to go to a day program or refusal to shower). Those who have been institutionalized may exhibit socially unacceptable behavior such as screaming and other noisemaking, begging for money, or approaching strangers (particularly children). Regressed institutionalized behavior, particularly behavior which is considered "disgusting," such as ruminating up gastric contents and chewing or smearing it or smearing feces contributes to social isolation. Although many mentally retarded individuals do not display these behaviors, socially unacceptable conduct contributes to difficulties in establishing group residences for mentally retarded individuals in neighborhoods and to attempts by neighbors to evict certain individuals or even entire residences. The psychiatric diagnoses and feeling states underlying these behaviors present a varied diagnostic and therapeutic challenge for the psychiatrist. Depression, in particular, is frequently underdiagnosed (23, 37).

Systems Characteristics

Mentally retarded individuals are often involved with multiple systems of care and caregivers. If the mentally retarded man or woman is not living and working independently, he or she is generally living in a residential program such as a group home or transitional apartment with varying levels of staffing. There is also generally a day program staff for the different day programs, from supervised "competitive" (regular) employment to day programs for dually diagnosed individuals too disturbed to function in a sheltered workshop environment. The individual may have been hospitalized or have been involved in a hospital diversion program as an alternative to hospitalization with its own staff. Residential and supervised employment programs often have their own consulting staffs. The mentally retarded individual may also be involved with a social service agency, an association for retarded citizens, and sometimes with the courts. Last and certainly not least, one or more concerned family members are also often involved with the mentally retarded patient.

Particularly with less verbal patients, history from observers assumes great importance and is most valid if the same history is obtained from multiple observers in different situations. The psychiatrist taking care of the mentally retarded individual in the community needs to communicate with and coordinate information from as many different sources as possible. One problem with multiple sources is that their definitions of "abnormal" may differ. Another is that their treatment philosophies may not be identical or even similar. Multiple "vendors" of services may not communicate well with each other, and some have their own histories of enmeshments and conflicts over policies, clients, money or "turf." These will combine with any positive or negative prejudices about psychotherapy and psychotropic medication to affect the information about the patient which is relayed to the psychiatrist. Some order may be imposed on this potential chaos through the use of agreed-upon checklists of observable behaviors. More specific information than the patient "had a bad week last week" may then be obtained. Knowledge of the history of service provision and philosophy of area service providers for that patient in that particular community is similarly helpful.

Philosophical disagreements over optimal therapy for mentally retarded individuals abound. They include the debate over rehabilitative versus clinical models, as well as the degree of commitment to normalization/promoting independence versus provision of structure. Also at issue is the controversy over whether mental retardation is a condition purely of developmental delay or whether issues of "difference" are also important.

Staff personnel who are extremely committed to normalization may see psychotherapy and particularly psychotropic medications as not "normal" and may therefore avoid recognition of significant mental illness. Even delusions may be explained as "stories he likes to tell." Fear of the effects and presumed power of psychotropic medications may lead staff members to avoid situations which might lead to requests for medication or to avoid giving medications if they are prescribed. The refusal may be direct or may be through talking about the medication to the patient ("You don't really need that poison"). The latter situation is more difficult to manage because it is often hidden from the treating physician. The mentally retarded individual is caught in the middle, often feeling trapped and helpless. The converse also applies: Personnel frequently hope that medication is more powerful than it is and may seek psychopharmacologic solutions to problems which can be addressed more effectively through environmental and behavioral techniques. One potentially successful approach is to point out that the ability to react to adverse circumstance with dysphoria is part of being "normal." If medications are used, information given by the staff regarding symptoms which may be side effects should be collected both before and after initiating treatment. The information that monitoring will be frequent and that the staff will play some role in decision making often allays fears. Behaviorally oriented staffs are accustomed to keeping detailed data, and information about target symptoms and side effects can easily be added to their procedure. In working with any mentally retarded person living in a staffed environment, prejudices about medications and psychotherapy need to be explored in the staff as well as in the individual and in his or her guardians.

The "development versus difference" controversy has existed in mental retardation literature for at least 25 years (38). Developmentalists have seen mentally retarded individuals as progressing over the same developmental territory more slowly—a position with some research support (39, 40). "Difference" theorists note additional specific defects in many mentally retarded individuals, such as attention deficit or language and communication retardation. IQ scores alone are relatively poor predictors of social functioning, suggesting that some other factor(s) besides cognitive delay interfere with adaptive behavior in some individuals and implying a need for separate evaluation of adaptation. This view is reflected in the AAMD and DSM-III-R requirements for demonstrated deficits in adaptive behavior as a criterion for the diagnosis of mental retardation. Many retarded adult individuals also lack the motivation, curiosity, or social abilities of the normal child at the equivalent cognitive level. This becomes more true as one moves down through the

IQ scale. Explanations of this phenomenon divide into those which argue that the observed differences are the result of psychologic reaction to years of experience of restricted opportunity, failure, and consequent loss of motivation (30, 41) and those which suggest that there may be additional differences based on neuropsychologic injury (42, 43).

The clinical consequences of a "pure" developmental position is the expectation that the deficits seen in individuals with mental retardation can be remedied by sufficient habilitation and teaching. A "difference" position suggests that some individuals will always need a more structured environment. Such theoretical differences also have clinical significance in considering whether, for example, oppositional behavior and tantrums in an adult represent a delayed normal developmental phase or a qualitatively different dysfunctional state. While it may be inappropriate to ignore temper tantrums in a 250 lb 30-year-old man regardless of theoretical position, the ways in which the behavior is understood affects therapist and community reaction and treatment options. It may be, however, that while mentally retarded individuals are developmentally delayed and progress along the same cognitive developmental path as nonretarded individuals, certain disabilities are more commonly associated with mental retardation on an organic basis (i.e., hyperkinesis, attention deficit, impulsivity). There may also be effects of viewing the world from a very young perspective for decades which leave the moderately–profoundly mentally retarded person not only developmentally delayed but also different. The two theories may not be as mutually exclusive as earlier debates suggest.

In addition to disagreements about treatment philosophy, community programs are often subject to unreliable funding and tend to change with successive turns of fashion and theory. These problems combine with the problems of staff and client turnover to leave mentally retarded individuals, who already have difficulty understanding and adapting to new environments and information, periodically having to cope with changing programs, changing rules, changing staff, and changing funding.

Finally, a very significant problem in the provision of outpatient-based care to the mentally retarded emotionally disturbed individual is a dearth of appropriate facilities to provide more intensive treatment should an inpatient stay be required (44). Dually diagnosed individuals tend to "fall between the cracks." Traditional psychiatric facilities feel they do not have sufficient expertise to cope with developmental delay; they are concerned about the effect on the milieu of the inpatient unit, particularly if the mentally retarded person in question is nonverbal or unable to self-toilet or self-feed. Similarly, units which are accustomed to rehabilitating developmental delay are uncomfortable monitoring psychiatric medications or coping with the relatively unpredictable and hostile interactions which may characterize an active psychotic process.

LEGAL ISSUES AND ETHICAL DILEMMAS

A multiplicity of civil and criminal issues have arisen with regard to mental retardation. Civil issues include individual rights with regard to education, housing, employment, guardianship, competency, marriage and child rearing, informed consent, and refusal of treatment. Criminal issues include competency to stand trial and criminal responsibility. These are not discussed in depth in this chapter because they involve the same principles as legal issues in other underprivileged groups (see chapter 44).

The psychiatrist treating dually diagnosed patients may be called on to contribute to evaluations regarding any of the above issues. He or she may be asked to provide a letter regarding community housing for a dually diagnosed patient who is currently asymptomatic in a structured setting but who has a prior history of inappropriate sexual behavior with children or of fire setting. The psychiatrist will have to explain the risk of tardive dyskinesia to a mildly–moderately retarded, verbal person with schizophrenia and determine the likelihood of a court finding that person competent to consent to medication. He or she will be asked to contribute to educational treatment plans, be called as a witness in litigation between parents and school systems, and be asked to assist in determining competencies from ability to stand trial to ability to own and drive a car.

Sexual rights and parenting constitute one area in which particular issues have arisen for mentally retarded persons. Eugenic arguments in the early part of the 20th century made the false assumption that mental retardation is almost always inherited. A case was then made, using public health arguments similar to those in the argument for compulsory vaccination, justifying compulsory sterilization in an attempt to limit the mentally retarded gene pool. Judges made statements such as "three generations of imbeciles is enough" (45), and by 1939 31 states in the United States had passed eugenic sterilization laws. Mentally retarded adolescents were often sterilized with no attempt to explain what was being done to them or why they could not have children. Within the past 20 years, policies of mainstreaming and normalization as well as increased awareness of individual civil rights have substituted education about sexuality and contraception for sterilization. Mentally retarded adults living in the community sometimes marry and have children. Subsequent research has noted that while IQ level does tend to cluster in families, children of mentally retarded adults are frequently not mentally retarded themselves. The feared effect on the gene pool does not seem to be occurring (46). Although individuals with low moderate to profound mental retardation (cognitive age 6 years or below) would not be expected to be able to function successfully as parents, they are often infertile. Discussions of the effects of mentally retarded parents on offspring generally refer to mild to high moderately retarded parents. Sterilization

may still be performed although problems of informed consent complicate voluntary sterilization, and involuntary sterilization is relatively difficult to secure even if a guardian is appointed. The AAMD has suggested guidelines for involuntary sterilization (47) in an attempt to urge a course between universal inappropriate sterilization and making sterilization virtually unobtainable. In many individuals, problems such as deficits in comprehension and adaptive ability or judgment, which make it difficult to obtain informed consent, are the same issues which compromise the ability to raise children.

The major concern about mentally retarded individuals functioning as parents has not been one of genetics so much as of ability to provide a stimulating, safe, and supportive environment for children. While most studies seem to indicate that many mentally retarded parents provide adequate parenting, difficulties in raising children for many other mentally retarded parents leave these children at a statistically greater risk for neglect, maltreatment, and developmental delay (48–50). The risk to children for behavioral and emotional problems is increased when mentally retarded individuals with major psychiatric disorders become parents. There is some risk to children of parents with major psychiatric disorders even in the absence of parental mental retardation (51–53). Disturbed parent–child interactions are felt to be the cause. In children of mentally retarded/mentally ill parents, a dual set of compromising factors may be present. Psychosocial retardation in children may also result from unstimulating home environments. On the other hand, mentally retarded adults have been shown to respond well to a teaching and behavioral model which instructs about parenting, emergency child care, and stimulation (54). Such parents are often better prepared for the tasks of parenting than many nonretarded individuals. This suggests, along with previous work (see reference 55 for review), that with intense social support and teaching, mentally retarded individuals can make quite adequate parents. There is no justification for removing children from mild to high moderately retarded parents who do not have emotional disorders simply because of their mental retardation. Love, marriage, sex, and having children are among aspects of normal life. Contraceptive information and education about sexuality are essential parts of education for mentally retarded adolescents. If individuals choose to become parents, extra support appears to be necessary to provide their children with normal opportunities, and this need should be addressed. When more pronounced levels of mental retardation are at issue, contraceptive education and occasionally sterilization should be provided.

THE CLINICAL INTERVIEW

Determining the Nature of the Problem

Some studies have suggested that clinicians tend to ignore debilitating psychiatric conditions in mentally retarded individuals which would be diagnosed and treated in nonretarded individuals, a phenomenon which has been called "diagnostic overshadowing" (56). This appears to be particularly true for anxiety disorders and depression. The suggestion is that clinicians tend to lump such disturbances together as "behavioral problems" associated with mental retardation. For the most part, the types of mental disorders seen in mentally retarded individuals are not different from those in nonretarded persons, and similar methods are used in diagnosis, particularly in mild–moderately retarded, verbal individuals. As the level of retardation deepens, communication difficulties increase, and diagnosis becomes more problematic. At all levels of mental retardation, exacerbation of previously learned, maladaptive behaviors may be exhibited under stress. In severe–profound mental retardation, certain behaviors become common which are uncommon in nonretarded individuals. These include rumination, smearing, and movement stereotypies. Severe self-injurious behavior, which is uncommon in nonretarded individuals, even in those with psychosis, is common enough in severe–profound mental retardation to be called by its acronym: SIB. Behaviors such as severe relationship difficulties, the need for sameness and resistance to change, and motor stereotypies which would be diagnosed as "autistic" in less retarded individuals also become more common in severe–profound mental retardation. Whereas underdiagnosis is often a problem with mild to moderate retarded individuals, care must be taken not to over diagnose regressed psychoses in the severe–profound group.

Mentally retarded adults often appear overly dependent or oppositional. This may occur as a consequence of their parents' reactions to the normal tasks of parenting. The normally narrow path between promoting independence in children and being negligent as parents or between appropriate supervision and being overprotective appears narrower to the parents of mentally retarded children. Comparisons with other parents' practices or guidance from "how to do it" books are more difficult to obtain. Most mentally retarded individuals have grown up more protected and with less encouragement of independent behavior than their peers. As adults, they often continue to mistrust their own judgment and will instead seek guidance from authority figures, thus appearing "overly dependent," whining, or clinging. Oppositional behavior may result from rebellion against the fear of being controlled. Adult mentally retarded people who were socially deprived as children, such as those who were institutionalized, may also use excessive dependence on adults in their current environment to try to fulfill needs which were not met in childhood.

Recognition of these common patterns allows the therapist working with the mentally retarded individual to address the current problem. It also allows the therapist working with families to develop a degree of empathy with the individual's parents. Concerned parents may infantilize their adult child out of appropriate concern rather than because of pathologic need.

Residential staffs, often young and dealing with their own issues of separation and independence, may become angered at the mentally retarded individual's parents for promoting dependence. Staff and parents may then find themselves at odds in treatment. The psychotherapist serves an essential purpose in helping all parties to see that despite their discrepant positions, all share mutual concern about the mentally retarded patient's welfare. By offering some validation to both positions, the therapist can then help develop and explain a more useful therapeutic plan.

Some clinical conditions occur with greater frequency in mentally retarded individuals than in nonretarded individuals. Psychotic symptoms on the basis of dementia are of particular concern in individuals with Down syndrome because of the increased incidence of Alzheimer's disease in that disorder (57, 58). Behavior which may be maladaptive for the individual's age and situation may also be part of a normal developmental progression. An example is a prolonged oppositional phase in a severely retarded person. Some idiosyncratic behaviors may be seen as learned behaviors in response to institutionalization and may even have been adaptive in that setting. Hoarding of possessions or food in odd places such as socks or extreme defensiveness about showering or being touched are examples of such behaviors.

Another phenomenon which should be considered in the diagnosis of behavioral disturbance in mentally retarded patients is the occurrence of unusual side effects and paradoxical effects of medications. Mentally retarded individuals may have difficulty describing side effects or even understanding that new symptoms after starting medication may be due to that medication. Target symptoms may increase or new symptoms may occur as reactions to the discomforts of side effects. For example, aggression as a response to akathisia has been described (59). Paradoxical response to sedative–hypnotics may be a significant problem (60) and should be considered if symptoms worsen or fail to improve. Similarly, physical discomfort due to illness may manifest as increased SIB, or decreased hearing due to cerumen may present as paranoid behavior. Physical evaluation is essential in evaluation of mentally retarded patients. One way to decrease unanticipated reactions is to avoid prescribing recently released medications for which the side effects are largely unknown. Residence staffs also need to be educated as to possible side effects as well as benefits of prescribed medications.

Retarded individuals require alterations in interview techniques (17). The examiner or therapist will probably need to be more directive and supportive and offer more structure, encouragement, and limits than usual. Receptive as well as expressive language problems are common in mental retardation. It is important not to confuse the patient's misunderstanding of the situation, questions, or requirements as delusional perception. The examiner's vocabulary will often need to be simplified and short sentences which lack subordinate clauses used. Open-ended questions may be very difficult for the mentally retarded person to process and answer; it may be more considerate to offer the patient simple two-choice answers. It may be necessary to allow more time for the mentally retarded person to form an answer to a question, but long silences generally indicate that the person has forgotten the question and is thinking about something else. Techniques of focusing attention may need to be used, such as including the patient's name in questions.

The tendency to dependency or oppositional behavior and expectation of failure which affect the mentally retarded individual's general adaptation also affect his or her reaction to the interview. Mentally retarded patients are very likely to view the interview as a test which they often expect to fail. This will lead some to be silent, others to withdraw, many to give answers which they think will please the examiner. This may result in denial of behavior or "I don't know" answers. Asking the patient whether "you don't know or you don't want me to know" will sometimes allow patients to admit their reluctance to discuss certain topics.

Reassuring the patient that "bad" feelings are not unique to him or her ("Most people I know get angry sometimes") may also allow some reluctant patients to discuss what they consider unpleasant or embarrassing feelings. Another way in which the individual may give answers in the hopes of pleasing the examiner is to repeat the last word of a question as the answer. This resembles echolalia ("Are you happy or sad?" "sad") but is not a manifestation of psychosis as evidenced by the absence of other symptoms of psychosis. Rephrasing questions to offer both endings ("sad or happy?" "happy") will indicate whether this is happening. The patient can then be asked which is the way he or she does feel. Reassurance and encouragement are often necessary, particularly if a formal cognitive examination is done. Difficulty with abstraction and proverbs is frequently found in persons with low IQ and does not indicate psychosis or other organic disorder. It is often helpful and may be necessary to see the mentally retarded individual in the presence of a supportive staff person. The individual can be asked whether he or she would feel better if the staff person were included. Many mentally retarded individuals view this not as an invasion of privacy but as an opportunity to bring an ally into the interview. Staff can then be used to help with choice of words or to remind the patient of concerns.

When evaluating nonverbal severely or profoundly retarded individuals, the means of communication as well as desire to communicate and relate to others become important aspects for assessment. Many nonverbal individuals can use sign language; some moderately retarded individuals can sign in long sequences. A staff person may become essential as an interpreter. Other nonverbal individuals use language boards; it is important to inquire if such aids are being used. In the case of severely–profoundly retarded individuals, the usual method of indicating wants and needs, such as pointing and leading,

should also be evaluated. Self-stimulatory behavior, such as rocking, may increase in the presence of anxiety and should not be overinterpreted. Nonverbal signs of dysphoria, such as biologic signs of depression also have increased significance in the psychiatric evaluation of nonverbal individuals. Some thought processes may need to be inferred, such as the possibility of hallucinations on the basis of sudden unexplained shifts of attention. While there are limits to the ability to make categorical diagnoses in this population (61), there are many questions which can help suggest possible treatment alternatives. What is the individual's day program and how has performance been? How easy or difficult is it for the staff to know what emotional state the mentally retarded individual is in? Would an outsider know? Many severely retarded individuals smile when happy and cry when sad, but as IQ level drops, happiness or sadness may instead be indicated by different types of vocalizations. Does the individual make eye contact? Do attention and mood seem to shift rapidly? Is the individual willing to make physical contact such as take an offered hand? Information about social withdrawal, confusion, and changes in task performance become more meaningful with this information. The possibility of error increases and reliability and validity of diagnosis decrease with greater use of inference and reliance on historical information. Standard or modified assessment scales are useful in providing more objective ways of monitoring progress, particularly when several informants are involved.

Developing and Maintaining a Therapeutic Relationship

Various prejudices discourage therapists from attempting psychotherapy with mentally retarded persons. One is the incorrect assumption that low intelligence keeps mentally retarded individuals from being aware of their deficits, understanding the need for change, or having motivation for change, a sort of "happy idiot" hypothesis. In fact, mentally retarded individuals are quite aware of the losses and pain which they have suffered (30). Verbal individuals may describe eloquently both the feelings they had at being called "retard" by their peers and the struggle to accept a self-identity which does not include the educational accomplishments of their siblings or the opportunities for romantic relationships of their nonretarded peers. Many mentally retarded individuals are acutely aware of their intellectual deficits and shortcomings in problem solving. They are often quite willing to learn more about themselves and to try alternative problem-solving methods if these are shown to them. This interest has been used to advantage in teaching parenting skills, for example (54).

Another prejudice is that skill deficits on an organic basis, such as impulse control, will prohibit behavioral change. Impulse control disorders, particularly those involving aggression are indeed problematic situations to manage. Before psychotherapy is considered, a diagnostic workup must be accomplished: The DSM-III-R, for example, lists over 20 diagnoses associated with aggression. Of these, diagnoses often seen in mentally retarded individuals include manic episodes, adjustment disorder with disturbance of conduct, attention deficit disorder with hyperactivity, oppositional and overanxious disorders, organic personality syndrome, personality disorders and the psychotic disorders. Aggression may also represent previously adaptive behavior (as, for example, in people who have previously lived in dangerous environments) or may result from physical discomfort. When a more specific diagnosis cannot be made, it is useful to teach patients that while difficulties in impulse control may not be their fault, they are still responsible for managing them. Verbal patients may be helped to recognize this through cognitive maneuvers. With intellectually concrete patients, one modification in therapeutic technique is to assume a teaching stance, similar to that used with children, in which the clinician reviews "good" and "not useful" behav-iors. Behavioral maneuvers, which offer the patient immediate and consistent feedback from the environment are also helpful. In the neighborhood, appropriate and normal consequences are often initially withheld through "consideration" for the individual's retardation followed by sudden and complete rejection from the environment when the behavior passes a threshold of tolerance. Work with the patient's environment to assure that natural consequences both occur and are not devastating is necessary. Therapists may also be reluctant to become involved in therapy with mentally retarded persons because of a feeling of lack of experience with mentally retarded persons who do not have emotional disorders. In the absence of a concept of "normal," reasonable goals for therapy seem elusive. This is currently an unavoidable difficulty. Increased training in this area in adult and child psychiatry training programs may help the situation in the future. Consultation with an individual with specialty training in the sphere should be helpful. Lack of research experience with and consequently lack of literature about the personality and relationship development, particularly of moderately–profoundly retarded individuals is another problem which is being addressed through increasing interest in this population.

One of the major problems in working with developmentally delayed patients is the development of trust. Many emotionally disturbed retarded adults react to the experience of multiple losses and expectation of failure by avoiding self-revelation or close relationships. They are often reluctant to trust a therapist or evaluator. Trust is developed over time, through consistency and continuity of care and by the therapist taking extra pains to show respect to the individual. In the case of nonverbal, severe–profound retarded patients this may take the form of quiet sitting and offering of a hand or walking the patient in the hall. In more verbal patients, potential feelings of humiliation are decreased by remembering to treat the mentally retarded person as an adult, with adult expectations and conflicts, despite a cognitive mental age which may be in single digits.

Finally, therapists with a retarded patient may find themselves recapitulating in modified form the grief and frustrations which the parents of a retarded child have felt. A retarded adult, even if living independently in the community and working competitively as a janitor, is still more limited than many other patients seen by outpatient psychiatrists. In helping patients accept themselves and be happy with limited goals, therapists may have to reexamine their own goals for their patients and their reasons for doing the work. For some, it may appear that the efforts are not worth what appear to be modest gains. This problem is not unique to mental retardation but is a common question for psychiatrists who work with chronically mentally ill patients.

Communicating Information and Implementing a Treatment Plan

The first approach appropriately taken by most therapists is to investigate any recent changes which might have occurred in the mentally retarded individual's life. Such changes as shifts in work assignment, clients moving into or out of the residence or workshop, staff turnover, physical illness, new medications, or even behavior of another client in the workshop may all affect the moods and behavior of the patient. Working with the system to modify the response to maladaptive behavior, with a behavioral or systems model, is often the most effective therapeutic maneuver.

When psychotherapy is indicated, cognitive, developmental, and psychodynamic approaches are all useful in working with mentally retarded persons. The need to feel "understood" by the therapist is particularly great in individuals who may have had difficulty in making themselves understood throughout life. Work on self-esteem and identity is also necessary for many mentally retarded individuals. Mentally retarded adults often have to accept a concept of self which includes the designation "mentally retarded" or "brain damaged." Mildly retarded men and

women may have read these phrases on their school or hospital records. Some will still be coping with the need to scale down their hopes of what they would be when they grew up or coping with the consequences of inability to obtain a driver's license or live independently. Helping the individual to look at accomplishments and strengths is very useful in also helping him or her to accept the limitations. Mental retardation is a handicap which is particularly difficult to deny, both for the individual and for those around him or her. Even a profound cognitive disorder, however, does not mean the individual is less worthwhile as a person.

Modified psychodynamic psychotherapy is also possible with many verbal mentally retarded individuals. These patients often benefit from the approach of learning to identify and label feelings followed by a trial of alternate responses to these newly labeled feelings. They may learn to look at the ways in which their internal dialog about a situation escalates and distorts it into anger or the expectation of failure. The adaptive and maladaptive nature of their defenses may also be examined with many individuals. In doing psychodynamic psychotherapy with mentally retarded individuals, the therapist may need to be more directive in suggesting alternative responses than is usual in work with nonretarded patients. The therapist must also remain aware of the sensitivity to criticism and need for support and reinforcement often seen in this population. For the therapist working in a community program, this approach may be combined with behavioral and cognitive techniques which reinforce adaptive behavior. In designing behavioral interventions, the use of social reinforcers such as individual time with staff, rather than concrete reinforcers such as food, will help to promote social skills through modeling and practice. Social interactions with staff (e.g., going for a walk, having a cup of coffee), also tend to raise self-esteem because they are "normal" activities undertaken with nonretarded people.

The use of medications with mentally

retarded individuals has gone through periods of overuse followed by periods of disfavor. Overuse has resulted in court intervention to mandate guidelines for the use of psychotropic medications with institutionalized mentally retarded individuals (62, 63). Some subsequent judicial decisions have taken on perogatives for decision making usually reserved to the physician, such as mandating drug-free periods or prohibiting the administration of neuroleptics in divided doses (64–66). In the past decade a more rational attempt to use psychotropic medications for specific indications, in conjunction with other interventions, has prevailed. Some of the earlier work suggesting that neuroleptics decrease learning and response to behavioral programming in mentally retarded people has recently come under criticism, both on methodologic and procedural grounds (21, 67). Several reviews of the literature suggest that psychotropic medications are helpful and appropriate when used for the same psychiatric indications for which they are useful in nonretarded patients (68–72).

Of the three most commonly studied neuroleptics in use with mentally retarded individuals (haloperidol, thioridazine, and chlorpromazine), none has been shown to be more effective than another in providing relief of symptoms. Similar indications and contraindications to choice of medication apply as in the nonretarded population, including the concern about possible development of tardive dyskinesia (73). Flexibility in prescription is necessary; some mentally retarded individuals respond to apparently small doses, while others require unusually high doses for response (22).

Depression is an underdiagnosed syndrome in mental retardation (23, 56, 74, 75) and responds well to combinations of psychotherapy and antidepressants. Heterocyclic antidepressants are easier to use with mentally retarded individuals than monoamine oxidase inhibitors because of the difficulty many mentally retarded individuals have in understanding and following a monoamine oxidase inhibitor diet.

Mentally retarded people living in residences also tend to eat meals communally, further complicating the problem of following a diet.

The manic phase of bipolar illness, generally manifested by irritability, excitability, and sleep disturbances rather than by grandiose ideation has been well described in mentally retarded individuals. This syndrome at all levels of of mental retardation, including severe–profound retardation, has responded well to lithium (25, 76–78). One problem in making a diagnosis of manic behavior in mentally retarded individuals is that many of the behaviors seen in mania—hyperactivity, distractibility, shortened attention span, impulse control problems—are frequently seen in association with mental retardation. Careful examination of history to show an increase in intensity or change in the behavior, particularly with cycling, is necessary before making the diagnosis. Obtaining a history from several sources is particularly helpful. Rapid-cycle variants and nonresponse to lithium are also a problem in this group, as in nonretarded persons.

Anxiety disorders, particularly agoraphobia and generalized anxiety disorder, occur in mentally retarded patients and respond to the same medications used by nonretarded patients. The use of anti-anxiety drugs on an as-needed basis is often prohibited in supervised residences, which are reacting against the older misuse of medications as "chemical restraints." Unfortunately, the global prohibition on as-needed medication schedules also applies to individuals who could self-medicate. One response is to avoid as-needed prescription and give all medications on regular schedules. This may result in patients' receiving greater amounts of medication than necessary and may increase the risks of addiction to drugs such as the benzodiazepines. Another option is to prescribe the medication on a regular schedule with the note that the patient should be asked whether he or she wants it at that time and has the right to refuse it. This effectively creates an as-needed schedule in which the patient is offered medication three or four times a day. This method does have disadvantages: It makes it difficult for medication to be requested at other than prescribed times, and the patient, repeatedly reminded of the existence of medication, may take it thinking it would please the staff. The method remains preferable, however, to regular prescription of medications when they are not necessary. Efforts to educate both staff and patients about the risks and benefits of proposed medications is generally successful in facilitating unusual medication schedules.

A more controversial area in work with mentally retarded patients is the use of medications for specific target symptoms, which may not be part of a recognized psychiatric syndrome. The two areas in which this most commonly occurs are in treatment of aggression and treatment of self-injurious behavior when no underlying psychiatric syndrome can be diagnosed. There have been numerous reports of successful use of neuroleptics or lithium for aggression; most of these have not made distinctions between aggression as a consequence of psychotic process versus impulse control disorder (68, 79–86). β-blocking drugs at cardiac doses have also been investigated with some success for use in aggressive behavior in patients with brain damage, including in mentally retarded patients (87–92). Severe SIB (detaching retinas by head banging, picking skin until it bleeds, self-biting, etc.) is more likely to be seen in severe–profound mental retardation than at higher levels of function (93, 94). The etiology of this behavior is unclear; it may be related to self-stimulation; however, normal infants who also self-stimulate rarely cause injury. Psychodynamic hypotheses used to explain SIB in nonretarded individuals, for example, self-cutting and burning by patients with borderline personality disorder, are probably not applicable in this severely–profoundly retarded population. Self-injurious behavior on the basis of more developmentally advanced concepts such as guilt would be more likely to be seen in mildly than in severely–profoundly retarded individuals. Among biologic hypotheses which have been considered are the attempt to decrease sympathetic arousal by depletion of cathecolamines following arousal by anxiety or other affective state (95) and abnormalities of the endorphin regulation system (60). Pharmacologic management may be avoided by protecting the individual from hurting himself through the use of mittens or headgear; however, this also limits exploration of the environment. Pharmacologic treatment generally proceeds from a search for an underlying medical or psychopathologic state (physical discomfort, anxiety, depression, agitation, psychosis, mania). Successful pharmacologic treatment is generally limited when no underlying cause for the target symptom(s) can be found. Some success has been reported, nevertheless, with neuroleptics, particularly when combined with behavioral treatments (96). Narcotic antagonists (naloxone) and lithium have also shown some promise (97).

Medications are useful as part of an integrated management approach to dually diagnosed individuals, but they are not a substitute for diagnosis, management of environment, consideration of intrapsychic process, adequate staffing, or appropriate residential and day programs. It is important to consider medications as an adjunctive therapy in a program in which environmental management and psychotherapy also play prominent roles.

Whatever the primary approach, interventions need to be flexible and to combine behavioral, environmental, systems, biologic, and psychodynamic approaches, reflecting the biologic, psychodynamic, and social stresses and vulnerabilities which lead to mental disorder.

CONCLUSIONS

The experience of being mentally retarded is a difficult one because of social experiences of stigma and decreased opportunity, psychological reactions to repeated failure and object loss, and biologic burden. In the face of these issues it is surprising that most mentally retarded people do not become seriously psychiatrically disturbed. For those who do develop emotional disorders, psychiatric intervention, particularly on an outpatient basis, is increasingly being requested and is potentially beneficial. With appropriate modification of technique, most of the modalities of currently practiced psychiatric technique may be successfully applied. Mentally handicapped people as much as anyone else can be helped to feel that they are accepted and valued members of society.

References

1. American Psychiatric Association: *Diagnostic and Statistical Manual of Mental Disorders (Third Edition-Revised)*. Washington, DC, American Psychiatric Association, 1987.
2. Doll EA: *The Measurement of Social Competence: A Manual for the Vineland Social Maturity Scale*. Minneapolis, Educational Test Bureau, 1953.
3. Nihirak K, Foster R, Shellhaasm, et al: *Adaptive Behavior Scales: Manual*. Washington, DC, American Association on Mental Deficiency, 1969.
4. Greenspan S, Shoultz B: Why mentally retarded adults lose their jobs: social competence as a factor in work adjustment. *Appl Res Ment Retard* 2:23–38, 1981.
5. Isett R, Roszkowski M, Spreat S, et al: Tolerance for deviance: subjective evaluation of the social validity of the focus of treatment in mental retardation. *Am J Ment Defic* 87:458–461, 1983.
6. Wolfensberger W: *The Principle of Normalization in Human Services*. Toronto, National Institute on Mental Retardation, 1972.
7. Skeels HM, Harms I: Children with inferior social histories: their mental development in adoptive homes. *J Genet Psychol* 72:283, 1948.
8. Skeels HM: Adult states of children with contrasting early life experiences: a followup study. *Monogr Soc Res Child Dev* 31:3, 1966.
9. Skodiak M: Adult states of individuals who experience early intervention. In Richardo BW (ed): *Proceedings of the First Congress, International Association Scientific Study of Mental Deficiency*. 1968.
10. Kugel RB, Wolfenberger W: *Changing Patterns in Residential Services for the Mentally Retarded*. Washington, DC, President's Committee for the Mentally Retarded, 1969.
11. Meyers CE, Macmillan DL, Yoshida RK: Regular class placement of EMR students, from efficacy to mainstreaming. A review of issues and research. In J Gottleib (ed): *Educating Mentally Retarded Persons in the Mainstream*. Baltimore, University Park Press, 1979.
12. Zigler E, Muenchow S: Mainstreaming: the proof is in the implementation. *Am Psychol* 34:993–996, 1979.
13. Zigler E, Balla D: The impact of institutionalized experience on the behavior and development of retarded persons. *Am J Ment Defic* 82:1–11, 1977.
14. Rutter M, Graham P, Yule W: A neuropsychiatric study in childhood. London, Heinemann Medical Books, 1970.
15. Corbett SA: Psychiatric morbidity and mental retardation. In James FE, Snaith RP (eds): *Psychiatric Illness and Mental Handicap*. London, Gaskell Press, 1979, pp 28–45.
16. Menaloscino FJ: Emotional disturbance and mental retardation. *Am J Ment Defic* 70:248–256, 1965.
17. Menaloscino FJ: The facade of mental retardation. *Am J Psychiatry* 122:1227–1235, 1966.
18. Szymanski LS: Psychiatric diagnostic evaluation of mentally retarded individuals. *J Am Acad Child Psychiatry* 16:67–87, 1977.
19. Parsons JA, May JG, Menaloscino FJ: The nature and incidence of mental illness in mentally retardated individuals. In Menaloscino FJ, Stark JA (eds): *Handbook of Mental Illness in the Mentally Retarded*. New York, Plenum Press, 1984, pp 3–43.
20. Tu JB, Smith JT: The Eastern Ontario survey: a study of drug-treated psychiatric problems in the mentally handicapped. *Can J Psychiatry* 28:270–276, 1983.
21. Aman MG, Singh NN: A critical appraisal of recent drug research in mental retardation: the Coldwater studies. *J Ment Defic Res* 30:203–216, 1986.
22. Menaloscino FJ, Wilson J, Golden CJ, et al: Medication and treatment of schizophrenia in persons with mental retardation. *Ment Retard* 24:277–283, 1986.
23. Kazdin AE, Matson JL, Senatore V: Assessment of depression in mentally retarded adults. *Am J Psychiatry* 140:1040–1043, 1983.
24. Kirman B: Drug therapy in the mentally handicapped. *Br J Psychiatry* 127:545–549, 1975.
25. Rivinus TM, Harmatz JS: Diagnosis and lithium treatment of affective disorder in the retarded: five case studies. *Am J Psychiatry* 136:551–554, 1979.
26. Matson JL: Psychotherapy with persons who are mentally retarded. *Ment Retard* 22:170–175, 1984.
27. Aman MG, Field CJ, Bridgman GD: City-wide survey of drug patterns among non-institutionalized mentally retarded persons. *Appl Res Ment Retard* 6:159–171, 1985.
28. Eaton F, Menaloscino FJ: Psychiatric disorders in the mentally retarded: types, problems and challenges. *Am J Psychiatry* 139:1297–1303, 1982.
29. Macmillan DL: *Mental Retardation in School and Society*, ed 2. Boston, Little, Brown, 1982.
30. Reiss S, Benson BA: Awareness of negative social conditions among mentally retarded outpatients. *Am J Psychiatry* 141:88–90, 1984.
31. Brown G, Chadwick O, Shaffer D, et al: A prospective study of children with head injuries, III: Psychiatric sequelae. *Psychol Med* 11:63–78, 1981.
32. Bear D: Interictal behavior changes in patients with temporal lobe epilepsy. In *American Psychiatric Association Annual Review*. Washington, DC,

American Psychiatric Press, 1985, vol 4, pp 190–210.

33. Roberts JK: Neuropsychiatric complications of mental retardation. *Psychiatr Clin North Am* 9:647–657, 1986.

34. Cantwell D, Baker L: Psychiatric disorders in children with speech and language retardation. *Arch Gen Psychiatry* 34:583–591, 1977.

35. Beitchman JH, Nair R, Clegg M, et al: Prevalence of psychiatric disorders in children with speech and language disorder. *J Am Acad Child Psychiatry* 25:528–535, 1986.

36. Richardson SA, Katz M, Koller H, et al: Some characteristics of a population of young adults in a British city. *J Ment Defic Res* 23:287, 1979.

37. Fraser WI, Leudar I, Gray J, et al: Psychiatric and behaviour disturbance in mental handicap. *J Ment Defic Res* 30:49–57, 1986.

38. Zigler E, Balla D (eds): *Mental Retardation: The Developmental–Difference Controversy*. Hillsdale, NJ, Lawrence Erlbaum, 1982.

39. Weisz JR, Zigler E: Cognitive development in retarded and nonretarded persons: Piagetian tests of the similar-sequence hypothesis. *Psychol Bull* 86:831–851, 1979.

40. Groff MG, Linden KW: The WISC-R factor score profiles of cultural–familial mentally retarded and nonretarded youth. *Am J Ment Defic* 87:147–152, 1982.

41. Zigler E: Developmental vs difference theories of mental retardation and the problem of motivation. *Am J Ment Defic* 73:536–556, 1969.

42. Spitz HH: Critique of developmental position in mental retardation research. *J Spec Ed* 17:261–294, 1983.

43. Trites RL: Neuropsychological variables and mental retardation. *Psychiatr Clin North Am* 9:723–731, 1986.

44. Marcos LR, Gil RM, Vasquez RM: Who will treat psychiatrically disturbed developmentally disabled patients? A health care nightmare. *Hosp Community Psychiatry* 37:171–174, 1986.

45. Buck v. Bell, 143 Va. 310, 130 S.E. 516 (1925).

46. Reed EW, Reed SC: *Mental Retardation: A Family Study*. Philadelphia, Saunders, 1965.

47. Vitello SJ: Involuntary sterilization: recent developments. *Ment Retard* 16:405–409, 1978.

48. Crain LS, Millor GK: Forgotten children: maltreated children of mentally retarded parents. *Pediatrics* 61:130–132, 1978.

49. Feldman MA, Case L, Townes F, et al: Parent education project I: the development and nurturance of children of mentally retarded parents. *Am J Ment Defic* 90:253–258, 1985.

50. Schilling RF, Schinke SP, Blythe BJ, et al: Child maltreatment and mentally retarded parents: is there a relationship? *Ment Retard* 29:201–209, 1982.

51. Beardslee WR, Bemporad J, Keller MB, et al: Children of parents with major affective disorder: a review. *Am J Psychiatry* 140:825–832, 1983.

52. Cytryn L, McKnew DH, Bartko JJ, et al: Offspring of parents with affective disorders II. *J Am Acad Child Psychiatry* 21:389–391, 1982.

53. Rutter M: *Children of Sick Parents: An Environmental and Psychiatric Study* (Maudsley Monograph No. 16). London, Oxford University Press, 1966.

54. Feldman MA, Towns F, Betel J, et al: Parent education project II: Increasing stimulating interactions of developmentally handicapped mothers. *J Appl Behav Anal* 19:23–37, 1986.

55. Feldman MA: Research on parenting by mentally retarded persons. *Psychiatr Clin North Am* 9:777–796, 1986.

56. Reiss SR, Levitan GW, Szysko J: Emotional disturbance and mental retardation: diagnostic overshadowing. *Am J Ment Defic* 86:567–574, 1982.

57. Burger PC, Vogel FS: The development of the pathologic changes of Alzheimer's disease and senile dementia in patients with Down's syndrome. *Am J Pathol* 73:457–468, 1973.

58. Reid AH, Aungle PG: Dementia in aging mental defectives: a clinical psychiatric study. *J Ment Defic Res* 18:15–23, 1974.

59. Kumar BB: An unusual case of akasthisia. *Am J Psychiatry* 136:1088, 1979.

60. Barron J, Sandman CA: Paradoxical excitement to sedative–hypnotics in mentally retarded clients. *Am J Ment Defic* 90:124–9, 1985.

61. Sovner R: Limiting factors in the use of DSM-III criteria with mentally retarded persons. *Psychopharmacol Bull* 22:1055, 1059, 1986.

62. Wyatt v. Stickney. 344 F. Supp. 373 (1972) (a)

63. Wyatt v. Stickney. 344 F. Supp. 387 (1972) (b)

64. Welsch v. Likens. 373 F. Supp. 487 (1974)

65. Welsch v. Likens. 550 F. 2d 1122 (1977)

66. Doe v. Hudspeth. Civil No. J75–36 (S.D. Miss., filed Feb. 17, 1977).

67. Holden C: NIMH finds a case of "serious misconduct." *Science* 235:1566–1567, 1987.

68. Freeman RD: Psychopharmacology and the retarded child. In Menaloscino J (ed): *Psychiatric Approaches to Mental Retardation*. New York, Basic Books, 1970, pp 294–368.

69. Sprague RL, Werry JS: Methodology of psychopharmacological studies with the retarded. In Ellis NR (ed): *International Review of Research in Mental Retardation*. New York, Academic Press, 1971, vol 5, pp 147–219.

70. Lipman RS, DiMascio A, Reatig, et al: Psychotropic drugs and mentally retarded children. In Lipman RS, Dimascio A, Killam KF (eds): *Psychopharmacology, A Generation of Progress*. New York, Raven Press, 1978, pp 1437–1449.

71. Rivinus TM: Psychopharmacology and the mentally retarded patient. In Szymanski LS, Tanguay P (eds): *Emotional Disorders of Mentally Retarded Persons*. Baltimore, University Park Press, 1980, pp 195–221.

72. Rogoff M: Psychotropic medications and mentally retarded patients. In Bernstein J (ed): *Clinical Psychopharmacology*, ed 2. Littleton, MA, Wright/PSG, 1983.

73. Gualtieri CT, Quade D, Hicks RE, et al: Tardive dyskinesia and other clinical consequences of

neuroleptic treatment in children and adolescents. *Am J Psychiatry* 141:20–23, 1984.

74. Sovner R, Hurley AD: Do the mentally retarded suffer from affective illness? *Arch Gen Psychiatry* 40:61–67, 1983.

75. Reiss S, Benson BA: Psychosocial correlates of depression in mentally retarded adults: I. Minimal social support and stigmatization. *Am J Ment Defic* 89:331–337, 1985.

76. Reid AH: Psychosis in adult mental defectives: I. Manic–depressive psychosis. *Br J Psychiatry* 120:205–212, 1972.

77. Hasan M, Mooney RP: Three cases of manic–depressive illness in mentally retarded adults. *Am J Psychiatry* 136:1069–1071, 1979.

78. Naylor GJ, Donald JM, LePoidevin D: A double-blind trial of lithium therapy in mental defectives. *Br J Psychiatry* 124:52–57, 1974.

79. LeVann LJ: Haloperidol in the treatment of behavioral disorders in children and adolescents. *Can Psychiatry Assoc J* 14:217–220, 1969.

80. LeVann LJ: Clinical experience with tarasan and thioridazine in mentally retarded children. *Appl Ther* 12:30–33, 1970.

81. LeVann LJ: Clinical comparison of haloperidol with chlorpromazine in mentally retarded children. *Am J Ment Defic* 75:719–723, 1971.

82. Kaplan S: Double blind study at state institution using thiorizadine in program simulating out-patient clinic practice. *Penn Psychiatry* 9:24–34, 1969.

83. Tischler B, Patriasz K, Beresford J, et al: Experience with pericyazine in profoundly and severely retarded children. *Can Med Assoc J* 106:136–141, 1972.

84. Lacny J: Mesoridazine in the care of disturbed mentally retarded patients. *Can Psychiatry Assoc J* 18:389–391, 1973.

85. Grabowski SW: Safety and effectiveness of haloperidol for mentally retarded behaviorally disor-

dered and hyperkinetic patients. *Curr Ther Res* 15:856–861, 1973.

86. Dale PG: Lithium therapy in aggressive mentally subnormal patients. *Br J Psychiatry* 137:469–474, 1980.

87. Elliott FA: Propranolol for the control of belligerent behavior following acute brain damage. *Ann Neurol* 1:489–491, 1977.

88. Yorkstone NJ, Zaki SA, Pitcher DR: Propranolol as an adjunct to the treatment of schizophrenia. *Lancet* 2:575–578, 1977.

89. Schreier HA: Use of propranolol in the treatment of postencephalitic psychosis. *Am J Psychiatry* 136:840–841, 1979.

90. Sheppard GP: High dose propranolol in schizophrenia. *Br J Psychiatry* 134:470–476, 1979.

91. Yudofsky S, Williams D, Gorman J: Propranolol in the treatment of rage and violent behavior in patients with chronic brain syndromes. *Am J Psychiatry* 138:218–220, 1981.

92. Ratey JJ, Morrill R, Oxenkrug G: Use of propanolol for provoked and unprovoked episodes of rage. *Am J Psychiatry* 140:1356–1357, 1983.

93. Bartak L, Rutter M: Differences between mentally retarded and normally intelligent autistic children. *J Autism Child Schizophr* 6:109–120, 1976.

94. Ando H, Yoshimura I: Prevalence of maladaptive behavior in retarded children as a function of IQ and age. *J Abnorm Child Psychol* 6:345–9, 1978.

95. Cataldo MS, Harris J: The biological basis for self-injury in the mentally retarded. *Analysis and Intervention in Developmental Disability* 2:21–39, 1982.

96. Singh NN, Millichamp CJ: Effects of medication on the self-injurious behavior of mentally retarded persons. *Psychiatric Aspects of Mental Retardation Reviews* 3:13–16, 1984.

97. Farber JM: Psychopharmacology of self-injurious behavior in the mentally retarded. *J Am Acad Child Adol Psychiatry* 26:296–302, 1987.

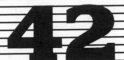

The Suicidal Patient

Linda Gay Peterson, M.D.
Bruce Bongar, Ph.D.

The earliest known writing about suicide came out of Egypt in 2000 B.C.:

Dialogue of a Weary Man with his Soul
  To whom can I speak today?
  I am laden with wretchedness
  For lack of an intimate (friend).
  To whom can I speak today?
  The sin which treads the earth,
  It has no end.
  Death is in my sight today
  (Like) the recovery of a sick man,
  Like going out into the open after a confinement. . .
  Death is in my sight today
  Like the longing of a man to see his house (again)
  After he has spent many years held in captivity. (1)

Over the centuries suicide has been variously regarded as a perverse oddity, (2) the result of an individual's tortured and tunneled logic in a state of intolerable emotion, (3) and the most serious philosophical problem that faces humanity (3). Explanations for suicide range from a biologic predisposition (4–6) to a reaction to humiliation, helplessness, hopelessness, and guilt (3); a manipulation, an escape from physical or psychologic pain, or an expression of violent rage (7); a reaction to separation from the family or from the loss of love (8); or an eroticization of death itself or aesthetic completion of patriotic sacrifice (9).

Suicide is the source of endless disquiet to the practicing clinician for it is one of the few fatal consequences of psychiatric illness (7). Among the survivors of the suicide, including the psychotherapist, the reaction is often shock, disbelief, shame, and anger (10).

"The central issue in suicide is not death or killing; it is rather the stopping of the consciousness of unbearable pain which—unfortunately—by its very nature entails the stopping of life. One of suicide's chief shortcomings is that it unnecessarily answers a remediable challenge with a permanent negative solution. By contrast, living is a long-term set of resolutions with often times only fleeting results" (11).

Suicidal behavior is the most frequently encountered of all mental health emergencies (12). At the same time, clinicians identify suicidal statements as the most stressful of all client communications (13). This is a reflection of the fact that the relationship between psychopathology, suicide attempting, and completed suicide is complex, dynamic, and not yet well understood. Recent studies show changes in the identity of high-risk groups (14), and follow-up studies demonstrate that risk factors among at-

569

tempters may be significantly different from those for the general population (15). Also, studies suggest that rates of suicide among the mentally ill (16) and physically ill (17) far exceed that of the population as a whole. However, the estimates of the rate of death by suicide due to psychiatric disorders vary greatly on the basis of such factors as country of origin and the diagnostic criteria used for the sample (e.g., a range of 15 to 55% as the number of manic depressives who die by suicide) (18). Clearly these variances mitigate against any unitary explanation of suicidal behavior or any single treatment approach.

MAJOR APPROACHES TO THE STUDY OF SUICIDE

The major research on suicide has focused on five approaches (19): (a) epidemiologic—population identifying; (b) psychologic—identifying psychologic states in suicide victims as well as the examination of cognitive components of suicidal acts (20); (c) sociocultural—assessing the impact of social and cross-cultural factors, or the correlation of social change with suicide (21); (d) biologic—looking at the relationship of psychiatric illness, genetics, and neurotransmitters to suicide; (22) and (e) prevention, intervention, and postvention (19). Other approaches of note have included the theologic, philosophic, constitutional, legal, global, political, and supranational (19).

One authority, Ronald Maris, has described the study of suicide as a "synergistic" blend of the theories and methods of the social sciences and psychiatry (2). Therefore, as a starting point, it may be helpful to examine the common conceptualization of suicidal behavior as a psychosocial response to separation and loss—particularly the loss of honor, social meaning, self-esteem, or of love (8). Cross-cultural research data on suicide can also illuminate the effects of particular sociocultural differences (23). Finally, attention must be directed toward the new biologic understandings of suicide.

Historical, Literary, Social, and Cross-Cultural Perspectives

Suicides to prevent humiliation or maintain honor can be seen in Biblical suicides and among the ancient Greeks and Romans. For example, Saul fell upon his own sword rather than be dishonored by capture by the uncircumcised Philistines. Samson provided the example of the classic suicide–murder when he pulled the temple down around him after being betrayed and humiliated by Delilah. Abimelach, after his skull was crushed by a millstone thrown by a woman from the parapets of the town that he was capturing, begged his swordbearer to kill him, so that he might not be disgraced by being killed by a woman. Judas hung himself after betraying Jesus. (Neither the Hebrew Bible nor the New Testament prohibits or condemns suicidal behaviors [24].)

Honor suicides were common among the ancient Greeks and Romans. Among the notable suicides, to avoid capture or humiliation, were Demonsthenes and Hannibal. There are also numerous instances of suicide and martyrdom among the early Christians (24).

Perhaps the best known of fictional suicides is Goethe's Werther. *The Sorrows of Young Werther,* published in 1774, was written by Goethe when he was 23 and was based in part on his own confused and disturbed emotional state. The novel tells a complex story of a young man's obsessive unrequited love that ends tragically in violent suicide. So powerful an influence was this book that a wave of imitative suicides ensued, with the completers often garbed in Werther's distinctive costume: a blue coat with yellow waistcoat and breeches (25). A contemporary parallel to this suicide phenomenon of contagion can be seen in the recent data indicating that the mere viewing of television news or dramas on teenage suicide may have an effect on raising a city's or country's adolescent suicide rate (26, 27).

The most cogent exponent of the sociologic view toward suicide was the French sociologist Emile Durkheim (28). *Le Sui-*

cide, first published in 1897, was Durkheim's comparative study of suicide in postindustrial society (29); this work continues to generate extensive research and discussion. Durkheim's general thesis states that the suicide rate varies inversely with external constraint and that external societal constraint has two dimensions: what Durkheim called integration and regulation (21).

An additional element in the sociologic approach to understanding suicide has included the concept of status integration, namely, that the suicide rate is inversely related to the stability and duration of social relationships (30). There may also be important social meanings in the way we calculate the rate of suicide; e.g., the reported suicide rates and specific criteria for reporting may have as many meanings and variations as there are coroners and medical examiners (31). An important social element in assessing risk is that of status loss, especially the loss of occupational status in males (21).

Important data have emerged from a study of suicidal biographies or "suicidal careers" (2) which point to the need to clearly understand the distinction between data obtained about suicide completers and that obtained about attempters (2). In his classic work, *Pathways to Suicide: A Survey of Self-Destructive Behaviors*, Maris found that early trauma, a multiproblem family of origin, negative interaction, and blocked aspirations were most characteristic of attempters and somewhat less so of completers. So numerous were the differences that Maris found between attempters and completers that it may be safe to say it is inappropriate to use the information obtained about suicide attempters as the basis for understanding the behavior of completers (2, 32). In fact, in a major prospective study of patients with affective disorders, while 68% of the patients who died from suicide had a positive history of suicide attempts, 32% had no history of suicidal behavior; in this same study there was no significant difference in frequency of suicide attempts between those who committed suicide and those

who did not commit suicide (33). Furthermore, it has been suggested that a 3rd category be studied, namely that of suicide ideators and threateners, who are hypothesized to be much more similar to attempters in their suicidal careers (32).

It is important to note that much of the data on suicide is based on information obtained from developed Western societies. All such data also need to be evaluated within culturally specific views of the self and the cultural organization of self concept (23).

Significantly, suicide may be one of the few expressions of frustration toward the social milieu left to oppressed minorities. Suicide attempts are often characteristic of groups of individuals who are dependent for their well-being on powerful institutions or persons. Making a suicide attempt, in such situations, is felt to be the only, or at least one of the few, acts that mobilize or influence others to take notice of one's grievances (34). This position is often characteristic of youth, women, and the unemployed (34).

For instance, in the Aguarana, a people along the Peruvian Amazon, the high rate of suicide is seen as part of a complex social process that links death threats, homicide, assertions of personal autonomy, and relations to dominance with an individual's inability to be part of a collective response to interpersonal conflict. Female suicides are particularly common. The local explanation for these suicides, from the Aguarana men, is that women lack the ability to control strong emotions (35). These women have little power in their community except for these threats of harm to themselves or others. This suggests that the use of suicidal behavior as an expression of frustration crosses cultural boundaries. In a contemporary American study of suicidal women and their relationships to husbands, boyfriends, or lovers, the suicide attempt often represented simultaneously a flight from an unhappy, sometimes physically violent, relationship and a desperate attempt to restore it on a different footing (36).

Suicide can also be a logical reaction to

(and outcome of) a traditional system of beliefs about gender. For example, among the Gainj, of the highlands of Papua New Guinea, female suicide is considered a viable option when women keep their part of a culturally defined marriage bargain and men do not (37). Suicide attempts, both fatal and nonfatal, may also be related to society's approbation towards particular sexual orientations or sexual life styles (2); e.g., young adolescent homosexuals may be at greater risk (38).

Some additional factors must also be considered. The first is the constantly shifting moral views of societies about the social acceptability of suicidal behavior. This has varied from viewing suicide as an appropriate social response to disgrace as seen in the Biblical examples quoted earlier, to the Japanese code of Bushido in the 17th century (which held that the disgrace of failure to one's lord could be expiated by the ritual taking of one's own life), to the Judeo-Christian ethos predominant through the first half of the 20th century, in which suicide has been viewed as an act against God. This attitude often served to deny a Christian burial to suicides. Membership in a particular religious group may effect suicide rates; e.g., the suicide rate of Protestants exceeds that of Jews, which in turn exceeds that of Catholics (2).

Biology of Suicide

From a biologic perspective, suicidal behavior has been viewed as the product of genetic predisposition, either related to or separate from hereditable mental illness with high rates of suicide (39, 40). Similarly, in the last 10 years evidence has accumulated on the biochemical changes in the brain which seem to be highly correlated with aggression, violent suicide attempts, and completed suicide, not necessarily related to a given psychiatric diagnosis (41, 42).

Some of these results can be summarized as follows (22):

1. Low levels of 5-hydroxyindoleacetic acid (5-HIAA; a metabolite of the neu-

rotransmitter serotonin, 5-HT) in the cerebrospinal fluid (CSF) are significantly correlated with a history of aggression, violent suicide attempts, and other nonviolent attempts (43, 44).
2. Traskman et al (45) have found that among patients with the lowest levels of 5-HIAA in the CSF (below 92.5 nmol/l) there was a 20% incidence of suicide in the following year.
3. Blunted thyroid-stimulating hormone thyrotropin-releasing hormone stimulation has been correlated with low CSF 5-HIAA and violent suicide attempts (44).
4. Plasma cortisol level higher than 20 mcg% may be positively related to suicide (46).
5. Mann et al. (47) have found lower levels of serotonin in the brains of completed suicides compared with those of a control group.

While these biologic findings are clearly of great significance, the practical meanings and applications of these findings to the daily practice of clinical psychiatry is not yet clear. Overall, these potential biologic markers of suicide risk constitute areas of continuing research rather than established clinical tools until much more substantiating data are available (48).

DEFINITION OF SUICIDE

The boundaries between self-mutilation, sensation seeking, and suicidal behavior are murky. There is a lack of clarity about whether consciously expressed suicidal desire accompanying the behavior should be requisite in order to classify the behavior as suicidal. Therefore, in undertaking this discussion of assessment and treatment, a reasonable definition of the problem being studied is necessary. While a truly comprehensive discussion of the issue is beyond the scope of this chapter, the reader is referred to *The Definition of Suicide* by Edwin Schneidman (19) and *Pathways to Suicide: A Survey of Self-Destructive Behaviors* by Ronald Maris (2).

In this chapter, the following definition

of suicide and suicidal behaviors proposed by the World Health Organization (WHO) is used:

Suicidal act—The self-infliction of injury with varying degrees of lethal intent and awareness of motive.
Suicide—A suicidal act with fatal outcome.
Suicide attempt—A suicidal act with nonfatal outcome.

The above definitions do not attempt to separate deliberate self-harm from suicide but instead suggest a continuum of lethality and intent, both of which may need to be assessed separately in terms of future risk. The same concept should probably also be extended to the area of suicidal ideation, that is, that both the level or intent and possible lethality of available means should be placed on a continuum.

The remaining goal of the chapter will be to examine suicidality in the context of the clinical interview, where the biopsychosocial context of suicidal behavior or statements can be explored and hypotheses about its etiology management and treatment examined.

CLINICAL ASSESSMENT

The assessment of suicide risk is a common and often urgent task for the practicing clinician (49). Through a psychiatric interview, a mental status examination, and an examination of past medical, social, occupational, and developmental history (49), a wealth of information can become available to assist the clinician in analyzing the nature of a suicidal communication. In addition, in a high-risk procedure such as suicide assessment, while it is clearly critical to collect and document as much data as possible, it is equally as important to take a realistic view of the subjective factors in the clinical risk assessment process and to acknowledge and recognize the competent patient's assumption of some share of the risk (50). The following, then, are some specific suggestions for conducting the clinical assessment.

First, the patient may communicate the matter directly to the clinician by her or his behavior or statements. Indirect data, such as data from informants, also add to the clinical picture. These same means of communication are open to the therapist in information gathering, hypothesis testing, and even for the stage of conflict resolution. There are two differing situations that the clinician may encounter and that need to be dealt with differentially. The first is the situation where suicidality becomes a central issue in an initial evaluation. The second is when suicidality becomes an issue in a case already in active treatment. Clearly, the meaning of the communication is vastly colored by the difference in the interpersonal context of these two situations. It is also of critical importance to note the intensity of the clinician's own personal reaction to the patient's suicidal communications, for it has been noted that countertransference feelings of anger, anxiety, and lack of control are common when interviewing suicidal patients. These feelings on the part of the clinician can, if not carefully monitored, cloud accurate clinical judgment and even impede the correct formulation of the treatment plan (51).

Structured instruments may be used to measured psychiatric symptomatology and/or suicide risk. These may serve as adjunctive tools in assessment (52) and include such commonly used measures as the Schedule of Affective Disorders, the DIS, the Hamilton, the Zung Depression Scale, the Beck Depression Scale, and the Hopkins Symptom Checklist. Instruments specifically designed to assess suicide risk include the Risk Estimator for Suicide, the Suicide Intent Scale, and the Risk–Rescue Rating Scale.

There are several limits on the use of these scales. For example, their impact on patient rapport must be considered when dealing with the patient who is in a state of great perturbation and psychologic pain and needs to talk about these feelings. Also, should the results of structured testing or questionnaires strongly conflict with the clinician's own clinical interview data, a state of cognitive dissonance and clinical uncertainty may develop. There is the additional problem of false positives, i.e., the overidentification of risk, with the suicide risk scales. For example, using the Risk–Rescue Rating on a large population, Bassuk found that 2000 at-risk individuals would need to be identified to actually identify one suicide completer (52). This is clearly an unacceptable false-positive rate for effective intervention.

The central problem in the refinement of these scales is the dilemma of making accurate clinical prediction with such a low base rate behavior as suicide (53, 54). Yet, if the clinician shifts her or his goal away from the specific prediction of a behavior to the area of the detection of imminent risk, the clinical task becomes much more manageable (54). In addition, it is critical to note that individual uniqueness suggests that when a clinical scale or risk assessment technique is not consistent with clinical judgment, clinical judgment should be given precedence (55).

The issue of liability prevention in the assessment must also be directly addressed through careful documentation of all objective data and subjective findings coupled with an informed consent, when the patient is competent (56). Such documentation needs to include a "thinking out loud for the record" determination of competency as well as dangerousness (56).

In the future an additional source of objective data may be laboratory testing. At this time, there are no specific biologic tests with high enough correlations with suicidal behavior to be practically used in the clinical setting (48). However, there is increasing evidence of increased suicidal risk in patients with low CSF serotonin and low CSF 5-HIAA, so that in the future there may be either a central or peripheral (blood) test to help in the assessment of suicide risk.

Overall, the goals of the clinical assessment, as in any interview, are threefold: diagnosis, the development of a therapeutic relationship, and education and treatment. In the case of the suicidal patient, diagnosis includes primarily the estimation of suicide risk. The development of a ther-

apeutic relationship may include intentional manipulation of the relationship to ensure patient safety, manipulation of the environment, and, possibly, hospitalization of the patient. Education would include assessing alternative behavioral approaches to the patient's situation, working with family members and the patient's support network, restructuring negative cognitions and teaching more appropriate problem-solving skills, and treating the underlying condition. In fact, it has been suggested that the inculcation of effective cognitive coping and problem-solving strategies may be the best form of primary prevention for suicide (57).

SUICIDAL COMMUNICATIONS

In order to satisfactorily assess patients who may be at risk for suicide, the clinician needs to be attuned to the diversity and variety of suicidal communicative styles. These are as follows.

Behavioral Messages

Patients may give direct behavioral messages apart from the obvious one of making a suicide attempt. These can include self-mutilatory behaviors such as wrist cutting or the tendency to make less contact than usual, for example, staring at the floor, decreased positive interaction, or desire to terminate the session early, or its reverse, oversolicitousness, thanking the therapist for trying to work with them or having a hard time terminating the interview when they usually finish promptly. Dramatic change in affect from previous sessions is also a warning sign. Any of these behavioral messages suggests the need to explore possible suicidal ideation.

Direct Communication

Patients may directly state that they are feeling suicidal, want to die, would rather be dead, wish they were dead, etc. They may also directly express their specific plan for taking their life. While it may seem a belaboring of the obvious, the careful and serious examination of any direct communications of suicidal ideation, impulse, and/or plan is critical.

Direct statements or behavioral cues need to be assessed for level of perturbation and lethality (19). It is not uncommon to have to assess and reassess these communications on an ongoing basis, regardless of whether similar statements by the patient have proved to be nonpredictive of an attempt. It is also important to at least conceptually separate the areas of previous self-inflicted sublethal acts from a serious attempted suicide, which the patient had not thought to survive. Indeed, instead of speaking of attempted suicide for nonlethal acts, it may be more accurate to see nonlethal, self-inflicted injurious suicide-like acts as having attempted parasuicide (19). One authority has even suggested that the phrase "attempted suicide" is a contradiction in terms, that, strictly speaking, a suicide attempt should refer only to those who sought to commit suicide and accidentally survived (19).

Furthermore, in assessing direct and behavioral communications, it is also essential to note that data from one study spanning a period of 10 years, suggest that only 1 of 20 who attempt suicide kill themselves, whereas of all those who kill themselves, 40% have made prior attempts (2).

At this point, the clinician may feel a sense of information overload from the massive literature on suicide and feel that predicting suicide risk, even in the clinical setting is an insuperable task (49). Yet, when confronted with a distressed patient who may or may not commit suicide, the clinician can draw comfort from the finding that any event which uses a suicidal modality is a genuine psychologic crisis and must be carefully managed, even though the event may not lead to a later completed suicide (19, 49).

The specifics of assessing direct communications involve establishing lines of inquiry to ascertain the presence of a plan, the availability of means for carrying out the plan and its potential dangerousness, the duration of suicidal ideation, and the intensity of the ideation. Precipitating factors need to be explored and other methods of dealing with the problem that the patient has used in the past can be reviewed. These same steps need to be taken even when the communication is indirect or the message is behavioral. However, in the latter two cases, additional groundwork may need to be laid in order to effectively initiate this dialogue.

Indirect Communication

Patients may communicate indirectly in a number of ways, such as saying goodbye at the end of a session when they usually do not, stating that they wanted to see you just one more time, bringing you a gift, giving away possessions to others, or telling you that they have been calling old friends or relatives they have not seen in a long time. Clearly, the affect of the patient when delivering these communications is critical in making an interpretation. Warning signs can involve the presence of depressed mood, decreased eye contact, slow or unusually soft speech, or inappropriately bright affect in a patient who has been very depressed or who one would expect to look sad because of external stressors.

Informants

In most cases, any time a friend or relative calls and reports suicidal ideation or behavior, this should be explored with the patient. Direct confrontation with this information is one option, or if this is usually ineffective in a particular patient, one might say that other people who feel like the patient or who are going through similar life situations often feel suicidal, so you wonder if the patient might feel this way.

No Communication

There are particular groups of patients who are probably at high risk in spite of no particular communication about suicide. These patients need to be specifically asked about suicidal ideation on a regular basis, if any true suicide prevention is to occur.

Data indicate that 70% of all people who complete suicides have seen a physician within the 3-month period prior to their death (58). This suggests that the assessment of suicidality by primary care physicians in medicine, family practice, and pediatrics might make a serious difference to the rate of completed suicides (57).

Statistical studies have indicated that a number of findings in a patient's history and social context predispose to suicide. These include history of a previous attempt, history of substance abuse, physical illness, recent loss of an important relationship, divorce or separation, suicide of a close relative, abuse as a child, homosexuality, living alone, and retirement (49).

The specific percentages for some particularly high-risk groups include patients with affective disorder (15% lifetime rate) (59); alcohol-dependent and abusing patients (20% lifetime rate in alcohol-dependent patients) (60); patients with other known major psychiatric disorders (61); the chronically mentally ill patient with a past history of a suicide attempt (this was the single best distinguisher of completed suicides, attempters, and natural deaths in Maris's study of Cook County deaths (2); patients with chronic physical illness (e.g., dialysis patients in the early days of dialysis had rates 400 times that of the general population (62); and psychiatric patients who are less than 1 month out of the hospital.

While each of these items can stand alone as an alerting factor, the risk is even greater when they occur in combinations in persons who bear a high-risk diagnosis, such as the schizophrenic, manic–depressive or alcohol/drug-abusing patient in a dangerous age group (e.g., the elderly or youth) (49).

Countertransference Communications

An important issue in exploring suicidal communications is the psychiatrist's own current feelings toward the patient and toward the suicidal communication (51). If the psychiatrist feels angry with a patient

(who, for example, has cut him- or herself superficially and phoned in the middle of the night), or if the psychiatrist feels as though she or he has failed because the patient makes a suicide attempt or continues to express suicidal ideation after significant therapeutic work, these attitudes and the patient's reaction can be a major obstacle to resolving the suicidal crisis. These issues are particularly important in the patient already in treatment, but should not be minimized in the patient seen for the first time in an emergency or office setting. Often patients who have made suicide attempts have already suffered the disdainful and punishing attitudes of medical personnel, who, in their frustration over caring for someone who hurts him- or herself intentionally or who, from their perspective, does not have real disease, act as though the only good suicide were a dead suicide.

There is also the suggestion in the literature that repeat attempts and successful suicides may follow low rather than high lethality attempts (63). This may indicate that the patient's sense of incompetence and unworthiness is magnified by the response of caregivers and significant others (64).

Thus, once a suicidal communication has been made, the clinician needs to thoroughly review general and individual risk factors, and try to interpret the meaning of the communication in the particular context. Simply put, the most effective way to reduce risk is to reduce the individual's anguish, tension, and pain (3). Risk reduction begins with sensitivity to the expressions of various forms of these feelings.

TEN CLINICAL QUESTIONS FOR RISK ASSESSMENT

As complex and difficult to determine as the causes of suicide are, there are basic guidelines for assessing risk, as summarized below:

1. Does the patient belong diagnostically to a high-risk group, e.g., history of

previous attempt, alcohol/substance abuse?

2. If the patient is in one of these groups, are there current changes in the course of illness or the environmental response to the patient's illness?
3. Has the patient suffered (or been threatened with) a major loss, either related to the above or of another type (65), such as the death of a spouse or child, loss of a job, loss of a residence, or other meaningful material object? Has she or he suffered from more subtle psychologic losses, such as humiliation (loss of honor), shame (loss of face), loss of hope, or loss of the feeling of being loved or being able to love another?
4. What is the patient's level of perturbation? Although hopelessness and helplessness are feelings most often encountered in both suicide attempters and in the histories of completers, a certain level of perturbation is necessary to carry out a suicidal act (11, 19). This is well understood in severely depressed patients, who often only become suicidal as they are successfully treated—only then do they have the level of energy and degree of concentration necessary to carry out a suicidal plan.
5. What are the specific parameters of the patient's suicidal intent? This includes whether suicidal thoughts are active or passive, how long they have been present, whether a specific plan has been made and how potentially lethal that plan is, and whether previous attempts have been made. Specific details about past attempts and about the patient's thoughts and feelings about them are particularly important.
6. What kind of support is available in the patient's environment, and can this support be mobilized to help get the patient through the suicidal crisis?
7. What means are available to the patient to commit suicide? Even if the patient states that she or he is planning to take pills, the presence of firearms in the home should still be

assessed, since in a moment of indecision or acute distress these are likely to be the real killers. For both men and women in the United States, firearms are the leading method used in suicidal death (66). For the patient already in treatment, and particularly one in high-risk conditions, the clinician should have already explored the issue of firearms in the home and encouraged their removal by both the patient and the family. Similarly, the clinician should already have attended to the issue of risk in her or his manner of prescribing. This means never giving more than a week's supply of antidepressant medication, and no more than a month's supply of sedative–hypnotic, anxiolytic, or antipsychotic medications. This also means keeping track of the frequency of refills and, if necessary, contacting the local pharmacist to see if the patient has been obtaining lethal medications from multiple physicians.

8. What additional information is available to the clinician from other people close to the patient? This is clearly an instance in which confidentiality may need to be breached in order to provide adequate care of the patient.
9. What resources does the patient have that keep him or her from committing suicide? Can the clinician mobilize any factors to strengthen the patient's will to live?
10. Finally, the clinician should explore what it would mean for the patient to be dead. For those who complete suicide the meaning of death is often narrowly seen as pain relief, without much thought to cessation of life or the implications of this cessation both for themselves and others. Patients may also have fantasies about being able to observe the grieving family at the graveside.

Once all of these factors have been assessed, the psychiatrist is left with the task of clarifying and dealing with the most critical question—Why now? This is particularly important in a patient in the midst of therapy, where a suicidal communication may be a signal that the therapeutic alliance is in serious difficulty or that the wrong diagnosis has been made or treatment given.

MANAGEMENT AND TREATMENT

Having thoroughly assessed the risk, the clinician must now establish an ongoing risk management system and treatment plan. For some patients, simply the careful exploration of their thoughts and feelings may cause them to feel less suicidal and, therefore, enable them to look at alternative ways of dealing with the perceived crisis that had precipitated their suicidal feelings. For those patients who continue to pose a risk, estimation of the level of risk can be determined by their responses to many of the above questions.

Patients experiencing an exacerbation of their illness (manic–depressive disorder, psychosis, alcohol/substance abuse) are clearly high risk and may require more intensive inpatient management. In this context it should be noted that alcoholic patients may have differing high-risk profiles when drinking as opposed to when sober (67). Similarly, patients with delusional depressions or major depressive episodes who feel that they are a source of shame and humiliation to their family or that they will be letting the family down should also be considered high risk. In a review of the cases seen by the University of Massachusetts Medical Center's Emergency Mental Health Service from 1984 to 1986 there were two cases where death followed within 1 week of contact. Both cases were males age 50 to 60 with major depressive episodes; both had supportive families, but each patient felt nonetheless that he was an inadequate provider for the family. Neither admitted continued suicidal thoughts at the end of his evaluation. In both of these cases, the issues of perceived loss of face, shame, and humiliation were key motivations to suicide.

Of particular importance in management and treatment is the careful assessment of certain psychologic problems—regression, low self-esteem, paranoid insecurity, and guilt (2). Most patients who commit suicide have been depressed for much of their life, and many of their reactions are adaptations to early ego faults (2, 68). It is also important to note that as crucial as ego problems, hopelessness, and depression are to an understanding of suicide, these are not sufficient conditions for suicide. It is also necessary to understand and to treat the anger, restlessness, irritation, and frustration that many suicidal patients express about the state of their lives (2).

Treatment and management should further help the patient acknowledge and help work through any recent loss or perceived loss, especially for patients who have limited social support or feel hopeless about resuming a meaningful life. Such patients are clearly in the high-risk category. An important subgroup of patients in this category are schizophrenic patients (not psychotic at the time) who have had a recent loss, such as of a place to live. These patients may not report suicidal thoughts without careful questioning, but are known to be the most frequent type of suicide in schizophrenia (69).

Successful management and treatment are facilitated the patient's ability to acknowledge and use social support, especially the support of the psychotherapist, without feeling further guilt and shame. The personal field between patient and psychiatrist can provide a "holding environment" in which previously unbearable feelings can be contained, and from which the patient can eventually differentiate extended life possibilities and a more adaptive sense of self (70). In addition, if the patient accepts the support of family, but sees it only as further evidence of his or her incompetence and worthlessness, this is not an adequate solution to the suicidal dilemma.

Extreme caution needs to be exercised with the patient with a high level of perturbation and easily available lethal means. This includes patients with poor impulse control who are in crisis and are unable to decrease their level of perturbation in the therapeutic encounter. This is why it is so important not to minimize the potential suicidality of character-disordered patients who are in crisis. On the other hand, patients who are less impulsive, more depressed, or psychotic, should be considered at higher risk if their suicidal ideation has been present for more than a few days and they have articulated any concrete elements of a plan.

Psychiatrists may need to consider hospitalization and the involvement of law enforcement agencies with the paranoid patient who has become overwhelmed by paranoid thoughts. These patients are at risk not only for suicide, but also suicide–murder; for if they feel that family members or other people in their immediate environment are part of conspiracies against them, suicide may be seen as the alternative (71).

From the viewpoint of the clinician, suicide is often the most feared outcome in psychotherapy; it may indicate a calamitous irrevocable failure in treatment (50). The anxiety that this situation evokes in the psychiatrist is a two-edged sword: It can either mobilize her or him to greater clinical alertness and therapeutic vigilance, or, if the psychiatrist becomes too preoccupied with the issue of suicidal risk alone, it can divert him or her from an accurate assessment of the total psychodynamic picture of the patient (50).

Shneidman's model of psychotherapeutic assessment and intervention is of particular value in the clarification of immediate treatment and management issues (3, 11, 19). This schema includes an understanding that the levels of perturbation and of lethality are separate and equally important factors in suicidal risk. Thus a patient who is both highly perturbed and highly lethal is at highest risk; conversely, one who is not perturbed or lethal is the lowest risk. Perturbation, be it psychotic or situational, is easily measured in a patient with impaired coping skills. Lethality is assessed by the level of planning, intent, and availability of means.

A further differentiation needs to be made when discussing suicide in an outpatient setting (70). This is the difference in assessing the acutely suicidal and the chronically suicidal patient. The chronically suicidal patient may fall in either the low-perturbation/high-lethality category or the high-perturbation/low-lethality category. In addition, the sense of negative feelings generated in the therapist by a patient who is persistently suicidal becomes a significant factor. The therapist may feel guilt, anger, frustration, impotence, and even hate (13). An awareness of the countertransference issues with these patients is essential to sound management and treatment.

Once again, as shown in Chapter 11, the goals of every interview entail assessment, the establishment of rapport, and education. This is just as true for the suicidal patient as for any other. As indicated by the preceding discussion, the development of rapport is also often a critical part of the assessment process, since the patient's ability to engage interpersonally indicates that he or she may be at a lower risk level. In this regard, suicide notes left by patients can be quite revealing: Attempters often leave notes with highly charged interpersonal content, whereas completers leave notes which at the most contain an apology and focus primarily on business left undone (2).

For suicidal patients, the formation of a therapeutic relationship must extend to the adoption of an active therapeutic stance, involving outreach and even home visits if necessary. The importance of continuity of care is critical since the suicidal individual is often rebounding from a loss experience. In both the outpatient and inpatient setting, having a single clinician or team working with the patient is essential. In order to decrease the immediate level of perturbation, a psychotherapist may even need, in the short run, to cater to the infantile idiosyncratic behaviors and excessive dependency needs of the patient (11).

The next step is the effective application of crisis intervention techniques. These include clarification of precipitating stress, correction of cognitive distortions, ventilation and labeling of affects, formation of new coping strategies and problem-solving approaches, and mobilization of environmental supports (72).

Finally, decisions must be made about the appropriateness of the use of medications and hospitalization. Diagnostic considerations, combined with crisis intervention procedures, often dictate the need to medicate the suicidal patient (73). If the patient's suicidality is largely a result of an ongoing depressive illness or psychosis, then clearly this must be treated. The psychiatrist must consider the patient's safety when prescribing; e.g., drugs used to treat schizophrenia, such as the phenothiazines, butyrophenones, loxapine, and molindone, are considered relatively safe because of the high level needed for a lethal dose (74). The correct prescribing policy is to prescribe small amounts of medication. In addition, the psychiatrist can enlist the help of a family member, or other responsible persons, to assist in dispensing medication. This can help reduce the risk of the patient's stockpiling medication or combining the prescribed medication with alcohol, other sedative–hypnotics, or anticholinergic drugs (74).

For the dangerous or disorganized patient, settings which offer containment, protection, and an active social environment may be essential (74). What are the indications for hospitalization of the potentially suicidal person? If after the initial intervention the patient is still at the moderate to high intent/lethality level, a hospitalization for further assessment, treatment, and immediate protection is indicated.

Hospitalization must also be actively considered when dangerousness is the issue and when one of the following is present: lack of an effective support system, disruption of attachments, significant psychopathology associated with increased risk (such as major affective disorders), suicidal symptoms in response to delusions and hallucinations, or pathologic identification with suicidal persons (19).

Other factors favoring hospitalization are the necessity of intense diagnostic evaluation and/or special treatments such as electroconvulsive therapy (ECT). In persons with treatment-resistant emotional disorders with a suicidal component, it has been estimated that suicide prevention efforts would be well served by a judicious increase in the use of ECT in depression and by a concerted effort to rule out any underlying physical disorders (48).

The Chronically Suicidal Patient

Unlike patients who have short-lived suicidal crises, related for example to sudden exacerbations of their psychiatric illness or to life crisis, there is a subgroup of patients, often carrying a diagnosis of a personality disorder, who are chronically suicidal. The suicidal borderline patient is a particularly difficult management problem since manipulations of the psychotherapeutic exchange and regression in the transference are common (74). Three brief clinical descriptions may underscore the problem:

1. A 19-year-old anorexic female who reports to always having suicidal ideations, and intermittently overdosing on a laxative, knowing that she may cause such extreme metabolic disturbances that she would die.
2. A 26-year-old dental student who reports that since her second depressive episode she has been stockpiling medications in case she just can't take it anymore.
3. A 48-year-old unemployed borderline-personality-disordered patient who revolves in and out of the state hospital using suicidal threats and attempts to gain admission on a frequent basis.

Careful and frequent assessment of changes in the level of risk must be made in these cases, and criteria must be decided on either by the therapist alone or by the therapist and the patient that will lead to hospitalization. It may be particularly useful to avoid defining these criteria in terms of suicidality, focusing instead on a need for additional support to help improve problem-solving skills. The psychotherapist thus avoids becoming punitive–protective.

Contracting with patients—e.g., that they call the psychotherapist before they do anything to harm themselves—has often been successfully used with suicidal patients. However, in effecting a contract the clinician must carefully weigh the unique psychodynamics of each patient. Some patients may interpret the contract to mean that they may call the therapist only when they are highly dysfunctional, perturbed, and contemplating a lethal act. It is also necessary for the therapist to understand that therapeutic concern cannot extend to an assumption of total responsibility for the patient's life, for in the final analysis, such responsibility is clearly impossible. The psychotherapist must avoid, in short, the trap of the omnipotent rescuer and instead convey to the patient a sense of enlightened caring and concern (70).

The implications of hospitalization may be very different, depending on whether the patient will be cared for by his or her own clinician on the inpatient unit or whether the patient is under the care of a different clinician. If the latter is the case, then the outpatient clinician must have a carefully negotiated plan for working with the inpatient clinician and the patient, to avoid "splitting" by the patient and other hazards of fragmented care.

Chronically suicidal patients may feel controlled by their emotions. Therefore, avoiding a crisis orientation and working with such patients to develop a structure for managing their emotions, in a long-term framework, is an important part of the therapeutic process. If these patients feel desperate, they may make frequent calls to the therapist. Management techniques can include limiting the number of calls, explaining the inability of the therapist to meet all the patient's needs, and planning with patients alternative ways to get support or deal independently with their feelings. When asked to take these responsibilities, some patients will seek another therapist. This is a point where it would be easy for the therapist to encourage the patient to leave because of his or her own frustration with the patient. In this instance, it is particularly important to encourage continuity, since these patients often have a pattern of leaving relationships to avoid dealing with interpersonal frustrations. One might instead suggest that the patient consider using the second therapist as a consultant. This can often provide the patient an opportunity to deal with intense negative feelings toward the therapist in a safe way and yet allow the therapeutic relationship to continue to grow. This may more realistically approximate the nature of relationships in life, where in fact multiple relationships of varying intensity are necessary to create a satisfying interpersonal sphere.

Commitment

An issue that often arises in making decisions about the management of the suicidal patient is the use of hospitalization for protection and treatment on an involuntary basis. Because of the often irrational nature of mental illness and its potentially lethal effects on the patient and on the rest of society, psychiatrists have been vested with the power to hospitalize people against their will (this issue is dealt with in more depth in Chapter 29). For example, commitment may be necessary for the suicidal patient, if the patient seems to have impaired judgment on the basis of an organic brain syndrome or an acute psychotic state which impairs the person's ability to appreciate the outcome of his or her actions and which precludes the patient's ability to participate in the decision-making process. This is most often true in the case of psychotic depression; e.g., patients believe their bodies are rotting or riddled with cancer and that death is preferable, when in fact they are actually in perfect health. Similarly, schizophrenic patients may believe they can jump off a bridge and live because they are invulnerable. Clearly, these are times when emergency hospitalization and treatment are required.

Postvention

Finally, there is the question of the role of the therapist after a patient commits suicide. This is a time to allow family and others the opportunity to process the effects of the death. These deaths are particularly difficult for the family because, as Shneidman has pointed out, "the suicide leaves his psychological skeleton in the closets of the survivors" (19). Along with the normal issues of grieving, the friends and family have a special survivor guilt and shame which is often incapacitating. Furthermore, postvention includes how the therapist deals with her or his own feelings.

A Case of Postvention

Mr. and Mrs. N and their sons, Bill and John, are now 2 years away from the suicide of their oldest son, Sam. Mr. N used to be close to John, the youngest son, but now hardly talks to him. Both Mr. N and Bill are drinking excessively. Mrs. N is so depressed she can hardly work. Mrs. N came seeking help for herself and her family. She described how Sam had talked about suicide intermittently from age 11 to age 19, when he finally took his own life. The day before his suicide, he told her his plan but she dismissed it as just adolescent talk. Mr. N insisted that Mrs. N not tell the other children it was a suicide and also that they tell everyone else that it was an accident, even though Sam left a note. Over the past 2 years both sons have become suspicious, and Mrs. N has finally told them that Sam committed suicide. She feels incapable of dealing with their feelings without the help of her husband.

Clearly this is the kind of situation where family therapy is indicated to allow the entire family to discuss their feelings about Sam's suicide and how it has affected the family. Since no one has talked about the death, there has been no opportunity to grieve and share the sadness and loss. This situation is not atypical, and in the case of the suicide of a patient whom the therapist was seeing, the therapist could call in a consultant to sit down with her- or himself and the family to process the death. The therapist may choose to work alone with the family, but this limits the therapist's own ability to work through her or his own feeling of loss. This is very important since often the therapist may have guilt feelings and feelings of professional failure that need to be dealt with (75, 76).

Perhaps nowhere in the practice of clinical psychiatry is the practitioner under more intense and significant stress than when he or she treats a suicidal patient (75). Clinicians often react to a patient's suicide with disbelief, shame, anger, vulnerability, guilt, and a loss of self confidence (19, 49). It has therefore been noted that there is no instance in a psychotherapist's practice when consultation with one's clinical peers is as important as when one is dealing with the suicidal patient (19, 49).

SUMMARY

The essential biopsychosocial risk factors in the etiology of suicide are psychiatric diagnosis; patient age; history of negative social interaction; drug and alcohol use; hopelessness, depression, and dissatisfaction; the number of suicide attempts; level of perturbation; and the use of lethal methods (2, 19). Secondary factors include sex, religion, early trauma, suicide in the family of origin, sexual deviance, work problems, physical illness, humiliation and shame, the suffering of an important loss, and conceiving of death as an escape (2).

Working with the suicidal patient involves an understanding of the formulation of suicidal risk, astute diagnostic skills, careful monitoring of behaviors and communications, consultation, attention to the transference, and the involvement of significant others (19, 49).

Thus the successful assessment, management, and treatment of the suicidal patient borrow heavily from the philosophy of crisis intervention, i.e., to see the focus of treatment not as the attempt to ameliorate the patient's entire personality or to cure all psychiatric illness, but rather to simply keep the person alive (19).

References

1. Pritchard JB (ed): *Ancient Near Eastern Texts*, ed 3. Princeton, NJ, Princeton University Press, 1969, p 407.
2. Maris RW: *Pathways to Suicide: A Survey of Self-Destructive Behaviors*. Baltimore, Johns Hopkins University Press, 1981.
3. Shneidman ES: Suicidal logic. In Sahakian WS (ed): *Psychopathology Today: The current status of Abnormal Psychology*, ed 3. Itasca, IL, Peacock Press, 1986, pp 00–00.
4. Asberg M, Bertillson L, Martensson B: CSF monoamine metabolites, depression, and suicide. *Adv Bioch Psychopharmacol* 39:87–97, 1984.
5. Brown L, Ebert MH, Goyer PF, et al: Aggression, suicide and serotonin: relationship to CSF amine metabolites. *Am J Psychiatry* 139:741–749, 1982.
6. Van Praag H: CSF 5-HIAA and suicide in nondepressed schizophrenics. *Lancet* 2:1256, 1983.
7. Nemiah JC: Foreword: In Bassuk EL, Schoonover SC, Gill AD (eds): *Lifelines: Clinical Perspectives on Suicide*. New York, Plenum, 1982, pp ix–x.
8. Richman J: *Family Therapy for Suicidal People*. New York, Springer Publishing, 1986.
9. Lifton RJ, Shuichi K, Reich MR: Mishima Yukio: the man who loved death. In *Six Lives/Six Deaths*. New Haven, Yale University Press, 1979.
10. Goldstein LS, Buongiorno PA: Psychotherapists as suicide survivors. *Am J Psychotherapy* 38:392–398, 1984.
11. Shneidman ES: Aphorisms of suicide and some implications for psychotherapy. *Am J Psychotherapy* 38:319–328, 1984.
12. Schein HM: Suicide care: obstacles in the education of psychiatric residents. *Omega* 7:75–82, 1976.
13. Deutsch CJ: Self-report sources of stress among psychotherapists. *Professional Psychology: Research and Practice* 15:833–845, 1984.
14. Boyd J: The increasing rate of suicide by firearms. *N Engl J Med* 308:872–898, 1983.
15. Frederick CJ: Current trends in suicidal behavior. *Am J Psychotherapy* 32:172–200, 1978.
16. Pokorny AD: Suicide rates in various psychiatric disorders. *J Nerv Ment Dis* 139:499–506, 1964.
17. Abram HS, Moore GI, Westervelt FB Jr: Suicidal behavior in chronic dialysis patients. *Am J Psychiatry* 127:1199, 1971.
18. Goldring N, Fieve RR: Attempted suicide in manic–depressive disorder. *Am J Psychotherapy* 38:373–383, 1984.
19. Schneidman, ES: *Definition of Suicide*. New York, Wiley, 1985.
20. Ellis TE: Toward a cognitive therapy for suicidal individuals. *Professional Psychology: Research and Practice* 17:125–130, 1986.
21. Maris RW: Sociology of suicide. In Perlin S (ed): *A Handbook for the Study of Suicide*. New York, Oxford University Press, 1976, pp 93–112.
22. Maris RW: Preface to the special issue: biology of suicide. *Suicide and Life Threatening Behavior* 16:v–viii, 1986.
23. Rubinstein D: Epidemic suicide among Micronesian adolescents. *Soc Sci Med* 17:657–665, 1983.
24. Rosen G: History of suicide. In Perlin S (ed): *A Handbook for the Study of Suicide*. New York, Oxford University Press, 1976, pp 3–29.
25. Auden WH: Foreword to Goethe's *The Sorrows of Young Werther*. (Mayer E, Bogan L, trans). New York, Modern Library, 1971.
26. Phillips DP, Carstensen LL: Clustering of teenage suicides after television news stories about suicide. *N Engl J Med* 315:685–9, 1986.
27. Gould MS, Shaffer D: The impact of suicide in television movies: evidence of imitation. *N Engl J Med* 315:690–694, 1986.
28. Maris RW: Sociology of suicide. In Perlin S (ed): *A Handbook for the Study of Suicide*. New York, Oxford University Press, 1976, pp 93–112.
29. Durkheim E: Suicide (Spaulding JA, Simpson G, trans). Glencoe, IL, *The Free Press* (original published in 1897).
30. Gibbs J, Martin T: *Status Integration and Suicide*. Eugene, OR, University of Oregon Press, 1964.
31. Douglas JD: *The Social Meaning of Suicide*. Princeton, NJ, Princeton University Press, 1967.
32. Farberow N: Foreword. In Maris RW (ed): *Pathways to Suicide: A Survey of Self-Destructive Behaviors*. Baltimore, Johns Hopkins University Press, 1981.
33. Fawcett J, Scheftner W, Clark D, et al: Clinical predictors of suicide in patients with major affective disorders: a controlled prospective study. *Am J Psychiatry* 144:35–40, 1987.
34. Baechler J: *Suicides* (Cooper B, trans). New York, Basic Books, 1979.
35. Brown MF: Power, gender and the social meaning of Aguarana suicide. *Man* 21:311–328, 1986.
36. Stephens BJ: Suicidal women and their relationships with husbands, boyfriends and lovers. *Suicide and Life-Threatening Behavior* 14:77–89, 1985.
37. Johnson PL: When dying is better than living: female suicide among the Gainj of Papua New Guinea. *Ethnology* 20:325–334, 1981.
38. *Youth Suicide in the United States, 1970–1980*. Atlanta, GA, Department of Health and Human Services, 1986.
39. Egeland JA, Sussex JN: Suicide and family loading for affective disorders. *JAMA* 254:915–918, 1985.
40. Rainer JD: Genetic factors in depression and suicide. *American Journal of Psychotherapy* 1984.
41. Asberg M, Bertillson L, Martensson B: CSF monoamine metabolites, depression, and suicide. *Adv Biochem Psychopharmacol* 39:87–97, 1984.
42. Brown L, Ebert MH, Goyer PF, et al: Aggression, suicide and serotonin: relationship to CSF amine metabolites. *Am J Psychiatry* 139:741–746, 1982.
43. Asberg M, Traskman L, Thoren P: 5-HIAA in the

cerebrospinal fluid: a biochemical suicide predictor? *Arch Gen Psychiatry* 33:1193–1197, 1976.

44. Van Praag HM: Affective disorders and agression disorders: evidence for a common biological mechanism. *Suicide and Life-Threatening Behavior* 16(2):21–47, 1986.

45. Traskman L, Asberg M, Bertilsson L, et al: Monoamine metabolites in CSF and suicidal behavior. *Arch Gen Psychiatry* 38:631–636, 1981.

46. Stanley M, Stanley B, Traskman-Bendz L, et al: Neurochemical findings in suicide completers and attempters. *Suicide and Life-Threatening Behavior* 16(2):204–218, 1986.

47. Mann JJ, Stanley M, McBride A, et al: Increased serotonin and β-adrenergic receptor binding in the frontal cortices of suicide victims. *Arch Gen Psychiatry* 43:954–959, 1986.

48. Motto JA: Clinical considerations of biological correlates of suicide. *Suicide and Life-Threatening Behavior* 16(2):1–20, 1986.

49. Maltsberger JT: *Suicide Risk: The Formulation of Clinical Judgment.* New York, New York University Press, 1986.

50. Gutheil TG, Bursztajn H, Hamm RM, et al: Subjective data and suicide assessment in the light of recent legal developments. Part I: Malpractice prevention and the use of subjective data. *International Journal of Law and Psychiatry* 6:317–329, 1983.

51. Smith K: *The Psychotherapy of Suicidal Patients.* Paper presented at the annual meeting of the American Association of Suicidology, 1986.

52. Bassuk EL: General principles of assessment. In Bassuk EL, Schoonover SC, Gill AD (eds): *Lifelines: Clinical Perspectives on Suicide.* New York, Plenum Press, 1982

53. Center for Disease Control, 1986.

54. Murphy G: The prediction of suicide. *Am J Psychotherapy* 38:341–349, 1984.

55. Motto JA, et al: Development of a clinical instrument to estimate suicide risk. *Am J Psychiatry* 142:680–686, 1985.

56. Gutheil TG, Bursztajn H, Brodsky A: The multidimensional assessment of dangerousness: competence assessment in patient care and liability prevention. *Bulletin of the American Academy of Psychiatry and Law* 14:123–129, 1986.

57. Berman AL: Adolescent suicides: issues and challenges. In Bronheim SM, Magrab PR, Shearin RB (eds): *Seminars in Adolescent Medicine: Adolescent Depression and Suicide.* New York, Thieme Medical Publishers, 1986, pp 269–277.

58. Robins E, Gassner S, Kayes J, et al: Communication of suicidal intent: a study of 134 cases of successful (completed) suicide. *Am J Psychiatry* 115:724–733, 1959.

59. Pokorny AD: Suicide rates in various psychiatric disorders. *J Nerv Ment Dis* 139:499–506, 1964.

60. Motto JA: Suicide risk factors in alcohol abuse. *Suicide and Life-Threatening Behavior* 10:230–238, 1980.

61. Pokorny AD: The prediction of suicide in psychiatric patients. *Arch Gen Psychiatry* 40:249–257, 1983.

62. Abram HS, Moore GI, Westervelt FB: Suicidal behavior in chronic dialysis patients. *Am J Psychiatry* 127:1199, 1971.

63. Card JJ: Lethality of suicidal methods and suicide rise: two distinct concepts. *Omega* 5:37–45, 1974.

64. Lazare A: Shame and humiliation in the medical encounter. *Arch Intern Med* 147:1653–1548, 1987.

65. Block LH: Personal communication, November 15, 1985.

66. Boyd JH: The increasing rate of suicide by firearms. *N Engl J Med* 308:872–989, 1983.

67. Mayfield DG, Montgomery D: Alcoholism, alcohol intoxication, and suicide attempts. *Arch Gen Psychiatry* 27:349–353, 1972.

68. Litman RE: Sigmund Freud on suicide. In Schneidman E (ed): *Essays in Self Destruction.* New York, Science House, 1967, pp 293–299.

69. Breier A, Astrachan BM: Characterization of schizophrenic patients who commit suicide. *Am J Psychiatry* 141:206–209, 1984.

70. Gill AD: Outpatient therapies for suicidal patients. In Bassuk EL, Schoonover SC, Gill AD (eds): *Lifelines: Clinical Perspectives on Suicide.* New York, Plenum Press, 1982, pp 71–82.

71. Allen NH: Homicide followed by suicide: Los Angeles, 1970–1979. *Suicide and Life-Threatening Behavior* 13(3):155–165, 1983.

72. Schoonover SC: Crisis therapies. In Bassuk EL, Schoonover SC, Gill AD (eds): *Lifelines: Clinical Perspectives on Suicide.* New York, Plenum Press, 1982.

73. Schoonover SC: Pharmacotherapy of the suicidal patient. In Bassuk EL, Schoonover SC, Gill AD (eds): *Lifelines: Clinical Perspectives on Suicide.* New York, Plenum Press, 1982, pp 59–68.

74. Schoonover SC: Intensive care for suicidal patients. In Bassuk EL, Schoonover SC, Gill AD (eds): *Lifelines: Clinical Perspectives on Suicide.* New York, Plenum Press, 1982, pp 137–153.

75. Kahn A: The stress of therapy. In Bassuk EL, Schoonover SC, Gill AD (eds): *Lifelines: Clinical Perspectives on Suicide.* New York, Plenum Press, 1982, pp 93–100.

76. Goldstein LS, Buongiorno PA: Psychotherapists as suicide survivors. *Am J Psychotherapy* 38:392–398, 1984.

43

The Chronic Mentally Ill

Jeffrey L. Geller, M.D., M.P.H.

The needs of the chronic mentally ill are profound and far reaching. In our efforts to deliver effective care to this population we swept them into segregated state asylums for the insane in the mid-19th century and swept them out of state hospitals in the mid-20th century. Our recent attempts to care for this population in the community have showed us that much of what we once believed to be the result of institutionalism and the social breakdown syndrome is more likely a result of chronic mental illness per se. Although we once thought that removing patients from long-term institutions would allow them to integrate into communities, we have instead created a population of homeless mentally ill, poorly equipped to survive without the room, board, and daily routine of state hospitals. We once believed that we could be true to the concept of individual liberty by "freeing" the mentally ill from long-term institutionalization; we now have a population of deinstitutionalized and uninstitutionalized individuals whose freedom is illusory at best.

In this chapter I shall examine the needs of the chronic mentally ill in the community and the roles those involved in outpatient psychiatry must play. The pervasive needs of this population call for a multidisciplinary approach to treatment, employing biologic, psychodynamic, behavioral, and sociocultural principles. All are re-quired to develop the necessary range of services for the care and treatment of the chronic mentally ill.

WHO ARE THE CHRONIC MENTALLY ILL?

"There are an estimated 2 million chronic mentally ill in America." Although this is an oft-quoted statistic, there is no consensus on an operational definition of the chronic mentally ill. This population is generally defined in terms of diagnosis, disability, and duration (1, 2).

Diagnostic categories included in chronic mental illness are schizophrenic disorders, major affective disorders, paranoid disorders, schizoaffective disorder, atypical psychosis, organic mental disorders, personality disorders and some of the substance use disorders.

Among individuals with these mental illnesses, there is a subpopulation with significant disability as defined by the limits of the individual's psychosocial functioning. Within this group, there is a further subpopulation whose duration of illness would qualify as "chronic." While in the past chronicity might have been determined by length and/or frequency of hospitalization, the use of alternatives to inpatient treatment require that we focus instead on duration of functional disability as the signpost of chronicity.

585

Using the 2 million estimate, what percentage of the chronic mentally ill might be seen in outpatient settings? Table 43.1 presents data from a report by the Public Citizen Health Research Group (3) on where this population lives. If we exclude those in hospitals and those in jails, we are left with almost 90%, or about 1,750,000 potential outpatients.

The development of the definition of the chronic mentally ill began by listing the diagnostic categories. As clinicians, we are used to labeling persons by diagnosis. The diagnosis that most often comes to mind when the term "chronic mental illness" is used is schizophrenia. Summers and his colleagues (4, 5) have found, however, that a considerable number of the chronic psychiatric patient population are not schizophrenic. They determined through a study of the postacute phase of illness that chronic patients have significant psychopathology, function poorly socially, are isolated, are highly recidivistic, and are vocationally dysfunctional. They found, however, no evidence that persons with chronic schizophrenia were more dysfunctional than chronic nonschizophrenic psychiatric patients. They suggested that "from a functional point of view, there might be something to be gained from a shift in the nosological frame of reference to viewing chronicity as the primary assessed disorder and the particular symptom pattern as the form which the disorder assumes in its acutely symptomatic state" (5). From another perspective, Harding et al (6) believe that repeated episodes of schizophrenic decompensation are not necessarily synonymous with chronic de-

bilitation. They argue that newer, longitudinal studies have found a heterogeneity in the long-term course and outcome of schizophrenia. To review, Summers et al. found that not all chronic mental illness is schizophrenia and Harding et al. indicated that not all schizophrenia is characterized by long-term deterioration and disability.

Brauchi and Kirby (7) developed an empirical typology of the chronic mentally ill which consists of five distinct types of patients: (a) "middle-aged female homemaker," (b) "mainstream chronically mentally ill patient," (c) "neurotically distressed and service-dependent chronics," (d) "institutionalized (ex-psychiatric hospital) clients," and (e) "young acting-out schizophrenics." The importance of this study is its use of typological strategies to delineate the heterogeneity of the chronic mentally ill and thereby to provide information for the useful development of clinical services.

The above discussion underscores the need for more empirical studies to help determine a meaningful definition of "the chronic mentally ill."

HOW DID THE CHRONIC MENTALLY ILL END UP IN THE COMMUNITY?

In colonial America the mentally ill were in the community. Those who were not local, who did not belong, were "warned out." Those who were local but unable to care for themselves were provided for (8). Mentally ill persons who were not dangerous or did not make "mischief" were cared for by families or in almhouses; those who endangered the social order were confined, not for treatment, but to prevent harm and/or disturbance (9). Confinement came without formal legal controls.

Colonial America also saw the birth of states' participation in the care of the mentally ill. Pennsylvania Hospital (1751) and New York Hospital (1771) were the first general hospitals to receive mental patients. The first hospital solely for mental patients was built in Williamsburg, Virginia in 1773. All three hospitals received state subsidies. The first hospital built and

Table 43.1 Location of the Chronic Mentally Ill

Site	Number	Percent
Own family	800,000	40
Nursing home	300,000	15
Foster group homes	300,000	15
By self	200,000	10
Hospitals	200,000	10
Public shelters/streets	150,000	8
Jail	26,000	1

operated by a state for the care of the mentally ill was established in 1822: the Eastern Kentucky Lunatic Asylum (10, 11).

Mid-19th century witnessed the beginning of two prevailing trends that substantially affected the locus of care of the mentally ill: the proliferation of state hospitals and the codification of commitment laws. Dorothea Dix, a Boston school teacher, crusaded throughout the United States for the establishment of state hospitals. She delivered lectures to state legislatures, pointing out that the "insane were presently confined in cages, closets, cellars, stalls, pens. . . [and that they were] chained, naked, beaten with rods and lashed into obedience." She argued for the establishment of institutions for the care and treatment of the insane not only on moral grounds, but also on economic grounds. In the age of curability in which she crusaded, hospitals reported cure rates approaching 100%. Establishing hospitals would return citizens to the work force and remove them from dependency status. Dix effectively caused the founding or enlarging of 32 psychiatric hospitals distributed across 20 states and Europe (10).

Concurrent with Dix's campaign, a system of procedural protections for the commitment of the mentally ill evolved (13). In many states those protections closely paralleled those of the criminal process. This movement was largely the result of exposés by Elizabeth Packard, a minister's wife who campaigned for reform following release from her own confinement (14).

As the 19th century came to a close, state hospitals, built for treatment in an era of optimism, became institutions for confinement in a more conservative and materialistic society (15). Shortly thereafter, the states reacted against the cumbersome legal procedures necessary for commitment, and commitment statutes became based simply on the need for treatment (16). State hospitals and their populations proliferated.

State and county mental hospitals reached their peak number of 352 in 1954

and their peak year-end census of 558,922 in 1955 (17). At this point, a number of factors came into play to begin the massive relocation of the mentally ill from state hospitals to communities. First, exposés were published, such as Mary Jane Ward's *The Snake Pit* in 1946, and Albert Deutsch's *The Shame of the States* in 1948. Second, the use of neuroleptic medication spread after its introduction for general use in state hospitals in New York State in 1955 (18). Third, President Kennedy delivered his Congressional Message and subsequently Congress passed the Community Mental Health Act of 1963 and Medicare and Medicaid in 1965. These represented a partial shift in financing of treatment of the chronic mentally ill from the states to the federal government. Finally, a series of legal cases addressed significant issues in mental health law—*Lake v. Cameron*, least restrictive alternative, 1966; *Wyatt v. Stickney*, right to treatment, 1971; *Lessard v. Schmidt*, procedural rights in commitment hearings, 1972; and *Addington v. Texas*, standard of proof in commitment hearings, 1979.

It is ironic that the arguments launched in favor of the demise, or at least curtailment of state hospitals, paralleled those employed by Dix for their establishment. The arguments were both moral and economic. They resulted in a sociopolitical reform known as "deinstitutionalization."

Viewed from the perspective of the physical movement of the chronically mentally ill out of hospitals providing long-term care, deinstitutionalization has been remarkably successful. By 1972, the state and county mental hospital year-end census had shrunk to less than 50% of its peak (17). By 1983, the year-end census was 117,084, or 21% of its 1955 peak (19). There resulted a marked shift from inpatient care of the chronic mentally ill to outpatient treatment (Fig. 43.1).

Viewed from the perspectives of quality of life, human dignity, and the provision of mental health services, however, deinstitutionalization has been far from successful.

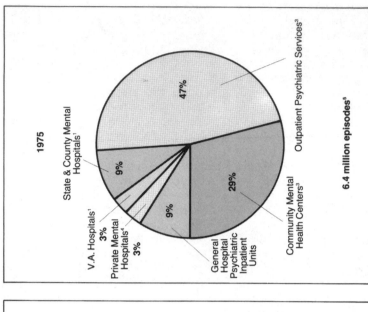

1975

State & County Mental Hospitals[1]

9%

V.A. Hospitals[1]
3%

Private Mental Hospitals[4]
3%

47%

General Hospital Psychiatric Inpatient Units

9%

Community Mental Health Centers[3]

29%

Outpatient Psychiatric Services[3]

6.4 million episodes[5]

[4] Includes residential treatment centers for emotionally disturbed children and inpatient services only of private psychiatric hospitals

[5] Excludes inpatient episodes of multiservice mental health facilities not shown in chart, all partial care episodes, and outpatient episodes of V.A. hospitals

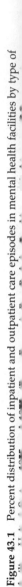

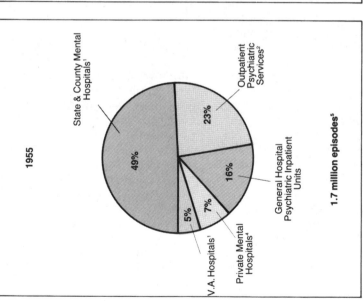

1955

State & County Mental Hospitals[1]

49%

Outpatient Psychiatric Services[2]

23%

General Hospital Psychiatric Inpatient Units

16%

Private Mental Hospitals[4]
7%

V.A. Hospitals[1]
5%

1.7 million episodes[5]

[1] Inpatient services only

[2] Includes free-standing outpatient services as well as those affiliated with psychiatric and general hospitals

[3] Includes inpatient and outpatient services of federally funded CMHC's

Figure 43.1   Percent distribution of inpatient and outpatient care episodes in mental health facilities by type of

SPECIAL SUBPOPULATIONS OF THE CHRONIC MENTALLY ILL

In the wake of deinstitutionalization, a number of subpopulations with special characteristics and/or service needs have emerged.

Young Adult Chronic Patient

The label "young adult chronic patient" came into common usage in psychiatry in the 1980s. The term defines a group of 18 to 35-year-olds who are the first generation of chronic patients to grow up in the era of deinstitutionalization. They are predominantly single, unemployed males who have never or have only briefly been institutionalized. Clinically they are seen as mobile, fragile, labile individuals with poor impulse control, poor functional and adaptive skills, and an inability or unwillingness to learn from experience. They are frequently diagnosed as having schizophrenia, but affective disorders, borderline personality, and multiple diagnoses are also well represented. Substance abuse, suicidal threats and gestures, and other self-injurious behavior are common. Natural supports are few; relationships are established only with great difficulty. The young adult chronic patient makes persistent but inappropriate demands on service providers, often engendering in those providers a sense of helplessness. Between periods when they use the entire range of mental health services and frequent general hospital emergency rooms, they may have periods when they use no services whatsoever (20–22).

The term "young adult chronic patient" is not without controversy. Bachrach has indicated that the "concept has outstripped systematic attempts to objectify the existence of young adult chronic patients as an empirical entity with clearly defined boundaries" (22). Estroff has called for the elimination of the term, indicating it is "misleading and ill-tempered." She indicates that the label is substantially pejorative and accusatory. She offers an alternative characterization of the population:

Younger persons who are defiant, who often prefer to take their own drugs rather than ours, who deeply value freedom, who often have not yet been broken in spirit by institutions or phenothiazines, and who refuse the role of "good patient." (23, p 5)

Regardless of what they are called, this population is different from the generation that preceded it, largely as a result of changed institutional practices. Appropriate services need to be developed to meet their needs as they age, for young adult chronic patients will soon become adult chronic patients.

Homeless Mentally Ill

The term "homeless mentally ill" is now replacing more colloquial destinations previously used for this population, such as "street people" or "bag ladies."

There is much disagreement over the number of homeless individuals in the United States; estimates range from a low of 250,000 (made by the U.S. Department of Housing and Urban Development) to 3 million (made by the Community for Creative Non-Violence) (24). Estimates of the percentage of those who are mentally ill vary almost as widely (25). Many of the mentally ill homeless cannot be located given their wanderings, their out-of-the-way haunts, and their disinclination to be recognized. Even determining who to count is difficult because the boundary between the domiciled and the undomiciled mentally ill is permeable, and the distinction between sheltered and unsheltered is fuzzy.

The homeless mentally ill are a heterogeneous group, but certain characteristics occur with frequency: an impoverished and highly stressful social network, a history of recidivism in both the mental health and the criminal justice systems, a high prevalence of physical illness, and a reluctance to accept traditional therapeutic offerings (26).

Engaging the homeless mentally ill in treatment has been a major challenge. It is clear that services must be brought to them as they will not come to the services, that a wide range of services are required, and that negotiating mutually agreed upon treatment strategies will be necessary for effective interventions.

Revolving Door Patients

This label describes individuals with multiple presentations to the emergency room, repeated admissions to the hospital, and/or frequent, unscheduled appearances at the outpatient department (27). Prior to the era of deinstitutionalization, most of these patients would have been long-term residents of state hospitals. Recidivism is an outgrowth of deinstitutionalization with its ethos of admission diversion and short term hospitalization.

Attempts to characterize this group to allow for preventive intervention have been thwarted by inconsistent findings. The most significant predictor of rehospitalization has been the evidence of prior hospitalizations (28). There are some indications that the population may be significantly represented by a subgroup of patients with schizophrenia and a subgroup of patients with severe personality disorders, two groups which require different clinical approaches (28).

Recidivists frequently engender anger in service providers, who feel their efforts are wasted. These patients require a carefully constructed, multidimensional, multidisciplinary treatment plan that incorporates all aspects of the service delivery system. Periodic hospitalization needs to be seen as an integral part of the overall treatment plan and not as evidence of outpatient failure (28).

Women

While it may appear inappropriate to label a subheading in this section "women," it is done to highlight the fact that women with chronic mental illness are different from and have a different course of chronic mental illness than their male counterparts. This observation, until recently, has been given little attention (29, 30). The

need of chronic mentally ill women for service, their utilization of facilities, their use of psychotropic medication, their response to psychotropic medication, their roles in the community, and the response they engender in mental health care providers are all different from chronic mentally ill men (29–32).

Elderly

The elderly are rarely focused on in the literature of chronic mental illness, despite the fact that they are a growing percentage of the population who have significant, and often untreated, psychiatric pathology. Rovner et al. found in a random sample of a large, intermediate care nursing home that 94% of the residents had dysfunctions that meet *Diagnostic and Statistical Manual of Mental Disorders (Third Edition)* (DSM-III) criteria for a mental disorder (33); Christenson and Blazer found that 4% of 997 elderly living in the community had generalized persecutory ideation and that many did not receive needed mental health services (34); and Bassuk et al. found that geriatric patients who presented in the emergency room with coexisting medical and psychiatric disorders would have the psychiatric pathology ignored if the medical disorder was treated (35).

While it is important for the outpatient clinician to be sensitive to the different presentations of psychiatric illness in the elderly and to understand the variations in standard treatments dictated by the age of the patient, the practitioner must also be cognizant of a disorder peculiar to this group—elder abuse. Elder abuse is defined as any action taken by an elderly person's family or caretaker that employs threats of violence, violence, disciplinary restraint, or neglect of basic needs in order to take advantage of the elder's bodily integrity, emotional well-being, or property. Cases of elder abuse are often missed by practitioners despite clinical evidence, perhaps because it is such an anathema. The outpatient clinician needs to be aware of the high-risk indicators—physical indicators such as bruises and welts, burns, multiple lacerations and abrasions, and head injuries; and behavioral indicators such as vigilance in the presence of caretakers and undue fear—in order to increase early detection. Appropriate interventions include short-term treatment of physical injuries and acute prevention of further harm and long-range interventions to alter the current environment or to permanently remove the elder person to a safe setting (36, 37).

Dual Diagnosis: Mental Illness and Mental Retardation

Deinstitutionalization of the mentally retarded is occurring, although it started later and has been more gradual than the exodus of the mentally ill from state hospitals (38). While the practitioner is quite likely to see mentally retarded individuals in outpatient psychiatric settings, he or she is prone to underdiagnose mental illness in the presence of mental retardation (39). The mentally retarded, however, have a greater than average risk to develop mental illness because of the high incidence of central nervous system pathology and diminished psychologic and interpersonal resources (40).

The mentally retarded are often more aware and more able to make informed decisions than the clinician unfamiliar with them might imagine. For example, mentally retarded individuals with affective disorders were quite able to report on their depressions (41), and dual diagnosis patients have been shown to be cognizant of and affected by negative social conditions (42).

The dual diagnosis patients require care and treatment for both chronic disorders. All too often they are rejected by each care system because they meet the criteria for the other (43) (see Chapter 41).

Dual Diagnosis: Mental Illness and Substance Abuse

Because the term "dual diagnosis" has been applied to individuals with substance abuse in conjunction with mental illness just as it has to individuals with mental retardation and mental illness, the clinician needs to ascertain which group of patients a colleague is referring to when the term "dual diagnosis" is used.

The individual with both substance abuse and chronic mental illness has long been the bane of the outpatient therapist. Many a supervisor has admonished that you can't treat the psychiatric disorder as long as the abuse continues, but the simultaneous treatment of the coexisting disorders can be achieved.

Kofoed et al. (44) treated 32 prior treatment failures at a Veterans Administration outpatient clinic for severe psychopathology and either significant alcohol abuse or alcohol and drug abuse. Although they had a high dropout rate, 11 patients remained 3 or more months and 7 of the 11 remained in treatment 1 year or more. Those who remained in treatment were significantly more likely to have had previous outpatient treatment than those who dropped out. The authors suggest that open-ended treatment of both disorders should go on simultaneously by one team of practitioners. They also indicate that the clinician may need to accept substance abuse in the early phase of treatment and that this issue may be a subject of prolonged negotiation between therapist and patient until abstinence can realistically be achieved (see Chapters 36 and 37).

TREATMENT MODALITIES APPLIED TO CHRONIC MENTAL ILLNESS

The needs of the chronic mentally ill are so far reaching that no single professional discipline and no single theoretical orientation can possibly meet them all. Providing outpatient mental health services to this population requires a multidisciplinary team of practitioners who can deliver to the patient biologic, psychodynamic, behavioral and sociocultural approaches in a coordinated fashion such that continuity of care is maximized, misuse of resources is minimized, and neither the patient nor any of the care providers feels misunderstood, misused, or abused.

Psychopharmacologic Treatments

The advent of psychotropic medication has led to impressive gains in the treatment of the chronic mentally ill. This, in turn, has altered the course of chronic mental illness and the types of services needed by this population. Yet we must apply psychopharmacologic treatment with caution. As Havens has said,

The rapid, haphazard advancement of deinstitutionalization resulted in part from the belief that psychotropic medications would do for schizophrenia and affective disorders what penicillin had done for syphilis and lobar pneumonia. . . . Such opinions . . . foster the continued rejection of the chronic mentally ill so readily fobbed off with medications perfunctionally administered. The great investment of energy, time, and imagination necessary for the care of chronic patients are being dismissed. (45)

In the psychopharmacological management of the chronic mentally ill, differentiating noncompliers from nonresponders has proved a difficult, often frustrating task. Noncompliance is a documented problem with the chronic mentally ill (46), and therefore practitioners tend to ascribe noncompliance to treatment failures. However, despite the efficacy of antipsychotic medication (47), there is a subgroup of chronic patients who are drug nonresponders, not noncompliers, and they require alternative interventions (48). The increased availability of blood level measurement should help the outpatient psychiatrist separate these two groups. However, the laboratory will never replace the constructive engagement of the patient by the clinician such that the two are involved in a cooperative venture aimed at minimizing the effects of chronic mental illness. If the patient's goal is to dupe the clinician into believing medication is being taken when it is not, the patient will find a way despite the laboratory.

For a more complete discussion of the psychologic problems of pharmacologic treatments, the reader is referred to Chapter 49.

Psychotherapy

Both individual psychotherapy and group psychotherapy can prove useful to patients with chronic mental illness (49, 50). The approach most commonly recommended is supportive psychotherapy (49–51). There have been masters of individual, insight-oriented psychotherapy, such as Elvin Semrad (52), Alfred Stanton (53), and Otto Will (54), who have applied this treatment to the chronic mentally ill. Application of this approach is now afforded only to the most well-to-do and only with those psychotherapists who work in institutions serving them. Even supportive psychotherapy is often unavailable in public sector institutions because of inadequate resources.

One caveat before proceeding. It is wrong to assume that we should strive to provide insight-oriented, psychodynamic psychotherapy to all. This treatment for some schizophrenic patients may be detrimental, hastening relapse for those who experience it as cognitively overwhelming (46, 55).

For further discussion of psychotherapy the reader is referred to Chapters 4 and 45.

Medical Treatment

The chronic mentally ill have a high rate of chronic medical illness (56). In some cases the medical problems may be closely linked to the mental illness, e.g., mental retardation, organic brain syndrome. In other cases, the relationship is less clear (56).

The chronic mentally ill tend to use those institutions they know best when they require medical treatment. For many, that facility is the state hospital. Since the state hospital has historically been a total-care institution, and since many of the deinstitutionalized have no recent experiences in receiving medical care in the community, they return to the state hospital for admission when they are medically ill (57).

Some of the chronic mentally ill may feel more comfortable about seeking treatment for medical problems at the state hospital rather than at traditional medical facilities where their complaints are less likely to be treated as valid. There is a tendency for medical facilities to react to the chronic mentally ill who present with a medical complaint as if that complaint was not physically based but rather a component of the psychiatric disorder, i.e., a delusion. For example, a 39-year-old female bursts into the general hospital emergency room in June with two overcoats on, three shopping bags in her left hand, and an open umbrella in her right hand. She screams "My ass is falling out, my ass is falling out" and continues to run frantically around the emergency room. Several interns react by saying she's crazy; one examines her and finds a prolapsed rectum. The chronic mentally ill have acute medical problems like everyone else and they should be evaluated like every one else. The physician needs to be sensitive to the patient's idiosyncratic verbal communications.

The provision of medical care to the chronic mentally ill has often been poor. In part this reflects both that much of their mental health care is provided in nonmedical facilities and that much of their mental health care is provided by nonphysicians. The case manager (see below) becomes crucial in the effort to get the chronic mentally ill to both scheduled and emergency medical care. For a review of the incidence of medical illness in psychiatric populations, the reader is referred to Chapter 17,

Social Skills Training

The observations that social dysfunction was a benchmark of chronic schizophrenia and that premorbid social adjustment correlated with the course of schizophrenia led to the pursuit of therapeutic efforts aimed at improving social functioning. Social skills training, also known as personal effectiveness training, assertiveness training, and structured learning therapy, has been developed over the past 20 years by psychologists with behavioral orientations (58–60).

An assessment of the appropriateness of social skills training for a patient proceeds by considering four questions: (a) Does the patient have an interpersonal dysfunction? (b) Is there an association between the dysfunction and a social skills deficit? (c) What are the circumstances in which the dysfunction occurs? (d) What is the specific nature of the skills deficit? (59). If the assessment indicates that social skills training is appropriate, a program tailored to the individual patient's needs is designed. Administered either individually or in groups, social skills training is a highly structured didactic exercise that utilizes instruction, role playing, modeling, positive reinforcement, homework, and repetition to produce changed behavior.

Reviews of social skills training published in 1980 (58, 60) questioned the maintenance, generalizability, and impact of this therapeutic approach. More recent works, however, hold out promise for social skills training as a technique capable of prolonging community tenure (61, 62).

Psychiatric Rehabilitation

A psychiatric rehabilitation program aims at changing the "client's" skills and/or changing the client's supports. As defined by Anthony, the mission of psychiatric rehabilitation is

to ensure that the person with the psychiatric disability can perform those physical, emotional, and intellectual skills needed to live, learn, and work in his or her own particular community, given the least amount of intervention necessary from agents of the helping professions. (63)

Psychiatric rehabilitation uses an atheoretical, eclectic approach that actively involves clients in their own rehabilitation process. The improvement of vocational functioning is a central outcome (64).

That aspect of psychiatric rehabilitation that focuses on clients' skill development is best exemplified by the social skills training discussed above. There are two note-worthy examples of programs focused on changing the client's environment—Fountain House and the Community Support Program (CSP).

Fountain House, the original clubhouse model in the United States, is a facility that provides to the chronic mentally ill a combination of services—a rehabilitation club, a range of community residential options, and an active vocational rehabilitation program. In the clubhouse model services are provided in a familylike network of relationships with blurring of staff–client distinctions and with clients providing useful services to the program itself. Fountain House serves as a prototype of the clubhouse model, now found throughout the United States.

The CSP was a National Institute of Mental Health pilot project, launched in 1977, to meet the comprehensive needs of the adult, chronic mentally ill. Community Support Programs were to include the following functions: identification of the target population and outreach to offer them services, assistance in applying for entitlements, crisis stabilization in the least restrictive alternative, psychosocial rehabilitation, supportive services as needed, medical and mental health care, backup support to families, inclusion of community members in planning and developing housing options and work opportunities, protection of client's rights, and case management.

The CSPs were an effort to create a system of comprehensive care, one that fostered the integration of health and human service systems beyond the traditional boundaries of the mental health system. Although inadequately funded from the outset, CSP did create models for well-integrated, far-reaching systems of care in some states. In many other states its lessons remain to be adopted (65).

For a further discussion of psychiatric rehabilitation, see Chapter 50.

Vocational Rehabilitation

Vocational rehabilitation is a key element of psychiatric rehabilitation. The out-patient clinician should be aware of three types of programs. Sheltered workshops allow individuals to do piecework contracted for by the agency. Each worker is paid by comparing his or her output to that of an average worker, and each worker's salary is that percentage of the minimum wage that his output warrants. Transitional employment programs place individuals in competitive work environments for defined periods of time while supported employment programs use competitive employment positions in an open-ended way, providing supports as necessary with a goal of weaning the worker off the supports. In this approach, staff may go with the client to the job site and remain there for as long as necessary.

Day Treatment

Day hospitals or partial hospitalization qualifies as outpatient treatment since patients live in the community and commute to the program site which may be in the hospital. Day hospitals are used to avoid inpatient admissions and as transitions from inpatient settings to less structured outpatient treatment. A recent study of this latter use demonstrated that the day hospital decreased readmissions, improved community integration, and succeeded in linking patients to long-term community treatment (66). Day treatment may be a useful adjunct for the outpatient therapist as an entry point for long-term services (66).

Group Treatment

Group therapy for the chronic patient may refer to any one of a heterogeneous array of services which have only their group context in common. Such groups include psychotherapy groups, task-oriented groups, peer groups, support groups, or medication groups. Each has been demonstrated to be effective in achieving its particular desired outcome. The outpatient therapist who plans on making a referral to outpatient group therapy needs to be explicit about the appropriate type of group (see Chapter 46).

Family Treatment

There has been an evolution in the thinking about the family's role in the production and/or maintenance of symptoms of chronic mental illness (usually schizophrenia). From earlier theories of the "schizophrenogenic mother"; disordered communication; and pervasively sick, disharmonious families, we have arrived at the period of "expressed emotion." "Expressed emotion" is "an operationally defined construct that is a measure of the extent to which relatives express critical, hostile, or overinvolved attitudes about a patient when discussing the patient's illness and family life with an interviewer" (67). It was observed, then empirically demonstrated, that families of schizophrenic patients showed high expressed emotion. This led to therapeutic efforts to reduce expressed emotion, the major effort being psychoeducation. Before defining psychoeducation it is worth noting, in the context of chronic mental illness, that there is nothing intrinsic to the concept of expressed emotion that limits it to schizophrenia (67).

Psychoeducation is grounded in the concept that providing information to families with a chronic mentally ill member can be therapeutically valuable. The program consists of a series of educational workshops in which parents learn to minimize certain environmental stressors to which their schizophrenic children are presumably biologically vulnerable (68).

An interesting expansion of psychoeducation has been its application to chronic mentally ill persons living in group situations without biologic family members (69). This application of psychoeducation raises the possibility of its widespread use in mental health agency sponsored residential programs.

Residential Programs

There is an array of residential programs with levels of supervision from minimal to continuous. Residential programs can provide a range of options from just a place to live to complete programming. Examples of the types and levels of residential programs are presented in Table 43.2. The data comes from the *Brewster v. Dukakis Consent Decree*, a United States District Court order based on the principle that "residents and clients are entitled to live in the least restrictive, most normal residential alternative and to receive appropriate treatment, training, and support suited to their individual needs" (70).

Crisis Intervention

Crisis intervention or psychiatric emergency services include a multitude of service delivery systems that have 24-hour, 7-day-a-week availability, prescreening functions for the public sector inpatient setting, and triage of all referrals. Services differ in four ways: location—general hospital emergency room, free-standing, component of community mental health centers; mobility—none (patient is brought to the service) or mobile team (staff can go out to the patient); clinical services available—only triage, outpatient management of crisis, beds for acute management; and staffing—psychiatrist available by phone only, psychiatrist can be called in, or psychiatrist on site.

In an era of admission diversion from inpatient to outpatient settings, the crisis team is seen as the keystone to success in the public sector. When state hospital censuses rise, the crisis team is usually the first component of the service system called to task.

Case Management

The chronic mentally ill in the community face myriad bureaucratic agencies and departments; they require assistance in negotiating the complexities of this system. The tasks of managing the chronic mentally ill person's accessing, utilizing, and integrating services belongs to the case manager. Often the junior member of the multidisciplinary outpatient treatment team, the case manager may have the most wide-reaching functions.

Case managers are generally individuals

Table 43.2   Continuum of Community Residential Services

Facility	Non-DMH[a]-provided or funded housing	Specialized home care	Supervised group home/supervised apt.	Transitional community residence/apt.	Group home/apt. with physical care	Group home/apt. with behavioral emphasis	Group home/apt. with physical care and behavioral emphasis
Definition	Own home, own residence, boarding house, single room occupancy, nursing home, resthome, cooperative apts	Supervised living; also called foster care	Provides room, board, supervision of daily living skills; residents have day programs at other sites	A 24-hr program supplying room, board, intensive training in daily living skills, supervision	Room, board, daily assistance, training in basic activities of daily living for persons with minimum of behavior problems and high activities of daily living needs	Room, board, intensive services within the residence for serious problems	Room, board, intensive behavioral program and physical care plus help with activities of daily living
No. of residents[b]	Variable	1/3	4/8	8/4	8/4	8/4	8/4
Funding source	Own resources, Social Security Income, Social Security Disability Insurance,	State	State	State	State	State	State
Per diem cost per resident[b, c]	Variable	$15.81	$31.21/$40.94	$40.05/$50.05	$46.12/$64.60	$52.81/$68.80	$56.65/$80.46
Annual average cost per resident[b, c]	Variable	$3,944.0	$11,392/$14,943	$14,620/$18,268	$17,084/$23,579	$19,276/$25,115	$20,679/$29,367

[a] Department of Mental Health.
[b] In each category, the number before the slash applies to group home, and the number after the slash applies to group apartment (apt.).
[c] In 1978 dollars.

who function solely in that role. There has been criticism of this structure because it may not allow the case manager to have an in-depth knowledge of the client. The case management system then becomes an impersonal bureaucracy. An alternative is to include the case management function in the job of the outpatient therapist (71).

SPECIAL-INTEREST GROUPS

There is a long history in the United States of interest groups concerned with chronic mental illness. Two early examples merit attention.

The National Association for the Protection of the Insane and the Prevention of Insanity, which was founded in 1880 and open to anyone with two dollars for membership, came into being with a rationale that sounds familiar:

The number of those more or less insane, who either do not go to public institutions, or cannot find room in, or be supported by them, is increasingly large, and for this class there is no systematic supervision or guardianship. There are multitudes of insane men and women in the United States for whom no special provision is made in the way of care and treatment. (72)

Although this Association lasted only 4 years, historians indicate that it did much good (10).

The National Committee for Mental Hygiene was founded in 1908 by Clifford Beers and had as its aims the prevention of mental disorders, improvement of mental health care, study of mental disorders, dispelling of notions that mental disorders are incurable, termination of the stigma of mental illness, and enlistment of the Federal Government in all these endeavors (10). Beers was himself an ex-patient, best known for his autobiography, *A Mind That Found Itself*. The National Committee for Mental Hygiene is the precursor of the National Mental Health Association, a group presently active.

Patient/Ex-Patient Groups

Currently, there are many groups of patients and/or ex-patients who are active in the United States. Many of these groups are "antipsychiatry." They often put out publications, rally at annual meetings, and protest. They have a long tradition of putting complaints about treatment into print (73). Organizations include Mental Patients Liberation Project, Network Against Psychiatric Assault, and Psychiatric Inmates Rights Collective. Publications include *Madness Network News* and *Mental Patients Liberation Front Newsletter*.

More recently, patient/ex-patients have formed groups that align themselves with mainstream psychiatry. An example is the National Depressive and Manic–Depressive Association, whose mission statement is, "The National Association recognizes the biochemical nature of bipolar and unipolar affective disorders and the disruptive psychological impact of the illness on patients and families."

Parents and Significant Other Groups

Parents of the chronic mentally ill are shedding their self-recriminating blankets of despair. They are expressing themselves in professional journals (74–77) and they are organizing advocacy groups. The most important of these is the National Alliance for the Mentally Ill—"a self-help organization of families of mentally ill persons, of mentally ill persons themselves, and of friends." Founded in 1979, NAMI now has hundreds of local and state chapters.

ISSUES IN THE CARE AND TREATMENT OF THE CHRONIC MENTALLY ILL

Present and future outpatient care and treatment of the chronic mentally ill pose many problems that must be addressed.

How Will Care and Treatment Be Financed?

Contemporary systems of financing mental health care and treatment dictate the nature of psychiatric services; outpatient treatment of the chronic mentally ill suffers as a result. In our current system states bear most of the cost for state hospital care and treatment but the Federal Government (through Supplemental Security Income, Social Security Disability Income, Medicaid, food stamps, housing subsidies, etc.) supports outpatients. Increasing state expenditure for mental health does not necessarily improve services (3). Systems work best where dollars follow patients, i.e., capitation. Diagnosis-related groups are useless in predicting outpatient mental health costs (78). In times of fiscal restraint, outpatient treatment is disproportionately underfunded (79).

Recent recommendations on financing the care and treatment of chronic mental illness include delivering SSI and SSDI funds to states as block grants (3) and creating a new federal entitlement program pooling all existing sources of dollars (80). These two approaches have in common the more rational expenditure of federal tax dollars.

How Do We Enhance Treatment Compliance?

The rate of noncompliance with long-term use of psychotropic medication averages 33% (81). Reasons for noncompliance have been well studied in schizophrenic (81, 82) and bipolar affective disordered (83, 84) outpatients. These reasons include premorbid personality traits; dysfunctional service delivery system; inadequate doctor–patient relationship; medication side effects including dysphoria, extrapyramidal side effects, akathisia, weight gain, sexual dysfunction, and cognitive impairments; concern about long-term side effects of medication, e.g., tardive dyskinesia, kidney damage; and a preference for the unmedicated state, i.e., schizophrenic existence, hypomania, mania.

Clinical management of noncompliance incorporates all the outpatient therapist's tools, including psychologic, somatic, psychosocial, and environmental interventions. From the psychologic perspective, the psychiatrists alter their stance from that of authoritarian prescriber to a prescriber allowing the patient to be an active participant; the process is grounded in concepts of negotiating with patients covered earlier in this text. Essentially, compliance follows from alliance. From the somatic perspective, it is often useful to honor patients' complaints about side effects by lowering the dosage of some medications and/or changing some medications. Another intervention that aids compliance is switching from oral to depot intramuscular medication. In the psychosocial sphere, it is often helpful to enlist the aid of family members in efforts to have the patient take his or her medication. For effective family cooperation, the practitioner should educate the family about the medications. From the environmental perspective, helping patients to develop systems for taking their medication correctly will often improve compliance in the nondeliberate noncomplier. For example, using an egg carton that the patient fills with the day's medication will assist those who can never remember how many pills they've taken. Enlisting the assistance of case managers for patient education about medication can be invaluable. Ancillary services like the Visiting Nurse Association can be employed. Sometimes, having the patient stop by the outpatient clinic every few days to pick up a few days' worth of medication can alter compliance.

We can devise many strategies to attempt to improve compliance. But if these strategies fail, can we impose treatment on chronic mentally ill outpatients?

How Do We Balance Patients' Rights and Patients' Needs?

We are in an era of the active promotion of psychiatric outpatients' rights (85, 86). But we are also in a time of the evolution of psychiatric service delivery, when the extent of outpatients' rights is being fundamentally questioned (87, 88).

The rallying cry of the promoters of community treatment has been the right to treatment in the least restrictive alternative (LRA). But LRA is a muddled concept and its application is rarely clear (89, 90). For example, how do you factor into an equation of restrictiveness the psychotic state, freedom to wander the streets, involuntary hospitalization, imposition of psychopharmacologic treatment, homelessness, and hunger? The point at which coercion is justified must be defined. Should the mayor of New York City, for example, be able to round up and shelter the homeless when the temperature goes below 32°F?

At present the battle between patients' rights and practitioners' imposition of treatment is being fought over outpatient civil commitment. Committing individuals to a treatment program in the community rather than to an institution holds both many promises for success and many perils (91, 92). The balance between autonomy of the chronic mentally ill in the community and the mental health practitioner's paternalistic interventions must be examined. The well-being of the chronic mentally ill in the community hangs in that balance.

How Do We Provide Continuity of Care?

As late as 1979, researchers were indicating that continuity of care for the chronic mentally ill in the community was infrequently studied (93). Since then, there has been a virtual explosion of interest in this issue.

Continuity of care can be conceptualized as consisting of seven dimensions: longitudinal nature, individuality, comprehensiveness, flexibility, relationship, accessibility, and communication (94). In essence, outpatients should have the opportunity to participate in a plan of care and treatment that is designed for them, encompasses all the services they need in an integrated fashion for as long as they need them, can change as their abilities/disabilities change, and will never leave them stranded.

Stone has indicated that the failure of continuity of care is the "greatest failing of the modern mental health system." (87). There have been many demonstration projects to remedy this shortcoming (95),

but their designs and achievements have yet to be generalized. Until continuity of care is achieved for the chronic mentally ill, the sad comment "he fell through the cracks" will continue to be heard.

How Do We Ensure Adequate Psychiatrists for the Task?

The problems of recruitment and retention of psychiatrists to work with the chronic mentally ill in the community are legion. Psychiatrists are often disinclined to work with chronic patients. They are pushed even further from the public sector by problems in the structure and pattern of mental health care delivery, such as constraints on the independence of the psychiatrist, the maintenance of responsibility and liability without authority, an openness to public scrutiny, and a lack of peer support. Yet, it is with the chronic mentally ill that the highest level of expertise in the broadest range of treatment modalities is needed.

If psychiatrists are to be recruited into the public sector, efforts must start during residency (96). Psychiatric residents must be taught to work with nonmedical interventions in nontraditional settings (97, 98). They must be provided with excellent role models, and they must know that mainstream psychiatry holds this kind of work in high regard.

The most promising prospects for training residents to work with chronic patients are the university–state collaborations (99). As federal dollars for training shrink, the liaison between state and university becomes more and more attractive.

Who Does What in Providing Outpatient Treatment?

Through the 1970s and early 1980s there was considerable blurring of the roles of the participants in delivering care and treatment. As indicated in Chapter 1, there also was a burgeoning of types of mental health practitioners whose various designations read like alphabet soup. The diversity of practitioners and the blurring of roles created a system which at its best was egalitarian teamwork, and at its worst was irresponsible confusion.

Concurrent with the changes in clinical personnel was a shift in managerial orientation. Clinics, once run by clinical professionals, began to be professionally managed, cost-effective operations whose application of technologies was heavily weighted by efficient application of resources.

Outpatient psychiatry for the chronic mentally ill now appears to be characterized by a reemergence of clinical leadership by clinically trained professionals in settings directed by professional managers who appreciate the mission of the agency. Multidisciplinary teams continue to exist but with greater specification of roles based on training. Increased specialization, such as geropsychiatry, law and psychiatry, and even public sector psychiatry, is available. Inpatient settings, and (sometimes) state hospitals are being reintegrated into the system of treatment.

What Are the Future Roles of State Hospitals?

What state hospitals were, are, and should be is the subject of considerable attention in professional publications (100–103). At this juncture the notion that state hospitals can be closed has waned since its zenith in the 1970s. Rather, issues now under study include integrating the state hospital into the community system of care and treatment, running excellent facilities in the public sector, better defining who benefits and who does not from institutional care and treatment, and ascertaining who needs asylum.

Asylum has become a more frequent topic of discussion as the care functions (as opposed to the treatment functions) of the state hospital are better appreciated (104–106). How do we create asylum for the chronic mentally ill who need it without resurrecting asylums? What role, if any, should state hospitals play in providing asylum?

As we struggle with the future of state hospitals, we must study their past. As Rosenblatt indicated, "Our predecessors who cared for psychotic patients were not quaint. Neither are we excessively wise" (107).

How Much "Treatment," How Much "Care?"

Moving patients from state hospitals to communities required the provision of extensive care to the population in the community so that they could even exist there. Contemporaneously with the change in the loss of care and treatment there occurred (a) the demedicalization of outpatient psychiatry; (b) the egalitarian approach to care and treatment, i.e., all staff, independent of training, have equal responsibility for making clinical decisions; (c) the belief that being "free" and "communitized" would improve chronic mental illness; (d) the belief that moving patients out of state hospitals and into other institutions ("transinstitutionalization") with less capacity for treatment was none-the-less liberating; (e) the notion that almost all acute mental illness could be handled by crisis intervention without recourse to institutions; and (f) the concept that better assessments of patients (called "clients" in the system) could somehow produce better treatment without having to independently fund treatment. Examination of documents from this era show little attention to treatment and considerable attention to care and management (70, 108).

Community mental health systems must be for care and for treatment. Paying little heed to the latter perpetuates the former. Few of the chronic mentally ill leave the system and the need for care facilities grows annually.

As indicated earlier, there appears to now be a shift back to professionalism in community mental health. While this will improve treatment, the movement should be accompanied by research so that we do not simply pendulously swing between service system designs without knowing what works for whom.

What About Research?

There have been extensive changes in the pattern of mental health services to the chronic mentally ill, with little investigation of what accounts for success and failure. State lunatic asylums were created and filled on ill-founded notions of curability, and state hospitals were emptied based on untested hypotheses, beliefs, and wishes.

As we proceed to modify the delivery of mental health services to the chronic mentally ill in the community, we must systematically examine what we are doing. We should have learned from Jarvis's demonstration in 1866 of an inverse relationship between use of the state hospital and distance from it (109) (a finding, incidentally, repeated in 1962 [110] and 1982 [111]) that planning for the chronic mentally ill requires the examination of many variables, some not apparent at first glance.

Systematic examination of outpatient services in the era of deinstitutionalization is beginning to appear (112, 113). We need considerably more study before we know what works for whom, where.

What About Stigmatization?

The literature on public opinions about mental illness (114) and on dangerousness of the mentally ill (115, 116) is complex and mired in contradictions. Nonetheless, the chronic mentally ill continue to be excluded from mainstream American life. There is much truth in the belief that the chronic mentally ill have gone from back wards to back alleys. It is the accounting for this journey that is yet to be made.

The mental health practitioner who works with the chronic mentally ill in outpatient settings must see as part of his or her job the education of the community, informing them about the nature of chronic mental illness and the qualities of those who are its victims.

Where Are We Now?

Even state-of-the-art treatment of the chronic mentally ill leaves much to be desired. Effective ministering to the needs of the chronic mentally ill continues to be a struggle. This is not only a consequence of resource allocation, it is also a result of our incomplete knowledge.

I see the chronic mentally ill warming themselves on heating grates. In a fast-food restaurant, I notice a chronically mentally ill person nursing the same cup of coffee for hours. As I walk the city streets, I observe a chronically mentally ill person who is pushing a shopping cart from trash receptacle to trash receptacle on a search for returnable soda cans. From these experiences, I painfully realize that the attitudes and practices of our society have allowed people to reach this state, and that we must address these attitudes and practices if we are to deliver effective outpatient care. The chronic mentally ill of each generation in this century have been abandoned. Only the setting has changed. This is not simply chronic mental illness. It is neglect.

References

1. Minkoff K: A map of chronic mental patients. In Talbott JA (ed): *The Chronic Mental Patient.* Washington, DC, American Psychiatric Association, 1978, pp 11–37.
2. Goldman HH: Epidemiology. In Talbott JA (ed): *The Chronic Mental Patient Five Years Later.* Orlando, Grune and Stratton, 1984, pp 15–31.
3. Torrey EF, Wolfe SM: *Care of the Seriously Mentally Ill.* Washington DC, Public Citizen Health Research Group, 1986.
4. Summers F: Characteristics of new patient admissions to aftercare. *Hosp Community Psychiatry* 30:199–202, 1979.
5. Summers F: Psychiatric chronicity and diagnosis. *Schizophr Bull* 9:122–133, 1983.
6. Harding CM, Zubin J, Strauss JS: Chronicity in schizophrenia: fact, partial fact, or artifact? *Hosp Community Psychiatry* 38:477–485, 1987.
7. Brauchi GN, Kirby MW: An empirical typology of the chronic mentally ill. *Community Ment Health J* 22:3–21, 1986.
8. Rothman DJ: *The Discovery of the Asylum.* Boston, Little, Brown, 1971.
9. Derschowitz A: The origins of preventive confinement in Anglo-American law. Part II: The American experience. *Cincinnati Law Review* 43:781–846, 1974.
10. Deutsch A: *The Mentally Ill in America.* New York, Columbia University Press, 1949.
11. Deutsch A: *The Shame of the States.* New York, Harcourt Brace, 1948.
12. Wilson DC: *Stranger and Traveler.* Boston, Little, Brown, 1975.
13. Appelbaum PS, Kemp KN: The evolution of commitment law in the nineteenth century. *Law and Human Behavior* 6:343–354, 1982.

14. Packard EPW: *Modern Persecutions: or Insane Asylums Unveiled.* Hartford, Anthoress, 1874.

15. Dain N: From colonial America to bicentennial America: two centuries of vicissitudes in the institutional care of mental patients. *NY Acad Med Bull* 52:1179–1196, 1976.

16. Curran WJ: Hospitalization of the mentally ill. *North Carolina Law Review* 31:275–298, 1953.

17. Goldman HH, Adams NH, Taube CA: Deinstitutionalization: the data demythologized. *Hosp Community Psychiatry* 34:129–134, 1983.

18. The introduction of chlorpromazine. *Hosp Community Psychiatry* 27:505, 1976.

19. State mental hospital inpatient population fell to 117,000 in 1983, NIMH report shows. *Hosp Community Psychiatry* 37:1273–1274, 1986.

20. Pepper B, Kirschner MC, Ryglewicz H: The young adult chronic patient: overview of a population. *Hosp Community Psychiatry* 32:463–469, 1981.

21. Schwartz SR, Goldfinger SM: The new chronic patient: clinical characteristics of an emerging subgroup. *Hosp Community Psychiatry* 32:470–474, 1981.

22. Bachrach LL: The concept of young adult chronic psychiatric patient: questions from a research perspective. *Hosp Community Psychiatry* 35:573–580, 1984.

23. Estroff SE: No more young adult patients. *Hosp Community Psychiatry* 38:5, 1987.

24. United States General Accounting Office: *Homelessness: A Complex Problem and the Federal Response* (GAO/HRD-85-40), Washington, DC, U.S. Government Printing Office, 1985.

25. Lamb HR: *The Homeless Mentally Ill.* Washington, DC, American Psychiatric Association, 1984.

26. Bachrach LL: Research on services for the homeless mentally ill. *Hosp Community Psychiatry* 35:910–913, 1984.

27. Geller JL, Munetz MR: The process of staff change: grappling with the needs of the high management patient. *Hosp Community Psychiatry* 37:1047–1049, 1986.

28. Geller JL: In again, out again: preliminary evaluation of a state hospital's worst recidivists. *Hosp Community Psychiatry* 37:386–389, 1986.

29. Test MA, Berlin SB: Issues of special concern to chronically mentally ill women. *Professional Psychology* 12:136–145, 1981.

30. Bachrach LL: Deinstitutionalization and women. *Am Psychol* 39:1171–1177, 1984.

31. Bachrach LL: Chronic mentally ill women: emergence and legitimation of program issues. *Hosp Community Psychiatry* 36:1063–1069, 1985.

32. Geller JL, Munetz MR: The iatrogenic creation of psychiatric chronicity in women. Nadelson C, Bachrach LL (eds): *Chronic Mentally Ill Women.* Washington, DC, American Psychiatric Press, 1988.

33. Rovner BW, Kafonek S, Filipp L, et al: Prevalence of mental illness in a community nursing home. *Am J Psychiatry* 143:1446–1449, 1986.

34. Christenson R, Blazer D: Epidemiology of persecutory ideation in an elderly population in the community. *Am J Psychiatry* 141:1088–1091, 1984.

35. Bassuk EL, Minden S, Apsler R: Geriatric emergencies: psychiatric or medical? *Am J Psychiatry* 140:539–542, 1983.

36. Rathbone-McCuan E, Goodstein K: Elder abuse: clinical considerations. *Psychiatr Ann* 15:331–339, 1985.

37. Rathbone-McCuan E, Voyles B: Case detection of abused elderly parents. *Am J Psychiatry* 139:189–192, 1982.

38. Braddock D: Deinstitutionalization of the retarded: trends in public policy. *Hosp Community Psychiatry* 32:607–615, 1981.

39. Reiss S, Levitan GW, Szyszko J: Emotional disturbance and mental retardation: diagnostic overshadowing. *Am J Ment Defic* 86:567–574, 1982.

40. Eaton LF, Menolascino FJ: Psychiatric disorders in the mentally retarded: types, problems, and challenges. *Am J Psychiatry* 139:1297–1303, 1982.

41. Kazdin AE, Matson JL, Senatore V: Assessment of depression in mentally retarded adults. *Am J Psychiatry* 140:1040–1043, 1983.

42. Reiss S, Benson BA: Awareness of negative social conditions among mentally retarded, emotionally disturbed outpatients. *Am J Psychiatry* 141:88–90, 1984.

43. Marcos LR, Gil RM, Vazquez KM: Who will treat psychiatrically disturbed developmentally disabled patients? A health care nightmare. *Hosp Community Psychiatry* 37:171–174, 1986.

44. Kofoed L, Kania J, Walsh T: Outpatient treatment of patients with substance abuse and coexisting psychiatric disorders. *Am J Psychiatry* 143:867–872, 1986.

45. Havens LL: Shooting ourselves in the foot. *Hosp Community Psychiatry* 36:811, 1985.

46. Hogarty GB, Goldberg SC: Drug and sociotherapy in the aftercare of schizophrenic patients. *Arch Gen Psychiatry* 28:54–64, 1973.

47. Davis JM: Overview: maintenance therapy in psychiatry. 1: Schizophrenia. *Am J Psychiatry* 132:1237–1245, 1975.

48. Goldberg SC, Schooler NR, Hogarty GE, et al: Prediction of relapse in schizophrenic outpatients treated by drug and sociotherapy. *Arch Gen Psychiatry* 34:171–184, 1977.

49. Epstein NB, Vlok LA: Research on the results of psychotherapy: a summary of evidence. *Am J Psychiatry* 138:1027–1035, 1981.

50. Wilson WH, Diamond RJ, Factor RM: A psychotherapeutic approach to task-oriented groups of severely ill patients. *Yale Journal of Biology and Medicine* 58:363–372, 1985.

51. Winston A, Pinsker H, McCullough L: A review of supportive psychotherapy. *Hosp Community Psychiatry* 37:1105–1114, 1986.

52. Adler G: The psychotherapy of schizophrenia: Semrad's contributions to current psychoanalytic concepts. *Schizophr Bull* 5:130–137, 1979.

53. Stanton AH (with Knapp PH): Intensive psychotherapy with schizophrenia patients: a preliminary manual. *McLean Hospital Journal* 9:1–30, 1984.

54. Will Jr OA: Schizophrenia and psychotherapy In Marmor J (ed): *Modern Psychoanalysis*. New York, Basic Books, 1968, pp 551–573.

55. Drake RE, Sederer LI: The adverse effects of intensive treatment of chronic schizophrenia. *Compr Psychiatry* 27:313–326, 1986.

56. McCarrick AK, Manderscheid RW, Bertolucci DE, et al: Chronic medical problems in the chronic mentally ill. *Hosp Community Psychiatry* 37:289–291, 1986.

57. Harris M, Bergman HL, Bachrach LL: Psychiatric and nonpsychiatric indicators for rehospitalization in a chronic patient population. *Hosp Community Psychiatry* 37:630–631, 1986.

58. Curran JP, Monti PM (eds): *Social Skills Training*. New York, Guilford Press, 1980.

59. Morrison RL, Bellack AS: Social skills training. In Bellack AS (ed): *Schizophrenia: Treatment, Management and Rehabilitation*. Orlando, FL, Grune and Stratton, 1984, pp 247–279.

60. Wallace CJ, Nelson CJ, Liberman RP et al: A review and critique of social skills training with schizophrenic patients. *Schizophr Bull* 6:42–63, 1980.

61. Hogarty GE, Anderson CM, Reiss DJ, et al: Family psychoeducation, social skills training, and maintenance chemotherapy in the aftercare treatment of schizophrenia. *Arch Gen Psychiatry* 43:633–642, 1986.

62. Liberman RP, Mueser KT, Wallace CJ: Social skills training for schizophrenic individuals at risk for relapse. *Am J Psychiatry* 143:523–526, 1986.

63. Anthony WA, Kennard WA, O'Brien WF et al: Psychiatric rehabilitation: past myths and current realities. *Community Ment Health J* 22:249–265, 1986.

64. Anthony WA, Cohen MR, Cohen BF: Psychiatric rehabilitation. In Talbott JA (ed): *The Chronic Patient Five Years Later*. Orlando, FL, Grune and Stratton, 1984, pp 137–157.

65. Turner JC, TenHoor WJ: The NIMH community support program: pilot approach to a needed social reform. *Schizophr Bull* 4:319–344, 1978.

66. Ferber JS, Oswald M, Rubin M, et al: The day hospital as entry point to a network of long-term services: a program evaluation. *Hosp Community Psychiatry* 36:1297–1301, 1985.

67. Keonigsberg HW, Handley R: Expressed emotion: from predictive index to clinical construct. *Am J Psychiatry* 143:1361–1373, 1986.

68. Anderson CM, Reiss DJ, Hogarty GE: *Schizophrenia and the Family*. New York, Guilford Press, 1986.

69. Drake RE, Osher FC: Using family psychoeducation when there is no family. *Hosp Community Psychiatry* 38:274–277, 1987.

70. *Brewster v. Dukakis* CA7604423-F (D Mass, Consent Decree, December 7, 1978).

71. Lamb HR: Therapist–case managers: more than brokers of services. *Hosp Community Psychiatry* 31:762–764, 1980.

72. Grob GN (ed): *The National Association for the Protection of the Insane and the Prevention of Insanity*. New York, Arno Press, 1980.

73. Geller JL: Women's accounts of psychiatric illness and institutionalization. *Hosp Community Psychiatry* 36:1056–1061, 1985.

74. Anonymous: First person account: a father's thoughts. *Schizophr Bull* 9:439–442, 1983.

75. Slater E: First person account: a parent's view on enforcing medication. *Schizophr Bull* 12:291–292, 1986.

76. Williams P, Williams WA, Sommer R, et al: A survey of the California Alliance for the Mentally Ill. *Hosp Community Psychiatry* 37:253–256, 1986.

77. Lamb HR, Hoffman A, Hoffman F, et al: Families of schizophrenics: a movement in jeopardy. *Hosp Community Psychiatry* 37:353–357, 1986.

78. Wood WD, Beardman DF: Prospective payment for outpatient mental health services: evaluation of diagnosis-related groups. *Community Ment Health J* 22:286–293, 1986.

79. Surber RW, Shumway M, Shadoan R, et al: Effects of fiscal retrenchment on public mental health services for the chronic mentally ill. *Community Ment Health J* 22:215–227, 1986.

80. Talbott JA, Sharfstein SS: A proposal for future funding of chronic and episodic mental illness. *Hosp Community Psychiatry* 37:1126–1130, 1986.

81. Kane JM, Borenstein M: Compliance in long-term treatment of schizophrenia. *Psychopharmacol Bull* 21:23–27, 1985.

82. Young JL, Zonana HV, Shepler L: Medication noncompliance in schizophrenia: codification and update. *Bull Am Acad Psychiatry Law* 14:105–122, 1986.

83. Van Patten T: Why do patients with manic-depressive illness stop their lithium? *Compr Psychiatry* 16:179–183, 1975.

84. Cochran SD: Preventing medical noncompliance in the outpatient treatment of bipolar affective disorders. *J Consult Clin Psychol* 52:873–878, 1984.

85. Allen P: A bill of rights for citizens using outpatient mental health services. In Lamb HR (ed): *Community Survival for Long-Term Patients*. San Francisco, Jossey-Bass, 1976, pp 147–170.

86. Lecklitner GL, Greenberg PD: Promoting the rights of the chronically mentally ill in the community: a report on the patient rights policy research project. *Mental Disability Law Reporter* 7:422–429, 1983.

87. Stone AA: Psychiatric abuse and legal reform: two ways to make a bad situation worse. *International Journal of Law and Psychiatry* 5:9–28, 1982.

88. Chodoff P: Involuntary hospitalization of the mentally ill as a moral issue. *Am J Psychiatry* 141:384–389, 1984.

89. Hoffman PB, Foust LL: Least restrictive treatment of the mentally ill: a doctrine in reach of its senses. *San Diego Law Review* 14:1100–1154, 1977.

90. Klein J: The least restrictive alternative: more about less. *Psychiatr Q* 55:106–114, 1983.

91. Geller JL: Rights, wrongs, and the dilemma of coerced community treatment. *Am J Psychiatry* 143:1259–1264, 1986.

92. Mulvey EP, Geller JL, Roth LH: The promise and peril of involuntary outpatient commitment. *Am Psychol* 42:571–584, 1987.

93. Tessler R, Mason JH: Continuity of care in the delivery of mental health services. *Am J Psychiatry* 136:1297–1301, 1979.

94. Bachrach LL: Continuity of care for chronic mental patients: a conceptual analysis. *Am J Psychiatry* 138:1449–1456, 1981.

95. Talbott JA (ed): *Unified Mental Health Systems.* San Francisco, Jossey-Bass, 1983.

96. Nielsen AC, Stein LI, Talbott JA, et al: Encouraging psychiatrists to work with chronic patients: opportunities and limitations of residency education. *Hosp Community Psychiatry* 32:767–775, 1981.

97. Cutler DL, Bloom JD, Shore JH: Training psychiatrists to work with community support systems for chronically mentally ill persons. *Am J Psychiatry* 138:98–101, 1981.

98. Minkoff K, Stern R: Paradoxes faced by residents being trained in the psychosocial treatment of people with chronic schizophrenia. *Hosp Community Psychiatry* 36:859–864, 1985.

99. Talbott JA, Robinowitz CB (eds): *Working Together: State–University Collaboration in Mental Health.* Washington, DC, American Psychiatric Press, 1986.

100. Talbott JA: *The Death of the Asylum.* New York, Grune and Stratton, 1978.

101. Morrissey JP, Goldman HH, Klerman LV: *The Enduring Asylum.* New York, Grune and Stratton, 1980.

102. Pepper B, Ryglewicz H: The role of the state hospital: a new mandate for a new era. *Psychiatr Q* 57:230–251, 1985.

103. Bachrach LL: The future of the state mental hospital. *Hosp Community Psychiatry* 37:467–474, 1986.

104. Bachrach LL: Asylum and chronically ill psychiatric patients. *Am J Psychiatry* 141:975–978, 1984.

105. Lamb HR, Peele R: The need for continuing asylum and sanctuary. *Hosp Community Psychiatry* 35:798–802, 1984.

106. Wasow M: The need for asylum for the chronic mentally ill. *Schizophr Bull* 12:162–167, 1986.

107. Rosenblatt A: Concepts of the asylum in the case of the mentally ill. *Hosp Community Psychiatry* 35:244–250, 1984.

108. Mental Health Action Project: *Final Report.* Boston, Commonwealth of Massachusetts, 1985.

109. Jarvis E: Influence of distance from and nearness to an insane hospital on its use by the people. *American Journal of Insanity* 22:361–406, 1866.

110. Person PH: Geographical variation in first admission rates to a state mental hospital. *Pub Health Rep* 77:719–731, 1962.

111. Breakey WR, Kaminsky MJ: An assessment of Jarvis' Law in an urban catchment area. *Hosp Community Psychiatry* 33:661–663, 1982.

112. Reynolds I, Hoult JE: The relatives of the mentally ill. A comparative trial of community-oriented and hospital-oriented psychiatric care. *J Nerv Ment Dis* 172:480–489, 1984.

113. Beiser M, Shore JH, Peters R, et al: Does community care for the mentally ill make a difference? A tale of two cities. *Am J Psychiatry* 142:1047–1052, 1985.

114. Rabkin J: Public attitudes toward mental illness: a review of the literature. *Schizophr Bull* 10:9–10, 1974.

115. Mulvey EP, Lidz CW: Clinical considerations in the prediction of dangerousness in mental patients. *Clin Psychol Rev* 4:379–401, 1984.

116. Mulvey EP, Lidz CW: Back to basics: a critical analysis of dangerous research in a new legal environment. *Law and Human Behavior* 9:209–219, 1985.

44

Legal Issues in Outpatient Psychiatry

Steven K. Hoge, M.D.
Paul S. Appelbaum, M.D.

The last two decades have seen the marked expansion of legal involvement in psychiatric practice. The era's major influences on mental health care—deinstitutionalization, the growth of psychopharmacology, and the diversification of mechanisms of third-party payment—have led to a shift of the primary locus for delivery of services from inpatient to outpatient settings (1). In response, mental health law itself has evolved, moving from its traditional focus on civil commitment and other aspects of inpatient care to encompass virtually every aspect of psychiatric practice.

The growth of outpatient psychiatric care, however, has been only partially responsible for the proliferation of legal regulation of mental health treatment. Patients and clinicians have been swept up with the rest of society in a general expansion of the role of law in modern life. Impersonal, but also impartial, law has replaced the web of personal relationships that in simpler times granted individuals some measure of control over their lives (2). Now, in an age when persons fear, above all, that broader forces in society will usurp their power to make decisions for themselves, law is looked to as the ally of the individual, the upholder of personal

rights. Just as this trend has brought us the flowering of civil rights law, consumer law, and privacy law in recent decades, so has it had a powerful influence on the development of the law of mental health care.

Nearly all of mental health law is preoccupied with a single subject: When negotiation fails to resolve conflict among the desires of lay persons, mental health professionals, and the state, whose wishes shall triumph? Once, the answer to this query was clear and unequivocal: The state's power, usually placed at the disposal of psychiatry, was supreme. The patient, presumed to be incapable of expressing meaningful desires, could do nought but submit. The contemporary expansion of mental health law, however, has rebalanced the scales, dissociating the interests of state and professions and returning a fair measure of autonomous judgment to patients (or those who would avoid being patients) themselves.

Although the effect of these changes is seen across all of psychiatric practice, outpatient psychiatry faces unique variations of its own. In attempting to carry out the basic functions of information gathering, diagnosis and treatment planning, and treatment, outpatient clinicians must adapt to legal regulation of their practice without many of the supports of their colleagues in inpatient settings. Clinician–patient interactions are often circumscribed; objective information about behavior outside the office may not readily be available. Decision making is frequently rushed, with access to consultation limited. The equities in resolving conflict between the wishes of patients and clinicians are often less clear than in inpatient facilities. And when control must be exercised over patients, the means of control may be difficult to exert.

Yet, this is not to suggest that outpatient clinicians are powerless. Indeed, it is the very potency of the interventions at their disposal—ranging up to involuntary hospitalization—that has precipitated the need for the establishment of some limits on their functioning. If outpatient clinicians are to perform their sensitive functions within the framework of law established by our society, an accurate understanding of the relevant legal architecture is essential. Unlike more comprehensive works (3), this chapter can provide only an introduction to this complex area. Thus, the emphasis shall be on principles rather than particulars, as we trace the issues that are likely to arise as the outpatient encounter develops.

LEGAL ISSUES AT THE INFORMATION-GATHERING STAGE

In the assessment of the outpatient, the initial concern of the clinician is to gather sufficient information on which to base diagnostic and treatment decisions. Although this process almost always begins with the patients themselves, it may soon move beyond them. Emergencies may require rapid additions to or verifications of patients' accounts with persons outside the therapeutic setting. Even in routine office evaluations, it may be desirable to involve outsiders such as family members or former therapists as informants. Both the process of acquiring additional information and the need to involve others in the patient's disposition may necessitate disclo-

sure of information gathered. Patients' understandable concerns about the degree of confidence attending their disclosures are therefore thrust to the forefront of the assessment process.

Principles of Confidentiality

The patient entering the psychiatric emergency room or office setting may have quite realistic concerns about the stigmatizing effect of others learning of his or her condition and treatment. Without at least implicit assurances of confidentiality, many patients would be unable to discuss the issues that brought them to seek care. Given society's interest in having its troubled members seek psychiatric care and, once in treatment, make optimal use of it, mechanisms have been developed to protect confidentiality, both prospectively and by allowing legal recourse to those whose confidentiality has been breached. Society, however, has other interests as well, and a second thrust of the law has been to define limitations to confidentiality, sometimes with actual obligations to disclose patients' communications. This has occurred when competing interests such as the safety of the public from foreseeable harm have been judged to outweigh individual interests in privacy. The tension arising from these competing values defines the ethical debate regarding confidentiality.

From a professional viewpoint, the doctor–patient relationship, the model on which other therapist–patient relationships are based, has been founded on the ethic of confidentiality since the time of the Hippocratic Oath (4). In modern times, the value of privacy of therapeutic divulgences has been more generally recognized. No longer is patients' confidentiality dependent solely on the ethical posture of the practitioner. State statutes and regulations prescribe the manner and circumstances in which patients may give consent to the release of their records or in which disclosure may take place without their consent. Most states have testimonial privilege statutes, of varying degrees of porosity, that allow patients to prevent therapists from offering testimony in court based on information given in confidence (5). In general, these laws have the effect of granting patients greater control over when and if disclosure occurs, with the exceptions to be discussed below.

Should breach of confidentiality occur despite these protections, legal recourse is available to the patient. Psychiatrists have been found liable for unconsented and unwarranted disclosure on a number of theories, including invasion of privacy, breach of implied contract, breach of fiduciary duty (the obligation to place the patient's interests above all), and failure to abide by professional standards (6). The holdings of these cases would likely apply to non-physician therapists as well. One recent case expanded the scope of liability to include both therapists who revealed information and those third parties who requested it, knowing of its confidential nature (7).

Yet, retrospective remedies such as these have provided relatively weak protection for patients' confidentiality. Litigation on the matter is uncommon for several reasons. Harms may be difficult to prove and to monetarize. Once compromising information is revealed, and the damage done, there may be little incentive for injured patients to take further action. And, of course, there is something inherently paradoxical about a remedy for breach of confidentiality that inevitably involves further public disclosure of the embarrassing material.

Thus, effective protection of patients' confidences rests, in the end, on the conceptualization of confidentiality as a matter of professional ethics, rather than an externally imposed duty. Clinicians' responsibilities also become clearer when confidentiality is linked to the professional responsibility to place patients' interests above one's own. Without patients' consent, patients' confidences should not be revealed unless the strong and urgent interests of the patient or significant danger to third parties requires otherwise.

Limitations on Confidentiality

The desire to uphold patients' confidentiality may sometimes conflict with other values, including the broader interests of patients and of society at large. These conflicts are examples of the struggle over decision-making power that characterizes mental health law. Courts and legislatures have defined four occasions in which countervailing interests overcome patients' rights to control the privacy of their communications: (*a*) emergencies, (*b*) when third parties are endangered, (*c*) when mandatory reporting laws exist, and (*d*) when the needs of third-party payers require disclosure.

Emergencies may necessitate sacrifice of confidentiality, even over patients' objections, when the patient's health or safety is threatened. When in clinicians' judgment additional information (e.g., whether there is a history of previous suicide attempts) is essential to the proper evaluation of a patient in an emergency setting, clinicians can seek those data, even if that will require disclosing some otherwise confidential information (e.g., that the patient is now in a psychiatric emergency room) in the process. Obviously, only the minimum amount of information necessary to obtain the relevant data should be revealed. Clinicians on the receiving end of such requests must recognize their obligation to provide the required information, despite the absence of patient consent. Similarly, when patients are transferred to the care of others, whether for hospitalization or further crisis care, good clinical practice demands that the transferring clinician provide the receiving facility with data pertinent to the circumstances of the transfer and the initiation of treatment.

Although the law sanctions in emergencies the surrender of patients' usual control over material they have revealed, the desire to sustain a therapeutic relationship despite this violation of autonomy demands that this power be assumed responsibly. Patients should be informed of clinicians' reasons for not respecting their wishes, and in particular that clinicians believe strongly that they are acting in patients' best interests. Patients may disagree with the action taken, but it is hoped that they will thereby recognize the essentially benevolent motivations of the clinician.

A more controversial exception to the ordinary requirements of confidentiality grows out of the landmark decision in *Tarasoff v. Regents of the University of California* (8). There the Supreme Court of California held that therapists who know or should know that their patients represent threats to third parties have a duty to take whatever steps are reasonably necessary to protect those parties from harm. Appellate courts in nearly half the states have considered *Tarasoff*-like cases, in general endorsing the duty to protect (9). Given the widespread acceptance of the doctrine, most authorities agree that therapists in all states are best advised to behave as if *Tarasoff* represented the law in their jurisdictions.

The furor over *Tarasoff*—based on the beliefs of mental health professionals that the duty is beyond their power to fulfill and that the threat of breaching confidentiality will keep patients with violent impulses from seeking therapy in the first place—has led to serious misunderstanding of the nature of the duty to protect enunciated in the case (10). The *Tarasoff* obligation is best understood as requiring a four-step process: gathering sufficient data to evaluate the patient's dangerousness, making a determination of likely dangerousness based on those data, selecting a course of action designed to protect the potential victim, and implementing that action appropriately (11).

Given the confusion over these obligations, it is equally important to recognize what *Tarasoff* does not require. Clinicians need take measures to protect potential victims only when they truly believe the threat is real. When patients report violent impulses or make overt threats, the clinician is obligated to conduct a careful assessment of the level of risk. The expression of aggressive thoughts occurs in a wide variety of clinical contexts, often divorced from any real intent of causing harm. Even if a conclusion is reached that a substantial risk of violence is present, confidentiality need not be breached. Any action that is likely to be reasonably protective of victims can constitute an appropriate response. Clinical maneuvers such as exploring the impulses, increasing the frequency of sessions, or adjusting medications may be sufficient to alleviate the threat. Potential victims, if intimates, as so many are, can be invited to join the therapy. Voluntary or involuntary hospitalization can be initiated. If breach of confidentiality is required for effective protection, it may be limited to family members who can be relied on to see that the patient neither has access to weapons nor comes into proximity with the potential victim. In some cases, however, these measures will be unavailing and notification of the victim and/or the police will be required.

Breach of confidentiality, though, does not necessarily imply an abandonment of a willingness to negotiate with the patient. Patients may have preferences as to which course of action (e.g., warning the victim versus hospitalization) is taken. When asked, they may be willing to talk directly with the object of their threats under the therapist's supervision or otherwise to aid the clinician in issuing a warning. Evidence suggests that patients are understanding of clinicians' obligations to protect third parties, and that chances for rupture of the therapeutic alliance are minimized when patients are involved in the process (12). Patients who participate in issuing warnings may thereby be encouraged to express anger verbally rather than acting on it. Even without their active participation, patients may benefit from observing clinicians' warnings, since opportunities for subsequent distortion are lessened, and patients may bring their reactions into the therapy for further exploration.

Mental health professionals' right to override patients' desires for confidentiality stems from the superior obligation to protect others in society. Such obligations are not new; physicians, for example, have long been required to report communicable diseases, regardless of patients' wishes. Codes of professional ethics have recognized this obligation (13). Further, to the extent that a violent act is prevented by the clinician's response to a threat, the patient benefits as well. It is clearly not in a patient's interest to commit a violent crime for which imprisonment is the likely consequence. Although the duty to protect is problematic in many ways and might well be recast in a form more in keeping with the limitations on clinicians' abilities to predict and prevent violence, (14) at its core it is morally sound and represents a permanent addition to clinicians' legal responsibilities.

The duty to protect might be thought of as a variant on other mandatory reporting obligations. Legislation has been enacted in every state requiring the reporting of suspected child abuse or neglect (15). Similar statutes in a growing number of jurisdictions mandate reporting of "elder abuse" (16). Again, clinicians are often concerned that reporting may rupture a fragile therapeutic relationship, particularly when a patient or family is new to therapy. The ambiguity of some statutes offers flexibility in regard to reporting cases in which the victim of abuse has not been seen by the clinician or when abuse occurred in the past and is unlikely to recur; other statutes, however, are more rigid in their demands. As in the situation of the duty to protect, sharing the dilemma with the patient is often useful. But the ultimate determination has been made by society: the protection of vulnerable persons must take precedence even over valid therapeutic concerns.

Mandatory reporting, however, does not extend in general to situations in which therapists become aware that patients have committed crimes in the past, unless those acts relate to the likelihood of future violent behavior (17). In almost every jurisdiction the idea has been rejected that previous crimes must be reported. Therapists who actively aid their patients in avoiding apprehension, however, may face legal consequences, but in almost every jurisdiction the idea has been rejected that previous crimes must be reported.

The final exception to confidentiality requirements involves transmittal of information to those third parties who pay for patients' care. In the present economic climate, with great emphasis placed on cost containment, patients are asked routinely to sign waivers allowing insurers access to information about their treatment. Although release of this information is technically not a breach of confidentiality, since consent is obtained, patients are often oblivious to the implications of the forms they sign. Information about their treatment may make its way back to their employers, particularly when claims are processed "in house," as many are these days in an effort to cut costs. Therapists should take the lead in discussing these issues with patients, since some patients may prefer to pay for treatment themselves rather than risk dissemination of the fact that they are seeking psychiatric care. Tighter concurrent review of longer term therapy has led to demands for increasing amounts of information to be released to insurers or their professional reviewers. Some consultation with the patient about the implications of responding to these requests is often indicated, allowing the patient to decide whether the benefit of continued coverage is worth the risk that their problems may become more widely known. Efforts to control fraud, particularly in public programs such as Medicaid, have resulted in subpoenas of therapists' records themselves, with the complete breach of confidentiality that implies. Courts have split on whether investigators may have access to such data in the absence of a particularized showing of its relevance to the inquiry at hand (18). But the risk is omnipresent.

LEGAL ISSUES AT THE STAGE OF DECISION MAKING AND TREATMENT PLANNING

Principles of Involuntary Commitment

The most crucial determination made by the outpatient clinician involves whether or not the patient's hospitalization is warranted. If so, and the negotiation process results in agreement on this course, state statutes governing voluntary hospitalization come into play. Psychiatrists (and in some states now, psychologists) who authorize patients' admission may be required to inform the patient of certain rights, and perhaps even to ascertain whether the patient is competent to consent to voluntary admission. But the process, consensual at its core, is relatively unproblematic.

Difficulties arise when negotiation fails. Unlike the situation that usually obtains in general medical settings, psychiatrists are endowed with the authority of the state to initiate proceedings aimed at the patient's involuntary detention. This nearly unique power (similar statutes have existed at one time or another for detention of patients with communicable diseases, including tuberculosis and leprosy) has existed since the first public institutions for the treatment of the insane were created in the 19th century. The overt premise for the exercise of this power was benevolent and unabashedly paternalistic: it was believed that the mentally ill would benefit from hospitalization and were unable to make reasonable decisions to seek their own care. Critics, however, have charged that the real goal was the containment of deviance in an increasingly disordered society (19).

The standards and procedures by which the power of involuntary commitment can be exercised have varied over time (20). The most recent cycle began in the late 1960s with the rejection of then-prevalent statutes based on vague criteria allowing hospitalization of all patients who "need treatment," with procedures largely in the hands of physicians. Civil libertarians challenged the historic basis for these laws, claiming that unbridled paternalistic intervention violated patients' liberty interests guaranteed by the constitution (21). The willingness of the courts to accept this argument was undoubtedly influenced by their recognition that many large state institutions merely warehoused patients with little or no treatment, often in shocking conditions. At the same time these issues were being pressed in the courts, widespread use of phenothiazines—the first really effective treatment for psychotic symptoms—was beginning, and the community psychiatry movement, with its emphasis on keeping people out of hospitals, was at its height.

The convergence of these influences led to substantial revision of the nation's civil commitment laws. New statutes were enacted in almost every state rejecting the idea that all patients who needed hospitalization could be admitted against their will. State intervention was seen as properly extending only to situations in which mentally ill persons posed a danger to others, or posed so serious a danger to themselves that their very existence was endangered. In a period of roughly a decade, nearly every state changed its statute to conform with this approach (22). At the same time, the procedures for commitment were tightened, with many new requirements drawn from the criminal justice model.

Although this is the situation that exists today, it is unlikely that the oscillations that have characterized commitment law will cease. Already dissatisfactions with the current system are being voiced; many relate to the difficulty of admitting patients who seem clearly in need of treatment but fail to meet narrow, dangerousness-oriented criteria. Equally significant has been the recognition of the limitations of pharmacotherapy and community care in the treatment of chronic mental conditions. Hospitalization is being acknowledged as essential for some patients, and less stringent commitment statutes are seen as vital to accomplishing that end. In response, some states have relaxed rigid procedures, while others have actually moved back to some modification of need-for-treatment criteria, usually emphasizing the likelihood of patient deterioration (22a). The American Psychiatric Association has published an influential Model Law on Civil Commitment, (23) which has served as a model for such changes.

Another proposed change that has attracted a good deal of interest involves the creation of new systems for outpatient commitment (24). Clinicians have grown impatient with a system in which patients cannot be compelled to receive care, particularly medications, until they have deteriorated to the point of dangerousness to themselves or others. The large number of "revolving-door" patients who are repeatedly hospitalized, only to stop their medications and deteriorate again soon after discharge, have stimulated suggestions for an alternative. Simultaneously, legal advocates, concerned that patients not be subjected to more restrictive conditions than necessary, have argued that some committed inpatients could be adequately treated as outpatient committees.

Two obstacles must be overcome before outpatient commitment can succeed. First, some consensus must be achieved on which patient group is really the focus of the procedure. Clinicians see outpatient commitment as a means of extending paternalistic control over a group of patients now outside their jurisdiction. Civil libertarians view it as a means of limiting the loss of liberty of patients now currently susceptible to inpatient commitment. Eligibility for outpatient commitment will vary markedly depending on whether statutes are written with one or the other group in mind; to a large extent the objectives appear to be mutually incompatible. Some states have resolved this issue in favor of committing frequent recidivists (25).

Second, effective means of enforcing outpatient commitment must be developed. Current statutes generally provide no sanctions for violations of the terms of commitment. This makes clinicians, who are at risk for being held responsible for untoward events, leery of attesting to a patient's incapacities and then requesting an intervention that does not permit effective control. To date, this problem has resisted resolution.

Responding to the Mandate of Involuntary Commitment

Many psychiatrists and psychologists are profoundly uncomfortable with the degree of coercive power afforded them by the civil commitment statutes; they shun situations in which such power might need to be exercised. The majority of clinicians recognize the problems attached to the involuntary hospitalization process, but believe strongly in the importance of intervening in the lives of mentally ill persons who by virtue of their illnesses cannot decide to accept care. They strive to find ways of accommodating civil commitment to a treatment process that evolved in an ethic of voluntary participation by patients.

In that regard, it must be recognized that the existence of the power to detain patients against their will does not imply that the process of negotiation between patient and therapist is moot. Commitment statutes are permissive, not mandatory—that is, they allow clinicians to initiate the commitment process in appropriate cases, but do not compel them to do so. A clinician who is persuaded of a patient's need for hospital care should (and in some states must) begin by attempting to elicit the patient's voluntary agreement to hospitalization. If the patient refuses, patient and therapist still retain the option of negotiating alternative interventions that might avoid commitment. For example, the patient might agree to accept depot medications or to come regularly as an outpatient for evaluation in place of hospitalization. It would be pretense to assert that this negotiation process is not affected by the clinician's power to effect hospitalization unilaterally. But the patient can still be afforded some measure of autonomy in choosing among courses of action.

As in any other circumstances where therapists exercise the power of decision on patients' behalf, attention to the long-term impact on the therapeutic alliance is required. Most severely ill patients manifest some degree of ambivalence about their need for care. Rarely does even the patient with the highest degree of denial not show some glimmer of recognition that a problem exists. The committing clinician must, in explaining the basis for commitment, appeal to that component of the patient's psyche that recognizes a need for care, with the hope that over time it will become dominant. Even when the process of negotiation is being short-circuited in the short run, efforts should be made to ensure that the chances are maximized for a long-term solution acceptable to both patient and therapist.

No less daunting is the task of determining when involuntary hospitalization is warranted. Almost all current statutes rely on clinical predictions of patients' future dangerousness to themselves or others. Sometimes these standards are modified by specification of the kind of evidence that can be considered by clinicians in making those judgments, e.g., overt acts of violence or self-destruction, threats of harm, reported fears of third parties. Yet, attempts such as these to structure clinicians' decision making run afoul of the very real limitations on clinicians' predictive abilities.

Predictions of dangerousness can be made in one of two ways: based on clinical judgment or on actuarial data. Studies of predictions of long-term dangerousness to others, though flawed methodologically, are unanimous in demonstrating that the rate of false-positive predictions exceeds that of true positives (26). In other words, when psychiatrists predicted that someone would commit a violent act if released, they were more likely to be wrong than right by a ratio of at least 2:1, and usually 4:1 or 5:1. Since these studies were based on clinical judgment, which was generally unstructured, efforts were directed toward seeing if predictions based on actuarial data—with all likely predictors factored into a regression equation—could do better. In fact, they did worse. Actuarial studies of the prediction of danger to self by suicide have shown similar results (27).

Clinicians faced with these data may be tempted to throw up their hands in despair. Since all states require that dangerousness be demonstrated at least by "clear and convincing evidence" and some states require proof "beyond a reasonable doubt," it might seem as though those standards could never be met. In fact, the

situation may not be quite so bleak. Experts have suggested that short-term prediction, which is more difficult to test empirically, may be more accurate than predictions of events in the distant future (28). In addition, the courts, whether rightly or wrongly, tend to take a commonsense approach to mental health professionals' testimony, rather than holding it to burdens of proof that are impossible to meet.

Clinicians can meet their obligations by relying on a system of prediction based on the best available data, considered in the context of a consistent and reasonably supportable theoretical framework. For danger to others, Monahan's classic study has identified a small set of factors that consistently correlate with violent behavior: a past history of violence, male gender, age in late teens and early 20s, black race, lower social class, history of opiate or alcohol abuse, low IQ, and residential and employment instability (26). These factors, however, are just a starting point, designed to enrich the base rate of violent behavior in the population about which more individualized predictions of violence will be made. Empirical data provide little assistance past this point, forcing clinicians to rely on a theoretical framework. This may come from theories that relate violence to social learning (29), frustration (30), or biologic factors (31), or from eclectic principles drawn from clinical experience (3, 26). The latter look generally toward the balance of factors promoting and reducing the risk of violent behavior, and have the additional virtue of pointing toward likely areas in which intervention might decrease the risk of violence.

Prediction related to other categories of behavior that permit involuntary commitment is equally problematic. Tests of actuarial prediction of suicidality have produced results of extremely low validity (27). Clinical predictions remain largely untested, primarily because of the ethical difficulty of allowing patients thought to be suicidal to go without intervention to test the accuracy of the prognostications. Existing empirical data point to depression and alcoholism as the major predisposing factors (32). Theories relate the predisposition to suicide to past and recent losses and particular character structures (33). It is of interest that prediction of suicide has received less attention until recently than prediction of violence toward others, perhaps because of the greater emotionality of the latter issue.

Even the third common ground for involuntary commitment—inability to care for one's basic needs (sometimes referred to as grave disability)—presents predictive problems. Although one might think that assessment of day-to-day functional capability would be more within the realm of mental health professionals, and therefore easier for them to predict, this too has been called into question (34). Commentators have pointed to the disjunction between symptomatology, on which clinicians usually focus, and functional ability. They encourage the use of structured evaluative techniques that focus on the latter (34). A number of such scales exist, and preliminary evidence suggests that they may indeed be useful for the purpose (35).

In sum, involuntary commitment is not a proceeding to be undertaken lightly. Careful attention needs to be paid both to the effects on the therapeutic relationship, and to systematic means of making the assessments required by the law.

LEGAL ISSUES AT THE STAGE OF TREATMENT

The Doctrine of Informed Consent

When the formulation of a treatment plan results in a recommendation for outpatient rather than inpatient treatment, as will usually be the case, the clinician faces the task of engaging the patient in treatment. The legal parameters of this delicate process have been defined by the doctrine of informed consent. The law of informed consent is often confusing to clinicians, who tend to view it as a legal intrusion on the clinical process, and reduce it to a meaningless, mechanistic ritual of form

signing. The idea of informed consent, however, is thoroughly consonant with our understanding of negotiation as the basis of doctor–patient interactions. If approached in this light, as a clinical tool, rather than a legal nuisance, informed consent can have powerful therapeutic influences of its own (36).

The underlying rationale of informed consent is that patients should have the right to participate actively in making decisions about their medical and psychiatric care. In ethical terms, this can be justified deontologically—that is, as a good in its own right—or consequentially—that is, because of the benefits derived from this approach. Among those benefits are a greater willingness by patients to cooperate with care that they have played an active role in selecting, and a greater likelihood that the treatment chosen will address patients' real concerns.

Historically, patients' right to participate in decision making was limited to the power to give or withhold consent to proposed treatment. To exercise this power they needed to be legally competent, and they had the right to decide without coercion. The Anglo-American common-law tradition held that any unauthorized touching, even when conducted with therapeutic intent, constituted a battery for which the perpetrator might be subject to criminal and civil penalties. But the giving or withholding of consent differs from actually working with the physician to select among therapeutic options. Under this historic approach, which can be characterized as a system of "simple consent," the patient had no right other than to hear a physician's recommendation of a proposed treatment and to "take it or leave it."

This approach began to change in the 1950s, as courts recognized that a serious commitment to patient participation in decision making could only come about if the nature of the doctor–patient interaction was altered. With alternative forms of treatment multiplying, many of them offering contrasting sets of benefits and risks, it seemed obvious to the courts that patients' interests could no longer be satisfied simply by the opportunity to accept or (rarely) reject the option selected by the physician. Rather, patients must be able to work with their physicians to select among available options, thus assuring that their peculiar needs, interests, and willingness to undergo risks would be reflected in the final decision (37).

Clearly, to accomplish this end, simple consent was insufficient. Patients needed to know more than just which procedure their physician was recommending. They needed, the courts agreed, information about the nature and purpose of the proposed treatment, its risks and benefits, and the availability of alternative treatments and their risks and benefits. Only then would their decision truly reflect their needs and values and thus be a genuine "informed consent." If this information were not supplied and an undisclosed risk materialized, patients who were able to prove that they would have foregone the treatment had they known of the risk would be able to collect monetary damages from the errant physician (Although almost all informed consent cases to date have involved physicians as primary caregivers, the principles of the doctrine apply to other disciplines that assume primary responsibility for patient care.)

Stating the requirement in this way belies the actual complexity of the doctrine. The inevitable question that follows a statement of the information that must be disclosed is, How much about each category must patients be told? Jurisdictions have varied in their responses. The largest number require clinicians to divulge that information that a reasonable practitioner would disclose; others look to the information that a reasonable patient would want to know; while a small number ask for disclosure of the data that *this* patient wants to know (38). In practical terms, when prescribing medication, regardless of the operative standard in a state, psychiatrists are on safest ground disclosing the most common risks (e.g., dry mouth and orthostatic hypotension with tricyclic antidepressants) and the most serious, as long as they are not generally considered to be rare

(e.g., one might disclose the risk of agranulocytosis with carbamazepine, but not with phenothiazines).

Several exceptions exist to the requirements to disclose information and to obtain consent (39). In *emergencies*, when the delay attendant on discussion of treatment options may result in harm to patients, the requirements of informed consent are suspended. The law is willing to presume that a reasonable person would consent in such circumstances. The doctrine of *therapeutic privilege* may be invoked if disclosure itself might cause harm to the patient; treatment can then proceed with only simple consent or perhaps even the substituted consent of a family member. It is important to note that therapeutic privilege does not justify withholding information simply because knowledge of risks might lead the patient to refuse treatment. That right of refusal, after all, is inherent in the idea of informed consent. Patients who so desire can invoke a *waiver* of their rights to disclosure and consent if they desire not to know of risks and options or to let the caregiver make the decision for them. When the patient is *incompetent*, as will be discussed further below, disclosure need not be made (although there may be some therapeutic benefit from doing so anyway) and the patient cannot give legally valid consent. In such circumstances, informed consent must be obtained from a substitute decisionmaker. Finally, involuntarily *committed patients* have historically been seen to represent a group exempted from the requirements of informed consent. This exemption is now being challenged by the movement to guarantee this group the right to refuse treatment. Given the complexity of the issue, and the current uncertain status of the right, the discussion that follows will focus exclusively on noncommitted patients.

In light of the tremendous emphasis placed by the courts on provision of information, two additional requirements that date from the doctrine of simple consent should not be neglected. First, the decision offered must be a voluntary one. This requirement is largely undeveloped in the civil law, in part because of its complexity and subtlety. Gross coercion, though easily identified, is rare. Certain patients, however, may be particularly vulnerable to less overt pressures. Very passive or dependent patients, for example, may feel obligated to accept treatment strongly urged by a therapist that they might otherwise refuse. The clinician, who has the responsibility of encouraging compliance with treatment that will be in the patient's best interests, must distinguish between legitimate exhortation in the negotiation process and illegitimate coercion. The latter is present when there is an overt or implied punishment for failure to comply.

The second requirement that must not be ignored is that the patient be competent to make the treatment decision. Psychiatric patients in particular may face problems in this area, given the wide variety of emotional and cognitive deficits they manifest. Unfortunately, little legal guidance has been available to clinicians who must screen for incompetence and decide if further action is required. Legal definitions tend to be vague or circular. In the absence of a legal standard to rely on, clinicians have formulated a variety of approaches toward structuring their evaluations. One commonly accepted model synthesizes suggested standards into a rough hierarchy that is useful for conceptual purposes. In increasing order of stringency, the evaluator can ask whether the patient can (*a*) evidence a choice concerning treatment, (*b*) achieve a factual understanding of the issues at hand, (*c*) rationally manipulate the information provided to him or her, and (*d*) appreciate the nature of the situation and the consequences of the decision (40). Failure on any of these standards may warrant a judicial determination of competence, with appointment of a substitute decision maker.

Informed Consent in Practice

For informed consent to be integrated into the process of negotiating treatment, it must be approached on an individualized basis. The process of providing information to the patient over time offers an opportunity to monitor the patient's responses and address concerns (36). As options are discussed and questions answered, the patient's understanding of the nature of the treatment and likely outcomes can be assessed. Just as in any other therapeutic encounter, distortions can be corrected and characterologically based responses clarified. A dependent patient, for example, whose therapy is based on encouraging her to take responsibility for her own decisions, can be helped to see that a waiver of her right to disclosure and consent—with its consequent reliance on the clinician—is another example of the pattern she is trying to break. In this manner, informed consent is part of and advances the therapy.

Whether because of their discomfort with discussing options with patients or simply lack of training in undertaking that task, many therapists employ quite a different model of informed consent. They see the consent interaction as an event, rather than as a process, focused on the signing of consent forms. The use of forms tend to restrict therapist–patient interaction, in that the form takes the place of an open interchange with its attendant monitoring of the patient's response. Merely presenting the patient with a consent form resembles more simple consent—with patients having only the option to accept or reject the proffered treatment—than it does informed consent—in which patients participate in the selection of treatment. Evidence suggests that forms are less effective than oral discussion in communicating information to psychiatric patients (41).

Forms also convey the message that once signed, informed consent has been completed and the negotiation process is over. In fact, variations in patients' conditions and responses to treatment, as well as their evolving attitudes toward the goals of treatment, make continued negotiation essential. The clinician needs to monitor patients' understanding and goals throughout treatment and respond accordingly. Needless to say, informed consent forms also have the drawback of being almost incomprehensible to most patients. They tend to be written in complex language, full of legal boilerplate and medical jargon (42).

Proponents of the use of consent forms argue that they immunize clinicians against lawsuits for failure to obtain consent. This is not necessarily the case. Consent forms may merely serve as evidence that certain crucial data were not disclosed to the patient or that information was provided in an unintelligible manner. Although their use may be acceptable if they are clearly limited to a subordinate role as documentation of a verbal interaction—rather than as a replacement for one—there is a preferable approach. Clinicians can write brief notes in patients' charts at the time of consent, briefly outlining the scope of disclosure and the patient's response. This approach is facilitated by the development of a standard "core disclosure" for each class of medications, to which particular elements can be added depending on patients' individual needs. The note need only indicate that the core disclosure, which the clinician should be able to describe in detail if need be, took place with modifications as noted. This may be just as protective in court (suits for lack of informed consent are exceedingly rare) and is much more in keeping with the interactive focus of the clinician–patient relationship.

A particular issue that concerns psychiatrists is the discussion of the risk of tardive dyskinesia (TD) when antipsychotic medication is prescribed. Many fear that disclosure of the risk of TD will lead patients, particularly those who are acutely ill, to refuse treatment to their detriment. Some psychiatrists have suggested, at the least, postponing the discussion of TD for several months, until the acute episode has resolved. This is justified on the basis that TD is unlikely to occur in the first few months of treatment and that the patient will be better able to understand the information after some clinical improvement has taken place (43). Others are reluctant to discuss the risk of TD even at that point,

for fear that a stabilized patient will go off the medication and relapse.

It is being increasingly recognized that this approach is not in keeping with the requirement to obtain patients' informed consent to treatment (44). The fear that patients will elect to refuse or discontinue medication if made aware of potential side-effects is not a justification for failure to inform; in fact, it is just such a choice that is protected by the doctrine of informed consent. If patients are incompetent to process the information, some form of substituted consent must take place. Otherwise, TD must be discussed. The level of the discussion, of course, can be adjusted to patients' ability to deal with the data. This may mean providing limited information about the nature of the risk early in treatment, with further elaboration as the patient is able to handle it. Even if some patients chose to discontinue their medication as a result of disclosure, society has elected to pay this price to protect the right of most patients to play a role in choosing their treatment.

A final practical issue related to informed consent deals with incompetent patients. These patients, as noted above, are not able to give legally binding consent and in theory should undergo formal adjudication of incompetence and have a substitute decision maker appointed by the courts. In some jurisdictions, under pressure from court decisions, this is increasingly taking place (45). Judges may appoint guardians to decide about psychiatric treatment (46) or, viewing neuroleptic medications as an extraordinary treatment beyond the power of guardians to approve (47), may reserve the decision to themselves.

In many jurisdictions, however, this procedure is rarely implemented. Initiating judicial competence determinations usually requires legal assistance, for which funding may not be available, and often rests on the presence of a person willing to serve as guardian, who may not exist. When recourse to the courts is unavailable, facilities dealing with large numbers of seemingly incompetent patients may, with the advice of counsel, elect to pursue other means of protecting their patients' interests. These may include obtaining second opinions about the use of medication or appointing informal "guardians" to look after patients' interests. Clinicians should not have to prescribe medication for incompetent patients without some such supports, which simultaneously protect patients' rights and minimize the risk of caregivers being accused of acting improperly.

MALPRACTICE AND OTHER FORMS OF LIABILITY

Concern about the possibility of suit for malpractice suffuses all stages of the therapist–patient relationship. Such a suit represents the ultimate breakdown of a relationship built on negotiation, involving as it does recourse to a third party—the court system—to obtain satisfaction that was not forthcoming within the relationship itself. With the media filled with stories of a "malpractice crisis," it is little wonder that clinicians manifest the level of concern they do about the chances of being sued. Nonetheless, some assurance can be provided at two levels: (*a*) Despite escalating numbers of malpractice suits, psychiatrists continue to be sued less frequently than any other medical specialty group, and suits against nonmedical therapists are even rarer; (48) and (*b*) some measure of protection against successful suits can be afforded by relatively simple measures.

The Legal Framework for Clinician Liability

Malpractice law must be understood within the context of the larger system for adjudicating disputes over civil wrongs— the tort system. A tort is an injury inflicted by one person on the body, property, or other interests of a second person (excepting breach of contract). Torts come in two broad categories, intentional and negligent, reflecting the degree of purposefulness behind the infliction of the injury. Malpractice is a negligent tort, one peculiar to professions with defined standards of conduct. But clinicians may commit intentional torts, too, including defamation, wrongful imprisonment, and battery.

The evolution of tort law has been guided by two major goals: deterrence of injury-causing behavior and compensation of victims (49). Deterrence is a straightforward goal in the case of intentional torts. As clearly volitional acts, they ought readily to be deterrable, assuming a sufficient level of sanction is applied. Punitive damages may therefore be recoverable by injured parties, above and beyond damages awarded for actual injuries. Given their morally reprehensible nature, intentional torts need not result in the infliction of actual physical or monetary harm to be compensible. For example, patients who receive electroconvulsive therapy without giving consent—thus becoming victims of a battery—may recover damages for dignitary harms even if benefited by the procedure. Deterrence is also a concern in negligent torts, the assumption being that, even though nonpurposeful, the behavior that resulted in harm could be prevented by sufficient attention and care.

Compensation of those injured by no fault of their own is the second major goal of the tort system. In most cases, the goal of compensation is circumscribed by the ability of victims to demonstrate that their injuries resulted from negligence or an intention to harm. The desire to afford compensation is limited by the need to identify and punish a wrongdoer. That need not be the case, of course, as some countries have created "no-fault" insurance systems in which all injuries are compensated, even those that result from "chance." Another means of achieving the same end is through the device of strict liability, in which the actor is held responsible for any harms causally linked to his or her behavior, regardless of intent or negligence. The theory of strict liability embraces insurance principles. Placing the cost of injuries on the actor—whether manufacturer, distributor, etc.—allows that party to pass on the costs of accidents to all persons who benefit from a particular activity, and to prevent ruinous losses by buying insurance for the purpose.

Strict liability per se does not apply to malpractice or other types of liability usually associated with mental health practice. These principles, however, have so suffused legal thought that they seem almost omnipresent in the courtroom. Juries are understandably sympathetic when faced with a demonstrably injured plaintiff. Rather than letting the victim bear the burden, the temptation is strong to gloss over relatively poor evidence of malpractice or tenuous causal links between the clinician's behavior and the injury, and to let the "deep pockets" of the insurance company bear the cost. Such reasoning on the part of juries and judges accounts for the inflation in the size of awards and some of the more questionable judgments.

Malpractice is the most common form of liability faced by clinicians. It rests on four principles: (*a*) the existence of a duty, (*b*) breach of that duty, (*c*) injuries suffered by the patient, and (*d*) a causal link between the breach and the injuries. A *duty* exists between clinician and patient when the clinician responds to the patient's request for help (or to the request of someone on the patient's behalf) with an indication that he or she will provide care. This is frequently an explicit agreement, but it need not be. A clinician working in an emergency room has an implicit responsibility to care for any patient who arrives, although not necessarily to offer ongoing treatment. Rather, as in an office or clinic setting where an agreement to evaluate the patient has been reached, the clinician is required only to assess the patient with sufficient care to enable an appropriate disposition to be made. That usually means ruling out the presence of a condition requiring emergency intervention and providing an appropriate referral. Ideally, the clinician should verify the willingness of the practitioner or facility to which the patient is referred to accept the patient. Failure to provide an appropriate referral may lead to charges of abandonment.

When a duty to care for a patient exists, its *breach* consists in a failure to live up to the standards of practice of the profession. Those standards are measured these days according the performance of a reasonabler practitioner under similar circumstances. In general, the reasonableness standards are drawn from a national reference group. The old "locality rule," in which defendant physicians were judged according to practice in their locale, has given way in the face of rapid dissemination of information in the profession to national standards of care. The patient plaintiff must suffer actual physical or emotional harm before a suit can be brought. Practices that constitute a breach of the standard of care, but from which the patient emerges unscathed, are not a basis for suit in malpractice.

Finally, for patients to prove that malpractice occurred they must demonstrate that the act or omission alleged to be negligent caused the injury. Proof of "proximate cause" does not always resemble scientific notions of proof. Juries, for example, must decide only whether it was more probable than not that the causal link existed. In the absence of data linking two phenomena, it is not uncommon for the jury to decide on its own that a causal relationship existed (50).

Two legal devices aid plaintiffs in establishing causal links between clinicians' behavior and the injury complained of. The first, the doctrine of "res ipsa loquitur," literally "the thing speaks for itself," applies when the instrument causing the harm was entirely under the control of the defendant and harm would not ordinarily result in the absence of negligence. For example, a patient who finds himself suffering a fractured vertebra after electroconvulsive therapy would, if he were successful in involving this doctrine, need to prove only that the injury did not exist prior to the treatment. The burden of proving nonnegligent care, often a difficult one, then falls on the psychiatrist. "Respondeat superior"—"let the master answer"— places responsibility on the physician for the misdeeds of those under his or her supervision. A clinician may thereby be vulnerable to suits arising from the acts of other mental health professionals, including students. In these times of increasing cost consciousness, when practitioners often find themselves supervising less well-trained clinicians, perhaps even by telephone, this is an important consideration. Therapists should accept these sorts of positions only when they can assure themselves of their ability to provide adequate supervision to those clinicians for whose patients they are ultimately responsible.

This discussion has focused on malpractice because it is the most common form of liability to which clinicians are subject. Allegations of intentional tort, however, are not uncommon. And the boundaries between the two categories are less clear than might be imagined. Sexual relations between therapists and patients, a growing source of litigation, were originally considered negligent torts and pursued as examples of malpractice. Increasingly, it is being recognized that this behavior is deliberate on the part of therapists, not merely negligent, and therefore ought to be dealt with as an intentional tort. This change has been supported by a professional consensus that having sex with one's patients, given the discrepancies in power and status and patients' emotional vulnerability, represents a gross breach of trust in a therapist–patient relationship and thus is always unacceptable. Ironically, since intentional torts are not usually covered by malpractice policies (though some have special riders covering allegations of undue familiarity with patients), so labeling this behavior may preclude injured patients from having access to the pool of insurance dollars for compensation.

Living with the Risk of Liability

Regardless of whether the many reforms to the tort system now being proposed are adopted, clinicians will continue to live in an environment in which the possibility of being sued is omnipresent. Although suits can be a highly traumatic experience for the clinician (51), they remain relatively rare. Fear of being sued probably has a more profound—and deleterious—effect on mental health care than the suits themselves. There is no set of practices that will guarantee immunity from suit, even from successful judgments. But several guidelines may provide reassurance and reduce the overall risk.

It is an axiom among malpractice attorneys that clinicians who maintain good relationships with their patients do not get sued, even in the face of unfortunate outcomes (52). Thus, the best preventive approach may be to adhere to a model of respect and concern for patients exemplified by the negotiated approach to patienthood and codified by the doctrine of informed consent. Defensive psychiatry, in so far as it involves creating an adversarial relationship between clinician and patient, is likely to lead to more suits rather than fewer. Among the reasons that psychiatrists are sued less than other medical specialists may be the stress that traditionally has been placed on the relationship with the patient, particularly in outpatient practice.

A corollary to this axiom is that when the practitioner is uncertain what to do in a particular situation—to release information or not, to commit a patient or not, to order a laboratory test or not—the best course is that which is consonant with the patient's therapeutic interests. Even if it leads to a poor result, or may actually violate legal rules of which the clinician is unaware, acting in the patient's interests will almost always be taken as evidence of good faith on the therapist's part. Too many clinicians become needlessly paralyzed in the face of difficult decisions with potential legal ramifications, when a return to first clinical principles is really all that is necessary.

Two other general principles are of help, as well. When perplexed by a difficult decision, the clinician should seriously consider seeking consultation from a respected peer. Calling in a consultant provides powerful evidence that the clinician did not act mindlessly, impetuously, or arrogantly. Further it suggests that the clinician was concerned with discovering the standard of care before proceeding, since the opinion of a reasonable colleague is the best evidence the clinician can ascertain of what constitutes the standard of reasonable practice.

Second, thorough documentation is essential in preventing and defending malpractice cases. Absence of notation as to the reasons that particular actions were taken will encourage plaintiffs and their attorneys to initiate suits, and give scope to their experts to speculate on the therapist's motives. Once a suit reaches court, contemporaneous documentation can tip the balance in what otherwise is a "my word against his word" situation in which everyone's assertions are subject to the accusation of self-interest. Notations should never be changed or added in retrospect; no single act so completely destroys the clinician's credibility in court. If evidence is missing from a chart that would be helpful in explaining the decision making that led to a poor outcome, it should be added after the fact only if dated accurately and its retrospective nature clearly indicated.

Documentation practices are not always logical. Clinicians in an emergency room or clinic, for example, are typically more careful in recording assessments of admitted patients than of those released. Yet the risk of suit for improper decisions to admit or commit is much less than for the unfortunate consequences of failing to admit. Similarly, facilities often require residents or nonphysician clinicians to receive supervisory approval for admission decisions, but not for decisions to release the patient. These sorts of practices ought to be rationalized, with at least equal care given to release decisions.

CONCLUSION

The impact of law on mental health practice cannot be denied, but it need not be feared. Clinicians need to remain current with changes in the law the same way they update themselves on new therapies or new additions to the pharmacopeia. In this self-education effort, they should emphasize principles that can be generalized to new situations, rather than blind rules that make little sense outside of the situation in which they are first applied. Above all, legal regulation must be seen in the context of the clinician–patient relationship. Law often becomes relevant when negotiation fails. An emphasis on the negotiated approach to patienthood keeps the most important principles before both patient and clinician, relegating law to its important, but secondary, role.

References

1. National Institute of Mental Health: *Mental Health, United States 1985* (DHHS Publication No (ADM) 85-1378). Rockville, MD, National Institute of Mental Health, 1985.
2. Friedman LM: *Total Justice*. New York, Russell Sage Foundation, 1985.
3. Gutheil TG, Appelbaum PS: *Clinical Handbook of Psychiatry and the Law*. New York, McGraw-Hill, 1982.
4. Reiser SJ, Dyck, AJ, Curran WJ: *Ethics in Medicine: Historical Perspectives and Contemporary Concerns*. Cambridge, MA, MIT Press, 1977.
5. DeKraai MB, Sales BD: Confidential communications of psychotherapists. *Psychother* 21:293–318, 1984.
6. Annotation: Physician's tort liability, apart from defamation, for unauthorized disclosure of confidential information about patient. 20 ALR 3d 1109.
7. *Alberts v. Devine*, No. N-3624 (Mass. Sup. Jud. Ct., June 4, 1985).
8. *Tarasoff v. Regents of the University of California*, 131 Cal. Rptr. 14, 551, P.2d 334 (1976).
9. Beck JC (ed): *The Potentially Violent Patient and the Tarasoff Decision in Psychiatric Practice*. Washington, DC, American Psychiatric Press, 1985.
10. Givelber D, Bowers W, Blitch C: *Tarasoff*, myth and reality: an empirical study of private law in action. *Wisconsin Law Review* 1984:443–497.
11. Appelbaum PS: Tarasoff and the clinician: problems in fulfilling the duty to protect. *Am J Psychiatry* 145:425–429, 1985.
12. Beck JC: When the patient threatens violence: an empirical study of clinical practice after Tarasoff. *Bull Am Acad Psychiatry Law* 10:189–201, 1982.
13. American Psychiatric Association: *The Principles of Medical Ethics, with Annotations Especially Applicable to Psychiatry*. Washington, DC, American Psychiatric Association, 1981.
14. Appelbaum PS: Rethinking the duty to protect. In Beck J (ed): *The Potentially Violent Patient and the Tarasoff Decision in Psychiatric Practice*. Washington, DC, American Psychiatric Press, 1985.
15. Holder AR: *Legal Issues in Pediatrics and Adolescent Medicine*, ed 2. New Haven, Yale University Press, 1985.
16. Salend E, Kane RA, Satz M, et al: Elder abuse

reporting: limitations of statutes. *The Gerontologist* 24:61–69, 1984.

17. Appelbaum PS, Meisel A: Therapists' obligation to report their patients' criminal acts. *Bull Am Acad Psychiatry Law* 14:221–230, 1986.

18. Appelbaum PS: Confidentiality: winning one for a change. *Hosp Community Psychiatry* 37:334–335, 1986.

19. Rothman DJ: *The Discovery of the Asylum: Social Order and Disorder in the New Republic.* Boston, Little, Brown, 1971.

20. Appelbaum PS: Civil commitment. In Michels R, Cavenar JO, Brodie HKH (eds): *Psychiatry.* Philadelphia, J. B. Lippincott, 1985, vol 3, chap 32.

21. Appelbaum PS: Is the need for treatment constitutionally acceptable as a basis for civil commitment? *Law, Medicine, and Health Care* 12:144–149, 1984.

22. Brakel SJ, Parry J, Weiner BA: *The Mentally Disabled and the Law.* Chicago, American Bar Foundation, 1985.

22a. Hoge SK, Appelbaum PS, Geller JL: Involuntary treatment. In Frances A, Hales R (eds): *American Psychiatric Association Annual Review* (Volume 8). Washington, DC, American Psychiatric Press, in press.

23. Stromberg CD, Stone AA: A model state law on civil commitment of the mentally ill. *Harvard Journal on Legislation* 20:275–396, 1983.

24. Appelbaum PS: Outpatient commitment: the problems and the promise. *Am J Psychiatry* 143:1270–1272, 1986.

25. Keilitz I, Hall T: State statutes governing involuntary outpatient civil commitment. *Mental and Physical Disability Law Reporter* 9:378–379, 1985.

26. Monahan J: *The Clinical Prediction of Violent Behavior.* Rockville, MD, National Institute of Mental Health, 1981.

27. Roy A: Risk factors for suicide in psychiatric patients. *Arch Gen Psychiatry* 39:1089–1095, 1982.

28. Monahan J: Prediction research and the emergency commitment of dangerous mentally ill persons: a reconsideration. *Am J Psychiatry* 135:198–201, 1978.

29. Bandura A: *Aggression: A Social Learning Analysis.* Englewood Cliffs, NJ, Prentice-Hall, 1973.

30. Dollard J, Doob LW, Miller NE, et al: *Frustration and Aggression.* New Haven, Yale University Press, 1939.

31. Mednick SA, Pollock V, Volavka J, et al: Biology and violence. In Wolfgang ME, Weiner NA (eds): *Criminal Violence.* Los Angeles, Sage Publications, 1982, pp 21–80.

32. Robins E, Murphy GE, Wilkinson RH, et al: Some clinical considerations in the prevention of suicide based on a study of 134 successful suicides. *Am J Pub Health* 49:888–899, 1959.

33. Weissman MM: The epidemiology of suicide attempts, 1960 to 1971. *Arch Gen Psychiatry* 30:737–746, 1974.

34. Nolan BS: Functional evaluation of the elderly in guardianship proceedings. *Law, Medicine & Health Care* 12:210–218, 1984.

35. Grisso T: *Evaluating Competencies.* New York, Plenum Press, 1986.

36. Appelbaum PS, Lidz CW, Meisel A: *Informed Consent: Legal Theory and Clinical Practice.* New York, Oxford University Press, 1987.

37. *Canterbury v. Spence,* 462 F.2d 772 (D.C. Cir. 1972).

38. President's Commission for the Study of Ethical Problems in Medicine and Biomedical and Behavioral Research: *Making Health Care Decisions: The Ethical and Legal Implications of Informed Consent in the Patient–Practitioner Relationship. Volume 3: Appendices.* Washington, DC, U.S. Government Printing Office, 1982.

39. Meisel A: The "exceptions" to the informed consent doctrine: striking a balance between competent values in medical decision-making. *Wisconsin Law Review* 1979:413–488.

40. Appelbaum PS, Roth LH: Competency to consent to research: a psychiatric overview. *Arch Gen Psychiatry* 39:951–958, 1982.

41. Munetz MR, Roth LH: Informing patients about tardive dyskinesia. *Arch Gen Psychiatry* 42:866–871, 1985.

42. Grundner TM: On the readability of surgical consent forms. *N Engl J Med* 302:900–902, 1980.

43. Sovner R, DiMascio A, Berkowitz D, et al: Tardive dyskinesia and informed consent. *Psychosomatics* 19:172–177, 1978.

44. Appelbaum PS: Question the experts: must chronic schizophrenic patients who have been stabilized on antipsychotic medication be told of the risk of tardive dyskinesia? *J Clin Psychopharmacol* 5:364–365, 1985.

45. *Rogers v. Commissioner of the Department of Mental Health,* 458 N.E. 2d 308 (Mass. Sup. Jud. Ct. 1983).

46. *Keyhea v. Rushen,* 178 Cal. App. 3d 526 (1st Dist. 1986).

47. Appelbaum PS: Limitations on guardianship of the mentally disabled. *Hosp Community Psychiatry* 33:183–184, 1982.

48. Tancredi L: Psychiatric malpractice. In Michels R, Cavenar, Jesse O. Jr., et al (eds): *Psychiatry* vol. 5. Philadelphia, J. P. Lippincott, 1985, pp 331–345.

49. Calabresi G: *The Costs of Accidents: A Legal and Economic Analysis.* New Haven, Yale University Press, 1970.

50. The Debendox saga. *Br Med J* 291:918–919, 1985.

51. Charles S: *Defendant.* New York, Free Press, 1984.

52. Three plaintiff attorneys tell why patient relations go wrong. *Malpractice Digest* 5(5):1, 4, 1978.

Section V

Aspects of Treatment in Outpatient Practice

45

The Individual Psychotherapies
Efficacy, Syndrome-Based Treatments, and the Therapeutic Alliance

John P. Docherty, M.D.

INTRODUCTION

The title of this chapter has been specifically chosen to be "The Individual Psychotherapies" rather than "Psychotherapy" to reflect a very important aspect of the current structure and practice of psychotherapy. Although there are extremely important generic elements that seem to be present in all psychotherapies, more important, from a contemporary standpoint, is the fact that there are now a number of diverse psychotherapies for different conditions. This does not mean simply that there are a number of different schools of psychotherapy. Indeed, at last count there were over 200 documented "brand-name" psychotherapies. However, this situation has been with us for some time. Rather, the title is intended to reflect an evolution which has occurred over the last decade in the field of psychotherapy.

The core of this evolution is colloquially characterized by the term "the manipulation of therapy." This term encompasses a major development. This development is the construction of techniques and methods for standardizing the practice of psychotherapy, that is, specifying exactly what the focus of a particular therapy is, what strategies and techniques will be used to accomplish that focus, and what strategies and techniques will or will not be used to achieve the aims of that therapy. This development has made possible and credible the application of the randomized clinical trial, a critical, scientific method of modern medicine, for the study of psychosocial treatment. The increased feasibility of such investigations has shifted scientific balance within psychotherapy. It has allowed it to make a quantum leap from observation to experiment.

This revolutionary development in psychotherapy has only begun to penetrate day-to-day clinical practice. The clinical practice of psychotherapy, to date, has not been organized in such a way as to permit the appropriate application to an individual patient the specific psychosocial procedure that would seem to be most beneficial to him or her. The patient, for the most part, has been offered the particular procedure with which the therapist feels most knowledgeable and comfortable. The basic tenet of this textbook's approach to treatment, however, calls for a change in that mode of practice. New developments in psychotherapy are highly consonant with those tenets. Specifically, it allows us to address the following principles which underly the approach to treatment proposed in this book.

Conceptual Clarity and Diversity

It has been emphasized throughout this book that the variations in patients' presentations for mental health care can be understood within a variety of different conceptual frameworks. Major frameworks that have been selected for attention in this book are the biologic, psychodynamic, behavioral, and social. Developments in contemporary psychotherapy and psychotherapy research have provided systematic elaboration and generation of conceptual systems both within and beyond these four domains to guide individual psychotherapeutic treatment.

Implicit in the therapeutic approaches characteristic of this development is the presence of a specific conceptual framework which organizes the patient's history and report of problems and assigns values and priority to different elements of the history. For example, in interpersonal psychotherapy of depression developed by Klerman, Weissman, and colleagues (1), depression is conceived of as a syndrome state resulting from a disruption in the individual's interpersonal world. Interpersonal psychotherapy provides a system for focusing on particularly salient forms of disruption of interpersonal experience and thus assigns relative therapeutic importance to different aspects of the individual's interpersonal life. Specific treatment interventions are then directed toward alleviating those disruptions. Thus, in a very basic way, the choice of a specific therapy represents the election of a specific conceptual approach and, linked to that conceptual approach, a defined body of therapeutic strategies and techniques.

Treatment Selection

The second major tenet of this book emphasizes the importance of precision of treatment selection, that is, selection of a particular treatment approach most acceptable to, applicable to, and available for the individual patient. Such a tenet presumes the availability of more than one alternative treatment approach. Developments in contemporary psychotherapy make possible the selection from alternative treatment approaches of the one approach or combination of approaches that would seem most suitable for an individual patient. For example, as shall be discussed later in this chapter, there are at least five different well-developed psychotherapies for depression which have all had the benefit of randomized clinical trials and have demonstrated efficacy. This gives the clinician extremely useful options for selecting an optimal treatment approach for an individual patient. Unfortunately, criteria and methods for the selection process are not well developed. Research in psychotherapy has not yet generated enough information to lay a firm, empirical basis for such selection. Current work which addresses this issue attempts to determine the indications and contraindications for particular treatments. In this regard some useful progress is being made. For example, it now appears that patients with significant cognitive dysfunction fare poorly in cognitive therapy, while those with significant social dysfunction fare poorly in interpersonal psychotherapy for depression. Thus, deficits in cognitive function would argue for the selection of some therapy other than cognitive behavior therapy such as interpersonal psychotherapy. Deficits in social function suggests the patient will be better placed in a therapy such as cognitive behavior therapy or one of the other alternative forms of treatment. In the treatment of agoraphobia, couples therapy is a useful adjunct if marital discord exists. If, however, agoraphobia is present without marital discord, the addition of couples treatment does not materially add to a successful outcome. Much more such work is needed to fully establish guidelines for the practicing clinician with regard to treatment selection. However, the groundwork for the conduct of such studies is clear, and with proper support much critically necessary information should be forthcoming in this and the next decade.

Above all, however, the essential point is that selection of treatment is not arbitrary. It is clear that patient choice and therapist competence must play a part in therapy selection. However, it is also becoming apparent that other variables are also important in facilitating successful treatment for an individual patient, such as the type of deficits accompanying a particular depressive disorder. Such data places a burden on the practicing clinician to be aware of all of the alternative psychotherapies available to facilitate the likelihood of matching an individual patient with the most appropriate of those treatments.

Negotiated Relationships

Another central principle for outpatient practice discussed throughout this book is the importance of developing a "negotiated relationship" between the therapist and the patient. This is a relationship which takes into account the patient's perspective on his or her illness, including the issues with which the patient wishes help, as well as the means through which the patient would like to see the help delivered. This principle is closely aligned to a major area of development in contemporary psychotherapy research, research on the therapeutic alliance. Such research has demonstrated that the therapeutic alliance is the single most important source of therapeutic gain across all different forms and modalities of psychotherapy. Processes and events that have a strong impact on the therapeutic alliance are carefully described throughout the chapters on the clinical interview. Particularly, Chapters 9 and 10 discuss one of the essential steps in forging the therapeutic alliance, namely identifying and resolving conflicts, implicit and explicit, which exist between patient and therapist. As noted, these conflicts will

involve the definition of the problem, goals, methods, and conditions of treatment. These conflicts also include substantive and affective aspects of the relationship between the patient and therapist. Discussed within the conceptual framework of negotiation strategy, major issues which we know are related to the formation, maintenance, and strength of the therapeutic alliance are identified, including (*a*) the communication of respect and care; (*b*) the establishment of trust and faith in the therapist's competence and experience; (*c*) establishment of a common framework of meaning; (*d*) clear and explicit communication; (*e*) flexibility; and (*f*) eliciting active participation from the patient.

Purposes of This Chapter

Material in this chapter is presented to highlight the place of these three principles in contemporary psychotherapy practice. Specifically, this chapter shall (*a*) review the current status of our understanding of the efficacy of psychotherapy both overall and for specific therapies for particular disorders; (*b*) review the basic advances and developments in the field that have fostered emergence of specific therapies for specific disorders; (*c*) review examples of therapies for each of the major disorders; and (*d*) review our current understanding about the therapeutic alliance and its components.

THE EFFICACY OF PSYCHOTHERAPY

A discussion of the literature on the efficacy of psychotherapy is included here for two reasons: first, to convey the knowledge that exists regarding the efficacy of this modality of treatment; and second, to highlight the approach toward the assessment of psychotherapeutic treatment out of which recent developments have emerged.

The question that is posed when one asks about the efficacy of psychotherapy is simply this: Does psychotherapy work?

From a contemporary perspective this is a naive question. It is tantamount to asking, Does surgery work? The question of true clinical interest is, What treatment is best suited for which patients suffering from what disorders, being treated in what context to achieve what outcomes? Nonetheless, the question of the overall efficacy of psychotherapy has been a lively and hotly debated one. Skeptics abound. It is important for the practitioner of this form of treatment to know the evidence. Critics include not only the policy makers, insurance companies, non-psychotherapy-inclined mental health professionals, but also patients. In the academic arena, the questions of the overall efficacy of psychotherapy have as its landmark reference point Eysenck's attack on the efficacy of psychotherapy almost 35 years ago (2). Since that time, the debate has continued with the other major critics of the efficacy of psychotherapy including Truax and Carkhuff (3), and most recently, Prioleau et al (4) who concluded that verbal psychotherapy seemed to show no major effectiveness over placebo control groups.

Fortunately, for the practitioner of psychotherapy, strong evidence exists to the contrary. Three major literature reviews have been undertaken which support the overall efficacy and outcome of psychotherapy, including that of Meltzoff and Kornreich (5), Luborsky et al. (6), and Bergin and Lambert (7). The most important and convincing reviews, however, have been published more recently. These reviews involve the use of a method of statistical analysis called meta-analysis.

There are three major types of literature reviews which provide a summary of the research investigations of the efficacy of psychotherapy. The first of these is an anecdotal summary reviewing the published literature. The second is a box-score method of summary in which the number of studies showing positive results is compared with a number of studies showing negative results. The third and most sophisticated type is the meta-analysis. This is a method of statistically summarizing and integrating information from a variety of different studies. It entails calculating a measure called the effect size. The effect size is obtained by dividing the mean difference in outcome scores between the treatment and control groups by the standard deviation (usually) of the control group (8). The resultant statistic is essentially a difference in standard (z) score means. The effect size is thus comparable for outcome measures originally expressed in different raw units (9). The effect size yields an estimate of the percentile of distribution of the control patients in which the average (that is the patient at the 50th percentile of the experimental group) would fall following treatment. This method has been used in a variety of different areas such as the assessment of the effect of social class on achievement, the effect of class size on attainment, and the effect of sex differences on conformity.

Recently, Smith et al (8) have applied the meta-analysis technique to research data on psychotherapy. They summarized the research literature from 1941 through 1976 including approximately 75 percent of all eligible studies. Four hundred and seventy-five controlled studies were included. These studies summarize the information deriving from 25,000 patients and yielded 1,766 treatment effects (that is, separate outcome assessments). Results of this analysis were examined to determine whether or not they were affected by rate of blinding, dropout rate, duration of therapy, or length of therapist's experience. None of these variables demonstrated a significant relationship to the main finding of the study which is that the effect size of psychotherapy is very large. Simply stated, psychotherapy is a very powerful treatment. Overall an effect size of .85 was obtained. This means that a patient who is only better off than 50% of his or her cohort prior to treatment would be better off than 80% of that cohort if the rest of the cohort remained untreated. Further, if placebo therapy is omitted from the untreated group, the effect size rises to .93; that is, as the more highly specified forms of therapy are examined the treatment seems to become more effective.

According to Rosenthal and Rubin (10), the effect sizes attributed to psychotherapy by Smith et al. are equivalent to reducing an illness or death rate from 66% to 34%—a clinically substantial feat.

Shapiro and Shapiro (11) adopted more rigorous selection criteria tnan those used by Smith et al., requiring that eligible studies must have involved the assignment of patients to two or more treatment groups and to one or more control groups. Reviewing research published during 1974 and 1979, the Shapiros identified 143 eligible studies—about 10% of all outcome studies actually published during that interval. Only 21 of the studies identified by the Shapiros overlapped with those of Smith et al. Thus, in toto, 597 controlled studies assessing the outcome of the psychotherapies have been analyzed by the meta-analysis procedure.

The results of the Shapiro and Shapiro review of outcome research were even more supportive of the potency of treatment than the study of Smith et al. The mean effect size found in their more carefully controlled sample of studies approached one standard deviation unit, that is, a treated group will evidence a full standard deviation unit of enhanced well-being compared to the untreated control group.

Andrews and Harvey (12) reported on a selected sample of the 475 studies examined in the Smith et al. review. They selected 81 studies of core mental disorders, that is, only those disorders which would generally be considered to be more serious manifestations of psychopathology. These patients were found to move from the 50th to the 77th percentile following treatment. There was also some suggestion that the behavior therapies are better than the dynamic therapies, which are better than the counseling therapies, and that increased duration of therapy is associated with increased efficacy.

In addition to these direct data supporting the efficacy of psychotherapy, there is some support for psychotherapy's effectiveness coming from another area as well. This is the area of the so called cost-offset. Work in this area measures the reduction in general medical and surgical costs found following the treatment of a group of patients with psychotherapy. This is a very interesting area of work which has suggested that patients, following treatment with psychotherapy, require less general medical and surgical services and accumulate less overall health care costs. A major review by Mumford, for example, found that 85% of 58 studies demonstrated a cost-offset effect (13). In addition, a second meta-analysis of 34 studies using brief psychotherapies or educational interventions for patients who had recently suffered a heart attack or who were scheduled for major surgery showed that these modest treatments merited strong significant effects reflected in more rapid recovery, a decreased need for pain and sleeping medications, and decreased length of hospital stay (14). Recent work based on an analysis of Blue Cross/Blue Shield data shows a general reduction in the overall health care costs over a 3-year period of time for those patients who have received psychotherapy (14); and one recent study of high utilization patients in a health maintenance organization setting showed that the treatment of 6-week brief group psychotherapy which focused on the identification of the relationship between feelings and physiologic responses decreased medical utilization by 47% in the subsequent 6 months (15).

All of these data, however, address the global efficacy of psychotherapy. None of this work addresses the question which has become the fundamental chant of contemporary psychotherapy research: What treatment for what disorder to achieve what outcome? The major event in psychotherapy of the last decade has been the development of a methodology which has permitted us to address this question.

SPECIFICITY AND STANDARDIZATION OF PSYCHOTHERAPY

For many years psychotherapy research has been plagued by a problem deriving from psychotherapy practice, the vaguery and ambiguity of the actual process of psychotherapeutic treatment. While this ambiguity has received ardent defense from some practitioners as a reflection of the inherent and necessary fluidity and spontaneity in the therapeutic process, it has posed obvious problems in terms of the development and evaluation of the relative efficacy of different kinds of approaches to different psychiatric problems. In effect, it was impossible to know exactly what transpired between patient and therapist. For example, in studies conducted as recently as 10 years ago, a typical description of the therapy procedure would be "this treatment was conducted by psychoanalytically oriented clinicians" or "five therapists trained in Gestalt therapy conducted the experimental treatment." Such descriptions are clearly insufficient to assure even a casually skeptical individual that a particular treatment approach has been adequately assessed.

Fortunately, this situation has changed dramatically over the last decade. The search for specificity which has characterized much of clinical psychiatric research and which has resulted in more precise and reliable diagnosis and assessment of outcome has become actualized within psychotherapy as well. These methods have included ways of addressing three fundamental questions. The first of these questions is, What is the therapy? This question has been answered through development of manuals which clearly describe the therapy including its rationale, strategies, and techniques and provides examples governing the application of these strategies and techniques. The manual not only describes the therapy, but also sets a boundary or limit around what may be included in such therapy.

The second question is, Are the therapists in the study competent to conduct the therapy? Techniques developed to answer this question represent a major breakthrough for psychotherapy research. Such techniques include the systematic training and supervision of therapists in the study therapy, the assessment through written examination and review of supervised videotapes of the competence of the therapist prior to beginning therapy, and the development of reliable rating scales for assessment of a therapist's competence in different components of the specific therapy. The development of these scales is in itself an important step. It establishes criteria which can be practically applied in order to determine the ability of the individual therapists to carry out the intended task. These scales not only assess the ability of therapists, but also serve to identify key variables and techniques constituting the therapy. Further discussion of such scale items appears later in the section on the psychotherapy of depression.

The third question is, Do the therapists continue to do the specific therapy during the course of the study? This question has been addressed by the development of monitoring techniques which allow for the continuous assessment of "adherence" of the therapists to the protocol of the specific therapies as well as ongoing assessment of the competence with which that therapy is practiced.

The development of specificity in psychotherapy has begun to erode the dominance of identification with one or another loosely defined theoretical "schools" of psychotherapy. Although therapists still tend to "be schooled" in one or another of these approaches, the development of specific therapies for particular disorders has led to increasing interest among practitioners in becoming "schooled" in these specific, operationally defined therapeutic approaches. For example, practitioners of various backgrounds have sought to obtain training in the interpersonal psychotherapy of depression following the establishment of its efficacy by controlled clinical trial.

As a result of the progressive standardization of specific psychotherapies, other interesting issues in the practice of psychotherapy have come to the fore. One of these is the adherence or "purity" of technique. The term "adherence" or "purity" has come to indicate the degree to which a psychotherapist actually practices the particular therapy that he or she purports to be practicing. Current observations indicate that therapists who do stay within the bounds of a particular therapeutic strategy seem to obtain better results. It is unclear whether this effect occurs because the therapy is maintained or because it reflects the capacity of the therapist to direct his or her behavior more precisely. It has also been noted that "patient difficulty," (the severity of disorder with which a patient presents) has a tendency to dislodge a therapist from the ability to maintain focus on a particular strategy. Unchecked, this process leads to progressive derangement of a therapist's competence. Furthermore, it does seem to be somewhat difficult to teach "old dogs new tricks." Therapists schooled within one particular perspective seem to find difficulty shifting perspectives. This is perhaps the most important observation to emerge from current work. The most difficult process in the instruction of a new therapist in a particular psychotherapy involves the ability of the therapist to grasp the conceptual framework guiding that therapy and to apply that framework in actual practice. In contrast, the learning of specific therapeutic techniques and procedures appears to be a very simple task. Thus it is relatively easy for the beginning cognitive behavior therapist to learn such techniques as reattribution, activity scheduling, graded task assignment, and so on. It is a far more difficult task to instruct the therapist in identifying and maintaining focus on the key cognitive disturbance in the patient (16).

SHORT-TERM PSYCHOTHERAPY

The nature of the practice of psychotherapy in the outpatient setting is primarily short term. In community mental health centers and in similar clinics, the average number of sessions per year per treated individual is 5.3 (17). In the private setting, the average number of sessions per treated individual per year is only 30, and this number is heavily influenced by a few individuals in intensive long-term therapy, thereby obscuring the very short-term nature of the work. Eighty-five percent of all patients are seen in less than 60 sessions per year and 78% of all patients are seen in fewer than 25 sessions per year. Furthermore, the work tends almost entirely to have a frequency of once per week (18). Only one percent of all treated patients in the private setting are seen three or more sessions per week. The relatively low frequency and short-term nature of such work has had progressive influence on the construction of psychotherapies for outpatient practice. Most therapies have become more modest in their goals. They tend to share an emphasis on selecting one major source of focus for the treatment intervention—even though multiple problems may be present. It is important to note, however, that this selection of a focus often becomes a critical task. It is the focus of much of the creativity of the short-term outpatient psychotherapies. In this sense, the selection of that focus is very much like the work of the master diamond cutter who is allowed one strike through the diamond to create the optimal cut.

This state of affairs has been reflected in the development of refined and sophisticated short-term psychodynamic psychotherapies. The work of four therapists has gained predominant recognition. These therapists are David Malan, Peter Sifneos, James Mann, and Habib Davanloo. There are very interesting differences in the structures of the four therapies developed by these therapists. However, more salient in terms of the general trend in the field is the remarkable similarity in structure and thrust in each of these therapies.

Malan (19) has developed a therapy called focal psychotherapy. This therapy is usually limited to 20 sessions. At its heart is the identification of a focal conflict, which forms the target of the treatment. It relies heavily for its technical intervention on precise interpretations directed toward the focal conflict. Furthermore, these are relationship-centered interpretations linking the focal relationship conflict to problems in the therapeutic relationship and to previous relationships in the patient's life.

Sifneos (20) has developed a therapy called anxiety-provoking psychotherapy. This term has been chosen in order to differentiate this treatment from supportive or "anxiety suppressive therapy." This term indicates the intent to bring about change of the fundamental psychologic structure of the individual, not simply to relieve anxiety. It too requires the ability to identify one specific area for therapeutic work. Criteria for entry into this therapy include the patient's ability to present one specific chief complaint as a priority for treatment. It is moreover preferable that this complaint reflects an oedipal conflict. Another criterion for therapy requires the patient to have experienced one *meaningful* relationship in his or her life.

Mann (21) has developed a therapy called time-limited psychotherapy. The focus of this therapy is on the principal source of separation/individuation anxiety in the individual's life. The constraint of the duration of treatment is thus seen as a positive therapeutic force in highlighting the efforts to focus on this conflict. The central target for treatment is identified as the patient's "chronic and enduring pain." This pain is characterized as the emotional constellation surrounding the patient's primary negative self-image. The treatment is limited to 12 hours.

Davanloo (22) has developed treatment called broad focus short-term dynamic psychotherapy. The main target for treatment in this therapy could either be an oedipal or pre-oedipal conflict. In general oedipal conflicts are felt to yield to short-term resolution, approximately 5 to 15 sessions; pre-oedipal, 20 to 40 sessions. In this treatment a specific focus must be identified. The treatment relies heavily for selection criteria on the patient's previous history of meaningful relationships, an indication of a motivation to change, not simply to achieve symptom or anxiety relief and demonstrated positive response to transference interpretations.

These therapies have in common an evaluation process to establish a specific and central focus for the treatment intervention. Multiple goals are eschewed. The central therapeutic task is relentlessly pursued. Thus, the evaluation process and the framing of the central focus of treatment is extremely important. These treatments also have in common the exclusion of patients from such therapy who demonstrate a strong potential for regression to psychotically decompensated, extremely dependent, or dysfunctional or suicidal states. Patients are also excluded from these therapies who demonstrate an inability to do the work of the therapy within the short-term frame. Criteria for exclusion of such patients are three: (*a*) a lack of motivation for change, (*b*) the inability to form a meaningful relationship with the therapist, and (*c*) a lack of the psychologic competence to carry out the work of the therapy, including insufficient intelligence, deficient psychologic mindedness, or inflexibility and rigidity of ego functions.

While this work represents an important advance in the field of psychotherapy, the area that has showed the most rapid progression is the development of specific therapies geared to the treatment of specific syndromes identified within the currently accepted diagnostic system.

SYNDROME-BASED PSYCHOTHERAPIES

In the following section current developments in the treatment of depression, anxiety disorders, and schizophrenia are reviewed.

Depression

Five major psychotherapies specifically directed at the treatment of depression have been developed. One is a psychodynamic form of therapy called interpersonal psychotherapy developed by Klerman, Weissman, and colleagues; (1) the second is a cognitive–behavioral therapy, developed by Aaron Beck (23); and the remaining are behavioral therapies: self-control therapy, developed by Lynn Rehm (24); social learning therapy, by Lewinsohn (25); and social skills training, by Hersen and Bellack (26). Approximately 25 controlled clinical trials have been undertaken testing one or another of these forms of therapy for depression. This represents by far the largest single body of research information currently available in the field. Results of these investigations clearly indicate that these treatments are effective methods for alleviating acute depression. Current issues receiving further study in this field involve the usefulness of these treatments to prevent the recurrence of depressive episodes and the systematic assessment of relative indications and contraindications for the use of one or another of these treatments.

Interpersonal Psychotherapy for Depression

Interpersonal psychotherapy for depression (IPT) is a short-term psychotherapy which is based on critical observations regarding the link between social factors and the occurrence of depression. The stability and quality of early attachments, the presence of trusting and confiding relationships in an individual's life, loss of important relationships and the presence of interpersonal stress, particularly marital distress, are closely linked with the onset of depression. A number of studies have now been carried out demonstrating the efficacy of interpersonal psychotherapy in alleviating both acute depressive episodes as well as in maintaining remission of depressive symptomatology. Research has also demonstrated the effectiveness of this treatment in alleviating the social functioning morbidity that accompanies depression.

The focus of IPT is on the production of symptom relief and the repair of interpersonal relationships. It specifically does not attempt to change long-standing personality problems. Its goals are essentially those of "supportive" psychotherapy: to bring about change in a disturbed current state of affairs by helping the patients to understand the nature of their distress through clarifying confused emotional states, rectifying distorted perceptions and increasing interpersonal coping competency. It does not attempt to restructure deeply rooted "intrapsychic patterns."

Conceptualization and Diagnosis. The patient's problem is conceptualized within an interpersonal framework. However, two diagnostic procedures are undertaken. The first is the diagnosis of the syndrome state. If the depressive syndrome state is found to exist, a secondary diagnostic process is undertaken to determine the exact nature of the interpersonal problem from which the individual is suffering. Four broad categories of problems have been developed for this therapy: grief and loss, role disputes, role transition, and interpersonal deficits. The patient is diagnosed as having one or more of these particular problem types. This problem type forms the major focus for the treatment intervention and dictates the major focus of the treatment intervention.

Grief refers, in the interpersonal therapy context, to an abnormal grief reaction such as the delay of onset of grief, the unusual persistence of grief or a severity of grieving that seriously interferes with functioning. *Interpersonal disputes* refers to a situation that can arise in a variety of interpersonal contexts where the patients and some other significant individual have nonreciprocal role expectations. This can occur between spouses, between parent and child, or in work situations. *Role transitions* refers to major change in individual's life role. This is typically the kind of situation that would occur with developmental changes such as leaving school, being promoted or demoted, changing place of residence, retiring, and so on. *Interpersonal deficits* refers to those individuals that are absent the skills for beginning or for maintaining interpersonal relationships. These individuals usually present with complaints of social isolation either related to the absence of relationships at all, or to the absence of depth or stability in relationships.

Strategies and Techniques. The treatment tends to be limited to 12 to 16 sessions, with a frequency of about once each week. There are three broad phases in the treatment. The first is assessment and negotiation of the treatment contract, the second is focus on a selected problem area, and the third is termination.

The assessment and negotiation phase entails the diagnosis of the syndrome state and the interpersonal problem. This phase also includes the process of helping the patient to deal with the depressive symptoms in the following ways: understanding the nature of these symptoms, clarifying the diagnosis, and presenting information regarding the nature of depression. An assessment is also carried out systematically of the person's interpersonal life. Essentially an inventory is conducted of all of the important interpersonal relationships and their current status. Following this, a therapeutic contract is established wherein the patient and the therapist agree to work on one specific focal interpersonal problem of the four identified in this therapy. Table 45.1 indicates some of the major goals of treatments for each of the problem areas. In addition to the specific goals of therapy noted in Table 45.1, interpersonal psychotherapy also involves the use of specific techniques which include attention to important administrative details to organize the ongoing therapy; the use of exploratory techniques such as nondirective exploration and supportive extension of the topic; the encouragement of the extension of

Table 45.1 Focus of Treatment for Each Problem Area in Interpersonal Therapy for Depression

Grief

1. Facilitate mourning.
2. Reestablish interest in relationships to substitute for one's loss.

Interpersonal disputes

1. Identify exact nature of dispute.
2. Choose plan of action.
3. Clarify patient's position in the dispute.
4. Modify expectations or faulty communication.

Role transition

1. Facilitate mourning and acceptance of loss of old role.
2. Regard new role as positive.
3. Restore self-esteem through a sense of mastery.

Interpersonal deficits

1. Recognize social isolation.
2. Encourage formation of new relationships.

affect in sensitive and key areas through the inquiry of feelings associated with reports of major life events; clarification and confrontation of interpersonal communications in the context of the therapy, including such techniques as restructuring and rephrasing; formal communication analysis and decision analysis; and the use of directive techniques such as advice giving and limit setting.

Major Issues. Interpersonal psychotherapy has demonstrated itself to be effective with regard to grief, interpersonal disputes, and role transition. Interpersonal-deficit patients seem to be the least responsive to IPT. It seems likely that such patients lack the social skills to adequately engage with the therapist within the short time frame.

Cognitive Behavioral Therapy

Cognitive behavioral therapy is a short-term psychotherapy for depression developed by Aaron Beck and elaborated in his work with Maria Kovacs and John Rush (23). This is a highly developed psychotherapy which has now had the benefit of a number of clinical trials which have demonstrated usefulness as a specific treatment for depression.

Cognitive behavioral therapy is based on a structural model of depression. It makes the assumption that the core difficulty in depression is a particular disorder of thought which in turn leads to associated emotional and behavioral symptoms of depression. This theory asserts that a depression is characterized by negative pleasureless views of the world, oneself, and the future. Examples of such negative thoughts are "I'm no good," "I can't get started," and "No one understands me." These negative thoughts are thought to derive from underlying negative schemas which are dysfunctional attitudes of which the individual is usually unaware. Examples of such dysfunctional attitudes are "If a person asks for help, it is a sign of weakness" or "Taking even a small risk is foolish because the loss is likely to be a disaster." It is thought that these dysfunctional attitudes are based on certain specific logical errors. Examples of some of the more important of these logical errors are the following:

1. Overgeneralizing: If it's true in one case it applies to any case even if it is only remotely similar.
2. Selective abstraction: The only events that matter are failures.
3. Excessive responsibility: I am responsible for all negative events and failures.
4. Assuming temporal causality: If it was true in the past, it will always be true.
5. Self-references: I cause all misfortunes.
6. Catastrophizing: Always think of the worst.
7. Dichotomous thinking: Everything is either one extreme or another.

Diagnosis. Diagnosis and conceptualization are essential to cognitive behavioral therapy. The diagnosis for this therapy consists of identifying the key negative cognitions and the key dysfunctional attitudes which characterize an individual patient's depressogenic cognitive complex. Therapy is then directed toward the alleviation of this specific "complex." Not all negative thoughts nor all dysfunctional attitudes are the focus of change. The cognitive therapy procedure partakes of the same recognition of reality which it attempts to convey, namely, the belief that not everything can be accomplished, that one should select his or her major goals and feel good about the effort to accomplish these goals.

Strategies and Techniques of Cognitive Therapy. Cognitive behavioral therapy uses three general approaches to treatment: didactic intervention, cognitive techniques, and behavioral techniques. There is also an important and specific focus on building and maintaining a therapeutic alliance.

The most essential features of the general strategy and specific techniques include three major areas. The first involves the personal characteristics of the therapist including such features as genuineness, warmth, accurate empathy, professional manner, and rapport. The second major area assessed is the general conduct of the interview including, (*a*) the establishment

of a sense of collaboration and mutual understanding; (*b*) the establishment of an agenda for each session; (*c*) the elicitation of reactions from the patient to the interview and the therapist; (*d*) efficient use of time in the therapy; (*e*) focus on the appropriate problem; (*f*) the appropriate use of questioning; (*g*) the provision to the patient of periodic summaries during the interview; and (*h*) the assignment of homework for the patient to carry out during the time between appointments.

The third area assessed is the use of specific cognitive behavioral techniques. These include (*a*) the use of a technique appropriate to the identified problem; (*b*) effective eliciting of automatic negative thoughts and the engagement of the patient in the identification of such thoughts through inductive questions, the use of imagery, and role playing; (*c*) the testing of automatic thoughts by helping the patient to pose specific hypotheses and collect valid evidence; (*d*) the identification and testing of underlying assumptions through the analysis of the validity of these assumptions; and (*e*) the flexible use of specific cognitive behavioral techniques such as reattribution, cognitive rehearsal, graded task assignment, and so on.

Major Issues. Cognitive behavioral therapy has been demonstrated to be effective. The interesting issues emerging in the use of this therapy now involve the identification of indications and contraindications for its use. In this regard, some new work does suggest that patients who are high on individual coping skills perform better with this therapy and do very poorly with a drug treatment, whereas patients who are low in individual coping skills do poorly with this therapy and selectively better with drug treatment. The other major issue of ongoing study is the degree to which this treatment protects against subsequent relapse and the appropriate follow-up interventions to improve its relapse preventing efficacy.

Behavioral Therapies of Depression

There are three major behavioral treatments which have been developed for depression. Self-control therapy, developed by Lynn Rehm (24); psychoeducational therapy, developed by Lewinson (25); and social skills training, developed by Hersen and Bellack (26). These treatments are discussed as a group because of the overlap in basic rationale and strategies and techniques that characterize them. Some of the specific differences between these therapies shall be highlighted.

Rationale. The essential feature which all of these therapies share is a dependence upon a behavioral formulation of depression proposed by Ferster (27). Ferster suggested that depression may be construed within a Skinnerian framework as a result of a loss of positive reinforcements. The reasons for the loss are mostly irrelevant and could result from death, separation, sudden environmental change, and so on. An associated hypothesis is that deficiency in social confidence and skill may be a vulnerability variable underlying chronic absence or repeated loss of positive reinforcement.

Strategies and Techniques. These therapies rely on a repertoire of techniques that have been developed within the framework of behavior therapy. These techniques include strategies for maintaining careful records of the amount of reinforcement activity, pleasant events, unpleasant events, and so on. They also involve focused strategies for developing attainable goals, to increase the number of reinforcing events, and to decrease those conditions preventing the occurrence of such events. These techniques also provide ways of tracking the accomplishment of such goals (monitoring and documentation techniques). The other major common area is skill-training techniques. These involve the training of social skills including communication skills and assertiveness accomplished through modeling, role playing, rehearsal, graduated task performance, relaxation training, time management training, stress reduction training, and cognitive skills training. Overall, the common goal of all of these treatments is to keep a clear and systematic focus, to enhance efficiency by precision and clarity

of intervention, and to carefully and reliably assess progress.

Specific Behavioral Therapies. *Self-Control Therapy.* Self-control therapy is based on Kanfer's learning theory model of self-control. Depression is thought to be related to a deficiency in an individual's ability to use self-control to deal with the loss or delay of reinforcement. According to the model there are three components of self-control: self-monitoring, self-evaluation, and self-reinforcement. Depressed patients may show deficits in one or more of these components.

Diagnosis within this therapy involves identifying the specific component of self-control demonstrating deficiency. For example, there may be a deficiency in self-monitoring with a selective attention to immediate and external events to the exclusion of internal consequences of behavior or selective attention to negative events. There may be deficits in self-evaluation due to unrealistic and perfectionistic goals, or there may be a deficiency in self-reinforcement with low rates of positive behavior permitted by the individual to him- or herself.

Self-control therapy involves utilizing a variety of behavioral techniques including monitoring techniques and goal-setting techniques to correct the deficit in self-control which has been identified. Therapy usually consists of six sessions, and homework is assigned to correct deficits between sessions.

Psychoeducational Treatment. Psychoeducational therapy is based on social learning theory. Depression is thought to represent a situation in which individual maladaptive patterns are identified: (*a*) Individuals allow themselves to remain in a life situation which is deficient in reinforcement; (*b*) the individuals are deficient in their ability to generate positive events or to cope with negative events; and (*c*) the individuals' internal response to positive events is attenuated or their individual response to negative events is exaggerated. This therapy focuses on the person–environment interaction. The intent is to correct the deficiencies in the individual which prevent a more positive interaction from developing so that the environment becomes more giving of positive reinforcement and the individual more able to generate the giving as well as to accurately perceive and react to its presence.

Social Skills Training. Social skills training focuses on the deficiency in social skills which may underlie depression in some patients. It identifies the specific area of deficiency either in the omission of important social skills such as positive assertion and conversational skills or in the ability of the individual to accurately interpret social cues. The diagnosis consists of identifying the specific area of deficiency. Treatment consists of using techniques to enhance social perception and prosocial behavior. The particular treatment also relies on the gradual movement of social skills through guided practice from the treatment setting into the natural environment.

Anxiety Disorders

Current developments in the psychotherapy of anxiety disorders have begun to reflect the newer diagnostic distinctions in this area of psychopathology. Yet far less work has been done with these disorders than with the psychotherapy of depression.

Agoraphobia

The psychotherapy of agoraphobia consists of four major forms of treatment: exposure-based behavioral treatment, psychodynamic psychotherapy, cognitive therapy, and marital therapy. Of these treatments the one which has demonstrated the greatest efficacy to date is exposure-based treatment. This treatment is based on the assumption that the patient's difficulty will persist without exposure to the anxiety-provoking situation. It is further assumed that if anxiety can be attenuated while the exposure occurs that the panic response and associated avoidance behavior will diminish. Exposure is carried out either through a process of systematic

desensitization in which the patient is gradually and progressively exposed to a series of anxiety-inducing situations or by flooding, in which there is a massive and continued exposure to an intensely anxiety-provoking situation until the fear response departs. Both of these techniques may be carried out either via imagery or in vivo. For in vivo exposure (exposure in the actual situation) the use of public transportation or a crowded shopping mall has proved to be quite effective. The administration of this treatment also partakes of the principles and techniques of behavior therapy, mentioned in the section on depression, and includes careful attention to record keeping, assessment of degrees of anxiety, homework assignments between formal therapy sessions, and methods for mastery of anxiety response such as relaxation training (28).

Psychodynamically based psychotherapy has not been demonstrated to be effective in controlled clinical trials, although case reports of efficacy have appeared. In general an approach carried out within this framework would attempt to uncover psychologic conflicts accounting for the agoraphobia. The patient will then be aided to deal with these conflicts directly so that the defenses of repression and displacement can be relinquished. In the anecdotal reports it is interesting to note that successful cases often involve the therapist's encouragement to the patient to engage in activities which progressively expose the patient to the feared situation.

One very interesting new development in the psychotherapeutic treatment of agoraphobia involves the use of marital therapy (29). The rationale for this treatment is based on three important observations. First, there is an increased prevalence of morbid jealousy among the spouses of female agoraphobics. Second, there has been a demonstrated inverse correlation between the level of marital satisfaction and the level of agoraphobia. As agoraphobia diminishes, marital satisfaction increases. Third, and perhaps most important, marital satisfaction has been demonstrated to be a predictor of outcome in agoraphobia, independent of severity of the disorder. Female agoraphobics in marriages with greater mutual dissatisfaction tend to have a poor outcome of treatment. These marriages seem characterized by two relationship patterns which may be simultaneously present. The unaffected spouse acts as "the protector" of the patient, keeping her out of the situations which she is symptomatically avoiding. The patient herself seems to seek certain kinds of gains from the dependency position in which the agoraphobic behavior places her. Recent work has demonstrated that marital therapy used as an adjunctive treatment to exposure based therapy improves outcome *in marriages in which there is a high level of marital dissatisfaction*. When marital satisfaction is high the adjunctive use of marital therapy does not contribute to an improved outcome beyond that achieved by the exposure based treatment alone.

Generalized Anxiety Disorder, Simple Phobia, and Obsessive–Compulsive Disorder

Treatment of generalized anxiety disorder, simple phobia, and obsessive–compulsive disorder has not been extensively investigated by formal clinical trial. Work that does exist suggests that relaxation training, psychodynamic psychotherapy and cognitive therapy may all be effective.

Psychodynamic treatment focuses on the ways of thinking that generate anxiety in situations where other people do not react with anxiety. It focuses on the development of these thought patterns and their roots in prior life experience. The focus of this treatment is on discrepancies between identified wishes, fears, and values and relevant current realities. An attempt is made to understand the origin of these conflicts in earlier important relationships of the individual and to facilitate the individual's understanding of repetitive unsuccessful ways of coping with these conflicts and the attainment of new and more successful strategies for resolving these conflicts.

Cognitive therapy for anxiety neurosis is a newly developed treatment (30). Beck has developed this treatment on the model of cognitive therapy of depression; that is, it focuses on identifying disturbed thought patterns which generate anxiety. There are, however, some salient differences between cognitive therapy for anxiety and for depression. These differences derive from the fact that the identification of anxiety-generating thoughts is technically more difficult than the identification of depressogenic thoughts. Anxiety-producing thoughts are more difficult to identify because the individual is often not anxious during the treatment session, the recollection of the anxiety-provoking thoughts tends to be state dependent and anxiety-producing thoughts tend to be of shorter duration than depressogenic thoughts. Some of the special methods used to identify these thoughts are assiduous attention to diary keeping and the use of imagery and role-playing.

One of the most interesting new developments in the treatment of anxiety disorders is the behavioral work which has been conducted in the treatment of obsessive–compulsive disorder. This work demonstrates that exposure to the stimulus which elicits the obsessive or compulsive behavior plus response prevention is a powerful psychotherapeutic intervention for producing a decrease of the obsessive and compulsive behaviors. It has further been determined that in order to maintain the gain obtained by the exposure and response prevention treatment, imaginal exposure to situations which might be encountered is a necessary additional treatment procedure (31).

Schizophrenia

The treatment of schizophrenia by psychotherapy has advanced considerably in the last decade. This has not been through the application of psychodynamic psychotherapy for schizophrenic patients. Rather, it has been primarily by the application of supportive psychosocial interventions and attention to the social (particularly familial) environment in which the remitted outpatient schizophrenic is living. Each of the three major therapeutic approaches shall be discussed: intensive psychodynamic, supportive psychotherapy, and family treatment.

Intensive Psychodynamic Psychotherapy

Treatment studies conducted to date have not yet satisfactorily demonstrated the efficacy of intensive psychotherapy for schizophrenic patients. It is important to note that there may be many salient reasons for this. The particular subgroup of patients responsive to this treatment may have not yet been identified; therapists engaged in these studies may not be sufficiently expert; sufficient attention may not have been paid to maintaining the "integrity" or adherence of the therapist to the therapy over the prolonged period of time necessary for this treatment; and the treatments may not have been conducted for sufficiently long enough periods of time to exert their effects. These important points notwithstanding, the practice of intensive individual psychotherapy for schizophrenic patients remains in a "gray zone" because of the lack of convincing evidence of its efficacy and proper application.

Nevertheless, intensive psychodynamic psychotherapy is the most highly developed and well-described therapeutic approach for dealing with this seriously disturbed patient group. The rationale for this approach is based on the assumption that the interaction between the mother and the child very early in life has been disturbed, leading to an early experience of "pain at being held, and pain at being laid down." This is thought to leave patients with a conflict in which they feel dependent on others by whom they feel persecuted and whom they further feel are unstable and unreliable (32).

Techniques and Strategies of the Treatment. The major strategy of intensive psychodynamic therapy involves using the relationship between the therapist and the patient to gradually rectify the core alienation and maladaptive ways of coping with this core conflict that has developed in a schizophrenic patient's life. In this thera-

peutic process, the attitude of the therapist toward the work of therapy and the patient is considered critical. This attitude is prescribed to be one in which the therapist is persistently aware of the healthy, human, and survival-oriented aspects of a patient's personality. It is also one in which the therapist is noncontrolling, optimistic, tolerant, and highly sensitive to the patient's autonomy. Strategies of treatment involve careful attention to establishing a relationship with the patient, with the understanding that a positive relationship may take far longer to establish with such patients than with nonpsychotic patients.

The work of the therapy consists in helping the patients to become aware of the full range of their feelings, teaching them how to bear those feelings, and gaining an analytic understanding of the feelings. The process of change in this therapy is thought to be brought about fundamentally through the maintenance of this relationship and, in that context, the use of multiple interpretations to bring into the awareness of the patient disavowed feelings and experiences in a way which integrates those with the patient's past, present and future. Gunderson and Frank (33) specifically differentiate intensive exploratory therapy from supportive therapy, as indicated in Table 45.2.

Supportive Psychotherapy

The major study of individual supportive psychotherapy which has been carried out is of major role therapy. This treatment was utilized as part of a large-scale study to assess the efficacy of phenothiazines in preventing relapse in discharged schizophrenic patients (34). This work demonstrated a twofold increase in relapse over a 2-year period in those patients who were on placebo rather than antipsychotic maintenance medication. It also demonstrated, however, that even minimal supportive psychotherapy, consisting of attention to helping the patient cope with and progressively engage more fully in major social and occupational role functioning, had a psychotoxic effect early in the treatment. During the first 6 months following dis-

Table 45.2 Comparison of Supportive and Exploratory Therapy for Schizophrenia (33)

	Supportive	Exploratory
Objectives	Symptom relief via drug management and strengthening of existing defenses	Self-understanding: how one feels and thinks and how these influence the course of one's life
Interview focus	Management, complaints, interpersonal problems, current situational problems	Relationship to therapist and significant others, exploration of feelings and conflicts
Psychic arena	Focus on what is already aware, no hidden agendas	Look for current meanings, hidden motivation, unconscious
Temporal focus	Present and future	Present and past
Techniques	Support, reassurance, limits, clarification, direction, suggestions for environment manipulation, use of community resources	Support, reassurance, limits, clarification, interpretation, catharsis
Transference	Encourage positive to further alliance, actively discourage negative	Accept positive and work through the negative
Countertransference	Positive feelings important and expressable; control negative	Mixed feelings expected and generally not disclosed

charge from the hospital those patients engaged in a supportive psychotherapy have a greater relapse rate. However, for those patients who survived the 6 months, the supportive psychotherapy had a salutary effect. Relapse was subsequently reduced in this group of patients. Furthermore, as time went on these patients showed a significant improvement in social functioning versus those patients who did not receive this therapy. This finding is consistent with the finding reported in the Gunderson and Frank study (33) of the psychotherapy of schizophrenia which showed enhancement of occupational functioning in those patients who receive supportive psychotherapy versus those who received an intensive exploratory psychotherapy. This work suggests the following consideration in designing an outpatient treatment for a schizophrenic patient.

1. Timing of particular psychosocial interventions for schizophrenic patients is extremely important. Specifically individual intervention even of a "supportive type" should be delayed until the patient has "consolidated" a recovery following a psychotic episode.
2. When such "consolidation" has occurred, gains can be expected by the addition of supportive therapy to standard maintenance medication treatment. Such patients will fare better than

those left to medication maintenance alone.

Family Treatment

The most exciting development in the psychosocial treatment of schizophrenic patients over the last decade has been the recognition that attention to the "family situation" in which the individual is living has a highly significant effect in preventing relapse of psychotic episodes. This body of work has demonstrated that the ability of a treatment to reduce the amount of expressed emotion, particularly hostility and criticism directed at the patient by significant others in that patient's life, *will* reduce the risk of relapse for that patient. At least two different methods have been shown to reduce the degree of expressed hostility. Falloon and colleagues (35) utilized a "behavioral strategy" in which the family members were schooled in a "rules of order" with regard to how they should speak with one another. There was specific training in the manner and way of addressing one another in the family setting which led to the reduction of disruptive, highly charged, negative emotions. The family members were also taught a highly structured formula for problem solving and were repeatedly practiced in this technique when dealing with family problems.

Hogarty and Anderson (36) have developed another method which involves a strong psychoeducational approach. This approach emphasizes instructing the family members in the nature of schizophrenic illness, its treatment, and its impact on social functioning and family relationships. The family members are then taught how to cope with aberrations in the schizophrenic patient's behavior, and an effort is made through a structural approach to maintain essential family boundaries, clarify family roles, and progressively increase the role competence of the schizophrenic patient. More recent work has shown that the dramatic improvement in relapse obtained by this treatment can be further enhanced by social skills training of the schizophrenic patient. It may seem somewhat odd that this treatment is included in a chapter on individual psychotherapy. This is not so odd as it may seem, since it is not clear at this point that the entire family needs to be present for this treatment to be effective. It may very well be that one key family member, seen in individual consultation, may be sufficient to exert this therapeutic effect. Current clinical experience certainly suggests that such an intervention should be undertaken if a full-scale family intervention is not feasible.

THERAPEUTIC ALLIANCE

The therapeutic alliance has been the focus of increasing interest in studies of psychotherapy. This focus has been generated more from accumulating empirical evidence of its importance than from persuasive theory. For example, although Freud noted that friendliness and affection are the vehicles for success in psychotherapy, the theoretical focus in psychodynamic psychotherapy has been on other areas.

Most of the rest of the field of psychotherapy practice has shared this bias. The importance of the relationship between therapist and patient has probably been most strongly advocated within client-centered psychotherapy and established through the work of Carl Rogers. Rogers described the critical facilitative conditions

for psychotherapy, as accurate empathy, nonpossessive warmth, and genuineness (37). This perspective on psychotherapy has also received strong support through the seminal work of Jerome Frank, who developed the conceptual framework of the "nonspecific sources of psychotherapy change efficacy." Frank (38) identified six nonspecific factors: (a) an emotionally charged confiding relationship; (b) a therapeutic rationale acceptable to the patient; (c) the provision of new information; (d) the strengthening of the patient's expectations for help; (e) the provision of success experiences; and (f) the facilitation of emotional arousal.

An emerging body of research, has over the last two decades, continued to support the enormous importance of the therapeutic alliance in the production of change through psychotherapy. It is now estimated that approximately 40% of the variance in outcome in all forms of psychotherapy can be accounted for by the strength and quality of the therapeutic alliance. More of the variance in outcome can be explained through the therapeutic alliance than by any other variable, including school of therapy and specific techniques. Thus, facilitating the development of a strong therapeutic alliance must be seen as the essential work for psychotherapy.

Edward Bordin has contributed to the most important current conceptual formulation of the therapeutic alliance (39). According to this formulation, the therapeutic alliance is conceptualized as consisting of three main components: affectional bonds, therapeutic tasks, and therapeutic goals. *Goals* refer to specific changes, particularly in interpersonal behavior, which are sought as a result of the therapy. *Tasks* refer to those specific techniques which are selected by the therapist to promote the work of the therapy. *Bonds* refer to the unavoidable emotional ties which develop between the therapist and the patient in the course of the work of the therapy. The formulation further describes three main phases of the therapeutic alliance: the formative phase, where initial trust is established which permits the work of the therapy to be undertaken; the working-through phase, which is characterized by fluctuations in the strength of the alliance and in which there is both progressive deepening of the alliance and therapeutic work on the repair of disruptions in the alliance; and the phase of termination. Progress in therapy is though to result from the ability to maintain a strong therapeutic alliance in the face of the strains, changes and potential disruptions introduced by the proper selection of therapeutic tasks (40). Notable about this conceptualization is that it provides the first coherent framework for resolving the hoary debate over the relative importance of relationship versus technique that has burdened the practice of psychotherapy.

Possibly the most important advance in the last several years in the empirical study of therapeutic alliance has been the development of useful and reliable measures for assessing the quality and strength of the therapeutic alliance. Six such measures have assumed prominence (41). These are the Penn Helping Alliance Scale, the Vanderbilt Psychotherapy Process Scale, the Vanderbilt Therapeutic Alliance Scale, the Therapeutic Alliance Rating System, the Working Alliance Inventory, and the Menninger Therapeutic Alliance Scales. These scales measure the alliance from the point of view of the patient, the therapist, and the interaction. Although these scales represent an important advance for the field, problems still exist with the scales in their current form. For example, there is the problem of sampling. We are not yet sure of the most useful unit of measure for these scales. Can we assess therapeutic alliance from 15-minute tape segments? Is the whole session necessary? Second, most of these systems assume a uniformity of the alliance over time. We know that this is probably not true, and a method for taking this variability into account must be developed. Finally, most of these scales assess different aspects of the patient's and the therapist's experience of the therapy. These different dimensions of experience are then condensed into a single measure of therapeutic alliance. The valid-

ity of this reduction of information needs to be established.

In reviewing the available empirical information on the nature of the therapeutic alliance, several findings seem to have some important stability. These findings are usually categorized under patient variables, therapist variables, and relationship or interaction variables. These are attempts to try to understand what is brought to the relationship by the patient, what is brought by the therapist, and what emerges in their interaction.

Patient Variables

The patient variables seem, by and large, to be more important than therapist variables in establishing a therapeutic alliance for short-term psychotherapy. Those features of the patient which seem related to the development of a positive alliance include: likability of the patient, a problem-solving attitude expressed on the patient's part, and the capacity of the patient to "experience," that is, to express a depth of feeling as well as an ability to reflect on those expressed feelings. In addition, recent work suggests that the quality of the relationships that the patient has experienced outside of the therapy are predictive of the relationship that will form with the therapist. This is no surprise. Those patients who do have a history of good relationships will tend to form good relationships in the therapy. Of great interest, however, from the point of view of improving the outcome of psychotherapy, is the finding that of those patients who have only mediocre relationships some will get well while others will do poorly in therapy. Clearly, overall outcome will be improved by understanding what permits some of these patients to establish a good therapeutic alliance (42).

Therapist Variables

There is a traditional triad of therapist's variables deriving from the early pioneering work by Carl Rogers and his group

(37). These included therapist's genuineness, warmth, and empathy. It has been demonstrated in a number of studies that therapist empathy *from the patient's perception* is positively correlated with good outcome (41). Another very interesting finding is that "freshness" of the therapist's language is also an important positive predictor. This appears to be the ability of a therapist to phrase issues in evocative, creative, and unusual ways which capture the patient's attention and imagination (44).

Recently, important work has demonstrated that technical competence is related to positive alliance and outcome. Strupp demonstrated that errors in technique are more predictive than patient or therapist variables in determining outcome (43). Other work by Luborsky has demonstrated that the adherence of the therapist to a particular form of therapy is also related to positive outcome (44). Foreman and Marmar (45) have also demonstrated that with patients who enter treatment with strong negative feelings, those therapists who address the defenses against the expression of feelings about relationships both outside and in the therapy seem able to help produce successful therapy experiences for these patients. It should be understood that this expression of feelings does not simply mean the expression of negative feelings, but the ability and competence to express the whole range of relationship feelings (46).

The Relationship Between the Patient and Therapist

The relationship between the patient and therapist has been demonstrated to be the most important in predicting outcome (47). This is especially true in longer term therapy. Interestingly, for less disturbed patients, if a positive relationship is not in place by six sessions then it is unlikely to develop (48). This is emphatically not the case for more disturbed patients. Important work by Frank and Gunderson (49) has shown that schizophrenic patients may take up to 6 months to demonstrate

the development of a positive relationship with the therapist. The positive relationship predictive of good outcome seems to be characterized by a caring attachment between the patient and therapist. The patient will experience this as feeling understood, as having a sense that the therapist regards him or her in a positive manner, as having a feeling that there is mutual understanding between the two of them, and by experiencing a subjective "good feeling" towards the therapist. In addition to the technical factors mentioned above, such a relationship is more apt to develop when patient and therapist demonstrate shared membership, that is, when there is some sense of the two belonging to the same group. Most important among the similarities between patient and therapist which assist this sense is shared mutual interests.

CONCLUSION

In closing, an important fact emerging from psychotherapy research should be kept in mind. Although there have been well over 600 studies examining the effectiveness of psychotherapy, there is little support for differences between therapy techniques. There is little evidence for differences between "schools of therapy." There is however, tremendous difference among therapists and their effectiveness as measured by patient benefits. A major basis for such differences between therapists appears to be in the capacity of therapists to develop positive therapeutic alliances. Thus, the best of current information suggests that this task must be the main, continuing and essential focus of a therapist's attention.

References

1. Klerman GL, Weissman MM, Rousaville BJ, et al: *Interpersonal Psychotherapy of Depression.* New York, Basic Books, 1984.
2. Eysenck H: The effects of psychotherapy: an evaluation. *J Consult Psychol* 16:319–324, 1952.
3. Truax, CB: Effective ingredients in psychotherapy: an approach to unraveling the patient–therapist interaction. *Journal of Counseling Psychology* 10:256–263, 1963.
4. Prioleau L, Murdock M, Brody N: An analysis of

psychotherapy versus placebo studies. *Behav Brian Sci* 2:275–309, 1983.

5. Meltzoff J, Kornreich M: *Research in Psychotherapy.* New York, Atherton Press, 1970.

6. Luborsky L, Singer B, Luborsky L: Comparative studies of psychotherapies. Is it true that "everyone has won and all must have prizes?" *Arch Gen Psychiatry* 32:995–1008, 1975.

7. Bergin AE, Lambert MJ: Evaluation of therapeutic outcomes. In Bergin AE, Garfield JL (eds): *Handbook of Psychotherapy and Behavioral Change,* ed 2. New York, Wiley, 1978, pp 139–189.

8. Smith ML, Glass GV, Miller TI: *The Benefits of Psychotherapy.* Baltimore, Johns Hopkins University Press, 1980.

9. Cohen J: *Statistical Power Analysis for the Behavioral Science.* New York, Academic Press, 1977.

10. Rosenthal R, Rubin DB: A simple, general purpose display of magnitude of experimental effect. *J Ed Psychol* 74:166–169.

11. Shapiro DA, Shapiro D: Meta-analysis of comparative therapy outcomes studies: a replication and refinement. *Psychol Bull* 92:581–604.

12. Andrews G, Harvey R: Does psychotherapy benefit neurotic patients? Analysis of the Smith, Glass and Miller data. *Arch Gen Psych* 38:1213–1218, 1981.

13. Mumford E, Schlesinger HJ, Glass GV: Problems of analyzing the cost offset of including a mental health component in primary care. In *Institute of Medicine: Mental Health Services in General Health Care.* Washington, DC, National Academy of Sciences, 1979.

14. Mumford E, Schlesinger HJ, Glass GV: The effects of psychological intervention on recovery from surgery and heart attacks: an analysis of the literature. *Am J Public Health* 72:141, 1982.

15. *The Boston Globe,* July 22, 1987.

16. Shaw B: Specification of the training and evaluation of cognitive therapists for outcome studies. In Williams JS, Spitzer RL (eds): *Psychotherapy Research.* New York, Guilford, 1984, pp 173–188.

17. Community Mental Health Center Panel Survey, 1978.

18. *Mental and Nervous Disorders Utilization and Cost Survey (Manual).* Washington, DC, Blue Cross/Blue Shield, 1977.

19. Malan DH: *The Frontier of Brief Psychotherapy.* New York, Plenum Press, 1976.

20. Sifneos P: *Short-Term Psychotherapy and Emotional Crisis.* Cambridge, Harvard University Press, 1972.

21. Mann J, Goldman R: *A Casebook in Time-Limited Psychotherapy.* New York, McGraw-Hill, 1982.

22. Davanloo H (ed): *Basic Principles and Techniques in Short-Term Dynamic Therapy.* New York, SP Medical and Scientific Books, 1978.

23. Beck AT, Rush AJ, Shaw BF, et al: *Cognitive Therapy of Depression.* New York, Guilford Press, 1979.

24. Rehm LP: A self-control model of depression. *Behav Ther* 8:787–804, 1977.

25. Lewinsohn PM, Anlonuccio P, Steinnetz J, et al: *The Coping with Depression Course: A Psychoeducation Intervention for Unipolar Depression.* University of Oregon, 1982.

26. Bellack AS, Hersen M, Himmellock JM: Social skills training compared with pharmacotherapy and psychotherapy in the treatment of unipolar depression. *Am J Psychiatry* 138:1562–1567, 1981.

27. Ferster CB: Classification of behavioral pathology. In Krasner L, Ullmann LP (eds): *Research in Behavior Modification.* New York, Holt, Rinehart and Winston, 1965, pp 6–26.

28. Barlow DH, Wolfe BE: Behavioral approaches to anxiety disorders—a report on the NIMH–SUNY, Albany Research Conference. *J Consult Clin Psychol* 49:448–454, 1981.

29. Barlow DH, O'Brian GT, Last CG: Couples treatment of agoraphobia. *Behav Ther* 15:41–58, 1984.

30. Gelder MG: Psychological treatment for anxiety disorders: a review. *J R Soc Med* 19:230–233, 1986.

31. Foa E, Stekettec GS, Milby MB: Differential effects of exposure and response prevention in obsessive–compulsive washers. *J Consult Clin Psychol* 48:71–74.

32. McGlashan TH: Intensive individual psychotherapy of schizophrenia (a review of techniques). *Arch Gen Psychiatry* 40:909–920, 1983.

33. Gunderson J, Frank A: Effects of psychotherapy in schizophrenia. *The Yale Journal of Biology and Medicine* 58:373–381, 1985.

34. Hogarty GE, Goldberg SC, Schooler NR, et al: Drug and sociotherapy in the aftercare of schizophrenic patients: II. Two year relapse rate. *Arch Gen Psychiatry* 31:603–608, 1974.

35. Falloon I, Boyd J, McGill CW, et al: Family management in the prevention of exacerbation of schizophrenia: a controlled study. *N Engl J Med* 306:1437–1440, 1982.

36. Gerald Anderson CM, Reese DJ, Hogarty G: *Schizophrenia and the Family: A Practitioner's Guide to Psychoeducation and Management.* New York, Guilford Press, 1986.

37. Rogers CR: The necessary and sufficient conditions of therapeutic personality change. *J Consult Clin Psychol* 21:95–103, 1957.

38. Frank JD: Therapeutic components of psychotherapy. *J Nerv Ment Dis* 159:325–342, 1974.

39. Bordin ES: The generalized ability of the psychoanalytic concept of the working alliance. *Psychotherapy* 16:252–260, 1979.

40. Bordin ES: *Of Human Bonds That Bind or Free.* Presidential address at Society for Psychotherapy Research meeting, Pacific Grove, CA, 1980.

41. Hartley DE: Research on the therapeutic alliance in psychotherapy. *Annual Review* 4:532–549.

42. Moras K, Strupp HH: Pretherapy interpersonal relations, patients' alliance and outcome of brief therapy. *Arch Gen Psychiatry* 39:405–409, 1982.

43. Suh CS, Strupp HH, O'Malley SS: The Vanderbilt Process Measures: The Psychotherapy Process Scale (VPPS) and the Negative Indication Scale (VNIS). In Greenberg LS, Pinsof WM (eds): *The*

Psychotherapeutic Process: A Research Handbook. New York, Guilford Press, 1986, pp 285–323.

44. Luborsky, McLellan AT, Woodly G, et al: Therapist's success and its determinants. *Arch Gen Psychiatry* 42:602–611, 1985.

45. Foreman SA, Marmar CR: Therapist actions that address initially poor therapeutic alliances in psychotherapy. *Am J Psychiatry* 143:922–926, 1985.

46. Frieswyk SH, Colson DB, Allen JG: Conceptualizing the therapeutic alliance from a psychoanalytic perspective. *Psychotherapy* 21:460–464, 1984.

47. Luborsky L, Auerbach A: The therapeutic relationship in psychodynamic psychotherapy: the research evidence and its meaning for practice. In *Psychiatry Update: American Psychiatric Association Annual Review.* Washington, DC, American Psychiatric Press, 1985, vol 4, pp 526–637.

48. Marziali E: Three viewpoints on the therapeutic alliance: similarities, differences and associations with psychotherapy outcomes. *J Nerv Ment Dis* 172:417–423, 1984.

49. Frank AF, Gunderson JG: The role of the therapeutic alliance in the treatment of schizophrenia: effects on course and outcome. Submitted for publication.

46

Group Psychotherapy

J. Scott Rutan, Ph.D.
Arnold Cohen, Ph.D.

"By the crowd they have been broken, by the crowd they shall be healed." (22)

GROUPS IN EVERYDAY LIFE

People live their lives in groups. We are born into a family group and from that time on we spend most of our lives in one group or another. The types of experiences we have in the various groups in which we participate have a profound impact on our functioning, our self-image, our self-esteem, and our fundamental psychologic health.

One needs only to observe the interaction between a mother and baby to see the powerful need to affiliate that is present from our earliest moments. We then move through school groups, religious groups, peer groups, work groups, and recreational groups as we mature and develop. The capacity to gain enjoyment and solace from others, as well as to give it, is a necessary prerequisite for a full life. Therefore, the acquisition of effective interpersonal skills is crucial to healthy functioning.

Modern society seems to be moving toward a renewed recognition of and appreciation of that basic fact. The "me generation" shows signs of fading, and we can perhaps describe our present time as a postnarcissistic era. In the Encounter Groups so popular in the 1960s, individuals used these groups to strengthen narcissism and the capacity for self-gratification. Today, as evidenced by the attention self-psychologists pay to the capacity to be empathic as a prerequisite for mental health, we see a renewed recognition of the importance of reciprocity and mutuality in relationships. In both intimate relationships and global politics, interdependence is viewed as more viable than independence.

Psychotherapy in groups is a relatively new phenomenon. In response to the great need for mental health care for vast numbers of individuals during World War II, psychodynamic therapists began seeing patients in groups (1). Initially this was done purely as an effort at efficiency, and the therapist essentially conducted multiple individual psychotherapies simultaneously. The group functioned largely as an audience, watching the therapist work with one or another member. Soon, however, group therapists began noting some specifically therapeutic functions of the group itself. These factors are considered below.

645

Gradually practitioners in most major schools of therapy began using groups. Today we have psychodynamic therapy groups, behavioral therapy groups, psychopharmacologic groups, and so on.

EFFECTS OF GROUPS ON PERSONALITY

Most major theories of personality include or imply the importance of others in the formation of personality (see Chapters 4 and 5). Therefore it follows that groups may have a profound effect on personality changes. As an example of this, let us consider three major schools of thought: psychodynamic, behavioral, and biologic theories of personality.

Psychodynamic Theories

In classical psychoanalytic theory (S. Freud) (2) the mother–child dyad is the foundation of personality. Psychologic structures originally develop out of the interactions between mother and child. A safe and trusting early relationship allows the infant to successfully pass through the first stages of development and help the infant come to view the world as essentially a safe and nurturing environment. Later and more advanced psychologic structures are based on the interaction of the growing child with ever-enlarging spheres of relationships with others. Inner conflicts between biologic drives and the society in which one lives result in the development of an ego, or a sense of self. This sense of self is highly influenced by the view the growing child has of the people he or she encounters as being benign or malevolent. The goal of therapy is to help the individual gain understanding regarding the traumatic and unacceptable memories, impulses, and feelings that are "repressed" and therefore made unconscious.

Ego psychology (A. Freud [3], Hartmann [4]) is a modification of classic psychoanalytic theory in which the classical definition of ego is expanded and elevated. The

importance of other people in the formation of one's ego is emphasized even more in this school of thought, and the goal of therapy is to strengthen the ego so that the defenses employed by the individual are more appropriate, effective, and flexible.

Self psychology (Kohut [5, 6]) places the self at the center of mental functioning. One's sense of self is derived through the relationships one has with the important others ("selfobjects") in development. One gains a healthy sense of who one is through seeing oneself mirrored empathically and accurately by others. Empathic failures by those important others result in narcissistic injury and failure to develop a healthy and accurate sense of self, including a flawed capacity to be empathic toward others.

Object relations theory (Klein [7], Fairbairn [8], Winnicott [9],) elevates the importance of relationships to the highest level. From this point of view, individuals cannot exist without others. The cornerstone of this theory is the importance of attachment to other people, and the drive toward attachment is considered primary. Thus, the relationships one has with others are both the total basis for psychological health or illness and at the same time the sole vehicle for change. The quality of one's personal relationships is the key to mental health. The role of therapy is to help the individual gain the ability to love and be loved more effectively.

Behavioral Theories

Behavioral theories (Skinner [10]) of personality are based on empirical evidence, and behaviorists distrust the subjective evidence cited by psychodynamic theorists to support their views. In this school of thought psychopathology is the result of learning, just as is psychologic health. The difference between health and pathology is that disturbed behavior is less socially adaptive and effective. One need not posit the existence of unobservable emotional states in order to understand behavior. Thus, the goal of therapy is not to "make the unconscious conscious," but rather to provide the client with more adaptive behaviors.

Behavior is learned through rewards. According to Skinner's "operant conditioning" theory, individuals "operate" on their environment by sending out many behaviors. Some of these behaviors are rewarded, and these then become more frequent. This is different from Pavlov's "respondent conditioning" theory, in which a stimuli which previously elicited behavior can be replaced by another stimuli if the second becomes associated with the first.

Without elaboration of the nuances of various behavioral theories, it is clear that for all behavioral theorists, other people are the primary stimuli which reward and do not reward various behaviors. Thus, in this theory as in those presented above, the groups to which individuals belong over lifetimes have powerful influence over the resulting behavior repertoires of the personalities of those individuals.

Biologic Theories

According to biologic approaches (Kraepelin [11]), clinical syndromes and personality can best be understood in terms of biologic processes. There is, however, considerable knowledge that clinical manifestations of major syndromes are affected by family behavior, that clinical response to psychopharmacologic agents are affected by the patient's relation to the therapist, and that the immunologic system is affected by psychosocial stress (see Chapters 3, 6, and 32 for discussion of the above). In sum, a person's biology is affected by psychosocial conditions, much of which are mediated through groups.

Conclusion

No matter where one places oneself on the widely varying spectrum of theoretical understanding of personality, the fundamental importance of other people in influencing psychologic well-being or illness is a given. How that influence is transmitted varies from theory to theory, but the influence itself does not. Consequently, the fact that groups can be uniquely helpful to individuals in distress should not come as a surprise. Nor should it surprise us that groups can work for individuals in a variety of different ways.

DIFFERENT MODELS OF HELPING PEOPLE THROUGH GROUPS

Mental health providers use many different types of groups to assist psychologically troubled individuals. It seems clear that simply putting individuals into groups under certain conditions has some beneficial effect in and of itself. A rudimentary understanding of different types of groups may help to place individuals in groups appropriate to their needs and stated goals. For now, we shall attempt to categorize some of the major ways in which groups are used to assist patients. We can begin by dividing groups into two types: (a) Ego supportive and (b) ego regressive.

Ego-Supportive Groups

Ego-supportive groups focus on supporting and nurturing the individuals who comprise them. The goal is to help people move ahead without having to resolve past conflicts and without having to reexperience painful situations or feelings. Some leaders who use this model do so because they do not believe it is necessary to understand history or to go through cathartic emotional experiences. They believe that supporting the ego is sufficient to help people grow. Others use this model because they feel it has beneficial effects even though they also believe in the beneficial effects of therapeutic regression. For such leaders, ego-supportive groups have special value in specific situations and/or with specific populations.

In ego-supportive groups members focus on the universal aspects of life, gaining recognition that they are not alone in their struggles and that their experiences are not entirely unique. They will work together to learn new ways of coping with situations, and they will focus on mirroring back to one another the positive aspects of self. Such approaches have many distinct advantages. For many individuals, the recognition that others share their worries and symptoms is very healing. Bulimic patients, for example, are often filled with shame and self-degradation over their symptom. The opportunity to speak openly with others who have the same symptom is healing.

The socially inept individual is uniquely served by such groups because they not only use the group as a mini-laboratory in which they practice interpersonal skills, but they also have the opportunity to "belong" to a community, which in itself is often a very new experience.

Probably the majority of groups run by mental health professionals are ego supportive in nature. They include but are not limited to psychoeducational groups, self-help groups, support groups, and inpatient community meetings.

Ego-Regressive Groups

Ego-regressive groups focus on encouraging regression and exploration of the past in the expectation that this will allow people to work out past conflicts. By resolving early conflicts an individual can move to a higher level of functioning. Several different theories of personality fall under the ego-regressive model (psychoanalytic, ego psychology, object relations, etc.). Each of these has implicit and explicit convictions abut how people change and grow.

Despite the many theoretical differences, ego-regressive approaches have important commonalities. They all emphasize emotionally charged interchanges and the consequent development of self-understanding as vehicles for change and growth (1). The focus of these groups is on characterologic change.

As opposed to the ego-supportive approach, the ego-regressive model defines the support and nurturing of individuals within the group differently. The goal is to encourage the open expression of affective responses to interactions in and out of the group. This sometimes means that people are not overtly warm and nurturing but rather are angry and confrontative. These expressions of affect are ultimately what makes the group work effectively. Members learn to work out relationships in the face of strong affective material. In such groups special attention is paid to the powerful transference reactions which occur. These include both vertical transference (transference relating to authority and parents) and horizonal transference (transference relating to peers and siblings). Transference phenomena are powerful regressive forces in groups. Ego-supportive groups attempt to minimize transference responses, while ego-regressive groups use transference as a stimulus for regression and as an opportunity for learning.

Ego-supportive and ego-regressive groups are both effective ways of working with our patients. Each has something to offer a person in distress. Next we shall explore the curative factors that are present in all groups.

CURATIVE FACTORS IN GROUPS

How does group therapy help patients? This question is no longer as elusive as it was 20 years ago. Current research and theory has elaborated the elements that help us understand what is curative about group therapy.

Yalom's (12) comprehensive study helps us understand the curative factors that operate in every type of therapy group (ego regressive or ego supportive). Rutan and Stone (1) discuss curative factors that operate in psychodynamic (ego-regressive) therapy groups. Below is a discussion of both sets of curative factors.

Yalom's Curative Factors

Yalom (12) divided the curative factors into 10 primary categories:

1. Imparting of information,
2. Instillation of hope,
3. Universality,

4. Altruism,
5. The corrective recapitulation of the primary family group,
6. Development of socializing techniques,
7. Imitative behavior,
8. Interpersonal learning,
9. Group cohesiveness,
10. Catharsis.

Yalom suggests that these factors assume a differential importance depending on the goals and compositions of specific groups. Though present to some degree in individual therapy, each of these curative factors is uniquely powerful in groups.

Imparting of information includes didactic instruction about mental health, mental illness or psychodynamics. It also includes advice, suggestions, or direct guidance about life problems. In individual therapy, the therapist is the sole source of such information, and in some traditions (e.g., psychoanalytic schools) the role of the therapist precludes much direct imparting of information. In groups the other patients become a resource of information. Often information offered by fellow patients is especially meaningful and useful to individuals.

Instillation of hope is essential for any group to be effective. This is true for all therapies, not just for group therapy. Research studies (13) have demonstrated that high pretherapy expectation is significantly correlated with positive therapy outcome. In group therapy an individual has the unusual opportunity to observe others get better. This often instills hope in patients still struggling with their problems.

As patients perceive their similarity to others and share their most intimate feelings, they experience a relief that they are not alone in their struggles. This *universalizing* experience is extremely helpful to patients who think that they are the only ones who have problems or that their acts or life experiences are shamefully different from all others. In group therapy an individual often hears fellow members going through familiar struggles. A patient often

experiences great relief to know that they are not alone.

People often feel better about themselves when they feel they can help another person. *Altruistic acts* set healing forces in motion in group therapy. Unlike individual therapy, a patient in group therapy has the opportunity to help others get better. When this occurs individuals often feel an increase in self-esteem.

A therapy group usually evokes many early memories of family life. The *corrective recapitulation of the primary family group* is an important element in how groups help people to get better. Group therapy offers the unique opportunity to reexperience the feelings of growing up in one's own family. The myriad relationships in group recapitulate family life and allow for a different and better way of working these relationships out. In psychodynamic groups this allows for reawakening of old memories, providing an opportunity for reworking painful historical material. In behavioral groups this allows individuals an opportunity to learn different behaviors from a different "family."

Social learning is present in any group experience. The *development of socializing techniques* varies greatly from group to group. The development of basic social skills is a curative factor in all therapy groups. The group is like a laboratory where an individual can observe various coping styles and try out new behaviors. The many different kinds of relationships in group therapy offer a unique opportunity to an individual needing to learn more effective socializing skills.

Imitative behavior, according to Yalom, is diffuse in groups because of the variety of people present to imitate. However, it is important in the therapeutic process. Although it may be short-lived, it often helps people to experiment with new sets of behaviors. The variety of relationships available in group therapy offers a person several different options of behavior to imitate and learn from.

Interpersonal learning and *group cohesiveness* are considered the two most important curative factors. Yalom sees interpersonal learning as an analogue to insight, working through the transference, and the corrective emotional experience in individual therapy. In the Sullivanian (14) tradition Yalom conceptualizes personality as the product of interpersonal interactions. Therefore, problems are worked out through interpersonal learning. The multiple horizonal transferences available in group therapy allow for a unique opportunity to work out interpersonal relationships.

Yalom uses the term "group cohesiveness" as an analogue to the therapeutic relationship in individual therapy. He suggests that the nature of the relationship in individual therapy is critical to the outcome of therapy. He believes this to be true for group therapy as well. If group cohesiveness is not present it is highly unlikely that an individual will benefit from the group experience. The sense of belonging, of being in a common endeavor, that one experiences in a group in unique and is an important part of the healing process.

Catharsis is a valuable part of the curative process in the psychodynamic traditions. Strong expression of emotion enhances the development of cohesiveness and a sense of belonging. This in turn creates an atmosphere where all the curative factors are more likely to exist. There is a reciprocal relationship between all the other curative factors and catharsis. In addition, one often feels safe in a group to express strong emotion because of the number of relationships available for support.

Rutan and Stone's Curative Factors

Rutan and Stone speak from a psychodynamic tradition regarding how groups affect change. Whether or not these dynamic processes are addressed in a particular group, they are nonetheless in operation.

They suggest that curative factors can be separated into mechanisms of change and processes of change (1). The psychologic mechanisms of prime importance are imitation, identification, and internalization. The important processes of change are confrontation, clarification, interpretation, and working through.

Mechanisms of Change

Much of early learning in groups is *imitative*. Patients can observe other members interact intensely and learn that they are not harmed by the expression of strong emotions. In fact, they see that members are often drawn closer by these exchanges. Patients see hope in the process and begin expressing feelings by imitating others' behaviors.

Identification can be defined in many ways. Rutan and Stone use the description by Loewald: "an unconscious process in which the subject takes on parts or aspects of the object" (15). By taking on aspects of another, the individual changes by altering his or her perceptions or affects.

Internalization is the most advanced and durable mechanism of change. In internalization, change is not the result of something taken in from the outside but rather is due to a shift in psychic structure. A person moves to a more mature level of functioning.

Processes of Change

The ways in which the mechanisms of change occur are through the processes of confrontation, clarification, interpretation, and working through.

Confrontations primarily address external aspects of behavior. They are usually observations or responses to interactions or comments about affects. In groups confrontations occur all the time by members as well as the leader. It should be mentioned that confrontations can be constructive, destructive, or both. It depends on the atmosphere that has been created in the group.

Rutan and Stone use Greenson's (16) definition for *clarification*: "Clarification refers to those activities that aim at placing the psychic phenomenon being analyzed in sharp focus. The significant details have to be dug out and carefully separated from extraneous matter." Clarification serves to organize and highlight important data that occurs in the group.

Interpretations are different from clarifications in that they are aimed at the unconscious. Interpretations attach meaning to an event or behavior. They attempt to help the patient gain an understanding of hidden motivations and conflicts. The timing of interpretations is critical. In groups there are several different kinds of interpretations. Knowing which to make when is the art of group therapy. In group therapy, some of the most poignant and powerful interpretations are made by patients.

Working through is the final essential element in enabling patients to change. In working through the emphasis is on increasing the patients' capacity to examine themselves, understand conflicts and areas of vulnerability, interpret their own behavior, and on helping them develop a more varied and flexible defensive system.

THE GROUP CONTRACT

In order for the curative factors to take effect a safe therapeutic environment must be developed. Groups can be dangerous and frightening places. One of the first scholars to study groups was Gustav LeBon (17), a French sociologist who began to study the power of groups in 1885. He was primarily interested in the destructive powers that groups had for the individuals who composed them. He described large crowds as regressive, primitive, and uncivilized. He stated:

By the mere fact that he forms part of an organized group, man descends several rungs in the ladder of civilization. Isolated he may be a cultivated individual; in a crowd he is a barbarian—that is, a creature acting by instinct. (17)

Making the group a safe place is a primary responsibility of the group therapist. The major foundation of creating a safe effective environment is the group contract. Clear goals and purposes are essential to the effectiveness of a group. William McDougall (18), an Englishman writing at the same time as LeBon, concurred with

LeBon about the power of groups. However, he saw the potential for groups to enhance the behavior of individuals. The key to turning the power of groups into a positive force was organization.

There is . . . one condition that may raise the behavior of a temporary and unorganized crowd to a higher plane, namely the presence of a clearly defined common purpose in the minds of its members. (18)

The group contract is the organizing principle of any group. It provides the basic structure, informs the members about how to use the group effectively, provides stability, contains and reduces anxiety, builds trust and predictability, and teaches and reminds members about responsibility. Rutan and Stone write,

The contract is the foundation for a productive and safe therapeutic environment. . . . We are convinced that any group needs a clear contract in order to be effective. (1)

The group contract is an essential curative factor. A therapist should give careful consideration to the type of contract he or she wants members to agree to before starting a group.

There are several essential elements that should be included as part of a group contract regardless of the orientation of the leader or the focus of the group (19). These essential elements are as follows.

Time, Place, and Fee

The time of the group, the place where the group will meet, and the cost of the group should all be presented and agreed to before an individual joins a group.

Attendance

A high priority must be placed on this element of the contract. The therapist should encourage as much continuity as possible in order to create a safe and trusting environment. Continuity is one of the cornerstones of the development of trusting relationships.

Nature of Relationships

This element of the contract offers guidelines to members about what types of behaviors are expected from them once they have become a part of the group. For example, therapists might have in their contract something about "no physical contact," or they might say that "socializing outside the group is discouraged." This aspect of the contracts helps prospective members develop a cognitive understanding of what to expect from the relationships in the group. This would also let prospective members know, for example, if they were entering an ego-supportive or ego-regressive experience.

Process

This aspect of the contract spells out what actually happens in a specific group session—how the group works. In other words, a therapist running a long-term psychodynamic psychotherapy group might tell prospective group members that they are expected to relate their memories, feelings, and associations as openly and spontaneously as possible during a group session. However, a therapist running a time-limited parent education group might tell a prospective member that the therapist will present information for the first half hour and then have responses to that material and open discussion for the last hour of the group.

Confidentiality

Confidentiality is a fundamental ingredient in the development of therapeutic relationships. All groups need an agreement about what can and cannot be repeated outside the group meetings. Depending on the nature of the group, these guidelines have varying degrees of strictness. Some therapists ask that nothing be communicated outside the group session. Others focus on protecting the identities of the members of the group, recognizing that it is probably impossible to require that members never speak of

their groups outside the group itself. What is important is that people feel that what they say in the group will be treated responsibly by the others. If it is discovered that a member has breached the confidentiality of another, the leader must address this in the group immediately.

Termination

Some agreement must be reached between the members and the therapist about when and how to leave the group. In time-limited groups this usually presents no problem because people are generally expected to attend each group session. In open-ended groups the issue becomes more complicated. Some therapists give a stated number of meetings that a person must attend after they announce they are leaving the group. Other therapists use a more general guideline, such as "members are expected to remain in the group until the problems that brought them to the group have been resolved." Again, what is important is that a clear procedure about how one is to leave the group is set forth from the beginning.

Within these categories there can and will be many variations. The nature of the group and the therapist's orientation will greatly influence the contract that will be presented to a prospective member. Nonetheless, it is important that a contract is clearly and overtly presented to members. A sample psychodynamic contract would be as follows: (1)

1. To be present each week, to be on time, and to remain throughout the meeting.
2. To work actively on the problems that brought you to the group.
3. To put feelings into words not actions.
4. To use the relationships made in the group therapeutically and not socially.
5. To remain in the group until the problems that brought you to the group have been resolved.
6. To be responsible for your bill.
7. To protect the identities of your fellow members.

REFERRING TO GROUP THERAPY

We believe the great majority of patients seen in psychotherapy can be helped by group therapy, either as the exclusive or a supplemental mode of therapy. The interpersonal setting of a group provides for generalized learning that translates naturally to the world at large. The interpersonal skills learned in a group provide immediate assistance in the life of the patient.

Referring patients to groups is not an easy process. While many individuals are eager to join groups, perhaps most patients come for individual therapy and the idea of sharing the therapeutic time with others is not a pleasant one. Further, the prospect of talking about one's feelings and one's "secrets" in public is difficult. Finally, groups do not offer the promise of a professional caretaker who will listen empathically to whatever a patient may choose to say. Rather, in groups there is always the possibility that another member will say something that will be hurtful (albeit possibly correct).

When referring a patient to a group it is important that the patient's presenting concern be directly linked to the specific effectiveness of group therapy. Thus, when individuals come to therapy to gain help in increasing self-esteem, or to achieve more gratifying relationships, or to gain understanding about why others react to them as they do, these are natural reasons to suggest that the interpersonal setting of a group might provide immediate and valuable information to these patients. It is our conviction that most patients seeking psychotherapy in this era do so, at least in part, in order to improve their capacity to relate better and more intimately with others. Thus, in a great many cases patients can be helped to see how therapy groups can assist them in gaining their goals.

Nonetheless, a patient should never be forced or manipulated into a group. The affective power of a group can be quite overpowering for some. And the honesty with which groups can quickly confront members on uncomfortable aspects of their behavior can be extremely painful to others. If a patient finds him- or herself in a painful situation in a group that the patient had not really wanted to join in the first place, the patient will probably not gain the full advantage of the group experience. Furthermore, this is exactly the type of patient who most readily quits the group prematurely, which not only does not make for a therapeutic experience for that patient but also hinders the work for all the other group members.

When a group is working well, it is a powerful healing force. For a group to be working at peak efficiency, the members should be committed to the group, should feel safe enough to take personal risks within the group, and should be willing to help others in the group even though at times that means putting self-needs second.

TRAINING IN GROUP THERAPY

It is tempting to begin group therapy by simply bringing together a group of patients and commencing. However, groups are complicated entities, and the ability to lead therapy groups is a skill that requires both extensive training and supervised experience. The American Group Psychotherapy Association has compiled a booklet outlining the prerequisites for training in group therapy (20). Therapists interested in becoming group therapists should consult that document and seek a senior member of that association for consultation and supervision before beginning groups.

There is growing research evidence that groups are uniquely helpful to our patients, irrespective of their pathology (21). With proper training therapists can unleash the powerful therapeutic forces inherent in groups and make them available to their patients.

References

1. Rutan JS, Stone WN: *Psychodynamic Group Psychotherapy*. New York, Macmillan Publishing, 1984.

2. Freud S: *The Standard Edition.* London, Hogarth Press, 1953–74.
3. Freud A: *The Ego and the Mechanisms of Defense.* New York, International Universities Press, 1936.
4. Hartmann H: *Ego Psychology and the Problem of Adaptation.* New York, International Universities Press, 1939.
5. Kohut H: *The Analysis of the Self.* New York, International Universities Press, 1971.
6. Kohut H: *The Restoration of the Self.* New York, International Universities Press, 1977.
7. Klein M: *Contributions to Psychoanalysis: 1921–1945.* New York, McGraw-Hill, 1964.
8. Fairbairn WRD: *An Object Relations Theory of the Personality.* New York, Basic Books, 1952.
9. Winnicott DW: *The Maturational Process and the Facilitating Environment.* New York, International Universities Press, 1965.
10. Skinner BF: *The Behavior of Organisms: An Experimental Analysis.* New York, Appleton-Century-Crofts, 1938.
11. Kraepelin E: *One Hundred Years of Psychiatry.* New York, Citadel Press, 1962.
12. Yalom I: *The Theory and Practice of Group Psychotherapy.* New York, Basic Books, 1975.
13. Goldstein AP: *Therapist Patient Expectancies in Psychotherapy.* New York, Pergamon Press, 1962.
14. Sullivan HS: *The Interpersonal Theory of Psychiatry.* New York, Norton, 1953.
15. Loewald HW: On internalization. *Int J Psychoanal* 54:9–17, 1973.
16. Greenson RR: *The Technique and Practice of Psychoanalysis.* New York, International Universities Press, 1967.
17. LeBon G: *The Crowd: A Study of the Popular Mind.* New York, Fisher, Unwin, 1920.
18. McDougall W: *The Group Mind.* New York, G. P. Putnam's Sons, 1920.
19. Englander T: *The facilitating environment and the contract in group psychotherapy.* Unpublished doctoral dissertation, Fielding Institute.
20. *Suggested Guidelines for the Training of Group Psychotherapists.* New York, American Group Psychotherapy Association.
21. Dies RR, MacKensie KR (eds): *Advances in Group Psychotherapy: Integrating Research and Practice.* New York, International Universities Press, 1983.
22. Marsh C: An experiment in group treatment at Worcester State Hospital. *Mental Hygiene* 17:406–407, 1933.

47

Family and Couples Therapy

William Vogel, Ph.D.

Family psychotherapy in the United States had its origin in the decade from 1950 to 1960; by the mid 1960s, family therapy was a familiar concept to all mental health professionals (1). The 1960s were a time of great technologic and intellectual ferment in the mental health field, and a time of great discontent with established approaches. Many professionals who worked in child guidance clinics, discouraged with traditional one-on-one techniques then commonly used with their child patients or with the children's mothers, found themselves "discovering" family therapy. The traditional child guidance technique, whereby one therapist worked intensively with the child patient while another worked intensively with the child's mother, with the two therapists occasionally meeting and exchanging views, seemed to lack efficacy in many cases. Clinicians discovered that whatever was being attempted by this traditional one-on-one approach might easily be negated, deliberately or inadvertently, by those family members who were not included in the treatment sessions.

Further, it gradually became apparent to the profession that the primary complaints of mothers who brought their children to child guidance clinics often had less to do with the child's "crazy" or "bad" behavior per se than with the nature of the interaction between the child and the mother (e.g., "he won't listen to me"; "I tell her a dozen times to bathe and it never gets done"; "I'm worried about him—he seems to have so few friends and to do so poorly in school"). It was, however, precisely that kind of presenting complaint—the troubled nature of the parent–child interaction—that was rarely addressed or even directly observed by traditional methods, since, prior to the advent of family psychotherapy, the mother and child would be separately evaluated and treated.

Yet another impetus to the family therapy movement was the troublesome observation of many workers that children in traditional individual treatment who were perceived by therapists as "getting better" were frequently perceived by their parents as "getting worse." This perception was presumably a result of the difficulty with which parents, in some troubled family systems, adjusted to the children's increased assertiveness and drive for independence.

A further impetus to the growth of family therapy was the women's liberation movement of the 1960s. The traditional child guidance treatment method (mother

655

and the "identified problem" child separately evaluated and treated in psychodynamically oriented psychotherapy) had remained unchanged and unchallenged for over 50 years. Those of us who were working in the decade of the 1960s will recall growing numbers of angry mothers who demanded to know why child guidance workers found it necessary to involve mothers of troubled children in intake and treatment sessions, but not fathers. Both parents, they reasoned, should share equal responsibility for child rearing.

The family therapy movement, then, was a phenomenon which grew both from professionals' dissatisfaction with traditional techniques and practice and with public demand for changes in these practices. These events corresponded in time with increased clinical and scholarly interest in group and family processes in general, an interest which grew considerably after World War II.

AIMS OF FAMILY THERAPY

The diverse group of workers who call themselves family therapists share the orientation that individuals' personalities and behavioral aberrations cannot be understood apart from the family context in which the individual currently operates (2). They believe that psychotherapy, to be effective, must of necessity involve the current family members. There is, however, wide diversity among family therapists as to what kind of family involvement is necessary for therapy to take place. Despite the diversity of theories and methods which characterize different schools, there are particular aims which characterize all family therapy, although the various theoretical schools and frameworks vary widely in the degree of emphasis given to achieving the particular aims (3). Some of these similar aims are as follows:

To Enhance and Facilitate Adaptive Verbal Communications Among Family Members. Members of dysfunctional families are characteristically polarized and unable to "hear" each other's communications. They may take refuge in silence and

noncommunication or, alternatively, engage in constant oppositional verbal squabbling. One aim of family therapy is to help the family members to listen, understand what others are trying to communicate to them, and respond with unambiguous communications of their own (2).

To Enhance and Facilitate Empathic Communication. In conflicted families the therapist often finds one or more family members either locked in conflict with or isolated and withdrawn from the other family members. At times, one or the other mode of interaction may characterize the entire family, or members of an entire family may alternatively battle each other and then withdraw. What one rarely finds in a conflicted family is an ethos of empathic communication. Typically, one or more members of the family are emotionally isolated from the others. They have difficulty both giving or receiving emotional support. The aim of the therapist is to end that emotional isolation by encouraging emotional vulnerability: The therapist assists family members in expressing their feelings (4) and receiving emotional expression from others.

To Redress Power Imbalances. A frequent complaint in troubled families is "powerlessness": a child may complain, "no one cares what I think, they just order me around"; a wife may complain that her husband makes decisions affecting the family without consulting her; a father–husband may complain that his wife and children are allied against him and that he has no voice in the family; the designated healthy family members may complain that a psychotic, alcoholic, or delinquent family member is controlling the family by disrupting the lives of everyone else; or the person who the family identifies as the "sick one" may be unhappy because the other family members "won't let me alone." A major focus of family therapy is to help the family address such feelings of powerlessness (5–8).

To Address the Problem of Roles Definition. Family roles (wife–mother, husband–father, child–sibling) alter as a function of social change (e.g., women's liberation—changing norms which result in wage-earner status for both husband and wife) or as a function of maturation (a person who is an "ideal baby" may become a "troublesome teen"). Dysfunctional families commonly require help in adjusting to changing role definitions. It becomes a central task of the therapist to supply such help (9).

To Adapt to Changes in Family Structure. Crises may occur as a function of changes in family structure (divorce, death, children leaving home for school or marriage, family members unilaterally changing their roles). An important goal of the therapist is to help the family adopt a structure that will respond to change (10,11).

To Meet Crises. Families frequently come to professional attention when experiencing difficulty in meeting a crisis (suicide attempt, death, retirement, job firings, arrests, etc.). Such families may or may not be dysfunctional in any chronic or structural sense; rather, the family may be seeking someone to provide guidance and support through the current difficulty.

To Eliminate Scapegoating. The majority of families who are seen in family therapy identify one of their members as the patient (the identified patient, or IP in family therapy parlance; the designation IP connotes that the identification is the family's, not the therapist's). The identified patients are typically seen by the family as, and often see themselves as, the source of the family's difficulty. Such an identification removes a sense of responsibility for the family's plight from the nonidentified family members. It makes complex issues seem to appear to be simple and solvable, if only the IP would "cooperate." This identification further serves to project the family's hostility and rage onto the IP. The IP, on the other hand, often is not simply a victim but someone who has been trained into the scapegoat role. This role carries definite rewards of its own. Not being expected "to behave," the scapegoat may be inadvertently "excused" from fulfilling social norms to which the other family members are held.

No one in the family is very surprised if the scapegoat does poorly in school, or on the job, or shows social "misbehavior." Consequently, the scapegoat is often ambivalently viewed by other family members, being at the same time both despised and envied. For many family therapists, a major goal of family therapy is eliminating the scapegoat role in the family (5–8, 10–12).

THE SUBJECT MATTER OF FAMILY THERAPY

One of the most important ways in which family and individual psychotherapy differ has to do with the problems with which each deals. The therapist who works with individual patients most commonly treats symptoms such as depression, anxiety, malaise, helplessness, and purposelessness, which tend to be pervasive and lack specific focus. Family therapy, on the other hand, typically deals with some specific issue which the family sees as posing a problem for the family as a whole, as well as for each of its individual members. The issues vary with the family's concept of what constitutes a problem. For example, an adolescent's school failure, a family member's arrest for commission of a crime, or drug or alcohol abuse, may be considered by some families as family problems.

THE ROLE OF FAMILY THERAPY IN A TREATMENT PROGRAM

There is disagreement among practitioners of family therapy as to whether family therapy is just one *technique* among many others, such as individual psychotherapy, psychopharmacology, or group psychotherapy, or whether it is on *orientation*, a framework within which all treatment should be performed (13–15). The latter view is held by those family therapists who adhere to a "systems theory" approach, which maintains that individuals cannot be understood apart from their functioning within the family system. For systems theory, any attempt to treat an individual, or identified patient, rather than the whole family system, is seen as scapegoating or as blaming the victim. In the systems view, individual treatment (psychotherapeutic, psychopharmacologic) or even any form of individual diagnosis may be not only counterproductive, but destructive, because it focuses blame on the patient rather than placing responsibility on the family unit. For a systems theorist, diagnosis should be employed, not as a descriptive analysis of a complex psychopathologic traits or behavior originating within the individual, but as a descriptive analysis of "the relationship between the family and the therapist."

No question so divides practitioners of family therapy than the question of whether family therapy is an orientation or a technique, and no question more clearly divides the main body of family therapists from other mental health professionals. As a general rule, health professionals who identify themselves primarily as family therapists tend to adopt a systems view of this matter, regarding family therapy as an orientation, whereas those who work in the family therapy field but who primarily identify themselves as psychiatrists, psychologists, social workers, psychiatric nurses, or pastoral counselors will tend to regard family therapy as a technique.

Family therapists differ vastly among themselves as to which family members should be seen in therapy and when. Some practitioners require the presence of the entire family ("family" being defined as all those family members who live together under one roof and share a common address) for all psychotherapy sessions (13); others prefer to shift attendance at the family sessions as the focus of the family changes (9, 10); still others, after an initial intake with a family during which one child is the identified patient, will work primarily with the parents (16,17). The question of which family members should be seen and when is a question of technique and of what method one regards as most efficacious; it is not a question of theoretical philosophy. Thus, some family therapists who regard themselves as "system theorists" may see the parents in therapy sessions, omitting the "identified

patient" child, even though they regard the family as the focus of treatment.

A complex and important clinical task for those who regard family therapy as a technique rather than as an orientation is the decision whether to use individual therapy or family therapy. Consider for example, the following cases:

1. A 40-year-old woman who has a B.S. in nursing science and is married and the mother of two children, ages 18 and 19, feels she no longer loves her husband. She wishes to divorce him and return to school part-time, to obtain her master's degree while supporting herself through full-time employment. Her husband and two children strongly oppose her plans for divorce and wish the family to be seen in family therapy. She rejects the idea and wishes to be seen in individual psychotherapy.
2. A 21-year-old college junior has greatly disturbed his parents and two older brothers with his announcement that he does not wish to join them in the highly successful and prosperous family business. The family wishes to be seen as a unit in family therapy. The young man wishes to be seen individually.
3. A 25-year-old schizophrenic male, currently in remission, wishes to leave his family and live independently. This family opposes the plan because several times in the past after following such a plan, he has deteriorated into a psychotic state, requiring a prolonged stay in a state hospital. The family wishes to be seen in family therapy. The young man opposes that plan, wishing instead to be seen in individual psychotherapy.

Each of these cases presents the practitioner with a dilemma. The cases clearly involve family conflict, but to accept the cases as family psychotherapy cases, in which all family members are present and the family is treated as a unit, may be to side with the family against the "identified patient." The "identified patient" would, in that instance, be forced to acknowledge membership in the very family system from which he or she wishes to dissociate. The practitioner for whom family therapy is but one technique among others will consider the use of family therapy (either by itself, or as one element in a treatment plan) in those situations in which the IP's problem arises from the dynamic interplay of forces within the family with whom the IP resides, rather than primarily from the IP's intrapsychic conflict, or from the IP's problems in relating to the world outside of the family (14).

In one sense family therapy is in accord with the feminist revolution of the 1960s and 1970s in that family life is viewed as an interactive enterprise for which husband and wife, mother and father, bear joint responsibility. In another sense, family therapy is in accord with the conservative social influences of our day, in that by its very nature, family therapy serves to affirm the philosophy and the values associated with the concept of the traditional nuclear family.

THE PROCESS OF FAMILY THERAPY

In the past two decades, there has been a rapid proliferation of theoretical frameworks for family therapy. However, there are some problems which all family therapies face, and there are certain stages through which virtually any course of family therapy passes, most especially outpatient family therapy. These are discussed below.

Initial Contact

Some families, a small although growing number, make contact with a clinic or a practitioner and request family therapy. The majority, however, come to the family therapist through one of two other channels.

Many are sent by other health professionals who have been consulted by the family about one of its members who is giving the family concern. The health professional, knowing something of family therapy and conceptualizing the problem as involving the family rather than just the individual member, makes the family therapy referral. Others are sent by institutional representatives of school systems, court systems, etc., who apply pressure on the family to seek help that the family would not have sought on its own. In all of these cases in which the family has been "sent" to the therapist rather than sought help on its own, the family therapist must engage in a considerable educational process if treatment is to have any hope of success. That educational process involves helping the family understand why family therapy is being considered rather than individual therapy for the identified patient.

For any family, whether self- or other-referred, the initial contact with the therapist involves helping the family to accept the process and rules of family therapy; e.g., many family therapists will refuse to allow confidential communications from one family member to the therapist, such as telephone calls that begin "I don't want the rest of the family to know this, but . . ." For the same reason, many therapists refuse any request from a family member for a private meeting while family therapy is ongoing. Should one family member demand confidential individual interviews, most family therapists' require that the request be processed through the family. If individual therapy is appropriate, the family therapist would refer that individual to an outside agency for individual help while continuing to treat the family.

During the initial contact, the therapeutic contract must be agreed on. In most cases, the contract calls for highly specific goals and time limits. The family has usually mobilized itself around the resolution of the crises which brought them to the therapist, and is motivated to continue treatment only until such time as the crisis is resolved or until the family members begin to feel that no further progress can be expected. Family therapy tends to be much shorter in duration than individual therapy, both because of its clearly defined goals and because of reality considerations. It is much more difficult to bring many individuals together in one place and one time to deal with issues that concern all of them partially, than it is to bring one therapist and one patient together in one place and one time to deal with issues that preoccupy one of them almost entirely.

It is during this period of initial contact that the family therapist addresses the question of diagnosis, formulation, and treatment plan. These will vary almost entirely as a function of the theoretical orientation of the therapist. There is as yet no generalized accepted taxonomy of family pathology or family dysfunction which is comparable to the *Diagnostic and Statistical Manual of Mental Disorders* (*Third Edition-Revised*) for individual psychopathology.

The Termination of Scapegoating

In the initial sessions, the family tends to focus discussion on the scapegoat (12, 15), or patient (as identified by family). For reasons discussed earlier, the family quite honestly sees one person as responsible for its problem, rather than perceiving the difficulty as issuing from the family dynamic. The therapist's task is to help the family redefine the presenting problem so that it involves them all. Thus a symptom such as enuresis, encopresis, school phobia, anorexia, bulimia, alcohol abuse or suicide attempt becomes not "his" or "her" but "our" problem. The techniques by which the therapist accomplishes this compose no small part of the armamentarium of the family therapist, and success or failure of this enterprise determines whether therapy may continue to the next stage or must end as a failure. Some of the techniques the therapist employs to gain these ends are (*a*) reducing the family's sense of guilt, since scapegoating is most often a means of attributing failure or responsibility for a perceived disaster to someone other than oneself; (*b*) helping the family to gain insight into the purpose of the scapegoating behavior and its futility as a means of dealing with the family's complaints, (*c*) empathizing with the family members' pain and frustration so that as they feel accepted and understood, there is less need to attribute blame, and (*d*) helping the family state precisely the source of their discontent, in terms of objectionable behaviors. The great majority of parents, given a choice, prefer to think of themselves as having raised a child who has specifiable objectionable traits, than as having raised a child who is a generally objectionable person.

Above all, the therapist must never make the same mistakes which the family makes, particularly by scapegoating any of the other family members for attributing blame to their children. Perhaps the most common single reason parents give for terminating family therapy sessions is that "the therapist *blamed us* for the problem and made us feel terrible about ourselves."

Encouraging Communication

There is sometimes a tendency, early in the course of family therapy, for family members to communicate only with the therapist, or with each other only through the therapist, rather than to each other directly. The more dysfunctional the family, the more pronounced may be this tendency. Such behavior results from "learned avoidance," attempts to communicate among themselves having too often failed or having led to increasing conflict and family stress. Their solution is to withdraw from each other and avoid both verbal and emotional communication, so that their communications with each other at home are most often trivial or of low emotional intensity. If the therapist makes the mistake of insisting too early in the therapy that the family members talk directly with each other, what follows is either tension-filled, embarrassed silence or strained, artificial interchanges. Better communication among family members comes as the therapist experiences success in helping them to listen and to respond to each other. As family empathy increases, the high levels of tension, anxiety, anger, and stress which previously characterized family interaction are reduced.

One initial hallmark of progress in family therapy is the observation by family members that "We've learned to talk to each other in therapy—why can't we do it at home?" In fact, learning to talk to each other in the therapy hour is the first step to communicating with each other at home.

The key for the therapist in this phase of therapy is known as "staying with the interaction." It is a common error among therapists who are first learning to become family therapists to focus their attention upon one family member, exploring that member's psyche, while the other family members sit and observe. Usually the object of this attention is the "scapegoat," and this kind of therapeutic error leads inadvertently to enhanced family scapegoating of the "scapegoat." On the other hand, the successful therapist who "stays with the interaction" focuses on events occurring between and among family members, rather than upon intrapsychic events occuring in the minds of any particular one of them.

"King Solomon"

There is a tendency on the part of the family members, once they have begun to effectively communicate, to solicit direction from the family therapist. They ask the therapist's advice, honor the therapist's expertise, and attempt to place responsibility for the solution to the family's problems upon the therapist. They come to treat the therapist as "King Solomon." The family therapist, like the individual therapist, must reject this role and place responsibility for attaining solutions upon the family. The temptation to accept the "Wise King Solomon" role is much greater for the family therapist than for the individual psychotherapist, since the positive regard of a group of attentive patients is more rewarding than that of just a single patient.

THE STAGE OF TASKS

As family therapy progresses and the aforementioned problems are more or less successfully faced, the family and therapist find themselves dealing directly with the content of those issues which have induced the family crisis. That may happen after very few sessions, or not until after many. It is at this point that the divergencies among therapists become most obvious, depending upon theoretical orientation. Nevertheless, there are commonalities. Most family therapists regard families as presenting a series of issues, which can be graded in terms of the degree of difficulty which their resolution presents to the family and to the therapist.

Thus, experience teaches us that enuresis is ordinarily fairly easily and quickly resolved; that wife or child abuse is less easily dealt with; and that treating an established cocaine habit is still more difficult. Most family therapists attempt to structure treatment so that the less complex issues are dealt with initially, so that the patients will be optimistic toward and confident in the family therapy process.

THEORIES OF FAMILY THERAPY

In part because family theory is such a recent and rapidly developing specialty, new theories and new theoretical frameworks are constantly being expounded and variations of older ideas constantly appearing. The student attempting to choose among these points of view will find little, if any, empirical evidence to aid in the choice. Further, there is constant cross-fertilization among the various viewpoints, so that lines of demarcation are unclear. One finds that it is frequently the case that proponents of the different theoretical points of view do much the same things in practice and differ mainly in the concepts and language which they use in discussing their practices. Choosing a theoretical framework, nevertheless, is essential for the student, both as a guide to conceptualization and to practice. Which framework one chooses will be more a matter of one's training and background than a question of any inherent superiority of one theory over another.

The essential and indispensible reference in family therapy is the comprehensive and encyclopedic guide, *Handbook of Family Therapy* (3). The difficulties of categorizing the various theories in clearly discrepant groups is clearly illuminated in the *Handbook,* which discriminates four major classes of theories, 14 subclasses, and numerous variations of the 14 subclasses. The distinctions among the four major classes or 14 subclasses is less than clear-cut. For example, the authors differentiate between "structural" and "strategic" approaches, but students of family therapy are aware that in clinical practice, there is much that is "structural" in the "strategic" approaches, and much that is "strategic" in the "structural" ones (18).

As a practical matter, I have found it to be generally the case that students seem to be most comfortable with those theoretical frameworks which have been developed by persons with a professional background similar to their own. Thus, as a general rule, psychologists are comfortable working within the behavioral framework profounded by Patterson (19, 20), while psychiatrists may be less so, but more comfortable with the frameworks of Ackerman (9), Bowen (16, 17), and Minuchin (10, 11). While this generalization may serve as a starting point for the beginning student, any practitioner should be acquainted with and have a working knowledge of all the major points of view.

DIFFERENCES AMONG FAMILIES AS A FUNCTION OF SOCIAL CLASS AND ETHNIC BACKGROUND

It is apparent to any practitioner of family therapy that there are major differences in the problems which families present and the manner in which they present them that are a function of social class and ethnic background. Working-class and middle-class families often have different child-rearing practices and value systems. As a result, there is always the danger that therapists of middle-class backgrounds will interpret working-class child-rearing

practices as pathologic simply because they are unfamiliar. Sensitivity training to class and ethnic differences, therefore, should be a major part of the training of any family therapist (21, 22). As a case in point, middle class professionals who were rarely spanked as children may regard such practices by working-class families as child abusive. The fact is that child discipline in many working-class as contrasted with middle-class families is comparatively more physical and less verbal. That difference, in and of itself, does not mean that the working-class families are any more child abusive than middle-class families.

Similarly, I have been impressed when viewing videotapes of therapists with a pronounced ethnic background (e.g., Jewish, Italian, Irish, Hispanic, or Black) who were working with families of the same background, that the therapist and clients often develop a spontaneous empathic communication. In the words of the old Irish song, they "speak a language that the strangers do not know." This is often true to a degree that even the participants themselves did not appreciate. Wherever possible, therefore, a family's request for a therapist who shares their background should be honored, and where such a request is not specifically made, an effort should be made to match families who show a distinct cultural heritage with a therapist who is familiar with and sensitive to that heritage.

MARRIAGE THERAPY

Marriage therapy has an older history than family therapy. Unlike family therapy, which from its inception has had cross-professional input from psychiatry, psychology, and so forth, marriage therapy until fairly recently was considered to be largely the domain of the social worker. The problems presented by marriage and family therapy are similar but by no means identical. For example, for obvious reasons, any worker who wishes to practice marriage therapy should have considerable familiarity with sex therapy (23), whether or not the marriage therapist plans to practice sex therapy. The same degree of familiarity with sex therapy is clearly not necessary for a family therapist who focuses exclusively on parent–child relationships. There are excellent texts on marriage therapy to which the reader is referred (24–27).

The practice of marriage therapy has undergone great changes in recent years, primarily because the institution of marriage has undergone such great changes. Thus, we no longer have universal conventions in regard to marriage roles, and it is no longer automatically understood as to which partner is responsible for wage earning, child care, homemaking, initiating love making, etc. In these regards, each couple must negotiate its own contract. Further, marriage is no longer assumed to be a permanent contract in a society in which, in some cultural settings, nearly 50% of recent marriages terminate in divorce. In our current society, families in which children are raised together who are products of three or more different marriages are not uncommon. The marriage therapist, like the family therapist, commonly sees classes of problems which were rare or nonexistent 10 or 20 years ago. In no area of psychiatry is intensive continued education more necessary, because in no area are the basic phenomena, the problems, and the techniques in such a state of rapid transformation.

For many workers the very term "marriage therapy" has fallen into disuse, to be replaced by the term "couples therapy." The reason is that many therapists treat couples of heterosexual, gay, or lesbian orientation who have established a family outside of the marriage convention and for whom marriage in any conventional or legal sense is not a consideration.

TRAINING IN FAMILY THERAPY

The American Association of Marriage and Family Therapists (AAMFT) was recognized by the former Department of Health, Education and Welfare as "the official agency designated to establish standards for certification of training programs in the field of marriage and family therapy" (1). Many programs accept AAMFT training criteria as a general guide. There is a general consensus among workers in the field that it is desirable for marriage and family therapists to have had academic work in the areas of child development; personality theory; and theory and practice of individual, couples, group, and family psychotherapy, and to have had very considerable and extensive supervised experience in interview and therapy techniques in each of these areas. Most persons who work to receive training as family and marriage (or couples) therapists begin with generalized training in one of the traditional mental health professions (e.g., psychiatry, psychology, social work, pastoral counseling, psychiatric nursing). They then enter into a specialized postgraduate training program which meets the accreditation standards of AAMFT; such programs exist now for members of most of these professions.

References

1. Broderick CB, Schrader SS: The history of professional marriage and family therapy. In Gurman AS, Kniskern DP (eds): *Handbook of Family Therapy*. New York, Bruner/Mazel, 1981, pp 5–35.
2. Foley VD: *An Introduction to Family Therapy*. New York, Grune & Stratton, 1974.
3. Gurman AS, Kniskern DP (eds): *Handbook of Family Therapy*. New York, Bruner/Mazel, 1981.
4. Satir V: *Conjoint Family Therapy*. Palo Alto, CA, Science and Behavior Books, 1964.
5. Haley J: *Strategies of Psychotherapy*. New York, Grune & Stratton, 1963.
6. Haley J: *The Power Tactics of Jesus Christ*. New York, Grossman, 1969.
7. Haley J: *Changing Families*. New York, Grune & Stratton, 1971.
8. Haley J: *Uncommon Therapy*. New York, Norton, 1973.
9. Ackerman NW: *Treating the Troubled Family*. New York, Basic Books, 1966.
10. Minuchin S: *Families & Family Therapy*. Cambridge, MA, Harvard University Press, 1974.
11. Minuchin S, Fishman HC: *Family Therapy Techniques*. Cambridge, MA, Harvard University Press, 1981.
12. Vogel EF, Bell NW: The emotionally disturbed child as family scapegoat. In Bell NW, Vogel EF (eds): *A Modern Introduction to the Family*. Glencoe, IL, Free Press, 1960.

13. Napier AY, Whitaker CA: *The Family Crucible*. New York, Harper and Row, 1978.
14. Vogel W, Mansfield L: Commentary on the "Family Crucible." *Int J Fam Ther* 5:54–60, 1981.
15. Haley J: Family therapy. In Sager CJ, Kaplan HS (eds): *Progress in Group and Family Therapy*. New York, Bruner/Mazel, 1972, pp 261–270.
16. Bowen M: The use of family theory in clinical practice. In Haley J (ed): *Changing Families*. New York, Grune & Stratton, 1971.
17. Bowen M: *Family Therapy in Clinical Practice*. New York, Jason Aronson, 1978.
18. Fish LS, Piercy FP: The theory and practice of structural and strategic family therapies: a delphi study. *J Marit Fam Ther* 13:113–125, 1987.
19. Patterson GR: *Families*. Champaign, IL, Research Press, 1971.
20. Patterson AR, Reid JB, Jones RR, et al: *A Social Learning Approach to Family Intervention: Families with Aggressive Children*. Eugene, OR, Castalia Publishing, 1975.
21. Minuchin S: *Families of the Slums: An Exploration of Their Structure and Treatment*. New York, Basic Books, 1967.
22. Minuchin S: The plight of the poverty-stricken family in the United States. *Child Welfare* 44:124–130, 1970.
23. Kaplan HS: *The New Sex Therapy*. New York, Bruner/Mazel, 1974.
24. Mudd EH: *The Practice of Marriage Counseling*. New York, Association Press, 1951.
25. Mudd EH, Stone A, Karpf MJ, et al (eds): *Marriage Counseling: A Casebook*. New York, Association Press, 1958.
26. Sager CJ: *Marriage Contracts and Couple Therapy*. New York, Bruner/Mazel, 1976.
27. Jacobson NS, Margolin G: *Marital Therapy: Strategies Based on Social Learning and Behavioral Exchange Principles*. New York, Bruner/Mazel, 1979.

48

Behavior Therapy*a*

Gene Richard Moss, M.D.
Robert Paul Liberman, M.D.

Psychiatrists are in a unique position among physicians and mental health professionals. By virtue of their training and experience, psychiatrists can combine biologic and behavioral advances in their treatment of mental and emotional disorders. As such, psychiatrists truly are biobehavioral clinicians.

Recent biologic advances in the understanding of psychiatric disorders have been astounding. Yet, as every clinician knows, biology by itself tells only half the story. The interactions between biologic endowment and environment, as manifested by a person's emergent behavioral repertoires, tells the rest. One without the other is incomplete.

Advances in behavior therapy have created a coherent approach based on specific, operational procedures—not merely isolated techniques—for biobehavioral clinicians to understand and treat the broad range of psychiatric disorders.

A principal distinction between behavioral and other psychotherapeutic approaches is the former's firm and systematic adherence to specification and

a The writing of this chapter was supported in part by National Institute of Mental Health Research Grant MH 30911 to the University of California at Los Angeles Research Center for Schizophrenia and Psychiatric Rehabilitation.

measurement. Behavioral analysis provides guidelines for assessing the nature, severity, and frequency of disordered behavior in an operational format that suggests specific treatment interventions. Description of the controlling environmental events is the "foundation" of behavioral analysis; measurement of behavioral change is the "cornerstone" of therapy. The "structure" of therapy is the functional relationship between the behavior of interest—the "target behavior"—and its environment antecedents and consequences. For the biobehavioral clinician it comes down to the ABCs—*Antecedents, Behaviors,* and *Consequences*—remote, recent, current, and future.

Medicine is art based on science. Most often, it is the art of applying science to one individual patient. Even more than the rest of medicine, the art of psychiatric treatment so often demands the cooperation and the collaboration of the patient. The biobehavioral approach is particularly well suited to these demands because treatment is individually tailored to each patient on the basis of mutual agreement. The biobehavioral clinician and the patient mutually agree on what constitutes the problem and the treatment goal. Together they survey the patient's relevant repertoire—an inventory of the patient's

665

behavioral assets, deficits, and excesses—with regard to treatment goals. They decide on specific treatment interventions, both biologic and behavioral, and establish measurement systems to determine progress toward treatment goals (1). This collaborative effort between clinician and patient has particular revelance to outpatient psychiatric treatment.

The biobehavioral clinician focuses on instrumental behavior, that is, the behavior of the individual in the context of a specified environment. This is not to say, however, that other aspects of behavior are ignored. For the biobehavioral clinician, behavior is described in broad, multimodal terms to include thought, emotion, sensation, verbal and nonverbal elements of social interaction, as well as biologic and physiologic events. If it can be discriminated, counted, observed directly or indirectly, reliably known to occur, reported, or measured in any way, then the event is of clinical interest. On the other hand, biobehavioral clinicians are less concerned with resolving hypothetical conflicts defined by abstract concepts, such as "psychic energy," or with diffuse, global aims such as restructuring the personality.

As do biologic treatments, behavior therapy rests upon a scientific foundation. Behavior therapy has been described as

the application of principles derived from research in *experimental psychology* (italics added) to alleviate human suffering and enhance human functioning. Behavior therapy emphasizes systematic monitoring and evaluation of the effectiveness of these applications. The techniques of behavior therapy are generally intended to facilitate improved self-control by expanding individuals' skills, abilities, and independence. (2)

The essential components of the behavioral approach are outlined in Table 48.1.

The biobehavioral clinician attempts to alleviate human suffering through both biologic intervention and behavioral change. The clinician often can provide speedy relief with medication followed by behavioral therapy aimed at changing the relationship between patient and environment. The phobic patient, for example, may be regulated on a monoamine oxidase inhibitor (MAOI) for panic attacks then de-

Table 48.1 Essential Components of the Behavioral Approach to Clinial Problems

The clinical strategy is framed as a series of questions that the clinician, patient, and significant others ask and answer in recurring cycles, first tentatively and later more definitely as progress occurs.

1. What behavior is maladaptive or problematic?
    Task: To specify concretely the observable behavior that should be increased or decreased. This procedure helps to clarify the therapeutic goals.
2. How often does the behavior occur?
    Task: To measure or record the frequency or intensity of the undesirable and desirable behavior. This procedure is necessary to follow therapeutic progress.
3. What environmental and interpersonal contingencies currently support the problem behavior and reduce the likelihood of more adaptive responses?
    Task: To specify the functional relation between behavior and those events and reactions which determine the frequency of the behavior. A retrospective analysis uncovers the conditioning history of the patient.
4. Which interpersonal transactions, particularly between clinician and patient(s), or other interventions can alter the problem behavior in a more adaptive direction?
    Task: To develop therapeutic tactics and strategy—using modeling, reinforcement, instructions, punishment, and counterconditioning—which effectively will modify behavior.

sensitized through graduated exposure to feared situations. The withdrawn schizophrenic may require longer term medication with a neuroleptic while receiving social skills training and vocational rehabilitation. The severely depressed patient may be aided by the use of a tricyclic antidepressant while, through family behavioral therapy, significant others learn to reinforce positive self-statements, care in grooming, and participation in family events. The suicidal patient suffering the torment of unrelenting depressive anguish may require immediate relief through electroconvulsive therapy (ECT) followed by medication and behavioral therapy. A hyperactive child may be weaned from stimulant drugs after his teacher and parents learn to use positive reinforcement to increase attention span during study and play.

Behavioral clinicians encourage their patients to take an active role in modifying their environments and the contingencies that impinge on them. Through behavior, biology and environment interact in a continuous interplay of dynamic forces:

$$\text{Biology} \leftrightarrow \text{Behavior} \leftrightarrow \text{Environment}$$

To a substantial degree, we create our own environments. Analysis of interpersonal sequences in controlled settings, for example, reveal that aggressive individuals, perhaps genetically predisposed, actualize through their conduct a hostile environment, whereas those who display friendly responsiveness, also perhaps genetically predisposed, produce an amicable social milieu (3). The individual can function both as an agent and as a target of behavioral change.

The biobehavioral clinician is interested in the dynamic interplay among biology, behavior, and environment and between different modes or levels of behavior. The man who suffers a loss and feels low, apathetic, and agitated may begin a "script" which leads to his talking to himself in ways such as "I am helpless," "The world is grim," "I can't do anything any more," and "I am worthless." These negative self-statements, in turn, aggravate dysphoria, agitation, and vegetative symptoms. The clinician working with this patient will focus on creating more positive "scripts" for the patient to use, especially when the patient is making self-evaluations of coping efforts. Similarly, a phobic patient may be taught to make coping self-statements such as "I can 'hang in' until the anxiety diminishes" or "By facing my fears, I will find out that nothing catastrophic will happen." Another example of how changing one level of behavior affects another is the benefit of relaxation training on hypertension and physiologic arousal (4). Another frequently replicated finding has been the improvement in mood, self-concept, and self-esteem accompanying therapeutic changes in social and instrumental behaviors (5).

Behavioral specification and measurement need not be confined to treatment methods subsumed under the rubric of behavior therapy. As an example, clinical and research strategies utilized behaviorally—e.g., specification of discrete behavioral problems and goals and repeated measurements of the behavior of interest using the patient as his own control by sequentially introducing and withdrawing treatment interventions until desired effects are produced—can be applied to psychopharmacology (6). In this manner, the confounding effects of interindividual differences in dose–response can be resolved by intensively monitoring individual patients as each is exposed to several dosage levels of a drug in sequence. This clinical and research strategy, capitalizing on the widely known fact of the uniqueness of each individual's response to medication, allows an assessment of latency, peak potency, duration of effects, and the interactions between chemotherapy and other modes of therapy.

Just as the environment influences the way in which genotypes are manifested, it is to be expected that future research will demonstrate the reciprocal influences of behavior and environment on biological substrates in patients. One example is biofeedback where information from the environment has been demonstrated to have an effect on physiologic functions. In this regard, Rioch (7) noted that "the behavioral approach, with its emphasis on operational formulation, gives promise for the development of a body of data in the future bridging the gap between the anatomical–biochemical analysis of the body on the one hand and the artistry of the clinic on the other."

As pointed out by the Task Force on Behavior Therapy of the American Psychiatric Association, a disorder with an organic or neurophysiologic etiology may be improved markedly by behavior therapy. Since behavior therapy is based on learning principles, it is particularly suitable for such problems, whatever their etiology, where retraining or learning new skills is necessary. Biologic treatments can reduce the symptoms and improve attentiveness and concentration, but they cannot produce directly the skills required for satisfactory adjustment and productivity in society. It is helpful in developing treatment strategies to view the various modes and levels of a person's behavior as representing the changing interface between the biologic substrate and the environment.

BEHAVIOR THERAPY AND THE THERAPEUTIC ALLIANCE

As is true for all psychotherapeutic approaches, the quality of the patient–therapist relationship is extremely important in behavior therapy. Without a positive, therapeutic alliance between clinician and patient, successful intervention becomes less likely. Behavioral interventions by the clinician may involve suggestions to generate specific activities and interactions; demonstrations by the clinician for modeling purposes; and differential feedback or reinforcement on directly observed or indirectly reported behaviors. The clinician is an effective instructor and reinforcer for patients to the extent that he or she is valued, respected, esteemed, and liked. The therapeutic relationship exerts a pervasive and profound influence on the process and outcome of any therapy, and behavior therapy is no expection. Indeed, research studies

have shown that major elements even in the efficacy of token economies are the social and symbolic approbation from staff mediated by the contingent dispensing of tokens, points, or coupons (8).

Clinicians have described the ingredients that go into this positive therapeutic relationship in many different ways, the terminology varying with the "school" of psychotherapy to which the clinician adheres. Some of the better known ingredients have been described as "nonpossessive warmth," "accurate empathy," and "genuine concern." The specific verbal and nonverbal components of the therapeutic alliance have begun to be teased apart by behavioral investigators with the results leading directly into programs for training individuals to become more effective therapists (9–11). The specific behavioral components of a reinforcing treatment relationship may vary with the type and age of the patient; for example, it has been shown with autistic children that strong aversive stimulation administered by the therapist paradoxically increases the child's preference for that therapist and the latter's reinforcing potency (12).

Psychiatrists long have been sensitive to the importance of quickly establishing a favorable relationship infused with mutual trust and regard and of maintaining it throughout the course of treatment. During the first few contacts, progress can be made in promoting the therapeutic alliance by the clinician's demonstrating acceptance, interest, and concern for the patient's problems, history, and apprehensions. By facilitating a catharsis and ventilation of negative feelings during the early stages of the evaluation and treatment periods, the clinician can minimize the patient's later resistance to the structured, active, and positive learning steps that are the basis of behavior therapy. Of great importance to outcome is the systematic way in which clinician and patient negotiate specific behavioral goals and allocate the responsibilities for achieving these goals. That this carefully structured mutual planning can facilitate the therapeutic alliance is evidenced by a comparative study of short-term behavioral and analytically oriented therapy. Process measures in this study of 61 patients treated by six experienced therapists indicated that the three behaviorally oriented therapists showed higher levels of accurate empathy, interpersonal contact, and therapist self-congruence than the three analytically oriented psychotherapists (13). Some behavioral investigators analyzed in behavioral terms the strategic interpersonal interventions used by "family therapists," such as paradoxical intentions and symptom scheduling (14). The goal of such endeavors was to specify the operations used by family therapists, making the evaluation and teaching of these operations more feasible. Similar applications can be made to other therapies, such as group therapy, art therapy, etc.

REVIEW OF APPLICATIONS OF BEHAVIOR THERAPY TO PSYCHIATRIC DISORDERS

The list of clinical problems in psychiatry which have been treated behaviorally is long and growing longer each year. To give a picture of the expansion by behaviorally oriented therapists into the psychiatric domain, a review was conducted of the major behavioral journals for selected years. The journals included *Behavior Research and Therapy*, *Journal of Applied Behavior Analysis*, *Behavior Therapy*, and *Journal of Behavior Therapy and Experimental Psychiatry* for the years 1968, 1970, 1972, 1975, 1980, 1983, and 1986. The results of this review are depicted graphically in Figure 48.1. It should be noted that some of the articles reported in the journals consist of pilot studies, some are well-controlled single case experiments, and some are large-scale, comparative group studies.

To do justice to the clinical and research literature in outpatient behavior therapy with a systematic and comprehensive evaluative review would require a book in its own right. As a compromise, clinical vignettes of a variety of outpatient cases treated using the biobehavioral approach shall be provided. The operational and empirical methods of behavior therapy shall be highlighted in the description of treatment. For readers with larger appetites for the facts, up-to-date and annual reviews of the behavior therapy literature are available such as *Progress in Behavior Modification* (15) and *Annual Reviews of Behavior Therapy* (16). The reader is also referred to Chapter 45 for a discussion of some of the short-term behavior therapies.

A sequential and systematic framework for assessment and therapy guides the biobehavioral clinician in carrying out comprehensive evaluation and treatment of psychiatric disorders. Assessment procedures are not completed at any particular point in time; rather, they are overlapping and reciprocating with treatment interventions. The regular monitoring of behavioral and symptomatic changes as treatment proceeds—through the use of self-report inventories and checklists, behavioral diaries, rating forms, direct observation, or biofeedback measurement—interconnects assessment and treatment in a functional way. Thus, biobehavioral assessment and therapy are inextricably linked in clinical decision making, intervention, and evaluation. The case examples that follow will illustrate this interplay. In Figure 48.2 is depicted the assessment–intervention framework that has served as an empirical template for biobehavioral clinicians in their work with various psychiatric disorders in the outpatient setting.

Panic Disorder

The results of many controlled clinical trials with exposure-based therapy for agoraphobics and panic cases throughout the world have demonstrated that 60 to 70% of those completing treatment will show substantial clinical benefit that endures up to 4-year follow-ups (17). While the use of behavior therapy for problems of anxiety, such as panic disorder, represents one of the success stories of psychotherapy, it is becoming increasingly clear that treatment efficacy is hampered by failures to improve, limited improvement, relapse, and drop-outs. The median dropout rate from exposure-based therapies is 12%, with rates from 25 to 40% recorded when drugs

	1965	1968	1970	1972	1975	1980	1983	1986
Sexual deviations	2	1	10	6	4	8	3	3
Phobias	1	2	10	7	13	14	26	28
Alcoholism	1	3	2	8	3	4	3	4
Eating disorder	1	1	3	4	5	11	9	12
Enuresis, encopresis	1	0	4	6	5	1	4	4
Speech disorder	1	6	1	2	1	1	2	4
Sleep disorder	1	0	2	1	3	4	5	3
Childhood autism		3	0	2	3	5	7	5
Depression		1	2	3	3	6	8	12
Pain		1	0	0	2	3	7	8
Drug addiction		1	1	3	2	0	0	1
Sexual dysfunction		1	1	2	0	3	2	3
Neurodermatitis		1	0	1	0	0	0	0
Adult psychosis		1	8	6	7	2	1	3
Gastrointestinal symptoms		1	3	2	2	1	0	0
Headache			2	0	2	3	5	2
Obsessive–Compulsive			3	7	5	7	9	6
Gilles de la Tourette			1	0	0	0	1	0
Hysterical conversion			1	1	2	2	0	1
Asthma			1	1	0	1	0	0
Mental retardation				4	0	26	13	9
Tics				1	0	1	1	1
Frequency of urination				1	1	1	1	0
Rage and crying				4	2	0	0	0
Muscle spasm				1	1	0	1	0
Vascular symptoms					2	1	0	2
Coprophagia and pica					1	0	0	1
Social deficits					2	13	6	6
Child behavior problems					4	11	15	7
Marital conflict					4	2	2	3
Anxiety						6	8	7
Tobacco dependence						6	7	8
Diabetes						1	1	1
Spina bifida						1	1	0
Myopia							2	0
Cancer							1	2
Post-traumatic stress disorder								5
Panic disorder								8
Herpes								1
Tinnitus								1

Figure 48.1 Number of behavioral articles published during selected years.

are added to the regimen (18). Graduated home-based and self-based exposure treatments appear to improve the cost-effectiveness of treatment especially when spouses are involved mediators (19).

Case Example

Mrs. O. was a 38-year-old, Caucasian, married woman who was self-referred with the chief complaint of "I can't go to meetings without feeling I'm going to pass out." This complaint had been fluctuating and continuous for many years and had increased markedly within the previous 2 years. Mrs. O. reported that she had suffered emotional discomfort for many years characterized by bouts of severe anxiety to the point of panic with dizziness, motor restlessness, perspiration, palpitations, and a sense of a loss of control. At the time of her first visit, Mrs. O. was taking 0.25 mg of alprazolam three times daily, which she had been taking for approximately 11 months and which had provided moderate

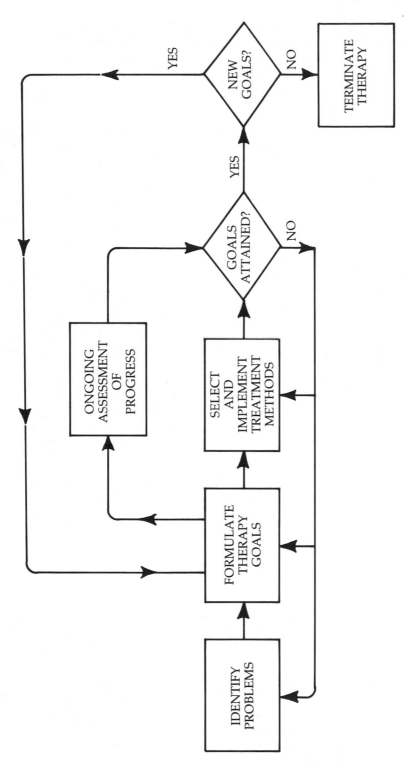

Figure 48.2.   Behavior therapy process.

relief; however, despite the benzodiazepine regimen, her panic episodes had increased in frequency and severity during the month previous. In the past, she had been given a variety of antidepressant medications, which she had discontinued because they had produced intolerable side effects.

Her recent exacerbation of symptoms was associated with her husband's more frequent traveling on business trips and arguments between the couple over trivial issues. She stated at her first visit, "I hate to be in the home alone." Mrs. O. reported experiencing bouts of panic in business meetings, in traffic, and most recently at home when her husband was away. She found that being around other people aggravated her symptoms. She also reported depression, which she attributed as secondary to the anxiety and to her impaired self-image related to having to take a medication. She reported that her sleep generally was "pretty decent"; however, during the 3 weeks previously she had experienced repeated awakening with bouts of anxiety accompanied by palpitations and rapid breathing.

Mrs. O. first had sought psychiatric treatment 12 years previously with similar complaints, for which she had had two previous psychiatric hospitalizations. During the 12 years, she had taken diazepam sporadically with only marginal relief and had seen a series of counselors at community mental health centers. She reported that she had had periods when she felt fairly well without medication. The change to alprazolam had improved her symptoms significantly. The patient reported that her daughter, age 18, also had experienced a bout of similar symptoms, which had remitted without treatment.

Mrs. O. stated that her general health was good. She denied any serious illnesses or surgery. In the past, she admitted to having consumed alcohol heavily but denied alcohol abuse for the past 3 years. She denied the use of illicit drugs or the use of medication other than alprazolam.

Mrs. O. was in her second marriage of 2 years. She characterized the marriage as a good one. Both Mrs. O. and her husband, age 38, worked for the same employer, a national firm with many sites throughout the nation. Unlike Mrs. O.'s job, her husband's job entailed a fair amount of travel away from home. Mrs. O. reported that she liked her job although she believed that her performance was inadequate in spite of receiving regular, substantial pay raises. "I think they just give them to everybody." She described her job as not very challenging.

Mrs. O. and her husband had moved across country approximately 2 years previously because of changes in the structure of the company. They both had received promotions. They were to remain away from their hometown for a total period of 3 years. Mrs. O. reported that she missed being away from her home town. "I'm getting accustomed to it, but I miss my friends and family." She had two children by her first marriage and none by her second. Her daughter, age 18, was employed full time and lived independently. Her son, age 16, lived with his father. He had gone to live with his father when Mrs. O. had suffered her first "nervous breakdown" 12 years previously. She had been married initially at age 19, and her first marriage had lasted for 7 years. She divorced shortly after her first "nervous breakdown."

Evaluation and Treatment Plan

Mrs. O. presented as a coherent, attractive, cooperative woman, appearing her stated age, who was dressed in a suit and was well groomed with minimal make-up. She showed signs of moderate depression, and her speech was somewhat pressured. Her intellect appeared high average. There was no gross evidence of psychosis nor organic brain disorder. Diagnostic impression was panic disorder and adjustment disorder with mixed emotional features of anxiety and depression.

The following problems were specified for treatment:

1. Avoidance of business conferences and meetings associated with panic attacks;

2. Increasing arguments with her husband and a decrease in social and recreational activities associated with feelings of mild to moderate depression; and

3. A deficit of assertive behaviors especially at work associated with self-reports of low self-worth and feelings of mild to moderate depression.

Her current behavioral assets relevant to each problem were the following:

1. A history of steady employment with the same company for several years, favorable evaluation reports, and an expressed desire to be effective at business conferences and meetings as she had been previously in spite of moderate anxiety and episodic panic attacks;

2. a. Stable marriage of 2 years to a husband who reported a genuine desire to assist her to improve, and

   b. A previous history of self-sufficiency

in social and recreational behavior; and

3. Previous history of some ability to assert herself in interpersonal situations as well as an ability to articulate and project appropriate emotional expressiveness during the initial psychiatric interviews.

In collaboration with Mrs. O. and after explaining a rationale for each of the elements of intervention, treatment planning was formulated (see Table 48.2).

Results

Pharmacologic intervention with alprazolam appeared effective at a relatively low dosage of 0.5 mg three times daily. Mrs. O. was able to attend all business conferences and meetings with self-reports of only mild to moderate anxiety and no panic attacks. After clinical stability had been achieved, the medication was tapered over several months without reported recurrence of

Table 48.2   Treatment Plan for Mrs. O.

Goals	Treatment Plan	Monitoring Progress
1. Attend all business conferences and meetings without suffering panic attacks.	1. Pharmacologic treatment with antipanic medication (alprazolam) in clinically effective dosage; relaxation training and systematic desensitization using a hierarchy of fear-eliciting situations at home and at work; and continued attendance at all scheduled business conferences and meetings to ensure in vivo exposure to anxiety-evoking stimuli.	1. Recording by patient of the percentage of business conferences and meetings attended and assessment of sense of well-being with regard to anxiety and panic using Target Complaint Scale (see Fig. 48.3).
2. Decrease frequency of arguments with husband and increase social and recreational activities with self-report of improvement of depression.	2. Development of a plan of social and recreational activities with her husband's involvement; cognitive restructuring to develop a more positive attitude about delay in returning to her hometown.	2. Recording by patient of social and recreational activities attended with and without her husband and assessment of sense of well-being with regard to depression.
3. Increase appropriate assertive behavior at work with report of improvement in self-image and depression.	3. Insight-oriented therapy to understanding historical factors leading to poor self-image and chronic depression; assertiveness training utilizing role rehearsal in work situation; and pursuit of more challenging and prestigious job with same firm to improve assertive skills and poor self-image.	3. Behavioral diary by patient documenting interpersonal situations demanding assertiveness and patient's response to those situations.

anxiety or panic attacks. The medication finally was discontinued without reported recurrence of symptoms over a 6-month follow-up interval.

The frequency of arguments with her husband decreased to the level prior to the move. Her social and recreational activities increased although the activities when her husband was away remained almost at the previous low level. The patient reported feeling less depressed about her situation and had less preoccupation with returning to her home town.

Mrs. O. reported asserting herself with her coworkers. A woman, for example, who shared the same office tended to chat socially with other employees on break, interfering with Mrs. O.'s work. The patient was able to confront this woman and to obtain the desired result without alienating her. More important, with her enhanced ability to assert herself, the patient sought and obtained a change of position, obtaining a more challenging and prestigious position, which, in turn, resulted in a reported increase in self-esteem.

Discussion

Mrs. O.'s case illustrates the harmonious blending of several treatment interventions through the biobehavioral approach. Because antipanic medications often are very effective in blocking panic attacks, they can allow more effective implementation of behavioral interventions. Once Mrs. O. felt secure that she would not suffer crippling bouts of panic, she felt more comfortable in fulfilling the behavioral aspects of the treatment plan to which she had agreed. It should be kept in mind that an attempt should be made to phase out the antipanic medication well before the end of treatment. If not, the risk of relapse after discontinuation of the treatment is increased (20).

Mrs. O.'s case also illustrates the role of the biobehavioral clinician in instigating specific aspects of behavioral interventions. Collaborating with the patient, the behavioral clinician instigates specified behaviors according to the mutually agreed on treatment plan. Mrs. O.'s treatment

plan, for example, called for shaping certain social behaviors by successive approximation toward specific treatment goals, making sure that each step was small enough to maximize chances for success. In this context, the biobehavioral clinician often makes use of the therapeutic alliance as a reinforcer for patient progress until sufficient gains have been made that reinforcers in the patient's own life situation take hold. Of note, one of the by-products of recent advances in behavior therapy has been the development of specific therapeutic aids available to the biobehavioral clinician. In Mrs. O.'s case, for example, use of a specific Guide to Recreational Planning proved helpful (21).

Obsessive–Compulsive Disorder

Well-controlled outcome studies of behavioral therapy with obsessive–compulsive patients in England, the Netherlands, Germany, and the United States have shown that 75% of cases treated markedly improve and maintain their benefit over a 2- to 3-year follow-up period (22). Results of response prevention of rituals coupled with prolonged exposure to the feared and dreaded stimuli reveal rapid improvement especially when patients are motivated to carry out the behavioral assignments on their own (23). Relapse occurs in approximately 20% of cases and seems more likely in patients who are only moderately improved at the end of treatment. Complacency with the effective procedures currently available is not warranted, however, since 25% of patients refused to partake in the treatment interventions and another 25% failed to benefit (24). Moreover, patients suffering from obsessions without rituals tend to be relatively refractory to current behavioral interventions.

Case Example

Mr. N. was a 21-year-old, single, Caucasian man referred by his personal physician with a chief complaint of ritualistic behavior interfering with his level of function for several years. During the initial session, Mr. N. was seen with his father since the patient himself refused to be examined without his father's being present. The father stated that the patient had had a long history of psychiatric problems first noted when the patient was of preschool age but becoming of increasing concern when the patient was 7 or 8 years of age. Initially, the problems were noted with the patient at play. They were characterized by poor cooperation and aggressive behavior. The patient's peers began to pick on him. In fact, he never had had any real friends. The patient's academic work was good. In the 4th grade, he was evaluated psychologically by the school with the recommendation for counseling. He was seen in counseling without improvement. There was no improvement with age.

The patient tended to concentrate on his academic tasks and achieved straight A's in middle school. His social problems, however, continued and were characterized by social withdrawal, nonparticipation in school activities, and difficulties in the family. As the patient concentrated on his academic tasks, he began to show increasing compulsivity; for example, arranging materials on his desk in a specific order. He also began to check his work over and over again until the early hours of the morning, which resulted in decreasing grades. His behavior at home became increasingly belligerent with occasional, outright, physical aggression. By the age of 15, the patient was noted to spend hours in the evening cleaning his school locker and even helping the janitors at school. He became preoccupied with the lack of cleanliness in the world and began to exhibit anger at other people for their lack of cleanliness.

He was referred to a clinical psychologist, whom he saw for several sessions without improvement. He then was referred to a psychiatrist, whom he saw for 6 months. He was given no medication at that time. The patient himself did not believe he needed help and did not want to attend sessions. He was forced to do so by his father, which resulted in more arguments. There was no improvement during the course of psychiatric treatment. The patient's rituals increased.

Mr. N. graduated high school and enrolled in college. He withdrew during the first semester because he was not able to achieve straight A's. Subsequently, he appeared miserable. He attempted to attend a junior college but withdrew when he found once again that he could not achieve straight A's. He then had no further treatment. Four months prior to his first visit, he had begun to admit to his family that indeed he did have a problem. He was seen by a nutritionist at a "bio-center" and given a number of vitamins and minerals but showed no improvement.

At the time of the evaluation, Mr. N. lived at home with his parents. He had not been working for approximately 2 months except part time for a coffee shop. When he did work he tended to show up a few minutes late every day regardless of the starting time, because of having to complete his rituals. He spent his leisure time sleeping, watching television, or staring at nothing.

Mr. N. was the younger of two, with a sister who was 1 year older. His father reported that the sister was the opposite of the patient and exhibited none of his problems. The patient was the product of an uneventful pregnancy and normal, full-term delivery. Early motor development appeared to be within normal limits. The patient tended to have episodes of screaming, however, before he developed speech. Toilet training was uneventful. Preschool social behaviors showed glimpses of problems to come. Within the family structure, the mother tended to be the buffer between the patient and the father and to serve as an apologist for the patient's problem behaviors.

The patient's general health had been excellent. There had been no surgeries nor were there known allergies. He had taken only vitamin and mineral supplements from the "bio-center." He denied the use of illicit drugs or alcohol.

Evaluation and Treatment Plan

Mr. N. presented as an alert, intelligent, young man, who was informally dressed and somewhat poorly groomed. He described his preoccupation with cleanliness and orderliness as abnormal and requested psychiatric assistance in gaining control over his intrusive and unwanted thoughts. He was restless, and his speech appeared moderately pressured but was logical and goal directed without loose association. He appeared of above average intellect. There was no gross evidence of psychosis nor organic brain disorder. Diagnostically, the patient was seen as having an obsessive–compulsive disorder and atypical conduct disorder of childhood and adolescence.

The following problems were specified for treatment:

1. Compulsions involving rituals of checking and arranging that were repetitive, purposeful, and intentional, which reduced the patient's reported feelings of anxiety and which the patient recognized as excessive and unreasonable;
2. Complaints of depression and demoralization related to his life situation;
3. Vocational behavioral deficits with failure to hold a job accompanied by excessive sleeping; and
4. Frequent arguments with parents, especially his father.

Mr. N.'s current behavioral assets relevant to each problem were the following:

1. a. Awareness of the unreasonable nature of obsessive concerns and compulsive rituals and
   b. an expressed desire to rid himself of these thoughts and rituals;
2. a. Expressed denial of suicidal ideation or intent and
   b. claimed willingness to cooperate with the treatment plan;
3. a. On the basis of the results of psychological testing, an intellect in the superior range, albeit with deficits in the verbal domain integrating social factors into higher cognitive processes, and
   b. previous superior performance in school; and
4. Ability to exert control albeit marginal

over aggressive impulses despite self-reports of sadistic, violent fantasies.

Mr. N. was seen in once weekly individual treatment sessions while his parents and he were seen once weekly in family therapy sessions for purposes of behavioral contracting. The treatment goals, treatment plans, and measurement systems are depicted in Table 48.3.

Results

Given the severity of Mr. N.'s problem, the resistance of his problem to treatment, and his difficulty in participating in treatment, it was anticipated at the outset that Mr. N.'s treatment would be prolonged. During the course of treatment, he reported the severity of his obsessive concerns and compulsive rituals decreased from "severe" to "mild" in that he believed they no longer interfered with his level of function. After one year of treatment, the MAOI was discontinued uneventfully. The patient reported his sense of well-being with regard to anxiety only slightly improved, a condition which did not change after the discontinuing of the MAOI.

With regard to depression, Mr. N. reported his sense of well-being improved from "poor" to "fair." He continued to report that he felt dissatisfied with his life situation, in general. During the course of treatment, he secured full-time employment doing unskilled, manual labor. After several months of stable employment, he moved out of his parents' home into an apartment he shared with two other men his age, also employed doing manual labor. The patient himself requested further treatment to improve his vocational status, hoping to return to college and also to improve his social skills. His father at that time, however, withdrew financial support for further treatment. The patient declined to seek counseling at the local community mental health center. Reports by both parents and patient revealed that prior to the patient's leaving his parent's home, arguments had decreased from at least once daily to once every 2 or 3 weeks. His parents reported his relations with them ap-

Table 48.3   Treatment Plan for Mr. N.

Goals	Treatment Plan	Monitoring Progress
1. Decrease frequency of compulsive behaviors to noninterfering level without increase in reported anxiety.	1. Direct behavioral interventions for compulsive behavior (such as thought stopping and response prevention) were refused by the patient; pharmacologic treatment with monoamine oxidase inhibitor (MAOI).	1. Global rating by patient of severity of compulsive rituals during the month previous on a scale from "much improved" to "much worse" since the patient had refused to record percentage of waking hours per day free from ritualistic behaviors; global rating by parents of severity of compulsive rituals during the week previous.
2. Improve sense of well-being with regard to depression.	2. Insight-oriented therapy to identify events in patient's life causing depression; pharmacologic treatment with MAOI.	2. Self-reports of his sense of well-being with regard to depression on a scale from "much improved" to "much worse"; reports by parents of level of patient's depressive behaviors during the week previous (e.g., complaints of depression, sad facies, negative self-statements).
3. Resume regular sleep schedule and obtain full-time employment leading to independent living.	3. Due to patient's refusal to follow a schedule of job seeking, a time limit was imposed to seek full-time employment or leave parents' home with sufficient funds to sustain him for 3 months.	3. Self-reports of job seeking specifying number of potential employers contacted previous week; reports by parents of patient's sleep patterns.
4. Decrease frequency of arguments with parents to a level acceptable to parents.	4. Using family therapy format, design a behavioral contract between patient and parents for patient to reside in parents' home.	4. Reports by patient of his view of quality of relations with his parents; reports by parents of the number of days per week free from arguments with patient.

peared to have improved superficially but basically were unchanged with regard to respective attitudes among the family members (i.e., patient's father remained demanding, the patient remained angry and resentful, and the mother continued to play the role of buffer.)

Discussion

Historically, obsessive–compulsive disorders have been considered very resistant to treatment (25). Even considering recent advances in behavioral interventions, outcome with these disorders remains uncertain. In Mr. N.'s case, the patient's reluctance to cooperate fully compromised even further chances for successful treatment.

Mr. N.'s case illustrates the need for cooperation and collaboration on the part of the patient. Biobehavioral therapy is not inherently coercive. Accordingly, treatment goals must take into account the patient's willingness and ability to participate in treatment. As Lazare has pointed out in this text, psychiatrists should adopt a "customer approach" to solicit the patient's participation in treatment. In the future, Mr. N. may return to treatment and more fully may "buy into the treatment plan" (e.g., response prevention, and in vivo exposure). Until such time, however, achievement of less than optimal treatment goals may yield significant and functional improvements.

Depressive Disorder

There have been few contributions of behavior therapy to the treatment of psychotic depression or bipolar disorders. Some years ago, Moss and Boren developed a model to analyze depressive behavior as a function of schedules of reinforcement (26). Of the therapeutic studies that have been published, there has been documentation that suggests specific behavioral interventions can be effective in the management of dysthymia and even major depression. Such studies have shown that social skills training and cognitive behavior therapy yield outcomes as favorable as antidepressant medication with 75% of patients or more exhibiting substantial clinical improvement or remission (27–29). Some studies have found a synergistic effect between antidepressant drugs and behavioral interventions (30); however, for those patients who cannot tolerate the side effects of antidepressants, behavior therapy may offer the biobehavioral clinician alternatives that are effective and that protect against leaving treatment against medical advice.

Case Example

Ms. T. was a 39-year-old, unmarried, Caucasian woman who was self-referred with a chief complaint of depression of many years duration recently exacerbated by a visit to her parents. Ms. T. reported that she previously had been in 16 years of continuous, outpatient psychiatric treatment for depression. When first seen, she was taking lorazepam 1 mg before sleep and believed herself psychologically dependent on the medication. She expressed anxiety about having the lorazepam taken away from her. Due to a move 3 months previously, the patient had discontinued with her previous psychiatrist but had continued the lorazepam.

The patient was employed in an executive position for a large corporation for the previous 4 years. Prior to the geographical relocation, the patient described having lived "in an old-age home" since the apartment complex in which she had resided contained mainly elderly people. With the move, she purchased a new home; however, she felt out of place in her new neighborhood because she was more educated and of higher socioeconomic circumstances than her neighbors.

Ms. T. suffered from mild craniosynostosis complicated by bilateral, recurrent dislocations of the patellae, which led to osteoarthritis of the knees with progressive pain and limitation. She had undergone knee surgery in the past without much improvement. Approximately 6 years previously she began to suffer increasing pain with decreasing function. When first seen, the limitations had increased to the point that she was unable to dance or to walk long distances. She also suffered from other congenital abnormalities—an extra rib on the left; a high, arched palate; and deformed teeth, which had been corrected somewhat. She denied any other serious illnesses, surgery, or substance abuse.

The patient reported a strong family history of psychiatric problems on her father's side. He had been hospitalized psychiatrically after retirement. His brother reportedly had had psychiatric problems also. The patient's paternal grandfather had committed suicide.

At the time of the evaluation, Ms. T. was doing well in her work and financially. Her immediate future occupationally and financially looked good. The patient reported that her social and recreational life had improved somewhat since the relocation. On the other hand, she viewed herself as limited by the chronic pain: "I hate my handicap."

The patient had been born and reared in a large Eastern city, the younger of two, with a sister 5 years older. Her father had retired, and the parents had moved out of state several months previously. The patient reported that her parents had argued a great deal during her childhood. She tended to side with her mother; the sister had sided with the father. The father was characterized as having been very distant while the patient was growing up. The mother was characterized as having been "changeable, overpowering, and controlling." The patient had had very few friends. She had been a good student in school. She graduated college and obtained a graduate degree in her field immediately thereafter. In her entire life, she had had only one serious, romantic involvement and that with a married man.

She expressed shame and depression about her life: "I think I'm a creep."

The patient was neither attractive nor ugly. When first seen, she was dressed in a tailored business suit and was moderately well groomed. She was tearful and had symptoms of moderately severe depression with sad facies, negative self-statements, and a reported sense of hopelessness and helplessness. She also complained of anxiety about her having to find a new psychiatrist and possibly having to discontinue lorazepam. Her speech appeared logical and goal directed without loose association. She appeared of superior intellect. There was no gross evidence of psychosis nor organic brain disorder. Diagnostic impression included dysthymic disorder; dependent personality disorder; craniosynostosis (mild) with recurrent, bilateral dislocations of the patellae complicated by chronic pain associated with osteoarthritis of the knees, and lorazepam abuse.

Treatment

The following problems were specified for treatment:

1. Complaint of depression with self-reports of low self-esteem and poor self-image associated with a deficit in social behavior;
2. Insomnia;
3. Lorazepam abuse; and
4. Recurrent, bilateral dislocations of the patellae resulting in limitation of social and recreational activities and associated with stated fear of becoming "crippled."

Ms. T.'s behavioral assets relevant to each problem were the following:

1. a. Successful achievement of a graduate degree in her vocational field with a strong, stable employment history and financial success and
   b. some effort toward increasing activities on her own;

2. a. Previous history of normal sleep pattern, albeit not for many years, and
   b. expressed desire to achieve normal sleep pattern free from sedative drugs;
3. a. Previous history of having functioned effectively in school and at work without antianxiety or other psychotropic medications and
   b. expressed willingness to discontinue lorazepam in spite of fear of doing so; and
4. a. Previous history of having followed prescribed exercises for her legs and
   b. expressed willingness to continue to follow prescriptive remedies.

Ms. T. was seen once weekly in outpatient treatment for a period of approximately 1 year. Treatment goals, treatment plans, and measurement systems are depicted in Table 48.4.

Results

Ms. T. successfully switched from lorazepam to temazepam with acceptable results then was withdrawn from temazepam, achieving 6 to 8 hours of sleep per night with self-reports of quality of sleep as "good" to "excellent." During the day she initially was regulated on small doses of alprazolam 0.25 mg twice a day with adequate relief. After discontinuation of the temazepam, Ms. T. was tapered off alprazolam. She reported her sense of well-being regarding anxiety as improved from "poor" to "moderate."

Ms. T. was referred to a physiatrist for consultation. He reported that she was adhering to an optimal treatment program. He provided her reassurance that she would not become "a cripple," although he could not rule out surgery for knee replacement eventually. Ms. T. reported less fear of the future regarding her disability. She remained reluctant, however, to use a wheelchair for activities requiring lengthy walking due to her not wanting to "advertise my disability."

All in all, Ms. T. reported that her sense of well-being regarding anxiety and depression improved from "poor" to "mod-

Table 48.4   Treatment Plan for M.

Goals	Treatment Plan	Monitoring Progress
1. Improve sense of well-being with regard to anxiety and depression; increase rewarding social and recreational activities; decrease dependence on psychiatric treatment.	1. Strengthening of therapeutic alliance recognizing potential for dependence; then after fulfilling other treatment goals, phase out psychiatric treatment; consideration of pharmacologic treatment with antidepressant medication.	1. Self-reports of sense of well-being with regard to both anxiety and depression; reports by patient of social and recreational activities pursued.
2. Improve sleep pattern without use of sedatives.	2. Pharmacologic treatment switching patient from lorazepam to temazepam for sleep to break symbolic attachment to lorazepam; then phase out temazepam; adjunctive use of alprazolam while withdrawing from temazepam, then phase out alprazolam.	2. Self-reports of number of hours slept per night and quality of sleep.
3. Discontinue all drugs of potential abuse.	3. Same as 2.	3. Self-reports of well-being with regard to anxiety and depression.
4. Achieve optimal level of physical function.	4. Physiatry consultation; specification of alternatives to generate increased social and recreational activities (e.g., using a wheelchair for activities requiring walking long distances such as museums, parks).	4. Report from physiatrist; self-reports of adherence to exercise regimen; alternatives used to generate increased social and recreational activities.

erate." She joined several social clubs and business organizations and became politically active in a lobbying group representing her profession. Use of antidepressant medication was discussed with the patient and rejected by her. Once treatment goals had been fulfilled to an extent found acceptable by her, the frequency of treatment sessions was decreased to every other week, then once monthly, then discontinued with agreement that she could make contact in the event that she felt the need.

Discussion

Affective changes and changes in self-concept generally move more slowly than do changes in overt behaviors. From the biobehavioral perspective, treatment planning generally calls for changes in overt behavior and schedules of the reinforcement first. Changes in affect and self-concept often follow thereafter. In the treatment contract with Ms. T., there was an implicit expectation on the part of the psychiatrist that she would increase her level of autonomy and decrease her reliance on him to the point that she could discontinue treatment entirely. Initially,

there was an immediate attack on her drug dependence through a medication change from lorazepam to an alternative with the goal of total discontinuation of medication entirely. Once that had been accomplished, treatment design centered around strengths already exhibited by Ms. T. especially in areas requiring cognitive restructuring of her self-image. Treatment was terminated while the patient was reporting an improvement in her sense of well-being from "poor" to "moderate" rather than to "good" or "excellent." In other words, Ms. T. exhibited substantial but not complete improvement. She had moved up to a level of function, however, that was considered within normal variation. It was hypothesized that future gains in her sense of well-being could be made by her on her own supported by the enriched schedules of reinforcement in her life situation.

Alcohol Abuse

Multimodal biobehavioral approaches to alcoholism have yielded the best outcome in terms of abstinence; reduced frequency of alcohol use; and improved affective, social, family, and vocational functioning. Treatment programs that include disulfiram, Alcoholics Anonymous, social skills training, and family therapy tend to have more durable efficacy (31). Patients with strong family or employment contingencies for obtaining and remaining in treatment and for maintaining abstinence generally have positive therapeutic outcomes (32, 33). Harnessing to the treatment program community and family reinforcers appears to improve long-term benefits to patients (34, 35).

Case Example

Mr. R. was a 38-year-old, married, Caucasian man, the father of a preadolescent daughter who was self-referred due to excessive consumption of alcohol of several years duration and a complaint of recurrent depression. Mr. R. was the founder and president of his own construction company. He had been in business for approximately 5 years and had been modestly successful. Despite severe competition, Mr. R. reported that his company had remained profitable.

Mr. R. complained of bouts of depression that had afflicted him for several years even before entering into his own business. In addition, he tended to binge-drink, which appeared to be associated with the bouts of depression. The drinking had become sufficiently severe that it was reducing his effectiveness as a businessman and leading to financial loss primarily because of the patient's inability to bid for new contracts. Although both he and his wife had admitted to his problem and agreed that he should abstain from alcohol, he was surrounded by others in his line of work who drank excessively and placed tremendous social and business pressure on him to use alcohol.

Mr. R. reported that his marriage was stable. He characterized his wife as supportive of him both in his work and his personal life. His wife consumed alcohol only moderately and had no history of drug abuse. Their daughter was doing well in school and appeared to represent no problem to her parents.

Mr. R.'s general health was good. There had been no previous surgery. There was no family history of alcohol or drug abuse or of psychiatric disorder or treatment.

Evaluation and Treatment Planning

Mr. R. presented as a well-developed, well-nourished, handsome man appearing his stated age of 38 who was dressed in work clothes covered with a bit of dirt and dust. His demeanor was affable although he reported feeling anxiety and depression. Speech was logical and goal directed. He appeared of above-average intellect. There was no gross evidence of psychosis nor organic brain disorder. Diagnostic impression include episodic alcohol abuse and dysthymic disorder.

After three evaluative sessions, one with the patient alone, one with his wife alone, and the third with both present, the following problems were specified for treatment:

1. Behavioral excess involving alcohol abuse; and
2. Complaints of bouts of depression with a suggestion of possible bouts of elation.

His current behavioral assets relevant to each problem were the following:

1. a. An expressed desire to remain abstinent from alcohol or other drugs with potential for abuse,
   b. a cooperative wife who agreed to participate as a mediator of treatment, and
   c. a successful business that was in jeopardy if alcohol abuse did not cease; and
2. a. Significant periods free from depression and
   b. expressed willingness to enter treatment and follow prescriptive recommendations.

Mr. R. was seen in individual therapy and occasionally in family therapy with his wife. Treatment goals, treatment plans, and measurement systems are depicted in Table 48.5.

Results

With regard to his alcohol abuse, Mr. R. remained on disulfiram for a period of 6 months and reportedly remained abstinent from all drugs of potential abuse including alcohol. He then discontinued disulfiram. Several months later, he began to abuse alcohol, and pursuant to the treatment plan specified previously, he resumed disulfiram for a period of 3 months. Then the disulfiram once again was discontinued. He remained abstinent for more than 1 year thereafter.

With regard to his complaint of depression, Mr. R. responded well to treatment with the tricyclic antidepressant. After 3 months, the antidepressant was tapered off. Mr. R. continued to measure his sense of well-being with regard to depression. It had been agreed during the treatment that after 3 months of consistent scores of 3 or greater without more than 3 consecutive days of a score less than 3, the patient would taper off the tricyclic antidepressant. Based upon continued self-monitoring of internal events, he would resume the tricyclic antidepressant if (*a*) he felt the urge to drink associated with the self-rating of less than 3 or (*b*) he suffered 5 consecutive days of a score less than 3. Based on his self-monitoring, it was found that Mr. R. exhibited a monthly cycle of moderate depression alternating with moderate hypomania. Consequently, his diagnosis was changed to cyclothymic disorder, and he was regulated on lithium carbonate, which smoothed out his cycle. The single bout of alcohol abuse suffered by Mr. R. appeared to be related to a specific job stress and not related directly to his sense of well-being with regard to depression. Subsequently, Mr. R. was followed in outpatient medication management for lithium maintenance.

Discussion

Mr. R.'s case illustrates a multimodal approach incorporating pharmacotherapy with antidepressant medication and disulfiram in combination with behavioral measurement through individual and family intervention. The pharmacologic and behavioral components were interactive in that behavioral measurement directly affected medication regimen. Particularly noteworthy was the change of diagnosis to cyclothymic disorder and of medication to lithium based on the patient's daily self-monitoring and graphing of an internal event, namely, his sense of well-being.

The use of family members and significant others in treatment as mediators of therapy is another distinctive aspect of the biobehavioral approach. In this regard, Mr. R.'s wife played a key role. While some psychotherapeutic approaches view the critical reinforcer in treatment as the relationship with the therapist, biobehavioral clinicians seek to identify alternate, critical reinforcers that can be harnessed to

Table 48.5   Treatment Plan for Mr. K.

Goals	Treatment Plan	Monitoring Progress
1. Abstain from alcohol and all other drugs with potential for abuse.	1. Recommendation that patient at least sample Alcoholics Anonymous, which he refused to do; pharmacologic treatment with disulfiram administered daily by his wife with discontinuation if patient remained abstinent for 6 months but reinstitution if patient resumed alcohol use.	1. Weekly report signed by wife of patient's adherence to disulfiram regimen and apparent abstinence from all drugs of potential abuse; after discontinuation of disulfiram, daily graphing by patient to measure days free from alcohol.
2. Improve sense of well-being with regard to depression without hypomanic or manic behavior.	2. Pharmacologic treatment with tricyclic antidepressant; insight-oriented therapy to identify events in patient's life causing depression.	2. Daily graphing by patient to measure his sense of well-being with regard to depression using a 5-point scale.

maximize potential for therapeutic success. The therapeutic alliance is not always the most potent reinforcer. In Mr. R.'s situation, his wife and his business appeared to be critical reinforcers available to treatment.

In treating alcoholism and substance abuse, the drug of choice cannot be taken away without substituting something in its place. In Mr. R.'s case, he was using alcohol in order to regulate his mood, a pattern prompted and reinforced socially by business associates. Treatment called for abstinence from alcohol and replacement of alcohol with a medication that would regulate his mood effectively without the adverse consequences of alcohol abuse. In this regard, an antidepressant and subsequently lithium carbonate were successful.

Relapses are a well-recognized part of the treatment of alcohol and substance abuse. Consequently, it is important to prepare the patient in advance for relapses in order to mitigate their potentially catastrophic effect. Marlatt, for example, has developed a specific behavioral procedure to prepare patients and family for relapses (36). For Mr. T., his relapse was handled smoothly in that the treatment plan already had included provisions for coping with relapse.

Schizophrenia

Major advances have been recorded in the treatment of schizophrenic patients outside hospitals, using behavioral and structured educational approaches. Carefully controlled studies of behavioral family management (37, 38), psychoeducational family therapy (39), and social skills training (39, 40), have documented reductions in relapse rates from 40 to 50% in 1 year to 20% or even lower. It now appears clear that the addition of structured behaviorally oriented interventions to judicious pharmacologic treatment with neuroleptic medication can provide substantial protection for patients against relapse as well as upgrade their level of social function and quality of life.

Commonly, patients suffering chronically from schizophrenia receive outpatient psychiatric treatment through clinics and community mental health centers. The case that follows illustrates treatment initially received in a day treatment center followed by treatment in the continuing care program of a community mental health center. The case illustrates the value of (a) combining social skills training to strengthen a patient's adaptive strengths and (b) contingency management procedures aimed at modifying bizarre, psychotic behavior. Ambulatory psychiatric settings including the psychiatrist's private office are ideal for mounting comprehensive, behavioral interventions for chronic and severe psychiatric disorders.

Case Example

Mr. F. was a 54-year-old, Mexican-American, who had six previous hospitalizations with a diagnosis of paranoid schizophrenia. Between hospitalizations, he continued to report persisting auditory hallucinations. The voices he heard told him to write incoherent phrases on the walls of his home. One month prior to his admission to a day treatment center, the nonsensical writing increased. Mr. F. began to withdraw from social contact, spending most of his time alone. He then began to write on the walls of the factory in which he worked. Mr. F.'s foreman placed him on extended sick leave without pay; nevertheless, his foreman had been impressed with Mr. F.'s previous ability to function as a worker. He told Mr. F. that if he could obtain satisfactory treatment and control his behavior, he could have his job back.

Mr. F. lived at home with his wife and two daughters, all of whom expressed concern about his condition and a willingness to assist in his treatment. With these supportive factors in the clinical picture, it appeared promising that through biobehavioral intervention Mr. F. could achieve a level of function acceptable to everyone.

Evaluation and Treatment Plan

Mr. F. was brought to the community mental health center by his wife and daughters. He appeared disheveled and distracted. He looked vacantly around and responded audibly to stimuli that were not apparent to others. When prompted with questions, he offered coherent responses and had a good fund of knowledge without any sign of memory impairment. He spoke openly about his "voices," which were women unknown to him giving him commands to write phrases on the walls of his home and worksite. While waiting for his initial appointment, he was observed writing on the bathroom walls at the mental health center. Diagnostic impression was schizophrenic disorder, paranoid type, chronic with acute exacerbation.

The following problems were specified for treatment:

1. Reported command hallucinations with acting out by writing nonsensical phrases on the walls of his home, worksite, and day treatment center; and
2. Social withdrawal and inadequate assertiveness with family members and foreman at work.

His behavioral assets relevant to each problem were the following:

1. a. Expressed dissatisfaction by the patient of his suffering auditory hallucinations and his recognition that they represented symptoms of a psychiatric disorder.
   b. expressed willingness by both patient and family to cooperate in psychiatric treatment, and
   c. previous acceptable level of function at work and at home; and
2. a. Previous high level of social activity in his local, Mexican-American community,
   b. previous ability to project personal warmth to others, and
   c. previous ability to engage others in personal relationships.

With the active involvement of patient and family, the psychiatrist at the day treatment center led a group of multidisciplinary mental health professionals in formulating therapeutic goals and specific treatment interventions (see Table 48.6).

Results

Mr. F. was placed on antipsychotic medication, trifluoperazine, at a moderate dosage of 20 mg daily. Even after titrating this dose upward and downward, Mr. F.'s reported hallucinations and nonsensical writing continued. He did report, however, that the hallucinations were less distressing and menacing to him. The psychiatrist decided that it would be preferable to add specific behavioral interventions than to increase the dosage of neuroleptic medication or add other medications as adjuncts. Accordingly, contingency management was introduced in that

Table 48.6   Treatment Plan for Mr. F.

Goals	Treatment Plan	Monitoring Progress
1. Reduce frequency and intrusiveness of reported hallucinations and acting out.	1. Titrate neuroleptic drug dose; contingency management of inappropriate writing with shaping less deviant writing behaviors.	1. Self-report of frequency and intrusiveness of hallucinations using Target Complaint Scale (see Fig. 48.3); frequency of "graffiti" appearing on walls.
2. Increase communication skills of the patient and receptivity of family to patient's verbal initiatives; improve patient's assertiveness with foreman regarding limits on his work capacity.	2. Social skills training and behavioral family management.	2. Completion of behavioral assignments and evidence of spontaneous generalization of skills; acceptance by employer for return to work.

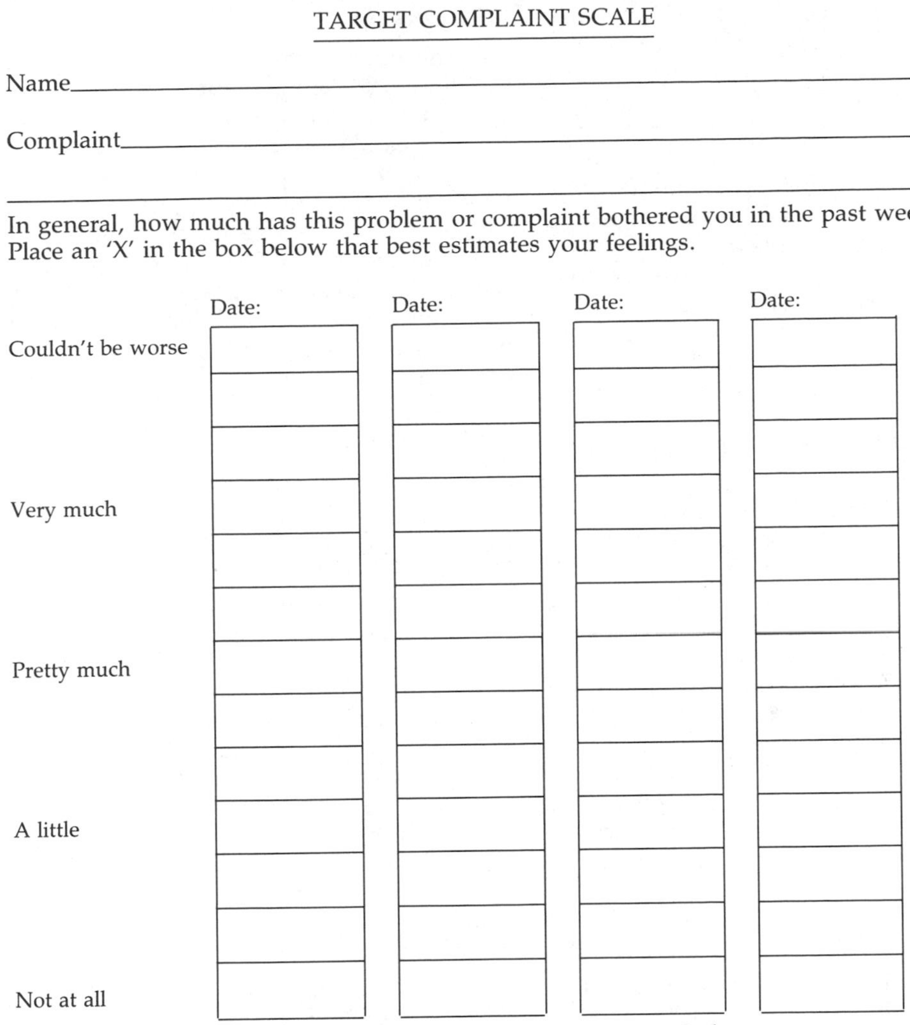

TARGET COMPLAINT SCALE

Name_____

Complaint_____

_____

In general, how much has this problem or complaint bothered you in the past week?
Place an 'X' in the box below that best estimates your feelings.

	Date:	Date:	Date:	Date:
Couldn't be worse				
Very much				
Pretty much				
A little				
Not at all				

Figure 48.3.   Target Complaint Scale.

Mr. F. was asked to carry a small notebook in which he was instructed to write down his nonsensical phrases. In addition, he agreed to surrender his daily supply of cigarettes and have them doled out to him by the staff contingent on his freedom from writing on walls. The contingency management program was quickly successful in eliminating his defacing of walls at the mental health center and was extended to his behavior at home. Within a month, his nonsensical writing had ceased, and the patient himself described a feeling of control over his hallucinations since he was able to chan-

nel the auditory commands to his notebook. The psychiatrist instructed Mr. F. to share the contents of the notebook only with the psychiatrist, which had the effect of reducing the social reinforcement he inadvertently had been receiving from his family for his psychotic behavior.

Behavioral analysis suggested the value of strengthening Mr. F.'s interpersonal skills both in relation to reestablishing his circle of friends and to helping him become more assertive at home with his family and at work with his foreman. Specific goals in social skills training were: (*a*) reestablishing social contact with friends, (*b*) taking wife and daughters to social outings, and (*c*) returning to work. Mr. F. joined a social skills training group at the day treatment center, which he attended four times weekly. The group consisted of 8 to 10 patients and focused on interpersonal goals that went beyond traditional concepts of "assertiveness." The group dealt with such social interactions as initiating, maintaining, and concluding conversations; meeting new people; getting information from others; and learning job-related interpersonal skills. The social skills training was carried out with the highly structured approach permitting individually tailored goals for each patient (41–42). The procedures for social skills training are outlined in Figure 48.4.

After 5 weeks at the day treatment center, Mr. F. had completed 80% of his assignments from the social skills group. The psychiatrist then met with the patient and family for family behavioral management sessions in which the patient and family were educated about the nature of schizophrenia, its effective treatments, and ways to communicate more successfully with one another. The family behavioral management sessions amplified the goals of the social skills training and enhanced generalization of skills learned by improving the receptivity of Mr. F.'s family to his newly learned assertiveness (43). With repeated practice, Mr. F. approached his foreman at work and negotiated a return to his previous job.

Over the course of behavioral interventions, the dosage of trifluoperaze was reduced to 5 mg daily associated with further reductions in patient's self-reports of hallucinations. The patient experienced no undesirable side effects at this dosage level. Mr. F. then was transferred to the continuing care program at the local community mental health center, where he was monitored monthly by a psychiatrist. His family attended monthly meetings of the local chapter of the Alliance for the Mentally Ill.

Discussion

Focal interventions such as providing contingency management of Mr. F.'s graffiti and a regular program of social skills training can be an efficient way to provide services and generate reconstitution as well as a return to social and vocational function in patients suffering from schizophrenic disorders. The importance of a careful biobehavioral analysis of the patient's needs, assets, and deficits cannot be overemphasized. In multidisciplinary settings such as clinics and community mental health centers, this analysis can be spearheaded best by the psychiatrist who provides clinical leadership for the multidisciplinary team.

CONCLUSION

Current psychiatric nomenclature, the *Diagnostic and Statistical Manual of Mental Disorders* (*Third Edition-Revised*), represents a shift over time from a nomenclature based primarily on psychodynamic theory to one based on phenomenologic observation and scientific findings. This shift highlights the multimodal dimensions required to describe fully the psychiatric disorders we diagnose and treat. Current nomenclature emphasizes the dynamic interaction between biologic process and environmental events.

Over the years, previous criticisms by psychodynamic theoreticians of biologic and behavioral treatments for psychiatric disorders have become less persuasive as psychodynamic therapies increasingly have been displaced by specific biologic and behavioral treatment interventions. Previous bugaboos such as "symptom substitution" have been debunked as concerns without foundation. As our case examples illustrate, successful biobehavioral intervention generally leads to generalization of therapeutic effect.

To some extent, psychodynamically oriented psychiatrists have incorporated the biobehavioral approach into their practices. On the other hand, biobehavioral clinicians have recognized the rich heritage of clinical description and therapeutic art

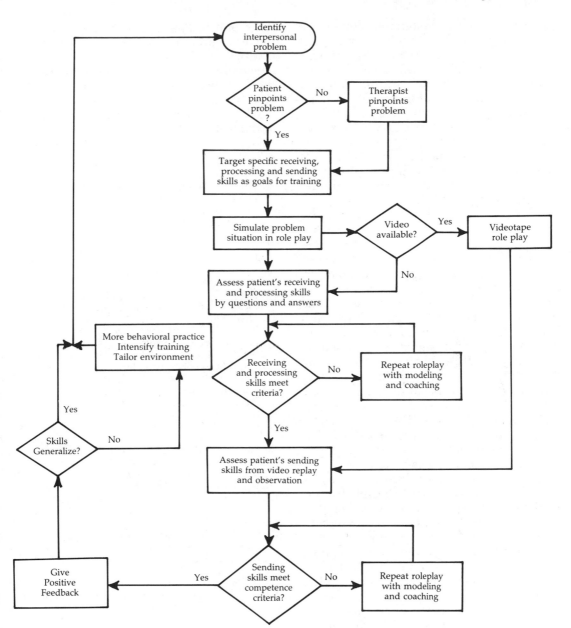

Figure 48.4.   Procedures for social skill training.

developed by psychodynamic therapists. The early claims by behavior therapists of quick and easy successes have given way to a maturity of sophistication regarding human complexity and the difficulties of applying scientific advancements through the healing arts. Accordingly, biobehavioral clinicians more readily recognize obstacles to treatment and feel comfortable specifying more modest treatment goals and more prolonged treatment plans.

Behavior reflects the conditions under which it occurs. As the conditions in the health care marketplace have become increasingly competitive among disciplines and among practitioners, the treatment behavior of psychiatrists has shifted increasingly toward the biologic accompanied by increasing professional identification with the rest of medicine. Unfortunately, the professional behavior of psychiatrists has shifted much less toward the behavioral, leaving that arena largely to nonmedical practitioners. If psychiatrists, who are the best suited to be biobehavioral clinicians, do not enter the behavioral arena more actively, they will leave it to others to develop and to harvest. The consequences will be to detract from psychiatry as an effective medical specialty and to decrease the quality of care available to patients. As government and other third-party payors demand increased out-of-hospital, outpatient care, psychiatrists will suffer professionally and financially. To some considerable extent, the responsibility lies with academic departments to promote teaching of biobehavioral psychiatry by psychiatrists who can function as models and mentors.

What of the future? In spite of treatment advances, large numbers of psychiatric patients remain relatively refractory to the best biologic and behavioral treatments available. From the biobehavioral perspective, change will come not only from advances in biologic description and treatments but from advances in behavioral assessment and therapies as well. One exciting area of future development, for example, is teaching patients effective self-monitoring and self-directed change using the rapidly advancing technologies of audiovisual programming and computerized instruction. Speed and extent of future developments will depend on advances in the empirical matrix of scientific inquiry and the effective amalgamation of biologic and behavioral approaches by those suited to the task.

References

1. Moss GR, Boren JJ: Specifying criteria for completion of psychiatric treatment. *Arch Gen Psychiatry* 24:441–447, 1971.
2. Brown BS, Weinckowski LA, Stolz SB (eds): *Behavior Modification: Perspective on a Current Issue* (DHEW Pub No. (ADM) 75-202). Washington, DC, U.S. Government Printing Office, 1975.
3. Rausch HL: Interaction sequences. *J Pers Soc Psychol* 2:487–499, 1965.
4. Jacob RG, Kraemer HC, Agras WS: Relaxation therapy in the treatment of hypertension—a review. *Arch Gen Psychiatry* 34:1417–1427, 1977.
5. Liberman RP: Behavior therapy in psychiatry: new learning principles for old problems. In Brady JP, Brodie HK (eds): *Controversies in Psychiatry*. Philadelphia, Saunders, 1977, pp 429–467.
6. Liberman RP, Davis J: Drugs and behavior analysis. In Hersen M, Eisler RM, Miller P (eds): *Progress in Behavior Modification*. New York, Academic Press, 1975, vol 1, pp 307–330.
7. Rioch DM: Personality. *Arch Gen Psychiatry* 27:575–580, 1972.
8. Liberman RP, et al: The credit-incentive system: motivating the participation of patients in a day hospital. *Br J Soc Clin Psychol* 16:85–94, 1977.
9. Willner AG, et al: The training and validation of youth-preferred social behaviors of child-care personnel. *J Appl Behav Anal* 10:219–230, 1977.
10. Jones FH, Frenouw W, Carples S: Pyramid training of elementary school teachers to use a classroom management "skill package." *J Appl Behav Anal* 10:239–253, 1977.
11. Sorcher M, Goldstein A: *Changing Supervisory Behavior*. Elmsford, NY, Pergamon Press, 1974.
12. Lovaas OI, Newsom CD: Behavior modification with psychotic children. In Leitenberg H (ed): *Handbook of Behavior Modification and Behavior Therapy*. Englewood Cliffs, NJ, Prentice-Hall, 1976, pp 303–360.
13. Sloane RB, et al: *Psychotherapy Versus Behavior Therapy*. Cambridge, MA, Harvard University Press, 1976.
14. Johnson S, Alevizos P: *Strategic interventions: a behavioral analysis*. Paper presented to Annual Convention of Association for Advancement of Behavior Therapy, 1975.
15. Hersen M, Eisler P, Miller PN (eds): *Progress in Behavior Modification*. New York, Academic Press, 1975–86.
16. Franks CM, Wilson GT (eds): *Annual Review of*

Behavior Therapy. New York, Brunner-Mazel, 1974–86.

17. Barlow DH, Waddell MT: Agoraphobia. In Barlow DH (ed): *Clinical Handbook of Psychological Disorders.* New York, Guilford Press, 1985, pp 1–68.

18. Klein DF, et al: Behavior therapy and supportive psychotherapy: are there any specific ingredients? *Arch Gen Psychiatry* 40:139–153, 1983.

19. Matthews AM, et al: A home-based treatment program for agoraphobia. *Behav Ther* 8:915–924, 1977.

20. Fyer AJ, et al: Discontinuation of alprazolam treatment in panic patients. *Am J Psychiatry* 144:303–308, 1987.

21. Liberman RP, et al: *Handbook of Marital Therapy.* New York, Plenum Press, 1980.

22. Steketee G, Foa EB: Obsessive–compulsive disorder. In Barlow DH (ed): *Clinical Handbook of Psychological Disorders.* New York, Guilford Press, 1985, pp 69–142.

23. Marks IM: Review of behavioral psychotherapy: obsessive–compulsive disorders. *Am J Psychiatry* 138:584–592, 1981.

24. Foa EB, et al: Treatment of obsessive–compulsives: when do we fail? In Foa EB, Emmel Kamp PMG (eds): *Failures in Behavior Therapy.* New York, Wiley, 1983, pp 10–34.

25. Fenichel O: *The Psychoanalytic Theory of Neurosis.* New York, Norton, 1945.

26. Moss GR, Boren JJ: Depression as a model for behavioral analysis. *Compr Psychiatry* 13:581–590, 1972.

27. Beck AT, Young JE: Depression. In Barlow DH (ed): *Clinical Handbook of Psychological Disorders.* New York, Guilford Press, 1985, pp 206–244.

28. Bellack A: Psychotherapy research in depression. In Beckham EE, Leber WR (eds): *Handbook of Depression.* Homewood, IL, Dorsey Books, 1985, pp 204–219.

29. Hoberman HM, Lewinsohn PM: The behavioral treatment of depression. In Beckham EE, Leber WR (eds): *Handbook of Depression.* Homewood, IL, Dorsey Books, 1985, pp 39–81.

30. Weissman MM: The psychological treatment of depression: an update of clinical trials. In Williams JB, Spitzer RL (eds): *Psychotherapy Research.* New York, Guilford Press, 1984, pp 89–105.

31. McCrady BS: Alcoholism. In Barlow DH (ed): *Clinical Handbook of Psychological Disorders.* New York, Guilford Press, 1985, pp 245–298.

32. Haynes SN: Contingency management in a municipally administered Antiabuse program for alcoholics. *Behav Ther Exp Psychiatry* 4:31–32, 1983.

33. Hore BD, Plant MA (eds): *Alcohol Problems in Employment.* London, Croom Helm, 1980.

34. Hunt GM, Azrin NH: A community reinforcement approach to alcoholism. *Behav Res Ther* 11:91–104, 1973.

35. McCrady BS, et al: Effects on treatment outcome of joint admission and spouse involvement in treatment of hospitalized alcoholics. *Addict Behav* 4:155–165, 1979.

36. Marlatt GA, Gordon JR (eds): *Relapse Prevention.* New York, Guilford Press, 1985.

37. Falloon IRH, et al: Family management in the prevention of exacerbations of schizophrenia. *N Engl J Med* 306:1437–1440, 1982.

38. Falloon IRH, et al: Family management in the prevention of morbidity of schizophrenia. *Arch Gen Psychiatry* 42:887–896, 1985.

39. Hogarty GF, et al: Family psychoeducation, social skills training and maintenance chemotherapy in the aftercare treatment of schizophrenia. *Arch Gen Psychiatry* 43:633–642, 1986.

40. Liberman RP, Mueser R, Wallace CJ: Social skills training for schizophrenic individuals at risk for relapse. *Am J Psychiatry* 143:523–526, 1986.

41. Liberman RP, et al: Social skills training for chronic mental patients. *Hosp Community Psychiatry* 36:396–403, 1985.

42. Hierholzer RW, Liberman RP: Successful living: a social skills and problem-solving group for the chronic mentally ill. *Hosp Community Psychiatry* 37:913–918, 1986.

43. Falloon IRH, Liberman RP: Behavioral family interventions in the management of chronic schizophrenia. In McFarlane W (ed): *Family Therapy of Schizophrenia.* New York, Guilford Press, 1983, pp 345–367.

49

Psychology of Psychopharmacology

Steven K. Hoge, M.D.
Thomas G. Gutheil, M.D.

Research has amply demonstrated the efficacy of clinical psychopharmacology in the treatment of a variety of mental illnesses, and therapists have faced the challenge of integrating these new treatments with traditional psychotherapeutic forms of treatment. Crucial to a successful blending of these treatment modalities is the ability of therapists to shift from one theoretical framework to a differing one. It has been noted that many therapists behave like "split brain preparations" alternating between these frameworks rather than successfully combining them. One important way in which the gap can be bridged between these two therapeutic modalities is to examine the psychology of prescribing medications. The psychology of psychopharmacology if understood by clinicians will result in greater therapeutic effectiveness. It is ignored at the risk of fracturing the doctor–patient relationship.

THERAPEUTIC ALLIANCE AND COMPLIANCE

The prescription of medication tends to promote an authoritarian posture in which the physician invokes his or her knowledge and expertise in biologic systems and success is measured in terms of the patient's compliance with prescribed treatment. Emphasis on the biologic substrates of mental illness promotes a subject–object relationship in which the patient's responsibility is conceived as complying with the doctor's orders (1). Indeed, the problem of noncompliance with prescribed medication has received considerable attention in the psychiatric and medical literature, and clinicians have been trained to impress the importance of compliance on their patients (2–4). This type of interaction leads to a relatively rigid and unyielding stance on the part of the prescribing psychiatrist. Though it is questionable whether such a relationship is appropriate in any branch of medicine, in psychiatry where issues of self-esteem and deficits of social and interpersonal interactions are common, there are serious countertherapeutic ramifications. Patients are encouraged to become more passive and dependent and to see the clinician as being responsible for clinical improvement. Such passivity may result in resentment when magical cures are not effected and in estrangement from treatment as a result of loss of confidence in the clinician. This passivity may then carry over to other aspects of the therapy

690

where it is clearly advantageous for the patient to take an active role.

The appropriate model for the doctor–patient relationship in regard to the prescription of medications is a specialized version of the therapeutic alliance—the pharmacotherapeutic alliance, which is characterized by a subject–subject relationship (1, 5). Under this model active efforts are made by the physician to enlist, recruit, and involve patients in a collaborative effort involving the use of medication. The psychiatrist shares the therapeutic goals as well as the uncertainty of treatment with the patient in a manner that conveys that the patient is an equal partner in the prescription of the medication. As a coequal the patient's strengths are reinforced, and responsibility is felt for therapeutic gains. The formation of a pharmacotherapeutic alliance gives the patient confidence to bring to the psychiatrist's attention adverse effects without fear that an authoritarian posture will be threatened. In order to form such an alliance, clinicians must accept that patients have their own concepts of medications, both rational and irrational, which must be respected (6). The reader is referred to Chapters 9 and 10 for related discussions of the "negotiated approach."

TRANSFERENCE

The pharmacotherapeutic alliance, like the treatment process in psychotherapy, is frequently strained and intruded upon by phenomena derived from transference aspects of the relationship. The physician may become the target of transference distortions of his or her role and intentions, either by prescribing or by not prescribing medications. In either case the transference may be positive or negative—a point often missed in discussions of this subject. Patients may establish a positive transference with the physician who prescribes medications and see him or her as giving, responsive, empathic, and nurturing. To some patients the act of prescribing medications conveys the sense that the doctor is taking the patient seriously and the illness or symptoms are validated (3).

Negative transference occurs in a variety of circumstances. Some patients may feel dismissed, fearing that the clinician does not want to hear about their suffering when medications are prescribed. Others may feel frightened by the passivity implied in accepting medication for treatment, or worse, may act out to counter such fears. Other patients feel degraded by having medications prescribed and interpret it to mean that they are more seriously ill than they had previously perceived (7). Patients who believe that the psychotherapies are somehow the higher forms of treatment may view medication as second-rate treatment.

Negative transference can take special or particular forms. Bipolar patients may view medication as attacking mania and therefore promoting depression. Patients who experience pleasurable, gratifying, or valued symptoms such as grandiose delusions may perceive medication in a negative light (8). Similarly patients deriving secondary gain from the sick role may feel threatened by medication.

The physician who does not prescribe medication either by failing to broach the subject spontaneously or by refusing to prescribe when asked to do so by the patient may be the subject of transference as well. Transference may be positive when the doctor's unwillingness to prescribe medication is seen as a refusal to be distracted from the patient as a person or, alternatively, as a vote of confidence in the patient's ability to solve his or her problems in other ways. The clinician may be viewed as being incorruptible and refusing to be diverted from the therapeutic work by those who value the talking therapies highly. Patients who hold such value systems may request medication when not really wanting it merely to see if the psychiatrist will "give in."

Failure to prescribe medication may be viewed negatively as well. Patients may view the absence of drug prescribing as a type of withholding; the doctor may be viewed as sadistic or uncaring or unwilling to help. Other patients may see the absence of drug prescribing as reflecting negatively on the seriousness and genuineness of their illness and feel that they are being accused of malingering. Patients may feel that the doctor is not taking them or their problems seriously if medications are not prescribed. In summary, both decisions—to prescribe or not to prescribe—may evoke a variety of transference reactions. These experiences may relate to the medication's effects but may also be quite independent of the specific pharmacologic indications, contraindications, or effects.

TRANSFERENCE TO MEDICATIONS

A unique aspect of psychopharmacology is a potential for transference to the medications themselves. While some may object that the term transference is not appropriately applied in this context, it is being used here to denote the use of a variety of psychic mechanisms including fantasies, displacement, and symbolizations about medications.

The placebo response is an example of a medication-related positive transference. The positive response is inexplicable either by the actual effects of the medications or by the known pharmacokinetics (9). Placebo effects that act in the desired direction go unchallenged, since questioning them serves no useful purpose. In some instances, however, such as the example of a patient who clings to a small dose of antipsychotic despite possible long-term side effects, positive transference is more problematic. This is particularly true of certain borderline patients with strong oral needs who typically seek to be medicated. Placebo side effects also occur, often a result of the fear of what the medication's effect would be.

Another aspect of transference to medications involves drug administration, i.e., scheduling dosage and the form in which the medication is administered. While there are empirical data to suggest that schizophrenic patients are relatively unaf-

fected by changes of "drug rituals" (10), it is a well-known clinical phenomenon nonetheless that such alterations in the form of administration may have profound symptomatic effects beyond what would be expected pharmacologically. For example, some patients with schizophrenia are known to experience both decompensation and recompensation merely around discussion of medication alterations without any actual change in the prescribed regimen.

Changes in drug rituals may have unexpected idiosyncratic effects. For example, some patients attach unusual meanings to the drug company's identifying markings on the tablets. One patient when he received his new medication became convinced that the markings "M.S.D." on each tablet indicated that his medication was analogous to L.S.D. and refused to take it.

Other patients may anthropomorphize the medication and act out their fantasies. One male patient with paranoid schizophrenia acted out his homosexual fears toward his male therapist when he complained of somatic sensations which he attributed to his medication. He divided antipsychotic medications into two groups, "male and female." He asked, "Why is it that medications are always named after people like Stella, Thor, and Mo?" He became fearful that his Moban was a "male medication" and that it was going to hurt him in some way. He requested a change to "Stelazine." The latent homosexual feelings toward his clinician were therefore expressed.

Another aspect of a patient's transference to medication that rests upon a personalized symbolization occurs when the medication is perceived as a personified intruder into the therapeutic relationship. Such patients tend to view the medication as a rival competitor for control of the patient's own positive treatment response or for efficacy over the patient. Patients may ask to be taken off the medication so that they may prove that they are responsible for getting better, not the medication.

MEDICATION AS A RELATIONSHIP EQUIVALENT

Prescribed medication may serve as a relationship equivalent. The most common example of this occurs on inpatient wards in teaching hospitals when physicians change over on an annual basis. The patient may be enormously attached to the departing physician, and the drug regimen serves as a souvenir or transitional object. In some cases the patient may energetically resist any alteration in this drug regimen because he perceives it as being disrespectful to his former relationship (11).

Requests for medication may represent the equivalent of a request for a relationship. Some patients feel unentitled to ask for conversation time or for a psychotherapeutic relationship unless they offer symptoms and accept medication. Because the patient views this as the only possible kind of relationship, it is easy for the physician to fall into the narrowed compass of possible relationships. Commonly such patients end up on multiple medications for their problems.

MEDICINE AS FOOD OR GIFT

Medication is frequently experienced as symbolic of food or gift. As food, medication may become a means of attempting to fill the patient's basic emptiness and inner impoverishment. Object hunger is acted out as drug hunger. In some instances patients may become frightened by these feelings, feel overwhelmed, and refuse the medications because of such overwhelming feelings of closeness.

Physicians generally speak of prescribing medication as "giving," and patients mirror this by saying I've been "taking" the medication. Clinicians need to be aware that patients often assume that gifts carry expectations. To give medication may be experienced by the patient as a demand to get better or to have the patient reciprocate in other ways.

Manifestations of transference phenomena in the prescribing of medications underscore the importance of a collaborative and flexible relationship that allows exploration in the context of a nonjudging alliance. In contrast, patients who are treated as being "noncompliant" in an authoritarian fashion will not feel inclined to provide the opportunities for such therapeutic exploration.

COUNTERTRANSFERENCE

Medication and its prescription may enter into countertransference in a number of ways. Each of the foregoing aspects of the prescription process discussed under transference may occur in the countertransference as well. The specific areas are usually quite idiosyncratic for the given physician–patient relationship. However, there are two difficulties in the area of countertransference that are common.

When patients reject or challenge the prescription of medication, the therapist may feel a certain helplessness. Clinicians more comfortable with an authoritarian stance may respond with anger and frustration that may impair open exploration of the issue.

A second common area of difficulty is exploration of medication related sexual dysfunction. Antipsychotic and antidepressants have effects on ejaculation and erection in the male and orgasm in the female. Cultural taboos and unresolved conflicts in patient and doctor conspire in many cases to prevent candid discussion about the side effects. The physician bears the added conflictive burden of recognizing that the dysfunction is a result of medication that he or she has prescribed. These situations are fraught with potential for countertransference issues of sadism and castration anxiety. From the patient's perspective, the fact that these potential side effects have not been spelled out in advance may lead to the conclusion that they are intentional and expected effects of the medication. Such problems are easily averted by frequent, systematic inquiry about all bodily functions including eating, eliminating, sleeping, and sexual functions. This practice tends to make both patient and physician more comfortable in discussing these difficult areas and grants permission to raise them in the therapeutic hour.

Another aspect of difficult countertransference manifestations involves the cost of medications. It has been noted that some patients would rather be "sick than poor" (12). These feelings are difficult for physicians to understand and unless the doctor feels free to explore such material in a collaborative fashion, resolution is difficult. By exploring and discussing with the patient the virtues of generic medications or the rationale for prescribing nongeneric medications when such may be indicated, the physician demonstrates that he or she has the patient's interest at heart. This serves to bolster the therapeutic alliance.

CONCLUSION

Drug prescribing is a legitimate subject for the therapeutic exploration and sensitivity typically applied in psychotherapeutic situations. The subject is as rich in potentially useful affects, fantasies, and associations as any other aspect of the therapeutic process; indeed, the correct use of medications requires such willingness to discuss and explore.

References

1. Docherty JP, Marder SR, VanKammen DP, et al: Psychotherapy and pharmacotherapy: conceptual issues. *Am J Psychiatry* 134:5, 1977.
2. Blackwell B: Drug therapy: patient compliance. *N Engl J Med* 289:249–252, 1973.
3. Gutheil TG: Improving patient compliance: psychodynamics in drug prescribing. *Drug Ther* 7:82–83, 87, 89–91, 95, 1977.
4. Gutheil TG: Drug therapy: alliance and compliance. *Psychosomatics* 19:219–25, 1978.
5. Gutheil TG, Havens LL: The therapeutic alliance: contemporary meanings and confusions. *Int Rev Psychoanal* 6:467–81, 1979.
6. Irwin S: How to prescribe psychoactive drugs. *Bull Menninger Clin* 38:1–13, 1974.
7. Ostow M (ed): *The Psychodynamic Approach to Drug Therapy.* New York, Psychoanalytic Research & Development Fund, 1979.
8. Van Putten T, Crumpton E, Yale C: Drug refusal in schizophrenia and the wish to be crazy. *Arch Gen Psychiatry* 33:1443–1446, 1976.
9. Shapiro AK: Semantics of the placebo. *Psychiatr Q* 42:653–95, 1968.
10. Burgoyne RW: Effect of drug ritual changes on schizophrenic patients. *Am J Psychiatry* 133:284–89, 1976.
11. Gutheil TG: The psychology of psychopharmacology. *Bull Menninger Clin* 46:321–330, 1982.
12. Havens LL: Some difficulties in giving schizophrenic and borderline patients medication. *Psychiatry* 31:44–50, 1968.

50

Psychosocial Rehabilitation

George L. Dion, Sc.D.

The purpose of this chapter is to acquaint the outpatient clinician with the field of psychosocial rehabilitation and provide a framework for developing effective use of rehabilitation services. To accomplish this goal, I shall discuss the need for rehabilitation, outcome in rehabilitation studies, psychosocial rehabilitation systems, clinical rehabilitation training models, barriers to successful collaboration between outpatient psychiatry and rehabilitation systems, and interdisciplinary collaboration with psychosocial rehabilitation systems.

THE NEED FOR REHABILITATION

The field of psychosocial rehabilitation has emerged in direct response to the tremendous, multidimensional needs of the psychiatrically disabled population. As most outpatient clinicians know, the era of deinstitutionalization produced vast numbers of patients who were discharged from institutions without the skills to survive effectively in the community. These patients create a number of unique problems for outpatient psychiatry. Psychiatrically disabled patients often exhibit a wide range of social and vocational dysfunction; fail to respond adequately to medication;

develop severe long- and short-term side effects to their medications; fail to comply with prescribed treatments; and are generally perceived to be difficult and not rewarding to treat.

The psychiatrically disabled patient often lacks the skills to acquire or maintain employment. The percentage of patients who become competitively employed following discharge has generally ranged from 10 to 30% (1). Dion et al. (2) reported that only 20% of a group of discharged bipolar patients were employed at premorbid levels 6 months after discharge. In a survey of well-educated, severely psychiatrically disabled family members of the National Alliance for the Mentally Ill (NAMI) the figures for employment were reported at only 6% for that point in time. Tessler and Goldman (3) reported employment rates of 11% for Community Support Program (CSP) patients in a cross-sectional survey. Farkas et al. (4) followed up 54 long-term state hospital patients over a 5-year period and reported a 0% employment rate.

Studies of recidivism of the psychiatrically disabled following deinstitutionalization also indicate poor outcome. Anthony et al. (1) in a review of extant outcome studies, reported that within 1 year of hospitalization, 40 to 50% of psychiatric pa-

695

tients are readmitted to the hospital at least once, and up to 75% of hospitalized patients are readmitted within 5 years of hospitalization.

OUTCOME IN REHABILITATION

Evidence supporting the need for rehabilitation services for the psychiatrically disabled is provided by the generally favorable outcome observed in studies of rehabilitation interventions. Dion and Anthony (5) reviewed rehabilitation outcome studies for the past 20 years and found that a majority of the experimental and quasi-experimental studies demonstrate a positive relationship between rehabilitation interventions focusing on skill development and functional outcome. The studies also validate the positive relationship between interventions focusing on the development of social and environmental supports and functional outcome. The review covered interventions including after-care programming, comprehensive rehabilitation center programming, case management, day treatment, social learning programs, vocational interventions, collaboration between service systems, and many other unique and innovative rehabilitation approaches. The findings generally supported the efficacy of rehabilitation in terms of increasing community tenure, vocational level of functioning, productivity, worker satisfaction, friendships, and role performance. A wide variety of interventions designed to teach or develop specific skills such as activities of daily living, transportation, community living, and social and psychologic skills also displayed a positive relationship to functional outcome. The reader is referred to Dion and Anthony (5) for a more comprehensive review of these studies.

Beyond the statistics related to recidivism and functional outcome, the effects of deinstitutionalization are evident in many areas. The so-called chronic patient is highly visible in the community. Although less frequently psychologically and psychomotorically uncontrolled, the chronic patient is easily identifiable by his or her inability to work or socialize adequately and by increasingly identifiable extrapyramidal symptoms, including tardive dyskinesia.

The outpatient clinician is also confronted with an increase in pressure from consumer groups, family organizations, and funding sources to respond to the needs of the psychiatrically disabled. These groups are demanding that the mental health system provide these patients with diverse programming such as vocational, social, and residential services. Given the fact that outpatient psychiatry has had little experience with providing these interventions, it has become clear that they must develop an understanding of the systems of psychosocial rehabilitation and develop collaborative relationships with practitioners within those systems.

PSYCHOSOCIAL REHABILITATION SYSTEMS

As a result of the frustrating consequences of deinstitutionalization, psychosocial rehabilitation systems utilizing one or more configurations of biologic, psychodynamic, behavioral, and sociocultural therapies emerged. These psychosocial rehabilitation systems began to evolve as a direct response to the particular needs expressed by the psychiatrically disabled population. They have evolved in a number of ways with a wide variation of theories, styles, techniques and approaches. As the reader shall see, there is much overlap and similarity among these approaches. Mental health delivery systems today may employ a number of these strategies. However, the differences in approaches can be very important when evaluating their utility in treating the individual patient. Certainly not all patients are helped by blanket administration of treatments and services, and some patients may be harmed by indiscriminate applications. By taking a closer look at these therapies and approaches, the clinician may be in a better position to evaluate and plan for an effective multidimensional utilization of rehabilitation services.

The Comprehensive Psychosocial Rehabilitation Center

Comprehensive psychosocial rehabilitation centers, often based on the psychosocial clubhouse model, lead the field in providing an integrated application of rehabilitation principles for the psychiatrically disabled. These centers provide a wide range of skill and support interventions including vocational, family, social, recreational, and residential services.

Many of the comprehensive, multiservice rehabilitation centers found throughout the nation evolved from the social clubhouse model pioneered by individuals at Fountain House in New York City and Horizon House in Philadelphia. The early social clubhouses were founded by groups of ex-patients to provide support for those disenfranchised by gaps in psychiatric services. Thresholds in Chicago, Hill House in Cleveland, Center Club in Boston, The Social Center in Virginia, and Fellowship House in Miami are examples of large urban centers using the essential principles of rehabilitation articulated in the early clubhouses. Community mental health centers throughout the nation are beginning to adopt the principles and program structures of comprehensive psychosocial rehabilitation centers in order to better serve the needs of the chronically mentally ill.

The goals of the psychosocial rehabilitation center often include preventing rehospitalization, increasing socialization skills, promoting independent living skills, increasing employment, and promoting basic educational skills (6, 7). Increasing skills and competencies while reducing dependence on the hospital underlies the philosophy of the psychosocial rehabilitation center.

The components of the comprehensive psychosocial center are by nature an extensive array of services and interventions. The following list of components is by no means exhaustive but is meant to illustrate the range of offerings by psychosocial centers.

Prevocational day programs encompass a very broad range of activities. These activities routinely are formulated on a continuum and include structured activities that utilize solitary, parallel or cooperative participation of members at graded stress levels. The activities may involve a physical task such as crafts or woodworking. Others may focus on group discussions of work issues, family issues or other topics which are perceived to have an effect on members' functioning and adjustment. Prevocational day programs often employ in-house cafeteria, maintenance, thrift shop, and clerical programs to provide increasing approximations of competitive employment. Other programs throughout the country are expanding on the range of these types of programs. Innovations include subcontracting work with local industry and developing prevocational programs that provide the specific skills needed to work in entry-level jobs that are required by employers in their region.

For those members who have successfully engaged in the prevocational day programs but may not yet be ready to attempt competitive employment, the Transitional Employment Program (TEP) provides an intermediate step. The TEP jobs are usually entry-level jobs located in local business establishments and pay at least the minimum wage. The jobs may be shared by a number of members, i.e., a full-time slot can be shared by two or more workers. The jobs are designed to last from 3 to 9 months although some programs are encouraging clients to stay in these jobs indefinitely if the worker and job are well matched.

Preparation for securing competitive employment may be accomplished through teaching specific skills or by intervening directly with prospective employers. Job placement services are often provided for members in the psychosocial rehabilitation center. Placement counselors develop relations with local industry and negotiate placement of individuals who have demonstrated acceptable levels of competence in prevocational activities and/or TEP jobs. Job-seeking skills such as finding job leads, filling out applications and responding to interview questions are often taught to members in groups or individually as needed.

Socialization skills may be addressed in a wide variety of ways within a psychosocial rehabilitation center. Activity groups such as leisure, homemaking, expressive arts, and athletics promote socialization through the process of the client's participation. Problem-solving and issues groups provide topical arenas for members to work through common concerns of socialization. Some psychosocial rehabilitation programs have begun to use specific social skills training curricula in an attempt to systematically improve member's social skills deficits.

Evening and weekend programs usually consist of social and recreational activities and are meant to address the problem of isolation that members often experience following discharge from the hospital. These programs also provide the opportunity for long-term contact and follow-up with members after they become employed or undertake other activities which prevent them from participating in the weekday activities.

Outreach programs have become a major component of the comprehensive psychosocial rehabilitation program. When a member has not attended the program for a number of days, both members and staff will call, visit, or write to communicate that the member has been missed and is expected and wanted to return. The reasons for the absence are explored and offers for assistance are extended to meet whatever concerns the member may communicate.

Many of the larger psychosocial rehabilitation centers provide residential services for their members. Transitional apartments, which have been leased from the community are often shared by two or three members with minimal supervision or contact with staff. The residences may or may not have restrictions in terms of length of occupancy depending on the philosophy and resources of the center. Besides community apartment programs, some centers have been pursuing the development of foster care placements and halfway houses.

Most comprehensive psychosocial rehabilitation centers make use of medical and psychiatric consultation services. Since most members are taking psychotropic medications and are often consumers of medical services, the centers recognize the importance of adequate medical services.

Community Support Programs

The National Institute of Mental Health (NIMH) created the CSP to address the massive void in services to the chronically mentally ill. The goals of CSPs in relation to serving their population have been described by NIMH (8) and summarized by Test (9):

1. To locate Community Support Systems (CSS) clients, reach out to inform them of available services;
2. Help CSS clients meet basic needs;
3. Provide adequate mental health care;
4. Provide 24-hour, quick-response crisis assistance;
5. Provide comprehensive psychosocial rehabilitation services;
6. Provide a range of rehabilitative and support housing options;
7. Offer backup support, assistance, consultation, and education to family and community;
8. Recognize natural support systems;
9. Establish grievance procedures and mechanisms to protect client rights;
10. Facilitate effective use by clients of formal and informal helping systems.

The objectives delineated by NIMH are broadly defined and have allowed state and local programs considerable flexibility in the manner in which they structure program services. Various geographic, demographic and resource variables influence the development of the CSP system in a particular area. Reinke and Greenely (10) have described three distinctive models of CSPs in Wisconsin that illustrate the ways that these systems can be molded to fit a community's needs.

The "caseworker model" makes use of the skills of social workers, rehabilitation counselors, nurses, and other related disciplines as case managers. Case managers offer direct service to the individual and relevant others in the client's social network. They may do outreach, advocacy, crisis intervention, basic life skills development, and coordination of other systems resources. Often, case managers carry specialized populations, e.g., geriatic or Hispanic, based on their unique skills and interests. This flexibility allows the system to adapt to fluctuations in the number, needs, and types of clients in the geographic area. The caseworker model may well be the most prevalent model of CSP service delivery. It is seen as providing the most direct service while serving the widest range of clients with the least cost (10).

An increasingly popular form of systems intervention is the "paraprofessional-extender" model. This system may use natural community and personnel resources in a variety of ways. A rural Wisconsin CSP employs program coordinators who recruit paraprofessional supervisors in the community. These supervisors in turn, recruit workers to provide individual services to each client. The workers basically provide front-line socialization, problem-solving, and monitoring contact. This particular system is well suited for rural areas with widely dispersed clients in a broad geographical area.

Another example of the paraprofessional model can be found in a program in Massachusetts which uses indigenous volunteers to be companions to persons with chronic mental illness. The volunteers may help with everyday issues, skill teaching, or just being available for normalized socialization. Another program within this system also uses trained paraprofessionals to directly intervene in crisis management. The workers may stay with the client in the client's home or augment staff at a detoxification center to help manage a client. They may also place the client in a supervised family care home or their own treatment service building to avert a costly and disruptive hospitalization.

The "team model" uses a number of mental health professionals of various disciplines and often focuses on the most recidivistic clients. They practice aggressive outreach with clients and become actively involved in the community with clients and the people with whom clients come into contact. Team members often share duties and work together in keeping track of difficult clients who are at risk for decompensation. This model employs a great deal of staff control over clients and their medication management and compliance. The team model appears to be most suited for urban areas with moderate to high concentrations of highly difficult or recidivistic clients.

Community Residential Services

The network of community residential services is an integral component of a psychosocial rehabilitation system. Perhaps the largest and most obvious sequelae of the deinstitutionalization movement is the glaring lack of housing and residential support for chronically disabled psychiatric patients. A greater than 60% cut in the state psychiatric hospital population resulted in a tremendous need for community residental alternatives. For many patients, this meant living in primarily low income housing such as rooming houses, single occupancy hotels and poorly maintained apartments. Other patients found refuge in nursing homes and board and care facilities which generally provided only custodial care. Still others could find no structured living arrangements and stayed on the streets and in shelters for the homeless.

Today, there is a far greater range of residential treatment options for the psychiatrically disabled patient. Cutler (11) described a range that includes crisis care at a state hospital, crisis respite centers, group homes, adult foster homes, satellite apartments, Fairweather Lodge model apartments, enhanced room and board, boarding homes, and hotels. Other innovations include more comprehensive half-way houses and a variety of supervised and cooperative apartments.

Crisis care at a state hospital usually involves only a brief amount of time on a designated unit of the hospital. The care is aimed at managing an acute exacerbation of symptomatic behavior. These programs usually employ 24-hour nursing care in high staff-to-patient ratios. Upon resolution of the acute crisis, the patient is returned to the original living arrangement or triaged to a more appropriate level of care.

Crisis respite centers generally attempt to serve the same function as state hospital crisis care, but in an alternative setting. These centers may be found in community mental health centers, psychosocial rehabilitation centers, or day hospital facilities. They also provide 24-hour supervision but may employ nonmedical and paraprofessional staff.

Group homes and halfway houses provide 24-hour supervision and in some cases day programming for clients in the community. They may vary greatly in the cost, census, and level of programming for the client. Quarterway houses are another permutation of this form of residence. These houses are often found on hospital grounds and employ a high staff-to-client ratio.

Foster care or family care programs are another form of alternative living arrangements for the psychiatrically disabled. These programs have been extremely popular in Europe and are increasingly employed in this country. The quality of placement is undeniably linked with the quality of the families involved.

Satellite, supervised, and/or cooperative apartments usually involve two to six residents sharing an apartment with various configurations of shared kitchen and day room arrangements. Residents usually have their own sleeping and bathroom facilities. Staffing may range from day staff involved in training residents in independent living skills; evening staff, who are available for administrative concerns and support; or night staff who are available for crisis intervention. Some apartment programs may employ staff only to do periodic visits, attend administrative meetings, or be on call for emergencies.

The Fairweather Lodge model (12) involves a group of residents living together in a quasi-family arrangement. They form a social unit and assume various household responsibilities such as cooking, cleaning, and shopping for the group. They may link with community support professionals or paraprofessionals to develop independent living skill training programs.

Boarding homes and single-occupancy hotels round out the continuum of community residential alternatives for the psychiatrically disabled. These arrangements obviously vary based on the landlords and people operating these facilities. They provide no formal supervision or training for residents but attempts are being made in some areas to provide support and consultation to managers of these operations by community support personnel.

The continuum of residential alternatives ideally provides a graded range of living arrangements based on the patient's need for supervision, structure and support. Unfortunately, there is much variation in the availability of these alternatives. Different geographic locations may yield a complete range of living environments or virtually none of them.

CLINICAL REHABILITATION TRAINING MODELS

The overwhelming evidence for the need for psychosocial rehabilitation has prompted funding sources such as the NIMH and the National Institute of Handicap Research to support the development of clinical training models of rehabilitation. Two research and training centers have been responsible for the development of current rehabilitation training models.

The Center for Psychiatric Rehabilitation at Boston University was funded in 1979 with the primary mission of developing, disseminating, and ensuring the utilization of rehabilitation research and technology.

In the past 8 years, Anthony (13) and his associates have developed a comprehensive clinical model of psychiatric rehabilitation which attempts to either teach the patients the skills they need to function in their particular community or modify the patient's community to be more supportive of the client's attempt to cope. The model consists of three phases of the treatment process: functional diagnosis, planning, and interventions. The functional diagnosis yields behavioral and descriptive information about the patient's current skills and the skill demands of the environment in which he/she chooses to function. The plan identifies which skills and resources the patient needs to develop in relation to the environment of choice, how those skills and resources will be developed, and which practitioners and systems will be responsible for carrying out the interventions. The primary interventions involved in skill and resource development are skill teaching, behavioral programming, resources coordination, and creation of new resources. Each phase utilizes an empathic counseling process described by Carkhuff (14), which is intended to maximize the involvement of the patient in his/her rehabilitation.

The process developed by the Center for Psychiatric Rehabilitation utilizes modules which have been developed, piloted, and evaluated to facilitate training in these skills. There are currently more than 50 sites utilizing this model nationally and internationally. The reader is referred to Anthony (13), Anthony et al. (15), and Anthony et al. (16) for a more in-depth examination of the psychiatric rehabilitation approach.

The Clinical Research Center for Schizophrenia and Psychiatric Rehabilitation at the University of California at Los Angeles School of Medicine has been the leader in developing social skills training technology for the rehabilitation of the psychiatrically disabled. The goal of social skills training is to facilitate coping and competence as a method of dealing with stress and vulnerability, reducing relapses and improving psychosocial functioning (17). Liberman et al. (17) state, "The basic model involves role playing by the patient and modeling, prompting, feedback and reinforcement by the therapist. A 'problem-solving' model of training provides general strategies for dealing with a wide variety of social situations." The model also focuses on developing the patient's ability to perceive and process the incoming messages and meanings of social interactions.

Liberman (18) also describes a "vulnerability–stress–coping–competence model" which provides a construct from which to conceptualize the onset, course and outcome as a set of biologic, environmental and behavioral interactions. From this model, interventions such as social skills training, family coping skills training, the development of vocational competencies, and psychopharmacologic treatment provide protection from stress and vulnerability. The reader is referred to Liberman et al. (19) and Liberman and Evans (20) for a more in-depth review of this training model.

BARRIERS TO COLLABORATION

Perhaps metaphorically, rehabilitation was not represented in the first edition of this book and is included as the last chapter in this second edition. In traditional models of outpatient treatment, psychosocial rehabilitation has been characterized as an afterthought or, unfortunately for many patients, often not thought of at all.

Historically, psychosocial rehabilitation has emerged as an entity quite separate from outpatient psychiatry. Psychosocial rehabilitation interventions evolved primarily as atheoretical responses to the pragmatic realities of living with a disability. The "clubhouse model" was developed by a group of ex-patients as a response to inadequate social and vocational opportunities following hospitalization. Drop-in centers have been developed as a response to those patients who are suspicious of or averse to receiving traditional psychiatric care. The latest psychosocial rehabilitation clinical technologies are "atheoretical and eclectic in principle"

(15) as a response to the diverse needs of this population.

Outpatient psychiatry on the other hand, has traditionally focused its efforts on symptom reduction through biologic, behavioral, or psychodynamic interventions. These interventions have usually evolved from the application of well-documented constructs developed in the study of psychoanalysis, behaviorism, and psychopharmacology.

As a result of these different "evolutions" outpatient psychiatry and psychosocial rehabilitation practitioners have developed different constructs, languages, and ideologies. These differences have fomented a number of myths and assumptions that have obstructed collaborative efforts between psychiatry and rehabilitation.

Many rehabilitation practitioners associate outpatient psychiatry with the "medical model," which is seen as being overly disease oriented and unresponsive to the functional and "everyday" needs of its "clients." Others view psychiatry as overly paternalistic and obsessed with control of the patient. Still others feel that psychiatric illness is a myth and that society is responsible for psychiatric disability rather than a disease process. Medication is often seen as only minimally effective and that side effects are often more disabling than the symptoms that the psychiatrist is treating. Finally many rehabilitation practitioners look upon treating this population in offices at clinic settings with disdain and feel that the clinician's motives are more directed at confirming his or her own theories than helping patients meet their basic needs.

Rehabilitation programs have been seen by psychiatry as naive and unsophisticated in their approach to treating people with very severe pathology. Outpatient clinicians are stymied by the wide array of rehabilitation models, programs and practitioners. The process of rehabilitation has somehow been seen as relegated to a number of professional disciplines, paraprofessionals and nonprofessionals. Many outpatient clinicians see rehabilitation as something that occupational therapists, recreational therapists and rehabilitation counselors do. This notion that rehabilitation is something that occurs "out there" has prevented the integration of the concept of rehabilitation as central to the treatment of the chronically mentally ill by outpatient psychiatry.

There are undoubtedly some truths inherent in both assumptions, but the result has been a fragmentation of service to the dysfunctional patient rather than a complementary or synergistic effect of treatments. The time has come for both groups to begin to understand each other.

INTERDISCIPLINARY COLLABORATION

By its very nature, rehabilitation demands the collaboration of all disciplines, families, and resources indigenous to the patient's environmental settings. Rehabilitation is not discipline specific. It is a fundamental mission that must guide interventions. Simply put, rehabilitation is concerned with what the patient can and can't do (skills) in relation to functioning within his or her range of environments; and what the patient has and doesn't have (supports) in relation to functioning in his or her range of environments. The mission of rehabilitation is to ensure that patients possess the skills and supports to succeed in their chosen environments. Understanding and supporting this mission is the single most important factor for the outpatient clinician in successfully collaborating with psychosocial rehabilitation systems.

In order to support this mission, the outpatient clinician must become better acquainted with their patients' level of functioning and the range of psychosocial rehabilitation services available in their particular community. It is critical that the primary clinician look beyond the focus of his or her particular area of expertise, e.g., family therapy, psychopharmacology, or psychodynamic psychotherapy, and to explore whether or not the patient is satisfied and successfully functioning at the appropriate vocational, educational, residential or social level.

By exploring patients' level of success and satisfaction with the specifics of their living, learning, working or treatment environments, the clinician can begin to assess areas that patients need help with and are motivated to work on. The clinician should also work with patients' significant others to elicit their perceptions of patients' success and satisfaction within those particular environments. This process helps to assess areas that the patient may be less aware of or less motivated to work on.

In exploring these environments with the patient and significant others, the clinician can begin to elicit some of the critical skills that the patient can or can't do in relation to succeeding in that environment. These skills may be very straightforward intellectual skills like balancing a checkbook, or they may be very complex psychologic skills like identifying and expressing negative emotions.

The clinician should also attempt to address some of the critical resources that the patient has or doesn't have in relation to succeeding in the environment of need. The patient may need disability income to meet financial needs, or a case manager to assist in coordinating services.

By assessing the resource and skill strengths and deficits in the patient's functional environments, the clinician is better able to assess the skills and supports impacting function that they may be able to provide directly, e.g., less sedating medications, family management training, and behavioral programs. The clinician may also begin planning for referrals to services that address the needs that they may not have the time, resources or expertise to deal with, e.g., case management, vocational training and placement, respite family care, and acquisition of social security disability.

Once the outpatient clinician is clear on which functional skills and supports he or she can address and which ones must be referred to other services, the clinician must begin to explore the range of psychosocial rehabilitation systems and services available. As noted before, there is wide variation from community to community in terms of services available. Clinicians need to know what services are available, what they do, and how to gain access to these systems for their patients.

For example, if the clinician is working with a patient whose illness is clearly exacerbated by troubling relationships within the family unit, that clinician may feel that the patient needs a family education intervention, crisis respite care, a halfway house or a combination of these. In determining the availability and appropriateness of these services in the community, the clinician must make both formal and informal contacts with potential providers. By gathering information about such things as the service's mission, goals, programs, and criteria for successful referral, the clinician is better able to ascertain the "goodness of fit" with patient and program. An additional benefit is the likely perception by the service provider that the clinician is interested in more than just "placing" or "dumping" the patient.

In initiating the referral process, it is important to provide the rehabilitation practitioners with all relevant historical and medical data. Providing information regarding the patient's functional strengths and deficits enhances the clinician's ability to identify critical service needs and facilitates the development of a "common ground" between outpatient clinician and rehabilitation practitioner.

In developing collaborative relationships with psychosocial rehabilitation services, it is also important to maintain regular contact with rehabilitation practitioners. This kind of contact continues to reinforce the clinician's commitment to treatment of the whole patient in the eyes of the rehabilitation practitioner. Regular contact also provides the clinician with continuous feedback regarding the patient's function and allows the clinician to provide feedback to program staff regarding issues in treatment. Frequent communication also provides an opening to enlist psychosocial rehabilitation staff in supporting the clinician's objectives, e.g., encouraging medication compliance, encouraging discussion of issues in therapy, and providing feedback regarding medication side effects.

Case Study

Michael is a 26-year-old, single male with atypical bipolar disorder. He has been hospitalized twice and has experienced a downward trend in psychosocial functioning. His problems include persistent delusions and worsening tardive dyskinesia that has prohibited treatment with a neuroleptic. Michael is seeing an outpatient psychopharmacologist (Dr. K.) who is treating him with lithium, clonazepam, and supportive psychotherapy. With consultation, Dr. K. began to do an assessment of Michael's psychosocial functioning and identified several critical strengths and deficits in skills and resource areas. Dr. K. first established that Michael wanted to stay at home and live in his present community. He then began to assess what Michael would need to stay there with some level of success and satisfaction.

In terms of skill strengths, the patient was very personable with professionals and patients with whom he had prior contacts. He was also quite athletic and enjoyed a number of sports. His skill deficits, however, included difficulty in initiating new social contacts in his home town, which had left him with virtually no socialization outside the home. Michael also had difficulty negotiating conflicts with his family. He would become enraged and act out verbally when his parents would ask him about medication compliance. Michael's other major skill deficit involved refraining from verbalizing delusional material in social situations, i.e., coffee shops. This deficit had caused people to withdraw from him and act somewhat warily around him which further exacerbated his delusions.

In terms of resource strengths, the patient was receiving Supplemental Security Income and disability support from a previous employer. Michael also has a very supportive family and feels fortunate that they have "stuck by him." The patient's primary resource deficit is a lack of daytime structure. Michael has clearly decompensated following the cessation of prior structured work and activity programs.

Following this assessment of critical skills and resources, Dr. K. called a number of professional contacts in the community. In conversations with a case manager at the local community mental health center, Dr. K. discovered that they funded a clubhouse model program that could address Michael's need for structure and provide him with social skill teaching groups. In later contacts with the case manager, Dr. K. identified the specific problems of negotiating conflicts with family and concealing delusional material. These deficits were dealt with directly by the case manager in the context of family management training and individual behavioral programming with the patient.

At this point, Michael is actively involved in the clubhouse and has a significantly larger social support network. He has participated actively in recreation groups and a prevocational program and is awaiting placement in the TEP program. Michael continues to experience troubling delusions but has been increasingly able to control their impact on his functioning. Michael also continues to have difficulty negotiating conflict with family members but they have become more sensitized to those topics that provoke anger in the patient. Dr. K. continues to see Michael monthly and continues his contact with Michael's rehabilitation practitioners.

Although this case study does not elaborate on the tremendous complexity of this process, it does provide some sense of the capacity of collaboration among outpatient clinicians and psychosocial rehabilitation professionals to have a positive impact on patient functioning and quality of life. By promoting the concept of a shared mission, the outpatient clinician can maximize the probability that all systems involved, (patients, families, community groups, rehabilitation and other disciplines), will create a synergistic effect in achieving the goal of optimal patient functioning.

References

1. Anthony WA, Cohen MR, Vitalo R: The measurement of rehabilitation outcome. *Schizophr Bull* 4:365–383. 1978.

2. Dion GL, Tohen M, Anthony WA, et al: Symptom and functional outcome in bipolar disorder. *Hosp Community Psychiatry*, in press.

3. Tessler RC, Goldman HH: *The Chronically Mentally Ill: Assessing Community Support Systems*. Cambridge, MA, Ballinger Press, 1982.

4. Farkas M, Rogers ES, Thurer S: Rehabilitation outcome of long term patients left behind by deinstitutionalization. *Hosp Community Psychiatry*, in press.

5. Dion GL, Anthony WA: Research in psychiatric rehabilitation: a review of experimental and quasi-experimental studies. *Rehabilitation Counseling Bulletin* 3:177–203, 1987.

6. Bond GR: An economic analysis of psychosocial rehabilitation. *Hosp Community Psychiatry* 35:356–362, 1984.

7. Beard JH, Propst RN, Malamud TJ: The Fountain House model of psychiatric rehabilitation. *Psychosocial Rehabilitation Journal* 5:47–52, 1982.

8. National Institute of Mental Health: *A Network for Caring: The Community Support Program of the National Institute of Mental Health* (ADM-81-1063). Washington, DC, U.S. Government Printing Office, 1982.

9. Test MA: Community support programs. In Bellack AS (ed): *Schizophrenia: Treatment, Management and Rehabilitation*. Orlando, FL, Grune & Stratton, 1984, pp 347–373.

10. Reinke B, Greenley JR: Organizational analysis of three community support program models. *Hosp Community Psychiatry* 37:624–629, 1986.

11. Cutler DL: Community residential options for the chronically mentally ill. *Community Ment Health J* 22:61–73, 1986.

12. Fairweather GW (ed): *The Fairweather Lodge: A 25-Year Retrospective* (New Directions for Mental Health Services, No. 7). San Francisco, CA, Jossey-Bass, 1980.

13. Anthony WA: *Principles of Psychiatric Rehabilitation*. Baltimore, MD, University Park Press, 1979.

14. Carkhuff RR: *Helping and Human Relations*. New York, Holt, Rinehart & Winston, 1969.

15. Anthony WA, Cohen MR, Cohen B: Psychiatric rehabilitation. In Talbott J (ed): *The Chronic Mental Patient: Five Years Later*. New York, Grune & Stratton, 1984, pp 137–157.

16. Anthony WA, Cohen MR, Farkas M: A psychiatric rehabilitation treatment program: Can I recognize one if I see one? *Community Ment Health J* 18:83–95, 1986.

17. Liberman RP, Mueser KT, Wallace CJ, et al: Training skills in the psychiatrically disabled: learning coping and competence. *Schizophr Bull* 12:631–649, 1986.

18. Anthony WA, Liberman RP: The practice of psychiatric rehabilitation: historical, conceptual and research base. *Schizophr Bull* 12: 542–559, 1986.

19. Liberman RP, Falloon IRH, Wallace CJ: Drug–psychosocial interventions in the treatment of schizophrenia. In Mirabi M (ed): *The Chronically Mentally Ill: Research and Services*. New York, SP Medical and Scientific Books, 1984, pp 175–212.

20. Liberman RP, Evans CC: Behavioral rehabilitation for chronic mental patients. *J Clin Psychopharmacol* 5:8s–14s, 1985.

Index

A